Critical Care Study Guide

Springer
New York
Berlin
Heidelberg
Barcelona
Hong Kong
London
Milan
Paris
Singapore
Tokyo

Critical Care Study Guide

Text and Review

With 249 Figures and 280 Tables

Editor

Gerard J. Criner, MD

Professor of Medicine
Division of Pulmonary and Critical Care Medicine
Temple University School of Medicine
Philadelphia, Pennsylvania

◆

Deputy Editor

Gilbert E. D'Alonzo, DO

Professor of Medicine
Division of Pulmonary and Critical Care Medicine
Temple University School of Medicine
Philadelphia, Pennsylvania

Illustrators

Susan E. Gilbert, CMI
Faith A. Cogswell

Springer

Gerard J. Criner, MD
Professor of Medicine
Division of Pulmonary and
Critical Care Medicine
Temple University School of Medicine
Philadelphia, PA 19140, USA

Gilbert E. D'Alonzo, DO
Professor of Medicine
Division of Pulmonary and
Critical Care Medicine
Temple University School of Medicine
Philadelphia, PA 19140, USA

Library of Congress Cataloging-in-Publication Data
Critical care study guide / [edited by] Gerard J. Criner, Gilbert E. D'Alonzo.
p. ; cm.
Includes bibliographical references and index.
ISBN 0-387-95164-4 (pbk. : alk. paper)
1. Critical care medicine. I. Criner, Gerard J. II. D'Alonzo, Gilbert E.
[DNLM; 1. Critical Care—Handbooks. 2. Critical Illness—Handbooks. WX 39 C9347 2002]
RC86.7.C754 2002
616'.028—dc2 2001049251

Printed on acid-free paper.

Production coordinated by Chernow Editorial Services, Inc., and managed by Terry Kornak; manufacturing supervised by Joe Quatela.
Typeset by Matrix Publishing Services, Inc., York, PA.
Printed and bound by Maple-Vail Book Manufacturing Group, York, PA.
Printed in the United States of America.

9 8 7 6 5 4 3 2 1

ISBN 0-387-95164-4 SPIN 10785270

Springer-Verlag New York Berlin Heidelberg
A member of BertelsmannSpringer Science+Business Media GmbH

Preface

Critical care medicine is a dynamic and exciting arena where complex pathophysiologic states requiring extensive knowledge and clinical acumen are commonly found. Caring for critically ill patients requires an extensive knowledge of basic pathophysiology, as well as awareness of the appropriate diagnostic tests and therapeutic interventions. Because this knowledge base crosses many different disciplines, introduction to caring for the intensive care patient, while exciting, may also be intimidating.

This textbook is designed toward making the dynamic environment of the critical care unit understandable and the approach to the patient both logical and successful. The book contains three components: (1) description of the procedural tasks commonly performed for the critically ill patient, (2) explanation of the most common pathophysiologic states encountered, and (3) description of specific disease entities with details of their differential diagnosis, diagnostic strategy, and therapeutic plan.

This book also uses several educational approaches that we have found useful in our own teaching sessions and prior textbooks. Clinical cases introduce chapters and highlight chapter segments to emphasize clinical relevancy. As an additional study aid, margin notes highlight important teaching points and facilitate easy review of chapter content. To consolidate the principles outlined in each chapter, review questions with full text explanations are provided at the end of each chapter. All these elements help reinforce the most important messages for the reader.

This textbook is the effort of many individuals across many disciplines who practice at Temple University School of Medicine. Nonetheless, only evidence-based literature is used to provide the basic concepts and therapeutic and diagnostic strategies presented; the content does not represent the convention of care endorsed by any single institution.

GERARD J. CRINER, MD

Acknowledgments

Writing textbooks is not easy; in critical care medicine, especially, it requires the efforts of many individuals. The editor wholeheartedly appreciates the efforts of all the contributors to this textbook and many others who made publication of this textbook a reality. These individuals include Darlene Macon for her secretarial support, Dr. Gilbert D'Alonzo for his editorial assistance, and the editorial staff at Springer.

Last but not least, I would like to acknowledge the everlasting support of my wife, Helga, and family. Their patience and help provides the necessary nurturing personal environment required to successfully accomplish professional endeavors.

Gerard J. Criner, MD

Contents

Part II Pathophysiologic Disease States Encountered in the Critically Ill Patient

Part IV Appendices

Contributors

MICHAEL BADELLINO, MD
Associate Professor of Trauma Surgery, Department of Surgery, Temple University School of Medicine, Philadelphia, PA 19140, USA

RODGER E. BARNETTE, MD
Professor of Anesthesiology, Department of Anesthesiology, Temple University School of Medicine, Philadelphia, PA 19140, USA

PHILLIP M. BOISELLE, MD
Department of Radiology, Beth Israel Deaconess Medical Center, Boston, MA 02215, USA

JOSEPH I. BOULLATA, MD
Associate Professor of Pharmacy, Temple University School of Pharmacy, Philadelphia, PA 19140, USA

KATHLEEN J. BRENNAN, MD
Assistant Professor of Medicine, Division of Pulmonary and Critical Care Medicine, Temple University School of Medicine, Philadelphia, PA 19140, USA

NEIL W. BRISTER, MD, PHD
Associate Professor of Anesthesiology, Department of Anesthesiology, Temple University School of Medicine, Philadelphia, PA 19140, USA

WISSAM CHATILA, MD
Assistant Professor of Medicine, Division of Pulmonary and Critical Care Medicine, Temple University School of Medicine, Philadelphia, PA 19140, USA

DAVID E. CICCOLELLA, MD
Associate Professor of Medicine, Division of Pulmonary and Critical Care Medicine, Temple University School of Medicine, Philadelphia, PA 19140, USA

FRANCIS C. CORDOVA, MD
Assistant Professor of Medicine, Division of Pulmonary and Critical Care Medicine, Temple University School of Medicine, Philadelphia, PA 19140, USA

GERARD J. CRINER, MD
Professor of Medicine and Director, Division of Pulmonary and Critical Care Medicine, Temple University School of Medicine, Philadelphia, PA 19140, USA

JOSEPH CROCETTI, MD
Fellow, Division of Pulmonary and Critical Care Medicine, Temple University School of Medicine, Philadelphia, PA 19140, USA

GILBERT E. D'ALONZO, DO
Professor of Medicine, Division of Pulmonary and Critical Care Medicine, Temple University School of Medicine, Philadelphia, PA 19140, USA

DAVID FRIEDEL, MD
Assistant Professor of Medicine, Division of Gastroenterology, Temple University School of Medicine, Philadelphia, PA 19140, USA

JAY HERMAN, MD
Professor of Medicine, Temple University Cancer Center, Temple University School of Medicine, Philadelphia, PA 19140, USA

HENRY H. HSIA, FACC
Cardiovascular Division, University of Pennsylvania Hospital, Philadelphia, PA 19140, USA

FREDERIC H. KAUFFMAN, MD
Associate Professor of Medicine, Temple University School of Medicine, Philadelphia, PA 19104, USA

SAMUEL KRACHMAN, MD
Associate Professor of Medicine, Division of Pulmonary and Critical Care Medicine, Temple University School of Medicine, Philadelphia, PA 19140, USA

L. JILL KRASNER, MD
Assistant Professor of Medicine, Department of Anesthesiology, Temple University School of Medicine, Philadelphia, PA 19140, USA

FRIEDRICH KUEPPERS, MD
Professor of Medicine, Division of Pulmonary and Critical Care Medicine, Temple University School of Medicine, Philadelphia, PA 19140, USA

MICHAEL S. LAGNESE, MD
Pulmonary Fellow, Division of Pulmonary and Critical Care Medicine, Temple University School of Medicine, Philadelphia, PA 19140, USA

YAROSLAV LANDO, MD
Pulmonary Associates of Lancaster, 555 North Duke Street, Lancaster, PA 17604-3555, USA

VADIM LEYENSON, MD
Assistant Professor of Medicine, Division of Pulmonary and Critical Care Medicine, Temple University School of Medicine, Philadelphia, PA 19140, USA

MARIA ROSELYN LIM, MD
Clinical Neurophysiology Fellow, Medical College of Pennsylvania, Philadelphia, PA 19132, USA

CATHY LITTY, MD
Director, Transfusion Medicine, St. Christophers Hospital for Children, Philadelphia, PA 19134, USA

NATHANIEL MARCHETTI, MD
Fellow, Division of Pulmonary and Critical Care Medicine, Temple University School of Medicine, Philadelphia, PA 19140, USA

UBALDO J. MARTIN
Assistant Professor of Medicine, Division of Pulmonary and Critical Care Medicine, Temple University School of Medicine, Philadelphia, PA 19140, USA

PAUL MATHER, MD
Assistant Professor of Cardiology, Division of Cardiology, Temple University School of Medicine, Philadelphia, PA 19140, USA

THOMAS NUGENT, MD
Fellow, Division of Pulmonary and Critical Care Medicine, Temple University School of Medicine, Philadelphia, PA 19140, USA

GERALD M. O'BRIEN, MD
Associate Professor of Medicine, Division of Pulmonary and Critical Care Medicine, Temple University School of Medicine, Philadelphia, PA 19140, USA

CLARKE U. PIATT, MD
Fellow, Division of Pulmonary and Critical Care Medicine, Temple University School of Medicine, Philadelphia, PA 19140, USA

GREGORY J. ROSSINI, MD
Fellow, Division of Pulmonary and Critical Care Medicine, Temple University School of Medicine, Philadelphia, PA 19140, USA

RONALD RUBIN, MD
Division of Hematology, Temple University School of Medicine, Philadelphia, PA 19140, USA

L.I. ARMANDO SAMUELS, MD
Assistant Professor of Medicine, Department of Nephrology and Kidney Transplantation, Temple University School of Medicine, Philadelphia, PA 19140, USA

ROBERT SANGRIGOLI, MD
Fellow, Division of Cardiology, Temple University School of Medicine, Philadelphia, PA 19140, USA

NOAH BRAD SCHREIBMAN, MD
Fellow, Division of Pulmonary and Critical Care Medicine, Temple University School of Medicine, Philadelphia, PA 19140, USA

SCOTT A. SCHARTEL, DO
Associate Professor of Anesthesiology, Department of Anesthesiology, Temple University School of Medicine, Philadelphia, PA 19140, USA

JOHN M. TRAVALINE, MD
Associate Professor of Medicine, Division of Pulmonary and Critical Care Medicine, Temple University School of Medicine, Philadelphia, PA 19140, USA

WALTER A. WYNKOOP, MD
Fellow, Division of Pulmonary and Critical Care Medicine, Temple University School of Medicine, Philadelphia, PA 19140, USA

PART I

Critical Care Procedures

CHAPTER 1

L. JILL KRASNER AND NEIL W. BRISTER

Airway Management

CHAPTER OUTLINE

LEARNING OBJECTIVES

After studying this chapter you should be able to:

- Perform a focused exam to assess a patient's oxygen and ventilatory needs.
- Know mechanisms available to assist oxygenation and ventilation.
- Identify the urgency of establishing an airway.
- Know anatomic classifications of the upper airway that identify a potentially difficult intubation.
- Understand equipment and resources needed to establish an airway in all categories of patients.
- Identify special medical and physical situations where establishing an airway requires skilled personnel.
- Know options of extubation versus tracheotomy.

EVALUATION FOR INTUBATION

Respiratory distress or disease may be a cause for a patient's admission to an intensive care unit (ICU). Reducing the work of breathing and providing supplemental oxygen for other systems such as the cardiovascular system is an integral part of critical care. Airway management is thus a central part of patient care and treatment. Before addressing the need to intubate for mechanical ventilation to support a patient's pulmonary system, it is important to review some concepts of respiratory function. The basic elements to evaluate are oxygen delivery and exchange and the work of breathing and ventilation.

The basic elements to evaluate for a patient with respiratory disease are oxygen delivery and exchange and the work of breathing and ventilation.

Oxygen Delivery and Exchange

Signs and symptoms of oxygen deprivation are evident in the neurologic, respiratory, and cardiovascular systems first. These changes may be noticed by family members earlier than by health care providers.

The most important drug that can be administered to a patient is supplemental oxygen. Oxygen is essential for the metabolism and function of all cells in the body. Clinical evidence of oxygen deprivation is a late sign of hypoxemia. Whatever the cause, oxygen deprivation results in rapid depletion of ATP, the primary energy source for most metabolic functions in the body.

Oxygen deprivation leads to clouded thinking, interrupted speech patterns, diaphoresis, and cardiovascular overdrive in an effort to compensate for hypoxic conditions. Thus, a quick evaluation entails assessing the neurologic, respiratory, and cardiovascular systems. First, a basic mental status evaluation includes looking for signs of anxiety, lethargy, change in thought process, hallucinations, or frank unresponsiveness. Subtle signs of hypoxia may be detected by family members earlier than by the health care providers. Decreased responsiveness, new bouts of confusion, or new combative behavior all may be signs of deteriorating oxygen supply to the brain. Next, a quick evaluation of the respiratory system involves observing the patient's respiratory pattern. Behavioral adjustments in an attempt to improve breathing may include sitting upright, nasal flaring, or strenuous use of the accessory muscles for breathing; these muscle groups include the abdominal and neck accessory muscles. Cyanotic changes are late signs of imminent respiratory failure. Finally, a patient's expected cardiovascular response to oxygen deprivation is tachycardia and hypertension. However, patients may be on beta-blockers or other medications, which may result in a nonspecific response to hypoxia; included are patients with heart failure and diabetes whose first cardiovascular response may include bradycardia and hypotension.

Pulse oximetry is the quickest and easiest way to assess oxygen status.

Pulse oximetry is the easiest tool to measure the patient's current oxygen status. Normal oxygen saturation should be greater than 95%. A saturation of 90% implies a PaO_2 of 60 mmHg, which borders on insufficient oxygen availability to meet cellular demands.

Broad categories of impaired oxygen delivery and exchange include the following:

- Low inspired fraction of oxygen
- Hypoventilation
- Diffusion impairment
- V/Q mismatch (areas of the lungs ventilated but not perfused)
- Pulmonary shunt (areas of the lungs perfused but not ventilated)

Work of Breathing and Ventilation

Normal respiratory rate is 16–20 breaths per minute. Increasing respiratory rate or change in tidal volume increases the work of breathing.

Ventilation allows exchange of oxygen into the lungs from the air and transfer of CO_2 from the blood into the lungs and out of the body. Normal respiratory rate is between 16 and 20 breaths per minute. Normal minute ventilation is 90–100 ml/kg. An increasing respiratory rate or changes in tidal volume outside normal values results in increased work of breathing. Changes in a patient's respiratory pattern may indicate pending respiratory failure. Although increased work of breathing is an attempt to meet these needs, it is in and of itself energy consuming and can contribute to respiratory collapse.

Prolonged elevated minute ventilation increases work of breathing and changes respiratory mechanics such that patient may not be able to sustain without assistance.

With a prolonged period of elevated minute ventilation, the work of breathing increases and respiratory mechanics change. Nonpulmonary causes of increased work of breathing include but are not limited to sepsis, cardiogenic shock, and anemia. In sepsis, the ventilatory demand on the cardiac output can increase from a baseline of 5% to as high as 25%. Although not a primary malfunction of the pulmonary system, the increased work of breathing is an attempt to meet increased oxygen requirements or removal of excess CO_2 from the body.

It may be necessary to establish an airway with intubation before determining the exact pulmonary or nonpulmonary causes of altered respiratory mechanics (Table 1-1). Apnea and total cardiovascular collapse require immediate action. However, in less desperate circumstances there may be sufficient time to further evaluate the ventilatory status of the patient before intubation. An arterial blood gas (ABG) may help in this evaluation. An ABG identifies metabolic and pulmonary determinants that contribute to normal or abnormal respira-

TABLE 1-1

CAUSES OF AIRWAY OBSTRUCTION

UPPER AIRWAY	LOWER AIRWAY
Laryngospasm: secretions	Bronchospasm: asthma, CHF
Tumor	Foreign body aspiration
Foreign body aspiration	Inspissated secretions
Tongue obstruction: obesity	Pulmonary embolus: blood, air, fat, or amniotic fluid
Soft tissue obstruction: sleep apnea	Pulmonary edema
External compression: neck hematoma, tumor, stab wound, carotid surgery; abscess	Endobronchial intubation
Vocal cord swelling/polyps	Kinked ETT
Tracheal stenosis	Aspiration
Bilateral recurrent laryngeal nerve injury	Tumor

CHF, congestive heart failure; ETT, endotracheal tube

tory patterns. The normal $PaCO_2$ value is 40 mmHg. Any large deviation from that baseline value requires further investigation. An increased respiratory rate should result in lower $PaCO_2$ values. Elevated $PaCO_2$ in the context of tachypnea indicates inadequate ventilation, respiratory fatigue, and pending respiratory failure.

The degree of respiratory distress and the patient's general medical condition impact the severity of the acute respiratory process and the need for mechanical ventilatory support.

Important considerations in evaluating respiratory distress are the degree of distress and any coexisting diseases that may influence the patient's condition. A patient with chronic obstructive pulmonary disease (COPD) and CO_2 retention may breathe comfortably with values of $PaCO_2$ of 50 mmHg and a PaO_2 of 55 mmHg. A patient with new-onset CHF, however, may have an increased risk for respiratory failure with the same set of parameters. Consequently, accurate assessment of the situation mandates determining the urgency of the need for mechanical ventilation (Table 1-2). It is also important to realize that, although it is easy to divide pulmonary problems into individual categories for discussion, a mixed combination of the aforementioned problems can lead to respiratory failure and the need for intubation and mechanical ventilation. Not all exams or tests will be available at the critical time when that decision must be made.

A quick assessment to evaluate the need for intubation includes observing the ABC's of an emergent situation: aberrations in airway, breathing, and circulation may mandate mechanical ventilation.

Without the luxury of a detailed medical history, a quick assessment for possible intubation includes evaluating the ABC's of an emergent situation: Airway (oxygenation delivery and exchange), Breathing (work of breathing and ventilation), and Circulation. The airway provides an unobstructed path for the delivery of oxygen and the exchange of CO_2. A patent airway is present when air movement can be detected at the nose or mouth. Air movement with noise, for example, snoring, may indicate the need to improve airway patency, which can be accomplished with various maneuvers such as repositioning the head, jaw thrust, and

TABLE 1-2

DISEASE PROCESSES THAT MAY REQUIRE INTUBATION

Trauma
Major thoracic or abdominal surgery
Postoperative: residual anesthetic, fluid overload bleeding, airway surgery
Acute mental status decline
Upper airway obstruction
Pneumonia
Pneumothorax
Pulmonary embolus: air, blood, fat, amniotic fluid
Severe asthma (status asthmaticus)
Flail chest
COPD
Congestive heart failure
Unstable hemodynamics, e.g., evolving myocardial infarction
  Shock: hemorrhagic, cardiogenic, neurogenic, or septic
Ischemic bowel
Acute renal failure with fluid retention

COPD, chronic obstructive pulmonary disorder

head extension or tilt (barring neck injury). Other techniques involve use of a nasal trumpet or oral airway, depending on the level of the patient's consciousness. An oral airway splints the tongue and keeps it from falling into the posterior pharynx, which can obstruct the airway. The splint is not well tolerated in awake patients, so it is best used when the patient has been adequately sedated or is already comatose. A nasal trumpet is better tolerated by a conscious patient; it too may open an obstructed airway by splinting the soft tissue in the oropharynx, thus permitting oxygen exchange. Its main potential problem is causing a nosebleed with its placement. Regardless of how an airway is established, it is important to maintain supplemental oxygen at all times. Delivery of supplemental oxygen can be via nasal cannula, venturi mask, nonrebreathing face mask, or an airway mask breathing unit (AMBU) bag.

The breathing pattern with respiratory distress is disordered. Rapid shallow breaths may indicate residual inhalation anesthetic following surgery, inadequate pain control, or respiratory muscle fatigue (panting). Also, sepsis can contribute to rapid breathing. Slow deep respirations may be indicative of systemic opioids or other sedatives. Narcotic reversal agents such as nalaxone may be helpful. Hand-ventilation with an AMBU bag may be necessary to achieve either adequate tidal volume or an appropriate respiratory rate for the patient. An AMBU bag is a device connected to a high-flow oxygen source with a mask that fits securely over the nose and mouth. Assisted ventilation requires synchronization with the patient's breathing pattern. Assisted ventilation also helps relieve the work of breathing until the patient improves or a more secure airway can be established, that is, intubation.

There are limited ways to provide noninvasive methods of supporting ventilation; these include continuous positive airway pressure (CPAP) or noninvasive positive pressure ventilation (NPPV) (see Chapter 34). Some patients tolerate noninvasive methods of ventilation during an acute phase of respiratory distress. Other patients become claustrophobic with nasal or face masks and do not tolerate this method of treatment for even short periods. If the patient appears to be worsening, then immediate intubation and mechanical ventilation are warranted. The etiology of the respiratory failure can be pursued after the patient is stabilized.

The hemodynamic profile (circulation) may be a contributing factor to the patient's status. Optimizing cardiac function with inotropes, vasodilators, or vasopressors may improve pulmonary status and eliminate the need for mechanical ventilation. Cardiac status and vital signs also help determine the type of sedative hypnotic and dosage most appropriate to facilitate intubation.

In summation, the initial evaluation of respiratory distress includes identifying the disease processes and assessing the ABC's of an emergent situation. A recent arterial blood gas (ABG) further helps assess the patient's level of oxygenation and ventilation status. Moreover, the physical assessment leading to intubation is critically important. The patient's symptomatic behavioral changes, physical exam, and other clinical criteria guide in the decision to proceed with intubation (Table 1-3).

TABLE 1-3

CRITERIA FOR INTUBATION OR ASSISTED VENTILATION

EXAMINATION/TEST	NORMAL	ASSIST RESPIRATORY EFFORT
Mental status	Oriented	Confusion/obtunded
Accessory muscle use	Minimal	Considerable activity
Nail beds	Pink	Cyanosis
Respiratory rate (bpm)	12–20	>30
SaO_2 (%)	>95%	<88%
PaO_2 (mmHg)	75–100 (room air)	<70 (facemask)
$PaCO_2$ (mmHg)	35–45	>45–55[a]
A-a gradient (mmHg)	10–25	>100
V_E (ml/kg)	90	150–200
NIF (cmH_2O)	<(−25)	>(−25)
Vital capacity (ml/kg)	65–75	<15

NIF, negative inspiratory force
[a] Check for underlying metabolic alkalosis

Checklist Before Intubation

Specific medical information helpful before intubation includes the following categories.

Medical Allergies

Most drug allergies do not interfere with the agents used for intubation. However, the rare history of pseudocholinesterase deficiency or malignant hyperthermia limits the use of succinylcholine as a muscle relaxant. There are also rare reported cases of allergy or porphyria associated with the use of pentothal.

Aspiration Risks

Full stomach precautions include trauma, small bowel obstruction, gastroesophageal reflux disease, hiatal hernia, pregnancy, obesity, diabetes, recent food ingestion ($<$8 h), and altered mental status. In an emergency intubation, it is reasonable to consider that the patient has increased aspiration risks.

Neurologic Status

The patient's mental status governs the technique and approach used to place an endotracheal tube (ETT). The obtunded patient may need little sedation or only topical oral anesthesia. The combative patient may require higher doses of sedative hypnotics to safely establish an airway. Intubation can be associated with temporary increases in intracranial pressure. Thus, any disease process associated with increased intracranial pressure needs to be considered, such as recent stroke, head trauma, or brain tumor.

Musculoskeletal Status

Musculoskeletal status influences the choice of medications as well as the technique used for intubation. Neuromuscular diseases impact the type and dosage of muscle relaxant agents used. Neck injury, arthritis, cervical stenosis, and a thick muscular neck raise concerns about the ease of intubation.

Coagulation Status

Severe liver disease and coagulopathy are strong contraindications to nasal intubation.

Previous Intubations or Tracheostomy

A history of tracheostomy may limit the diameter or size of ETT that will pass into the tracheal lumen. Although rare, a prior history of difficult intubations raises considerable concerns about establishing an airway quickly.

Obesity and Generalized Body Edema

These conditions can contribute to respiratory distress. As airway tissue swells, it can create partial or total upper airway obstruction. Recent failed attempts at intubation can also create significant edema or injury, making subsequent attempts more difficult. Finally, obesity can lead to redundant tissue in the airway, creating obstruction. Obese patients may experience no problems or may manifest chronic obstruction in the form of sleep apnea. In any of these situations, the immediate availability of this information helps the operator performing the intubation decide which technique and medications are most appropriate in establishing an airway.

> Gathering additional information through a physical exam and pertinent history while preparing to intubate help determine the technique to be used to establish a patent airway.

Obtaining the information just described can be done in a short period of time while preparing the patient for intubation. The person planning the intubation should be develop-

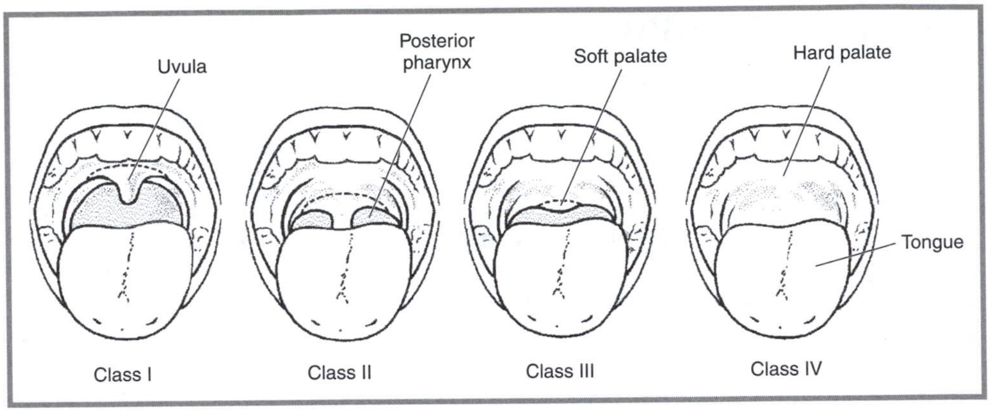

FIGURE 1-1

Maximal opening of oral cavity (*left to right*, class I–class IV) provides visualization of structures in the oropharynx. In class I, structures are easily identified, and in class IV the tongue obstructs view of posterior pharynx. (Modified from Mallampati SR, Gatt SP, Gugino LD, et al. A clinical study to predict difficult tracheal intubation. A prospective study. Can J Anaesth 1985;32:429–434.)

ing more than one plan. Intubation is not a benign procedure and carries with it certain inherent risks, even when done by the most skilled operator. Any information that suggests possible complications or difficulty with placing an endotracheal tube directly impacts the method and technique used.

INTUBATION

General Approach

Assessing the anatomy of the upper airway, the Mallampati scale, and the range of motion of the neck helps distinguish the easy airway from the difficult airway.

While preparing to intubate a patient, one assesses airway anatomy. The upper airway includes the nose, mouth, oropharynx, mandibular space, and neck. Evaluation of nasal anatomy is not routine but is pertinent in the presence of head and neck injury. Range of mouth opening affects the ability to place a laryngoscope and view the oropharyngeal structures. Anesthesiologists have designed a classification system known as the Mallampati scale that defines the relationship of the tongue to the oropharynx (Figure 1-1). When the patient opens the mouth and extends the tongue, visualization of the soft palate and uvula is easy and the structures of the posterior pharynx are easily identified; this is considered class one. In class four, the tongue occupies most of the oral cavity and none of the aforementioned structures can be visualized. Class one indicates that routine intubation is likely to be easily performed, whereas class four suggests that significant difficulties may be encountered and requires special considerations and technique.

Further, during laryngoscopy, the structures of the larynx in the oropharynx have also been classified into four grades based on anatomic structures visualized. Grade I permits vi-

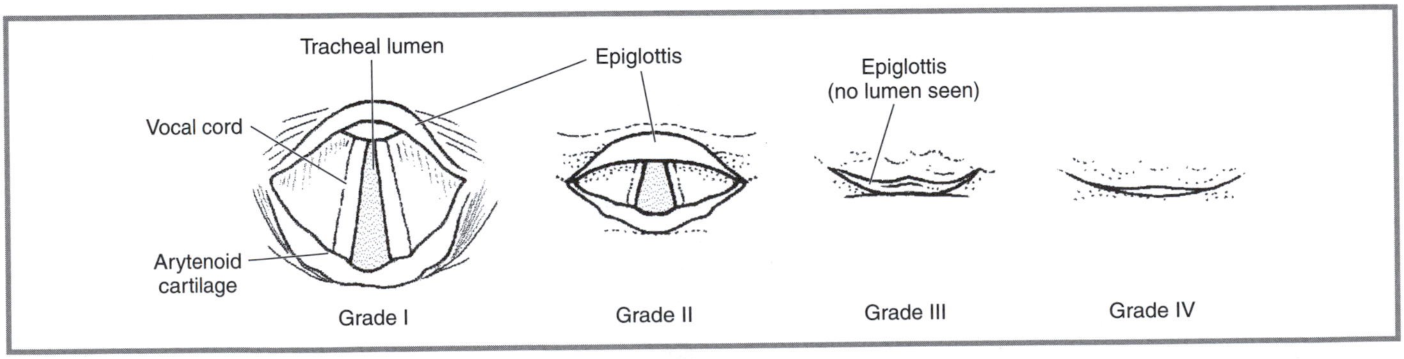

FIGURE 1-2

Grade I: optimal view of vocal cords during laryngoscopy. With a grade III view only the epiglottis can be clearly identified and the tracheal lumen cannot be visualized. (Modified from Mallampati SR, Gatt SP, Gugino LD, et al. A clinical study to predict difficult trachael intubation. A prospective study. Can J Anaesth 1985;32:429–434.)

sualization of the epiglottis, arytenoid cartilage, and the entire vocal cord structure (see Figure 1-2). These grades may be affected by the structures in the mandibular space, which is the area between the mental aspect of the mandible and the superior midline portion of the thyroid cartilage. With the head extended, this space is known as the thyromental distance, which can be measured in fingerbreadths or centimeters (normally three fingerbreadths or greater than 6 cm) (Figure 1-3). The larynx and the tongue fit into a portion of this anatomic space. Crowding of the mandibular space is best illustrated by the Pierre–Robin syndrome, which is characterized by micrognathia and macroglossia. Patients with this syndrome are extremely difficult to intubate with common methods. A more common example of crowding within this space is obesity, which also produces redundant tissue in the upper airway, both in the mandibular space and in the posterior pharynx. Finally, head, neck, and mouth mobility is important for optimal positioning of the patient before intubation. Limited range of motion of both the mouth and the neck may limit laryngeal visualization of the epiglottis and vocal cords.

Reviewing the diagrams of Figure 1-4 shows that three different axes require alignment to provide maximal exposure of the glottic opening by direct laryngoscopy. These axes are the

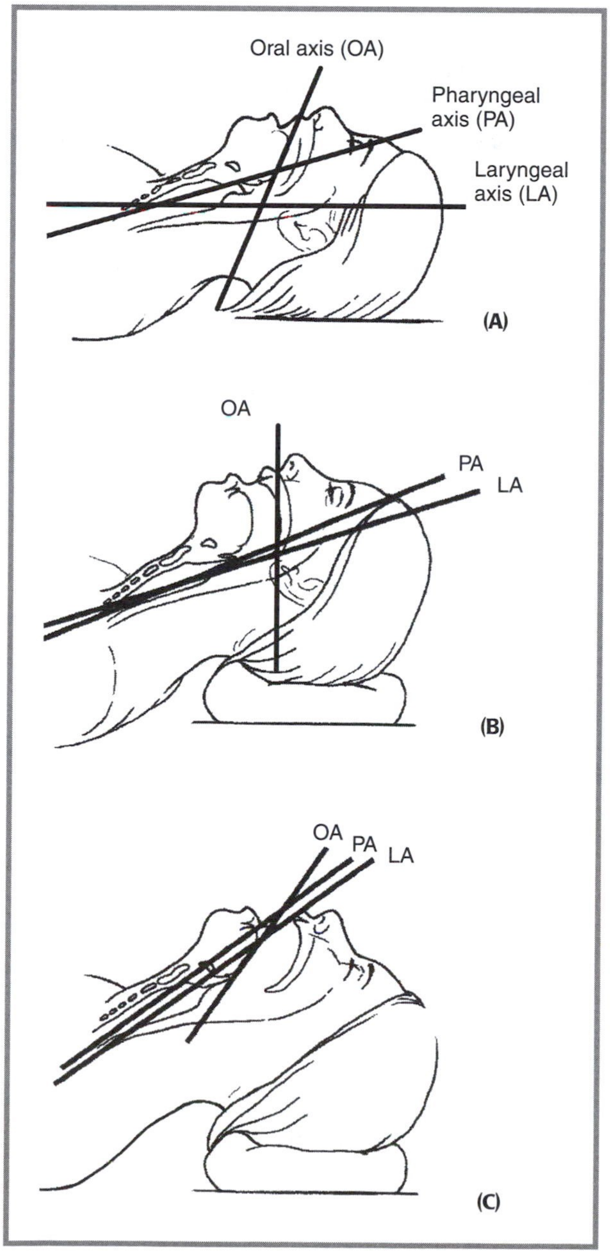

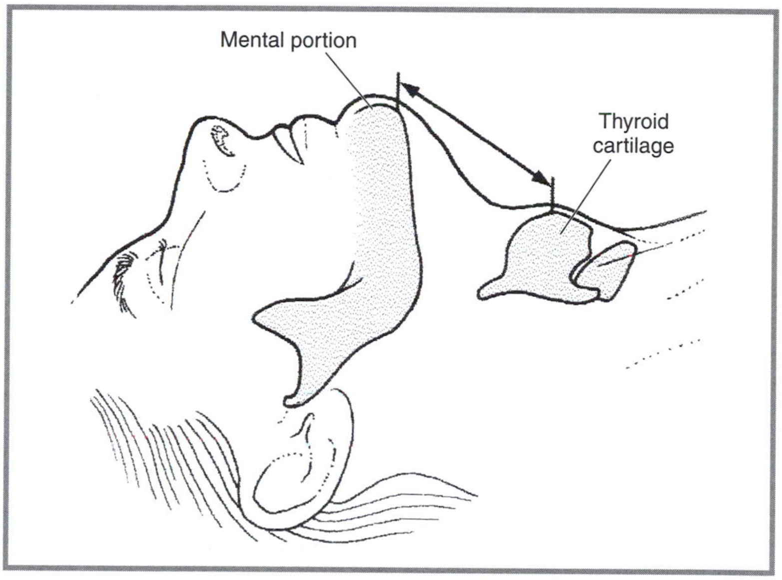

FIGURE 1-3

The distance from the mental portion of the mandible to the thyroid cartilage notch is known as the thyromental distance.

FIGURE 1-4

Schematic representation of the oral axis (*OA*), pharyngeal axis (*PA*), and laryngeal axis (*LA*) in three different head positions. In position A, the head is resting on a pillow with the head slightly flexed to align the PA and LA; however, the OA is not aligned. In position B the head is in neutral position with divergence of each axis. Position C is optimal for laryngoscopy, with the head on a pillow and neck extended (sniff position), thus aligning the OA, PA, and LA.

oral axis, the pharyngeal axis, and the laryngeal axis. Positioning of the head, neck, and shoulders can facilitate optimal position for laryngoscopy and successful intubation (Figure 1-4).

Monitors

Monitoring equipment normally available while performing an intubation includes a pulse oximeter to monitor oxygen saturation, EKG for rhythm and rate, blood pressure check, and a stethoscope for auscultation of breath sounds.

Equipment and Materials

Supplemental oxygen and appropriate equipment and medications are required for intubation.

Oxygen Delivery System

The ability to perform intubation quickly and efficiently depends on having the appropriate equipment available. Supplemental oxygen is mandatory.

Frequently, the patient already is receiving supplemental oxygen via nasal cannula or face-mask. An AMBU bag provides a method to deliver maximal oxygen outside the operating room setting; it also allows the operator to ventilate the patient, either assisting the patient or breathing for the patient when the patient becomes apneic. Other types of breathing circuits are available that balance augmentation of oxygenation with CO_2 removal. However, the AMBU bag circuit meets the needs of most adult patients and has gained popularity over time.

An established intravenous (IV) access allows fluids to be given, as well as medications that aid in the placement of an endotracheal tube (ETT) or correction of hemodynamic changes which can occur after intubation.

Suction System

The airway may be full of secretions or blood. Suction needs to be available to remove any secretions or debris in the airway during laryngoscopy to enhance visualization and minimize aspiration risk.

Airway Support Devices

Oral airway, nasal trumpet, laryngeal mask airway (LMA), and combitube are the airway support devices.

Endotracheal Tubes of Several Sizes

Endotracheal tube size is primarily determined by patient age. In most adult individuals, a #8 ETT is routinely used. With adolescents and children, however, a smaller tube size is required. Another consideration for using the largest acceptable tube size is the ability to perform bronchoscopy with a suction port large enough to accommodate lavage and removal of debris in the bronchial tree. It is much more important to establish an airway and safely place an ETT, even if the ETT is too small to accommodate a bronchoscope.

Laryngoscope

Several types and sizes of blades should be available. Distinct anatomic differences exist among patients.

Medications

Medications most commonly used during intubation are narcotics, sedative-hypnotics, and muscle relaxants; these may be used individually or in any combination, taking into consideration their indications, hemodynamic profile, and side effects. Details about these agents can be found in Chapters 44 and 46.

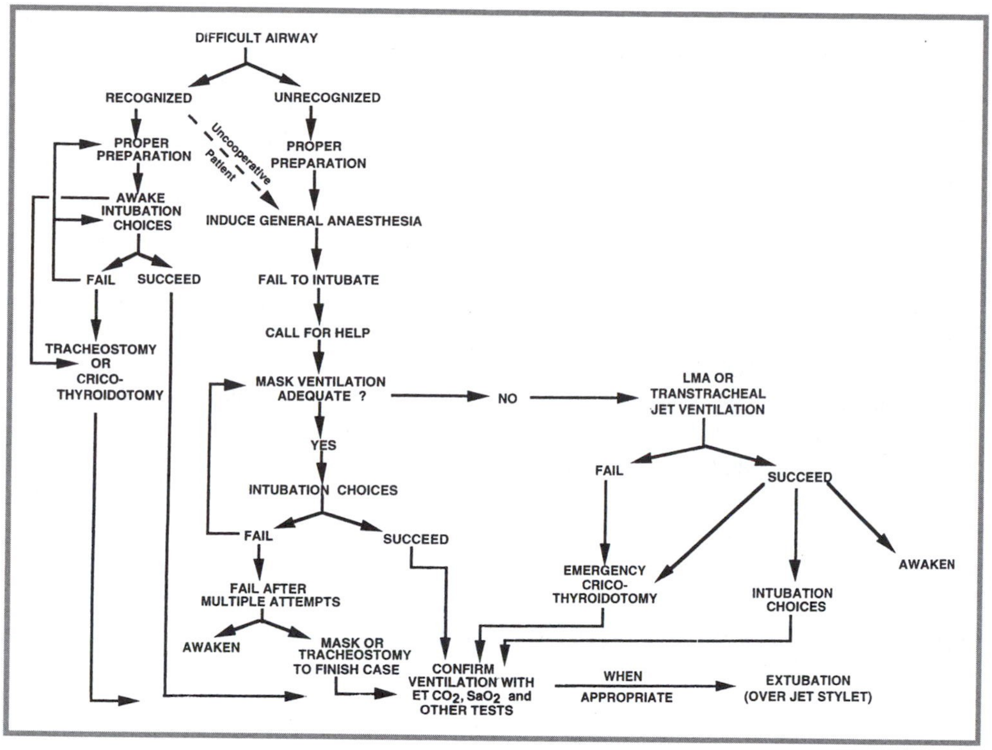

FIGURE 1-5

American Society of Anesthesiologists (ASA) Difficult Airway Algorithm.

Fiberoptic Scope

The fiberoptic scope is a thin, flexible optic device that allows visualization of the oral anatomy which is inaccessible by other means. The device needs a light source and has a port that allows either suctioning of secretions or insufflation of oxygen. The operator must have good working knowledge of airway anatomy and skill in manipulating equipment controls. Fiberoptic scopes are available in various sizes. The larger scopes provide larger suctioning ports and increased rigidity, which facilitates threading the ETT over the scope into the trachea. In most instances, the scope is not immediately available outside the operating room.

Once having decided to proceed with intubation, most individuals classify the situation into three basic categories based on their airway assessment: easy, somewhat difficult, and extremely difficult. The American Society of Anesthesiologists has developed a pathway for establishing an airway in each of these situations (Figure 1-5). In most instances, however, this procedure is readily performed.

Act of Intubation

The most commonly used and easiest technique is orotracheal intubation, which can be done quickly and efficiently with a laryngoscope and an ETT. In many situations, the patient is given medications to induce a brief state of unawareness to place the ETT. The disadvantage with medications is that the patient usually becomes apneic for a brief period. However, awake intubation with direct laryngoscopy can also be performed with the same result. Which method of intubation is performed is partially operator dependent and partially dependent on the status of the patient. It requires a minimal amount of equipment and further can be performed in almost any setting. Awake intubation entails totally anesthetizing the oropharynx with a topical anesthetic (lidocaine). A laryngoscope is then used to view the anatomy of the airway, and additional topical anesthesia is applied to the epiglottis and vocal cords. This method is popular because the patient maintains spontaneous ventilation and the airway is never lost. Anesthesiologists traditionally withhold muscle relaxants after sedative-hypnotics have been given until they are able to confirm the ability to ventilate the patient.

Orotracheal intubation is the most commonly used and easiest technique for establishing an airway.

Intubation is facilitated by optimizing patient position.

To intubate the patient, the height of the patient's bed is adjusted to a level comfortable for the operator. The operator must be able to reach the head of the patient easily to adjust head position and gain access to the airway. The patient is supine. Occasionally, with severe respiratory failure, the patient is in the sitting position, and changing that position toward the supine position creates extreme anxiety for the patient. Therefore, oxygenation and ventilation are controlled with the patient in the sitting position. Sedation is titrated to effect. Then the patient is moved to the supine position quickly and the airway is established. The optimal position for intubation is the sniffing position (see Figure 1-4). In an adult, a #8.0 ETT is preferable in the intensive care unit (ICU) setting. Smaller-diameter tubes cause more resistance and increase the work of breathing. Once the ETT is placed and the cuff portion of the ETT inflated, it is necessary to confirm its placement by listening to the chest for equal breath sounds and determining CO_2 return with litmus analyzers or CO_2 detectors. Continuous end-tidal CO_2 return is the best indicator of proper ETT placement. It is important to auscultate the abdomen to ensure that the ETT is not in the stomach. Breath sounds in both the abdomen and the chest most likely indicate esophageal intubation. Continuous end-tidal CO_2 is absent in this setting. Phonation may also indicate incorrect location of the tube. Other methods that identify appropriate ventilation include observing chest wall motion and humidity in the endotracheal tube with expiration.

Rapid Sequence Induction and Intubation

When a full stomach is suspected, rapid sequence is used to minimize the risk of aspiration.

One associated technique used in emergency intubations is known as rapid sequence induction and intubation. This technique, compressing the cricoid cartilage (located below the thyroid cartilage) posteriorly against the esophagus (Sellick maneuver), prevents gastric contents from reaching the posterior pharynx, thus minimizing the risk of aspiration. The technique requires preoxygenation, induction of deep sedation, and simultaneous use of muscle relaxants without confirming ventilation before intubation; this is the standard technique routinely used to prevent aspiration. Adequate bedside suctioning equipment still must be present.

When ventilation is established, air leaks eliminated, adequate tidal volumes and oxygenation established, and the tube secured, the patient can be placed on a mechanical ventilator for supportive care. There are a number of ways to secure the ETT. Regardless of the method used (benzoin, tape, umbilical tape, or endotracheal tube holders), the tube must be carefully secured, as it is now a lifeline for the patient. A chest x-ray helps confirm the ETT position within the bronchial tree. Optimal position of the tip of the ETT is approximately 2–3 cm above the carina or slightly below the level of the clavicular heads, with the patient's head midline and in a neutral position. Flexion or extension of the head can move the distal end of the ETT 2–5 cm either proximally or distally, respectively.

Nasotracheal Intubation

Another technique employed is nasotracheal intubation. This procedure can be done in conjunction with direct laryngoscopy and a pair of Magill forceps, which can help guide the ETT into the trachea with direct vision. Another approach is to insert the endotracheal tube through the nose into the pharynx and then into the trachea without visual confirmation, which is accomplished by adjusting head position, changing tube direction, and advancing the tube while listening to breath sounds, thus performing a "blind intubation." Vasoconstrictors, lubricant, and topical anesthetic are used to prepare the nares for nasal intubation, thus requiring more preparation time than for the oral route. The size of the ETT is limited by the size of the nasal passages; an ETT that is smaller than that used for an oral intubation may be required. The risk of bleeding is notably higher, given the smaller space and the number of superficial blood vessels. Nasotracheal intubation can be done relatively efficiently, however, and is preferred for some patients if the intubation is to continue for more than a few days. From the patient level of comfort, a tube in the nose is better tolerated than in the mouth. One major problem with the nasal route, however, is that sinusitis can develop with prolonged intubation. Subsequently, this technique is quietly falling out of favor if a

Nasotracheal intubation is used primarily in the OR setting now, given the recognized risk of sinusitis with a nasotracheal tube in situ for more than a few days.

prolonged intubation is anticipated. However, it is commonly used for certain types of surgery in the operating room.

Difficult Intubation

If the initial attempt at intubation fails, then the setting is transformed from an easy to a somewhat difficult intubation. Alternative solutions need to be identified. Most important to keep in mind is that so long as the patient can be easily ventilated there is time to make decisions about the next steps. These steps can be as simple as changing patient head or neck position or suctioning to clear debris. Equipment changes such as changing the laryngoscope blade or size may provide better visualization of the anatomic structures of the airway. Smaller ETTs may facilitate passage of the tube through a stenotic area and into the trachea. Another problem may be the responsiveness of the patient such as considerable movement or combativeness, which prohibits intubation. Additional sedation may be needed in this particular situation. Muscle relaxants may be added to facilitate tracheal intubation, although it is important to keep in mind that the resultant apnea may result in loss of the airway. Finally, changing the operator is an option. In most of these situations, altering approach with any one or two of these maneuvers results in successful intubation.

An intubation may be difficult for one of several reasons. So long as it is possible to ventilate the patient, there is time to make decisions about the next steps.

Repeated manipulation and attempts to intubate the airway result in bleeding and swelling of the airway, making oxygenation and ventilation increasingly difficult or impossible, with sudden and unexpected loss of airway. The American Society of Anesthesiologists derived the difficult airway logarithm to "reduce the likelihood of adverse outcomes (see Figure 1-5). The principal adverse outcomes associated with the difficult airway include (but are not limited to) death, brain injury, myocardial injury, and airway trauma." This algorithm attempts to maintain a patent airway at all times. The algorithm's initial assessment is divided into three areas: difficult intubation, difficult ventilation, and difficulty with patient cooperation or consent. Primary and alternative strategies deal with each difficult situation.

The ASA algorithm defines the pathway to follow with both the recognized and unrecognized difficult airway.

Support Devices That May Improve Oxygenation or Ventilation

Laryngeal Mask Airway

The laryngeal mask airway (LMA) can be used in difficult intubation circumstances so long as it is possible to ventilate the patient. This device provides a means of establishing an airway and allows a conduit for fiberoptic intubation (Figure 1-6). The LMA is a tube with a masklike structure that fits into the oropharynx and covers the laryngeal outlet, thus allowing ventilation without directly viewing the laryngeal anatomy. The LMA is not tolerated by a conscious patient because of the stimulation of the oral airway. Adequate sedation is required when inserting this device as well as during its use.

Support devices are available that may improve oxygenation or ventilation if routine intubation is not possible.

Combitube

The combitube, which is used for emergency intubations, usually in the field outside the hospital, is a double lumen tube blindly placed into the oral cavity and advanced into either the esophagus or trachea. Inflation of the two balloons and ventilation of each port allows the identification of the port that communicates with the trachea, thus establishing adequate ventilation and oxygenation (Figure 1-7).

If the airway seems difficult secondary to anatomy, excess swelling, or tissue injury, fiberoptic intubation may be the technique of choice. This procedure can be done via the oral or nasal route, but, in addition to topical anesthetic for the oropharynx and vasoconstrictors, a fiberoptic scope with a light source is required. This technique requires more time, so the degree of respiratory distress affects the decision to use it. If the airway appears difficult, then the ASA algorithm for a difficult airway may be followed (see Figure 1-4). Fiberoptic intubation requires preparation and additional equipment to adequately intubate

Fiberoptic intubation may be used in controlled difficult intubations.

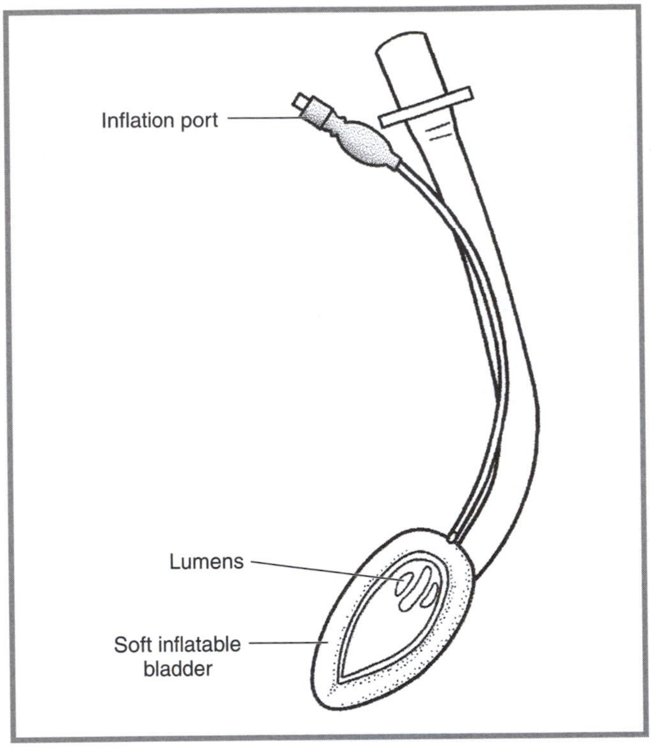

FIGURE 1-6

Laryngeal mask airway (LMA). The LMA is inserted into the oropharynx with the soft inflatable bladder deflated. When the LMA is in position at the laryngeal outlet, the bladder is inflated.

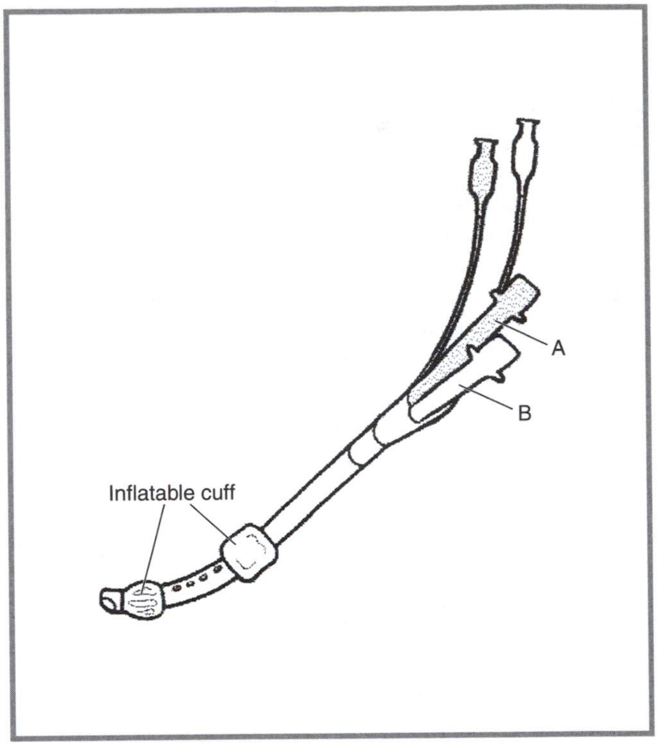

FIGURE 1-7

Combitube. Either port can be used to ventilate the lungs, depending on the final placement of the device. A, esophageal lumen; B, tracheal lumen.

the patient. If the nasal approach is used, the nares need to be adequately prepared. Some believe that when a fiberoptic scope is required the nasal approach is easier and more expeditiously performed. With the oral approach, a specially designed oral airway (ovassapian) helps guide the fiberoptic scope around the tongue into the posterior pharynx. If several intubations have been attempted, there is likely to be airway swelling. If an LMA is available, it may help establish an airway and maintain easy ventilation until a more stable airway is established, that is, an ETT or tracheostomy. By using a fiberoptic scope to visualize and confirm vocal cord, tracheal, and carinal anatomy, a smaller ETT (6.0) can be advanced over the scope and through the LMA lumen into the trachea. After the LMA is removed, the tube can be changed to a larger size; this is facilitated by using a endotracheal tube exchanger, which is a long, semirigid catheter placed through the lumen of the ETT.

Other methods of establishing an airway are described, such as a lightwand or retrograde intubation, but operator experience is imperative if these techniques are attempted.

Other modes of establishing an airway include the illuminating intubating stylet (a.k.a. lightwand) and retrograde intubation. The lightwand technique uses transillumination of the midline neck to guide an intubation without direct visual confirmation of the airway anatomy (blind intubation). Retrograde techniques involve threading a wire or catheter through the cricothyroid membrane up the trachea and out through the oropharynx; this then serves as a guide for a stiffer hollow catheter, which then is used to guide the ETT into the correct position. In the ICU setting, the special equipment needed is frequently inaccessible. Operator experience may also be a limiting factor. When intubation is not possible and ventilation becomes difficult or impossible, a surgical airway needs to be established. If no surgical personnel are immediately available, cricothyroidotomy with a large-bore IV catheter, followed by transtracheal jet ventilation, can temporize the situation until a surgery team can arrive. Commercial cricothyroidotomy sets are available that provide a more substantial temporary airway which can be converted to a formal tracheotomy at a later time.

TABLE 1-4

COMPLICATIONS OF INTUBATION OR LARYNGOSCOPY

Laryngoscopy
Mucosal lacerations of lips, cheeks, tongue
Dislodged tooth, increases risk of aspiration
Neck extension results in nerve damage or exacerbation of nerve injury
Vagal response causes lowered BP or HR
Esophageal intubation
Esophageal perforation
Indwelling Tube
Endobronchial intubation
Aspiration
Glottic and subglottic edema
Vocal cord paralysis
Excessive/inspissated secretions
Pneumonia/tracheobronchitis
Nasal bleeding from nasal intubation
Perforation of ethmoid sinuses
Tracheal tear
Tracheomalacia
Inominate artery perforation
Tracheal stenosis
Vocal cord granulomas
Kinked ETT

Worsening respiratory distress overburdens the cardiovascular system. Heart rate (HR) and blood pressure (BP) are frequently elevated secondary to sympathetic nervous system stimulation from anxiety or increased work of breathing. Another contributing factor may be elevated carbon dioxide and borderline hypoxia. Vagal stimulation may occur with laryngoscopy, causing a precipitous drop in HR and then BP. Laryngoscopy can also markedly increase HR and BP. Whether marked elevation or decrease in hemodynamics occurs, the procedure may need to be interrupted to correct or blunt these responses. After intubation, there is generally a decrease in BP and HR because of a drop in the sympathetic response. Postintubation hemodynamic instability can occur with correction of hypoxia and hypercarbia, as well as the effect of positive pressure ventilation on preload. With complete cardiovascular collapse, there is insufficient perfusion to the lungs. Even if the ETT is in the correct position, there will be no evidence of CO_2 return as a result of the lack of pulmonary blood flow. The alveoli are ventilated but not perfused. In the constant evaluation and reevaluation process of establishing an airway, the ABC's of an emergency must always be at the basis of treatment until the patient's condition can be stabilized.

Although respiratory distress may overburden the cardiovascular system before intubation, hemodynamic instability may occur after intubation as a result of several factors.

Table 1-4 indicates some of the complications associated with the act of intubation, laryngoscopy, or tracheostomy. From the table, it is clear that intubation should be performed only if indicated. It is generally understood that the longer the artificial airway is maintained, the higher the likelihood of complications associated with its use. The risk/benefit ratio must be assessed repeatedly to determine the benefits of prolonged airway cannulation.

PHARMACOLOGIC AIDS FOR INTUBATION

Numerous agents to induce a state of unconsciousness and keep the patient from fighting procedural maneuvers during intubation include barbiturates, etomidate, propofol, ketamine, narcotics, and benzodiazepines. Choice of the specific induction agent is influenced by cardiovascular and neurologic status at the time of intubation. Neuromuscular blocking agents facilitate tracheal intubation but provide absolutely no sedation or hypnotic effect. Metabolism and excretion of all these agents are influenced by liver and renal disease.

Numerous pharmacologic agents are available to aid the process of establishing an airway. Choice of agent is decided by the known pharmacodynamic and pharmacokinetic effects and by the patient's physiologic status.

The medications chosen for facilitating intubation are potent sedative-hypnotics that have rapid onset times. These medications induce unconsciousness. Due to their pharmacokinetics, they are redistributed away from vessel-rich organs (brain, heart, liver, kidney) into vessel-poor tissues. During the period of unconsciousness, the ability to ventilate the patient should be confirmed. Anesthesiologists use these types of agents after preoxygenation with 100% O_2 because, in the case of an unexpected difficult airway, the patient should be able to wake up within 5 min and resume spontaneous ventilation.

The uncooperative patient with a difficult airway presents the most problematic situation for intubation. Use of sedative-hypnotics and neuromuscular blocking agents eliminates spontaneous ventilation but does not guarantee ventilation. The resultant situation could be an unconscious, nonbreathing patient who cannot be ventilated. It is important to reassess the neurologic status of the patient once an airway has been established to ensure that no neurologic injury has occurred during the procedure. Once this has been established, sedation can be instituted to keep the patient comfortable and to minimize the tendency to fight against the sensation of a foreign object in the throat. Sedation may also blunt the initial discomfort associated with positive pressure ventilation. A full explanation of sedative/hypnotic and neuromuscular blocking agents is provided in Chapters 44 and 46, respectively.

SPECIAL SITUATIONS

> Some special situations, such as epiglottis, facial, or airway trauma and mediastinal mass, significantly affect the style and method of establishing an airway.

Certain conditions that may or may not be related to airway anatomy affect the method and style of intubation. Some of these conditions include full stomach, increased intracranial pressure, myocardial ischemia, neck injury, mediastinal mass, and trauma. A skilled intubator can quickly assess a situation while preparing to perform the procedure. While observing and asking various questions, the person preparing to intubate should be developing several plans. These plans are affected by information the health care providers can offer before intubation.

Full Stomach, Nausea, or Vomiting

A patient with a "full stomach" has a higher risk of aspirating stomach contents into the lungs with intubation. It is important to minimize this potential problem by use of clear antacids (Bicitra), awake intubation, or rapid sequence induction (previously described). Histamine receptor type 2 blocking agents limit the harmful acidity of the gastric contents. However, their onset of action is too slow to be effective in an urgent situation. Most patients requiring intubation in the intensive care unit have some risk factor associated with "a full stomach."

Other risk factors for full stomach include pregnancy, obesity, gastroparesis (diabetic neuropathy), bowel obstruction, emergency surgery, trauma (blunt or penetrating), enteral nutrition, and upper GI bleeding.

Increased Intracranial Pressure

Increased intracranial pressure (ICP) may be secondary to head trauma, brain tumor, or subarachnoid hemorrhage. Sedative agents and methods used to minimize change in ICP during intubation include induction of general anesthesia, controlled hyperventilation, and adequate oxygenation. Noting pupil size before and after intubation provides an initial neurologic assessment.

Myocardial Ischemia

Cardiovascular status impacts the choice of medications used to induce a state of unconsciousness. Most induction agents are myocardial depressants. Both myocardial ischemia and cardiomyopathy (reduced ejection fraction) may cause a low flow state. Reduced dosage and delayed onset time characterize the pharmacodynamics of these agents. Laryngoscopy and sympathetic excess may induce or exacerbate significant arrhythmias.

Neck Injury

Patients who require a restrictive neck brace have limited neck motion, and this factor may limit optimal positioning and subsequent airway visualization. With direct laryngoscopy, an assistant is required to maintain inline stabilization. With neck injury, it may be possible to ventilate the patient without being able to intubate. Fiberoptic intubation may be the technique of choice. Tracheotomy may also be an option.

Mediastinal Mass

An anterior mediastinal mass can compress and collapse either the trachea or mainstem bronchi. Spontaneous ventilation is maintained by the patient's muscle tone, negative pressure ventilation, and postural changes. Changes in any one of these supportive maneuvers may result in collapse of the airway below the vocal cords. A smooth induction with sedatives and neuromuscular agents may allow correct placement of the ETT. However, it may not be possible to oxygenate and ventilate the patient as a result of collapse of the airway with positive pressure ventilation. Typically, these patients are intubated using awake fiberoptic technique while maintaining spontaneous ventilation; this allows confirmation of the ETT placement and, more important, visualization of external compression of the trachea or bronchi. Occasionally, the only way to oxygenate and ventilate a patient in this situation is by using cardiopulmonary bypass.

Oropharyngeal and Facial Trauma

If facial injuries are substantial, a surgical airway may be required immediately. Blind nasal intubation is contraindicated because of unknown facial injury and the possibility of a placing an ETT into the cranial vault. The ability to open the mouth may also be significantly compromised with mandibular fractures. Forcing the mouth open after muscle relaxation may result in a large hematoma or uncontrolled bleeding into the oral cavity. Such trauma is another circumstance in which tracheostomy may be the best option to secure the airway.

Self-Extubation

Many patients who extubate themselves may not always need immediate reintubation. Patients who are alert and self-extubate are more likely to remain extubated than patients who have been accidentally extubated. The patient's oxygenation and ventilatory pattern determine whether an airway needs to be reestablished. However, reintubation may be difficult because of airway edema and other pathophysiologic changes.

Independent Lung Ventilation

Indications for one-lung ventilation using a double lumen endotracheal tube (DLT) in the operating room are classified as absolute and relative. Absolute indications include isolation of a healthy lung to prevent contamination from infection or bleeding, controlled distribution of ventilation to one lung only, or unilateral lung lavage. Relative indications are related to the need to improve surgical exposure. With the increasing use of video-assisted thoracoscopy, the need to have a nonmoving collapsed lung is increasingly important. The DLT has a large external diameter and requires more skill in establishing its proper positioning. The distal bronchial lumen is curved to allow placement into the mainstem bronchus. Its placement routinely is confirmed with fiberoptic bronchoscopy. In the operating room, changing the patient's position can result in dislodging the DLT from its proper position. In the intensive care setting, a patient with a DLT must remain sedated and paralyzed. Independent lung ventilation is usually related to unilateral infection, bronchopleural fistulas, or ruptured pulmonary artery. There are certain instances in which the compliance of each lung is sub-

FIGURE 1-8

The double lumen tube (DLT) can be right- or left-sided. Because of the likelihood of obstructing the right upper lobe bronchial orifice when using the right-sided DLT, the left-sided DLT is used most frequently in both the ICU and operating room setting.

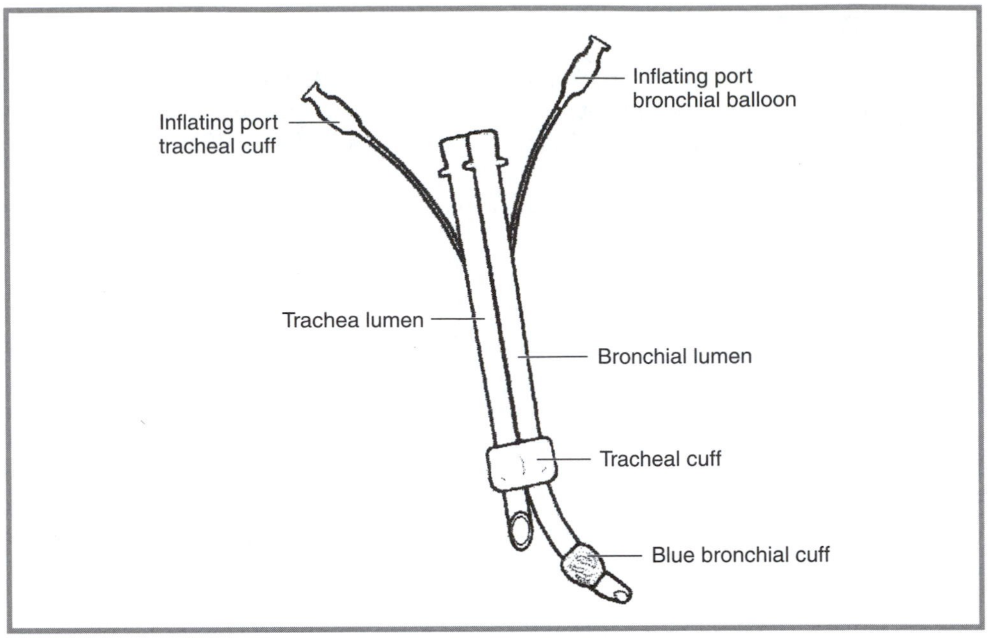

stantially different so as to require two ventilators to optimize ventilation in each lung. A double lumen ETT is the only way to establish this kind of support (Figure 1-8).

Withholding Intubation

There are times not to establish an airway in the face of respiratory distress; this is usually in a situation in which there is an established "do not resuscitate" (DNR) order. If the patient's prognosis is so poor that life expectancy is limited, then it is reasonable to question whether this therapy is indicated. Keeping the patient comfortable with analgesics and sedatives may be the better alternative. The final decision is best made by the individuals responsible for the primary care of the patient.

WHEN TO EXTUBATE

The underlying process that induced respiratory distress must be improved before considering extubation.

Numerous criteria have been developed for extubation over the years. Weaning parameters are performed with variation of frequency, depending on the length of intubation and institutional policies. There is considerable debate about the best weaning protocol even within an institution. Exact definitions of specific indicators are beyond the scope of this chapter. Regardless of the criteria used, the initiating process that brought about respiratory distress must be adequately corrected before considering extubation.

WHEN TO PROCEED WITH TRACHEOTOMY

Timing of tracheotomy is based on the patient's condition, the anticipated need for mechanical ventilation, and the demonstrated progress, or lack thereof, while intubated.

Timing of tracheotomy is based on clinical judgment. Tracheotomy requires thoughtful consideration rather than adherence to overly simplistic and unsubstantiated rules. The literature supports proceeding with tracheotomy within 2 weeks to as long as 6 weeks. Patients with only pulmonary disease usually do not proceed to a tracheostomy. There is usually a compounding disease process that exacerbates the marginal pulmonary status. For example, a patient with end-stage pulmonary disease who has developed concomitant cardiac failure may benefit from early tracheotomy. However, if the patient appears to be improving with therapy, then waiting longer may allow the patient to heal without a tracheostomy. The decision when to proceed with tracheostomy should be tailored to the patient's medical requirements. Patients who have been intubated for more than 1 month have been successfully weaned from the ventilator without proceeding to tracheotomy. Surgical cases involving median sternotomy may lead to maintaining the oral ETT airway for a longer period of time rather than proceeding to tracheostomy; this decision is related to concerns about potential wound infection of the chest with secretions from the tracheostomy.

Proceeding with tracheotomy should be presented as a positive step in the patient's medical therapy. Frequently, patients wean from ventilatory support much more quickly once the deadspace and resistance of the endotracheal tube have been eliminated. Pulmonary toilet is easier. Patients are more comfortable without a tube in the posterior oropharynx. It is considerably easier to reconnect a patient with a tracheotomy to the ventilator if weaning trials fail than to reestablish an airway with an ETT. Therefore, although it is a surgical procedure and in most cases requires exposure to an anesthetic, the overall advantages of the procedure usually outweigh the basic risks of the surgery.

It is well recognized that with certain types of strokes patients have limited ability to protect the airway due to loss of airway reflexes. In bone marrow patients, neutropenia may be significant and cause early pneumonia. Early tracheostomy may be helpful in this patient group. Other advantages of tracheotomy include accelerating the process of weaning and thus reducing the duration of ventilation, length of hospitalization, and costs. On the other hand, tracheotomy may provide no benefit to patients with respect to survival and duration of mechanical ventilation and may increase airway injury. Tracheostomy does require proper care such as maintaining patency by frequently changing the inner cannula and limiting cuff pressures to reduce tracheomalacia and tracheal stenosis. One small but serious risk of tracheostomy is inominate artery perforation caused by erosion of the tracheal wall by a chronically overinflated tracheal cuff.

> Tracheostomy is performed when the overall benefits outweigh the risks of the procedure.

MANAGING THE CHRONICALLY INSTRUMENTED AIRWAY

Tracheal Tube Designs

Several types of endotracheal tubes are used for airway management. Most common in the intensive care setting are tubes composed of polyvinyl chloride (PVC). In some instances, an armored or anode tube may be used to prevent kinking or obstruction of the established airway. Cuffed endotracheal tubes have either high-pressure, low-compliance or low-pressure, high-compliance cuffs. Excessive pressure on the trachea with inflated cuffs can lead to ischemic tissue and tracheomalacia with prolonged intubation. A cutoff of 25 mmHg is the suggested pressure limit of the cuff. The goal is to inflate the cuff with the minimum amount of air needed to provide an adequate seal for adequate mechanical ventilation.

Finally, given the rising incidence of ventilator-associated pneumonia (VAP) with prolonged intubation, a new endotracheal tube design includes one that allows suctioning of secretions from above the pilot balloon (subglottic secretions); this appears to diminish the incidence of VAP (Valles et al.).

MAINTENANCE OF ENDOTRACHEAL TUBES

Once placed, the endotracheal tube is subjected to the dynamic changes of patient pathophysiology as well as medical therapy. Although this statement seems obvious, it is important to remember that the piece of plastic serving as an airway is prone to complications if not well managed. Inspissated secretions can block the tube, inhibiting exchange of oxygen and carbon dioxide. The endotracheal tube can slip down into the right mainstem bronchus with neck flexion or can slip out of the trachea with neck extension. The amount of air in the pilot cuff can be too little, allowing for an air leak and decreased tidal volumes. Conversely, the pilot balloon can be inflated too much, leading to tracheal ischemia and subsequent tracheal complications.

> Maintenance of indwelling endotracheal tubes is mandatory to ensure patency and proper position.

Several steps can be taken to minimize potential problems:

- Suctioning: Suctioning helps minimize secretions in the ETT and mucous plugs.
- Cuff Pressures: Ideally, cuff pressures should be less than 25 mmHg to minimize ischemic changes to the trachea.
- Tape Changes: Frequent taping of the ETT can produce excoriation of the face and neck. It is important to ensure the security of the endotracheal tube. If the patient remains intubated for long periods of time, there may be less injury with cloth tape or IV tubing. Additionally, the lips can sustain pressure necrosis if the ETT tube is always taped in the same position in the mouth.
- Nasotracheal Tubes: Nasotracheal tubes can eliminate some of the discomfort felt with oral ETTs, but sinusitis can occur if the tube remains in place for a prolonged period. Fever of unknown origin must be evaluated to exclude severe sinusitis from nasal intubation.

Tracheal irritation begins as soon as the endotracheal tube is placed.

Another significant potential problem with prolonged intubation is development of postintubation laryngotracheal stenosis. Tracheal irritation begins as soon as the endotracheal tube is placed. Short periods of intubation are usually well tolerated without major complications. Factors leading to laryngotracheal stenosis include direct pressure necrosis from the cuff material and high pressures, duration of intubation, macro- and microtrauma during intubation, the intubation technique used for placement of the ETT, the degree of respiratory failure, infection, and poor tissue perfusion.

Endotracheal Tube Changes

Endotracheal tube changes should be done only when necessary and only under the supervision of experienced personnel.

Endotracheal tubes should be changed carefully and only by experienced personnel. Changing an ETT may be required secondary to the following:

1. Leaking pilot balloon.
2. Thick secretions obstructing the lumen of the tube.
3. Changing from a typical PVC tube to an armored, more rigid tube to minimize kinking.
4. Placing a larger tube for bronchoscopy.
5. Placing a smaller tube to minimize vocal cord granulation formation.
6. Changing a single lumen tube to a double lumen tube for independent lung ventilation.
7. Changing a double lumen tube to a single lumen tube when independent lung ventilation is no longer needed. Double lumen tubes have narrow lumens and are more easily affected by secretions than are single lumen tubes. Pulmonary toilet is thus hampered, and resultant mucous plugging and hypoxia can occur. Therefore, once sufficient lung healing has occurred, it is best to reestablish a single lumen tube with a larger lumen; this technique enables the caregiver to more adequately remove excess secretions through suctioning techniques.

Frequently, these patients have been intubated for a long time, and the upper airway may be swollen. Direct laryngoscopy should be performed to evaluate the oropharynx and vocal cords. If minimal edema is present or if the vocal cords are easily visualized, then the tube can be easily removed and another tube easily placed. However, if there is too much edema, then the tube needs to be replaced using a smaller catheter. The catheter acts as a guide, and oxygen can be insufflated through it. The ETT in situ can then be removed and a new one placed over it; this maintains an airway while allowing a necessary procedure to be performed.

SUMMARY

When a patient is critically ill, respiratory compromise is frequently either a cause of the illness, or a consequence of the underlying problem. Our role in the intensive care setting is to attempt to alleviate the cause of the acute respiratory distress or to ensure that oxygen delivery and exchange, ventilation, and the work of breathing are optimized to meet the demonstrated demands of the patient's condition.

Airway management might be conservative or it might be aggressive and invasive. Conservative management may be offered if the inciting problem clears quickly or if the patient's condition has deteriorated to the point that no medical intervention can change the course of the patient's outcome. Any condition between these two ends of the spectrum mandates a focused examination and assessment of the need for mechanical ventilation. If the decision is reached that an artificial airway needs to be established to improve the patient's chances of survival, the urgency for proceeding forward can be established by running a quick checklist of the patient's condition; this can also be done even more quickly by observing the ABC's of an emergency situation. Should an intubation be required to establish mechanical ventilation, basic monitoring equipment should be available. Adequate intubation equipment and adjunct medications enable establishing an airway quickly and efficiently in most settings.

The difficult airway is handled based on the ability to oxygenate and ventilate. If it is possible to assist ventilation, then there is time to consider reasonable options for establishing a patent airway. Should the situation deteriorate to an inability to accomplish these goals, then emergent surgical airway is the appropriate approach to the problem. Initiating mechanical ventilation does not necessarily mean that the patient will always require this medical intervention. Once mechanical ventilation has been instituted, however, it is important to continue until the underlying process that led to the respiratory compromise has been addressed and corrected. Then, the ability to wean from mechanical ventilation or the need for tracheostomy can be fully assessed.

A chronically instrumented airway needs attention to prevent plugging from secretions, to maintain patency, and to change the airway when needed to provide optimum support for the patient. The longer the period of intubation, the more likely the need for tracheostomy, and the higher the potential for complications.

REVIEW QUESTIONS

1. **Signs of hypoxia in a medical or surgical patient can include which of the following:**
   - **A.** Changes in the patient's mental status
   - **B.** Patient changing from the supine position to a sitting position
   - **C.** Tachycardia or bradycardia
   - **D.** Hypertension or hypotension
   - **E.** Cyanosis

2. **A medical patient whose arterial PCO_2 is 55 mmHg requires which of the following:**
   - **A.** Immediate endotracheal intubation
   - **B.** Assessment of their medical history
   - **C.** Repeat arterial blood gas measurements
   - **D.** Assessment of physical exam and vital signs
   - **E.** Supplemental oxygen

3. **Evaluation of the airway before an urgent intubation should include which of the following:**
   - **A.** Assessment of the maximal opening of mouth and visualization of structures in the oropharynx
   - **B.** Amount of edema or fat tissue in the neck region of the patient
   - **C.** Conditions such as hiatal hernia, pregnancy, obesity, or recent food ingestion that may contribute to aspiration of stomach contents
   - **D.** History of previous vascular surgery
   - **E.** Knowledge of patient's pulmonary artery pressures

4. **Equipment that is absolutely necessary for intubation of a patient in the critical care setting includes which of these:**
   - **A.** Ventilator
   - **B.** AMBU bag (airway mask breathing unit)
   - **C.** Nasal cannula or face mask oxygen source
   - **D.** Suctioning equipment
   - **E.** Bronchodilator agents

5. **Effects of laryngoscopy can include which of the following:**
   - **A.** Increase in heart rate
   - **B.** Decrease in heart rate
   - **C.** Asystole
   - **D.** Ventricular arrhythmias
   - **E.** Increase or decrease in blood pressure

ANSWERS

1. The answer is A, B, C, D, E. Signs of hypoxia can masquerade as any of these changes. The initial signs of hypoxia (tachycardia and hypertension) may not be appreciated or attenuated by other medications such as beta-blockers or analgesia and sedative medications. Changing from the supine to sitting position is a compensatory behavior in an attempt to improve oxygen exchange.
2. The answer is B, D. Assessment of the patient's history focuses on chronic obstructive pulmonary disease, the associated retention of CO_2, and concomitant metabolic alkalosis. Previous sedative or narcotic medications may result in an acute increase in PCO_2. Supplemental oxygen theoretically may inhibit respiratory drive.
3. The answer is A, B, C. Answers A and B are concerned with the anatomic structures that may change the level of difficulty associated with laryngoscopy and correct placement of an endotracheal tube. Conditions that increase the likelihood of regurgitation and aspiration should also be assessed.
4. The answer is B, D. An AMBU bag is necessary for maximal preoxygenation of the patient as well as permitting hand-ventilation of the patient before intubation. Hand-ventilation may be required by the patient's medical condition or medications used before intubation. Suction equipment is always necessary and should be immediately available next to the patient's head when manipulation of the airway is anticipated.
5. The answer is A, B, C, D, E. Induction of anesthesia, use of muscle relaxation, and endotracheal intubation can induce significant sympathetic stimulation. Intubation is also associated with vagal stimulation. Most sedative-hypnotic agents used for induction can cause vasodilation.

SUGGESTED READING

Barash PG, Cullen BF, Stoelting RK. Clinical Anesthesia, 3rd Ed. Philadelphia: Lippincott–Raven, 1997.

Benumof J. The American Society of Anesthesiologists' Management of the Difficult Airway algorithm and explanation-analysis of the algorithm. In: Benumof J (ed) Airway Management: Principles and Practice. St. Louis: Mosby, 1996:142–156.

Benumof J. Definition and incidence of the difficult airway. In: Benumof J (ed) Airway Management: Principles and Practice. St. Louis: Mosby, 1996:121–125.

Berry AM, et al. The laryngeal mask airway in emergency medicine, neonatal resuscitation, and intensive care medicine. Int Anesthesiol Clin 1998;36(3):91–109.

Blot F, Guiguet M, Antoun S, et al. Early tracheotomy in neutropenic mechanically ventilated patients. Support Care Cancer 1995;3: 291–296.

Boerner TF, Ramanathan S. Functional anatomy of airway. In: Benumof J (ed) Airway Management: Principles and Practice. St. Louis: Mosby, 1996:3–21.

Christie JM, Dethlefsen M, Cane RD. Unplanned endotracheal extubation in the intensive care unit. J Clin Anesthiol 1996;8:289–293.

Deem S, Bishop MJ. Evaluation of the difficult airway. Crit Care Clin 1995;11(1):1–27.

Ferdinande P, Kim DO. Prevention of postintubation laryngotracheal stenosis. Acta Oto-rhino-laryngol Belg 1995;49:341–346.

Gursahaney AH, Gottfried SB. Weaning from mechanical ventilation. In: Stock MC, Perel A. (eds) Mechanical Ventilatory Support, 2nd Ed. Philadelphia: Williams & Wilkins, 1997:Chapter 23.

Heffner JE. Timing tracheotomy. Chest 1998;114(2):361–363.

Joshi GP, Smith I, White PE. Laryngeal mask airway. In: Benumof J (ed) Airway Management: Principles and Practice. St. Louis: Mosby, 1996:353–373.

Kowk HC. Airway management in the intensive care unit, Resident Reporter 1999;4(4):8–12.

Mallampati SR. Recognition of the difficult airway. In: Benumof J (ed) Airway Management: Principles and Practice. St. Louis: Mosby, 1996:126–142.

Mallampati SR, Gatt SP, Gugino LD, et al. A clinical study to predict difficult tracheal intubation. A prospective study. Can J Anaesth 1985;32:429–434.

Maziak DE, Meade MD, Todd TR. The timing of tracheotomy, a systematic review. Chest 1998;114(2):605–609.

Petruzelli GJ. Extrinsic tracheal compression from an anterior mediastinal mass in an adult: the multidisciplinary management of the airway emergency. Otolaryngol-Head Neck Surg Case Rep 1990; 103(3):484–486.

Stock MC, Perel A (eds). Mechanical Ventilatory Support. 2nd Ed. Baltimore: Williams & Wilkins, 1997:Chapter 23.

Valles J, Artigas A, Rello J, et al. Continuous aspiration of subglottic secretions in preventing ventilator-associated pneumonia. Ann Intern Med 1995;122:179–186.

Yao FF. Aspiration pneumonitis and acute respiratory failure. In: Yao FF, Artusio JF. (eds) Anesthestiology: Problem-Oriented Patient Management, 3rd Ed. Philadelphia: Lippincott, 1993:47–74.

CHAPTER 2

WISSAM CHATILA

Oxygenation Without Intubation

CHAPTER OUTLINE

LEARNING OBJECTIVES

After studying this chapter you should be able to:

- Identify different devices for supplying oxygen therapy.
- Describe the mode of function of different oxygen-supplying devices.
- Select specific devices to deliver oxygen in different patient populations.
- Adjust the oxygen delivery devices to ensure adequate oxygen supplementation.

Oxygen therapy, a lifeline for many critically ill patients, can be delivered in nonintubated patients via several devices. Unlike patients with chronic hypoxemia, the long-term comfort or cosmetics of the patient are not a concern of intensivists; instead, the goal is to ensure adequate oxygen delivery to prevent hypoxemia. Although hypoxemia is often corrected with oxygen therapy, care should be taken to understand the pathophysiology leading to hypoxemia. The appropriate management of hypoxemia should include treatment of the underlying pathology to prevent any complication and progression of the disease. For example, many patients with postoperative atelectasis develop hypoxemia responsive to oxygen therapy. Treatment of postoperative hypoxemia with oxygen supplementation alone without initiating lung reexpansion measures to treat atelectasis is insufficient. This chapter covers noninvasive modes of supplying oxygen and does not discuss other means of correcting hypoxemia.

SUPPLYING SUPPLEMENTAL OXYGEN

There are three main components of oxygen supplementation: (1) the control component, which includes regulators (reducing valves that buffer high pressures from bulk oxygen systems to a lower pressure patient point of access) and flowmeters (which control and indicate flow) (Figure 2-1), (2) the blending of air and oxygen, and (3) the administration of oxygen through devices that include cannulas and masks. Respiratory care therapists are usually responsible to ensure proper functioning of the first two components, but physicians who order oxygen supplementation tend to specify the mode of oxygen delivery; therefore, physicians should familiarize themselves with indications of available devices for oxygen administration.

The goal of oxygen supplementation is to ensure adequate oxygenation regardless of mode of delivery.

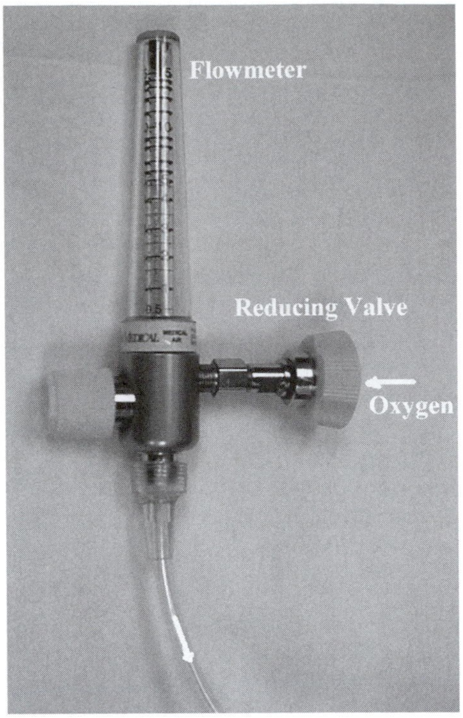

FIGURE 2-1

A flowmeter that regulates the flow of oxygen from a central source while simultaneously displaying the oxygen flow rate.

Do not confuse low-flow devices with low concentration of oxygen supplementation.

The oxygen delivery devices can be divided into two major groups. Low-flow oxygen systems comprise one group. Nasal cannulas, simple masks, and reservoir masks are examples of low-flow systems that are used when consistency in fraction of inspired oxygen (FiO_2) delivery is not crucial. In contrast, high-flow oxygen systems, the second group of devices, are capable of delivering at least 40 liters per minute (l/min) of conditioned gas, providing a precise and consistent FiO_2 regardless of the patient's breathing pattern. Venturi masks and oxygen tents are examples of high-flow systems. Accordingly, when prescribing oxygen, the desired range of FiO_2 and the patient's ventilatory pattern need to be considered to ensure effective oxygen supplementation. Both low-flow and high-flow systems can deliver a wide range of FiO_2; the terms "low" and "high" do not reflect the delivered FiO_2 but describe the flow of gas delivered through the system. A detailed description of each device follows in the next section (Table 2-1).

DEVICES THAT PROVIDE SUPPLEMENTAL OXYGEN

Nasal Cannula

The nasal cannula is the most common oxygen delivery system, used both for hospital inpatients and for outpatients (Figure 2-2). It consists of two small prongs inserted about 1 cm into each nare through which flows 100% oxygen, with the oxygen flow adjusted by the flowmeter. Although nasal cannulas are well tolerated in the majority of patients, there is a great variability in the final FiO_2 because of admixture with entrained ambient air. Thus, this system is valuable for patients who require up to 40% of uncontrolled oxygen, or those who do not tolerate facemasks. Nasal cannula use is discouraged with flows greater than 6 l/min because of drying of the nasal mucosa, crusting of secretions, epistaxis, and septal perforation or in patients who have significant nasal obstruction and are mouth breathers.

Simple Mask

Similar to the nasal cannula, the simple mask does not allow precise control of delivered oxygen concentration because of dilution with ambient air that is drawn in and inspired from

TABLE 2-1

OXYGEN CONCENTRATIONS FOR LOW- AND HIGH-FLOW DELIVERY SYSTEMS

DEVICE	OXYGEN FLOW RATE (L/MIN)	FiO_2
Nasal cannula	1	0.21–0.24
	2	0.23–0.28
	3	0.27–0.34
	4	0.31–0.38
	5–6	0.32–0.44
	6–8	Up to 0.50
Simple masks	5–6	0.30–0.45
	6–10	0.35–0.55
Venturi masks[a]	4	0.28
	6	0.28
	6	0.31
	8	0.31
	8	0.35
	12	0.40
	12	0.50
Partial-rebreathing masks	7	0.35–0.50
	≥8	≥0.60
Nonrebreathing masks	≥10	≥0.80

[a] The final FiO_2 varies according to the oxygen flow and to the total gas delivered, which is a function of the diluter jet and flow settings

the exhalation ports (Figure 2-3). However, the mask can deliver higher FiO_2 (to 55%), especially with higher flows (7–10 l/min), and produces a good seal around the patient's nose and mouth. Another advantage of the mask compared to the nasal cannula is improved humidification and fewer drying side effects. On the other hand, care should be taken not to order low flows (<5 l/min) when using the simple mask because of the potential for rebreathing exhaled carbon dioxide when mask deadspace is not continuously flushed by flowing oxygen.

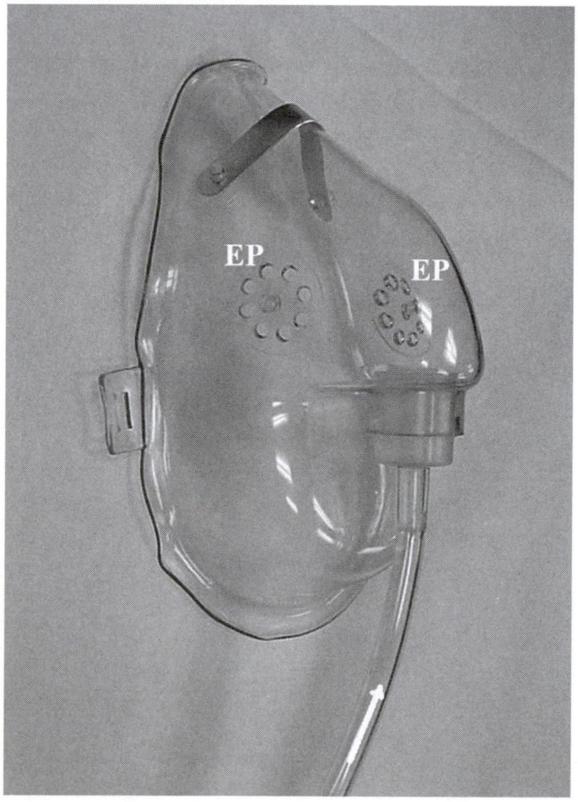

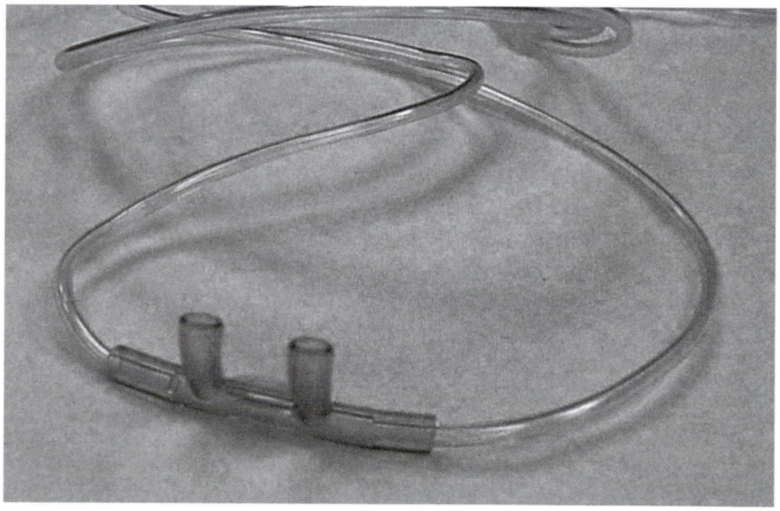

FIGURE 2-2

A nasal cannula used to deliver supplemental oxygen.

FIGURE 2-3

A simple facemask for oxygen delivery that has portholes for expiration (*EP*).

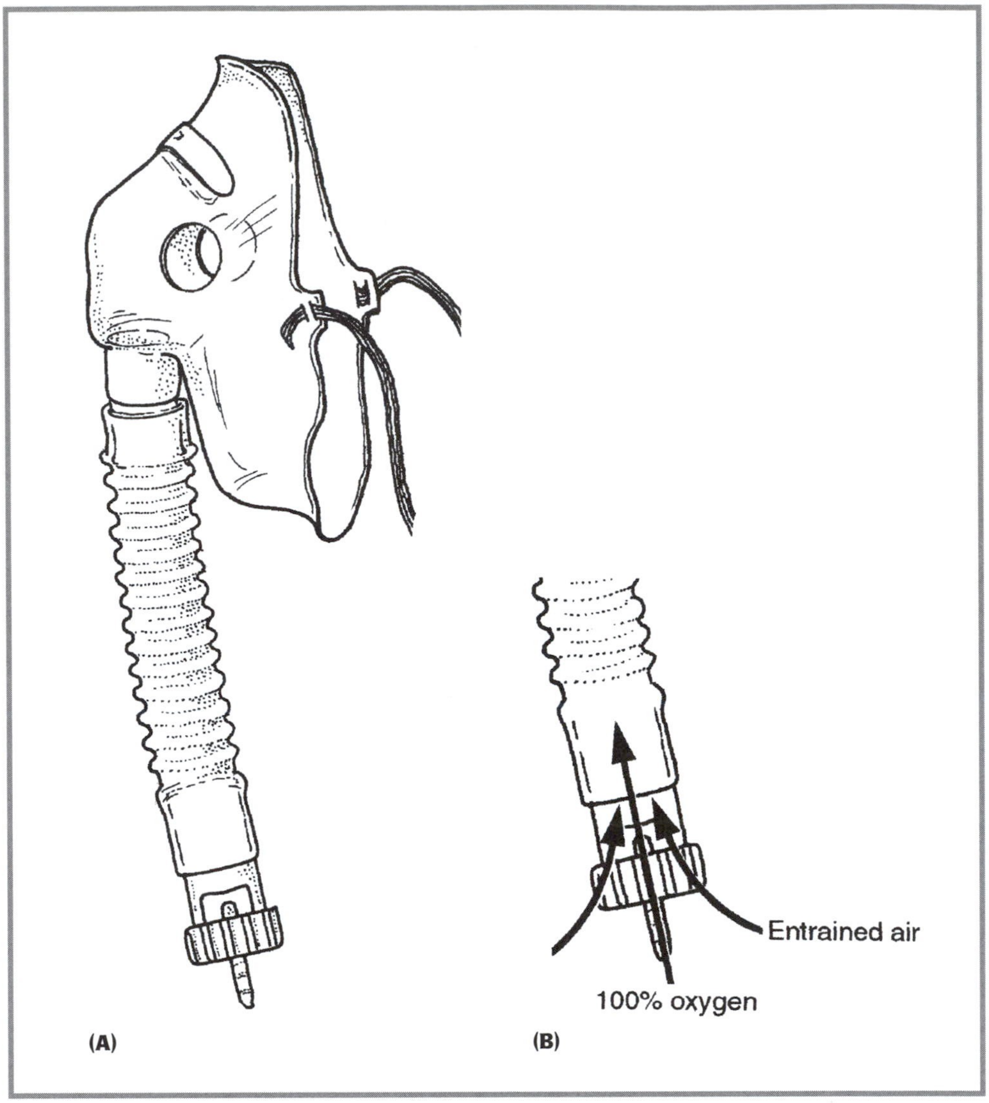

FIGURE 2-4

(A) A disposable venturi mask that allows more precise control of delivered oxygen. Gas passes through a small opening exit with a high velocity generating subatmospheric pressure that also entrains room air from the side ports. **(B)** Different diluter jets specify the amount of delivered oxygen and entrained room air mixtures that are used to vary the inspired oxygen concentration.

Venturi Mask

In nonintubated patients, the venturi mask is the only mask that delivers controlled high-flow oxygen concentration.

The venturi mask is characterized by its accurate delivery of oxygen concentration; its accuracy is within 2% of the set FiO_2 (Figure 2-4). Hypercapnic patients who are at risk for developing respiratory depression while on oxygen supplementation are good candidates for this mask. Although the venturi mask has exhalation ports similar to the simple mask, it is designed to generate very high velocity flows of 100% oxygen through a narrow orifice that limits entrained ambient air from the base of the mask; hence, the patient's inspiratory flow rate will not affect the ratio of inspired oxygen to entrained room air. This mask is constructed on the Bernoulli principle; the high-velocity flows of oxygen going through the narrow orifice generate a subatmospheric pressure around the stream of oxygen, which in turn entrains a specific proportion of room air.

Partial-Rebreathing Mask

Except for a reservoir bag, the partial-rebreathing mask is comparable to the simple mask. The oxygen source directly feeds into the reservoir bag, and when the patient inhales gas is drawn from the bag and from the exhalation ports. As the patient exhales, the first third of the exhaled tidal volume returns into the reservoir and the rest dissipates through exhalation ports. So long as the bag does not collapse by maintaining high oxygen flow rates, the partial-rebreathing mask may deliver up to 60% inspired oxygen concentration, depending on the breathing pattern of the patient.

Nonrebreathing Mask

The nonrebreathing mask can deliver up to 100% FiO_2.

Two valves, added on the inhalation and exhalation ports, distinguish the nonrebreathing mask from the partial-rebreathing mask (Figure 2-5). These two one-way valves allow the patient to inhale oxygen from the reservoir, but prevent the backflow of expired volume into the bag during exhalation and thereby avoid entraining ambient air through the exhalation ports during inspiration. The nonrebreathing mask can deliver close to 100% oxygen when adequate flow is maintained and the mask has a good seal on the patient's face. Manufacturers of nonrebreathing masks avoid placing valves on the two exhalation ports as a precautionary measure in the event of inspiratory valve malfunction, which would interrupt the flow of oxygen (note one exhalation port is covered in Figure 2-6). To avert potential valve problems, some intensivists make up reservoir masks by adding large deadspaces to simple masks (Figure 2-7). These reservoir masks, known as tusk masks, still require high flows of oxygen to flush all exhaled air from the mask deadspace and minimize the entrainement of the ambient air during inspiration.

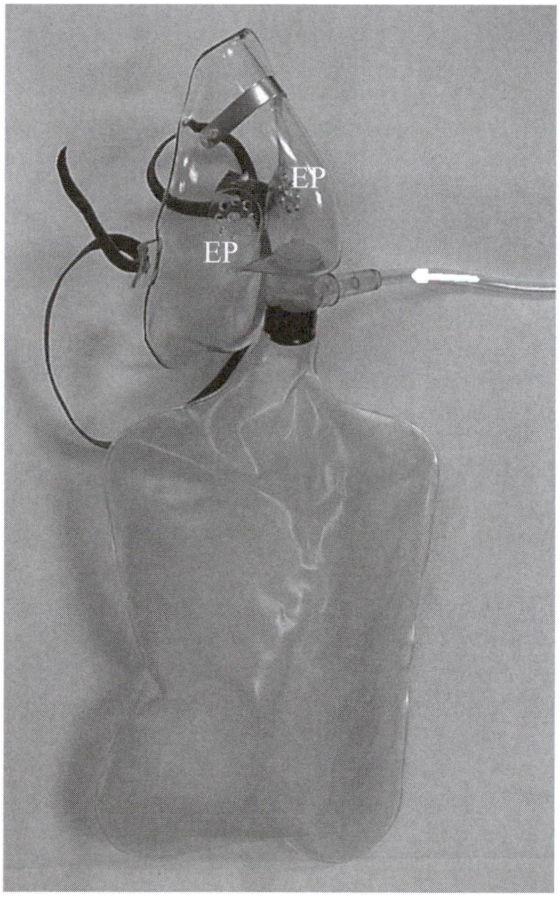

FIGURE 2-5

A partial-rebreathing facemask that delivers high levels of oxygen. The inflatable bag acts as an oxygen reservoir from which the patient can rebreathe high concentrations of supplemental oxygen. The patient expires through expiration ports (*EP*), as illustrated.

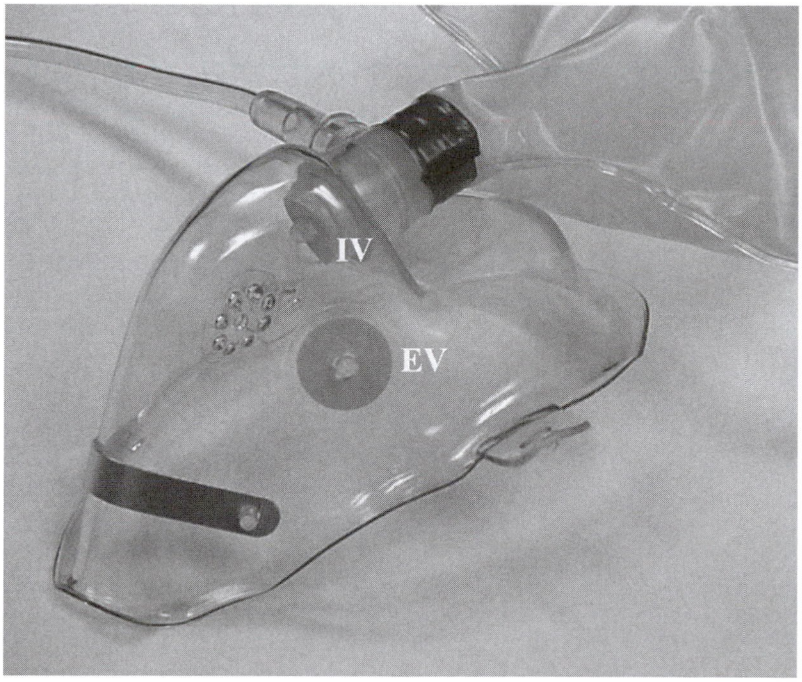

FIGURE 2-6

A nonrebreathing facemask. A one-way valve at the inhalation port (*IV*) prevents expired gases from refilling the oxygen reservoir bag. The presence of a one-way exhalation valve (*EV*) prevents room air from being inspired during inhalation.

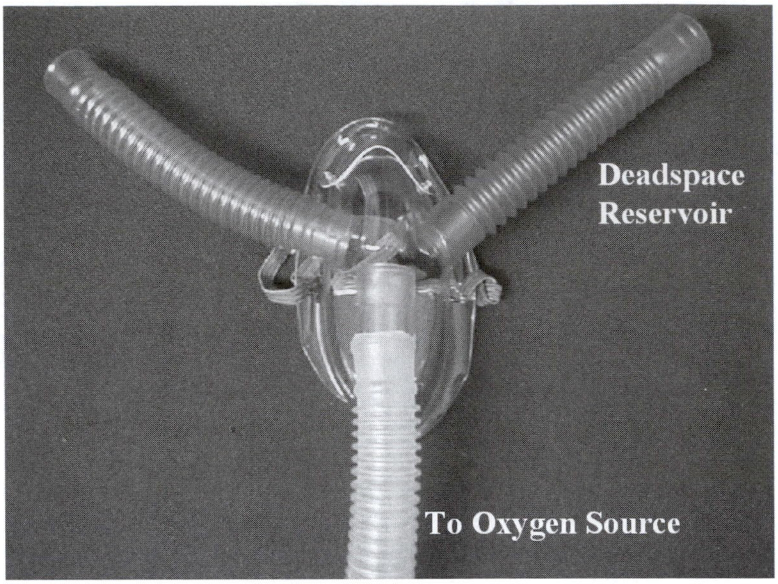

FIGURE 2-7

Modification of a facemask with 6-in. tubing substituted for exhalation valves to prevent entrainment of room air during inspiration. The mask is also known as a "tusk mask."

AMBU (Airway Mask Breathing Unit) Bag and Mask

Bag and mask ventilation is usually reserved for patients with decompensated respiratory failure, or after cardiopulmonary arrest, while preparing the equipment required for intubation. The majority of patients can be adequately supported with bag–mask ventilation as long as a tight seal between the patient's face and mask is maintained. A variety of masks are available, but a clear mask should always be used to observe for vomiting and potential aspiration.

Oxygen-Conserving Devices

Recently, newer devices for delivering oxygen have been introduced for patients on long-term oxygen therapy. Known as oxygen-conserving devices, these systems are used mostly in outpatients; these systems are not available in many hospitals and are not suited for the management of acute hypoxemia.

There are two main mechanisms for oxygen conservation. One mechanism is based on collecting 100% oxygen during exhalation in a reservoir. The reservoir is either mechanical, such as the nasal reservoir cannula or a pendant reservoir cannula that then empties on inspiration (Figure 2-8), or anatomic via a small catheter inserted into the trachea (Figure 2-9). The transtracheal oxygen system uses the proximal trachea as an expanded anatomic reservoir; oxygen flowing into the trachea washes out the anatomic deadspace, thereby also reducing work of breathing. Hence, it has the added advantage when compared with the rest of the oxygen-conserving devices of improved compliance, comfort, and functional capacity. On the other hand, this device requires higher maintenance to prevent infection at the site and obstruction of the catheter by dried secretions, which restricts its use to a minority of patients.

The second mechanism for oxygen conservation is based on the pulsation of oxygen during the first quarter to one-half of each inspiration. With these devices, as in the pendant reservoir cannula, nasal prongs are used to deliver the oxygen.

CONTINUOUS POSITIVE AIRWAY PRESSURE

Continuous positive airway pressure (CPAP) is often confused with noninvasive ventilation (bilevel positive airway pressure [BiPAP®] or pressure support ventilation). Although both modes of ventilatory support can be delivered via nasal or oronasal masks, they have different functions.

CPAP is not considered a mode of noninvasive ventilation.

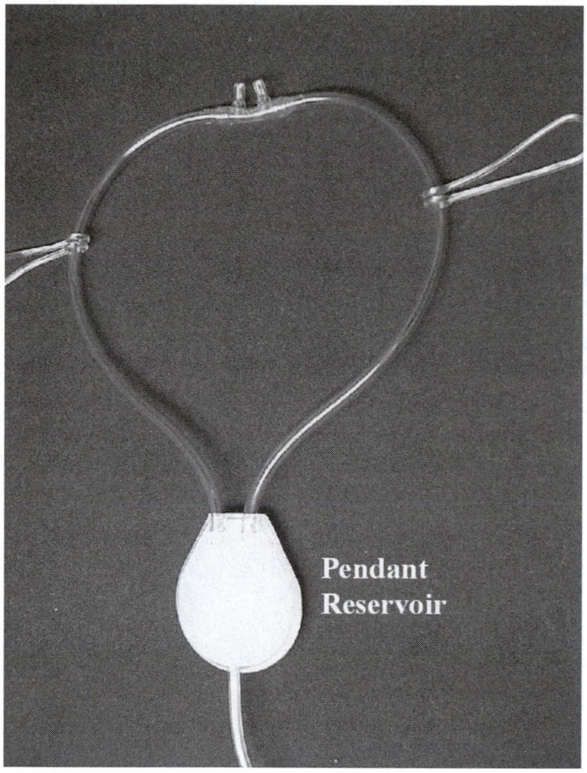

FIGURE 2-8

Nasal cannula capable of delivering high filled oxygen with the use of an oxygen reservoir. The pendant reservoir device serves as a repository of enriched oxygen from which the patient can breathe with each inhalation. The nasal cannula and tubing are larger than conventional nasal cannula to allow a higher flow of inspired gas.

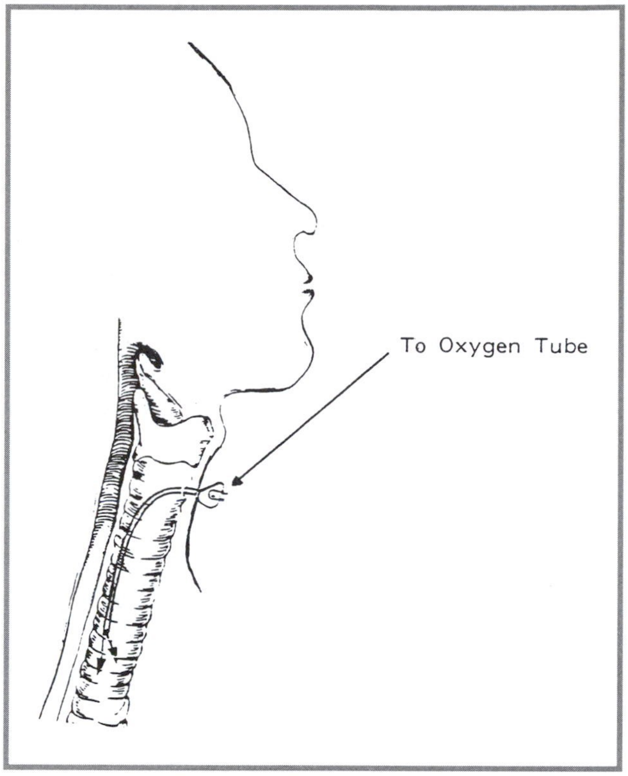

FIGURE 2-9

Proper placement of a transtracheal catheter for oxygen administration. The transtracheal oxygen delivery system uses the proximal trachea as an anatomic reservoir.

CPAP works by generating a continuous airflow that maintains a continuous positive pressure to the respiratory system during inspiration and expiration, thus preventing airway and alveolar collapse. By expanding end-expiratory lung volume, CPAP increases functional residual capacity, thus reducing the degree of intrapulmonary shunt caused by both atelectasis and fluid. In addition, through complex heart–lung interactions, the applied positive pressure may have favorable hemodynamic effects in patients with compromised cardiac function. CPAP improves left ventricular performance by reducing left ventricular preload and afterload. Obviously, CPAP can be applied in intubated patients in the form of CPAP or positive end-expiratory pressure (PEEP), but when used in spontaneously breathing nonintubated patients it serves as a pneumatic splint of the airway, which makes it a very effective method to treat obstructive sleep apnea. In the hospital, the role of CPAP is limited to patients known to have obstructive sleep apnea and selected patients with decompensated heart failure (who are hemodynamically stable and cooperative) to prevent intubation. Nevertheless, although CPAP has been shown to reduce the work of breathing in patients with chronic obstructive lung disease, many physicians elect to use noninvasive ventilation, such as BiPAP® support, because of the added advantage of delivering inspiratory support as well as PEEP while on this mode of ventilation. CPAP may improve alveolar ventilation and oxygenation by preventing airway obstruction and reversing atelectasis, but often oxygen is bled in the apparatus, that is, added to its tubing, to treat refractory hypoxia. However, one should keep in mind that in both CPAP and BiPAP® the final oxygen concentration will be uncontrolled because of patient's breathing pattern, mask fit, and, most important, the machine setting.

MONITORING

Transcutaneous pulse oximetry is effective to monitor adequate oxygenation but can be inadequate in certain subgroups of patients.

Hospitalized patients requiring oxygen supplementation should be monitored with transcutaneous pulse oximetry to ensure adequate oxygen delivery and oxygenation. However, oxygen saturation is not the only parameter that needs to be closely observed in critically ill patients with impending respiratory failure. Other clinical parameters (unstable vital signs, physical findings such as altered mental status that suggest organ dysfunction) that characterize severe illness dictate the frequency and the intensity of monitoring. A subgroup of patients with chronic hypoventilation, for example, obesity hypoventilation and some patients with chronic obstructive pulmonary disease (COPD), may experience respiratory depression with supplemental oxygen resulting in worsening hypercapnia. These patients are better monitored with arterial blood gases to better assess the level of carbon dioxide retention.

It is also important to be aware of other limitations of the transcutaneous pulse oximetry measurements. Patients suffering from various hemoglobinopathies and poisonings, such as carbon monoxide inhalation or cyanide toxicity, can have normal transcutaneous oxygen saturation values but still be severely hypoxemic.

SUMMARY

A wide variety of devices are available to deliver oxygen therapy for inpatients. Although the nasal cannula route is most widely used, critically ill patients often require other devices to meet their oxygen needs. Breathing pattern, underlying mechanism of hypoxemia, and tolerability should all be considered when choosing an oxygen delivery device, keeping in mind that the primary goal of management is adequate oxygenation.

REVIEW QUESTIONS

1. **Which of the following oxygen devices delivers precise FiO_2?**
   - **A.** Partial rebreathing mask.
   - **B.** Venturi mask.
   - **C.** AMBU bag and mask.
   - **D.** CPAP.

2. **A patient with chronic obstructive pulmonary disease (COPD) on home oxygen, set at 2 l/min and delivered via a nasal cannula, was admitted to the intensive care unit for monitoring of an upper gastrointestinal bleeding. The patient is comfortable with an oxygen saturation of 95% while on oxygen at 2 l/min via nasal cannula. While the patient is monitored with continuous pulse oximetry, it is recommended to do the following:**
   - **A.** Increase the FiO_2 to 4 l/min using the nasal cannula.
   - **B.** Change the nasal cannula to a venturi mask to deliver 30% FiO_2.
   - **C.** Continue the current oxygen setting.
   - **D.** Continue oxygen at 2 l/min but change from nasal cannula to a partial-rebreathing mask.

3. **A 70-year-old man, with a past medical history of severe chronic obstructive lung disease on chronic oxygen therapy at 2 l/min via nasal cannula, presents to the emergency room in respiratory distress, diaphoretic, and agitated. He gives a history of progressive dyspnea associated with a worsening productive cough, fevers, and chills. On arrival to the emergency room, his vital signs were blood pressure 150/90 mmHg, pulse rate 130 beats/min, temperature 38.5°C, and respiratory rate 33 breaths/min; and his oxygen saturation measured by transcutaneous pulse oximetry was 80%. He was placed on oxygen supplementation at an FiO_2 of 30% delivered with a simple facemask, and he was treated with repeated doses of nebulized bronchodilators. While waiting for the rest of his workup, the patient's transcutaneous pulse oximetry was reading 90% but his breathing was becoming more labored and he was difficult to arouse. What is the most appropriate step in the management of this patient?**
   - **A.** Discontinue the simple mask and place him back on nasal cannula at 3 l/min of oxygen flow.
   - **B.** Keep the simple mask and increase the FiO_2 to 50%.
   - **C.** Change the simple mask to a nonrebreathing mask to try to deliver an FiO_2 of 100%.
   - **D.** Start AMBU bag-mask ventilation and prépare to intubate the patient.

ANSWERS

1. The answer is B. The most precise delivery devices are the high-flow air-entrainment devices such as the venturi mask. The rest are dependent on mask seal and patient ventilatory pattern.
2. The answer is C. Because the patient is hemodynamically stable and there is no evidence of hypoxemia, there is no need to change the oxygen delivery system or FiO_2.
3. The answer is D. The patient is in acute respiratory failure showing deterioration of his clinical status despite aggressive conventional therapy; therefore, he needs to be intubated for ventilatory assistance and protection of his airway. Remember that the primary goal to therapy is to ensure adequate oxygenation. Although the change in his mental status may be related to CO_2 retention, if FiO_2 is lowered he will become more hypoxemic.

SUGGESTED READING

American Association of Respiratory Care. Clinical practice guidelines: oxygen therapy in the acute care hospital. Respir Care 1991;36: 1306–1311.

Cairo JM. Administering medical gases: regulators, flowmeters, and controlling devices. In: Mosby's Respiratory Care Equipment, 6th Ed. St. Louis: Mosby, 1999.

Phillip Y, Kristo D, Kallish M. Writing the take-home oxygen prescription for COPD patients. Document hypoxemia, then aim for a target oxygenation level. J Crit Illness 1998;13(2):112–120.

CHAPTER 3

JOSEPH CROCETTI AND SAMUEL KRACHMAN

Blood Gas Sampling

CHAPTER OUTLINE

LEARNING OBJECTIVES

After studying this chapter, you should be able to:

- Know the indications for obtaining an arterial blood gas.
- Understand the techniques used to measure an arterial blood gas.
- Have an understanding of the acid–base status and buffering system of the body.
- Identify sources of error in arterial blood gas measurements.
- Know how to identify the presence of a simple and mixed acid–base disorder.
- Know the causes of a simple acid–base disorder.
- Understand the measurements of arterial oxygenation.
- Know the components that can affect mixed venous oxygenation.

Critically ill patients require intensive monitoring during their care, both to detect and access acute changes that might occur and to determine the response to a therapeutic intervention. Blood gas sampling, which includes both arterial and mixed venous blood, is a modality that provides important information on a patient's metabolic status as well as their overall oxygenation (Table 3-1). Clinical decision making based on the analysis of the blood gas data often leads to changes in patient care, which may have a significant effect on their survival. This chapter discusses both arterial and mixed venous blood gas analysis and the implications.

INDICATIONS FOR ARTERIAL BLOOD GAS ANALYSIS

Acid–base status is determined by measuring arterial pH and $PaCO_2$.

Arterial blood gas sampling provides for the assessment of two important measures in the care of a critically ill patient: the systemic acid–base status and the total body oxygenation. The systemic acid–base status is determined by measuring the arterial pH and partial pressure of carbon dioxide ($PaCO_2$) and calculating the serum bicarbonate [HCO_3^-], using specific electrodes in a blood gas analyzer. Arterial partial pressure of oxygen (PaO_2) is also determined using a blood gas analyzer whereas the arterial oxygen saturation (SaO_2) is measured with a co-oximeter. Although this chapter discusses acid–base status and arterial oxygenation separately, the reader must be aware that these two entities are closely associated

TABLE 3-1

INDICATIONS FOR BLOOD GAS SAMPLING

Arterial blood gas
Assess acid–base status
Assess systemic arterial oxygenation
Determine response to therapeutic intervention
Mixed venous blood gas
Identify alteration in oxygen delivery or consumption
Determine response to therapeutic intervention
Determination of systemic acid–base status
Determination of systemic arterial oxygenation
Assess response to therapeutic intervention

under physiologic conditions. For example, decreases in oxygenation can lead to tissue hypoxia, which will affect overall acid–base status. Conversely, acid–base disorders can shift the oxyhemoglobin dissociation curve and thus affect regional or systemic oxygenation or both. Arterial blood gas analysis allows for an accurate and immediate determination of these two important entities, which are often crucial in the care of the critically ill patient.

Arterial PaO_2 is determined using a blood gas analyzer.

ACID–BASE STATUS

Measurement of Acid–Base Status

The HCO_3^-–CO_2 system is the principal buffer utilized by the body to maintain the arterial pH within the normal physiologic range. The arterial blood pH and $PaCO_2$ are directly measured from the arterial blood gas using a blood gas analyzer. $[HCO_3^-]$ is calculated from the blood gas analyzer and not directly measured, utilizing the relationship between pH, $PaCO_2$, and $[HCO_3^-]$ as expressed in the Henderson–Hasselbalch equation:

The HCO_3^-–CO_2 system is the principal buffer utilized by the body.

$$pH = 6.1 + \log ([HCO_3^-]/(0.03 \times PaCO_2)) \qquad (3\text{-}1)$$

Another approach in evaluating the acid–base status of the patient utilizes the measured serum $[HCO_3^-]$ rather than the calculated $[HCO_3^-]$ obtained from the relationship expressed in the foregoing equation. The total serum CO_2 is actually measured from the venous blood sample, but because serum $[HCO_3^-]$ makes up about 95% of the total CO_2, the two measures are used interchangeably. However, because venous blood is used, the measured $[HCO_3^-]$ is 1–3 mmol/l higher than that obtained in an arterial sample. Therefore, more errors are made with measurement of the serum $[HCO_3^-]$, and thus assessment of an acid–base disorder is made with the calculated $[HCO_3^-]$.

The acidity of body fluids is measured in terms of the hydrogen ion concentration $[H^+]$. The important relationship between the $[H^+]$ and the HCO_3^-–CO_2 buffer system can also be expressed in a modified form of the Henderson–Hasselbalch equation as:

$$[H^+] = 24 \times PaCO_2/[HCO_3^-] \qquad (3\text{-}2)$$

The serum $[H^+]$ is about three million times less than the serum sodium concentration, yet because of its small size it is highly reactive and thus tight regulation is needed. The pH is defined as the negative log of $[H^+]$:

$$pH = -\log [H^+] \qquad (3\text{-}3)$$

and is normally maintained between 7.35 and 7.45. pH and $[H^+]$ are inversely related, and thus estimation of $[H^+]$ can be made from pH. Between pH 7.2 and 7.5, for each 0.1 unit change in pH there is a 10 mmol/l change in $[H^+]$ in the opposite direction. This correlation is lost at a pH above 7.5 or below 7.2.

pH is normally maintained between 7.35 and 7.45.

Acid production in the body occurs in two major ways. The first pathway involves CO_2, which is produced during oxidative metabolism and then hydrated by the cytoplasmic enzyme carbonic anhydrase to produce carbonic acid (H_2CO_3). This volatile acid is then disposed of by the elimination of CO_2 by the lungs. The second pathway involves nonvolatile metabolic acids that are produced by aerobic and anaerobic metabolism and includes sulfuric, phosphoric, and lactic acids. Because these nonvolatile acids are not in equilibrium, they must be metabolized and excreted by the kidneys.

Buffer Systems

Changes in acidity can be stabilized by the body's buffers.

Derangement in the body's pH can have severe effects on cellular and physiologic function and thus tight regulation of acid–base status is imperative. Changes in acidity can be stabilized but not totally corrected by the body's buffers, which are molecules that accept or donate hydrogen ions. As already mentioned, the major buffer in the body is HCO_3^-; less important roles are played by phosphates, protein, and hemoglobin. Thus, both the lungs and kidneys play a major role in the regulation of the body's acid–base status, and there is major interdependency between the respiratory and metabolic systems in maintaining the body's pH.

Both the lungs and kidneys play a major role in regulating acid–base status.

There are, however, two standard metabolic measurements that are independent of the respiratory system, the standard HCO_3^- and the base excess. The standard HCO_3^- is the plasma HCO_3^- concentration present in a blood sample that is fully saturated with oxygen and equilibrated in vitro at 38°C with a $PaCO_2$ equal to 40 mmHg. The normal standard HCO_3^- is 24 nM/l. Standardization of the blood oxygen level is important because the level of oxygenation will alter hemoglobin buffering capacity. When hemoglobin releases oxygen, it becomes less acidic and accepts more protons, thus increasing its buffering capacity; the opposite occurs after oxygen is taken up by hemoglobin.

The base excess is the amount of acid or alkali that must be added to a liter of fully oxygenated blood exposed in vitro to a $PaCO_2$ of 40 mmHg at 38°C to obtain a normal pH. When alkali is needed to achieve a normal pH, the sample being evaluated is said to have a base deficit. When added acid is needed to achieve a normal pH, a base excess is present. Although these parameters are independently calculated, neither the standard HCO_3^- nor the base excess has been shown to offer any advantage over plasma bicarbonate level in the determination of a metabolic disturbance.

Sources of Error

Body temperature can affect arterial blood gas.

Although the blood gas analyzer is considered the gold standard instrument for the evaluation of the acid–base status and oxygenation in a patient, errors can occur (Table 2-2). A patient's body temperature can affect arterial blood gas analysis, yet arterial blood gas samples are routinely analyzed with the electrodes heated to a constant temperature of 37°C. Temperature correction refers to the adjustment of the values measured at 37°C to that of the patient's actual temperature. For instance, if a patient's temperature is below 37°C, the temperature-corrected $PaCO_2$ and PaO_2 are lower because the solubility of CO_2 and O_2 is decreased at lower temperatures. The temperature-corrected pH is higher than the 37°C value because water is less dissociated into $[H^+]$ and $[OH^-]$ at lower temperatures. The clinical significance of changes caused by temperature is uncertain, however, and it is recommended that clinical decisions be based on measurements obtained at 37°C.

An air bubble in the arterial blood gas can affect PaO_2 and $PaCO_2$.

Air bubbles in the arterial blood gas sample will affect the PaO_2 and $PaCO_2$. CO_2 diffuses from the blood into the bubbles and decreases the $PaCO_2$ and increases the pH. The effect of air bubbles on PaO_2 measurement in the blood depends on the concentration gra-

TABLE 3-2

SOURCES OF ERROR IN ARTERIAL BLOOD GAS MEASUREMENTS

Changes in body temperature	Time left in syringe
Air bubbles	Elevated WBC count
Heparin	Elevated platelet count

dient between blood PaO_2 and the oxygen tension of room air (PaO_2, 159 mmHg). If the blood concentration is higher than that in the surrounding atmosphere and therefore in the air bubble, the PaO_2 measured in the blood will be falsely lowered; the opposite will occur if the gradient is reversed.

Heparinization of the blood sample limits the deposition of protein on the electrodes. However, excess heparin can affect blood gas analysis by lowering the $PaCO_2$ and calculated HCO_3^- due to a dilutional effect. Although heparin is an acid, the pH is usually not affected because of the buffering effects of the blood. The PaO_2 can also be falsely elevated.

The time during which the arterial blood gas sample remains in the syringe will also affect the results. Ongoing metabolism by the white blood cells and platelets will tend to decrease PaO_2 and increase $PaCO_2$, resulting in a decrease in pH. Thus, it is important to place the arterial blood gas sample on ice to slow metabolism. At room temperature, the rate of change caused by metabolism is about 0.1 mmHg/min for $PaCO_2$ and 0.001 unit/min for pH. The PaO_2 will fall more rapidly when the blood is fully saturated than for venous blood. Because the rate of change for these parameters is proportional to leukocyte and platelet counts, significant changes can be seen in patients with substantial leukocyotosis with leukemia or thrombocytosis. For instance, an entity known as "leukocyte larceny" has been described in which the high WBC seen in acute leukemia severely decreases the measured PaO_2 in the arterial blood gas whereas the oxygen saturation seen on the pulse oximeter is normal.

"Leukocyte larceny" can affect the measured PaO_2 in patients with leukemia.

SIMPLE ACID–BASE DISORDERS

The term acidemia refers to an increase in $[H^+]$ and a decrease in the pH of the arterial blood, whereas acidosis refers to a process that causes acid to accumulate in the body. The term alkalemia refers to a decrease in the $[H^+]$ and increase in the pH of the arterial blood, whereas alkalosis refers to a process in which alkali accumulates in the body.

Metabolic Acidosis

A metabolic acidosis occurs when there is either an increase in acid accumulation or a decrease in extracellular bicarbonate, with a resulting decrease in both serum pH and $[HCO_3^-]$. As a compensatory response, there is an increase in alveolar ventilation leading to a decrease in $PaCO_2$. Maximal respiratory compensation results in a $PaCO_2$ of 10 mmHg. The expected compensatory $PaCO_2$ can be calculated using the Winters equation:

A compensatory response to a simple metabolic acidosis is a decrease in $PaCO_2$.

$$PaCO_2 = 1.5[HCO_3^-] + 8 \pm 2 \quad (3\text{-}4)$$

Thus, with a simple metabolic acidosis, the patient's minute ventilation will increase and $PaCO_2$ will decrease to a value calculated from the Winters formula (Table 3-3). If the cal-

TABLE 3-3

ACID–BASE CALCULATIONS: SECONDARY COMPENSATION

Metabolic acidosis:	$PaCO_2 = 1.5 \times [HCO_3^-] + 8 \pm 2$
Metabolic alkalosis:	$PaCO_2 = 0.7 \times \Delta\ [HCO_3^-]$
Respiratory acidosis:	
Acute	Decrease in pH $= 0.008 \times \Delta PaCO_2$ Increase in $HCO_3^- = 0.1 \times \Delta PaCO_2$
Chronic	Decrease in pH $= 0.003 \times \Delta PaCO_2$ Increase in $HCO_3^- = 0.3 \times \Delta PaCO_2$
Respiratory alkalosis:	
Acute	Increase in pH $0.008 \times \Delta PaCO_2$ Decrease in $HCO_3^- = 0.2 \times \Delta PaCO_2$
Chronic	Increase in pH $= 0.003 \times \Delta PaCO_2$ Decrease in $HCO_3^- = 0.4 \times \Delta PaCO_2$

TABLE 3-4

COMMON UNMEASURED ANIONS AND CATIONS

Unmeasured anions (negative charges)	Unmeasured cations (positive charges)
Albumin	Potassium
Proteins	Magnesium
Paraproteins (multiple myloma)	Calcium
Sulfate	
Phosphate	

culated and observed $PaCO_2$ are different, then a mixed acid–base disorder is present (see following).

Metabolic acidosis can be separated on the basis of whether there is an anion gap:

$$\text{Anion gap} = [Na] - ([Cl] + [HCO_3^-]) = 12 \pm 4 \text{ mEq/l} \quad (3\text{-}5)$$

The anion gap is based on the principle of electroneutrality, in which the total serum cations equal the total serum anions. Because the normal reference range for the anion gap is 12 ± 4 mEq/l, it more accurately reflects the amount of unmeasured anions in the plasma, the majority of which are plasma proteins. Common anions and cations are listed in Table 3-4.

Albumin is the major anion in the blood.

Despite the wide use of the anion gap, it has many limitations that must be appreciated before it can be utilized. Albumin is the major anion in the blood, and thus changes in the serum albumin will have a major effect on the anion gap. For every 1 g/dl decrease in albumin, there is a 2–3 mEq/l decrease in the anion gap. Thus, in patients who are severely hypoalbuminemic the normal anion gap may be as low as 4–5 mEq/l. Other common causes of a decreased anion gap are paraproteinemias, hyponatremia, lithium toxicity, profound hyperkalemia, hypercalcemia, hypermagnesemia, or halide poisoning (Table 3-5). Recognition of factors that reduce the anion gap is important because patients with a "normal anion gap" may actually have a low anion gap with a concomitant severe metabolic acidosis. Finally, the blood pH can alter the anion gap by affecting the anionic charge of serum proteins and by altering the quantity of organic acids; this can lead to a 1–3 mEq/l decrease in the anion gap in acidemic states and a 3-5 mEq/l increase in alkalemic states.

With an anion-gapped acidosis, there is 1 mEq/l decrease in HCO_3^- for every 1 mEq/l increase in the anion gap.

In a pure anion gap metabolic acidosis, for every 1 mEq/l increase in the anion gap there is a reciprocal decrease of 1 mEq/l in the serum HCO_3^-. For instance, if a patient has a calculated anion gap of 20 mEq/l, this is 8 mg/l above the normal value of 12 mEq/l. This difference (calculated anion gap − normal anion gap) is referred to as the "delta gap." A reciprocal decrease in the serum $[HCO_3^-]$ should occur (24 − 8), resulting in a $[HCO_3^-]$ of 16. If the actual HCO_3^- differed from 16 mEq/l, it would suggest the presence of a mixed acid–base disorder. Another way to look at this is to simply add the delta gap to the measured HCO_3^-. If the sum is less than 24 mEq/l, it suggests the presence of an associated nongapped metabolic acidosis. If the sum is greater than 24 mEq/l, it suggests a coexisting metabolic alkalosis. This approach is very useful in excluding the presence of a mixed acid–base disorder. The causes of an anion gap acidosis are listed in Table 3-6.

Nongapped acidosis can be categorized into those disorders with a normal or elevated serum potassium level and those with hypokalemia (Table 3-6). A nongapped acidosis can result from (1) the loss of $[HCO_3^-]$ from the body, (2) the inability to replace the $[HCO_3^-]$ used during the day to neutralize acids produced by the body, (3) the administration of an acid, or (4) the administration of fluid that does not contain $[HCO_3^-]$, also known as a dilu-

TABLE 3-5

CAUSES OF A DECREASED ANION GAP

Hypoalbuminemia	Hypercalcemia	Lithium toxicity
Hyponatremia	Hypermagnesemia	Acidemia
Hyperkalemia	Paraproteinemia	Halide poisoning

TABLE 3-6

METABOLIC ACIDOSIS

- High anion gap
  - Ketoacids
    - Diabetes
    - Alcoholic (ethanol)
    - Starvation
  - Lactic acidosis
  - Uremia
  - Toxins
    - Methanol
    - Ethylene glycol
    - Propylene glycol
    - Salicylates
    - Paraldehyde
- Normal anion gap
  - Hypokalemic
  - GI loss of HCO_3^-
    - Ureteral diversion
    - Diarrhea
    - Ileostomy
  - Renal loss of HCO_3^-
    - Proximal renal tubular acidosis
    - Carbonic anhydrase inhibitors
  - Normokalemic/hyperkalemic
  - Renal tubular disease
    - Acute tubular necrosis
    - Chronic tubulointerstitial disease
    - Distal renal tubular acidosis (types I and IV)
    - Hypoaldosteronism, aldosterone inhibitors
  - Pharmacologic
    - Ammonium chloride
    - Hyperalimentation
    - Dilutional acidosis

tional acidosis. The urine anion gap can often be useful in differentiating the cause of a nongapped acidosis. Defined as:

The urine anion gap can help define the cause of a nongapped acidosis.

$$[Na^+] + [K^+] - [Cl] = \text{urine anion gap} \qquad (3\text{-}6)$$

the urinary gap is normally negative as a result of the excretion of ammonium into the urine. If the urine anion gap is positive, it reflects an impairment in ammonium excretion, as is seen in patients with renal tubular acidosis (RTA). The urinary pH can then be helpful in differentiating the type of RTA that is responsible for the nongapped acidosis. If the pH is high (>6.0), a distal RTA is present. If the urinary pH is low, and remains low even with HCO_3^- infusion, a proximal RTA is suggested. In patients with a hyperkalemic distal RTA, as seen with aldosterone deficiency, the urinary pH can be variable.

The clinical manifestations associated with a metabolic acidosis depend on the underlying cause. Patients usually develop rapid, deep respirations to compensate for the metabolic acidosis (Kussmaul's respiration).

Metabolic Alkalosis

A metabolic alkalosis can develop when there is either an increase in serum $[HCO_3^-]$ or a loss of acid from the body with a relative increase in the serum $[HCO_3^-]$. A metabolic alkalosis leads to an increase in serum pH, associated with an increase in serum $[HCO_3^-]$. Compensation for metabolic alkalosis includes a decrease in alveolar ventilation, resulting in an increase in the $PaCO_2$. The appropriate compensatory increase in $PaCO_2$ can be calculated by the equation:

Metabolic alkalosis results from an increase in serum HCO_3^- or loss of acid from the body.

$$PaCO_2 \cong 0.7\ \Delta[HCO_3^-]$$

TABLE 3-7

METABOLIC ALKALOSIS

Chloride-responsive/hypovolemic
Renal Cl loss
Loop diuretics
Early distal diuretics
Posthypercapnic states
Gastrointestinal Cl loss
Vomiting
Gastric suction
Villous adenoma
Congenital chloridorrhea
Alkali administration
High-dose carbenicillin
Chloride-resistant/hypervolemic
Mineralocorticoid excess
Primary aldosteronism
Cushing's syndrome
Renin-secreting tumors
Renovascular disease
Pharmacologic hydrocortisone/mineralocorticoid excess
Bicarbonate overdose
Massive blood transfusion
Milk-alkali syndrome
Miscellaneous
Glycyrrhizinic acid (licorice)
Liddle's syndrome
Severe potassium depletion
Bartter syndrome

Metabolic alkalosis can result in seizures or an altered mental status.

The maximal compensatory response in measured $PaCO_2$ is 65 mmHg (see Table 3-3). A metabolic alkalosis can be categorized as either being chloride responsive or chloride unresponsive, and thus measurement of urine chloride can differentiate between the two conditions (Table 3-7). In a chloride-responsive metabolic alkalosis, the loss of urinary chloride has played a significant role in producing the alkalosis, and the urine chloride will be low (<10 mmol/l). Metabolic alkalosis is corrected with the administration of chloride as NaCl. In chloride-unresponsive metabolic alkalosis, the urine chloride will be greater than 10 mmol/l and will not respond to NaCl administration. Some of the clinical manifestations of metabolic alkalosis include decreased cerebral blood flow, seizures, and altered mental status. Metabolically, it will result in a decrease in ionized calcium and cause hypokalemia.

Treatment is aimed at the underlying cause, and chloride-responsive alkalosis usually responds to repletion with normal saline, which contains 154 mEq/l of chloride. The chloride-unresponsive disorders are usually associated with either primary or secondary mineral-corticoid excess, hypokalemia, or certain inherited disorders. Treatment is directed at the underlying cause.

Respiratory Acidosis

Respiratory acidosis causes increased $PaCO_2$ and decreased pH.

Under normal conditions, alveolar ventilation removes the metabolically produced CO_2 and maintains a normal $PaCO_2$ of 40 mmHg. If this balance is not maintained, because of either an ineffective alveolar ventilation or an increase in CO_2 production, $PaCO_2$ will increase, resulting in a respiratory acidosis. The normal response to an increase in $PaCO_2$ is to increase alveolar ventilation, mediated by changes in the $[H^+]$ of the cerebrospinal fluid, which affects medullary chemoreceptors. A respiratory acidosis causes a decrease in pH and an increase in $PaCO_2$. Common causes are listed in Table 3-8.

Compensation for a primary respiratory acidosis is metabolic. The acute phase for compensation occurs almost immediately when $PaCO_2$ increases. Nonbicarbonate tissue buffers such as hemoglobin bind with $[H^+]$, resulting in a rapid generation of $[HCO_3^-]$. This initial increase in $[HCO_3^-]$ is modest, with 0.1 mEq/l increase in HCO_3^- for every 1 mmHg increase

TABLE 3-8

RESPIRATORY ACIDOSIS

Airway/pulmonary parenchyma disease
- Upper airway obstruction
- Lower airway obstruction
- Pulmonary alveolar process
  - Cardiogenic pulmonary edema
  - Pneumonia
  - Acute respiratory distress syndrome (ARDS)
- Pulmonary perfusion defect
  - Pulmonary emboli
  - Fat emboli

Normal airway/lung parenchyma
- Central nervous system depression
- Neuromuscular impairment
- Ventilatory restriction

in $PaCO_2$ (see Table 3-3). The maximal increase in HCO_3^- during acute compensation is 31–32 mEq/l. In addition, with a respiratory acidosis the pH also decreases by 0.008 units for every 1 mmHg increase in $PaCO_2$ (Table 3-3). With chronic compensation, the kidneys play a major role. Proximal reabsorption of filtered HCO_3^-, and excretion of $[H^+]$ in the form of ammonia, result in a 0.3 mEq/l increase in HCO_3^- for each 1 mmHg increase in $PaCO_2$, with a maximal increase in serum HCO_3^- of 45 mEq/l (Table 3-3). pH also decreases by 0.003 units for each 1 mmHg increase in $PaCO_2$ (Table 3-3).

The clinical manifestations of a respiratory acidosis depend on the acuity of the event leading to the acidosis and the degree of hypoxemia that is present. In patients with acute hypercapnia, there can be profound changes in mental status and hemodynamics. In patients with chronic hypercapnia, such as with severe chronic obstructive pulmonary disease (COPD), however, the $PaCO_2$ may rise into the 50–60 mmHg range without central nervous system (CNS) or cardiac changes. In response to an increase in $PaCO_2$, cerebral blood flow increases secondary to cerebral vasodilatation, leading to a concomitant increase in intracranial pressure. The hemodynamic changes associated with hypercapnia are tachycardia, hypertension, supraventricular arrhythmias, and peripheral vasodilation.

An increase in $PaCO_2$ results in cerebral vasodilatation.

Treatment is directed at the underlying cause (see Table 3-8). Because most causes of respiratory acidosis are associated with ineffective ventilation, treatment often consists of supportive care such as intubation and mechanical ventilation. In some cases, noninvasive ventilation can be used in a hemodynamically stable patient who is alert enough to protect their airway. Both these forms of ventilatory support increase alveolar ventilation, resulting in a decrease in $PaCO_2$ and an increase in pH. Posthypercapnic alkalosis is associated with rapid correction of a respiratory acidosis, in which the elevated $PaCO_2$ is lowered to normal but the compensatory increase in HCO_3^-, which takes longer to resolve, remains.

Respiratory Alkalosis

A respiratory alkalosis develops because of an increase in alveolar ventilation, resulting in a decreased CO_2 tension in the body. Alveolar ventilation is controlled by several factors, including (1) chemoreceptors in the medulla that are sensitive to changes in $[H^+]$, (2) carotid body receptors that are sensitive to changes in PaO_2, (3) voluntary cortical input to the respiratory control center, and (4) mechanicoreceptors in the lung and chest wall. Activation by any of these receptors can result in hyperventilation and a respiratory alkalosis. Table 3-9 lists the common causes of a respiratory alkalosis. The metabolic compensation for a respiratory alkalosis consists of both an acute component, utilizing nonbicarbonate buffers, and a more chronic compensation, through the renal loss of $[HCO_3^-]$. Serum $[HCO_3^-]$ will decrease 0.2 mEq/l and 0.4 mEq/l for every 1 mmHg decrease in $PaCO_2$ during the acute and chronic compensatory phases, respectively (see Table 3-3). The change in pH can be calculated based on the change in $PaCO_2$, with an increase in pH of 0.008 and 0.003 during acute and chronic compensation, respectively, for every 1 mmHg decrease in $PaCO_2$ (see

Respiratory alkalosis is the result of hyperventilation.

TABLE 3-9

RESPIRATORY ALKALOSIS

Central nervous system stimulation
Fever
Pain
Cerebrovascular accident
Hypoxemia or tissue hypoxia
Pneumonia
Pulmonary edema
Severe anemia
Stimulation of chest receptors
Pulmonary emboli
Pulmonary edema
Pneumonia
Drugs or hormones
Medroxyprogesterone
Catecholamines
Salicylates
Miscellaneous
Sepsis
Pregnancy

Compensation for chronic respiratory alkalosis can result in normalized pH.

Table 3-3). With a chronic respiratory alkalosis (more than 2 weeks in duration), compensation may eventually result in a normalized pH.

Clinical manifestations with a respiratory alkalosis include CNS symptoms such as confusion, seizures, parasthesias, and circumoral numbness. Muscular cramping and spasms may also be seen. Metabolically, hypokalemia and hypophosphatemia may result, as will a decrease in ionized calcium. Alkalosis also shifts the oxyhemoglobin dissociation curve to the left, which decreases the release of oxygen at the tissue level.

MIXED ACID–BASE DISORDERS

An inappropriate compensatory response suggests the existence of a mixed acid–base disorder.

It is important when determining the acid–base status of a patient that there are not two primary processes present at the same time; this is referred to as a mixed acid–base disorder. It should be made clear that the normal compensatory response to a primary acid–base disorder should not be considered as a secondary process. To determine the presence of a secondary process, the physician should make certain that the patient has the appropriate compensatory response to account for the observed laboratory values. As already discussed, a patient with an anion-gapped metabolic acidosis should have a delta gap that, when added to the serum [HCO_3^-], results in a normal [HCO_3^-]. A significantly lower [HCO_3^-] would suggest the coexistence of a nongapped metabolic acidosis. In a patient with a chronic respiratory acidosis, a serum [HCO_3^-] that is significantly higher than expected based on the aforementioned compensatory equation or that is greater than 45 mEq/l suggests the coexistence of metabolic alkalosis. Thus, it is important to assure that the compensatory response is appropriate and does not suggest the existence of a mixed acid–base disorder.

ARTERIAL OXYGENATION

The driving pressure and solubility of oxygen in the plasma determine the PaO_2.

In addition to determining the systemic acid–base status, the arterial blood gas provides an accurate measurement of arterial oxygenation. The arterial partial pressure of oxygen (PaO_2) is a measurement of the quantity of oxygen that is dissolved in the blood. Both the driving pressure and solubility of oxygen in the plasma determine the PaO_2. The driving pressure is dependent on the partial pressure of oxygen in the alveolus (P_AO_2). If the alveolus is considered a fixed space, and the nitrogen present is disregarded, the only two gases that are present are oxygen and carbon dioxide. The P_AO_2 is then equal to the amount of O_2 inspired into the alveolus minus the amount of CO_2 of the alveolar space. The fraction of inspired oxygen (F_iO_2) must be multiplied by the barometric pressure at which the measurement is taken (760 mmHg at sea level). In addition, inspired air is warmed and becomes humidified in the upper airway; therefore, the partial pressure of water in the trachea (47 mmHg) must be subtracted from the barometric pressure. Thus, the P_AO_2 is determined by the following equation:

$$P_AO_2 = F_iO_2 \text{ (barometric pressure} - \text{partial pressure in the trachea)} - PaCO_2/R \quad (3\text{-}7)$$

The P_AO_2 at sea level while breathing room air ($F_iO_2 = 0.21$) can be calculated as:

$$P_AO_2 = 0.21(760 - 47) - 40/0.8 \quad (3\text{-}8)$$

where the $PaCO_2$ is assumed to be equal to the tension of $PaCO_2$ in the alveolus, and 0.8 is the respiratory quotient, which assumes an "ideal" relationship between ventilation and perfusion.

The PaO_2 is normally less than the P_AO_2 resulting from the presence of physiologic shunting of blood from the bronchial veins emptying into the pulmonary veins and from the thesbian veins that originate in the coronary sinus and empty into the left atrium. Thus, blood passes from the venous circulation into the arterial circulation without being exposed to oxygen in the pulmonary capillaries. This difference ($P_AO_2 - PaO_2$) is referred to as the alveolar–arterial oxygen tension gradient, or A-a gradient. In young adults this is normally 8–12, with values increasing with age into the twenties. A correction factor (age/3 + 3) can be used to calculate the age-adjusted A-a gradient. This gradient is often elevated in disease states that cause hypoxemia (ventilation–perfusion inequality, shunting, and diffusion impairment), except in cases that are secondary to hypoventilation, where the A-a gradient is normal.

In disease states that cause hypoxemia, the A–a gradient is elevated except when hypoxemia is caused by hypoventilation.

When interpreting the arterial blood gas, it must be remembered that the amount of oxygen dissolved in the blood, the PaO_2, makes up only a small component of the arterial oxygen content. The oxygen content of arterial blood (CaO_2) consists of two components, the oxygen bound to hemoglobin and the oxygen dissolved in blood. The CaO_2 is provided by this equation:

PaO_2 contributes only a small amount to the overall oxygen content of the blood.

$$CaO_2 = (1.3 \times Hb \times SaO_2) + (0.003 \times PaO_2) \quad (3\text{-}9)$$

where Hb is hemoglobin and SaO_2 is the arterial oxygen saturation. Thus, each gram of hemoglobin binds 1.3 ml of oxygen when completely saturated ($SaO_2 = 100\%$). As can be seen in the latter part of the equation, only a fraction of oxygen is dissolved in the blood and contributes little to the overall CaO_2. Thus, the SaO_2 is the most important blood gas variable for assessing the CaO_2 because the majority of oxygen is carried in the blood bound to hemoglobin.

MIXED VENOUS BLOOD SAMPLING

Following oxygen extraction by the peripheral tissues, blood returns to the right side of the heart and is referred to as the mixed venous blood. True mixed venous oxygenation measurements are taken from the pulmonary artery, because the inferior vena cava and superior vena cava differ in their O_2 content. Factors that can affect the mixed venous O_2 content ($C\bar{v}O_2$), and thus the mixed venous oxygen saturation (SvO_2), can be appreciated by rearrangement of the Fick equation:

Mixed venous oxygen saturation is measured from the pulmonary artery.

$$\dot{V}O_2 = CO \times (CaO_2 - C\bar{v}O_2) \quad (3\text{-}10)$$

$$C\bar{v}O_2 = CaO_2 - \dot{V}O_2/CO \quad (3\text{-}11)$$

where $\dot{V}O_2$ is oxygen consumption and CO is cardiac output. Thus, a decrease in hemoglobin, an increase in $\dot{V}O_2$, a decrease in SaO_2, and a decrease in CO can lead to a decrease in $S\bar{v}O_2$.

Mixed venous blood is routinely sampled from the distal port of the Swan–Ganz catheter, located in the pulmonary artery. The sampled blood is then run through the blood gas analyzer and co-oximeter, similar to an arterial blood gas sample. Under normal conditions the mixed venous PaO_2 is 40–45 mmHg, which corresponds to a $S\bar{v}O_2$ of 75%.

At the present time, $S\bar{v}O_2$ can be continuously measured using a pulmonary artery oximetry catheter. Overall, there is a variability of ±6%; this must be considered both when monitoring stable patients and when determining when a rising or falling trend is significant. Thus, a persistent drop in $S\bar{v}O_2$ from 77% to 70% should be considered significant. At the same time, if the goal of therapy is to maintain a $S\bar{v}O_2$ greater than 65%, keeping the $S\bar{v}O_2$ greater than 71% assures that this goal will be met with a 95% accuracy. Because the normal value for $S\bar{v}O_2$ of 75% is on the steep portion of the oxyhemoglobin dissociation curve, a linear relationship exits between $P\bar{v}O_2$ and $S\bar{v}O_2$, with a 1 mmHg change in $P\bar{v}O_2$ being associated with a 2% change in $S\bar{v}O_2$. Overall, cardiopulmonary instability is seldom seen with a $S\bar{v}O_2$ greater than 60%. A reduction of $S\bar{v}O_2$ to less than 50% is commonly associated with development of anaerobic metabolism. Changes in $S\bar{v}O_2$ have been utilized by clinicians to identify an alteration in the balance between oxygen delivery and consumption. For instance, a significant drop in $S\bar{v}O_2$ in a patient with congestive heart failure may indicate an associated decrease in CO. However, it has been demonstrated that in this patient population, as well as in those with postcoronary artery bypass grafting (CABG), there is a relatively poor correlation between CO and $S\bar{v}O_2$. In addition, no threshold values for $S\bar{v}O_2$ that predict survival have been identified in patients with septic shock or postmyocardial infarction. In patients with septic shock or the acute respiratory distress syndrome (ARDS), the $S\bar{v}O_2$ can be normal to elevated, despite a significant decrease in tissue oxygenation, as a result of decreased extraction at the cellular level or the shunting of blood to organs that do not require the increased oxygen delivery. In addition, a decrease in $S\bar{v}O_2$ may reflect a change in the SaO_2 rather than a change in CO. Thus, the $S\bar{v}O_2$ should never be used as a single parameter, but must be utilized in conjunction with other measurements, such as CO, PaO_2, SaO_2, and $\dot{V}O_2$, to determine the etiology of a change in tissue oxygenation.

> A 1 mmHg change in $P\bar{v}O_2$ is associated with a 2% change in $S\bar{v}O_2$.

> Anaerobic metabolism may occur with a $S\bar{v}O_2$ <50%.

SUMMARY

Blood gas sampling is an important modality in the assessment of the critically ill patient. Arterial blood gases are valuable in the determination of the patient's acid–base status as well as their arterial oxygenation. Mixed venous blood sampling, including the use of continuous monitoring of $S\bar{v}O_2$, can assess changes in the oxygen delivery–consumption relationship. Proper interpretation of both arterial and mixed venous blood gas samples allows appropriate clinical decision making, which may have an impact on patient outcome.

REVIEW QUESTIONS

1. **Which one of the following factors will not affect the results of arterial blood gas measurement?**
   - **A.** Too much heparin
   - **B.** Too much blood
   - **C.** Hypothermia
   - **D.** Air bubbles

2. **Which of the following statements regarding the anion gap is not true?**
   - **A.** If the pH is greater than 7.5, albumin becomes more negatively charged and the anion gap will increase secondary to an increase in unmeasured anions.
   - **B.** The anion gap can increase if there is a decrease in unmeasured cations or if there is an increase in unmeasured anions.

C. For every 1 g/dl decrease in albumin, a 2–3 mEq/l decrease in the anion gap will occur. Thus, the anion gap should be corrected for hypoalbuminemia.
D. Common causes of a increased anion gap include paraproteinemias, hyponatremia, lithium toxicity, profound hyperkalemia, hypercalcemia, hypermagnesemia, and halide poisoning.

3. **In which of the following clinical situations will the A-a gradient be increased?**
   A. A 23-year-old medical student who has had too much to drink and is found unconscious.
   B. A 45-year-old man with multiple trauma-related injuries who is in respiratory failure with adult respiratory distress syndrome (ARDS).
   C. A 22-year-old dental student who has been complaining of shortness of breath and is newly diagnosed with asthma.
   D. A 65-year-old woman with idiopathic pulmonary fibrosis.

4. **Which of the following is false concerning mixed venous blood?**
   A. The normal $S\bar{v}O_2$ is between 70% and 75%, which reflects a $P\bar{v}O_2$ of 40–45 mmHg.
   B. The normal $P\bar{v}O_2$ and $S\bar{v}O_2$ lie on the steep portion of the oxyhemoglobin dissociation curve, so large changes in the mixed venous blood are needed to reflect changes in the mixed venous oxygen saturation.
   C. The major determinants of the mixed venous saturation are cardiac output, oxygen consumption, arterial oxygen saturation, and hemoglobin.
   D. A change in the $S\bar{v}O_2$ of ±4% is needed before a rising or falling trend can be considered significant.

ANSWERS

1. The answer is B. Heparin, hypothermia, and air bubbles will all affect arterial blood gas measurements. Heparin can affect blood gas analysis by lowering the $PaCO_2$ and calculated HCO_3^- by a dilutional effect. The pH is usually not affected due to the buffering effects of blood. Air bubbles in the sample will affect the PaO_2 and $PaCO_2$. CO_2 will diffuse from the sample into the bubbles, decrease the plasma $PaCO_2$, and increase the pH. The effect of air bubbles on PaO_2 depends on the concentration gradient between the blood and the PaO_2 in the bubble (PaO_2 159 mmHg). If the blood concentration is higher, it will falsely lower the concentration, and if it is lower it will raise the concentration. If a patient's temperature is below 37°C, temperature-corrected $PaCO_2$ and PaO_2 will be lower, due to decreased solubility at lower temperatures. The pH will be higher because of the decreased dissociation of H_2O at lower temperatures. Thus, only the amount of blood in the syringe will not affect the arterial blood gas.
2. The answer is D. The blood pH can affect the anion gap by altering the anionic charge of proteins (including albumin), as well as changing the amount of organic acids that are present. An alkalemic state can thus increase the anion gap by 3-5 mEq/l. Because albumin is the major anion in the blood, a decrease in albumin will lead to a decrease in the anion gap. The normal anion gap of 12 ± 4 mEq/l basically reflects the amount of unmeasured anions in the blood. An increase in albumin will thus lead to an increase in the anion gap, as will a decrease in unmeasured cations, such as potassium and calcium. Therefore, paraproteinemias, hyperkalemia, and hypercalcemia all result in a decrease rather than an increase in the anion gap.
3. The answer is A. Of the four major causes of hypoxemia, only hypoventilation is associated with a normal A-a gradient, because at the alveolar level there are no anatomic abnormalities that would lead to hypoxemia. Rather, a decrease in ventilation decreases the alveolar oxygen concentration, which results in a decrease in the arterial oxygen content. Ventilation–perfusion (V/Q) inequality account for the hypoxemia that is seen with an acute exacerbation of asthma. Shunt and V/Q inequality are the major mechanisms for hypoxemia in patients with ARDS. Patients with end-stage pulmonary fibrosis have diffusion impairment that leads to hypoxemia.
4. The answer is B. The normal values for $P\bar{v}O_2$ and $S\bar{v}O_2$, 45 mmHg and 75%, respectively, do sit on the steep portion of the oxygen–hemoglobin dissociation curve and thus small changes in $P\bar{v}O_2$ are associated with major changes in the $S\bar{v}O_2$. A change in $P\bar{v}O_2$ of 1 mmHg will result in a 2% change in $S\bar{v}O_2$. Although changes in cardiac output, oxygen consumption, arterial oxygen concentration, and hemoglobin concentration may all lead to a change in the $S\bar{v}O_2$, a ±6% change is needed before it can be considered significant.

SUGGESTED READING

Adrogue HJ, Madias NE. Arterial blood gas monitoring: acid–base assessment. In: Tobin MJ (ed) Principles and Practice of Intensive Care Monitoring. New York: McGraw-Hill, 1998:217–241.

D'Alonzo GE, Dantzker DR. Respiratory failure, mechanisms of abnormal gas exchange, and oxygen delivery. Med Clin North Am 1983;67(3):557–571.

Narins RG, Emmett M. Simple and mixed acid-base disorders: a practical approach. Medicine (Baltim) 1980;59(3):161–187.

Tobin MJ. Respiratory monitoring in the intensive care unit. Am Rev Respir Dis 1988;138:1625–1642.

CHAPTER 4

UBALDO J. MARTIN AND SAMUEL KRACHMAN

Hemodynamic Monitoring

CHAPTER OUTLINE

LEARNING OBJECTIVES

After studying this chapter, you should be able to do the following:

- Understand the indications for placing arterial, central venous, and pulmonary artery catheters.
- Select catheter placement sites, based on patient characteristics and relative risk for complications.
- Establish a differential diagnosis based on the pulmonary artery catheter measured and derived parameters.
- Understand the role of the pulmonary artery catheter in managing and diagnosing specific critical care conditions.
- Interpret pulmonary artery waveforms and their significance.
- Understand the controversies associated with pulmonary artery catheter use.

Many patients admitted to the intensive care unit (ICU) become hemodynamically unstable, with the cause often difficult to discern by physical examination alone. Invasive monitoring is often utilized in these patients to help diagnose the cause of hemodynamic instability, as well as to assess the patient's response to therapy. This chapter reviews the use of hemodynamic monitoring, specifically, the indications, complications, and interpretation of data associated with the use of arterial, central venous, and pulmonary artery (PA) catheters.

PRECAUTIONS FOR CATHETER INSERTION

Before placing any catheter, several steps must be taken to reduce the risk of complications:

- Obtain appropriate laboratory tests, including BUN (blood urea nitrogen), creatinine, electrolytes, ions, platelet count, and coagulation profile (prothrombin time, partial thromboplastin time).

- Correct abnormalities whenever possible. Consider using desmopressin (DDAVP) for uremic patients that may have platelet dysfunction and using blood products (fresh-frozen plasma, platelets, etc.) for a bleeding diathesis. Correct electrolyte abnormalities.
- Consider intravenous sedation or analgesia, or both.

ARTERIAL CATHETERS

Indications

The placement of an arterial catheter is indicated in clinical conditions where there is a need for the precise and continuous measurement of arterial blood pressure. Such conditions include hypertensive crisis, where intravenous vasodilator therapy is used, cardiogenic shock requiring inotropic therapy, and septic shock that requires continuous vasopressor support.

Placement of an arterial catheter is indicated whenever precise or continuous measurements of blood pressure are needed.

Other indications for the insertion of an arterial catheter include the need for frequent arterial blood gas analysis, such as in patients with acute respiratory failure requiring mechanical ventilation. Arterial acid–base status, as well as systemic oxygenation, can be accurately assessed, thereby allowing prompt adjustment in ventilator settings or measurement of the response to certain therapeutic interventions (i.e., addition of PEEP [pulmonary end-expiratory pressure], effects of inotropes on oxygen delivery).

Hypertensive crisis, cardiogenic shock, and septic shock are important indications for arterial cannulation.

Contraindictions

The insertion of an arterial catheter is a relatively safe and inexpensive procedure that has no absolute contraindications. Relative contradictions include bleeding diathesis, current anticoagulation, or the use of thrombolytic agents. Severe occlusive arterial disease with distal ischemia, poor collateral circulation (confirmed by Allen's test; see following), and the presence of a vascular prosthesis, local infection, and full-thickness burns are site-specific contraindications.

Bleeding diathesis, anticoagulation, and use of thrombolytics are relative contraindications to arterial line placement.

Insertion Technique

Several anatomic sites are suitable for arterial cannulation. The radial artery is preferred because it is relatively superficial, easy to access, and carries a lower incidence of complications. Other sites include the pedal, femoral, and brachial arteries. The selected artery can be cannulated via two different methods: (1) inserting the catheter directly into the artery over a needle, or (2) using the Seldinger technique, in which a guidewire is inserted through the needle after the artery is entered, the needle is then removed, and the catheter is placed over the wire into the artery. The choice of technique depends on the anatomic site selected, the depth of the artery, and the operator's familiarity with the procedure.

Because of its superficial location and low incidence of complications, the radial artery is the preferred site for arterial cannulation.

When an anatomic site has been selected and aseptically cleaned, the operator localizes the artery with the index finger of the nondominant hand and the trajectory of insertion is palpated with the index and third fingers. Only slight pressure is applied to avoid collapsing the artery. The needle hub is held like a pencil with its bevel up.

- Radial artery cannulation: The arm is immobilized in the supine position with a dorsally placed armboard. The wrist is partially extended by placing a gauze roll underneath. The armboard is secured with tape at the level of the metacarpal bones and arm. The needle is inserted 0.5–1.0 in. proximal to the wrist and advanced at a 30° angle (Figure 4-1).
- Brachial artery cannulation: The arm is immobilized in the supine position with an armboard, preventing elbow flexion. The needle is inserted at an angle of 30° and directed toward the pulsation in the antecubital fossa above the elbow crease (Figure 4-2). Because of the paucity of collaterals and the risk of damage to the median nerve, this approach should be reserved for patients in whom other approaches are unsuccessful.

Because of possible damage to the median nerve, brachial artery cannulation should be used only when other approaches have failed.

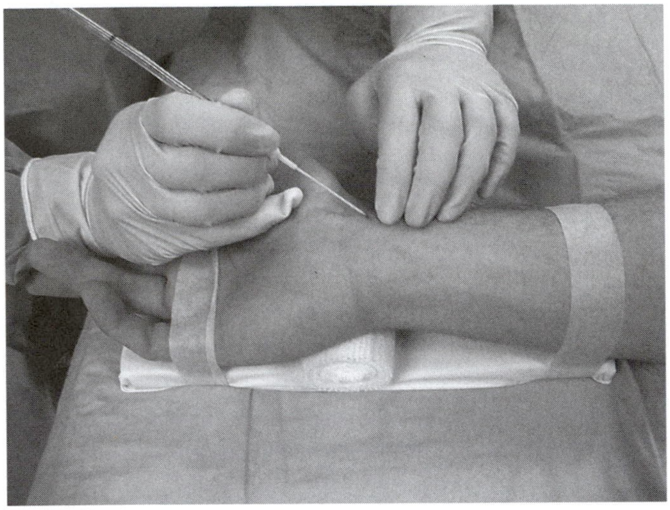

FIGURE 4-1

Radial artery cannulation. The arm is immobilized in the supine position with an armboard. The wrist is partially extended by placing a gauze roll underneath. The operator locates the pulse with the index finger of the nondominant hand and follows the trajectory of the artery with the third finger. The catheter is held like a pencil, with the needle bevel up. The catheter is inserted 0.5–1 in. proximal to the wrist and advanced at a 30° angle.

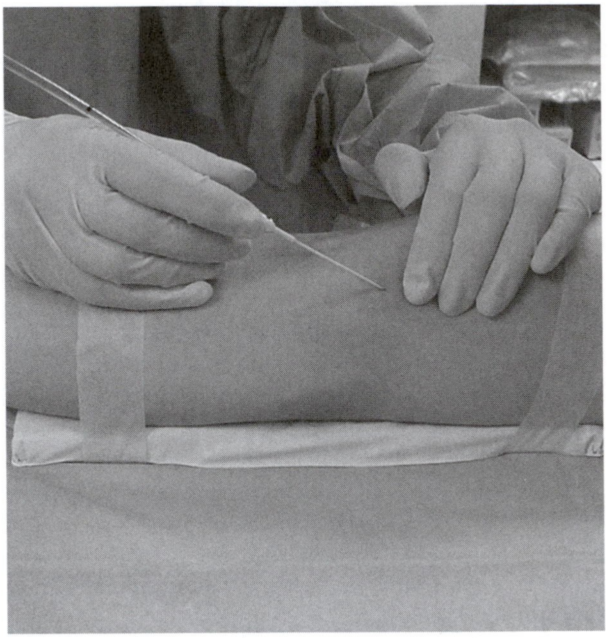

FIGURE 4-2

Brachial artery cannulation. The arm is immobilized, preventing elbow flexion. The operator palpates and localizes the artery in the antecubital fossa, following its trajectory with two fingers. Using the dominant hand, the catheter is inserted at a 30° angle toward the pulsation above the elbow crease.

- Femoral artery cannulation: The needle is inserted at a 45° angle 2–5 cm below the inguinal ligament at the inguinal crease (Figure 4-3). Once blood is retrieved, the angle of entrance can be lowered to facilitate introduction of the catheter or a wire if the Seldinger technique is being used.
- Dorsalis pedis artery cannulation: The artery runs over the dorsum of the foot, usually lateral to the tendon of the extensor hallucis longus. The artery is palpated and entered midway along the dorsum of the foot. It is important to remember that systolic pressures at the dorsalis pedis artery tend to be 5–20 mmHg higher than those measured at the radial artery (Figure 4-4).

> Systolic pressures at the dorsalis pedis artery are generally 5–20 mmHg higher than radial artery pressures.

The presence of blood in the hub signals the entrance into the vessel; when the artery has been found, the needle–cannula system is advanced 1–3 mm beyond the point of initial flash to ensure that the tip of the cannula is inside the vessel. While the needle is held steady, the cannula is advanced into the artery. If the Seldinger technique is used, the needle is inserted and the guidewire is advanced. The guidewire should advance with ease. The catheter is then advanced over the guidewire when the needle has been withdrawn.

Complications

The rate of clinically relevant complications for arterial cannulation ranges from 2% to 5%; specific complications are listed in Table 4-1.

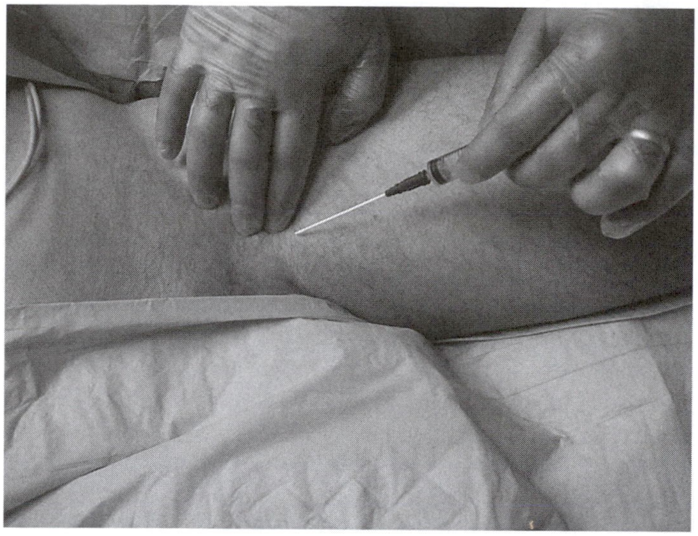

FIGURE 4-3

Femoral artery cannulation. Using the index finger of the nondominant hand, the operator locates the femoral artery pulse at the inguinal crease. The catheter is inserted at a 45° angle, 2–5 cm below the inguinal ligament at the inguinal crease. Once blood is retrieved, the angle is lowered to facilitate passing the catheter or a guidewire if the Seldinger technique is employed.

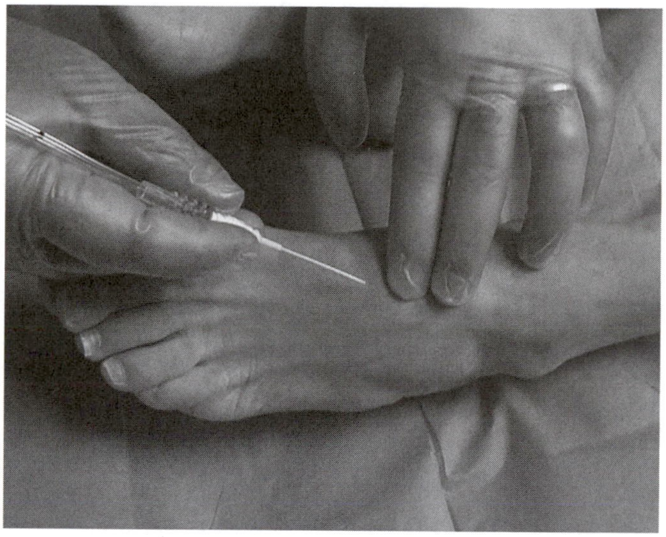

FIGURE 4-4

Dorsalis pedis artery cannulation. The artery is palpated, generally lateral to the tendon of the extensor hallucis longus. After locating the arterial pulse and following the trajectory of the artery with the index and third fingers of the dominant hand, the operator inserts the catheter at a flat angle. The artery is entered midway along the dorsum of the foot.

CENTRAL VENOUS CATHETERS

Indications

The use of central venous pressure (CVP) catheters has increased over the past few decades, paralleling advances in ICU technology. There has been an increased recognition of the usefulness of central hemodynamic monitoring in the ICU. Some of the most common uses of CVP catheters in ICU include the following:

- Rapid administration of intravenous (IV) fluids. It is important to note that the rate at which IV fluids are administered depends on the radius and the length of the catheter. In some instances a large-bore, short peripheral catheter is better suited for rapid administration of IV fluids then a long, thin central venous catheter. (For example, a peripheral 16-gauge venous catheter can infuse fluid more rapidly than a triple lumen catheter inserted into the superior vena cava.)
- Administration of specific medications such as chemotherapeutic agents or antibiotics that may be irritants to the peripheral veins, as well as vasoactive agents that may cause peripheral vasoconstruction and skin necrosis if extravasated.
- Administration of hyperosmolar fluids and total parenteral nutrition (TPN).
- Emergency venous access.

Large-bore peripheral lines are more suitable for fluid resuscitation than long, thin central vein catheters.

Vasoactive agents should be delivered via central venous catheter.

TABLE 4-1

COMPLICATIONS OF ARTERIAL CANNULATION

Hemorrhage	Thrombosis and emboli	Distal necrosis
Hematoma formation	Arterial laceration	Infection

- Monitoring central venous pressure.
- Long-term IV access.
- Placement of PA catheter.
- Placement of temporary transvenous pacemaker.
- Access for right heart catheterization or arteriogram.
- Access for hemodialysis or plasmapheresis.

Contraindications

There are no absolute contraindications to placement of a central venous catheter.

There are no absolute contraindications for the placement of a central venous catheter. The availability of multiple access sites allows the operator to choose a site that has the lowest risk for complications. Contraindications can thus be categorized as those related to securing central venous access in general and site-specific complications.

General contraindications for central vein cannulation:

- Distortion of local anatomy from previous trauma, surgery, or radiation.
- Injury to the vessels as a result of prior trauma or previous cannulation efforts.
- Bleeding diathesis or coagulopathy.
- Uncooperative or combative patients.
- Patients unable to tolerate the Trendelenburg (i.e., head-down) position.

Site-specific contraindications to central vein cannulation:

- Chest wall deformities that make subclavian vein insertion more difficult.
- Inability to tolerate a potential pneumothorax (limited pulmonary reserve).
- Superior vena cava lesions or superior vena cava syndrome, preventing insertion of the catheter into the central vein after cannulation.
- Penetrating abdominal wounds, so that central venous access should only be attempted above the diaphragm.
- Full-thickness burn or skin infection at the access site.
- Specific for internal jugular vein cannulation: severe carotid artery disease, contralateral hematoma from previous attempt (to avoid bilateral hematoma that may compromise the upper airway).

In patients with abdominal wounds, central venous access should only be attempted above the diaphragm.

Insertion Technique

The choice of central venous access should be based on patient characteristics.

The choice of a central venous access site should be based on patient characteristics. Certain anatomic characteristics are likely to influence placement site, such as a short neck, which favors a subclavian approach, as well as obesity or indistinct landmarks. Other factors that are taken into account are the risk of bleeding, a patient's ability to tolerate the supine position, and the operator's familiarity with a particular approach.

Several venous sites can be chosen for access. The more commonly used sites are the internal jugular, subclavian, and femoral veins. Other access sites that can be used are the external jugular, axillary and brachial veins, but these sites have many limitations that make them less desirable. We focus on the three central venous access sites most commonly used.

Internal Jugular

The internal jugular vein is an easily compressible vessel, which makes it the preferred site in patients with an abnormal coagulation profile.

The internal jugular vein descends in the neck within the carotid sheath, which also contains the carotid artery and the vagus nerve. It traverses the neck and drains into the subclavian vein to form the innominate or brachiocephalic vein behind the head of the clavicle (Figure 4-5). The internal jugular vein offers several advantages, including easy compressibility in case of bleeding and a lower incidence of pneumothorax compared to the subclavian approach. Disadvantages include an increased risk of carotid artery puncture, an increased risk of infection (especially in patients with a tracheostomy tube), and an increased risk of air embolism. The three different approaches to cannulating the internal jugular vein are based

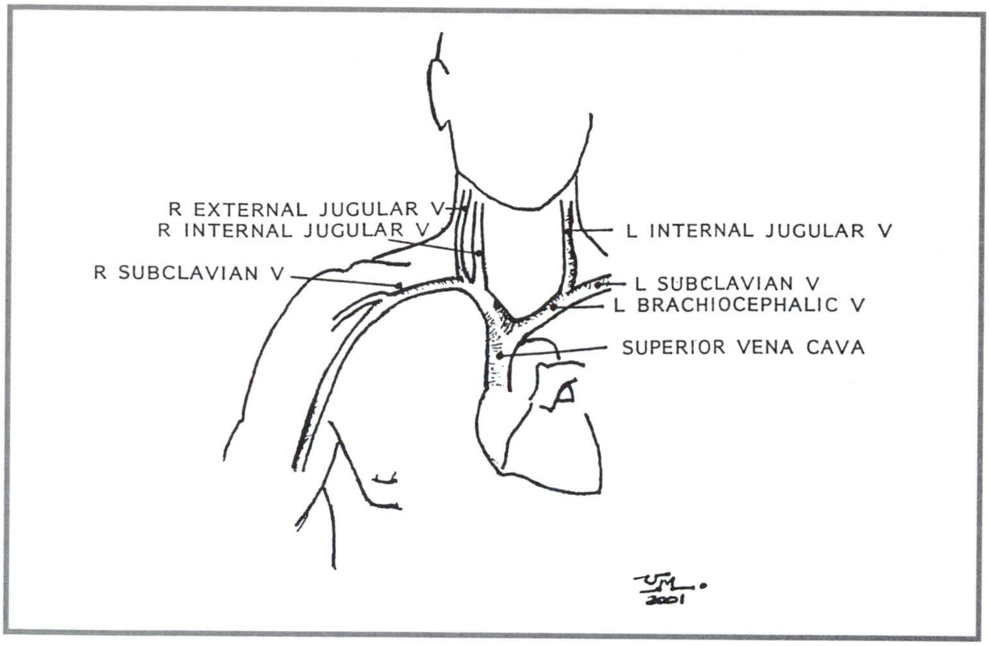

FIGURE 4-5

Anatomy of the neck veins.

on accessing the vein along the anterior, middle, or posterior aspect of the sternocleidomastoid muscle. The right internal jugular vein is usually preferred because of its straight trajectory toward the superior vena cava. However, the apex of the right lung is slightly higher than the left, which may increase the rate of pneumothorax of right-sided cannulation. When using the anterior approach, the operator localizes the space between the trachea and the median head of the sternocleidomastoid (SCM) muscle at the level of the cricoid cartilage. The carotid artery is palpated and the needle is inserted into the space between the carotid and the medial head of the sternocleidomastoid muscle, pointing toward the ipsilateral nipple or shoulder. The anterior approach has been associated with an increased risk of carotid artery puncture. The middle approach requires the operator to localize the triangle formed by the medial and lateral heads of the sternocleidomastoid muscle with the clavicle. The internal jugular vein runs parallel to and below the lateral head of the SCM. The carotid artery is situated medial to the vein. The needle is inserted at the apex of the triangle (Figure 4-6) and directed toward the ipsilateral nipple. It is important to palpate the carotid artery to establish its position, but excessive pressure may collapse the internal jugular vein, making cannulation more difficult. The vessel can usually be located at a depth of 2–4 cm.

The internal jugular vein approach carries a higher risk of carotid artery puncture.

Because the carotid artery and the internal jugular vein share the same sheath, care must be exercised not to collapse the vein while palpating the artery.

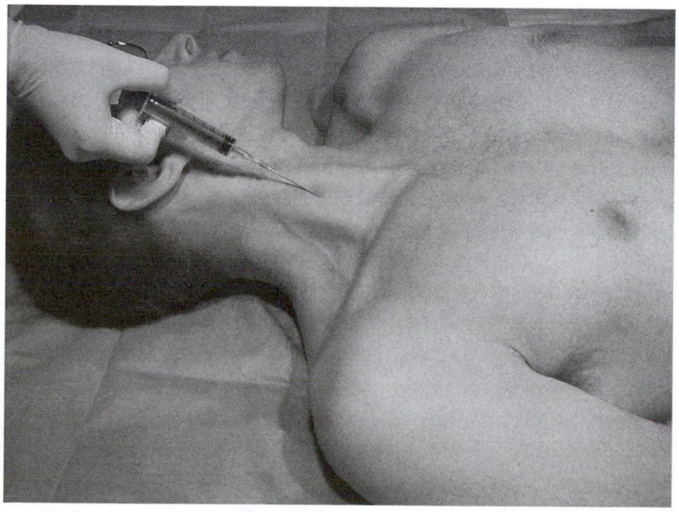

FIGURE 4-6

Internal jugular vein cannulation. When using the middle approach, the apex of a triangle formed by the medial and lateral heads of the sternocleidomastoid muscle (SCM) with the clavicle is localized. The vein runs parallel to and below the lateral head of the SCM. Applying gentle pressure (to avoid collapsing the vein that lies in the same sheath), the operator locates the carotid artery pulse with the index finger of the nondominant hand. The needle is inserted at the apex of the triangle and directed toward the ipsilateral nipple.

The posterior approach requires the operator to identify the posterior aspect of the lateral head of the sternocleidomastoid muscle, which can be done holding both bellies of the muscle between the index and thumb finger. The needle is inserted above the point where the external jugular vein traverses the sternocleidomastoid muscle and is directed under its lateral belly toward the suprasternal notch. The vein is usually entered at a depth of 3–5 cm (Figure 4-7).

Subclavian Vein

The placement of a pillow behind the patient's shoulders during subclavian cannulation may decrease the space between the first rib and the clavicle, making cannulation more difficult.

The subclavian vein originates from the axillary vein and ends posterior to the medial head of the clavicle where it joins the internal jugular vein to form the innominate (brachiocephalic) vein (see Figure 4-5). The usual approach to the subclavian vein is via the inferior route. The patient is positioned supine with the head lowered 15°–30°. Although a common practice, placing a pillow or towel roll between the scapulae can actually decrease the space between the first rib and clavicle, making access to the vein more difficult. The needle is inserted 1 cm below the junction of the middle and medial thirds of the clavicle and directed toward the suprasternal notch (Figure 4-8). The left subclavian vein is longer and follows a straighter pathway than its right counterpart, making it easier to insert the central line through this approach. Because the subclavian vein cannot be compressed, this approach should be avoided in patients with a bleeding diathesis. It also carries a higher risk of pneumothorax and air embolism as compared to the internal jugular vein approach. On the other hand, the landmarks are easier to identify, and there seems to be a lower incidence of catheter-related infections, especially if the patient is intubated or has a tracheostomy in place. In addition, most conscious patients report less discomfort with a subclavian line.

The subclavian approach should be avoided in patients with a bleeding diathesis (noncompressible site).

Femoral Vein

The femoral vein lies medial to the femoral artery.

At the level of the inguinal ligament, the femoral vein lies medial to the femoral artery. To access the vein, the patient's lower extremity should be positioned in complete external ro-

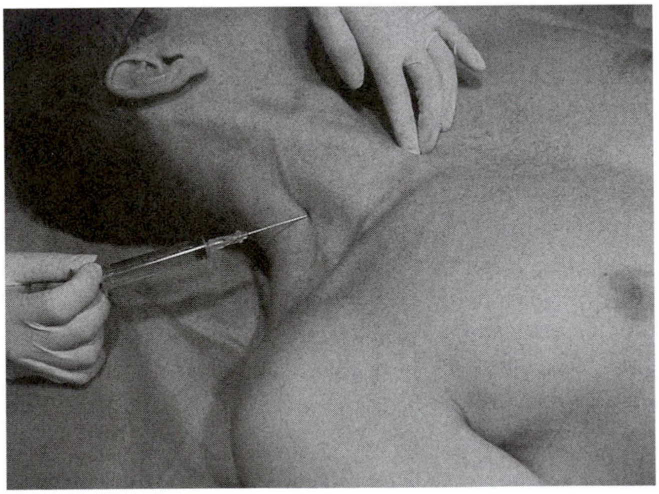

FIGURE 4-7

Internal jugular vein cannulation. When using the posterior approach, the operator locates the posterior aspect of the lateral belly of the sternocleidomastoid muscle. The needle is inserted above the point where the external jugular vein traverses the lateral belly of the sternocleidomastoid muscle and is directed (underneath the muscle) toward the suprasternal notch.

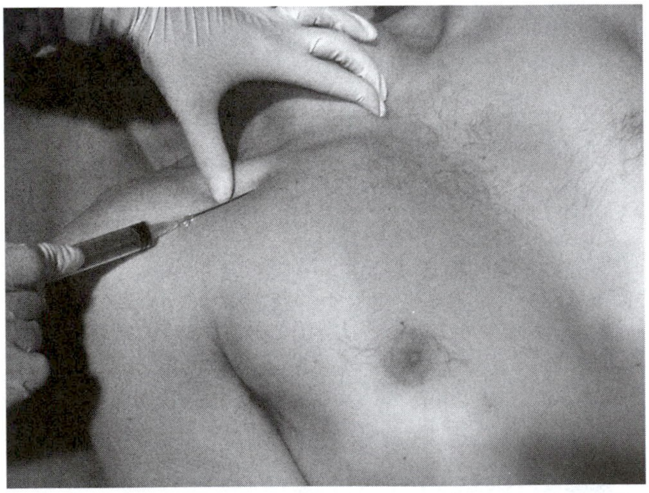

FIGURE 4-8

Subclavian vein cannulation. The operator locates the junction of the middle and medial thirds of the clavicle. The needle is inserted 1 cm below this point and directed toward the suprasternal notch, which is marked by the operator's nondominant hand's index finger. The needle is maintained as parallel to the skin as possible.

tation. The operator should palpate for the arterial pulse and insert the needle medial to it. The needle should be angled about 45° from the skin plane toward the head and slightly toward the midline (about 15°). The vein is usually entered at a distance 3 and 5 cm from the skin surface. The risk of complications is much lower with femoral lines. The site can be easily compressed. During the first 72 h, the incidence of catheter-related infection is not different from that of other sites if the inguinal area is adequately prepared.

During the first 72 h, there is no increase in the incidence of catheter-related infections with femoral catheters.

Clinical Utility

A properly placed central venous pressure (CVP) catheter can be used to measure right atrial pressure (P_{RA}). In the absence of tricuspid valve disease, the CVP closely mirrors right ventricular end diastolic pressure (RVEDP). RVEDP can be used as a surrogate for right ventricular end diastolic volume (RVEDV) and thus preload. CVP is decreased in patients with hypovolemia and increased in patients with tricuspid regurgitation, right ventricular failure or infarction, and pericardial tamponade. In patients with normal cardiac function, a CVP greater than 10 cmH_2O signals an adequate intravascular volume. The absence of inspiratory variation in the CVP waveform correlates with a lack of further increase in cardiac output with continued fluid resuscitation. The CVP measurement, however, may not be an accurate assessment of cardiac function in critically ill patients, especially those with severe pulmonary hypertension, mitral valve dysfunction, or with right ventricular abnormal compliance or dysfunction. In these patients, there is a poor correlation between right- and left-sided pressures.

The absence of inspiratory variation in the central venous pressure waveform correlates with a lack of further increase in cardiac output with fluid resuscitation.

The CVP should always be attached to an electronic pressure transducer that displays the CVP waveform and its different components. Analysis of the waveform can give valuable insight into the underlying pathology in patients with cardiovascular disorders. The CVP waveform should always be interpreted with the influence of respiratory variation taken into account, and be examined during end-expiration for consistency.

PULMONARY ARTERY CATHETER

History

Pulmonary artery wedge pressure (PAWP) was first measured nearly 50 years ago. Before 1970, hemodynamic monitoring was not done outside of the *catheterization* laboratory. It was reserved for patients with congenital cardiac abnormalities and patients undergoing valvular surgery. The catheters that were employed initially were rigid and their insertion was frequently associated with bleeding and arrhythmias. In 1970, Swan and colleagues described the use of a flow-directed, balloon-tipped catheter that could be placed into the pulmonary artery at the patient's bedside without the need for fluoroscopy.

Description of the Pulmonary Artery Catheter

The pulmonary artery catheter (PAC) has undergone several modifications since its introduction in the 1970s. Modern catheters now allow for pressure monitoring, measurement of cardiac output, fluid and vasopressor infusion, and even therapeutic interventions such as cardiac pacing. The general design is very similar among the different catheters. The PA catheter is 110 cm long and heparin bonded throughout its entire length to decrease the incidence of catheter-associated thrombosis and microbial adherence. The four-lumen version allows for continuous measurement of cardiac pressures, as well as determination of the cardiac output (CO) using the thermodilution technique. The five-lumen catheter offers an additional port in the right atrium for fluid administration (Figure 4-9).

The pulmonary artery (PA) catheter is heparin bonded to reduce the incidence of thrombosis and microbial adherence.

Modifications in the catheter have allowed for continuous monitoring of variables that in the past were only intermittently obtained, such as mixed venous oxygen saturation. The development of a fast-response thermistor has enabled the continuous measurement of CO or

FIGURE 4-9

The pulmonary artery catheter.

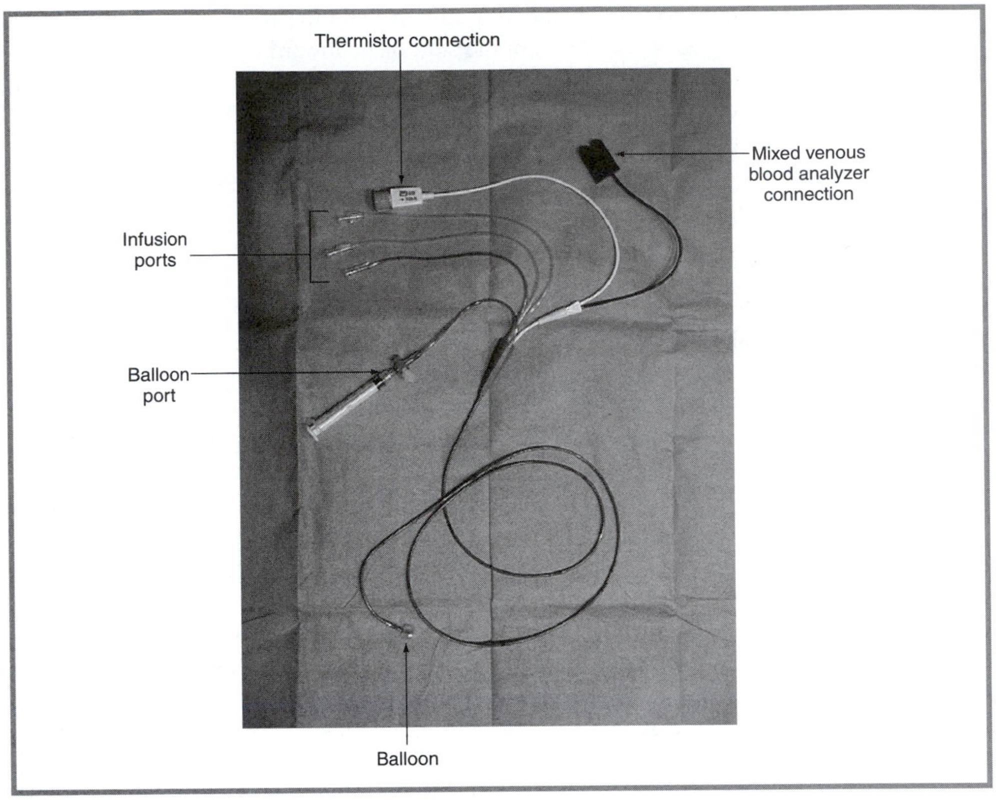

the right ventricular ejection fraction. Another modification allows for atrial or ventricular pacing.

What Does the Pulmonary Artery Catheter Measure?

The PA catheter directly measures right atrial pressure, right ventricular and pulmonary artery systolic and diastolic pressures, and pulmonary artery occlusion pressure.

The PA catheter directly measures the P_{RA}, right ventricular, and PA systolic and diastolic pressures, as well as the PAWP (Table 4-2). In addition, cardiac output (CO) can be intermittently obtained and mixed venous oxygenation and core body temperature can be continuously measured. With these measured variables, several calculated indices are obtained, including oxygen delivery and consumption and the oxygen extraction ratio (Table 4-3). Calculation of systemic and pulmonary vascular resistance, left and right ventricular stroke work, and work rate can also be obtained (Table 4-4).

In the "wedge" position, the measured pressure reflects the hydrostatic pressure of the blood column at the confluence of the pulmonary veins.

To obtain the PAWP, the PA catheter is wedged into an interlobar pulmonary artery, while the balloon is inflated with full volume. Wedging of the catheter with a partially inflated balloon (air volume less than 1.5 ml) indicates "overwedging" or too distal placement of the catheter end. The measured pressure reflects the hydrostatic pressure of the column of blood

TABLE 4-2

MEASURED HEMODYNAMIC VARIABLES

VARIABLE (ABBREVIATION)	UNIT	NORMAL RANGE
Systolic blood pressure (SBP)	mmHg	100–140
Diastolic blood pressure (DBP)	mmHg	60–90
Pulmonary artery systolic pressure (PASP)	mmHg	15–30
Pulmonary artery diastolic pressure (PADP)	mmHg	4–12
Right ventricular systolic pressure (RVSP)	mmHg	15–30
Right ventricular end-diastolic pressure (RVEDP)	mmHg	0–8
Central venous pressure (CVP)	mmHg	0–8
Pulmonary artery occlusion pressure (PAOP)	mmHg	2–12
Cardiac output (CO)	l/min	Varies with size

TABLE 4-3

DERIVED HEMODYNAMIC VARIABLES

TERM	ABBREVIATION	DEFINITION	NORMAL RANGE
Arterial blood oxygen content	CaO_2	Volume of gaseous oxygen/dl blood	16–22 ml/dl
Arterial blood oxygen content	DO_2	O_2 volume ejected from left ventricle: $DO_2 = CI \times CaO_2 \times 10$	500–650 l/min/m^2
Oxygen consumption, ml/min/m^2	VO_2	O_2 volume used by tissue: $VO_2 = CI \times C(a–v)\ O_2 \times 10$	110–150
Oxygen uptake, ml/min/m^2	–	O_2 volume taken up by lungs	110–150
Extraction ratio	ER	$ER = VO_2/DO_2$	0.22–0.30

CI, cardiac index (l/min/m^2); CaO_2, arterial oxygen (ml/dl blood); C(a–v) O_2, arterial venous oxygen content difference (ml/dl blood); BSA, body surface area (m^2)

at the confluence of the pulmonary veins (Figure 4-10), allowing the clinician to estimate (not measure) two important parameters, the hydrostatic pressure gradient for pulmonary edema formation and the LVEDV.

Indications

Differentiation Between Cardiogenic and Noncardiogenic Pulmonary Edema

Attempting to clinically discern between cardiogenic and noncardiogenic pulmonary edema is a common scenario encountered in the ICU. In both cases, patients present with bilateral alveolar infiltrates, hypoxemia, and decreased lung compliance. Obtaining a thorough history, physical examination, and chest radiographs are the initial steps. However, several stud-

TABLE 4-4

OXYGEN TRANSPORT VARIABLES

TERM	ABBREVIATION	CALCULATION	NORMAL RANGE
Mean arterial pressure	MAP	MAP = DBP + ((SBP – DBP)/3)	70–105 mm Hg
Mean pulmonary artery pressure	MPAP	MPAP = PADP + ((PASP – PADP)/3)	9–16 mm Hg
Cardiac index	CI	CI = CO/BSA	2.8–3.2 l/min/m^2
Stroke volume	SV	SV = CO/HR	Varies with size
Stroke index	SI	SI = CI/HR/beat/m^2	30–65 ml
Left ventricular stroke work index	LVSWI	LVSWI = CI × (MAP – PAOP) × 0.0136	44–64 g · m/m^2
Right ventricular stroke work index	RVSWI	RVSWI = CI × (MPAP – CVP) × 0.0136	7–12 g · m/m^2
Systemic vascular resistance index	SVRI	SVRI = ((MAP – CVP)/CI) × 80	1600–2400 dyne · s · cm^{-5}/m^2
Pulmonary vascular resistance index	PVRI	PVRI = ((MPAP – PAOP)/CI) × 80	250–430 dyne · s · cm^{-5}/m^2

PADP, pulmonary artery diastolic pressure (mm Hg); PASP, pulmonary artery systolic pressure (mm Hg)

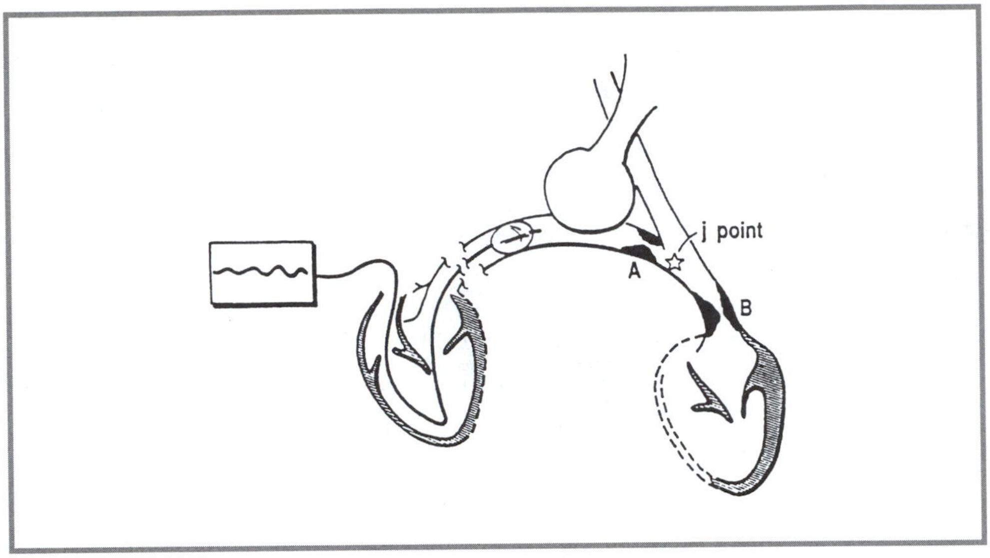

FIGURE 4-10

Principle of the pulmonary artery wedge pressure (PAWP) measurement. When the balloon is inflated, the catheter records the pressure at the junction of the static and free flowing channels, the j point. An obstruction distal to the j point at B will cause the PAWP to overestimate left atrial pressure. (From O'Quin R, Marini JJ. Pulmonary artery occlusion pressure: clinical physiology measurement and interpretation. Am Rev Respir Dis 1983;128: 319–326, with permission.)

The ability to discern between cardiogenic and noncardiogenic pulmonary edema by clinical assessment alone is limited.

ies have shown that, in the ICU, physicians are limited in their ability to distinguish between cardiogenic and noncardiogenic pulmonary edema. Based on clinical assessment alone, physicians were able to determine PAWP and cardiac index (CI) correctly in only 30%–69% of the patients. In addition, using a PA catheter led to a change in therapy in 40%–60% of the cases.

There are noninvasive alternatives to the PA catheter in determining the etiology of pulmonary edema. Using a long suction catheter, a lavage can be performed to determine the protein concentration in pulmonary edema fluid. The ratio of the pulmonary edema fluid protein concentration to the serum protein concentration can help differentiate cardiogenic from noncardiogenic pulmonary edema. A ratio greater than 75% is associated with increased permeability (noncardiogenic) pulmonary edema; a ratio less than 65% is highly suggestive of hydrostatic (cardiogenic) pulmonary edema. This technique is useful only if performed very early in the course of edema formation. In addition, because this technique is not performed routinely in the ICU, the results may not be reproducible. Despite the noted limitations in identifying a cause for pulmonary edema, the initial clinical impression by the physician should direct therapy. Insertion of a PA catheter should be considered in patients who do not respond to initial therapy or have a rapid clinical deterioration. Traditionally, an elevated PAWP is taken to indicate a significant component of hydrostatic pulmonary edema, whereas a low PAWP is usually indicative, but not diagnostic, of noncardiogenic pulmonary edema. An American-European Consensus Statement recognizes a PAWP less than 18 mmHg as one of several criteria in the diagnosis of the acute respiratory distress syndrome (ARDS).

The American-European Consensus recognizes a wedge of less than 18 mmHg as one of the diagnostic criteria for the acute respiratory distress syndrome (ARDS).

Diagnosis of Shock

The PA catheter can be used to help establish the etiology of shock; the most common causes include hypovolemic, septic, and cardiogenic shock. Hypovolemic shock is suggested when there is a recent history of trauma, bleeding, or protracted volume loss from diarrhea or emesis. Physical examination reveals enophthalmos, dry mucous membranes, loss of skin turgor, and flattened neck veins. In addition, hypotension and postural changes in heart rate or blood pressure or both can be seen. Laboratory findings may demonstrate an elevated blood urea nitrogen (BUN) and creatinine, as well as hypernatremia and hemoconcentration. The diagnosis of hypovolemic shock is usually made on the basis of clinical information.

In certain cases, it is difficult to differentiate between septic and cardiogenic shock. Echocardiography is an alternative to PA catheter placement in establishing the presence of left ventricular dysfunction. Nevertheless, septic shock can be associated with abnormal left ventricular function, and a more definitive diagnosis can be established with placement of a PA catheter. Patients with cardiogenic shock characteristically demonstrate a low CO and high systemic vascular resistance. In contrast, patients with septic shock have an abnormally high CO and low systemic vascular resistance. In addition to establishing the etiology of a patient's shock, the PA catheter is very useful in managing fluids as well as for monitoring the effects of inotropic and vasoactive agents.

Patients with cardiogenic shock have a low cardiac output and a high systemic vascular resistance.

Management of Acute Respiratory Distress Syndrome

In patients with ARDS, a PA catheter is useful not only in establishing an accurate diagnosis but also in directing therapy. Possible therapeutic interventions include adjustment of vasoactive medications or a change in the rate of fluid infusion to minimize edema formation in the presence of capillary leak. The PA catheter also can be useful in titrating the amount of positive end-expiratory pressure (PEEP) in patients with ARDS. Recently, focus has increased on the use of higher levels of PEEP combined with lower tidal volumes to minimize the risk of ventilator-induced lung injury. PEEP will recruit collapsed alveoli and increase end-expiratory lung volume, decreasing ventilation–perfusion mismatch and shunt. Unfortunately, higher levels of PEEP increase intrathoracic pressure and decrease venous return, resulting in a decrease CO. With a PA catheter, the effects of PEEP on CO can be monitored, with a decrease corrected with intravascular volume or the initiation of an inotropic agent.

The PA catheter can be useful in titrating pulmonary end-expiratory pressure (PEEP) in patients with the acute respiratory distress syndrome.

MANAGEMENT OF MYOCARDIAL INFARCTION AND CARDIOGENIC SHOCK

Shock may be one of the presenting manifestations of an acute myocardial infarction (MI). Patients can present with evidence of hemodynamic compromise, including hypotension, pulmonary edema, and oliguria. Shock may be secondary to relative hypovolemia with a decreased preload or to a low CO state. The use of a PA catheter in patients with an acute MI should be reserved for those with clinical signs of shock. A PA catheter guides preload and afterload reduction and the use of diuretics, as well as inotropic support. The PA catheter may also be useful in the diagnosis and management of right myocardial infarction. Right myocardial infarction occurs in about 30% of patients with an inferior wall MI. Patients generally present with precordial pain, associated with hypotension and clear lung fields. Kussmaul's sign (engorgement of the jugular veins during inspiration) and the hepatojugular reflex may be present. The diagnosis is made by electrocardiographic changes in the right precordial leads and elevation of cardiac enzymes. Placement of a PA catheter shows elevated mean right atrial pressure (see following). The PA catheter may also be useful in managing fluids in these patients, whose right ventricular preload can be compromised.

Patients who present with an acute myocardial infarction (MI) and signs of shock should be managed with a PA catheter.

The presence of elevated right atrium pressure and systemic hypotension are characteristic in patients with an acute right ventricular MI.

The PA catheter also allows diagnosing some of the complications of acute MI. Papillary muscle ischemia or rupture results in acute mitral regurgitation, which can be assessed by the presence of giant v waves in the pulmonary artery wedge tracing (see following). A rupture of the interventricular septum can be diagnosed by establishing the presence of an increase in the O_2 saturation in the blood samples from the right ventricle. Patients with advanced heart failure may also benefit from PA catheter insertion during episodes of decompensation. These patients often need similar therapeutic interventions that require close hemodynamic monitoring.

Papillary muscle ischemia or rupture results in acute mitral regurgitation, which will manifest as large "v" waves in the pulmonary artery wedge tracing.

Perioperative Management

The role of the PA catheter in the perioperative setting is controversial. High-risk surgical patients, for example, those with decompensated heart failure and history of a MI in the previous 3 months, are likely to benefit from PA catheter insertion. There is little evidence to support the use of PA catheters in patients undergoing coronary artery bypass graft surgery. An exception may be the subgroup of patients with left main coronary artery disease. In one

Patients with left main coronary artery disease may benefit from perioperative PA catheter monitoring.

retrospective study, these patients had a 17% decrement in mortality when managed with a PA catheter in the perioperative period.

The use of the PA catheter has been evaluated in patients undergoing peripheral vascular surgery with associated comorbidities. Despite a reduction in intraoperative hemodynamic complications, overall mortality did not differ between the group that was monitored with a PA catheter and the group that was not. In patients undergoing elective abdominal aortic aneurysm repair, no difference in morbidity and mortality was noted between patients monitored with a CVP catheter and those patients with a PA catheter.

In a study by Shoemaker et al. (1988), patients who underwent surgery for high-risk conditions (abdominal catastrophe, multiple trauma, etc.) were randomized to three different groups. Groups 1 and 2 were monitored with CVP and PA catheters, respectively. A third group was monitored with PA catheters, but therapy was guided to increase CI and DO_2 to supraphysiologic levels, based on prior data collected from survivors of high-risk surgical interventions. The third group showed a significant reduction in mechanical ventilator days, ICU/hospital days, and hospital costs. The results of this study were not reproduced when supraphysiologic parameters were used in high-risk medical patients. In summary, only patients with a history of recent MI, decompensated heart failure, and left main coronary artery disease are likely to benefit from PA catheter monitoring in the perioperative period. Patients who undergo high-risk surgical procedures may benefit from PA catheter monitoring and the use of augmented circulatory responses (CI and DO_2).

Insertion Technique

Preliminary Steps

In addition to the general precautions and preliminary steps undertaken each time an intravenous catheter is placed, the placement of a PA catheter warrants several particular measures such as continuous electrocardiographic monitoring, frequent blood pressure measurements (manual or automatic devices), and oxygen saturation monitoring with pulse oxymetry.

When venous access has been obtained, an introducer is placed. The PA catheter is placed through the introducer and advanced to about 15–20 cm. From this point, it is important that the operator is able to recognize the different waveforms that will be displayed on the monitor. The PA catheter balloon is inflated and the catheter is slowly advanced, observing the changes in waveforms on the monitor (Figure 4-11). On entering the right ventricle from the right atrium, a sharp increment in systolic pressure is observed. The catheter is then advanced into the PA. Diastolic pressure increases, and a dicrotic notch is noted in the PA waveform. As the catheter is advanced further into the PA, progressive dampening of the waveform is observed.

The wedge position is characterized by a sine wave that oscillates with respiration. The wedge position is usually reached 10–15 cm after passage through the right ventricle or at 45–55 cm from the skin when the right internal jugular approach is used for access. Failure to detect a wedge waveform should prompt the operator to deflate the balloon and retract the catheter to the right atrium to attempt to refloat the PA catheter. Advancing the catheter beyond the expected distance that a wedge waveform should be obtained can result in coiling or knotting. The balloon should always be deflated before retracting the catheter. It is important to realize that the term wedge is a misnomer that relates to the way pressures were measured with stiff catheters before the advent of the flow-directed, balloon-tipped catheters. Stiff catheters had to be introduced deep into the PA until the catheter wedged, which increased the incidence of complications. In contrast, modern PA catheters need only to be advanced into an interlobar artery, and they allow for easier placement by using balloon flotation and minimize arterial rupture and overwedging by measuring pressures at an interlobar artery.

> The balloon should always be deflated before retracting the pulmonary artery catheter.

> Modern PA catheters are placed in an interlobar artery.

If there is difficulty advancing the catheter into the PA (patients with pulmonary hypertension, cardiomyopathy, enlarged right ventricle), several maneuvers can be attempted. If the patient is awake, a deep inspiratory effort will increase venous return and help float the catheter into position. Placing the patient in the supine position with a slight elevation of the

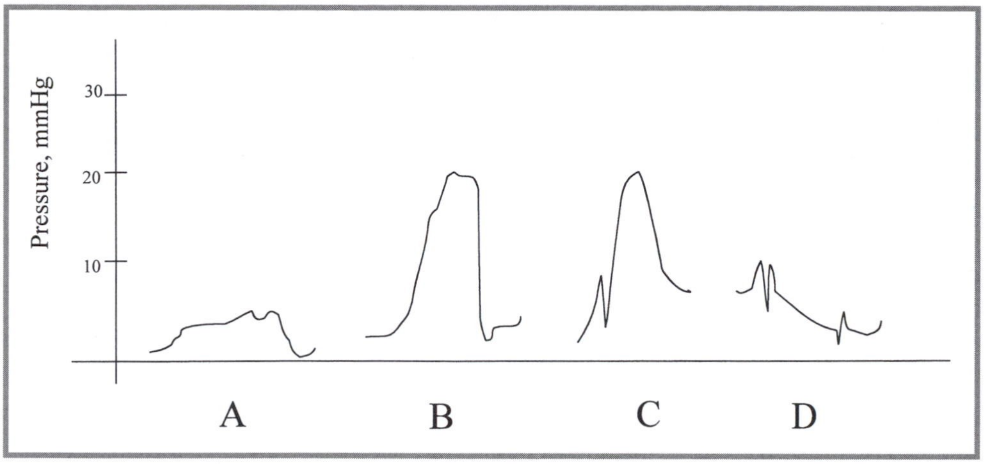

FIGURE 4-11

As the pulmonary artery catheter is inserted, the different waveforms and pressures should be carefully observed. As the catheter is inserted, a central venous pressure tracing **(A)**, characterized by a and v waves, is seen. On entering the right ventricle from the right atrium, a sharp increment in systolic pressure is noted **(B)**. The catheter is then advanced to the pulmonary artery, characterized by an increment in diastolic pressure and the presence of a dicrotic notch, the waveform **(C)**. As the catheter is advanced further into the pulmonary artery, a progressive dampening of the waveform is noted. The "wedge" position is characterized by a sine wave that oscillates with respiration **(D)**.

head, or turning to the left lateral decubitus position, may also help. If the catheter is in the circulation for several minutes, it may warm up and become more compliant. In that case, infusing a small amount of ice-cold saline may increase the stiffness of the catheter. Stiffer catheters are available, but the operator must be aware that there may be an increased risk of perforation. If these maneuvers are not successful, the catheter should be placed under fluoroscopy. Once the wedge position is reached, the balloon should be deflated and the PA waveform should return. A chest radiograph should always be obtained to confirm the catheter's position and to rule out a pneumothorax.

A chest radiograph should always be obtained to verify catheter position and rule out the presence of pneumothorax.

Measurement of Cardiac Output

Measurement of CO plays an important role in clinical decision making in the intensive care unit. CO reflects a measurement not only of pump function but of overall circulatory function as well and is important in determining the cause of hypotension. In conjunction with other parameters measured with the PA catheter, CO enables the physician to diagnose and treat shock regardless of its etiology.

CO is directly related to the metabolic rate and thus oxygen consumption ($\dot{V}O_2$). The relationship in normal individuals is linear, with an increase in $\dot{V}O_2$ (as during exercise) resulting in a parallel increment in CO. This linear relationship allows CO to be calculated with a margin of error of only about 5%. A decrement in CO is not necessarily related to a decrease in $\dot{V}O_2$. For example, in patients who develop CHF (congestive heart failure), a decrease in CO will not affect $\dot{V}O_2$ because of an increase in oxygen extraction at the tissue level. In other disease states, such as ARDS, the tissues are not able to increase their extraction of oxygen and thus the $\dot{V}O_2$ can be very dependent on CO.

Cardiac output is directly related to oxygen consumption.

The relationship between blood pressure and CO is best expressed by the formula:

$$\text{Blood pressure} = \text{CO} \times \text{SVR} \qquad (4\text{-}1)$$

where SVR is systemic vascular resistance. In other words, the development of hypotension can be directly related to a decrement in CO (e.g., cardiogenic shock) or a decrease in SVR

Measurement of cardiac output can be obtained by thermodilution or the Fick method.

(e.g., septic shock). Commonly, CO in the ICU can be measured by the Fick method or by thermodilution.

Fick Method

Measurement of CO by the Fick method requires an indicator that is added at a constant rate. Oxygen is a very good indicator because oxygen uptake and the arterial and venous oxygen contents can be measured with relative ease. The formula for cardiac output using oxygen as an indicator is:

$$CO = \dot{V}O_2/(CaO_2 - C\bar{v}O_2) \quad (4\text{-}2)$$

where CaO_2 is the arterial oxygen content and CvO_2 is the mixed venous oxygen content. $\dot{V}O_2$ can be determined from the difference between oxygen content in inspired and expired air as measured by a gas analyzer. The arterial content of oxygen can be calculated from the following formula:

$$CaO_2 = 1.36 \times Hb \times SaO_2 \quad (4\text{-}3)$$

where Hb is hemoglobin, 1.36 is a constant that gives the amount of oxygen bound to each fully saturated molecule of hemoglobin, and SaO_2 is arterial oxygen saturation, which can easily be determined by arterial blood gas analysis.

The mixed venous oxygen content can be calculated from the formula:

$$C\bar{v}O_2 = 1.36 \times Hb \times SvO_2 \quad (4\text{-}4)$$

where SvO_2 represents the mixed venous oxygen saturation. A sample of mixed venous blood should be obtained from the distal port of the PA catheter. Equation 4-2 can then be rewritten as:

To avoid errors in measurement of cardiac output with the Fick method, mixed venous blood samples should be obtained from the right ventricle or the pulmonary artery.

$$CO = \dot{V}O_2/1.36 \times Hb \times (SaO_2 - S\bar{v}O_2) \quad (4\text{-}5)$$

Several sources for error can occur when using the Fick method to calculate cardiac output. The mixed venous blood sample must come from the RV or PA. The presence of an intracardiac shunt can alter the oxygen content of the sample. Although dissolved oxygen in the arterial blood (PaO_2) normally contributes little to the overall oxygen content (not even included in Eq. 4-4), at a high FiO_2 its contribution can be underestimated. Errors may also occur as a result of inaccurate measurement of $\dot{V}O_2$ from the exhaled gases.

Changes in pulmonary gas volume, performing a Valsalva maneuver, or receiving a transfusion can all affect the measurement of CO using the Fick method. In addition, inflammatory disorders in the lungs, such as pneumonia, increase the consumption of oxygen by the lungs before it reaches the blood, leading to an overestimation of $\dot{V}O_2$ by as much as 15%.

Thermodilution Method

The thermodilution technique has become the method most commonly used to determine CO in the ICU. The technique involves injecting either 10 ml of ice-cold dextrose in water, or dextrose in water at room temperature, through the proximal port of the PA catheter into the RA. The change in temperature is sampled by a thermistor located in the distal end of the PA catheter that is located in the PA. A computer records the change in temperature from baseline and the cardiac output is calculated by the integration of temperature over time (Figure 4-12). Traditionally, an ice-cold injectate was used, but more recent studies have demonstrated room temperature injectates to be as accurate and more convenient. Sources of error using this technique include inaccurate baseline temperature measurements and injecting the wrong volume. During respiration, variation in lung temperature may occur, resulting in fluctuations in the thermistor's baseline temperature reading. Volumes smaller than

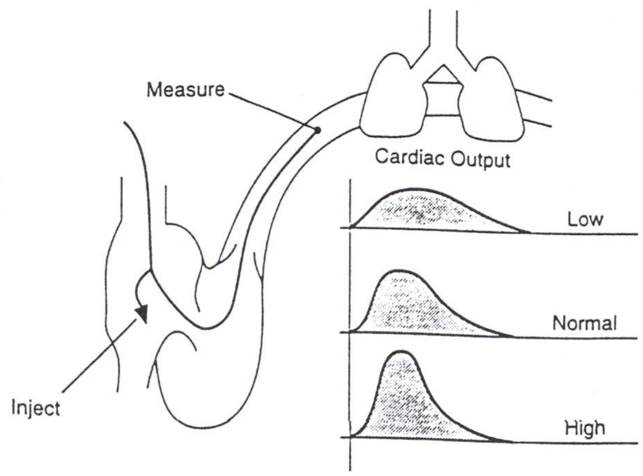

FIGURE 4-12

Cardiac output (CO) measured by thermodilution. A bolus of crystalloid solution is injected into the central venous circulation, and temperature is measured by a thermistor at the tip of the pulmonary artery catheter. Typical thermal dilution curves are shown. (From Bartlett, RH. Blood volume. In: Critical Care Physiology. Little Brown and Company, 1996:33, with permission.)

10 ml are associated with a greater magnitude of error. Other sources for error include arrhythmias, tricuspid regurgitation (which may under or overestimate CO), intracardiac shunts, and a low cardiac output.

Arrhythmias, tricuspid regurgitation, and low cardiac output may result in an erroneous estimation of cardiac output by thermodilution.

Modern pulmonary artery catheters allow for continuous measurements of CO, which can be accomplished by two methods. A continuous CO derived from the Fick equation can be obtained by measuring oxygen consumption using indirect calorimetry and the analysis of inspired and expired gases, continuous pulse oximetry for the assessment of arterial oxygen saturation, and continuous mixed venous oximetry for the assessment of mixed venous oxygen saturation. When the outputs of these three devices are computed using the Fick's equation, a near real time assessment of CO can be obtained. The second method is based on the thermodilution theory. Instead of measuring changes in an injectate temperature, CO is calculated using thermal boluses generated by a heating filament on the catheter to produce temperature changes.

Interpretation of Pressures

Right Atrial Pressure

The normal range for P_{RA} is 2–8 mmHg. P_{RA} reflects right ventricular end-diastolic pressure (RVEDP) if tricuspid regurgitation or stenosis is not present. P_{RA} is usually lower than PAWP, but with normal cardiac function there is a good correlation between these pressures. In patients with left ventricular hypertrophy, CHF, or ischemia, this close correlation may not be present. In these cases, PAWP may be markedly elevated with only a modest elevation in P_{RA}. P_{RA} will be higher than PAWP in the presence of pulmonary hypertension, such as with massive pulmonary embolism or tricuspid regurgitation. In patients with normal cardiac function, a P_{RA} greater than 10 mmHg indicates an adequate intravascular volume. The P_{RA} normally falls during inspiration because of transmission of the negative intrathoracic pressure. The absence of a decrement in P_{RA} during inspiration indicates that CO cannot be further increased by volume infusion.

A poor correlation between pulmonary artery wedge pressure and right atrial pressure is observed in patients with heart failure, ischemia, and left ventricular hypertrophy.

Pulmonary Artery Pressure

The normal values for pulmonary artery pressure (PAP) are a systolic pressure of 15–30 mmHg, a diastolic pressure of 4-12 mmHg, and a mean of 9–18 mmHg. The difference between the PA diastolic pressure and the PAWP is normally 1–4 mmHg, and this difference can often narrow the differential diagnosis of an elevated PAP. A PA diastolic − PAWP greater than 5 mmHg suggests increased pulmonary vascular resistance, as in patients with acute (ARDS) and chronic (pulmonary fibrosis) hypoxemia, or pulmonary emboli. In contrast, pul-

A gradient >5 mmHg between the pulmonary artery diastolic pressure and the wedge pressure suggests the presence of increased pulmonary vascular resistance.

monary hypertension resulting from increased downstream pressures (elevated PAWP in patients with CHF) usually maintains a normal gradient.

Pulmonary Artery Wedge Pressure

One of the most common indications for insertion of a PA catheter is to measure the PAWP. By occluding a branch of the pulmonary artery, a static column of blood is created distal to the occluded vessel. The hydrostatic pressure at the confluence of the pulmonary veins can then be determined. PAWP is the pressure measured at the point at which the vascular segment of the pulmonary vein that is occluded joins the rest of the pulmonary veins which contain free flowing blood; this point is also known as the j point. It is therefore clear that PAWP estimates, but does not measure, two parameters: the hydrostatic pressure gradient for edema formation at the pulmonary capillaries and the left ventricular end-diastolic volume.

Several technical problems that can result in an erroneous reading of the PAWP must be considered.

Invalid Waveform

The validity of the waveform needs to be assessed in several ways. The first is to make sure that when the balloon is deflated a PA waveform tracing is observed. On wedging, the tracing should have characteristics typical of a left atrial pressure waveform. The mean PAWP pressure should be less than mean PA pressure and generally less than PA diastolic pressure (tracings with cannon a waves may be an exception).

Inaccurate Zero Pressure Reference

Alterations in the zero hydrostatic pressure reference can cause important errors in measuring PAWP. A deviation of 10 cm from the true zero point will cause a change (in the opposite direction) of 10 cmH_2O, or about 7.5 mmHg, in the measured PAWP. There are two ways to set the zero pressure reference level. In the first, the pressure transducer is leveled at the midaxillary line using a ruler with a leveler. The transducer is then opened to air, and thus atmospheric pressure, at that level and zeroed. In the second method, the more distal three-way stopcock going to the PA port is placed at the midaxillary line, opening it to air, adjacent to the patient. The catheter is thus zero referenced at this level. There is a greater chance for movement from the zero referenced mark using the first technique because the catheter is not stabilized to a pole and can inadvertently be moved.

Catheter Tip Not in Zone III

To accurately measure intravascular pressures, the tip of the PA catheter must be in a position where zone 3 conditions prevail.

Regional differences in pulmonary perfusion result from the interactions of several factors, including gravity, PA pressure, pulmonary venous pressure (PVP), and alveolar pressure (P_{ALV}). Three different zones can be identified within the lung, with zone 1 at the apex, zone 2 in the midlung field, and zone 3 at the base. Zone 2 is characterized by PAP $>$ P_{ALV} $>$ PVP and zone 3 by PAP $>$ PVP $>$ P_{ALV}. For practical purposes, when the balloon is inflated, PAP becomes irrelevant because pressure is measured distal to the balloon. When PVP exceeds P_{ALV} (zone 3), intravascular pressure is recorded. If P_{ALV} is greater than PVP, the measured pressure will reflect alveolar pressure (zone 2) (Figure 4-13). In clinical practice, the effects from zone 2 are relatively uncommon because the catheter is flow directed and has a tendency to find its way to a position lower than the left atrium. It is theorized that applied PEEP to the airway in patients with ARDS results in increased alveolar pressure and non-zone 3 placement. Zapol and Snider (1977) found no significant change in PA and PAWP readings when PEEP was reduced from 20 to 0 cmH_2O in 10 patients with ARDS; this may result from the decreased lung compliance in ARDS, causing poor transmission of airway pressure to the intravascular compartment.

It is important to read the PAWP at the end of expiration, a point at which there is the least effect of intrapleural pressure changes on transmural cardiac pressure measurements.

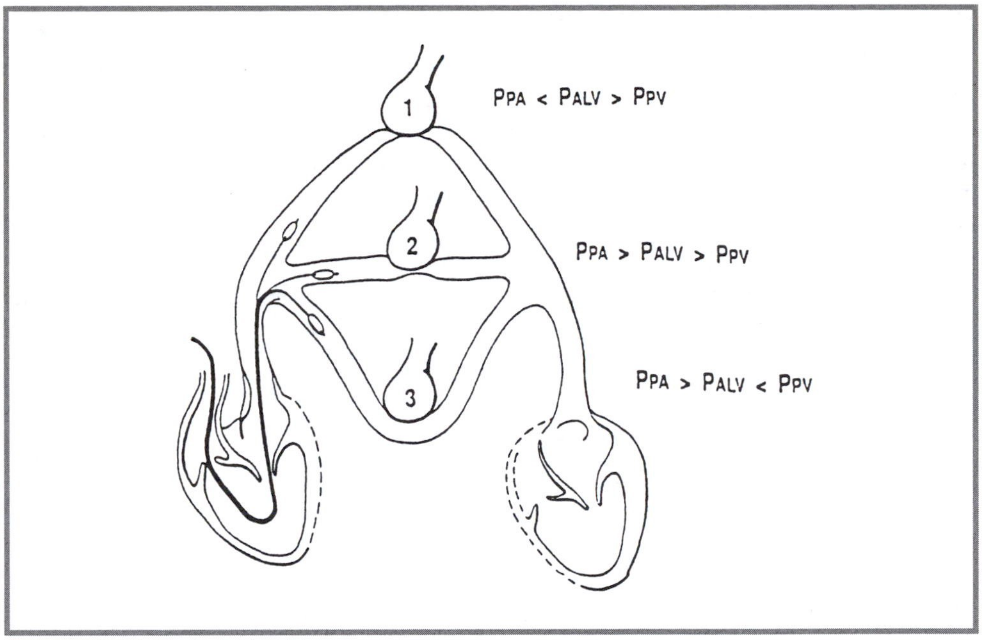

FIGURE 4-13

Physiologic lung zones, based upon the relationship between pressures in the pulmonary artery (PPA), alveolus (PALV), and pulmonary vein (PPV). (From O'Quinn R, Marini JJ. Pulmonary artery occlusion pressure: clinical physiology measurement and interpretation. Am Rev Respir Dis 1983;128:319–326, with permission.)

Failing to accurately identify the point of end-expiration is the most common error in measuring PAWP. End-expiration can be identified by careful examination of the patient or, if that fails, by using an esophageal balloon.

It is also important to determine the contribution of increased intrathoracic pressure caused by tachypnea or asynchrony with the ventilator. Increased intrathoracic pressure occurs with conditions such as pneumothorax, applied PEEP, or intrinsic PEEP. These problems should be addressed and corrected before the PAWP is measured. Increased intrathoracic pressure will increase juxtacardiac pressure. The effect of PEEP on juxtacardiac pressure can be estimated as follows. The change in pleural pressure (PPL) for a given change in airway pressure (PAW) has been shown to be a function of the relative compliances of the lung (CL) and the chest wall (CW):

Increased intrathoracic pressure will cause an increment in pleural or juxtacardiac pressure.

The change in pleural pressure for a given change in airway pressure is a function of the relative lung and chest wall compliances.

$$\Delta P_{PL}/\Delta P_{AW} = C_L/C_L + C_W \text{ or} \quad (4\text{-}6)$$

$$\Delta P_{PL} = \Delta P_{AW} \times (C_L/C_L + C_W) \quad (4\text{-}7)$$

In normal lungs the relative contributions of CW and CL are similar in magnitude. Equation 4-7 can be rewritten as:

$$\Delta P_{PL} = \Delta P_{AW} \times 1/(1 + 1) \text{ or}$$

$$\Delta P_{PL} = \Delta P_{AW}\,(0.5) \quad (4\text{-}8)$$

In other words PPL will increase by about one-half the increase in applied PEEP. In the setting of ARDS, CL is substantially lower than CW. For example, if CL is reduced to 25% of its normal value,

$$\Delta P_{PL} = \Delta P_{AW} \times 0.25/(0.25 + 1) \text{ or}$$

$$\Delta P_{PL} = \Delta P_{AW}\,(0.2) \quad (4\text{-}9)$$

In this particular case, the application of 10 cmH_2O PEEP would result in an increment of 2 cmH_2O in PPL, which is equivalent to 1.47 mmHg (using 1.36 to convert cmH_2O to mmHg).

Hydrostatic Gradient for Pulmonary Edema Formation

Under normal conditions, the pulmonary capillary bed is the most important site where fluid filtration can occur in the lungs. According to the Starling relationship, two kinds of pressure determine fluid filtration across the capillary vessel wall, hydrostatic and osmotic pressures. The balance of these forces is determined by the pressure differences between the microvascular and interstitial compartments. An imbalance between these forces will result in net movement, or filtration, of fluid from one compartment to the other. For example, in a patient with CHF, in whom the microvascular pressure (P_{MV}) is increased, fluid moves from the intravascular to the interstitial compartment. The value of PAWP is that it serves as a minimum estimate for P_{MV} and can be monitored after therapeutic interventions aimed at decreasing the hydrostatic pressure gradient are implemented.

PAWP as an Index of Left Ventricular Preload

Left ventricular preload is defined as left ventricular end-diastolic volume.

The PA catheter reflects left ventricular end-diastolic pressure (not volume); hence, it does not always reflect preload.

In patients with cardiovascular disease, left ventricle (LV) preload cannot be accurately estimated by measuring RV preload, as assessed by a CVP catheter. The use of the PA catheter to estimate LV preload remains controversial. It is important to recognize that LV preload is defined by LVEDV and not by LVEDP. Although LVEDP is correlated to LVEDV, LVEDP can be influenced by other factors, such as ventricular compliance and intrapleural pressure changes, making the relationship between pressure and volume inaccurate. Alterations in left ventricular end diastolic compliance can occur with LV hypertrophy or fibrosis. Because juxtacardiac pressure determines LV transmural (distending) pressure, factors that affect juxtacardiac pressure, such as pericardial tamponade, PEEP, and autoPEEP, will also alter the LVEDP–LVEDV relationship. Therefore, a relationship between LVEDP and LVEDV can only be inferred after careful consideration of factors that may alter LV compliance. The juxtacardiac pressure can be measured by subtracting esophageal pressure (as measured by an endoesophageal balloon) from PAWP.

The correlation between PAWP and LVEDV can also be affected by the presence of valvular heart disease. PAWP measures the pressure at the confluence of the pulmonary veins; it is generally in good agreement with LAP. In the absence of valvular disease, LAP correlates with LVEDP. In mitral stenosis, PAWP overestimates LVEDP because of the pressure gradient between LA and LV. In aortic regurgitation, PAWP underestimates LVEDP because of early closure of the mitral valve from retrograde filling of the LV.

Normal Waveforms

Right Atrium

The onset of the right atrial waveforms follows the appearance of the p wave on the EKG (Figure 4-14). Several waveforms can be identified in the right atrial tracing. The first positive wave is the a wave, which is caused by the contraction of the right atrium; this is followed by the x descent, which signals the relaxation of the right atrium after systole. The x descent can be interrupted by a positive deflection called a c wave, which is the result of closure of the tricuspid valve. During ventricular systole, the atrium is filled passively, creating the second major positive wave, called the v wave. The v wave is followed by the y descent, signaling the opening of the tricuspid valve.

Pulmonary Artery

The pulmonary artery wave has a systolic pressure wave and a diastolic trough. The systolic wave can have an indentation or dicrotic notch caused by the closure of the pulmonic valve.

Pulmonary Artery Wedge

The waveforms obtained with the balloon inflated, and the PA catheter advanced into the interlobar artery position, are similar to those seen in the right atrium.

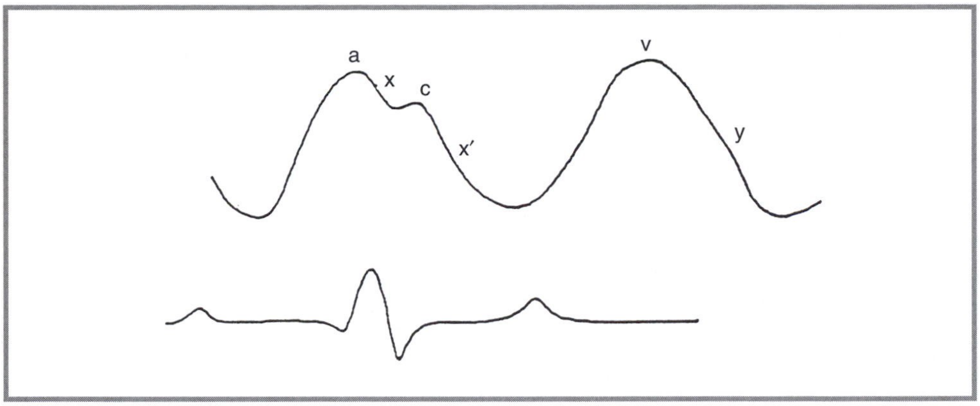

FIGURE 4-14

Schematic drawing of the right atrium waveform. The first positive wave is the *a* wave, caused by contraction of the right atrium; this is followed by the *x* descent, which signals the relaxation of the atrium after atrial systole. The x descent can be interrupted by a positive deflection, the *c* wave, which is the result of the closure of the tricuspid valve. The second major positive wave, the *v* wave, occurs during passive filling of the atria during ventricular systole. The v wave is followed by the *y* descent, signaling the opening of the tricuspid valve.

Waveform Analysis: Pitfalls

Overdamping

Overdamping decreases systolic and increases diastolic pressures, resulting in an inaccurate PAP measurement. Overdamping can be the result of air bubbles in the tubing, clots at the tip of the catheter, or a partially occluded or kinked catheter (Figure 4-15). Flushing the catheter should generate a very high pressure reading, followed by a rapid fall in pressure, or overshoot, after the flush is stopped. The absence of a sharp decrement in the pressure reading and lack of an overshoot should raise the suspicion of an inappropriately dampened catheter.

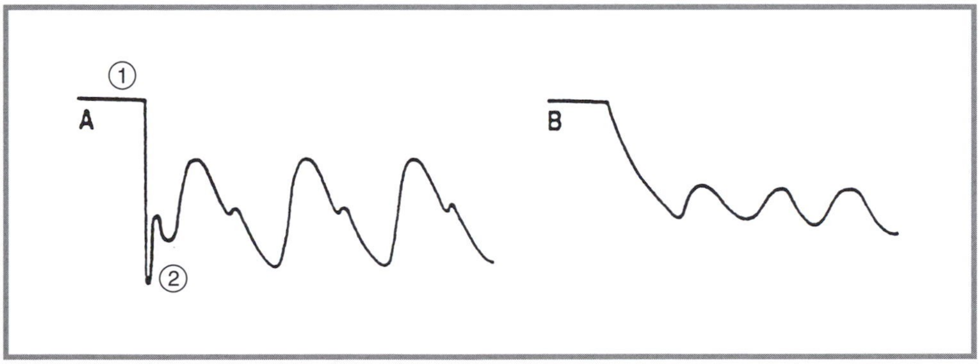

FIGURE 4-15

Overdamping can be caused by a kinked catheter, air bubbles in the transducer, or a fibrin clot. Flushing the catheter helps in determining the presence of overdamping. **(A)** Normally, flushing the catheter results in high pressure at the transducer (*1*); when flushing is stopped, a rapid fall in pressure results in an overshoot (*2*), followed by a return to the waveform. **(B)** An overdamped system lacks the overshoot seen in A and shows a flattened waveform.

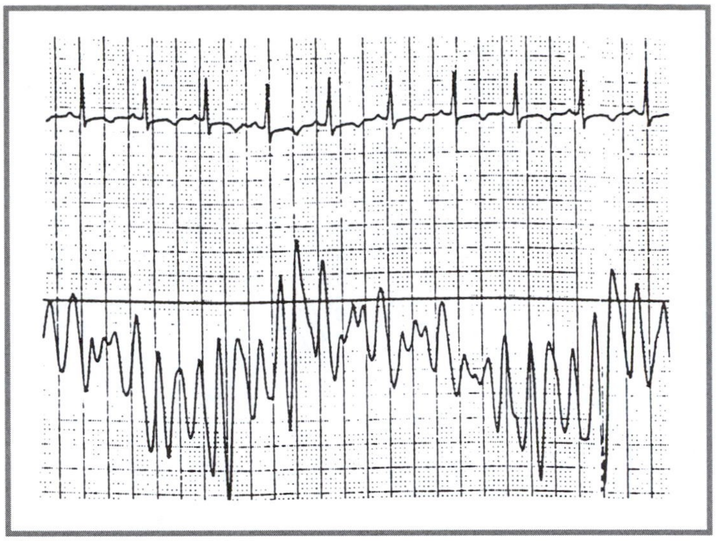

FIGURE 4-16

Catheter whip. Right ventricle contractions are transmitted to the pulmonary artery catheter, resulting in prominent excursions.

Whip Artifact

Cardiac contractions and the resulting changes in intracardiac pressure cause whip artifact (Figure 4-16). When prominent, this artifact can lead to difficulty in interpreting pressure waveforms, causing a fictitious rise in systolic pressure and an underestimation of the diastolic pressures.

Overwedging

Overwedging most commonly occurs when catheters migrate too far distally. In these cases, the catheter needs to be withdrawn to a more proximal position in the PA and refloated. Rarely, overwedging occurs when the balloon protrudes over the catheter tip or pins the tip against a vessel wall (Figure 4-17).

Abnormal Waveforms

Acute Mitral Insufficiency

Acute mitral insufficiency can occur with papillary muscle rupture or ischemia. The incompetent valve allows blood to enter the left atrium during ventricular systole, causing a prominent v wave in the PAWP tracing. The PA waveform will acquire a bifid shape (Figure 4-18).

Tricuspid Regurgitation

Tricuspid regurgitation can result from pulmonary hypertension or endocarditis. A prominent v wave can be seen in the RA tracing, as well as a broad c-v wave (Figure 4-19).

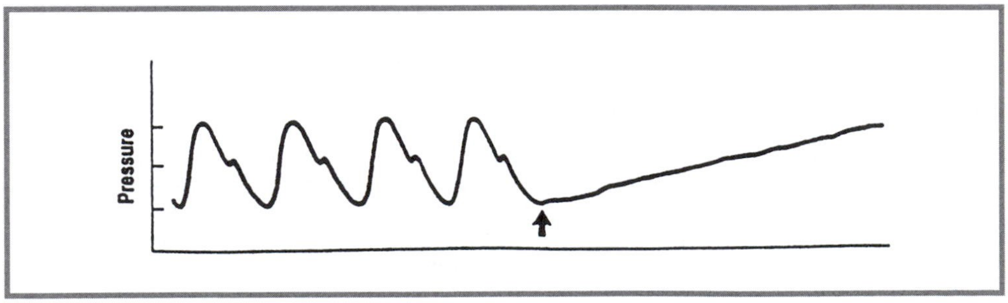

FIGURE 4-17

Overwedging. The *arrow* indicates the point at which the balloon is inflated. A sustained increment in pressure reading can be seen.

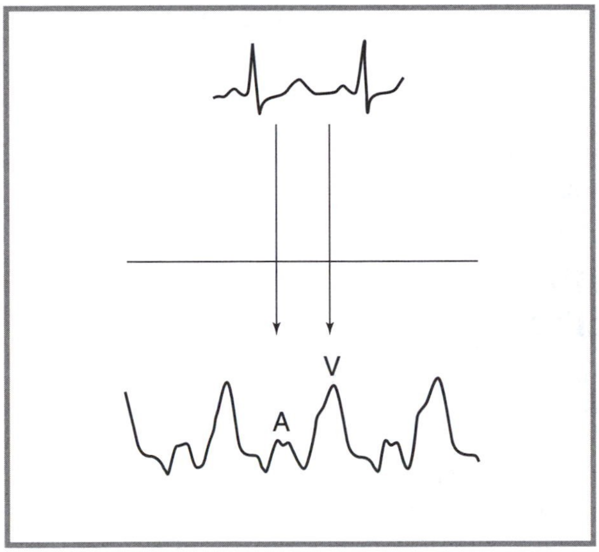

FIGURE 4-18

Acute mitral insufficiency. The incompetent valve allows blood to enter the left atrium during ventricular systole, resulting in a prominent *v* wave.

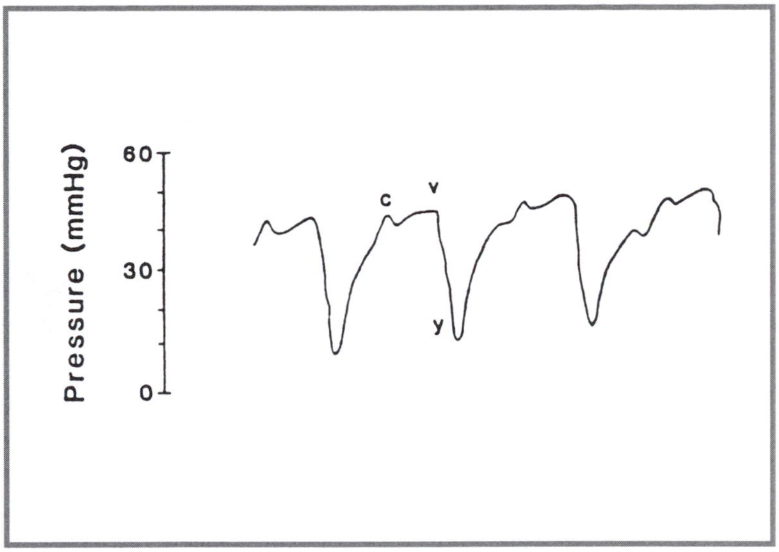

FIGURE 4-19

Tricuspid regurgitation. A broad *c–v* wave can be observed.

Right Ventricular Infarction

Right ventricular (RV) infarction complicates about 30% of patients with an inferior myocardial infarction. RV infarction should be suspected in patients with a positive hepatojugular reflex, engorged internal jugular during inspiration (Kussmaul sign), and clear lung fields. Right precordial leads are useful in identifying this entity. The RA waveform shows deep x and y descents, causing the RA waveform to resemble the letter W (Figure 4-20.).

Pericardial Tamponade

Accumulation of fluid in the pericardial space can result in pericardial tamponade, which is a limitation of cardiac filling during diastole. The pericardium is able to accommodate large amounts of fluid if accumulation occurs gradually, but rapid accumulation of fluid does not allow for changes in pericardial compliance, resulting in tamponade even with relatively small amounts of fluid. As intrapericardial pressure rises, it equalizes with RA and then with LA pressure. At this point the RA pressure and PAWP are determined by intrapericardial pressure, accounting for the equalization of pressures seen in pericardial tamponade. The RA waveform usually has a preserved x descent and a blunted y descent.

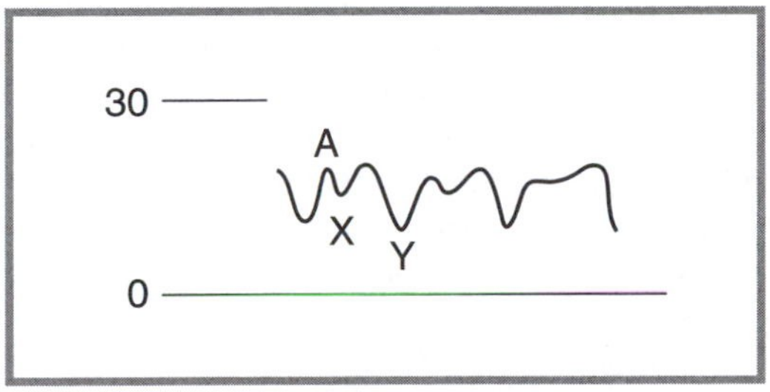

FIGURE 4-20

Right ventricular infarction often results in marked acute dilatation of the right ventricle. Acute dilatation is limited by the pericardium. Deep *x* and *y* descents, resembling the letter W, characterize the waveform.

Constrictive Pericarditis and Restrictive Cardiomyopathy

The pathophysiologic abnormality in constrictive pericarditis and restrictive cardiomyopathy is limitation of ventricular filling. In both cases there is a marked elevation of the RA pressure and PAWP. In restrictive cardiomyopathy, the PAWP is usually greater than the RA pressure whereas in constrictive pericarditis the pressures are similar. Constrictive pericarditis is associated with prominent x and y descents, with the y descent usually being deeper.

Complications Associated with Pulmonary Artery Catheters

Complications of PA catheter placement can be divided into those occurring during catheter insertion and those occurring once the catheter is in place.

Pneumothorax The incidence of pneumothorax varies from 1% to 3%. Risk factors associated with the formation of a pneumothorax include multiple attempts at needle insertion, an inexperienced operator, patients with respiratory distress, cachectic or extremely obese patients, and catheter placement under emergent conditions. The risk is greater when using a subclavian and middle internal jugular approach when compared to other sites. Forcing the guidewire can also result in a pneumothorax. A chest radiograph should always follow the procedure.

Arterial Puncture and Hemorrhage Arterial puncture has been reported to occur in up to 15% of central venous catheter placements. In most cases, applying pressure to the area for 5–15 min easily controls the bleeding. Rarely, hemorrhage into the area may result in the formation of a hemothorax or cause an expanding hematoma that compromises the airway. Inadvertent arterial cannulation can result in cerebral ischemia and infarction. The catheter should ideally be removed by vascular surgery in the operating room to repair the artery. Correcting abnormal coagulation defects and replacing platelets can minimize the risks of arterial hemorrhage. If a coagulopathy cannot be corrected, ultrasound/doppler can be used to localize the appropriate vein. The subclavian approach should be avoided because this is a noncompressible site.

Miscellaneous Complications Other complications reported to occur in less than 1% of patients include knotting of the catheter, fragmentation, and cardiac perforation.

Complications During Catheter Insertion

Transient cardiac arrhythmia is the most common complication of pulmonary artery catheter insertion.

Arrhythmias Cardiac arrhythmia is the most frequently cited complication of PA catheter insertion, with a prevalence of 10%–80%. Arrhythmias are thought to arise from mechanical irritation of the right atrium or ventricle. They are usually transient and quickly disappear after advancing the catheter beyond the right ventricle or withdrawing it. The incidence of minor arrhythmias, including premature atrial or ventricular contractions, have been reported to occur in 4%–69% of all PA catheter insertions. The incidence of transient ventricular tachycardia or fibrillation is between 0.5% and 63%, with sustained ventricular arrhythmias being uncommon. Despite a low incidence of tachyarrhythmias, an effort should be made to prevent their development by correcting conditions that increase myocardial irritability, such as hypoxemia, hypothermia, acidosis, alkalosis, and electrolyte abnormalities. There is no evidence that prophylaxis with antiarrhythmic drugs such as lidocaine are useful.

A right bundle branch block can occur with PA catheter insertion, but it is usually transient. In patients with a preexisting left bundle branch block (LBBB), the formation of a right bundle branch block during PA catheter insertion will result in complete heart block. The risk of complete heart block is small, however, and the placement of a temporary pacer before PA catheter insertion is not recommended.

Complications After PA Catheter Insertion

Infection Infection is the most common cause for clinical intervention once PA catheters are in place. Infectious complications range from colonization with pathogenic organisms to overt sepsis and shock. As author definitions have varied from study to study, it is difficult to establish the overall prevalence of catheter-associated infection. Infection of the insertion site has been reported to occur in 0%–22% of all patients. The prevalence of sepsis is much smaller, ranging from 1% to 3% in large series. Coagulase-negative *Staphylococcus* is the most frequently isolated pathogen, followed by *Staphylococcus aureus* and enteric gram-negative bacteria. Several steps may reduce the incidence of infection, including sterilizing the skin at the insertion site, use of full barrier precautions (wearing masks, hats, gowns, and gloves), minimal manipulation of infusions, use of antibiotic-coated catheters, and reducing the time the catheter is left in place (ideally less than 5 days).

Thrombosis The overall incidence of thrombosis is uncertain. Although mural thrombus has been reported in 30%–60% of patients, the clinical significance of this finding is uncertain. Furthermore, because special studies such as venography and doppler ultrasound are needed to diagnose this entity, it may be underreported. Interestingly, complications of thrombotic events, namely pulmonary embolism, superior vena cava syndrome, and thrombosis of the internal jugular vein, are rare, with an incidence ranging from 0.1% to 6%. In addition to the physical findings, dampening of the PA waveform and difficulty withdrawing blood from the catheter should alert the physician to the possibility of thrombus formation. Modern PA catheters are heparin bonded throughout their entire length, which reduces the incidence of thrombosis. Treatment consists of anticoagulation and removal of the catheter. Prevention of thrombosis is extremely important and entails limiting dwell time, especially in patients at high risk for thrombotic events (cancer patients and those with hypercoagulable disorders).

Rupture of Pulmonary Artery Although the incidence of rupture or perforation of the PA is low (less than 1%), it is associated with a high mortality (45%–60%). Several mechanisms have been proposed to explain PA rupture, such as overinflation of the balloon in a proximal vessel, normal inflation in a distal vessel, and direct perforation while placing the catheter. Manifestations of PA rupture include hemoptysis, hemothorax, or a new asymptomatic parenchymal infiltrate. Treatment depends on the presentation; hemoptysis should be managed by positioning the patient with the affected side down. Localization should be attempted with chest radiography or bronchoscopy if needed. Options to stop the hemorrhage include bronchial balloon tamponade or embolization performed by interventional radiology. Hemothorax should be managed with chest tube placement and blood products. Surgery becomes an option if bleeding persists or the patient is unstable. The formation of a false aneurysm should be considered when a "halo sign" is seen on chest x-ray adjacent to the distal tip of the PA catheter. These aneurysms lack an endothelium and contain clot and are considered unstable. Diagnosis often requires a pulmonary angiogram. Regularly checking the position of the catheter with radiographs, avoiding overinflation of the balloon, and avoiding inflation if resistance is met can minimize rupture and perforation.

Mortality in pulmonary artery rupture ranges from 45% to 60%.

Miscellaneous Complications Other complications include pulmonary infarction, intracardiac injury, and air embolism and balloon rupture. Finally, death directly attributable to catheter-related complications has been reported in less than 0.1% of patients.

CONTROVERSIES

In 1996, Connors et al., seeking to determine whether placement of a pulmonary artery catheter improved survival in the ICU, evaluated previously collected data from more than 5000 patients in five U.S. hospitals. Right heart catheterization was performed in 2184 patients within the initial 24 h of ICU stay. The control group consisted of ICU patients who did not have a PA catheter in place. Cases were matched for baseline characteristics and prognosis. Following adjustment, the PA catheter group showed an increased relative risk of death at 30 days. PA catheter use was associated with a significantly higher relative risk of death among patients with acute respiratory failure and multiorgan failure. Subgroup analysis did not reveal an association between increased mortality and elderly patients, women, shock, sepsis, and postoperative care. Following this article, a large meta-analysis of mortality data from randomized trials showed a nonsignificant trend toward reduced mortality in patients managed with a PA catheter. Recently, in a meta-analysis of 12 randomized trials, the use of PA catheter was associated with a mean protective effect of 21.9% in terms of morbidity risk. An ongoing randomized, controlled, multicenter trial should answer questions regarding PA catheter safety and effectiveness.

SUMMARY

In the ICU, critically ill patients often require invasive monitoring for diagnostic purposes as well as to assess the response to therapeutic interventions. Arterial catheters enable continuous monitoring of systemic blood pressure and blood sampling to assess arterial oxygenation and acid–base status. Central venous access, with either a CVP line or a PA catheter, allows for important hemodynamic monitoring, including an assessment of cardiac function and measurement of intravascular filling pressures. Further studies are needed to determine whether therapeutic interventions based on an assessment of hemodynamic data affects patient survival.

REVIEW QUESTIONS

1. **Regarding central venous pressure (CVP) catheters, all the following are correct, except:**
   - **A.** CVP catheters can be used to measure right atrial pressure.
   - **B.** In the absence of tricuspid disease, CVP mirrors right ventricular end diastolic volume.
   - **C.** CVP is decreased in patients with right ventricular infarction.
   - **D.** In patients with normal cardiac function, adequate intravascular volume is considered when CVP is greater than 10 mmHg.

2. **Regarding placement of the pulmonary artery catheter, all the following statements are correct, except:**
   - **A.** The left subclavian vein has a straighter trajectory than the right subclavian vein, making insertion of the PA catheter easier.
   - **B.** The PA catheter is generally placed into an interlobar artery.
   - **C.** To obtain an accurate measurement, the catheter trip should be placed in zone 3 of the lung.
   - **D.** The inability to fully inflate the catheter's balloon signals that the catheter is in the "wedge" position.

3. **All the following statements regarding measurement of cardiac output with a PA catheter are correct, except:**
   - **A.** Measurement of cardiac output with the Fick method can be affected by blood transfusions and changes in pulmonary gas volume.
   - **B.** Inflammatory processes, such as pneumonia, may cause an overestimation of VO_2.
   - **C.** Ice-cold injectates are necessary to measure cardiac output using the thermodilution method.
   - **D.** Arrhythmias, intracardiac shunts, and tricuspid regurgitation may result in an erroneous measurement of the cardiac output by the thermodilution method.

4. **Regarding PAWP measurement, which of the following statements is correct?**
   - **A.** It should be measured at the end of expiration.
   - **B.** The application of PEEP results in increased intrathoracic pressure and generation of zone 3 conditions.
   - **C.** The transmission of PEEP to the vascular compartment is independent of lung and chest wall compliance.
   - **D.** PAWP closely reflects left ventricular preload.

ANSWERS

1. The answer is C. The CVP catheter can be used to measure right atrial pressures. In patients without tricuspid disease, it reflects right ventricular end diastolic volume and right ventricular preload. Patients with right ventricular infarction typically present with chest pain, hypotension, and clear lung fields. Kussmaul's sign and hepatojugular reflex are usually present. Characteristically, CVP is elevated in these patients.
2. The answer is D. Because modern PA catheters are flow-directed, balloon-tipped catheters, they generally "float" to an area where zone 3 conditions ($P_V > P_{ALV}$) exist. The PA catheter is generally inserted into an interlobar pulmonary artery, where the balloon can be inflated. The inability to fully inflate the balloon should alert the physician to the possibility of a too-distal positioning of the catheter tip. Because this error may increase the risk of complications (such as pulmonary infarct), no further attempts to inflate the balloon should be made before radiographic confirmation of the catheter's position.
3. The answer is C. Measurement of cardiac output with the Fick method requires an indicator that is added at a constant rate. Oxygen is a good indicator because oxygen uptake and arterial and venous oxygen content can be measured with relative ease. The major determinants of the Fick equation are hemoglobin and oxygen uptake. The thermodilution method allows measurement of the cardiac output by recording the change in temperature of an injectate. The technique involves injecting 10 ml of an injectate through the proximal port of the PA catheter. The change in temperature is sensed by a thermistor at the tip of the PA catheter, and cardiac output is calculated by integration of temperature over time. Arrhythmia, intracardiac shunt, and tricuspid regurgitation distort the flow of the injectate and cause temperature changes by admixing blood, resulting in erroneous estimations of cardiac output. Although ice-cold injectates were used in the past, recent studies have demonstrated that room temperature injectates are more accurate and easier to handle.
4. The answer is A. The measurement of PAWP should be performed at the end of expiration when the influence of intrathoracic pressure is the least. The presence of PEEP and autoPEEP will result in generation of zone 2 conditions ($P_{ALV} > P_V$). The transmission of PEEP or PAW in general has been shown to be a function of the relative compliances of the lung and the chest wall. Preload is defined as left ventricular end-diastolic volume (LVEDV). The PAWP is not a measurement of LVEDV but an estimate of left ventricular end-diastolic pressure. Therefore, preload can only be estimated, taking into careful consideration factors that may alter LV compliance (LV hypertrophy, pericardial effusion, high PEEP).

SUGGESTED READING

Connors AF, Speroff T, Dawson NV, et al. The effectiveness of right heart catheterization in the initial care of critically ill patients. JAMA 1996;276:889–897.

Gattinoni L, Brazzi L, Pelosi P, et al. A trial of goal-oriented hemodynamic therapy in critically ill patients. N Engl J Med 1995;333:1025–1032.

Lodato RF. Use of the pulmonary artery catheter. Semin Respir Crit Care 1999;20:29–42.

O'Quinn R, Marini JJ. Pulmonary artery occlusion pressure: clinical physiology, measurement, and interpretation. Am Rev Respir Dis 1983;128:319–326.

Pepe PE, Marini JJ. Occult positive end-expiratory pressure in mechanically ventilated patients with airflow obstruction: the auto-PEEP effect. Am Rev Respir Disease 1982;126:166–170.

Shoemaker WC, Appel PL, Kram HB. Prospective trial of supranormal values of survivors as therapeutic goals in high risk surgical patients. Chest 1988;94:1176–1186.

Swan HJ, Ganz W, Marcus H, et al. Catheterization of the heart in man with use of a flow-directed, balloon-tipped catheter. N Engl J Med 1970;283:447–451.

Zapol WM, Snider MT. Pulmonary hypertension in severe acute respiratory failure. N Engl J Med 1977;296:476–480.

CHAPTER 5

MICHAEL S. LAGNESE AND JOHN M. TRAVALINE

Drainage Tube Management

CHAPTER OUTLINE

LEARNING OBJECTIVES

After studying this chapter you should be able to do the following:

- Know the most common indications for various drainage tubes used in the management of critically ill patients.
- Know the methods of insertion of various drainage tubes and how to maintain their proper function.
- Recognize the potential complications associated with drainage tubes used in critical care.

This chapter describes mangement of the more commonly used drainage tube systems in the critical care setting.

CHEST TUBES

The insertion of tubes into the thorax has been a technique in medicine since ancient times. Hippocrates used metal tubes in the pleural space to drain "bad humors." Hewett in 1876 applied closed chest drainage tube with an underwater seal. During World War II there was widespread use of tube thoracostomy for traumatic hemopneumothorax and empyema. Current practices include tube thoracostomy for many different indications.

Indications

There are a variety of indications for the placement of a thoracostomy tube. In general, the indications can be divided into placement for the drainage of air from the pleural space or for drainage of fluid. In the critical care setting, chest tubes are generally placed because of

TABLE 5-1

INDICATIONS AND CONTRAINDICATIONS FOR CHEST TUBE INSERTION

Indications
- Traumatic hemothorax or pneumothorax
- Hemopneumothorax
- Pneumothorax with or without tension
- Pneumothorax in patient on positive pressure ventilation
- Pyothorax
- Complicated parapneumonic effusion
- Bronchopleural fistula
- Chylothorax
- Postthoracic surgery

Contraindications
- Coagulopathy (relative)
- Large bullae mistaken for pneumothorax
- Large pleural effusion or pneumothorax with mainstem bronchial occlusion (relative)
- Hemidiaphragm elevation (relative)
- Massive hemothorax when accumulated blood may aid in hemostasis (relative)

the presence of air or fluid or both in the pleural space. Tubes placed during thoracotomy procedures are inserted in anticipation of air and fluid remaining in the pleural space following an operative procedure. Table 5-1 lists the indications and contraindications for chest tube insertion.

In general, chest tubes are placed for the drainage of air or fluid from the pleural space.

Insertion Techniques

Once the need for a chest tube is established, the next steps are to determine the size of the chest tube needed and the insertion method. The size of the tube depends largely on the indication for the tube. For example, a small (12–22 Fr.) tube is sufficient to drain air from a simple pneumothorax. On the other hand, a much larger tube (e.g., 36–40 Fr) (Figure 5-1) is likely needed to manage the thick, viscous material usually found in an empyema.

The size of the chest tube and the insertion site depend on the indication for placing the chest tube.

The insertion site and method are generally determined by the indication. For example, if the tube is being placed for free air in the pleural space, the tube is directed apically from the fifth intercostal space in the midaxillary line (Figure 5-2) or the second intercostal space in the midclavicular line (on the right only). For free fluid, the sixth intercostal space with

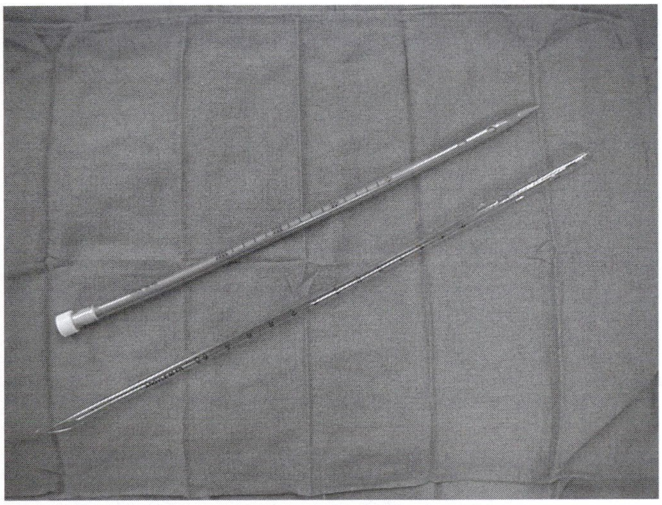

FIGURE 5-1

Two 36 Fr. chest tubes. The top tube has an introducer catheter within it to facilitate placement of the chest tube over a guidewire. The tube shown below is typically placed using a blunt dissection technique.

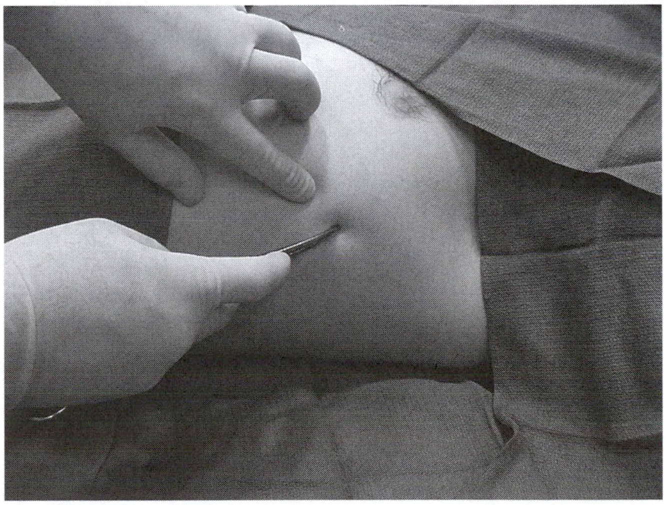

FIGURE 5-2

Chest tube insertion site as shown here is the fifth intercostal space in the midaxillary line.

FIGURE 5-3

An introducer needle and syringe, guidewire, dilators, and 14 Fr. chest tube with an introducer catheter within it.

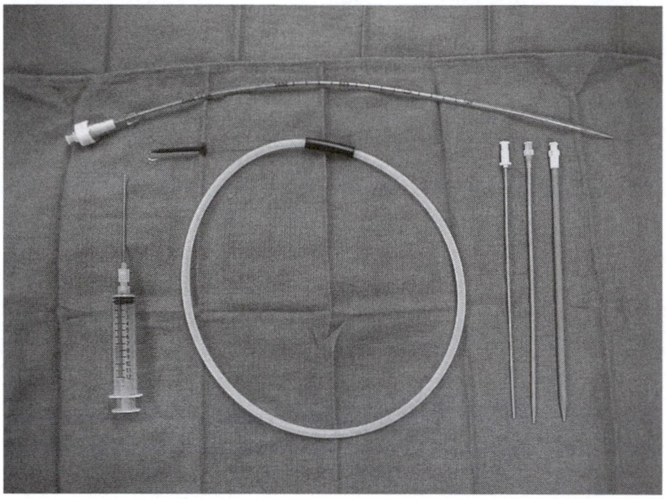

the tube directed posterobasally may be more suitable. For loculations of fluid or air, tube placement is based upon the location of the loculations.

Specific insertion methods include the use of a trocar, blunt dissection, and guidewire technique. The use of a trocar to establish an opening in the chest wall through which a tube is placed may be associated with more complications and is generally not favored. Tube thoracostomy using a blunt dissection is probably the most commonly employed technique. Guidewire placement of a chest tube is perhaps the least traumatic for a patient but is limited by the size of the tube that can be placed in this fashion and the inability to digitally palpate the lung away from the tract of insertion. Moreover, if there are pleural adhesions present, the blunt dissection technique allows the physician to palpate for such adhesions and thus avoid malpositioning of the tube and injury to the underlying lung.

The guidewire technique involves entering the pleural space with an introducer needle. A guidewire (0.89 mm in diameter) is placed through the introducer needle, and the introducer is removed. A small skin incision is made around the wire, and then dilators are placed over the guidewire into the pleural space to create a tract for the tube to eventually be inserted. Dilators of increasing size are sequentially inserted and removed to progresssively dilate the tract. Finally, the chest tube is inserted with the last dilator (Figure 5-3). The wire and dilator are then removed, and the tube is connected to a collection device and secured.

Maintenance

Pleural collection devices contain three compartments: a suction control chamber, a water seal chamber, and a collection chamber.

Once the chest tube is inserted and properly secured, it is connected to a pleural collection device (Figure 5-4). These collection devices have three distinct compartments. The first is a suction control chamber that allows for the regulation of negative pressure applied to the pleural space via the tube. The second is a water seal chamber that allows for the determination of air leakage in the system. The third is a chamber that collects any fluid material that may drain from the pleural space. Once the chest tube is inserted, secured, and attached to a collection device, usually little maintenance is required. Table 5-2 suggests a checklist guide for the ongoing assessment and care of a patient with a chest tube.

Antibiotics

Pleural space infection caused by a chest tube is rare.

Antibiotic prophylaxis for chest tube insertion is not recommended.

Antibiotic prophylaxis with chest tube insertion is sometimes considered; however, available data generally do not support this practice. Although some studies have shown a lower incidence of infection in groups of patients such as those with penetrating chest wounds, for other indications, such as spontaneous pneumothorax, antibiotic prophylaxis may be associated with increased complications. Antibiotic therapy should be based on suspected or proven infection. The routine use of antibiotic prophylaxis is not warranted in the management of chest tubes.

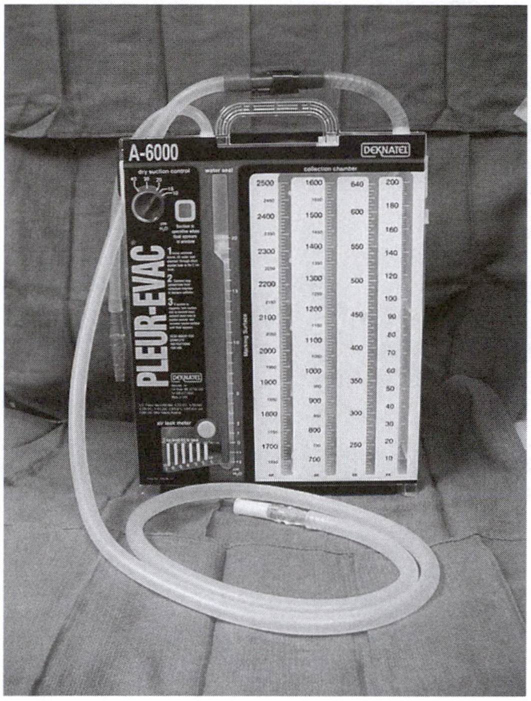

FIGURE 5-4

Pleural collection device.

Fibrinolytic Therapy

In the management of complicated parapneumonic effusions and empyema, intrapleural streptokinase may be useful. This agent may be used to liquefy viscous material that is sometimes present in pleural infections and hemothoraces. The typical dose for streptokinase is 250,000 U diluted in 50–100 ml normal sterile saline solution instilled via the chest tube. The tube is typically clamped for 2–4 h before opening it again to drain. There are no systemic effects of the fibrinolytic agent on the systemic coagulation profile when administered intrapleurally. This technique generally results in a dramatic improvement in about one-third of patients, a slight improvement in another third, and no significant effect in the remaining third.

Instillation of a fibrinolytic agent into the pleural space may facilitate drainage through a chest tube.

Bronchopleural Fistulae

The presence of air in the pleural space most commonly results from a disruption of the lung parenchyma such that air entering the lungs via the bronchi is in direct communication with the pleural space; this defines a bronchopleural fistula. Although a chest tube may effectively evacuate air from the pleural space, if the defect in the lung parenchyma remains, air flow through the fistulous tract will continue. A chest tube may help to diagnose this problem by allowing observation of bubbling in the water seal compartment of the pleural collection device (Figure 5-5). Table 5-3 describes grading the degree of air leakage from a bronchopleural fistula.

TABLE 5-2

KEY ASPECTS IN EVALUATION OF A PATIENT WITH A CHEST TUBE

Patient assessment (chest sounds, site, etc.)
Look for air leak
Assess chest radiograph
Tube inspection (respiratory variation)
Output assessment

FIGURE 5-5

Closer view of pleural collection device and the water seal chamber used in the determination of air leakage.

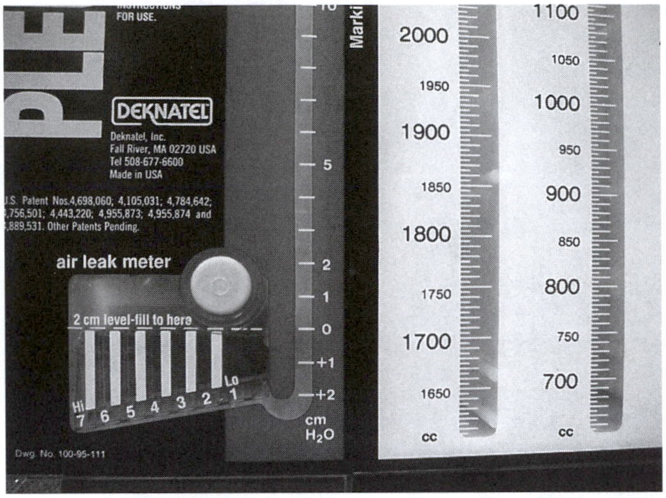

Complications

The incidence of complications related to chest tubes is about 5%–25%. Table 5-4 lists many of these complications. Pleural space infection after a chest tube is removed is less than 5% and probably relates to the underlying process. Another rare complication sometimes associated with chest tubes is reexpansion pulmonary edema, which results from the removal of a large volume of fluid or air from the pleural space. The clinical manifestations of this rare complication include pernicious cough and chest tightness during or immediately following the procedure. The chest x-ray may show unilateral changes consistent with pulmonary edema, although contralateral pulmonary edema has also been reported. Generally the symptoms are progressive over 24–48 h, and there is usually complete recovery. The incidence is unknown, but the condition is thought to be uncommon.

The risk for reexpansion pulmonary edema is higher when lung reexpansion occurs following the removal of air (more so than fluid), following a long duration (>3 days) of lung collapse, and following the use of negative pressure devices to remove the air or fluid. To avoid this complication, it is generally recommended to remove less than 1 l of fluid within the first 30 min of pleural drainage.

The pathogenesis of reexpansion pulmonary edema is thought to involve anoxic damage to the pulmonary capillary endothelial cells during chronic lung collapse followed by an increased permeability after reexpansion and restoration of blood flow. A sudden and large increase in negative pleural pressure may then lead to transudation and exudation across the capillaries. Reperfusion injury involving free radical formation may also be involved in promoting lung injury.

Removal

Chest tubes are usually removed when an air leak has resolved for at least 24 h or fluid drainage output is less than 100 ml in a 24-h period.

General guides to help determine when a chest tube is no longer needed include air leak resolved for at least 24 h on water seal or fluid or blood drainage of less than 100 ml in a 24-h period. These guidelines, however, are not absolute, and removal of chest tubes depends on a patient's particular situation.

TABLE 5-3

GRADES OF AIR LEAKS

Grade 1: infrequent with cough
Grade 2: with every cough
Grade 3: present with some spontaneous breaths
Grade 4: present with every spontaneous breath

TABLE 5-4

COMPLICATIONS OF CHEST TUBES

Improper position
Soft tissue bleeding, intercostal vessel injury
Intercostal nerve damage
Long thoracic nerve (serratus anterior) damage "winged scapula"
Visceral organ and diaphragm damage
Pulmonary edema
Bronchopleural fistula
Infection

Ideally, a chest tube should be removed when pleural pressure is positive. For a patient on positive pressure mechanical ventilation, pleural pressure is maximum during the inspiratory phase of an assisted breath so that an inspiratory hold to withdraw the tube may be utilized. In a spontaneously breathing patient, one asks the patient to inspire to total lung capacity, then to perform a valsalva maneuver to maximize pleural pressure while the tube is removed. Once the tube has been removed, one should establish an airtight seal of the skin and subcutaneous tissue and apply a gauze dressing to the site.

NASOGASTRIC TUBES

Indications

Perhaps the biggest role for the nasogastric tube in the critical care setting is in the management of acute gastrointestinal bleeding (Table 5-5). Generally, a nasogastric tube should be placed in all patients with gastrointestinal bleeding, even if the suspected site of bleeding is in the lower gastrointestinal tract. In upper gastrointestinal tract bleeding, the stomach acts as a pool for blood accumulation from the esophagus, the stomach itself, or even the duodenum because blood will reflux back into the stomach in most cases. Placement of the tube in the stomach, therefore, serves as a means to diagnose this problem, allows the monitoring of ongoing bleeding and detection of recurrent bleeding, and, in a limited way, can serve as a means for therapy. Gastric lavage may help to determine the rate of bleeding or whether bleeding has stopped. In addition, decompression of the stomach (or evacuation) will allow the stomach walls to collapse and possibly aid in hemostasis of a gastric bleeding site.

Generally, nasogastric tubes should be placed in all patients with suspected gastrointestinal bleeding.

Other uses of the nasogastric tube in critical care include a means for gastric lavage in certain toxic or drug ingestions, decompression of the stomach in cases of gastric distension from air, a means for medication delivery, and a route for nutritional support. In situations in which it is important to clear the stomach of pills or pill fragments, a large diameter tube (Ewald) may be used. For decompression or medication delivery, a Levine tube is advised (Figure 5-6). For enteral feeding, a duotube is recommended.

Contraindications to nasogastric tube placement include a bleeding diathesis that may result in uncontrollable nasal bleeding, sinusitis, and maxillofacial fractures. In such cases, the tube may be inserted via the oropharynx.

Orogastric tube placement is sometimes necessary in patients with bleeding diathesis, sinusitis, or maxillofacial fractures.

Insertion Technique

Placement of a nasogastric tube is generally achieved most effectively with the patient in an upright position. Prior to insertion, a lubrication substance should be applied to the distal

TABLE 5-5

USES OF NASOGASTRIC TUBES IN THE MANAGEMENT OF GASTROINTESTINAL BLEEDING

Determining bleeding source	Gastric lavage
Monitoring rate of bleeding	Gastric decompression

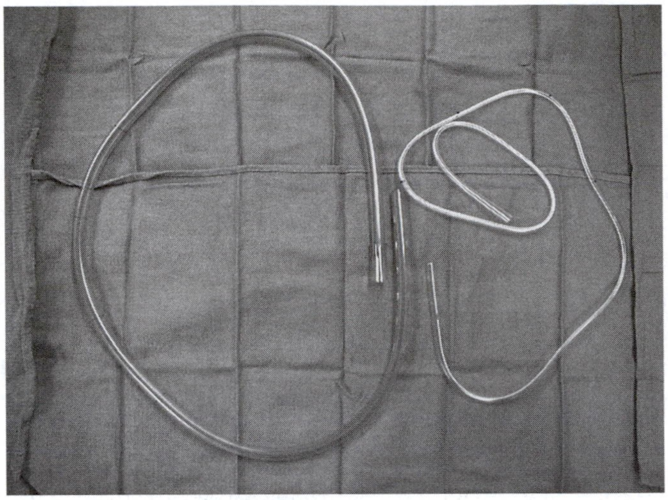

FIGURE 5-6

Nasogastric tubes: Ewald tube (*left*); Levine tube (*right*).

portion of the tube. Next, an assessment should be made as to which side of nose is most patent, or least obstructed. This can be done by simple visual inspection of the nares with the use of a flashlight. The nasogastric tube is then gently and slowly inserted through the nares. If it is possible to position the patient's head in a semiflexed position, this may facilitate the placement of the tube into the hypopharynx and then esophagus. The tube is then advanced to approximately 60 cm from the tip of the nose. Tubes are marked to indicate the length of tube already advanced. Resistance to tube advancement is not usual, and if encountered, indicates that the tube is not passing freely into the esophagus and stomach. If resistance is encountered, the tube should not be forcefully advanced. Rather it should be removed, the patient repositioned, and reinsertion attempted again.

Once the tube is advanced into the stomach, confirmation of its position can be obtained by the instillation of a 50 cc bolus of air into the tube with simultaneous auscultation over the patient's stomach listening for a loud gurgling sound indicating proper placement. In addition, aspiration of gastric contents through the tube indicates its position in the stomach, as does the tube's presence in the stomach as shown on a radiograph.

Complications

Table 5-6 lists common complications associated with nasogastric tubes.

URINARY CATHETERS

Indications

The chief indication for urinary catheters in the critical care setting is the need to closely monitor urine output in the critically ill patient. Other indications include urinary obstruction from uretheral stricture or prostatic obstruction. The need to keep the perineum clean and dry because of the presence of surgical wounds in the area is also an important use of a urinary catheter.

TABLE 5-6

COMPLICATIONS OF NASOGASTRIC TUBES

Nasal and throat discomfort	Exacerbating existing bleeding site
GE reflux	Nosocomial pneumonia
Aspiration	Sinusitis
Mucosal trauma	

Insertion Technique

Urinary catheters are available in single use kits that ensure the sterility of the catheter and provide the necessary drapes, antiseptic swabs, and lubricant needed to place the catheters. Insertion of the catheters involves the use of sterile technique for placement. This begins with the application of an antiseptic cleansing solution to the urethral meatus. Appropriately placed sterile drapes and the use of sterile gloves then allow the lubricated catheter to be advanced through the urethral meatus into the bladder. Placement in the bladder is confirmed by the flow of urine through the catheter. Once positioned in the bladder, a distal balloon at the tip of the catheter is inflated with approximately 10 cc of saline to provide an anchor effect so that the catheter remains in place.

Complications

Complications associated with urinary catheters include trauma to the urethra either from a traumatic insertion or a patient inadvertently pulling the catheter, patient discomfort, and urinary tract infection.

RECTAL TUBES

Indications

Rectal tubes are used in critically ill patients in many clinical situations (Table 5-7). Traditionally, they serve mainly to relieve the discomfort associated with bowel ileus and subsequently retained gas and stool. These conditions can be associated with a variety of medical and surgical diseases seen in the critical care setting. Interestingly, most of these process are nongastrointestinal in origin.

Perhaps one of the most common uses of the rectal tube is in the presence of diarrhea. Frequent or watery stool can be extremely irritating to the perineum and pose significant risk of breach of the skin in this area, thus predisposing to infection; this can occur even when diarrhea is not voluminous. In addition to collection of stool to avoid potential problems related to diarrhea in the bedbound patient, at times it is important to quantitate the amount of stool expelled, and a rectal tube attached to a reservoir bag can facilitate this process.

> Frequent and watery stool, particularly in a bedbound patient, is a common indication for the use of rectal tubes.

Although rectal tubes are generally considered to be among the safer of the procedures performed in the modern intensive care unit, often being used at the discretion of the critical care nurses, there are contraindications to their use that need to be considered (Table 5-8). Generally, contraindications to rectal tubes involve local anatomic or functional abnormalities that might be worsened by an invasive catheter, especially given the nature of the material it is intended to drain. Any real or suspected perianal infectious processes, including abscesses, cellulitis, and fistulae, generally require that the lesion be explored and drained surgically. Adequate drainage of these lesions can be impeded by the placement of a rectal tube, even when tubes of small caliber are used. Likewise, most anatomic disorders involving the anus or rectum represent relative contraindications to the placement of a rectal tube.

TABLE 5-7

INDICATIONS FOR RECTAL TUBES

- Symptomatic abdominal distension
  - Retained flatus
  - Retained stool
  - Large bowel ileus
    - Medical/surgical disease
    - Medication side effects
- Stool control
  - Voluminous diarrhea
  - Stool quantification

TABLE 5-8

CONTRAINDICATIONS TO RECTAL TUBES

Absolute	
	Acute surgical abdomen
	Paralytic ileus
	Staff convenience
Relative	
	Local infections of the perineum or rectum
	Abscess
	Cellulitis
	Fistulae
	Anatomic or functional disorders
	Hemorrhoids
	Perforations
	Fistulas
	Perineal irritation
	Perineal edema
	Rectosigmoid obstruction
	Stool
	Tumor

These processes include hemorrhoids, perforations, irritations, edema, or rectosigmoid obstructions of any cause. When any of these disorders is suspected or present, risk/benefit ratio must be carefully considered before a rectal tube can be safely inserted. Rectal tubes are also contraindicated following any rectal or prostatic surgery unless, of course, a tube has been placed perioperatively by the surgical team as part of the procedure. Last, rectal tubes should not be placed as a mere convenience to spare the time and effort required to care for patients who have voluminous diarrhea or frequent gas or stool expulsion.

Insertion Technique

Although commercial rectal tube kits are available, any soft, flexible catheter of sufficient diameter can be used. Foley urinary catheters are commonly used. Usually, a 22–32 Fr. catheter is optimal for adults. After determination that a rectal tube could benefit the patient, careful examination of the anus and perineum should be done to ensure that no obvious contraindications exist, including a digital rectal examination to verify that the rectal vault is empty. Manual disimpaction of any formed stool should be performed to facilitate tube insertion. The abdomen should also be examined for signs of acute obstruction or other urgent processes that may require a surgical intervention and possibly preclude rectal tube insertion.

Following inspection and palpation of the anus and rectum, a generous amount of water-soluble lubricant should be placed on the tip of the rectal tube. The tube is then introduced gently into the anus. If the patient is conscious and can perform a Valsalva maneuver as the tube is inserted, this will reduce the anal sphincter tone and usually result in a less uncomfortable experience. The tube should be advanced 5–10 cm with the tip directed toward the patient's umbilicus. The ideal position of the tip is just proximal to the rectal vault, as this will help prevent stool and gas from entering and uncomfortably distending the rectum. The tube should be then secured with adhesive tape, and the distal end can be connected to a reservoir collection container. If a catheter with a retention balloon is used as the rectal tube, this should be left deflated, as inflation usually results in eventual expulsion of the catheter by normal rectosigmoid peristalsis.

Maintenance

The length of time the rectal tube is left in place is determined by the specific indication. For intermittent relief of retained gas associated with abdominal distension, the tube should be removed after no more than 30 min, and reapplied at regular intervals or as needed for patient comfort. If the tube has been inserted for stool evacuation or quantification, it may be left in place for longer periods; however, careful and frequent evaluation of the tube's placement and monitoring for mucosal irritation, ulceration, or perforation are required.

Complications

Rectal tubes are not without inherent complications and, as their application becomes more prevalent in the intensive care unit, an increase in the absolute number of complications can be expected. The most common complication is patient discomfort. Sedation and anxiolysis often minimize discomfort, but as the patient becomes more conscious, pain and discomfort may become more prominent. Other real but relatively uncommon complications include rectal mucosal irritation, ulceration, perforation, and necrosis. Infection introduced by a rectal tube is probably very uncommon; however, secondary infection of a breached rectal wall mucosa can occur. Daily reassessment of the indication for the rectal tube is important. The tube should be removed when there is no longer an indication for its use.

Daily reassessment of the need for continued use of a rectal tube is important. The tube should be removed when there is no longer an indication for its use.

SUMMARY

The practice of critical care frequently involves the use of various tubes placed into patients. These procedures are performed mostly for therapeutic indications, as is most evident in the use of chest tubes. Similarly, nasogastric tubes have an important therapeutic role but are also useful in diagnostic monitoring in some cases of upper gastrointestinal bleeding. Rectal tubes also play an important role in both monitoring patients and facilitating their management in the critical care setting.

REVIEW QUESTIONS

1. **A patient with pneumonia is found to have a free-flowing pleural effusion. A thoracentesis reveals serosanguinous fluid that is not particularly viscous. You determine that a chest tube is needed for this patient. Which chest tube size would you select?**
   - **A.** Large-bore (42 Fr.) chest tube
   - **B.** 28 Fr. chest tube
   - **C.** Any size but with a trocar
   - **D.** 12 Fr. chest tube

2. **Which of the following are complications of chest tube insertion?**
   - **A.** Bleeding
   - **B.** Pulmonary edema
   - **C.** "Winged scapula"
   - **D.** All the above

3. **Indications for nasogastric tubes include all the following except:**
   - **A.** Gastric lavage in the case of toxic substance ingestion
   - **B.** Gastric decompression
   - **C.** Minimization of gastroesophageal reflux and aspiration
   - **D.** Diagnostic adjunct for gastrointestinal bleeding

4. **Which of the following statements regarding rectal tubes is false?**
   - **A.** The most common indication is convenience for the staff.
   - **B.** Paralytic ileus is a contraindication to their use.
   - **C.** Patient discomfort is the most common complication.
   - **D.** If a catheter with a retention balloon is used, the balloon should be kept deflated.

ANSWERS

1. The answer is B. For free-flowing, nonviscous fluid in the pleural space, generally a relatively small to medium-sized tube is appropriate. A large tube is not necessary in this case, and trocar insertion techniques are not recommended. A 12-Fr. tube may work but, because of its small lumen, may be prone to obstruction.
2. The answer is D. Bleeding, reexpansion pulmonary edema, and injury to the long thoracic nerve producing a "winged scapula" are all reported complications from chest tube insertion.
3. The answer is C. Gastric lavage, gastric decompression, and the use of a nasogastric tube in the management of gastrointestinal

bleeding are all important indications for nasogastric tubes. Gastroesophageal reflux and aspiration are potential complications of the use of nasogastric tubes.

4. The answer is A. The presence of a paralytic ileus is a contraindication to rectal tube insertion. Patient discomfort is the most common complication of rectal tubes. Often sedation is helpful, but as a patient becomes more awake, discomfort from the tube is more prominent and limits its continued use. When a catheter with a retention balloon is placed in the rectum, if the retention balloon is inflated, it may facilitate the expulsion of the catheter secondary to normal peristalsis. Therefore, when such catheters are used, the retention balloon should be kept deflated. Rectal tubes should never be used simply for convenience.

SUGGESTED READING

Light, RW. Chest tubes. In: Pleural Diseases, 3rd Ed. Baltimore: Williams & Wilkins, 1995:327–337.

Smeltzer S, Bare B. Brunner's Textbook of Medical-Surgical Nursing. Philadelphia: Lippincott Williams & Wilkins, 1996.

Smith-Temple J, Young J. Nurse's Guide to Clinical Procedures, 3rd Ed. Baltimore: Lippincott Williams & Wilkins, 1998.

CHAPTER 6

HENRY H. HSIA

Implantable Devices for Cardiac Pacing and Defibrillation

CHAPTER OUTLINE

LEARNING OBJECTIVES

After studying this chapter, you should be able to do the following:

- Know the coding of implantable pacemakers and ICDs.
- Understand the basic operations of implantable devices.
- Know the indications of implantable pacemakers and ICDs.
- Systematically evaluate possible device malfunctions.
- Better manage patients with implantable devices.

This chapter introduces the basic concepts of implantable pacemakers and implantable cardioverter-defibrillators (ICDs). We discuss indications and management of patients with implantable devices. The purpose of this discussion is not to provide a comprehensive review of pacemakers and ICDs but rather to provide a knowledge base for systematic evaluation for possible device malfunctions as well as issues relevant in an ICU setting.

BASIC PRINCIPLES

To evaluate patients with implantable devices, the physicians must consider the implantable system. The system consists of the pulse generator (pacemaker or ICD), the lead(s), the myocardium, and the connections between the lead(s) and generator. Evaluations should include all components of the system involving both the hardware (leads, myocardium, generator) and the software (device parameters). A careful, systematic approach is required to deter-

The implantable system:
- The device: pacemaker or ICD
- The lead(s)
- The lead–heart interface and lead connections

mine the appropriateness of pacemaker behaviors, or ICD responses, and to prevent potentially devastating consequences.

Obtain a history that includes:
- Underlying cardiac and arrhythmia diagnoses
- Indications of device implantation
- Brand name and model of the device
- Symptoms of possible device malfunction

It is important to be familiar with the patient's underlying cardiac diagnoses and arrhythmia history. Multiple medical conditions may exist in critically ill patients that can either induce new arrhythmias or exacerbate preexisting arrhythmias. Because the prognosis of these patients is mostly determined by the underlying cardiac and medical conditions, a holistic management approach is recommended. Various factors such as hypoxia, electrolyte imbalance, cardiac ischemia, sepsis, heart failure, or drug toxicity must be considered. The physician should be familiar with the patient's bradycardia indications (for pacemaker implantation) or their tachyarrhythmia indications (for ICD implantation). The manufacturer and model number of the device must also be available for interrogation using the dedicated programmer. Inability to communicate or reprogram the device in an emergency can be disastrous. Last, a careful history should be obtained; the questions are geared to detect any symptoms that may suggest possible device malfunctions or inappropriate interactions, such as pacemaker syndrome, palpitations, dizziness, syncope, or shock delivery.

The physical examination should start with the patient's basic vital signs. An elevated body temperature may suggest an underlying infection with an appropriate sinus tachycardia. An elevated resting heart rate may reflect new onset of atrial fibrillation/flutter, an inappropriate pacemaker activity response, or pacemaker-mediated tachycardia (PMT). A high respiratory rate can induce tachycardia in patients with minute ventilation-based rate modulation devices. An examination for signs of local venous obstruction, AV dissociation, high filling pressure, or congestive heart failure is also crucial. The device pocket should also be evaluated for signs of inflammation, infection, hematoma, and erosion.

Electrocardiography:
- 12-lead ECG
- Free-running rhythm strip
- Rhythm strip with magnet application

The 12-lead ECG may provide information on patient's underlying heart disease (prior myocardial infarction, transmural scar, ventricular hypertrophy), intrinsic rhythm (sinus rhythm, sinus bradycardia, atrial fibrillation or flutter), underlying conduction disturbances (PR prolongation, bundle branch block, heart block), and the current operating mode of the device. For patients with permanent pacemakers, a free-running rhythm strip should be obtained in addition to a rhythm strip with magnet application. Magnet application causes a temporary asynchronous (nonsensing) operation of the device (both pacemaker and ICD). It is used to perfom a threshold margin test (TMT) to verify capture and to display the programmed pacing mode and intervals. Magnet application can also cause specific beginning-of-life (BOL), elective replacement index (ERI), or end-of-life (EOL) pacing rate responses used to check battery status. Each model of pacemaker has its unique ERI and EOL rate responses that can be referenced. Although the magnet test is a part of routine evaluation in patients with pacemakers, it is generally avoided in patients with implantable ICDs because the asynchronous magnet mode renders the ICD unable to detect arrhythmia. Furthermore, a prolonged magnet application could permanently deactivate some models of ICDs.

Magnet operation:
- Asynchronous operation
- Perform threshold margin test
- Verify capture
- Check battery status
- Indicate programmed pacing mode and intervals

It is important to recognize that the patient's arrhythmias and device–rhythm interactions may be intermittent, such as a mode switch induced by paroxysmal atrial fibrillation, antitachycardia pacing triggered by ventricular tachycardia, or pacing for intermittent heart block and bradycardia. As abnormalities are usually transient and difficult to demonstrate, continuous electrocardiographic monitoring is essential in all patients with suspected device malfunction.

MANAGEMENT OF PATIENTS WITH PACEMAKERS

NBG Code

To manage patients with pacemakers, it is necessary to have a basic understanding of pacemaker therapy. Some pacing systems are single chamber, limited to either atrium or ventricle, or they may be dual-chamber systems. They may sense in one chamber and pace the other, sense one and pace both, or sense and pace both chambers. Their operation can vary from beat to beat depend on the programmed mode and the underlying rhythm. As a result of a joint approach of NASPE (North American Society of Pacing and Electrophysiology) and the BPEG (British Pacing and Electrophysiology Group), an NBG (NASPE and BPEG

TABLE 6-1

NASPE/BPEG GENERIC (NBG) CODE

POSITION/ CATEGORY	I: CHAMBER PACED	II: CHAMBER SENSED	III: RESPONSE TO SENSE	IV: PROGRAMMABILITY RATE MODULATION	V: ANTI-TACHYCARDIA FUNCTION
	O, none	O, none	O, none	O, none	O, none
	A, atrium	A, atrium	T, triggered	P, simple	P, pacing
	V, ventricle	V, ventricle	I, inhibited	M, multiprogrammable	S, shock
	D, dual	D, dual	D, dual	C, communicate	D, dual
	S, single chamber	S, single chamber		R, rate modulation	

generic) code was developed (Table 6-1). This is a three- to five-position code to designate the programmed functionality of the device. The first letter designates the chamber(s) paced; *A* stands for atrium, *V* for ventricle, *D* for pacing capability in both atrium and ventricle, and *O* if the unit is deactivated without pacing. The position II letter designates the chamber(s) sensed; *O* stands for asynchronous operation without sensing. The third letter describes the unit's response to a sensed signal; *I* indicates that the pacemaker pacing is inhibited by a sensed event, *T* indicates a pacing stimulus is triggered by a sensed event, and *D* represents an operating mode that a stimulus may be triggered by a sensed event in one chamber and inhibited by a sensed event in the other. For example, a *DDD* pacemaker senses an atrial signal that triggers a ventricular pacing output; however, a sensed ventricular signal will inhibit the pacing stimulus in the ventricle. The fourth letter most commonly describes the degree of programmability and rate-modulation capability. Position V of the NBG Code is reserved for devices with antitachycardia functions and is only applicable to the current generation of ICDs.

Since the development of pacemakers in the early 1960s, the goals of pacing therapy have evolved from basic pacing support to sustain life to optimizing physiologic functions using rate-responsive pacing. The pacemakers have developed from VOO to DDDR systems. Most pacemakers today have activity-responsive, rate-modulating capability that reacts to a patient's physiologic demand. An example of an activity-response curve is illustrated in (Figure 6-1). Many activity sensor technologies have been developed, but only a few have been deployed successfully. The most popular activity sensors are based on the piezoelectric effects. Distortion of piezoelectric crystals can generate electric signals as indirect measures of the patient's physiologic rate demand. In response to chest muscle contractions (arm movement) or body motion (changes in momentum), a vibration sensor or an accelerometer adjusts the pacing rate according to the programmed threshold and the slope (Figure 6-2). An alternative activity sensor is based on minute ventilation (MV) measured by the changes in

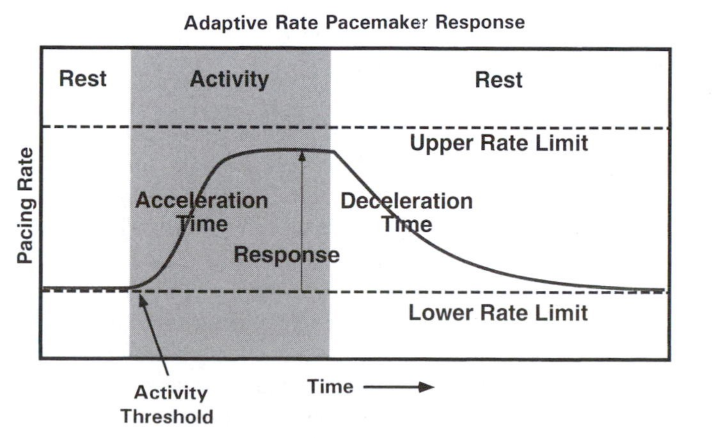

FIGURE 6-1

Activity response. As the activity sensor signals rise beyond the activity threshold, the pacing rate increases from the lower rate limit toward the upper rate limit, following acceleration and deceleration time profiles.

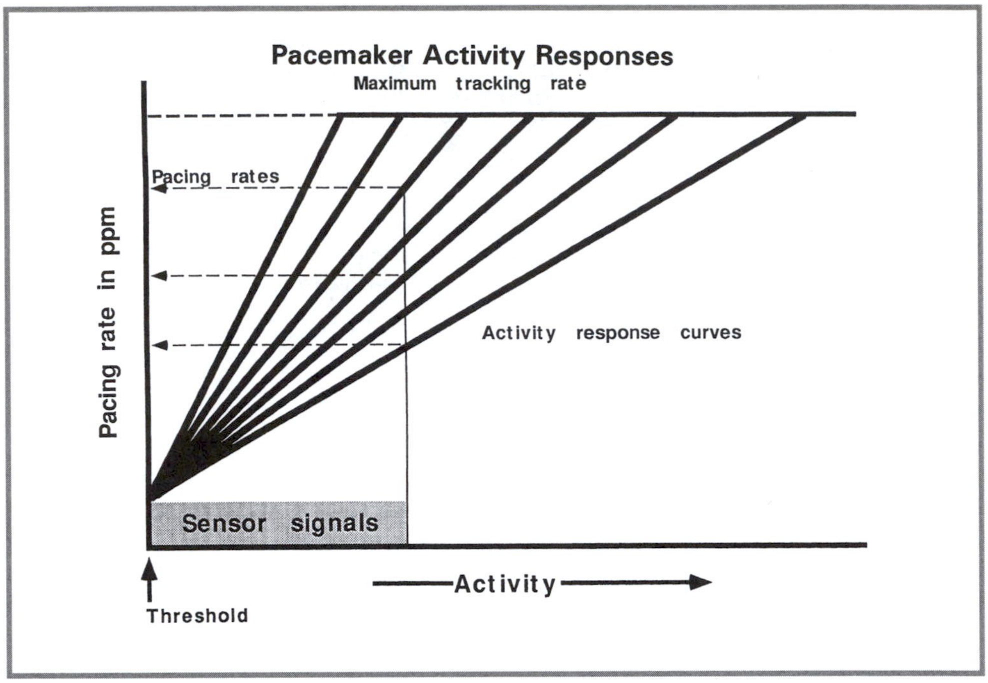

FIGURE 6-2

Activity response curves. The *x*-axis is the activity level and the *y*-axis is the delivered pacing rate. As the sensor signals rise beyond the threshold, different pacing rates result depend on the amplitude of sensor signals and the slopes of the activity response curves.

the transthoracic impedance over time. An increased minute ventilation is translated to an increased physiologic demand and pacing rate.

Indications for Pacemaker Implantation

Indications for permanent pacemaker implantation can be grouped into several categories, including (1) acquired AV block, (2) chronic fascicular block, (3) AV block associated with acute myocardial infarction, (4) sinus node dysfunction, and (5) carotid sinus hypersensitivity and neurally mediated syncope. Other newer indications for pacing are continually expanding, such as pacing for tachyarrhythmia termination and prevention. Clinical studies involving pacing for symptomatic, hemodynamic benefits in patients with heart failure, dilated cardiomyopathy, or hypertrophic cardiomyopathy have demonstrated mixed results at this time. In general, the decisions about the need for a pacemaker are influenced by the presence and absence of symptoms that are directly attributable to bradycardia or heart block. Other considerations for pacing therapy are prophylactic, such as in patients with chronic multifascicular block who present with syncope.

The long-term prognosis of survivors of acute myocardial infarction who develop conduction defect is related primarily to the extent of myocardial damage. Indications for pacing in this setting do not necessarily depend on the presence of symptoms. The risk of developing complete heart block following acute myocardial infarction can be predicted on the basis of the results of several large studies. The presence (new or preexisting) of any of the following conduction disturbances was considered as a risk factor: first-degree AV delay, second-degree AV block (Mobitz I or II), hemiblock (left anterior or posterior), or right or left bundle branch block. Each electrocardiographic risk factor was assigned a score of 1, and a risk score can be calculated as the sum of all risk factors. The incidence of complete heart block occurred as follows: risk score 0, 1.2%–6.8%; risk score 2, 25%–30.1% incidence; the risk increased to greater than 36% for higher scores (Figure 6-3). The decision to implant a pacemaker for conduction defects complicating an acute infarction depends on the *location* of myocardial infarction and the *type* of conduction disturbances. An inferior infarction is usually associated with an increased vagal tone and AV node ischemia with a lesser degree of myocardial conduction system necrosis (see Chapter 15). Even in the presence of complete heart block, the conduction disturbance is generally at the nodal level and

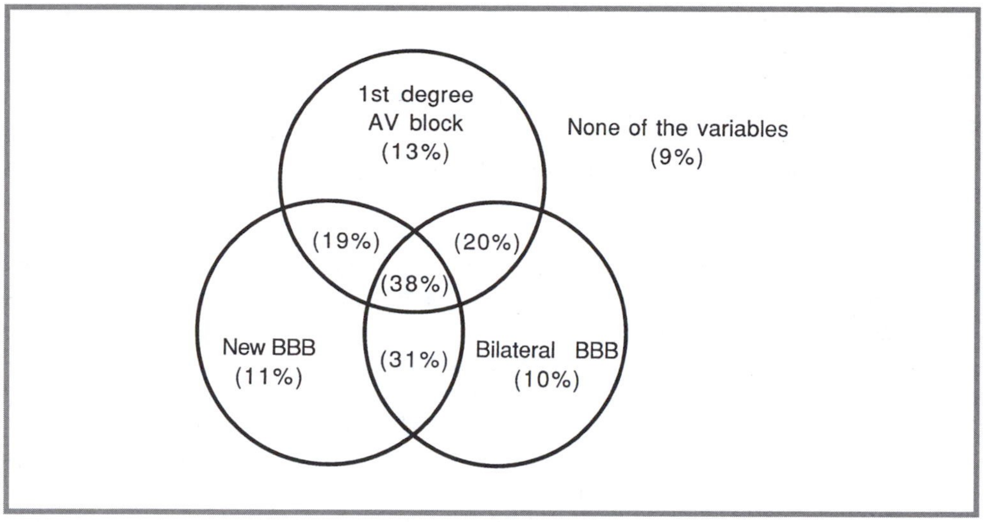

FIGURE 6-3

Risk of developing complete heart block in acute myocardial infarction. Bilateral BBB includes either RBBB+LAFB, or RBBB+LPFB; new BBB includes the development of any new bundle branch aberrancy associated with an acute myocardial infarction.

improves with time. An adequate escape rhythm is usually available and responds to autonomic maneuvers such as atropine administration. An anterior myocardial infarction causes necrosis of the His bundle or bundle branches in addition to predominant left ventricular damage. Complete heart block may develop suddenly with a wide, bizarre QRS complex escape rhythm and severe bradycardia that frequently does not respond to atropine. A pacemaker is indicated in patients who develop a *new* high-grade AV block complicating anterior myocardial infarctions.

Although periinfarction conduction defects have been associated with an unfavorable outcome and an increased incidence of sudden death, pacing therapy has not demonstrated a definitive improvement in a patient's prognosis, which probably reflects the overwhelmingly negative impact on mortality by the extensive myocardial damage. The presence of conduction defect in the setting of acute infarction identifies patients with large myocardial necrosis and ischemic burden. These patients are at risk not just for the development of complete heart block but also for ventricular tachyarrhythmia.

Pacing Mode Considerations

The most widely utilized pacing modes in the United States include single-chamber ventricular pacing (VVI), dual-chamber pacing (DDD), and physiologic rate adaptive pacing (VVIR, DDDR). Choices of pacing mode depend on many factors. The chronotropic response, status of the AV conduction, ventricular function, and presence of chronic versus paroxysmal atrial arrhythmias should be considered. In patients with chronotropic insufficiency, that is, inadequate heart rate response to activity or demand, a rate-adaptive, activity-responsive pacing mode is recommended. In patients with AV block, dual-chamber pacing is the mode of choice because AV synchrony is maintained. Data strongly support the benefits of preserving AV synchrony so as to reduce the risk of atrial fibrillation, strokes, and congestive heart failure. In patients with paroxysmal atrial arrhythmias, atrial pacing may be effective in preventing arrhythmia recurrence. Thus, the DDD or DDDR mode is preferred over ventricular pacing alone. Dual-chamber pacing also has been shown to provide an improved cardiac output and exercise tolerance and to avoid A-V dissociation and pacemaker syndrome. Conversely, VVI pacing is ideal in patients with chronic atrial fibrillation and an adequate ventricular rate response for their physiologic demand. VVIR pacing is recommended for the subset of patients who are active and would benefit from activity-responsive pacing because of "relative" bradycardia for their physiologic demands.

Choices of pacing mode considerations:
- Atrial:
  - Chronic atrial arrhythmias
  - Chronotropic incompetence
  - Paroxysmal atrial arrhythmias
- Ventricular:
  - Diastolic dysfunction
  - Systolic function
  - Hypertrophy

AMS (automatic mode switch) is a function available in the newer generations of dual-chamber pacemakers. In patients with paroxysmal atrial arrhythmias, the device can detect the "inappropriate" atrial high rate and mode-switches from DDD/DDDR to either VVI/VVIR or DDI/DDIR functionality to avoid rapid atrial sensing and tracking during episodes of atrial fibrillation, flutter, or atrial tachycardia.

Pacemaker Malfunction

Pacemaker malfunction:
- Undersensing
- Oversensing
- Failure to pace
- Failure to capture
- Altered pacing rate
- Undesirable interaction

In patients with suspected pacemaker malfunction, physicians must consider all components of the pacing system, including the generator, the lead(s), the myocardium, and the connections between the lead(s) and generator. A methodical evaluation is required for both the hardware and software of the system. Pacemaker malfunction can be categorized to (1) undersensing, (2) oversensing, (3) failure to pace, (4) failure to capture, (5) altered pacing rate, and (6) undesirable interactions.

Proper evaluation of a patient with suspected pacemaker malfunction begins with the understanding of the indications of pacemaker implantation and the underlying intrinsic rhythms (atrial arrhythmias, chronotropic competence, status of AV conduction) of the patient. A 12-lead ECG with magnet application and a long rhythm tracing should be obtained and analyzed. Interrogation of the programmed parameters and the measured data is essential. Inappropriate device programming must be ruled out. A high lead impedance (resistance) suggests obstruction of current flow, such as in the case of lead (conducting wire) fracture. Conversely, a low lead impedance with high current drainage suggests "leakage" of current, such as in the case of lead insulation failure. In devices with intracardiac electrogram (EGM), high-frequency noise during manual manipulation of the pacing system may imply lead fractures or defective/loose connections with "make–break" contact potentials. Abnormal, variable amplitude and morphology of the intracardiac electrogram may indicate an unstable lead position or dislodgment. In addition, a chest x-ray should be obtained to confirm lead position and examine lead integrity. A discontinuity in the conducting element implies lead fracture, and a lead lucency may represent a breach of insulation.

Undersensing

Undersensing: inappropriately timed pacing spikes resulting from nonsensing of intrinsic signals
- Lead dislodgment
- Poor electrogram signals
- Inappropriate programming
- Lead insulation or conductor defect
- Connector defect
- Component failure

Undersensing refers to presence of inappropriately timed pacing artifacts due to "non-sense" of intrinsic P or R waves, which results in a faster than expected heart rate with more pacing events. The problem may be intermittent or persistent. This asynchronous pacing could result in induction of new arrhythmias such as atrial fibrillation, ventricular tachyarrhythmia from premature atrial depolarization, or R-on-T phenomenon. The most common cause of undersensing is lead dislodgment with failure to sense the intracavitary signals. Other causes of inadequate electrogram amplitude include infarction, scarring, and local fibrosis at the lead tip–tissue junction. Some drug effects or electrolyte imbalance may also influence the signal quality. Occasionally, improper programming of inadequate sensitivity or inappropriately long refractory periods may also result in apparent undersensing. During sinus tachycardia, intermittent atrial undersensing may occur as rapid atrial signals encroach upon the atrial refractory periods (Figure 6-4); this is described as "pacemaker Wenckebach" or "upper rate behavior" of dual-chamber pacemakers.

Oversensing

Oversensing: absence of pacing caused by inhibition of "inappropriately" sensed signals
- Inappropriate programming
- Lead fracture: make–break potentials
- Skeletal muscle artifacts
- Electromagnetic interference (EMI)
- Lead dislodgement
- Repolarization potential

Oversensing refers to the absence of pacing artifacts resulting from inhibition of inappropriately sensed signals or artifacts, which results in a slower than expected heart rate with fewer pacing outputs. Oversensing may be caused by lead dislodgment or poor positioning with sensing of far-field signals. A dislodged atrial lead or an atrial lead placed too close to the tricuspid valve may sense far-field ventricular signals with subsequent atrial inhibition. Oversensing is frequently intermittent, and one must exclude the possibility of a lead fracture (Figure 6-5). Sensing of the make–break potentials generated by intermittent contacts of fractured wires can be provoked by manipulations of the generator or surrounding tissues (arm movement).

Extracardiac or nonphysiologic signals can also contribute to oversensing inhibition. In general, unipolar leads are more prone to oversensing than bipolar leads because of the large sensing field (Table 6-2). Unipolar leads sense and pace between the intracardiac distal tip

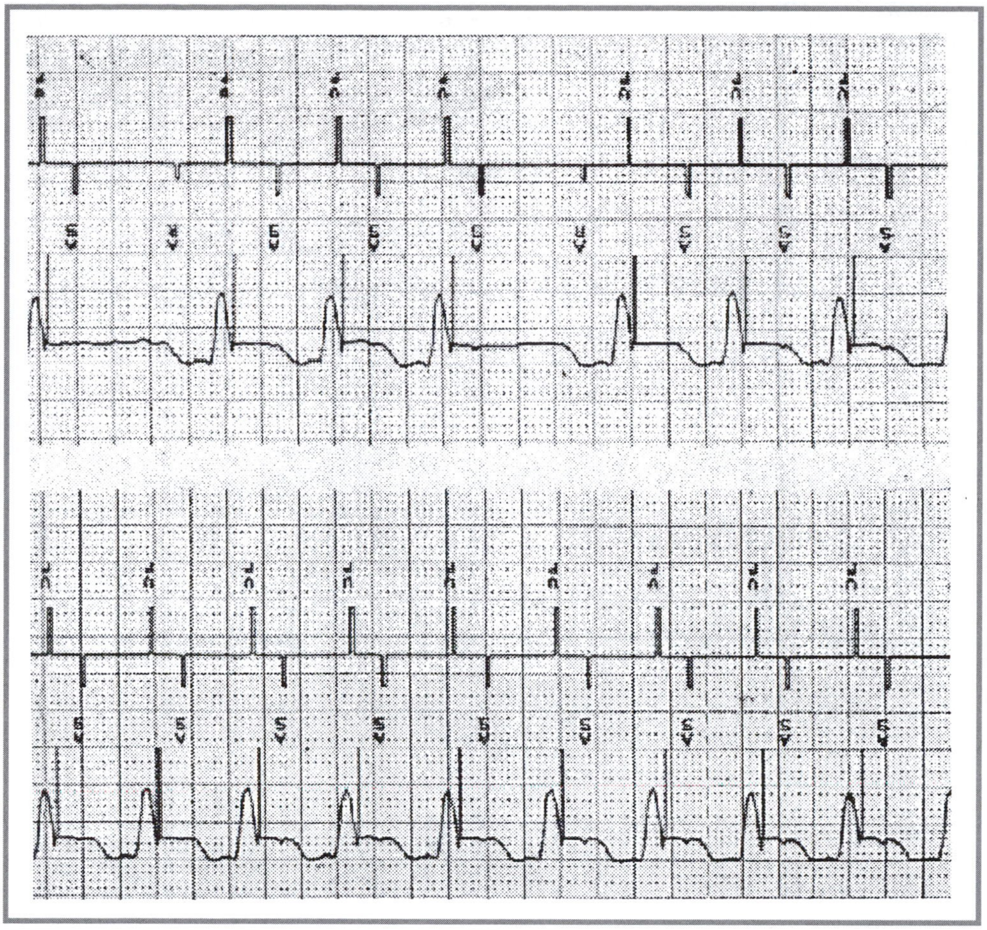

FIGURE 6-4

Apparent undersensing in a pacemaker Wenckebach behavior. The rapid atrial signals impinge on the atrial sensing refractory periods and resulted in atrial drop-outs and intermittent atrial undersensing with P waves in the T waves. The intracardiac markers demonstrated atrial sensing (AS) with ventricular pacing (VP). The *top tracing* showed 1:1 atrial sensing and tracking; the *bottom tracing* showed intermittent atrial undersensing in the refractory periods (AR).

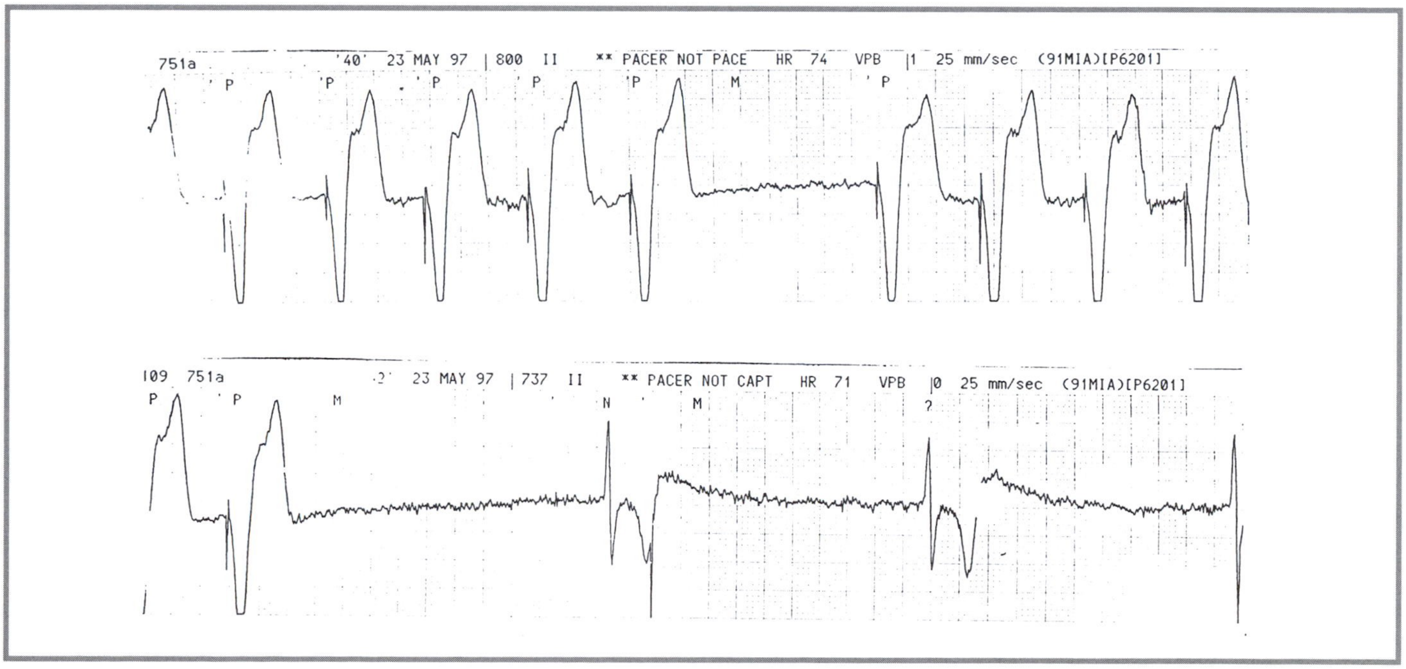

FIGURE 6-5

Oversensing associated with a lead fracture. Intermittent make–break potentials generated by contacts of the fractured lead elements were sensed as intrinsic signals. The pacing intervals were reset and pacing outputs were inhibited. The pauses were not multiples of a basic pacing interval, which suggests oversensing rather than failure to pace.

TABLE 6-2

UNIPOLAR VERSUS BIPOLAR LEADS

UNIPOLAR	BIPOLAR
Large artifact	No pocket stimulation
Less stiff	No muscle inhibition
More reliable	Less crosstalk
Simple connector	EMI protected
Smaller lead body	Smaller T waves

EMI, electromagnetic interference

of the lead and the pulse generator. Bipolar leads have both electrodes located at the distal tip. Myopotential oversensing of skeletal muscle artifacts with pacing inhibition and asystole is almost exclusively observed in patients with unipolar lead systems (Figure 6-6). Again, this phenomenon may be elicited by arm movement or chest muscle contraction. Electromagnetic interference (EMI) is another important cause of nonphysiologic signals; this is a crucial topic relating to both pacemaker and ICD and is discussed at the end of this chapter.

Occasionally, repolarization potentials following either spontaneous or paced complexes may be oversensed, particularly in patients with prominent T waves or unipolar lead systems. This phenomenon may be further exacerbated by electrolyte imbalance, antiarrhythmic drugs, and high rate pacing at high outputs (Figure 6-7). Similar to the issues in undersensing, oversensing may occur with inappropriate programming. A too-sensitive setting or an inappropriately short refractory period may result in T waves or muscle potential interference.

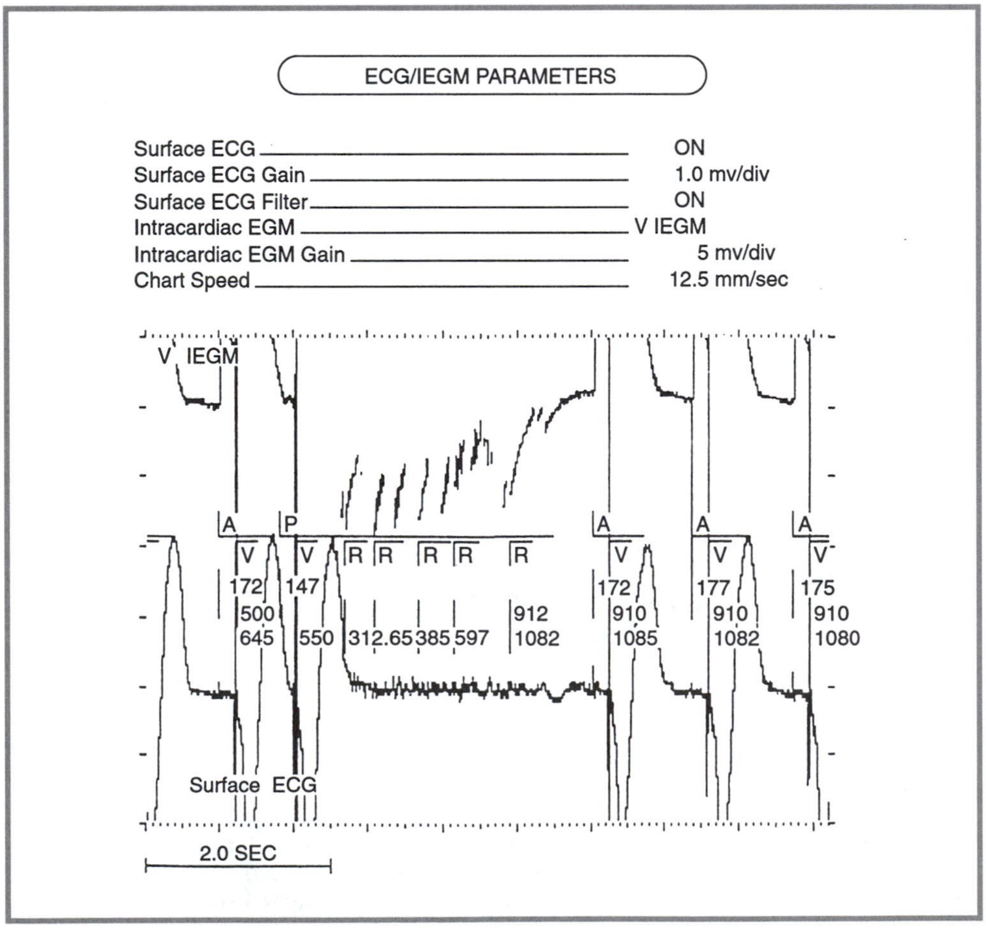

FIGURE 6-6

Myopotential oversensing of skeletal muscle artifacts with pacing inhibition. The surface ECG showed motion artifacts with muscle contraction and a long pause. The intracardiac recordings demonstrated multiple myopotential signals that were sensed by the pacemaker as intrinsic R waves and inhibited pacing outputs.

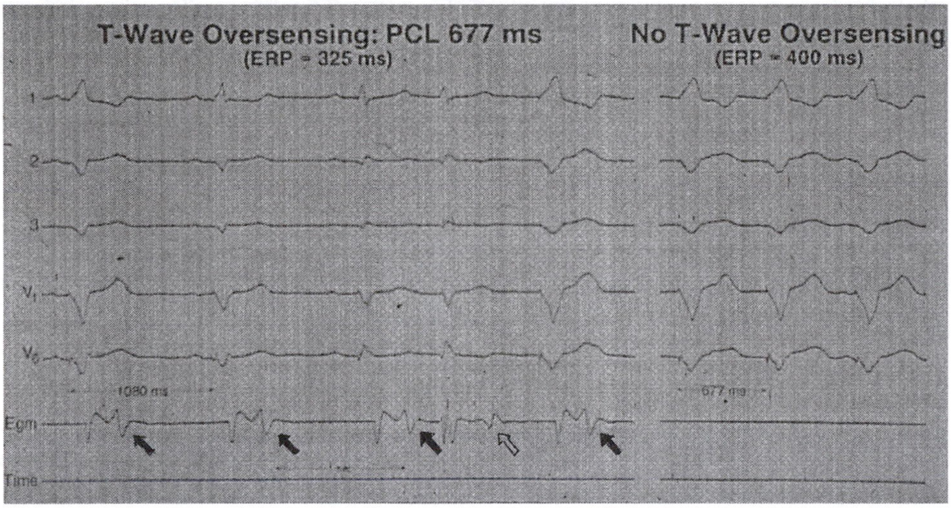

FIGURE 6-7

Intermittent T-wave oversensing. The intracardiac electrogram (EGM) showed prominent repolarization potentials that resulted in intermittent oversensing (*solid arrows*) at an refractory period (ERP) of 325 ms. This problem was corrected by increasing the refractory period to 400 ms.

Failure to Pace

Failure to pace indicates absence of pacing stimulus at the expected time interval. The most common cause is oversensing inhibition or misinterpretation of the electrocardiographic tracings. Often, hysteresis or sleep function of the device may be activated, and the pacemaker appears to fail to pace or pace at a slower than expected rate (see Altered Rate). Other reasons for failure to pace include complete lead fracture without current flow (Figure 6-8) or battery depletion. Rarely, component defects or error in connecting the leads to the generator at implant can result in absence of stimulus artifact.

Failure to pace: absence of pacing stimulus at the expected interval
- Lead and generator not connected
- Complete lead fracture
- Battery depletion
- Hysteresis, sleep rate
- Oversensing
- Component failure

Failure to Capture

Failure to capture indicates a failure to generate a localized tissue depolarization (P or R waves) despite the presence of a pacing stimulus. The stimulus artifacts are present but ineffective. The most common cause of failure to capture is an elevated pacing threshold. Many factors influence the capture threshold for generating tissue depolarizations (Tables 6-3 and 6-4). In the early postimplant period, the possibility of lead dislodgment must be excluded. The newly implanted lead induces a localized inflammatory process that significantly elevates the pacing threshold (up to four times of the implant threshold value). This lead maturation process may last up to 8 weeks postimplantation as the local inflammation resolves (Figure 6-9). With the development of new technology, such as steroid-eluting leads, the acute elevation of thresholds soon after implantation may be blunted. For chronic lead systems, antiarrhythmic drug use, lead damage, exit blocks with local scarring at the lead–

Failure to capture: ineffective pacing stimuli that fail to capture
- Lead dislodgment
- Myocardial perforation
- Insulation defect: low impedance and high current flow
- Conductor failure: high impedance
- Threshold elevation
- Inappropriate programming: output too low

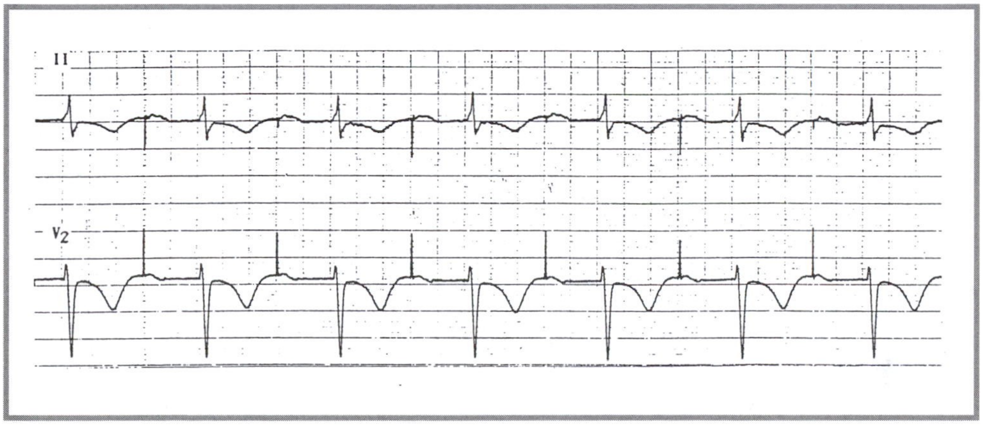

FIGURE 6-8

An example of failure to pace caused by a complete lead fracture. Interrogation of the device revealed a dual-chamber pacemaker in an AV sequentially paced rhythm. Atrial pacing output was present without ventricular pacing artifacts.

TABLE 6-3

FACTORS INFLUENCING PACING THRESHOLDS

Lead maturation process: trauma, inflammation, fibrosis
Lead technology:
- Steroid eluting lead
- New metallic element
- Factured lead with high surface area

Drug effects
Electrolyte imbalance
Infarction, local scar
Excessive fibrosis: exit block

tissue junction or interim myocardial infarctions should be considered when physicians encounter high pacing thresholds. Other reasons include a poor lead–tissue contact, such as lead dislodgment or myocardial perforation, or inadequately programmed pacing outputs. As always, careful evaluation of the lead integrity must be performed because lead insulation defect or fracture can progress and produce devastating consequences.

Altered Rate

Altered pacing rate:
- Battery depletion (EOL)
- Rate drift in old pacemaker
- Activity responses
- Hysteresis
- Recorder defect:
  - Altered paper speed
  - Holter battery depletion

One other manifestation of pacing system malfunction is altered pacing rate. The pacemaker paces at a rate other than the programmed rate, either faster or slower, commonly as a result of pacemaker battery depletion. As the device reaches the elective replacement index (ERI) or end-of-life (EOL) status, the pacemaker automatically decreases its pacing rate to conserve the battery, and occasionally asynchronous pacing at a slow rate can be observed. Another common cause for a pacemaker to pace at a slower rate is the hysteresis function. Hysteresis is defined as a slowing of pacing rates in response to sensed events (Figure 6-10). A less common observation is a faster than expected pacing rate, which is usually related to inappropriate programming of an activity-responsive pacemaker (DDDR, VVIR). Rarely, defective recording instruments with *slow* paper speed can create an apparent accelerated heart rate.

Undesirable Interactions

Undesirable interactions:
- Infection
- Hematoma
- Erosion
- Extracardiac stimulation
- Inappropriate programming

A discussion of malfunction of implantable devices would not be complete without mentioning the undesirable interactions, which can be divided into acute versus chronic. The acute interactions are related to surgical complications that include infection, hematoma, pericarditis, cardiac perforation, and tamponade; the chronic adverse side effects include erosions of the lead or the generator and venous thrombosis or vascular obstruction. Furthermore, physicians should be cognizant of the fact that apparent device malfunctions are frequently related to the undesirable interactions between the programmed parameters (outputs, sensitivity, intervals, and rates) and the individual patient's rhythm.

TABLE 6-4

DRUG INFLUENCES ON PACING THRESHOLDS

INCREASE	DECREASE
Flecainide, class IC	Glucocorticosteroid
Procainamide, class IA	Catecholamine
Propanolol	
Amiodarone/class III	

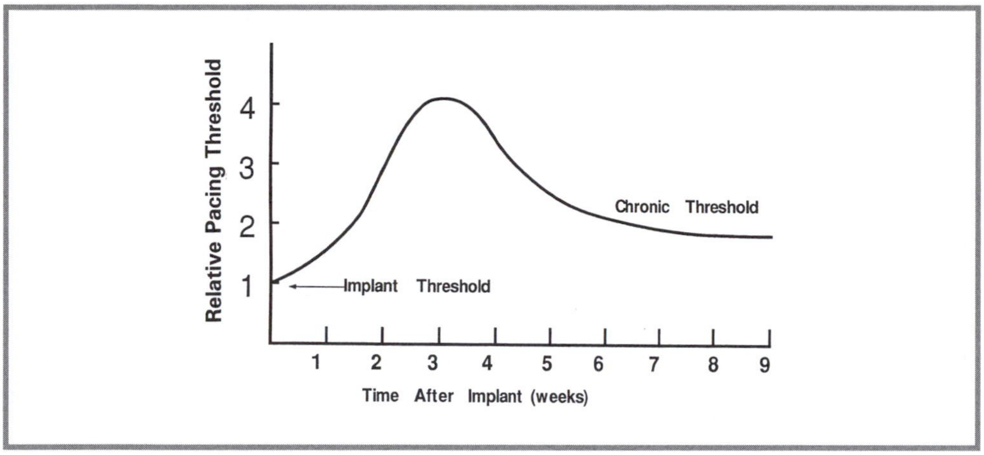

FIGURE 6-9

Maturation of implanted leads. The pacing threshold increases and peaks approximately 3–4 weeks postoperatively to three to four times the initial implant value. The threshold gradually decreases and reaches a chronic threshold level at approximately twice the implant value. The maturation process may last up to 8 weeks postimplantation as local inflammation resolves. Similar changes may be observed with sensing function.

PACEMAKER SYNDROME

Pacemaker syndrome is a clinical complex of signs and symptoms related to the adverse hemodynamic and electrophysiologic consequences of ventricular pacing caused by asynchronous, inadequate timing of atrial and ventricular contractions. It is most commonly described in patients with single-chamber ventricular pacemakers but has been reported in those with dual-chamber pacing systems. The pathophysiology is based on the loss of AV synchrony. A properly timed atrial contraction (atrial kick) accounts for a minimal 20% of the cardiac output. The loss of positive atrial kick may significantly decrease cardiac output with inadequate preload, especially in patients with structural heart disease and abnormal chamber compliance. The negative atrial kick associated with retrograde VA conduction results in systemic and pulmonary venous regurgitations and pressure overload. Furthermore, augmented atrial distension can induce a reflex vasodepressor effect with decreases in peripheral resistance and hypotension. Manifestations of pacemaker syndrome include near or frank syncope, fatigue, dyspnea with exercise intolerance, heart failure, orthostatic symptoms, palpitation, "pounding," and a sensation of throat fullness. Patients who suffer from pacemaker syndrome frequently present with signs of VA dissociation with large cannon A waves and variable liver pulsations. The abnormal hemodynamic sequales may be confirmed by an echocardiographic color doppler study that demonstrates tricuspid or mitral regurgitations with reversal of venous blood flow during VVI pacing. Treatment is aimed at restoration of

Pathophysiology of pacemaker syndrome:
- Loss of AV synchrony
- Loss of positive atrial kick:
  - Decreased cardiac output
- Negative atrial kick:
  - Venous regurgitations, pressure overload
  - Atrial distension: reflex vasodilation

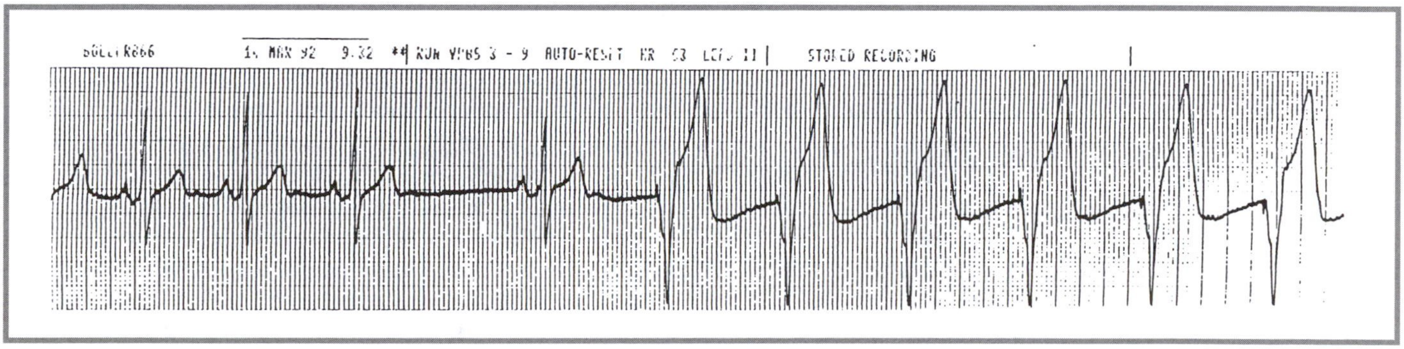

FIGURE 6-10

An example of pacemaker hysteresis. The pacemaker is programmed to a pacing rate of 60 ppm and hysteresis rate is programmed to 40 ppm.

AV synchrony with atrial or dual-chamber pacing, reduction of ventricular pacing rate, or activation of hysteresis function.

TEMPORARY PACING

Indications for temporary pacing:
- Bradyarrhythmia
- Prophylactic therapy for anticipated bradyarrhythmia
- Hemodynamic
- Tachyarrhythmia:
  - Termination
  - Prevention
- Acute myocardial infarction

The primary objective of temporary pacing is for short-term hemodynamic support in unstable patients. Indications for temporary pacing include (1) symptomatic bradycardia and AV block, (2) prophylactic therapy for anticipated bradycardia or AV block, such as after an acute myocardial infarction, and (3) acute tachyarrhythmia termination and prevention, such as in patients with either drug-induced or bradycardia-related torsade de pointes. Occasionally, temporary pacing may be instituted in postoperative patients to improve hemodynamics. In a setting of acute myocardial infarction, temporary pacing is advisable in certain patients because of the high risk of developing complete heart block, including patients with *new* bilateral (bifascicular) bundle branch block (for example, right bundle branch block with left anterior or posterior hemiblock), *alternating* bundle branch block, and first-degree AV block (Figure 6-3). Temporary pacing support can be achieved with transvenous pacing wire placement or occasionally with noninvasive external pacemakers.

The clinician must keep in mind that as many as 10%–20% of patients may develop complications related to insertion of temporary pacing wires. Complications associated with central vascular access (pneumothorax, hemothorax), arrhythmias, cardiac perforation, and local infection occur in 1%–5% of cases depending on the operator. In experienced hands, a temporary pacing wire can be safely advanced into the right ventricle at the bedside using electrocardiographic guidance (Figure 6-11).

A transthoracic external pacing system can be used to maintain a heart rate until a transvenous pacing wire can be inserted. It is also reserved as a prophylactic standby in high-risk patients. It is generally safe and does not cause any myocardial damage. However, because of the relatively high current delivery, significant cutaneous nerve stimulation and skeletal muscle contraction will result. The degree of discomfort is related to the amount of energy required to capture the heart. In patients with obesity, large chest wall size, pulmonary disease, and high pacing threshold, substantial pain may result. A major limitation of the use of an external pacemaker is the intolerable discomfort patients experience, especially when the pacemaker is used for a prolonged period of time at a fast rate.

TRANSESOPHAGEAL PACING AND RECORDING

Esophageal electrocardiography is a useful noninvasive technique to diagnose arrhythmias. The esophagus is posterior and in close proximity to the left atrium. A catheter electrode can be inserted into the patient's esophagus without significant discomfort. These esophageal electrodes can record atrial signals and pace the left atrium with variable success. The optimal electrode position for atrial pacing is generally within 1 cm from the site at which the maximum amplitude of the atrial electrogram is recorded. Patients can also easily swallow a small pill or capsule electrode attached on a string for continuous, long-term atrial recordings with minimal discomfort and complication. The esophageal atrial electrogram is most useful in differentiating SVT with aberrant conduction from ventricular tachycardia. Ventriculoatrial relations can be easily identified, and RP or PR intervals can be estimated. The esophageal atrial recordings are also helpful to define the mechanism of supraventricular tachycardias, especially in atrial flutter with 2:1 AV block. In addition, transesophageal pacing may terminate reentrant SVTs, although high current outputs may be needed with moderate discomfort.

CARDIOVERSION AND DEFIBRILLATION

The occurrence of hemodynamically unstable, sustained ventricular tachycardia (VT) or ventricular fibrillation (VF) is a catastrophic event that demands immediate response. Multiple

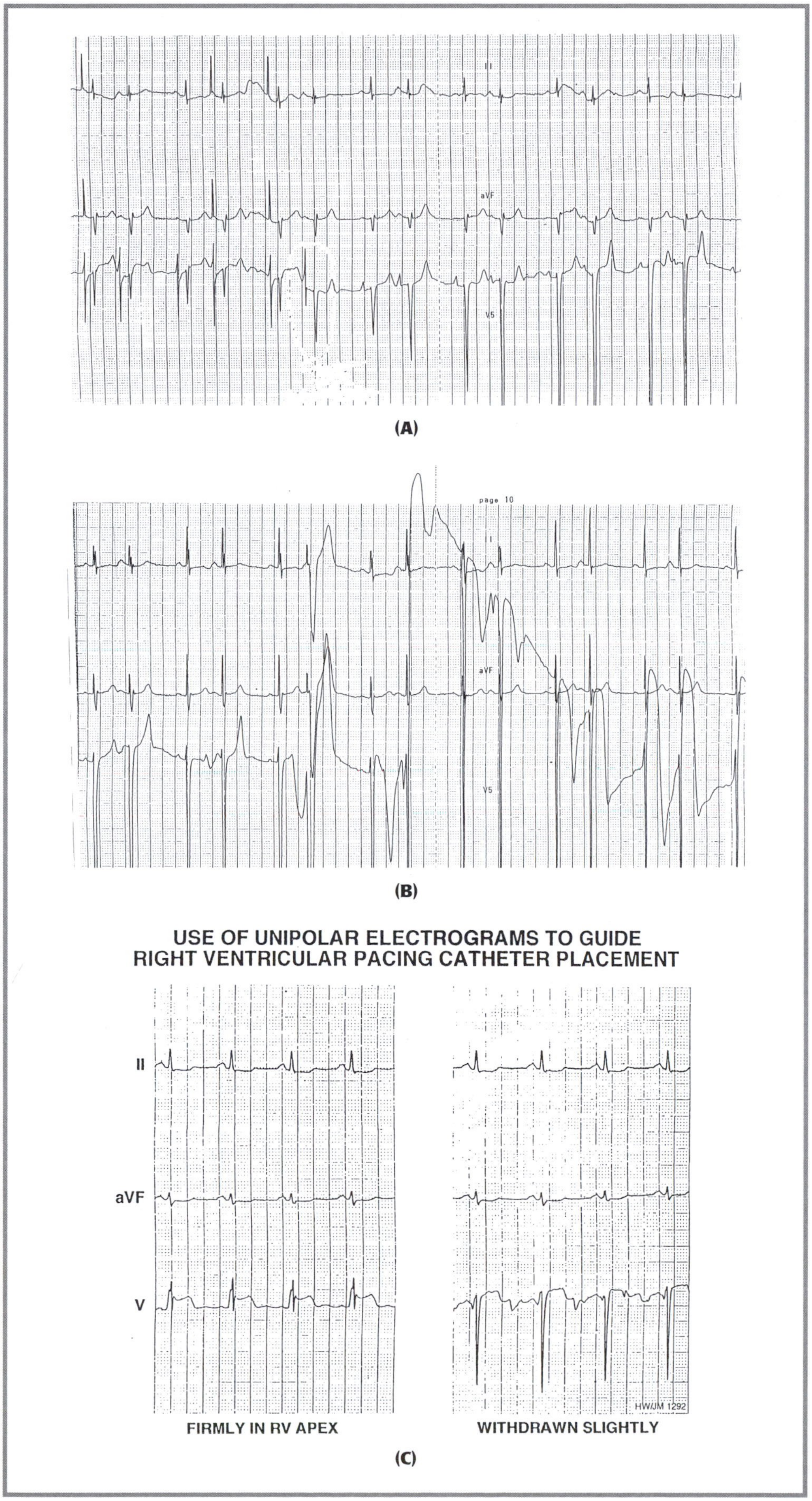

FIGURE 6-11

Temporary pacing wire placement using electrocardiographic guidance. The distal tip of the pacing wire is connected to lead V-5 of an ECG machine in an unipolar configuration. **(A)** The unipolar electrogram showed large atrial signals on the *left side* of the tracing with a large ventricular signal on the *right side* of the tracing as the catheter was advanced from the right atrium into the right ventricle. **(B)** The unipolar electrogram showed large injury potentials as the catheter made contact with the ventricular myocardium. **(C)** Final placement of the pacing catheter to achieve a stable position.

high-energy shock delivery is generally safe and does not cause any significant myocardial damage. The cardioverter-defibrillator (either external or implantable) charges the capacitors to create a voltage (V) gradient between the electrodes (paddles or leads). Current passage between the electrodes through the myocardium (either intracardiac or transthoracic) down the voltage gradient and is described as energy delivery per time (joules). However, it is the *transmyocardial current flow* that actually induces cellular membrane changes that terminate propagations of arrhythmia wavefronts. The defibrillation threshold (DFT), or the cardioversion energy requirement (CER) is related to the underlying arrhythmias (VT versus VF), electrolyte/metabolic milieu, ischemic burden, current pathway resistance, and the duration of arrhythmia.

For successful external defibrillation resuscitations, one must ascertain the proper placement of electrode paddles and establish a firm skin contact (greater than 10 pounds of pressure) with gel application to minimize resistance. Rapid recharging of the defibrillator for repeated shock delivery is recommended immediately after a discharge to minimize the time delay, total arrhythmia duration, and hypotensive period.

In patients who have failed repeated defibrillation/cardioversion attempts, one *must* distinguish a failed shock from immediate arrhythmia reinitiation following successful terminations. In patients with frequent arrhythmia reinitiations, other factors such as drug toxicity, ischemia, and metabolic and electrolyte derangement must be excluded. Excessive bradycardia following tachycardia termination can also promote arrhythmia initiation, and temporary pacing may be indicated in such special circumstances. In addition, judicious use of a low-dose beta-blocker to counteract the high catecholamine state may be considered for incessant arrhythmia recurrences in an acute setting. In patients with implantable defibrillators, resuscitative efforts should *not* be altered due to presence of the device. Patients should always be treated regardless of the ICDs. However, paddle positions directly over the pulse generator should be avoided.

Since the advent of implantable cardioverter-defibrillators (ICDs) in the 1980s, device therapy has evolved from a last-resort effort to a primary treatment option in management of patients with tachyarrhythmias (VT, VF, or sudden cardiac death). The growth of ICD has been exponential (Figure 6-12) and is currently in its fifth generation of device development (Table 6-5). Early observational reports and recent prospective and randomized trials have uniformly documented the benefit of ICD therapy in reduction of sudden cardiac death, both in survivors of cardiac arrest (secondary prevention) (Figure 6-13) and in high-risk patients

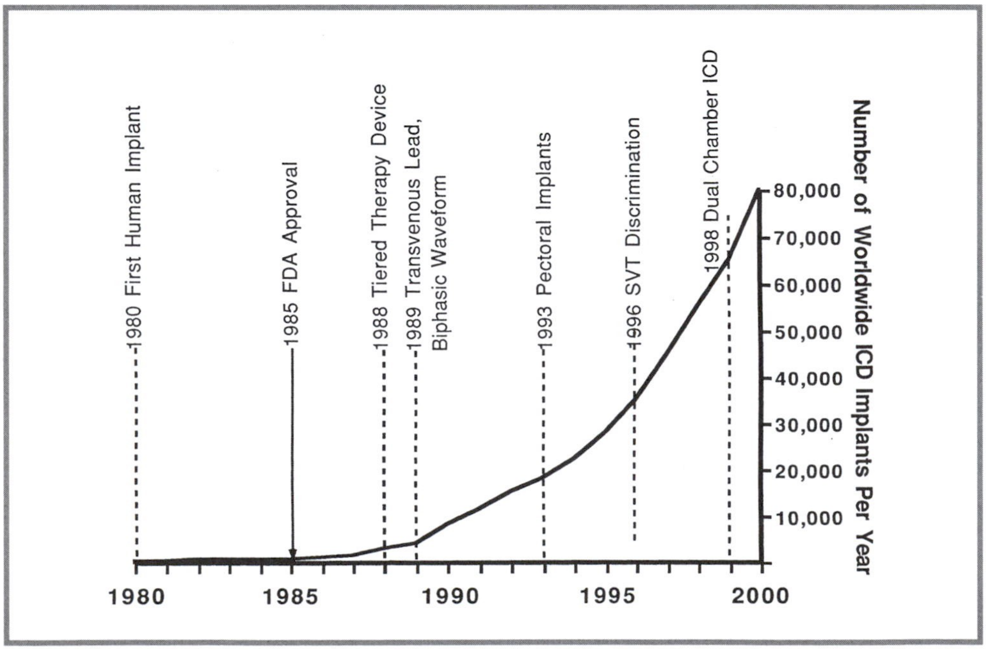

FIGURE 6-12

Evolution of ICD therapy. Major landmarks include the development of transvenous lead and biphasic waveform energy, smaller size for pectoral implantations, and the dual-chamber devices. It is estimated that 80,000 ICDs will be implanted worldwide in the year 2000 with approximately 30,000 units implanted in the United States.

TABLE 6–5

COMPARISON OF IMPLANTABLE CARDIOVERTER-DEFIBRILLATORS (ICDS)

	FIRST GENERATION	SECOND GENERATION	THIRD GENERATION	FOURTH GENERATION	FIFTH GENERATION
High-energy shocks	+	+	+	+	+
Programmable rate	−	±	+	+	+
Programmable detection	−	±	+	+	++
Tiered therapy	−	−	+	+	+
Low-energy cardioversion	−	+	+	+	+
Waveform	M	M	M/B	B	B+
Antitachycardia pacing	−	−	+	+	+
Brady pace	−	−	+	++	++
Stored electrogram	−	−	±	+	+
Noninvasive electrophysiology	−	−	+	+	++
Dual chamber	−	−	−	−	+

M, monophasic; B, biphasic

for future arrhythmic event (primary prevention) (Figure 6-14). In addition, ICD therapy may also be associated with a lower total health care cost and better quality of life (QOL) for patients.

ICD CONFIGURATIONS

Physicians in an ICU setting should be familiar with the basic design and function of ICDs and be able to troubleshoot in an emergency. An electrophysiologist should be consulted for device interrogation, reprogramming, and follow-up. In general, an ICD consists of a sensing circuit, a detection algorithm, and a therapy delivery system. In contrast to pacemakers with a fixed, programmed *sensitivity* (usually 2.0–10.0 mV for ventricular leads and 0.5–4.0 mV for atrial leads), the sensing circuit of ICDs can automatically enhance and adjust its *sensitivity* or *gain* on a beat-to-beat basis to track low-amplitude signals (as low as 0.2–0.5 mV) accurately during arrhythmia episodes. Although this "auto-gain" or auto-adjusting sensitivity function is fundamental to the operation of ICDs, the highly sensitive algorithm

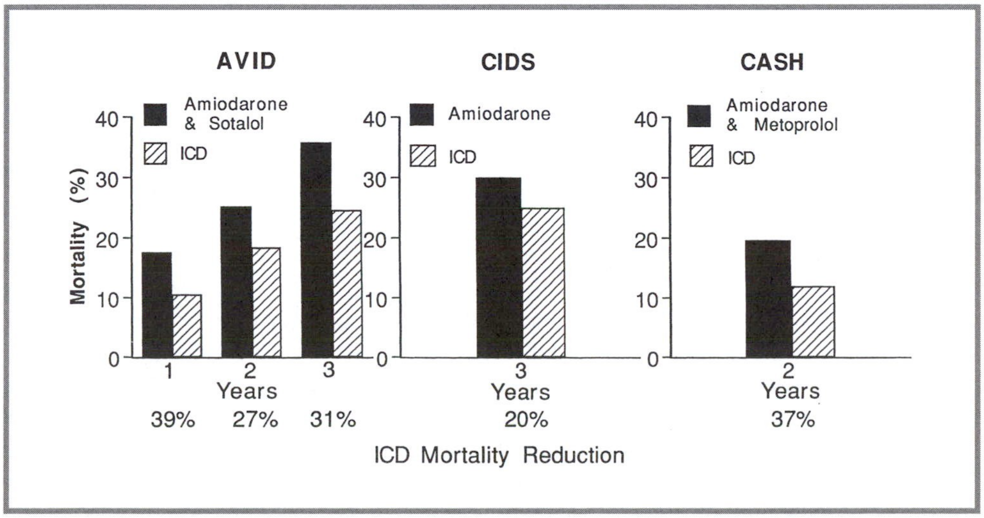

FIGURE 6-13

A summary of major secondary prevention trials in sudden cardiac death survivors. *AVID* (Antiarrhythmics Versus Implantable Defibrillators), *CIDS* (Canadian Implantable Defibrillator Study), and *CASH* (Cardiac Arrest Study Hamburg) trials clearly demonstrated significant mortality reductions with ICD therapy compared to antiarrhythmic medications for ventricular fibrillation or life-threatening ventricular tachycardia.

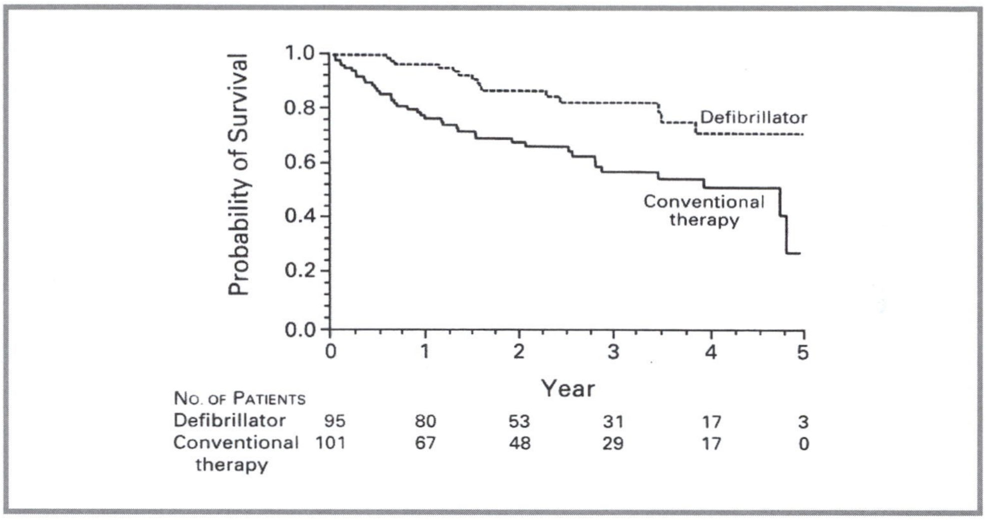

FIGURE 6-14

The MADIT (multicenter-automatic defibrillator implantation trial) enrolled a group of high-risk patients with previous MI, nonsustained VT, LVEF <35%, and inducible VT that is nonsuppressible with IV procainamide during EP study. Patients were treated with either ICD or conventional pharmacologic therapy (mostly with amiodarone). Patients randomized to ICD therapy had a 54% reduction in all-cause mortality compared to patients receiving conventional therapy.

can also detect inappropriate signals or artifacts with adverse oversensing consequences. Once a tachyarrhythmia is sensed with a heart rate above the programmed rate cutoff, ICDs employ a detection algorithm to confirm and declare the presence of a sustained episode before therapy delivery. Either a fixed number of heart beats or an averaged heart rate above the rate cutoff is required, or a rolling window algorithm is utilized (for example, 12 of 16 or 18 of 24 intervals are faster than the rate cutoff). These basic features have been present since the first-generation automatic implantable defibrillator (AID) developed by Drs. Mirowski and Mower.

In contrast to the first-generation ICDs, the current devices have far more programmable options. Multiple detection inhibitors or modifiers have been developed to improve the ability of the device to distinguish supraventricular (most often atrial fibrillation/flutter or sinus tachycardia) from ventricular tachyarrhythmias. Once an episode of tachycardia (SVT or VT) is detected, programmable options such as sudden onset or heart rate stability can inhibit therapy delivery and minimize inappropriate treatment for supraventricular arrhythmias. In addition, extensive recording and data storage capability have been incorporated into the newer generations of devices. To enhance detection specificity, intracardiac electrogram (EGM) characteristics such as width or morphology can be processed for automatic, real-time analysis and templates comparison. Other safety features such as sustained rate duration (SRD) or extended high rate (EHR) are designed to counteract potential delay in therapy with inappropriately programmed inhibitors of detection. After a predetermined time period, the ICD will deliver therapy regardless of the nature of the tachycardia (VT versus SVT).

All ICDs have charge-capacitor systems for delivery of high-energy defibrillation shocks or low-energy cardioversion shocks. In addition, antitachycardia pacing (ATP) has been incorporated in ICD for potential painless termination of ventricular tachycardias. Current generations of ICDs are capable of delivering tiered therapies for multiple tachyarrhythmias detected in different zones, for example, ATP for a relatively slow ventricular tachycardia and defibrillation shocks for a fast tachycardia or fibrillation. All ICDs have bradycardia backup pacing, originally in the VVI mode, designed to prevent bradycardia after shock termination of VT/VF and bradycardia-induced tachycardia. With the recent development of dual-chamber devices, the role of ICDs have expanded from a pure antitachycardia platform to hemodynamic support and arrhythmia prevention (VVIR, DDDR).

Given the similarities of ICDs and pacemakers, the initial approach of a possible ICD malfunction is similar to that of a pacemaker. However, some problems are unique to patients with ICDs. Frequent ICD discharges, inappropriate interactions with permanent pacemakers, and antiarrhythmic drug effects on ICD performance represent major challenges in patient management.

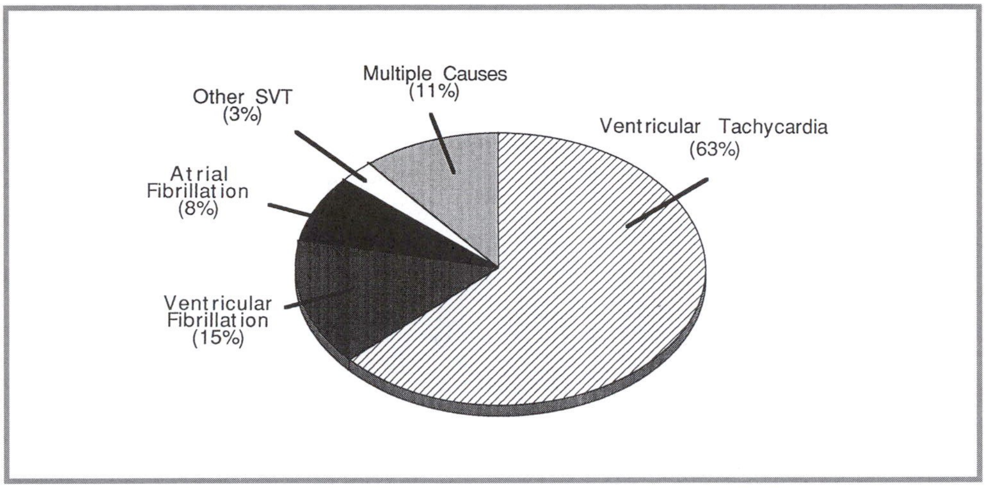

FIGURE 6-15

Patterns of frequent ICD therapy delivery from data collected at Temple University Hospital in 1996. The most common cause of frequent ICD shocks was ventricular tachyarrhythmias that triggered "appropriate" ICD response. Of all the causes of "inappropriate" ICD shocks, atrial fibrillation or sinus tachycardia were most often encountered.

FREQUENT ICD THERAPY

It is important to remember that patients may have multiple causes of ICD discharges (Figure 6-15). The potential causes for frequent ICD shocks include (1) increased frequency of VT/VF, either sustained or nonsustained episodes, (2) increased frequency of supraventricular arrhythmias, such as sinus tachycardia, atrial fibrillation/flutter, or other reentrant SVTs, (3) sensing malfunction, and (4) phantom shocks. The first step in proper management is to establish the correct diagnosis; treatment strategy must be individualized (Table 6-6). The most common cause of frequent shocks is recurrent ventricular the arrhythmias with appropriate ICD responses, which may be caused by changes in arrhythmogenic substrate such as new infarction, scar formation, ischemia, metabolic derangement, or worsening heart failure. Addition or withdrawal of antiarrhythmic drugs may also promote arrhythmia recurrences or convert nonsustained to sustained episodes. Improper programming of detection criteria with a short NID (number of intervals detected) slows rate cutoff and can lead to frequent, premature therapy delivery for nonsustained episodes, especially in a committed device. Management of recurrent episodes of VT/VF should first be focused on improving the underlying substrate, such as optimizing heart failure therapy and eliminating ischemia.

Causes of frequent ICD discharges:
- Increased frequency of VT/VF episodes
  - Sustained vs. nonsustained
- Increased frequency of supraventricular arrhythmias
  - Sinus tachycardia vs. atrial fibrillation/flutter vs. SVT
- Sensing malfunction
- "Phantom" shocks

TABLE 6-6

MANAGEMENT OF FREQUENT ICD THERAPY DELIVERY

ICD interrogations:
- Episode history:
  - Delivered vs. aborted therapy
  - Reconstruct event sequences: therapy efficacy
- Recorded intracardiac electrogram:
  - SVT vs. VT (inappropriate vs. appropriate therapy)
  - Tachycardia initiation and termination
- Real-time intracardiac electrogram
  - Lead stability, noise
  - Respiration, lead manipulation
- Lead impedance
  - Low: insulation failure
  - High: lead fracture

Ambulatory Holter monitor, event recorder:
- AF/flutter, atrial tachycardia, sinus tachycardia
- Nonsustained ventricular arrhythmias

Chest radiography/fluoroscopy:
- Lead dislodgment, lead fracture

Electrolytes/drug levels

Environmental interference

Causes of increased frequency of supraventricular arrhythmias:
- Changes in substrate
- Addition/withdrawal of antiarrhythmic drugs
- Nonsustained episodes in a "committed" device
- Programming error
- Lead dislodgment: mechanical stimulation

Indiscriminate use of antiarrhythmic drugs should be avoided because of the potential complex proarrhythmia interactions in unstable patients. Last, lead dislodgment can also induce frequent arrhythmias by mechanical stimulation, especially in patients with recently implanted devices.

Causes of increased frequency of supraventricular arrhythmias:
- Up to 30% of "inappropriate" ICD therapy
- Addition/withdrawal of antiarrhythmic medications/AV nodal blocking agents
- Worsening LV dysfunction and hemodynamics
- Exertion, fever, pneumonia, pericarditis

Up to 30% of ICD shocks were caused by supraventricular arrhythmias, most often sinus tachycardia or atrial fibrillation. Conditions such as fever, pneumonia, pericarditis, exercise or exertion, mental stress or anxiety, or worsening heart failure can cause rapid heart rates and trigger ICD shocks. The inappropriate therapy may in turn induce ventricular arrhythmias and result in a vicious cycle of incessant shocks. A magnet application in this situation renders the ICD "non-sense" and avoids inappropriate therapy. In most patients with recurrent supraventricular arrhythmias, the device can be reprogrammed to a higher rate cut-off or longer detection intervals to delay SVT detection. Detection inhibitors such as rate stability or sudden onset can also be activated to enhance discrimination between supraventricular and ventricular tachycardias. Furthermore, judicious use of antiarrhythmic agent(s) may be considered to reduce episode recurrences (class I or III agents) or impose better rate control (AV nodal blockers) in atrial tachyarrhythmias.

INTERACTIONS OF ANTIARRHYTHMIC DRUGS AND ICDS

The use of antiarrhythmic drugs in patients with ICDs is associated with a multiplicity of complex interactions (Table 6-7). Although antiarrhythmic drugs may decrease the frequency of sustained or nonsustained episodes of arrhythmias, careful considerations of the risk–benefit ratio must be given before therapy initiation. A rapid polymorphic ventricular tachycardia or fibrillation may be converted to a slower monomorphic tachycardia in the presence of antiarrhythmic drugs. Although this may improve the hemodynamic tolerance and enhance the efficacy of termination by antitachycardia pacing (ATP), the slowed arrhythmia rate can fall below the programmed detection parameters with underdetection and no therapy delivery. Antiarrhythmic drugs can also induce aberrant conduction or bundle branch block with QRS widening. During supraventricular arrhythmias, the abnormally wide QRS may negate the discrimination algorithms of ICDs and result in inappropriate therapy delivery. In addition, antiarrhythmic drugs can provoke AV conduction disturbances or heart blocks, which may exacerbate the pacemaker–ICD interactions (see following), as well as produce adverse hemodynamic decompensation. Finally, the risk of proarrhythmia (induction of new arrhythmias or development of incessant episodes) must be considered, especially in a patient population with arrhythmogenic substrates and unstable triggering factors.

Effects of antiarrhythmic drugs on defibrillation thresholds:
- Class IA: minimal effect on DFT in therapeutic dosage
- Class IB: mild elevation of DFT
- Class IC: significantly elevate DFT
- Class II: minimal effect on DFT
- Class III: variable amiodarone: depends on dose, duration, and route of administration

The influence of antiarrhythmic drugs on the defibrillation thresholds (DFT) has been examined. Approximately 15%–50% of ICD patients require antiarrhythmic drug treatment for

TABLE 6-7

POTENTIAL INTERACTIONS OF ANTIARRHYTHMIC THERAPY AND ICDS

- Decrease the frequency of sustained VT/VF
- Decrease/eliminate nonsustained episodes of arrhythmia
- Minimize supraventricular arrhythmias to reduce "inappropriate" device therapy
- Increase (or potentially decrease) defibrillation thresholds (DFTs)
- Alteration of VT rate:
  - Underdetection by the ICD due to slowing of VT rate
  - Improved hemodynamic tolerance with slowing of VT
  - Slower VT may improve the efficacy of termination by cardioversion or pacing
- Conduction disturbances:
  - QRS widening may confuse the detection criteria of ICD and deliver therapy for SVT
  - AV conduction disturbances that necessitate pacing and potentiate pacemaker–ICD interactions
- Proarrhythmia with frequent arrhythmias

management of frequent arrhythmia recurrences. In general, membrane-active drugs such as Vaughan William's class I and class III agents can affect the defibrillation energy requirement. No consistent effect on DFT was observed with the use of class IA drugs in therapeutic dosages. Class IB drugs (lidocaine and mexiletine) cause a concentration-dependent, reversible mild increase in defibrillation energy requirement. The use of class IC drugs should be avoided because significant elevation in DFT can result in addition to proarrhythmia. The effects of class III drugs can be variable. It appears that amiodarone lowers the DFT when administered acutely (intravenous or orally) but that chronic use of amiodarone may significantly elevate the defibrillation energy requirement. Therefore, repeated evaluation of ICD function is recommended after initiation of antiarrhythmic drugs. This should include induction of new arrhythmias, assessment of detection accuracy, efficacy of antitachycardia pacing and defibrillation threshold determination. Other drugs, including D-sotalol, *N*-acetylprocainamide (NAPA), and catecholamines may facilitate ventricular defibrillation and decrease the DFT.

In an increasing number of ICD patients with recurrent arrhythmias and frequent shocks, radiofrequency (RF) catheter ablation should be considered as a treatment option. Catheter ablation can be curative for elimination of SVTs such as atrial tachycardia, atrial flutter, AV nodal reentry, or orthodromic tachycardia utilizing a bypass tract. AV nodal modification or ablation provides an effective method for palliative rate control in patients with drug-refractory rapid atrial fibrillation. In patients with ventricular arrhythmias, although catheter ablation is rarely curative, it appears to be an effective and safe therapy to reduce the incidence of arrhythmia recurrences and perhaps ICD shocks.

ICD SENSING MALFUNCTIONS

Sensing abnormality is a potentially disastrous complication of ICD therapy. In addition to the usual device malfunctions associated with pacemakers such as lead dislodgment or insulation failure, several sensing problems are unique to ICDs. In patients who present with asymptomatic shocks, an ICD lead fracture must be excluded. Intermittent lead contact with make–break potentials can generate high-frequency electric noise that is sensed as ventricular fibrillatory signals with subsequent spurious shocks (Figure 6-16). A suspected lead fracture requires immediate attention and surgical revision because effective ICD therapy cannot be delivered during VT/VF.

Because of the robust sensing function of the ICDs, occasional double-counting of cardiac or extracardiac signals can be observed. During sinus tachycardia or high rate pacing, T-wave oversensing can result in an apparent fast heart rate with ensuing therapy delivery, especially in patients with metabolic abnormalities, electrolyte imbalance, or antiarrhythmic drug use (conditions that augment repolarization abnormalities). Occasionally, noncardiac signals such as myopotentials can also produce oversensing and inappropriate therapy. This phenomenon can be minimized by prudent reprogramming of the sensitivity or the refractory period of ICDs.

Causes of sensing malfunction:
- Adaptor malfunction
- Lead fracture
- Lead migration
- Double counting of cardiac/extracardiac signals:
  - Cardiac T-wave oversensing in sinus tachycardia or pacing
  - Noncardiac myopotentials sensing
- Electromagnetic interference (EMI)
- Sensing circuit component malfunction
- Interaction with other devices

ADVERSE DEVICE INTERACTIONS

Adverse ICD interactions with other devices such as a pacemaker or a neuromuscular stimulator unit have been documented. In a patient with a separate implanted pacemaker and an ICD, oversensing inhibition during ventricular tachyarrhythmias must be carefully excluded. During ventricular tachycardia or fibrillation, the pacemaker frequently undersenses the low-amplitude VT/VF signals and behaves asynchronously. The large pacing artifacts (several volts in amplitude) are detected as sinus rhythm by the auto-adjusting sensing function (0.2–0.5 mV in sensitivity) of ICDs, and the underlying ventricular fibrillatory signals are ignored; this may result in significant delays in VT/VF detection and inhibition of life-saving therapy.

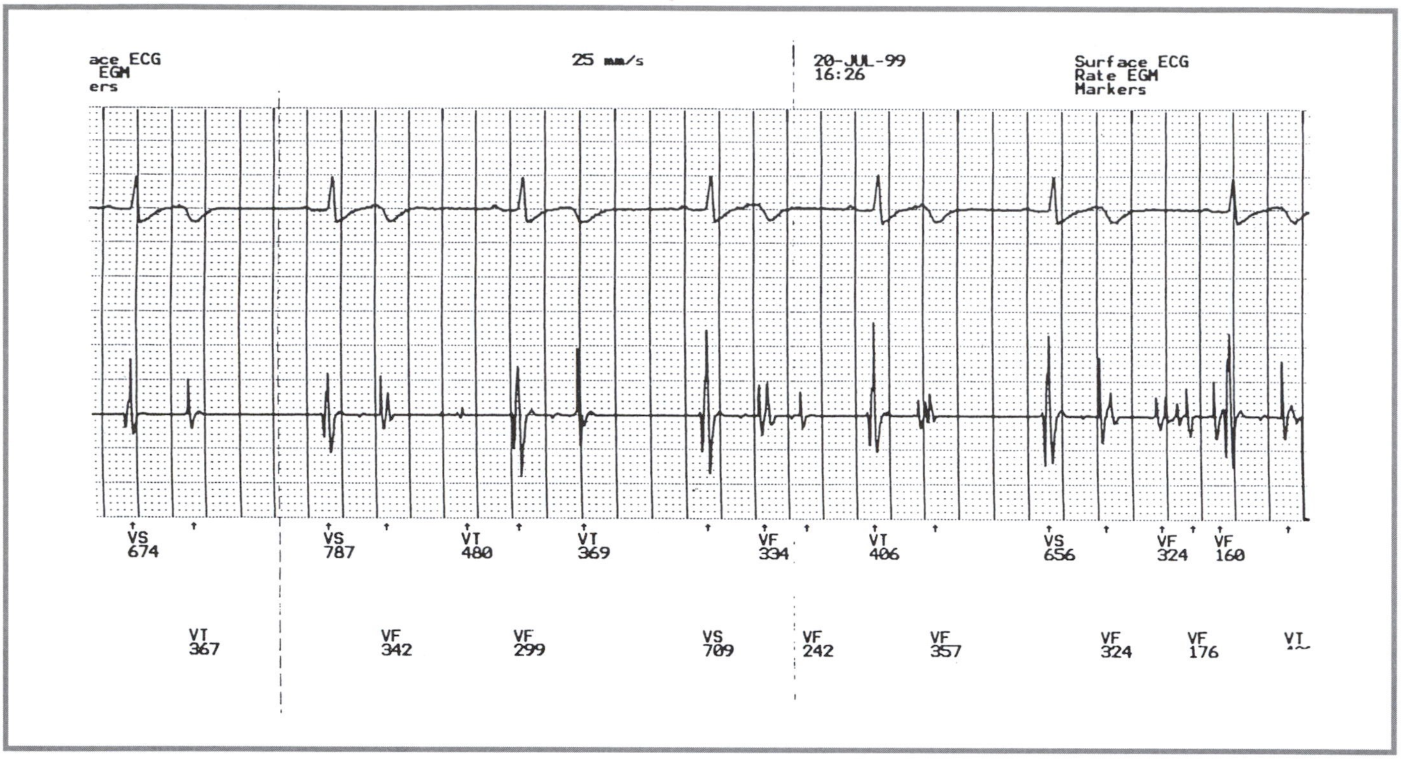

FIGURE 6-16

Spurious intracardiac signals generated by a fractured lead. The intrinsic regular signals represent sinus rhythm (VS) and correspond to surface QRS. The high frequency make–break signals were detected as (VT, VF) by the device and may result in inappropriate ICD shocks.

ELECTROMAGNETIC INTERFERENCE

Given the expanding indications of ICDs and pacemakers, electromagnetic interference (EMI) is a growing concern for patients (Table 6-8). Fortunately, it is usually not a clinically significant problem with proper precaution. Any strong electrical or magnetic field should be avoided. In a hospital environment, EMI is most frequently encountered with high-energy defibrillation/cardioversion shocks, or when direct electric current is applied to the patient, such as electrocautery (Bovie) machines or neuromuscular stimulator units (TENS). Magnetic resonance imaging (MRI) can also cause interference by generating secondary electrical currents from the magnetic field.

Low-amplitude, high-frequency electric current passage can be sensed by the implanted leads as either rapid intrinsic cardiac signals or noise (depending on the frequency and the specific device tolerance). This type of EMI can cause pacing inhibition and asystole in patients with implanted pacemakers. In patients with ICDs, the high-frequency signals may be detected as ventricular fibrillation with subsequent shock delivery. These situations are most commonly encountered intraoperatively and can be easily circumvented by applying a magnet over the device; this causes the ICD to behave asynchronously and ignore the electrical interference.

Potential adverse effects of shocks on implanted system:
- Irreversible damage to the pulse generator
- Reprogramming: reversion
- Stimulation thresholds:
  - Acute rise with loss of capture
  - Chronic rise with "exit block"
- Transient undersensing

The physician should also be familiar with the adverse effects of high-amplitude electrical surges (shocks) on implanted pacemakers and ICDs. Irreversible damage to pulse generators or leads is uncommon, albeit possible with direct electrode contact. Occasionally, reprogramming of the pacemakers with reversion to a nominal parameter setting can be observed. Direct effects of shocks on the myocardium also can cause changes in thresholds. An acute rise in

TABLE 6-8

ELECTROMAGNETIC INTERFERENCE (EMI)

In home and work environment:
- Electric arc welding, induction furnace
- Cellular phones, CB/amateur radios
- Large magnets
- Ignition cables, power tools
- Microwave ovens
- Antitheft devices

In hospital and clinic environment:
- Defibrillation, cardioversion
- Electrosurgery, electrocautery
- Diathermy
- Ultrasound therapy, lithotripsy
- Magnetic resonance imaging

stimulation threshold with loss of capture or a transient undersensing can occur immediately after shocks; this may facilitate arrhythmia recurrence as a result of asynchronous pacing (R-on-T phenomenon) or bradycardia-induced tachycardia. Occasionally, a chronic rise in pacing threshold with progressive scarring at the distal lead–tissue interface can be observed. Therefore, it is important to interrogate implanted devices after electrocautery, shock delivery, or other EMIs to exclude reversion or alteration of thresholds. In addition, ionizing radiation can also cause direct damage to the electronic circuitry of the implanted devices. The portals for radiation therapy should not include the generator and should be as far away from the implantable system as possible. A cardiologist or radiation oncologist, as well as the device manufacturer, should be consulted before initiation of treatment.

SUMMARY

The management of patients with implantable devices should include a thorough understanding of indications of pacemaker or ICD implantation, the device hardware and electronics, and a systematic evaluation to identify the potential causes of device malfunction. A combination of medical history, physical examination, and careful analysis of the interrogation data enables one to establish the correct diagnosis and develop a treatment strategy. Most patients can be managed with medication adjustment, device reprogramming, or a combination of these approaches. Occasionally, surgical revision of the generator or the lead(s) may be necessary. For those patients who present with frequent ICD shocks due to arrhythmia recurrences, catheter ablation is a viable option that can be performed safely with good efficacy.

REVIEW QUESTIONS

1. **With magnet application, the implanted pacemaker will do the following:**
   A. Slow the pacing rate
   B. Be deactivated
   C. Perform a threshold test
   D. Pace asynchronously

2. **A 73-year-old woman with a history of sinus node dysfunction, heart failure, and paroxysmal atrial fibrillation presented with complete heart block and syncope. The best selection of pacing mode is which of these:**
   A. VVI
   B. DDDR
   C. VVIR
   D. AAIR
   E. DDD

3. **In a patient with suspected pacemaker malfunction, what information is essential for proper evaluation?**
   - **A.** Brand name (manufacturer) and model number of the device
   - **B.** Indications for pacing therapy
   - **C.** Electrocardiographic monitoring
   - **D.** All the above
   - **E.** A and C

4. **A 70-year-old man has coronary artery disease, prior myocardial infarctions, renal insufficiency, and paroxysmal atrial fibrillation on procainamide. The patient also has an implantable defibrillator for ventricular tachycardia. He presented with five consecutive shocks while mowing the yard. What is the least likely cause of his ICD shocks?**
   - **A.** Rapid atrial fibrillation
   - **B.** Recurrent ventricular tachycardia
   - **C.** Lead fracture
   - **D.** Generator malfunction

5. **An elderly patient with renal insufficiency presented with an acute anterior myocardial infarction and underwent successful thrombolysis. He developed alternating bundle branch blocks on ECG with variable PR interval. Nonsustained ventricular ectopy was also noted on telemetry. What should you do?**
   - **A.** Administer procainamide for his ventricular ectopy
   - **B.** Insert a temporary pacing lead
   - **C.** Start beta-blocker therapy
   - **D.** Implant a defibrillator

ANSWERS

1. The answer is D. A magnet application will cause the pacemaker to pace asynchronously and not sense the intrinsic rhythm. Most pacemakers will pace at a specified "magnet rate." The magnet rate is usually faster than the programmed lower rate and may change when the battery is near the elective replacement index (ERI) or end-of-life (EOL) status. Few pacemakers will automatically perform a threshold test, and none will be deactivated as a consequence.
2. The answer is B. The patient requires ventricular pacing support for symptomatic heart block. A dual-chamber device should be considered to maintain atrioventricular synchrony in patients with heart failure. Rate responsiveness of the pacemaker is desirable in patients with sinus node dysfunction. Atrial pacing may also reduce the incidence of recurrent atrial fibrillation.
3. The answer is D. In a patient with suspected pacemaker malfunction, continuous monitoring is necessary because the device malfunction may be intermittent. The name and model number of the device are essential for proper interrogation of the battery voltage, lead impedance, and sensing and pacing thresholds. Knowing the indications for pacemaker implantation will facilitate patient management. For example, a pacemaker-dependent patient with complete heart block should receive the highest priority, with immediate intervention.
4. The answer is D. The defibrillator detected a fast heart rate while the patient was physically active. The patient has structural heart disease with ventricular and atrial tachyarrhythmias. The heightened adrenergic state during activity may have triggered recurrent ventricular tachycardia or rapid atrial fibrillation. The use of procainamide in patients with renal insufficiency is always a concern because procainamide clearance is determined by renal function. Toxic levels of antiarrhythmic drugs can also be proarrhythmic and must be excluded. Because most defibrillator systems utilize subclavian or cephalic veins for vascular access, a lead fracture is always a possibility when arm movements trigger defibrillator discharges. Device generator failure is rare.
5. The answer is B. In a setting of an acute myocardial infarction, prophylactic pacing is indicated in patients with high risk of developing complete heart block. These risk factors include: *new* bilateral (bifascicular) bundle branch block (for example, right bundle branch block with left anterior or posterior hemiblock), *alternating* bundle branch block, and first-degree AV block. Nonsustained ventricular ectopy in the periinfarct period is a concern. However, procainamide is contraindicated in the setting of infranodal conduction disturbances. Although beta-blocker therapy is recommended in postinfarction patients, it should be avoided at this time because of conduction disturbances. Further electrophysiologic evaluation may be required to define the patient's need for pacemaker or defibrillator implantation.

SUGGESTED READING

ACC/AHA Guidelines for implantation of cardiac pacemakers and antiarrhythmia devices: executive summary. Circulation 1998;97:1325–1335.

Allessie MA, Fromer M (eds) Atrial and Ventricular Fibrillation: Mechanisms and Device Therapy. Armonk, NY: Futura, 1997.

Dillon SM, Kwaku KF. Progressive depolarization: a unified hypothesis for defibrillation and fibrillation induction by shocks. J Cardiovasc Electrophysiol 1998;9:529–552.

Ellenbogen KA (ed) Cardiac Pacing. Oxford: Blackwell, 1992.

Hillis LD, Lange RA, Wells PJ, Winniford MD. Manual of Clincial Problems in Cardiology. Boston: Little, Brown, 1992.

Ideker RE, Zhou X, Knisley SB. Correlation amoung fibrillation, defibrillation, and cardiac pacing. PACE 1995;18[pt II]:512–525.

Kroll MW, Lehmann MH (eds) Implantable Cardioverter Defibrillator Therapy: The Engineering-Clinical Interface. Dordrecht the Netherlands: Kluwer, 1996.

Levine JH, Kadish AH, Reiter MJ. Transesophageal pacing and recording. In: Zipes J (ed) Cardiac Electrophysiology: From Cell to Bedside. Philadelphia: Saunders, 1992.

Podrid PJ, Kowey PR. Handbook of Cardiac Arrhythmia: Baltimore: Williams & Wilkins, 1996.

Strickberger SA, Man C, Daoud EG, Morady F. A prospective evaluation of catheter ablation of ventricular tachycardia as adjuvant therapy in patients with coronary artery disease and an implantable cardioverter-defibrillator. Circulation 1997;96:1525–1531.

DAVID E. CICCOLELLA

Enteral Feeding Tubes

CHAPTER OUTLINE

LEARNING OBJECTIVES

After studying this chapter, you should be able to do the following:

- Be familiar with the various methods for delivering enteral feeding.
- Know the indications and contraindications for using enteral feeding tubes.
- Know the complications associated with enteral feeding tube insertion.

The use of enteral nutrition dates from the ancient Egyptians and Greeks, who instilled nutrient directly into the rectum. Although the concept of enteral nutrition to treat disease and foster health remains the same, the delivery route has been modified only during the last century. The current consensus among intensivists is that nutritional support should be initiated early in the course of the critically ill patient. Early nutritional support is thought to shorten hospital stay and to support the increased metabolic demand resulting from illness or injury.

The initiation of nutrition in the intensive care unit can begin as either enteral or parenteral feeding or both. Parenteral feeding is considered in patients who are not suitable for enteral feeding. It is generally agreed, however, that enteral nutrition is superior to parenteral nutrition because it is associated with fewer complications and is more cost-effective (Table 7-1). In general, enteral nutrition should be started in patients with current or potential malnutrition caused by inadequate oral intake, with absence of clinical shock and an intact gastrointestinal tract. More specific indications and contraindications for enteral nutrition have been published by several medical and surgical societies. Some general indications and contraindications for enteral nutrition are shown in Table 7-2. In certain cases the legal guardian and physicians may decide that feeding is not to the patient's benefit, so long as this is within applicable hospital policy and laws. Some patients with certain clinical conditions may be considered for partial enteral support. Moreover, partial enteral support with low-volume feedings may help maintain gastrointestinal (GI) integrity. Considering the foregoing, to determine if a patient can safely tolerate enteral feeding, GI function should be evaluated.

Clinical indicators of GI function, such as bowel sounds and flatus, are nonspecific and do not portend tolerance of enteral feeding. Patients should be able to tolerate enteral feeding if the GI output is less than 500 ml/24 h. In intensive care unit (ICU) patients, some conditions that may produce excessively high GI outputs and therefore preclude the use of

Bowel sounds and flatus passage do not predict enteral feeding tolerance.

TABLE 7-1

ADVANTAGES OF ENTERAL COMPARED TO PARENTERAL SUPPORT

GI tract structure/function preservation
More efficient nutrient use
Avoiding central venous catheter insertion/postinsertion complications
Fewer infectious/metabolic complications
Easier administration
Lower cost

enteral nutrition are gastroparesis, intestinal obstruction, paralytic ileus, high-output enteric fistulas, *Clostridium difficile* colitis, severe idiopathic diarrhea, short-bowel syndrome (early stage), and severe GI bleeding. Enteral liquid feeding may buffer gastric acid and improve mild GI bleeding, however, and usually does not exacerbate mild lower GI bleeding. Therefore, if enteral nutrition is clinically indicated and in the absence of contraindications such as clinical shock and significant GI disease (e.g., abdominal distension, excessively high GI output, intractable vomiting, diffuse peritonitis, obstruction prohibiting use of bowel, ileus, ischemia, severe malabsorption, and massive GI bleeding), a trial of enteral nutrition should be attempted to determine if the GI tract can be safely used for feeding.

ENTERAL FEEDING TECHNIQUES

For short-term feeding and in the absence of contraindications, nasal or oral feeding is easy and convenient.

Once the decision for enteral nutrition is made, the physician must decide on the type of enteral feeding tube to deliver the nutrition. There are two possible approaches to enteral feeding: nasal or oral tube insertion (gastric or postpyloric) placed bedside, endoscopically, or fluoroscopically and tube enterostomy placed endoscopically, fluoroscopically, or surgically (Table 7-3). The anticipated duration of enteral feeding, tube preference, patient illness, GI condition (patency and motility), aspiration risk, and presence of intubation and mechanical ventilation will affect the type of approach. Primarily, the nasal/oral approach is considered for expected short-term use while tube enterostomies are considered for expected long-term use. Generally, for several reasons, gastrostomy and jejunostomy are preferred for patients with longer requirements for nutrition, usually more than 4 weeks.

TABLE 7-2

INDICATIONS AND CONTRAINDICATIONS TO ENTERAL FEEDING

- Indications: consider full support
  - Patients with current or potential malnutrition with inadequate oral intake
  - Full-thickness burns
  - Following massive (up to 90%) small bowel resection
  - Enterocutaneous fistula (low output <500 ml/day)
- Indications: consider partial support only
  - Partial bowel obstruction
  - Severe, unrelenting diarrhea
  - Enterocutaneous fistula (output >500 ml/day)
  - Severe pancreatitis or pseudocyst
  - Help maintain GI integrity
- Contraindications: full or partial support
  - Clinical shock
  - Gastrointestinal disease
    - Complete bowel obstruction
    - Intestinal bowel ischemia
    - Ileus
    - Massive GI bleeding
      - Short bowel syndrome
      - Intractable vomiting
      - Peritonitis
  - Within hospital policy/laws, legal guardian does not desire nutritional support

TABLE 7-3

SELECTING THE METHOD OF TUBE DELIVERY

A. Nasal/oral insertion: unguided bedside, endoscopic, or fluoroscopic
  - Nasal route preferred for nonintubated patients
  - Oral route preferred for mechanically ventilated patients
  - Gastric or postpyloric position

B. Transabdominal insertion: percutaneous, fluoroscopic, laparoscopic or surgical
  - Gastrostomy
  - Jejunostomy
  - Transgastric Jejunostomy

NASAL/ORAL GASTRIC/ENTERAL FEEDING TUBES

Generally, if the need for enteral feeding is thought to be short term (<4 weeks), the use of a nasally or orally inserted tube is easy and convenient so long as there are no specific contraindications. Some specific indications and contraindications for insertion of a nasal or oral feeding tube are shown in Table 7-4. The indications for nasoenteric feeding include patients with neurologic or psychological disorders that prevent adequate oral intake and patients with certain GI tract disorders from the mouth to the colon that prohibit eating. Indications for other conditions include burns, weakness due to acquired immunodeficiency syndrome (AIDS), and undergoing chemotherapy or radiotherapy. Nasoenteric tube feedings also may be used as supplementary nutrition to parenteral nutrition in patients with GI fistulas, by bypassing the fistulous tract, and during the transition to oral intake to decrease the risk for parenteral nutrition-associated complications. Nasoenteric tube feeding is contraindicated in

TABLE 7-4

INDICATIONS AND CONTRAINDICATIONS TO NASOENTERIC TUBE FEEDING

- Indications:
  - Neurologic disorders
  - Psychological disorders
  - Oropharyngeal/esophageal disorders
    - Neoplasms
  - Gastrointestinal disorders
    - Enteric fistulas (selected)
    - Short bowel syndrome
    - Inflammatory bowel disease
  - Pulmonary disorders
    - Intubation and mechanical ventilation
  - Total parenteral nutrition (TPN)
    - TPN transition to oral intake
    - Enteric fistulas: adjunctive feedings to TPN
  - Unspecified
    - Acquired immunodeficiency syndrome
    - Chemotherapy/radiation therapy
    - Burns
- Contraindications (some):
  - Absolute contraindications
    - Facial/cranial abnormalities or injuries (some)
    - Nasopharyngeal obstruction
    - Esophageal obstruction (stricture or malignancy)
    - Complete gastric or intestinal obstruction
    - Incomplete gastric or intestinal obstruction (controversial)
    - Ileus (fluid and electrolyte abnormalities, infection, narcotics, sepsis, or trauma)
    - Recent GI surgery (i.e., fresh suture lines)
    - Long-term enteral feeding requirement (>4–6 weeks)
  - Some relative contraindications:
    - Coagulopathy/thrombocytopenia
    - Esophageal varices
    - Acute GI hemorrhage
    - Inflammatory bowel disease (very active)

TABLE 7-5

RISK FACTORS FOR NASAL/ORAL EF TUBE INSERTION-RELATED COMPLICATIONS

Neurologic
Altered mental status: coma, delirium
Neuromuscular blocking drugs
Nasal/oropharyngeal/laryngeal/tracheal
Septal deviation/nasal polyps
Impaired gag reflex
Decreased laryngeal sensitivity
Recent endotracheal intubation
Gastroesophageal
Esophageal stricture/web/obstruction
Gastric obstruction

patients with complete gastric or intestinal obstruction. In partial obstruction, patients typically have nausea, vomiting, and bloating, and the use of enteral feeding is controversial.

In critically ill patients requiring a nasal/oral feeding tube, tube insertion may result in significant complications. Before a feeding tube is inserted, the physician should carefully assess the patient for an intact GI tract and risk factors for complications during nasal/oral insertion. These factors can be grouped into neurologic, nasooropharyngeal, and pulmonary-related risk factors (Table 7-5).

In the ICU, the nasal route is preferred for nonintubated patients and the oral route preferred for intubated patients on mechanical ventilation in either the gastric or more preferable postpyloric duodenal position. However, initially a large-bore nasogastric tube is usually inserted to start enteral feeding; this allows for regular aspiration of stomach contents, which is important to evaluate for adequate absorption of feedings and possibly for bleeding. The larger-bore nasogastric tube (14–18 Fr.) is usually made of stiff polyvinyl chloride (PVC) and is easy to insert. However, this large-bore tube is usually replaced by a smaller-bore (8–12 Fr.) polyurethane or silicone tube designed to enable transpyloric passage to deliver nutrients into the proximal duodenum theoretically to reduce the risk of aspiration.

Nasal or orally inserted tubes may be placed in the gastric or transpyloric position or duodenal or jejunal positions.

The nasoenteric small-bore tubes available from a variety of manufacturers vary in length, diameter, material, stylet type and lubrication, and the presence of a weighted tip. There are also combination enteral tubes, composed of stiff outer, large-caliber PVC tubing and a more pliable inner small-caliber silicone tubing, that may help with insertion or gastric decompression. The choice of tube diameter and length depends on its use and placement: gastric, ~33 in.; duodenal, ~43 in.; jejunal, ≥48 in. Weighted tips may help with gastric insertion in the presence of cuffed endotracheal tubes but probably provide no advantage in attaining transpyloric passage. Otherwise, there are no major differences and tube choice should be based more on familiarity, ease of use, and cost.

Procedure for Feeding Tube Insertion

The approximate length of the tube for nasal insertion can be individually estimated by placing the tip of the tube on the xiphoid process and then wrapping the tube around the patient's ear and extending it to the tip of the nose. For oral insertion, the tube is extended to the corner of the mouth. A longer tube guided by endoscopic or fluoroscopic methods may be considered for placement beyond the pylorus. After selection of the feeding tube, the tube may be inserted using the following procedures:

Nasal Feeding Tube Insertion

1. Place the patient in a comfortable, semiupright position.
2. Put a small amount of water-based lubricant around the nasal vestibule to facilitate passage.
3. Start the insertion of the tube along the inferior aspect of the nose and advance it slowly until it is in the posterior pharynx.

4. Request the patient to swallow repeatedly to promote esophageal placement.
5. The tube should be advanced to approximately 40–45 cm for placement into the stomach.
6. The tube is taped to the nose with a loop of tubing approximately 5–10 cm left to allow for migration into the small intestine. Taping the tube to the nose by anchoring a tube loop to the ipsilateral cheek base will help to avoid upward tension and pressure on the anterior nare.

Oral Feeding Tube Insertion

1. The tube should be directed posteriorly through the mouth using the index finger to negotiate the bend in the posterior pharynx into the esophagus.
2. The tube is advanced to 40 cm from the incisors.
3. To assess position, approximately 100 ml of air should be instilled while auscultating over the stomach, as this distends the stomach and promotes transpyloric migration.
4. The patient should then be placed on their right side; the tube advanced another 15 cm and secured with tape.
5. An x-ray should be taken after the patient has remained on the right side for 1 h.

Assessing Tube Placement

The methods for assessing tube placement include physical signs and roentgenography (Table 7-6). Physical signs can be helpful during the initial insertion procedure of a feeding tube. One method to help evaluate tube placement in the gastrointestinal tract is by measuring the pH of aspirated gastric material. Physical signs such as auscultation after insufflation of air into the tube, observing for cough, and testing the patient's ability to speak are helpful but more unreliable in confirming tube position. Because physical signs are not reliable in confirming tube position and the complications of tube misplacement are significant, confirmation of tube placement by abdomen and/or chest roentgenogram is required. If the location of the feeding tube is still unclear, injection of the tube with a small amount of radiopaque liquid (e.g., meglumine diatrizoate) can confirm its location; this is especially helpful in distinguishing between gastric and proximal duodenal placement.

Physical examination signs of tube placement are helpful but unreliable to confirm tube placement.

Enteral tube placement requires confirmation by radiography.

Postpyloric tube feeding, especially distal to the ligament of Treitz, may be preferred theoretically over gastric feeding because this may reduce the risk of gastric feeding residua and aspiration, but spontaneous transpyloric passage of the feeding tube (usually within 8–24 h) in critically ill patients is usually unsuccessful because gastric atony is common. To promote the transpyloric placement of feeding tubes, promotility agents, stylets, and guided insertion can be used. The promotility agents include metoclopromide, 20 mg, or erythromycin, 200–400 mg intravenously, which are administered approximately 30 min before tube insertion. However, use of prokinetic agents alone is usually ineffective in critically ill patients, and methods to guide insertion into the correct position are needed. Some literature suggests use of inner stylets by an experienced and proficient operator may facilitate transpyloric placement of feeding tubes. If duodenal placement does not occur after several hours, fluoroscopic or endoscopic guidance may be used.

Transpyloric placement of feeding tubes may be aided by promotility agents, stylets, and guided insertion.

TABLE 7-6

ASSESSING NASAL/ORAL FEEDING TUBE PLACEMENT

Physical signs
Aspiration of gastric contents
Air insufflation and abdominal auscultation
Observe for cough and patient's ability to speak
Submerge tube end under water and observe for air bubbles
Color and pH testing of aspirates
Roentgenography
Abdominal x-ray
Injection of radiopaque liquid (5–10 ml) if needed to verify gastric versus proximal duodenum

Accordingly, the American College of Chest Physicians (ACCP) recommends using fluoroscopic guidance to place small-bore feeding tubes transpylorically for the early initiation of feeding, especially in those patients requiring feeding for more than 3 weeks, unconscious or mechanically ventilated patients, and those with significant gastric residua despite use of promotility agents. Alternatively, endoscopic placement of the feeding tube is recommended as it is usually successful and allows immediate initiation of enteral feeding.

Complications

Tube insertion-related complications are usually related to tube misplacement and generally to the anatomic areas traversed.

Intubated patients on mechanical ventilation are at significant risk of tube misplacement because of cuff compression of the esophagus and ability of small feeding tube to pass into the trachea.

Long-term use of oral/nasal feeding tubes may result in nasopharyngeal and laryngeal stenosis and pharyngeal and vocal cord paralysis.

Enteral feeding tube complications may be divided into insertion- and postinsertion-related complications (Table 7-7). These complications are related to the anatomic areas traversed and can be further grouped into nasopharyngeal-otic-sinus, gastrointestinal, pulmonary, and metabolic complications. The complications of enteral feeding tube insertion, especially using small-bore tubes with stiff guidewires, are usually secondary to tube misplacement; these include perforation of the esophagus and of the lung into the pleural space. Patients on mechanical ventilators with inflated endotracheal tube cuffs are at significant risk, probably owing to cuff compression of the esophagus posteriorly and the ability of the stiffened feeding catheter to slide past the cuff into the trachea.

The postinsertion tube complications include GI tract erosion and ear and sinus infections. Aspiration is a major complication of enteral feeding tubes, whereas prolonged use of nasal tubes may result in nasopharyngeal and laryngeal stenosis as well as pharyngeal and vocal cord paralysis. Other complications related to the amount and type of tube feedings such as underlying metabolic disorders are not within the scope of this chapter.

TABLE 7-7

NASAL/ORAL ENTERAL FEEDING TUBE COMPLICATIONS

A. Insertion-related complications
   - Nasal-oropharyngeal
     - Nasal trauma
     - Pharyngeal irritation-induced vomiting
   - Gastroesophageal
     - Esophageal perforation/hemorrhage
   - Respiratory
     - Feeding tube perforation into lung/pleural space
     - Hemoptysis
     - Hydrothorax/pneumothorax
     - Bronchopleural fistula
     - Pneumomediastinum
     - Subcutaneous emphysema

B. Postinsertion-related complications
   - Nasal-oropharyngeal-oto-sinus
     - Ear, nasal/sinus infections
     - Nasopharyngeal stenosis
     - Laryngeal stenosis
     - Pharyngeal/vocal cord paralysis
   - Gastroesophageal
     - Tube dislodgement/migration (especially esophagus)
     - GI mucosal tract erosion (by tube tip)
     - Esophageal stricture
   - Respiratory
     - Infused solution aspiration
     - Enteral feeding pneumonia/pleural effusion
     - Bacterial pneumonia/empyema
   - Intrinsic tube problems
     - Bursting/breakage
     - Kinking
     - Obstruction

TRANSABDOMINAL TUBE ENTEROSTOMIES: GASTRIC, JEJUNAL, AND TRANSGASTRIC JEJUNAL

The long term use of nasal feeding tubes (>4–6 weeks) may lead to nasopharyngeal and laryngeal stenosis and suppurative sinusitis. Nasal feeding tubes can be dislodged or obstructed. In patients requiring long-term nutritional support, access in the form of gastrostomy or jejunostomy is required. These tubes have a larger diameter, with less tendency to clog and easier and more rapid feeding and medication delivery. Gastrostomy and jejunostomy tubes are more convenient and aesthetically acceptable. The tubes have less tendency to migrate, which may decrease the aspiration risk.

Gastrostomy Tubes

Transabdominal gastrostomy can be placed surgically, laparoscopically, endoscopically, or fluoroscopically. Percutaneous gastrostomy can be placed with endoscopic or fluoroscopic guidance. Alternatively, gastrostomy can be placed surgically. Usually surgical gastrostomy is a simple procedure performed during another abdominal surgical procedure. However, the laparotomy exposes the patient to the risk of ileus, wound infection, and dehiscence. Furthermore, major complications are more common (2.5%–16%) and may reflect poorer patient condition (elderly, high-risk, general anesthesia) compared to those patients undergoing percutaneous gastrostomy. In acceptable patients, the method of choice for gastrostomy tube placement is percutaneous endoscopic gastrostomy (PEG) because it is safe, technically easier, cheaper, and postoperatively less painful than surgical gastrostomy. Although experience with laparoscopic techniques is limited, laparoscopic gastrostomy may be indicated if PEG technically cannot be performed. Fluoroscopic percutaneous techniques may be an alternative to PEG in which endoscopy cannot be performed.

In acceptable patients, the preferred method for gastrostomy tube placement is percutaneous.

The specific indications and contraindications for PEG tube placement are listed in Table 7-8. It can generally be considered in patients who have an inability to eat, normal gastric emptying, low risk for pulmonary aspiration, and absence of near total pharyngeal or esophageal obstruction to allow for performance of endoscopy. Contraindications include patients at risk for aspiration in such conditions as gastric outlet obstruction, gastric atony, documented gastroesophageal (GE) reflux, and prior history of aspiration. These patients may

Consider a PEG tube for patients who have an inability to eat, normal gastric emptying, low risk for pulmonary aspiration, and an absence of bowel obstruction, especially nearly complete pharyngeal or esophageal obstruction, which prevents endoscopy.

TABLE 7-8

PERCUTANEOUS ENDOSCOPIC GASTROSTOMY: INDICATIONS AND CONTRAINDICATIONS

- Indications
  - Prolonged need (usually >4 weeks) for enteral feeding
  - Impaired swallowing or access/obstructive conditions
    - Oropharyngeal dysphagia
    - Partial esophageal dysphagia or oropharyngeal obstruction
    - Neurologic conditions
    - Neoplastic disease (oropharynx, larynx, esophagus)
  - Head/facial trauma
- Contraindications
  - Absolute
    - Functional impairment/obstruction of GI tract
    - Documented gastroesophageal reflux
  - Technical (absolute)
    - Inadequate transillumination
    - Inability to approximate anterior abdominal and gastric walls
    - Near-total esophageal or oropharyngeal obstruction
    - Subtotal gastrectomy
  - Technical (Relative)
    - Uncorrectable coagulation abnormalities
    - Gastric wall disease (inflammatory, infiltrative, neoplastic)
    - Ascites
    - Prior abdominal surgery

be considered for gastrojejunostomy. Other contraindications include large esophageal varices, sepsis, left upper quadrant skin burns, and anterior abdominal or gastric wall malignancy or infection, as well as technical aspects such as uncorrectable coagulopathy, inability to pass the endoscope (e.g., upper GI obstruction) or to approximate the anterior abdominal and gastric walls (e.g., because of massive ascites, prior gastric surgery, intestinal loop interposition resulting from prior adhesions or musculoskeletal abnormalities). Massive ascites, especially after large-volume paracentesis, obesity, and previous abdominal surgery, are relative contraindications.

There are several variations on the original technique for percutaneous gastrostomy tube placement. Although a detailed description of these techniques is beyond the scope of this volume, the original and most popular of these is performed through a pull technique described in 1980 by Gauderer and others. Briefly, the technique entails insertion of a endoscope through the esophagus and into the stomach, after which air is insufflated, resulting in stomach distension with approximation of the anterior gastric and abdominal walls and transverse colon displacement distally. The optimal insertion site, which is identified by maximal transillumination, is along the left lateral rectus muscle and below the left lobe of the liver. This site is transilluminated endoscopically, confirmed by digital palpation, and followed by a 1-cm incision and insertion of a catheter needle. Under continued endoscopic observation, a heavy suture with a looped distal end is passed through the catheter and snared with a polypectomy loop. Both the endoscope and suture are then drawn up the gastrointestinal tract and out of the patient's mouth. The PEG catheter is then securely tied to the suture, drawn into the esophagus and, under endoscopic guidance, through the gastroesophageal junction and juxtaposed to the anterior wall. After endoscopic stomach decompression and endoscope removal, the inner and outer bumpers are secured.

Complications with PEG tube placement are uncommon, with a mortality rate approximately 0.3%–1% and a morbidity rate of 3%–5.9% in the largest series. Overall and serious complication rates have been reported as 15% and 3%, respectively. Complications include infection of the cutaneous insertion site, which is the most common complication, necrotizing fasciitis, peritonitis, septicemia, aspiration, peristomal leakage, tube dislodgement, bowel perforation, pneumoperitoneum, gastrocolocutaneous fistula and internal bumper irritation/erosion into the abdominal wall, and GI bleeding (Table 7-9). A gastrocolocutaneous fistula may be caused by inadvertent needle puncture of a displaced colon loop. Pneumoperitoneum due to gastric wall puncture is usually not clinically significant, but if fever and abdominal pain develop, a gastrograffin study should be performed to exclude a leak. Excessive tension on the tube may result in gastric wall necrosis leading to GI bleeding or to separation of the anterior gastric/abdominal walls during feeding, leading to peritonitis. Use of prophylactic antibiotics may reduce peristomal wound infection; antibiotics are needed only in those patients not receiving appropriate antibiotics for other infections. Excessive tension between the inner and outer bumpers may cause pressure necrosis of the wall caus-

TABLE 7-9

PERCUTANEOUS ENDOSCOPIC GASTROSTOMY (PEG): COMPLICATIONS

- Infection
  - Insertion site wound infection
  - Necrotizing fasciitis
  - Septicemia
  - Peritonitis
- GI hemorrhage
- Gastrocolocutaneous fistula
- Pneumoperitoneum
  - Bowel perforation
- Aspiration
- Peristomal leakage
- Tube dislodgment
- Internal bumper irritation/erosion into the abdominal wall

TABLE 7-10

JEJUNOSTOMY: GENERAL INDICATIONS AND CONTRAINDICATIONS

- Indications
  - Repeated tube feeding-related aspiration
    - Severe gastroesophageal reflux
    - Gastroparesis
    - Neurologic disorders
  - Previous gastric resection
  - Gastrocutaneous fistula
  - Postoperative laparotomy (required gastric decompression/enteral feeding)
- Contraindications
  - Regional or radiation enteritis
  - Small bowel ischemia (especially needle-catheter jejunostomy)
  - Ileus
  - Postjejunal obstruction
  - Short bowel syndrome
  - Intermittent or bolus feedings

ing tube dislodgment. Nonendoscopic replacement of a dislodged tube can only be considered in a mature fistulous tract; otherwise, this is performed endoscopically.

Jejunostomies and Transgastric Jejunostomies

Jejunal tubes can be placed using endoscopic, fluoroscopic, laparoscopic, or surgical methods. However, for jejunostomy tubes, surgical and fluoroscopic techniques are better. The small intestine is small and narrow, making it difficult to insert a jejunal feeding tube percutaneously. The laparoscopic indications and techniques are still evolving and may be an alternative to the percutaneous endoscopic procedure. Specific procedures include the surgical jejunostomies: needle-catheter jejunostomy (NCJ) and subserosal tunnel jejunostomy (Witzel procedure), percutaneous endoscopic jejunostomy (PEJ), or a transgastric jejunostomy (TGJ). Although still controversial, the most common indication for jejunal tube placement is to help prevent repeated feeding-related aspiration, especially in medical conditions with high aspiration risk such as severe gastroesophageal reflux, gastroparesis, and neurologic disorders. The other indications include patients with prior gastric resection or gastrocutaneous fistula, and also in postoperative abdominal surgery because small intestinal motility is usually restored more quickly than gastric motility (Table 7-10). Some contraindications to jejunostomy tube placement include ileus, distal bowel obstruction, radiation and regional enteritis, and anesthetic considerations. Furthermore, jejunal feedings must be continuous because bolus feeding is not tolerated as well as when the stomach is used as a reservoir. General complications of jejunostomy are included in Table 7-11. Some complications are more specific to the type of procedure.

> Some jejunostomy variations include percutaneous endoscopic or fluoroscopic, needle-catheter and subserosal, a combination of gastric and jejunal access, and transgastric.

> Proposed indications for jejunostomy include possible prevention of aspiration, prior gastric resection, and postoperative gastroparesis.

> Jejunal feedings must be continuous because bolus feeding is not well tolerated.

The NCJ is the method of choice in many centers and is usually performed at the time of laparotomy for another indication. The procedure does require a proficient and experienced operator. It involves the insertion of a needle into the small intestine, after which a polyethylene catheter is inserted through the needle and then through the anterior abdominal wall. Other than catheter leakage, tube obstruction, catheter displacement, and diarrhea,

TABLE 7-11

JEJUNOSTOMY TUBES: COMPLICATIONS

- Wound infection
- Proximal/distal tube migration
- Intestinal obstruction
- Intraabdominal leak
- Small intestine ischemia/infarction
- Tube malfunction: clogging

complications specific to NCJ include small bowel ischemia, pneumatosis intestinalis (1%), and small bowel obstruction (<1%). Feedings should be held for patients at risk for bowel ischemia, which include those who are hypotensive or receiving vasopressors.

Percutaneous endoscopic jejunostomy (PEJ) is a method to obtain access to the stomach and jejunum for decompression and jejunal feeding. The procedure, which is technically difficult, essentially involves the initial placement of a large-bore PEG tube followed by coaxial insertion of a smaller jejunal tube. However, the gastric and jejunal portions may be ineffective for decompression and jejunal feeding, respectively, because of tube problems. Transgastric jejunal tubes provide better and easier access to the stomach and small intestine than the PEJ tube, allowing gastric decompression and jejunal feedings. These tubes are especially useful in critically ill patients who undergo laparotomy and commonly require gastric decompression and enteral nutritional support. The transgastric jejunal tube procedure can be performed radiologically or surgically, but the endoscopic technique has not been perfected.

SUMMARY

Enteral feeding appears to be superior to parenteral nutrition because it is associated with fewer complications and is more cost-effective. Although there are specific indications and contraindications to enteral tube feeding, in general enteral feeding should be started in patients who have an intact GI tract, no obstructions, GI output less than 500 ml/day, and are at risk for malnutrition. Methods of feeding discussed in this chapter may be able to circumvent some of these contraindications. Some conditions in ICU patients such as intestinal obstruction, ileus, enteric fistulas, *Clostridium difficile* colitis syndrome, and severe GI bleeding can produce high GI output and preclude the use of enteral tube feeding. Accordingly, GI tract function should be carefully evaluated for safe use in ICU patients before tube placement.

There are two general approaches for delivering enteral tube feeding: nasal/oral feeding tubes and tube enterostomies such as gastrostomy and jejunostomy performed by fluoroscopic, laparoscopic, endoscopic, or surgical methods. Nasal or oral enteric feeding tubes are primarily used for patients requiring short-term feeding while the more invasive procedures are required for patients requiring long-term feeding. For nasal or oral enteric feeding tubes, many types of small-caliber tubes are available. Some tube characteristics such as lubrication, stylet type, weighted tip, and promotility agents may help with insertion or postpyloric tube placement because the main goal for small-caliber tube placement is the small bowel. Fluoroscopic and endoscopic guidance methods have been used for postpyloric tube placement in the duodenum and jejunum. Confirmation of correct tube placement requires interpretation of radiographic plain films. The long-term use of nasal or oral feeding tubes may lead to complications, especially in the upper airway, and generally patients needing long-term enteral feeding will require tube enterostomy such as gastrostomy and jejunostomy.

Gastrostomy can be generally considered in patients who have an inability to eat, normal gastric emptying, low risk for pulmonary aspiration, and absence of bowel obstruction. A percutaneous endoscopic technique cannot be technically performed in the presence of nearly complete pharyngeal or esophageal obstruction due to inability to pass the endoscope. Otherwise, PEG is generally the procedure of choice. Other indications for gastrostomy include patients who have access problems or facial trauma, pharyngeal or esophageal obstruction, and oral pharyngeal dysphagia. Contraindications include patients at risk for aspiration, but these patients may be considered for gastrojejunostomy; it carries a low complication rate, especially compared to surgical placement. Although still controversial, the most common indication for jejunostomy placement is to help prevent repeated feeding-related aspiration, especially in medical conditions with high aspiration risk. Other indications include prior gastric resection and postoperative abdominal surgery. The types of feeding jejunostomy tubes include surgical jejunostomies such as needle-catheter jejunostomy (NCJ) or subserosal tunnel (Witzel procedure), percutaneous endoscopic jejunostomy (PEJ), and transgastric jejunal tubes. Jejunostomy feedings must be continuous because bolus feeding is not tolerated well.

The clinician has a number of available techniques and tubes, each with their own indications, contraindications, and associated risk for complications to provide safe enteral nutrition for patients. Further ongoing refinements in tube technology and techniques will continue to expand and improve the options for enteral nutrition.

REVIEW QUESTIONS

Each of the questions below has one best answer.

1. **Which statement regarding enteral feeding is false?**
   - **A.** Should be avoided in patients with paralytic ileus.
   - **B.** Should be avoided in all patients with gastrocutaneous fistula.
   - **C.** Is cheaper and associated with fewer complications than parenteral nutrition.
   - **D.** Helps to prevent intestinal atrophy.
   - **E.** May increase gastric pH and improve mild gastrointestinal bleeding.

2. **A 60-year-old man with diabetes mellitus and amyotrophic lateral sclerosis develops respiratory failure secondary to pneumonia and requires mechanical ventilation. After 4 weeks of nasoduodenal feeding for persistent gastric atony, the patient develops nasopharyngeal stenosis. Of the following, the most appropriate method to provide nutrition is:**
   - **A.** Total parenteral nutrition (TPN)
   - **B.** Nasogastric tube feeding
   - **C.** Open gastrostomy
   - **D.** Nasojejunal tube
   - **E.** Jejunostomy
   - **F.** Percutaneous endoscopic jejunostomy
   - **G.** Transgastric jejunal

3. **Contraindications to enteral support in any amount include all except:**
   - **A.** Clinical shock
   - **B.** Complete bowel obstruction
   - **C.** Intestinal bowel ischemia
   - **D.** Paralytic ileus
   - **E.** Enterocutaneous fistula (output 700 ml/day)

4. **Complications that can occur during nasal or oral enteral feeding tube insertion/placement include all except which of the following:**
   - **A.** Esophageal perforation
   - **B.** Esophageal variceal rupture
   - **C.** Pericardial effusion
   - **D.** Pneumothorax
   - **E.** Fatal intracranial placement

5. **In assessing the patient for a nasal feeding tube, *known* factors increasing risk for complications associated with feeding tube insertion include all the following except:**
   - **A.** Delirium
   - **B.** Septal deviation
   - **C.** Esophageal web
   - **D.** Gastric obstruction
   - **E.** Impaired gag reflex
   - **F.** Congestive cardiomyopathy

6. **The most reliable methods to distinguish between gastric and duodenal placement of a enteral feeding tube are:**
   - **A.** Testing pH and color of aspirated fluid
   - **B.** Air insufflation and abdominal auscultation
   - **C.** Plain abdominal roentgenogram
   - **D.** Aspiration of bile

7. **An absolute contraindication to percutaneous endoscopic gastrostomy (PEG) is:**
   - **A.** Ascites
   - **B.** Oropharyngeal dysphagia
   - **C.** Previous abdominal surgery
   - **D.** Partial (25%) esophageal obstruction
   - **E.** Prior subtotal gastrectomy

ANSWERS

1. The answer is B. A nasoenteric tube can be placed more distally to bypass the fistulous tract. Compared to parenteral nutrition, enteral feeding is cheaper, associated with fewer complications, and helps to prevent intestinal mucosal atrophy even with as little as 10 ml/h.
2. The answer is G. At this time the patient continues to have persistent gastric atony that would preclude oral, nasogastric tube, and open gastrostomy feeding. Although nasaljejunal tube feedings are suitable for short-term use, the patient has been on nasal tube feeding for 4 weeks and has also developed a complication of prolonged nasal tube feeding. Other jejunal feeding methods would be appropriate, and several can be considered, such as percutaneous endoscopic jejunostomy (PEJ), jejunostomy (by laparotomy, laparoscopic, or fluoroscopic methods), and trans-gastric jejunostomy (by surgical or fluoroscopic methods). Jejunostomies are usually indicated for patients with temporary gastric reflux or atony. PEJ can provide simultaneous access to the stomach and jejunum for decompression and jejunal feedings. However, the technique is difficult, the gastric component often provides ineffective decompression, and the jejunal component frequently returns to the stomach. Transgastric jejunostomy has advantages over the PEJ or jejunostomy as it can provide more effective gastric decompression and enteral feeding until gastric dysfunction resolves, and then, if needed, provide for directly administered gastric feeding.
3. The answer is E. Although enteral nutrition can be administered to patients with enterocutaneous fistula, they should be monitored carefully. Enteral feedings during clinical shock may cause bowel ischemia and infarction, especially in those patients with acute risk for bowel ischemia. Intestinal bowel ischemia may result in bowel infarction. Further evaluation would be required to determine if feeding could be given. Complete bowel obstruction is an absolute contraindication. For paralytic ileus due to a wide variety of reversible and nonreversible causes, the physician should evaluate and treat the cause while parenteral nutrition is administered.
4. The answer is C. The insertion of small-bore feeding tubes has less risk for complications than the insertion of central venous lines for parenteral nutrition. Despite improvements in enteral feeding tube technology for more accurate insertion and placement (e.g., better radiopaque tube quality, self-lubrication, and less rigid stylets), a number of misplaced tubes have resulted from increased use of small-bore tubes. Placement of small-bore feeding tubes should be performed carefully, especially in intubated patients on mechanical ventilation. Pericardial effusion has not been noted as a complication directly associated with nasal or oral tube insertion. To help avoid intracranial placement, exercise more caution in patients with maxillofacial or basilar skull fractures and use oral insertion or endoscopy. In general, if resistance is met during tube insertion, discontinuation of tube placement may help avoid a number of complications such as esophageal perforation, esophagitis, gastrointestinal perforation, and pneumothorax. The risk of esophageal variceal rupture may be reduced by using a smaller, softer tube and caution with guidewires.
5. The answer is F. Congestive cardiomyopathy is not a known risk factor for feeding tube insertion. The other factors have been described in the literature.
6. The answer is C. A plain roentgenogram of the abdomen is very reliable. However if the location (stomach or proximal duodenum) of the feeding tube is still not clear, injection of a radiopaque liquid can help verify the location. Of the physical signs, testing pH and color of aspirated fluid is more reliable than the other physical signs, but both have some problems.
7. The answer is E. Depending on the amount of residual stomach present, other surgical techniques may be helpful; all the others are relative contraindications. Massive ascites was initially an absolute contraindication, but if the ascites is drained and the bowel is not interposed between the anterior gastric and abdominal walls, the technique can be performed. Previous abdominal surgery may cause technical problems, but the abdomen needs further evaluation including CT scan imaging. For partial (25%) esophageal obstruction, PEG can be performed if the obstruction is less than near total to allow endoscopy to be performed.

SUGGESTED READING

American Society of Parenteral and Enteral Nutrition. Board of Directors. Guidelines for the use of enteral nutrition in adult and pediatric patients. J Parenter Enteral Nutr (JPEN) 1993;17(Suppl 4).

American Society of Parenteral and Enteral Nutrition. Board of Directors. Guidelines for the use of enteral nutrition in adult and pediatric patients. Enteral access devices. J Parenter Enteral Nutr (JPEN) 2001 (in press).

Cerra FB, Benitez MR, Blackburn GL, et al. Applied nutrition in ICU patients. A consensus statement of the American College of Chest Physicians (ACCP). Chest 1997;111:769–778.

Klein S, Kinney J, Jeejeebhoy K, et al. Nutritional support in clinical practice: review of published data and recommendations for further research directions. J Parenter Enteral Nutr 1997;21:133.

Napolitano LM, Bochicchio G. Enteral feeding of the critically ill. Curr Opin Crit Care 2000;6:136–142.

Souba WW. Nutritional support. N Engl J Med 1997;336:41–48.

Zaloga GP. Bedside method for placing small bowel feeding tubes in critically ill patients. Chest 1991;100:1643–1646.

World Wide Web Sites

American Society for Parenteral and Enteral Nutrition: www.clinnutr.org

American Society for Clinical Nutrition: www.faseb.org/ascn

American Gastroenterological Association: www.gastro.org

CHAPTER 8

Vadim Leyenson

Common Procedures in the Intensive Care Unit: Thoracentesis, Lumbar Puncture, Paracentesis, and Pericardiocentesis

CHAPTER OUTLINE

LEARNING OBJECTIVES

After studying this chapter, you should be able to do the following:

- Know the general methods of aseptic and local anaesthesia techniques in most common ICU procedures.
- Know the most important indications and contraindications for thoracentesis, lumbar puncture, paracentesis, and pericardiocentesis.
- Know how to diagnose and treat complications associated with the described procedures.
- Know the common methods of performing thoracentesis, lumbar puncture, paracentesis, and pericardiocentesis.

Several general conditions should be fulfilled before performing any type of invasive procedure. First, the benefits and nature of the procedure and possible complications should be explained in full to the patient and their family member. An informed consent, preferably written, should always be obtained before performing any procedure.

Second, care should be taken to minimize patient discomfort during the performance of any intervention. Much psychological comfort can be provided by reassuring and communicating with the patient before and during the procedure. A well-organized procedural plan includes the proper number and types of instruments, available monitoring equipment, and intravenous access—all to be prepared beforehand. Proper planning shortens the time of an intervention and provides a sense of comfort to both the patient and the operator.

Third, the correct type and dose of anesthetics have great value in the conduct of any procedure. In most cases, especially for the procedures discussed in this chapter, local anesthesia, usually with topical infiltration of lidocaine, is suggested. However, in some ICU patients undergoing procedures, the systemic use of analgesic, sedative, or paralytic agents may be employed on occasion to control agitation or discomfort.

Informed consent, patient comfort, and sterile technique are important for any type of procedure.

Finally, optimal positioning not only facilitates the performance of a procedure but also may help avoid complications. Because infection is a common complication of a variety of procedures, special attention should be devoted to performing procedures with aseptic, sterile technique. Generally, the skin over the procedural site is carefully and thoroughly cleansed with an antiseptic solution over an area that extends at least 4 to 6 in. in all directions from the selected site. A sterile drape with the center hole taped around the site of skin entry is required, and the operator is appropriately gowned and gloved to ensure sterile operator technique.

In this chapter, we discuss the diagnostic and therapeutic procedures that are commonly used in ICU patients. Special attention is given to the indications, the technique of performance, and the adverse effects of the procedures most commonly performed.

THORACENTESIS

The pleural cavity is a potential space for accumulating fluid resulting from different pathophysiological conditions. There is always a small amount of fluid in the pleural space. This thin layer of fluid acts as a lubricant and helps the visceral pleura to move efficiently along the parietal pleura during respiratory excursions. The normal amount of pleural fluid has not been formally established; however, it is agreed that up to 3–5 ml of fluid may normally be present in each pleural space at any given time.

Indications

Indications for thoracentesis can be divided in two major categories: diagnostic and therapeutic. A diagnostic thoracentesis is performed to sample the pleural effusion to evaluate the type and character of the fluid and to confirm or exclude certain pathophysiologic states. A therapeutic thoracentesis serves to remove fluid that may represent a nidus for persistent infection (e.g., empyema) or to drain an excessive amount of effusion to avoid respiratory compromise secondary to the restrictive effects of a large pleural effusion on thoracic performance.

Contraindications

The major contraindication for thoracentesis is coagulopathy.

The main contraindication to thoracentesis is the presence of a coagulopathy or hemorrhagic diathesis. We recommend measuring not only prothrombin time but also partial thromboplastin time and a platelet count before the procedure. Also, blood urea nitrogen and creatinine should be measured in patients with suspected renal insufficiency because patients with azotemia may have serious platelet dysfunction. If necessary, coagulopathy or platelet abnormalities should be corrected or minimized before the procedure. A thoracentesis should be avoided in areas of cutaneous infection. Obviously, if the patient is hemodynamically unstable, stability should be restored before the procedure.

Site Selection

Before any attempts at thoracentesis, the amount and location of pleural effusion should be confirmed, at least by chest x-ray imaging. It is important to establish whether the pleural effusions are free flowing or located. One of the simplest diagnostic tests is a supine and bilateral decubital chest x-ray. If the position of the pleural effusion changes, a free-flowing pleural effusion is most likely present. Ultrasound imaging can also be used and is especially helpful in cases of smaller or loculated pleural effusions as it allows the operator to locate and measure the collection of pleural fluid more precisely. However, ultrasound is more expensive and sometimes more difficult to obtain. Physical findings such as percussion dullness, reduced or absent breath sounds, and loss of tactile fremitus are all very helpful in the identification and localization of pleural effusions. Thoracentesis should be performed one interspace below the spot where percussible sounds become dull, several inches posteriorly from the supine, a location where the ribs are wider and more easily palpated. The precise location for penetration of the skin should be just superior to a rib (Figure 8-1). This location avoids the arteries, veins, and nerves that run just inferior to the rib, thereby minimizing the risk of pleural bleeding and intercostal nerve injury.

Thoracentesis should be performed with the needle advanced into the pleural cavity over the superior aspect of a rib.

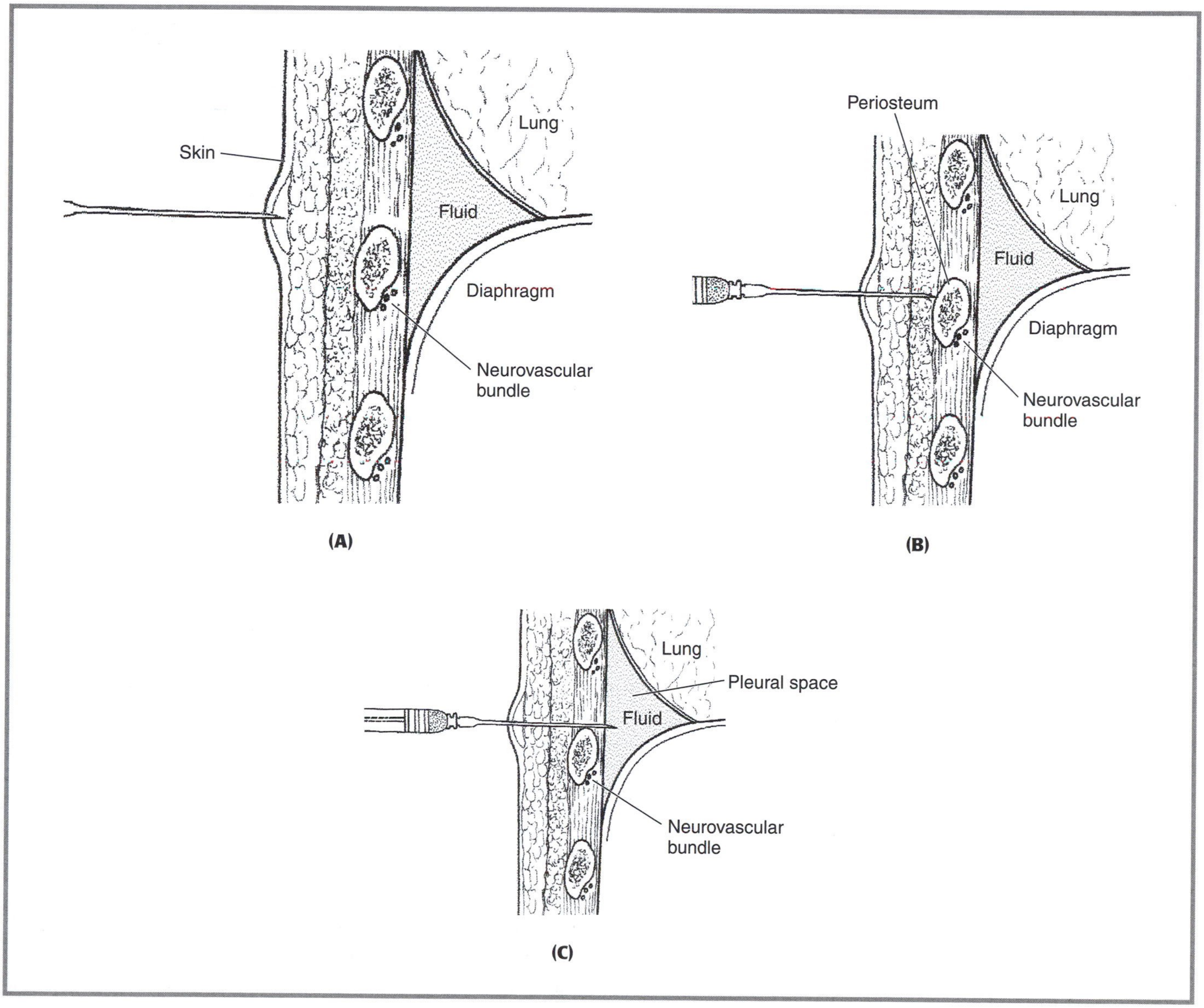

FIGURE 8-1

Thoracentesis technique. **(A)** The skin is injected with 1% lidocaine. **(B)** The periosteum is injected with 1% lidocaine. **(C)** The pleural space is entered above the rib to avoid injury to the vessels and nerve. (From Light RW. Pleural Diseases, 3rd Ed. Baltimore: Williams & Wilkins, 1995:313, Figure 23–2.)

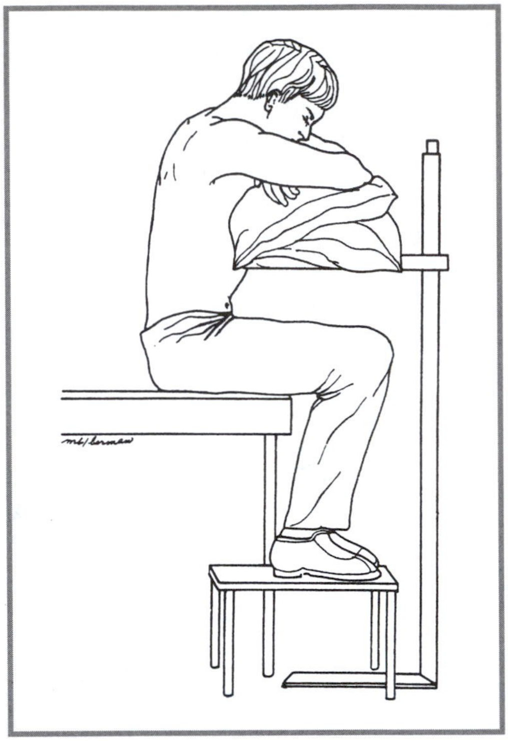

FIGURE 8-2

Positioning for thoracentesis. The sitting position, with the arms supported by the bedside table and feet resting on a footstool, is recommended for thoracentesis. (From Light RW. Pleural Diseases, 3rd Ed. Baltimore: Williams & Wilkins, 1995:312, Figure 23–1.)

Patient Position

In the intensive care unit, thoracentesis may be performed while the patient lies recumbent with the head of the bed elevated close to 90°. In this case, thoracentesis is performed in the midaxillary line.

Correct positioning of the patient has a significant role in the successful performance of a thoracentesis. Usually, the patient is placed in the sitting position with the arms supported on the bedside table and the feet resting on a footstool (Figure 8-2). It is recommended that the patient be positioned with the back vertical so that the pleural fluid remains posteriorly and dependent second to gravitational effects. For an ICU patient too ill to sit erect, a thoracentesis may be performed in the supine position with the head of the bed elevated close to a 90° angle. In this position, thoracentesis is performed in the posterior axillary line after localization by ultrasound.

Technique

The materials required to perform a thoracentesis (Table 8-1) should be assembled before starting the procedure. Once the thoracentesis puncture site is identified and sterilely prepared, the skin is anesthetized with a 25-gauge needle, connected to a 5-ml syringe, and filled with 1% lidocaine solution, creating a skin wheal. Then, with a 20-22-gauge needle, the operator should anesthetize the deeper subcutaneous tissues, the rib periosteum, and the parietal pleural (see Figure 8-1). The needle, positioned above the rib, may be slowly advanced into the pleural space with continuous aspiration followed by the injection of about 0.2–0.3 ml of lidocaine every 1–2 mm. This technique guarantees anesthesia of the parietal pleural and avoids accidental injection of lidocaine into the skin or intercostal vessels. When pleural fluid is aspirated back into the syringe, the syringe and needle should be withdrawn from the pleural space and a thoracentesis catheter should be inserted. Pleural fluid is withdrawn by a 50-ml syringe connected via a three-way stopcock to the pleural catheter and sampling container (Figure 8-3).

Sometimes no pleural fluid is obtained when the 1.5-in., 22-gauge needle is inserted into the pleural space. In this situation, the needle should be slowly withdrawn with constant aspiration. The reason is that the rim of the pleural fluid is sometimes thin and may be missed as the needle is inserted. If there is no fluid obtained even after the needle is withdrawn, we suggest changing the point of skin penetration one interspace inferiorly. If penetration is still

TABLE 8-1

MATERIALS AND EQUIPMENT REQUIRED TO PERFORM THORACENTESIS

MATERIALS FOR LOCAL ANESTHESIA AND STERILE TECHNIQUE	MATERIALS FOR PLEURAL FLUID DRAINAGE	MONITORING EQUIPMENT
Lidocaine, 1%	Thoracic needle and catheter ($n = 1$)	Pulse oximeter
25-gauge needle ($n = 1$)	Three-way stopcock ($n = 1$)	Inflatable blood pressure cuff
20-gauge needles ($n = 2$) 5-ml syringe ($n = 1$) 10-ml syringe ($n = 1$)	50-ml syringe Tubes for pleural fluid ($n = 3$) Sterile bag or container for pleural fluid	
Sterile gloves Sterile gauze pads Sterile drape with center hole Band-aids Aseptic solution Alcohol swabs		

unsuccessful, ultrasound localization may be helpful. After the procedure is completed, it is important to obtain a chest x-ray to exclude pneumothorax. The skin wound is covered by a sterile dressing at the end of the procedure.

Pleural Fluid Analysis

If thoracentesis is performed for diagnostic reasons, pleural fluid should be collected in special tubes, which are usually provided by almost all types of thoracentesis kits, and sent for chemistry analysis, which includes protein, glucose, LDH. Cytology, bacterial Gram stain, and aerobic and anaerobic cultures should also be done. We recommend sending at least 50–100 ml of pleural fluid for cytologic examination, an amount of fluid that may increase the diagnostic sensitivity for cytologic analysis. A separate specimen may be needed for pleural fluid pH analysis. For pH sampling, we recommend that the pleural fluid be placed

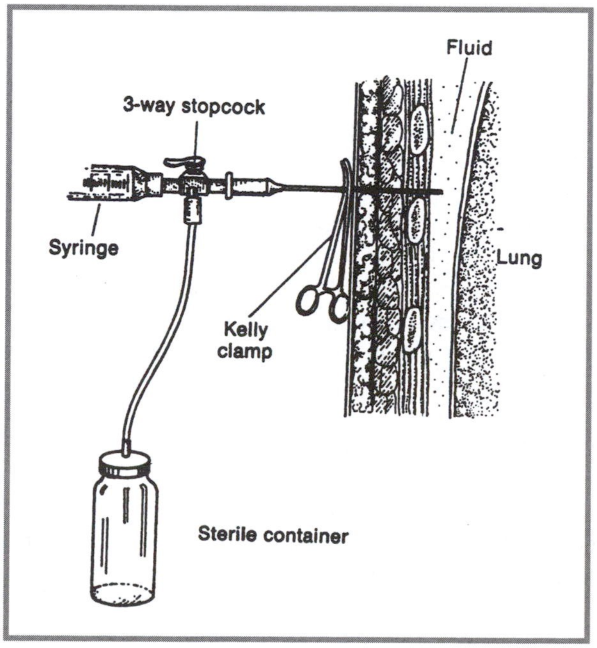

FIGURE 8-3

Final step of thoracentesis. Pleural fluid is withdrawn by a 50-ml syringe connected via a three-way stopcock to the pleural catheter and sampling container. (From Civetta JM, Taylor RW, Kirby RR. Critical Care, 3rd Ed. Philadelphia: Lippincott, 1997.)

in an arterial blood gas syringe with the specimen inserted in ice and delivered to the lab as soon as possible. Delays in pleural fluid processing may significantly alter the pH.

Complications

Pneumothorax is the most common complication of thoracentesis.

The most common complication of thoracentesis is pneumothorax. The incidence of pneumothorax after thoracentesis varies significantly, ranging from 5% to 20%. However, serious pneumothorax requiring chest tube placement occurs relatively rarely and probably occurs in less than 5% of all cases of pneumothorax resulting from thoracentesis.

Another complication of thoracentesis is hemothorax, which usually occurs as a result of injury to the intercostal artery. This complication can usually be avoided if thoracentesis is performed just superior to a rib, as previously described. However, in certain conditions, such as severe pulmonary hypertension or bronchiectasis, or in older patients, the intercostal arteries may be tortuous and hemothorax can result even when proper technique is performed. An infection of the pleural space is a rare complication of thoracentesis. About 2% of all pleural infections are caused by infection of the pleural space during thoracentesis. Strict enforcement of sterile technique during thoracentesis is necessary to help prevent this complication.

Postthoracentesis reexpansion pulmonary edema is a rare, although potentially serious, complication. The etiology and pathogenesis of this complication are complex and not well established. It may occur when the lung is reexpanded too rapidly and stretch lung injury causes noncardiogenic pulmonary edema. However, this complication is preventable and almost never occurs when the pleural fluid is withdrawn slowly. For this reason, we do not recommend using vacuum bottles for thoracentesis and prefer to aspirate the pleural fluid slowly by manual methods. The amount of fluid that is safe to remove while avoiding reexpansion pulmonary edema is controversial. However, it is generally believed that up to 1500 ml of pleural fluid can be safely withdrawn without causing reexpansion pulmonary edema.

The patient may also develop a vasovagal episode during thoracentesis, which is characterized by bradycardia, decreased cardiac stroke volume, and a fall in blood pressure. A vasovagal reaction occurs secondary to stimulation of the parietal pleura if not properly anesthetized. This reaction can be treated and prevented by intramuscular administration of 1 mg atropine. Other rate complications of thoracentesis include splenic and hepatic puncture, soft tissue infection, and adverse reactions to the local anesthetic.

PARACENTESIS

Indications

The major indication of paracentesis is to evaluate the etiology of ascites or remove excessive amounts of fluid.

Indications for paracentesis can be also divided into therapeutic and diagnostic categories. A diagnostic paracentesis is particularly important in patients with ascites, unexplained fever, or leukocytosis or suspicion for peritonitis. Diagnostic paracentesis can also be used to rule out intraabdominal hemorrhage in patients with a rapid increase in ascitic fluid that previously was well controlled by medical therapy. Therapeutic paracentesis is usually performed in patients with respiratory compromise secondary to the restrictive effect of severe, massive ascites. Paracentesis is also occasionally recommended in patients with hepatorenal syndrome with the intention of decreasing intraabdominal pressure and increasing renal artery perfusion.

Site Selection

The best site for paracentesis is the left flank of the lower abdomen lateral to the rectus abdominis muscle.

The most important aspect of site selection is choosing an avascular site on the abdominal wall. The usual point for penetration is the lower abdominal wall, just lateral to the rectus abdominis muscle in the left lower abdominal quadrant; other sites can also be used (Figure 8-4).

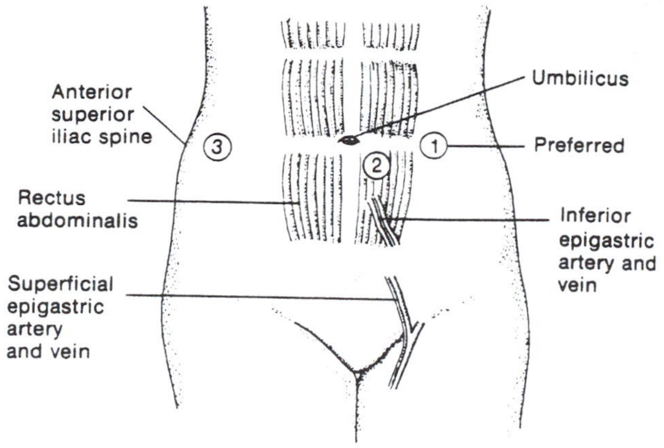

FIGURE 8-4

Possible sites for paracentesis. The preferred site is on the left side of the lower abdomen, lateral to the rectus abdominis muscle. (From Civetta JM, Taylor RW, Kirby RR. Critical Care, 3rd Ed. Philadelphia: Lippincott, 1997.)

Procedure

The patient is placed in the supine position. Before the procedure, it is very important to ensure that the urinary bladder is well drained to avoid accidental bladder injury. Also, before the procedure the operator should confirm the presence of ascitic fluid at the site of intended paracentesis, which is usually done by percussion of the anterior abdominal wall. On occasion, ultrasound guidance may be used. In most cases, however, physical examination suffices. The skin in the area of the intended procedure must be cleaned and sterilely draped. Skin anesthesia is achieved by creating a skin wheal with injection of 1% lidocaine, using a 25-gauge needle. Lidocaine is then injected with a larger needle (e.g., 20-gauge needle), first through the skin wheal and then through the fascia and peritoneum. When the peritoneal space is entered, a "pop" or decrease in tissue resistance is felt. Every time the needle is advanced, aspiration should be applied until ascitic fluid is returned. At this point, the needle is removed, and a 20-gauge angiocatheter attached to at least a 20-ml syringe is entered through the anesthetized area into the peritoneal space. When ascitic fluid returns, the catheter is advanced over the needle, the needle is then removed, and a 5-ml syringe is connected to the catheter. Care should be taken to avoid pulling the catheter back over the needle because this may shear off the catheter tip into the peritoneal space.

The total amount of ascites fluid that can be safely withdrawn remains unknown. However, probably as much as 2 l of fluid can be withdrawn without creating any significant side effects. The ascitic fluid should be sent for specific gravity, protein, cell count, cytology, Gram stain, and culture. If there is a clinical suspicion of pancreatitis, a sample can also be sent for amylase. The gross appearance of ascitic fluid may also play a significant role in the differential diagnosis of various disease states.

Complications

Complications of paracentesis, which are uncommon, include bleeding, injection, bowel or bladder perforation, and a persistent leak of ascitic fluid. Occasionally, hypotension may develop after therapeutic paracentesis if an excessive volume of fluid is withdrawn.

LUMBAR PUNCTURE

Indications

The major indication for lumbar puncture of the ICU patient is to obtain spinal fluid for chemical and microbiological analysis, as well as opening pressure measurements, to diagnose or exclude CNS infection, subarachnoid hemorrhage, or increased intracranial pressure

The major indication for the performance of lumbar puncture is for diagnostic purposes.

states. Occasional indications may include administration of analgesics following surgery or trauma, or for pain relief in conditions such as reflex sympathetic dystrophy. Lumbar puncture can also be used as a route to administer antibiotics.

Contraindications

Absolute contraindication for lumbar puncture is full anticoagulation or severe coagulopathy, because of the significantly increased risk of epidural hematoma formation with severe neurologic sequelae. Cutaneous infection of the site of the procedure also represents an absolute contraindication. Lumbar puncture should be avoided if there is evidence of increased intracranial pressure secondary to a space-occupying lesion. In these circumstances, withdrawal of spinal fluid may lead to brainstem herniation. Therefore, it is very important to exclude an intracranial mass or abscess by physical exam or head CT scan before performing this procedure.

Technique

The fetal position is optimal for the performance of lumbar puncture in the ICU setting.

Before attempting lumbar puncture, one should clearly identify bony markings and properly position the patient. The operator should remember that the space between the vertebrae varies depending on the patient's position, weight, and height. Occasionally, osteoarthritis and spinal fusion can completely obliterate the space between the vertebrae and make the procedure extremely difficult. Positioning of the patient is absolutely critical for success in performing this procedure. The lateral decubitus position is used more frequently in the ICU because most critically ill patients are not able to sit. The patient should assume the fetal position, which is achieved by flexing the knees to the chest and flexing the neck. This position allows greater separation between the vertebrae and, therefore, facilitates penetration of the invertebral space (Figure 5A,B). If the patient is in the flexed lateral decubitus position, a line projected between the iliac crests crosses over the L4 vertebra or L4–L5 interspinal space. In most cases, the spinal cord terminates at the level of L2. Therefore, a lumbar puncture procedure performed at level of L4–L5 rarely causes any spinal cord injury.

Assistance may be necessary for this procedure, especially in the ICU setting. An assistant facilitates patient positioning and monitors vital signs. Different commercial lumbar puncture kits can be used with care to ensure aseptic technique. The choice of the kit depends on local preference and economics. Any kit used should include the items listed in Table 8-2.

Method

Several approaches may be used to perform a lumbar puncture. A midline approach is most commonly used during lumbar puncture and is considered the preferred method. After skin infiltration with a few milliliters of a local anesthetic, a special needle with an introducer is inserted into the interspinal ligament at the L3–L4 or L4–L5 interspace (Figure 8-6). The spinal needle is passed through the introducer and carefully and slowly advanced in a slightly cephalad direction. A typical decrease in resistance occurs as the needle traverses the ligamentum flavum and approaches the subarachnoid space. When spinal fluid is seen in the needle hub, a manometer is attached to measure spinal fluid pressure. Normal spinal fluid is "tear-clear" in gross appearance. After measuring pressure, a sample of spinal fluid is collected for cytology and cell count, protein and glucose determinations, serology, and microbiology. At the end of the procedure, the point of entry is closed with a sterile bandage and the patient is placed in the supine position.

Complications

Headache is the most common complication following a lumbar puncture. It can be prevented by maintaining the patient in the supine posture several hours after performance of the procedure.

Headache is probably the most common complication of lumbar puncture and is believed to be due to persistent cerebrospinal fluid (CSF) leak. The onset of headache may not occur until several hours after the procedure and worsens if the patient does not maintain the supine

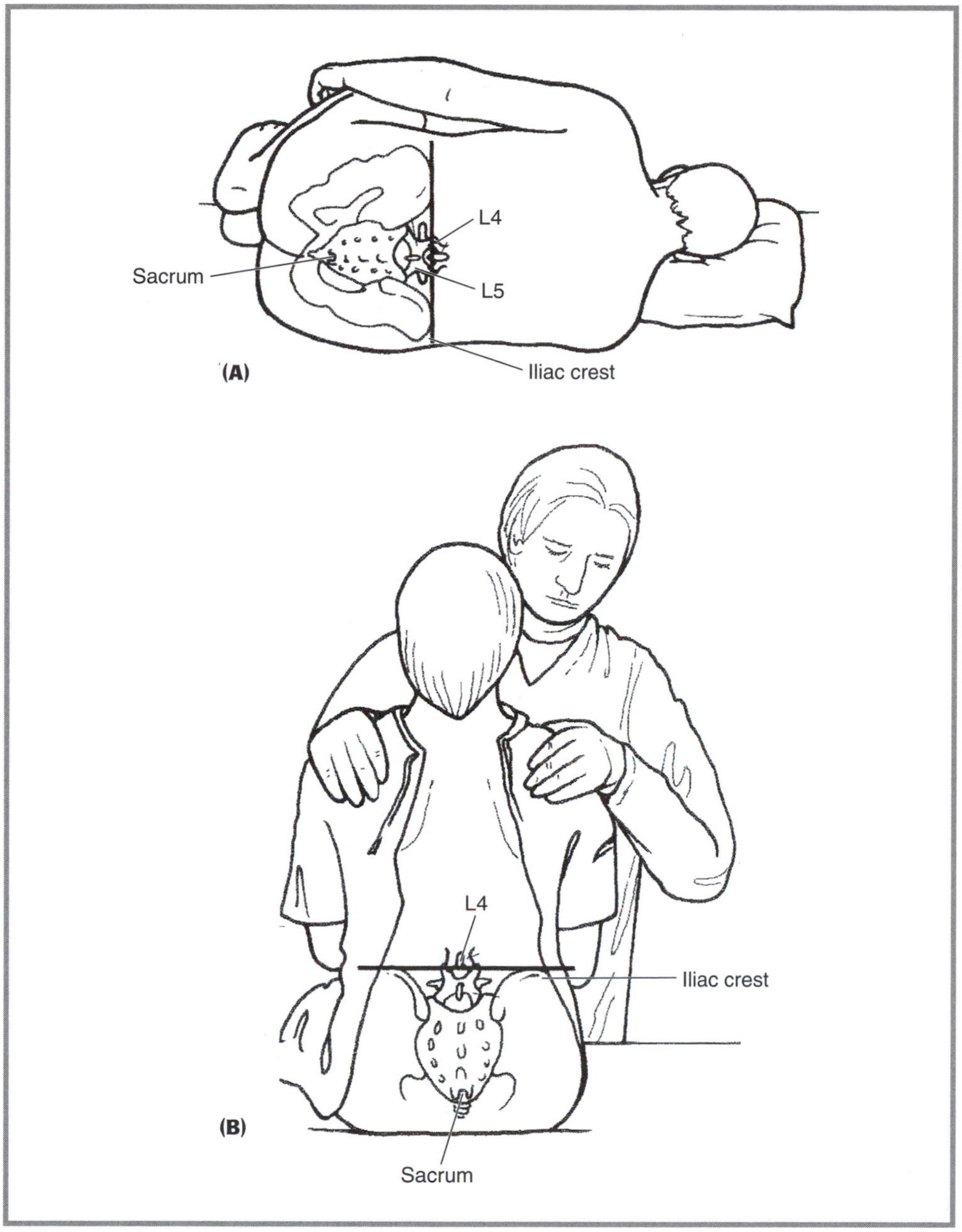

FIGURE 8-5

Positioning for lumbar puncture. **(A)** Lateral decubitus position. **(B)** Sitting position. A line connecting the iliac crests crosses over L4 or the L4–L5 interspace.

TABLE 8-2

MATERIALS REQUIRED TO PERFORM LUMBAR PUNCTURE

MATERIALS FOR LOCAL ANESTHESIA AND STERILE TECHNIQUE	MATERIALS FOR OBTAINING SPINAL FLUID
Aseptic solution	Spinal needle
Sterile gloves	Spinal fluid collection tubes (*n* = 4)
Sterile gauze pads	Manometer tubing
Sterile drape with center hole	
Sterile gauze pads	
Lidocaine, 1% solution	
25-gauge needle (*n* = 1)	
10-ml syringe (*n* = 1)	
Bandage	

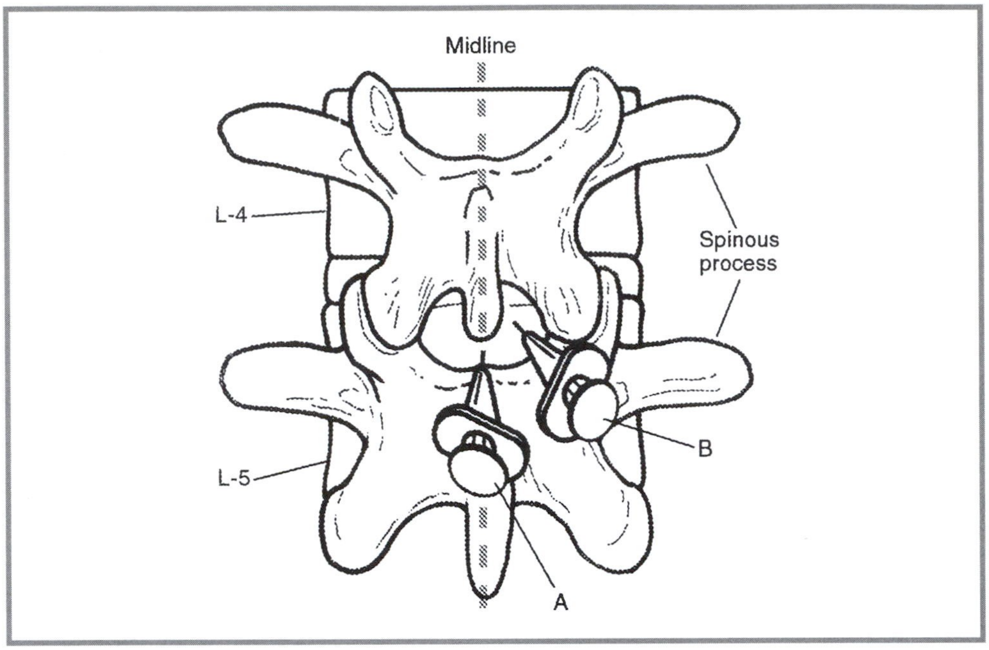

FIGURE 8-6

Lumbar puncture approaches. **(A)** Midline approach. **(B)** Paramedian approach. A midline approach is recommended.

position. Headache usually resolves with bed rest, fluids, and analgesics. However, in severe cases of headache, an epidural block patch can be applied. (The description of this technique is beyond the scope of this chapter.) The occurrence of headache after a lumbar puncture is prevented in most cases by 6–8 h of bed rest.

The most common cause of neurologic damage following lumbar puncture is needle trauma, which usually affects a single spinal nerve. The risk of trauma to the spinal cord is very remote, especially if the lumbar puncture is performed below the level of the conus medullaris. Any complaints of pain from the patient during insertion of the lumbar puncture needle must be taken seriously and evaluated immediately. Any suspicion of spinal cord injury should lead to immediate termination of the procedure.

Epidural hematoma in most cases follows anticoagulant therapy. The main symptom is severe backache with progressive paraplegia. This complication is a surgical emergency. The treatment of choice is surgical decompression. Epidural abscess is also a life-threatening complication and surgical emergency. The usual presentation is fever, leukocytosis, pain, and paraplegia. The diagnosis requires a high level of clinical suspicion and CT or MRI confirmation. Adhesive arachnoiditis is a serious but rare complication that can lead to severe disability. The symptoms are pain, paralysis, and impairment of bowel function. The abscess rarely occurs with a simple lumbar puncture; it usually follows accidental injection of an irritant solution into the arachnoid space. The disorder is characterized by fibrosis and distortion of the arachnoid space. Unfortunately, clinical symptoms and signs may not be evident for weeks after the procedure. There is no definite treatment for this complication.

PERICARDIOCENTESIS

Normally, as much as 50 ml of fluid can be contained in the pericardial space. The composition of the fluid is very similar to serum. An accumulation of fluid in the pericardial sac may be caused by a variety of reasons, including trauma, inflammation, neoplasms, and renal failure. Pericardial tamponade is caused by restriction in ventricular diastolic filling secondary to a significant accumulation of fluid, which leads to a reduction in cardiac ejection fraction and mean arterial blood pressure. Pericardial tamponade is a life-threatening condition, requiring immediate intervention.

Indications

Pericardiocentesis is indicated for treatment of cardiac tamponade or for the etiologic diagnosis of pericardial effusion.

Pericardial tamponade is the major indication for emergent pericardiocentesis.

Contraindications

There are no absolute contraindications for an emergent therapeutic pericardiocentesis. Coagulopathy and skin infection are considered to be the two major contraindications for a diagnostic pericardiocentesis.

Technique

The patient is placed in the supine position with the chest and shoulders elevated at least 30°. Routine sterile precautions are followed. One percent lidocaine is used as the local anesthetic. Figure 8-7 demonstrates two approaches to perform pericardiocentesis: the paraxiphoid subcostal approach and the left parasternal approach. We describe here only the paraxiphoid subcostal approach. It is the most commonly performed technique because it is relatively simple and avoids both the pleura and major vessels.

For this approach, a long, large-bore (~18 cm, 18 gauge) cardiac needle, connected to a syringe and the V lead of the EKG (Figure 8-8), penetrates the skin just underneath the costal margin next to the xiphoid and is advanced carefully at a 45° angle, beneath the ribs toward the midpoint of the left clavicle. Suction is continuously applied to the syringe as the needle is advanced while monitoring for a cardiac injury current. ST segment elevation is seen with ventricular epicardial contact, and atrial epicardial injury is manifested by PR segment elevation. If any of these are noted on the EKG, the needle should be slightly withdrawn and redirected. When fluid is returned, the needle is secured to prevent accidental overpenetration by attaching a hemostat at the skin level or taping the needle to the skin. Removal of even a small amount of fluid may bring a rapid improvement in hemodynamic status if the procedure is performed for pericardial tamponade.

Monitoring should be provided while performing pericardiocentesis to exclude the development of a cardiac injury current.

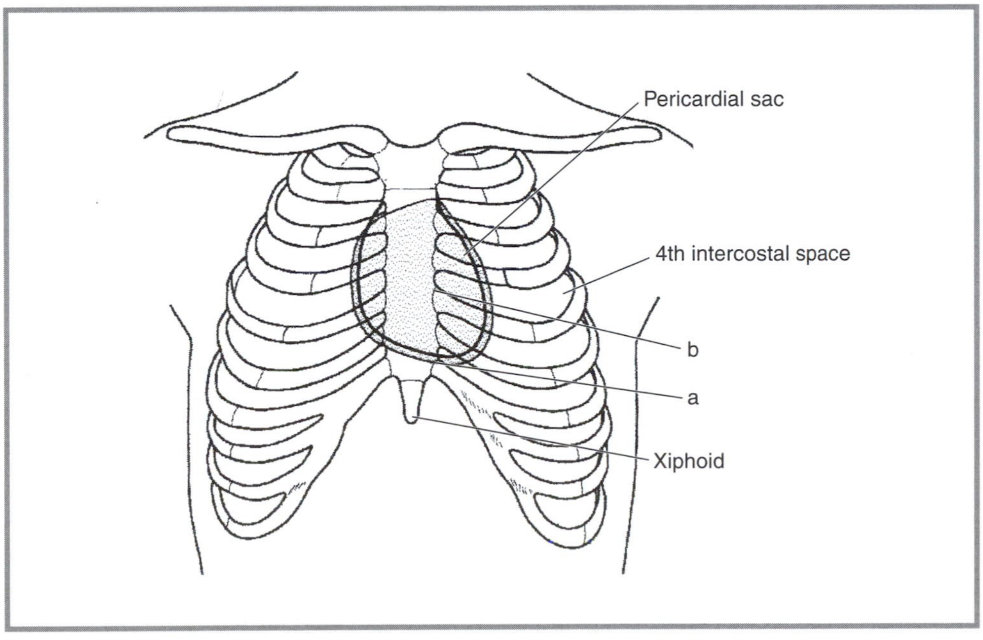

FIGURE 8-7

Two approaches to perform pericardiocentesis: the paraxiphoid subcostal approach **(A)** and the left parasternal approach **(B)**. (From Civetta JM, Taylor RW, Kirby RR. Critical Care, 3rd ed. Philadelphia: Lippincott-Raven, 1997.)

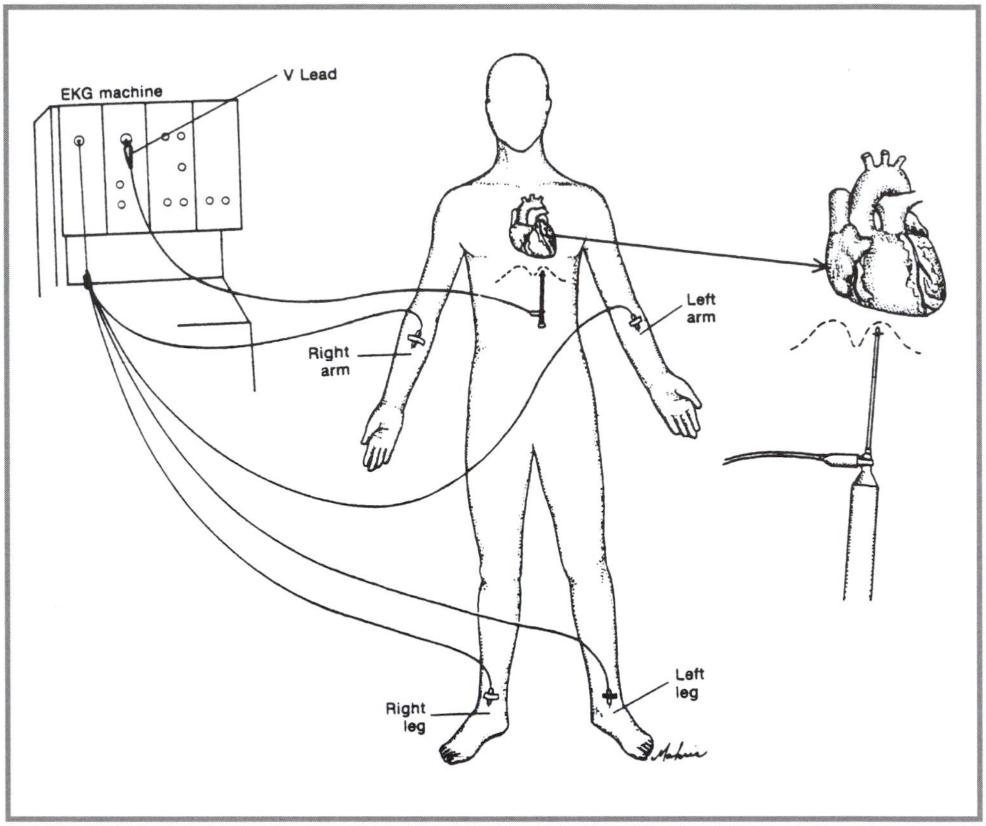

FIGURE 8-8

Pericardiocentesis technique. A cardiac needle is connected to the V lead of the EKG to monitor for a cardiac injury current. (From Civetta JM, Taylor RW, Kirby RR. Critical Care, 3rd Ed. Philadelphia: Lippincott-Raven, 1997.)

Complications

Cardiac arrhythmias and coronary artery laceration are potential complications of pericardiocentesis, as well as hydrothorax and pneumothorax. However, both coronary artery laceration and pleural space injury seldom occur with the paraxiphoid subcostal approach. Ventricular tachycardia may occur during the procedure as a result of ventricular puncture. If ventricular puncture occurs, the patient should be watched for possible intrapericardial bleeding.

SUMMARY

The procedures of thoracentesis, paracentesis, lumbar puncture, and pericardiocentesis can often be performed safely at the bedside using standard sterile techniques. It is imperative that the physician understands the indications and contraindications for each procedure to minimize the risk of adverse events.

REVIEW QUESTIONS

1. **Which of the following is the major reason why thoracentesis should be performed above the rib?**
   - **A.** It is easier to perform.
   - **B.** It is more comfortable for the patient.
   - **C.** It is safer.

2. **The most important factor for choosing a site for paracentesis is:**
   - **A.** The least amount of adipose tissue
   - **B.** Proximity to umbilicus
   - **C.** Finding an avascular site

3. **A patient developed fever, leukocytosis, pain, and paraplegia 12 h after lumbar puncture. The most likely diagnosis is:**
   - **A.** Epidural abscess
   - **B.** Epidural hematoma
   - **C.** Arachnoiditis

4. **During pericardiocentesis, the patient developed PR segment elevation in the V lead on the EKG. What is the most likely reason for this observation?**
   - **A.** Ventricular epicardial injury
   - **B.** Ischemia
   - **C.** Atrial epicardial injury

ANSWERS

1. The answer is C. A neurovascular bundle is located on the inferior surface of the rib; therefore, approach above the rib is associated with less chance of an injury to this structure.
2. The answer is C. Paracentesis has a relatively low incidence of complications. One of these is bleeding from the site of needle insertion, because many patients with ascites have coagulopathy. Therefore, finding an avascular site is very important. An area on the left flank of the lower abdomen, adjacent to the rectus abdominis, meets this criterion.
3. The answer is A. Epidural abscess is a complication secondary to introduction of infection into the epidural space. It usually has hematogenic origin but occasionally may occur as a result of lumbar puncture. It has typical symptoms of infection (fever and leukocytosis) as well as severe neurologic deficit and pain.
4. The answer is C. ST segment elevation would be characteristic for ventricular epicardial injury. PR segment elevation during pericardiocentesis is typical for atrial epicardial injury and not for ischemia.

SUGGESTED READING

Davidson RI. Lumbar puncture In: Vandersalm TJ (ed) Atlas of Bedside Procedures, 2nd Ed. Boston: Little, Brown, 1988.

Runyon BA. Paracentesis of ascitic fluid: a safe procedure. Arch Intern Med 1986;146:2259.

Spodick DH. The technique of pericardiocentesis. J Crit Illness 1995; 10(11):807–812.

CHAPTER 9

FRANCIS C. CORDOVA AND NATHANIEL MARCHETTI

Noninvasive Monitoring in the Intensive Care Unit

CHAPTER OUTLINE

LEARNING OBJECTIVES

After studying this chapter, you should be able to do the following:

- Know the different noninvasive monitoring techniques commonly used in the ICU setting.
- Know the advantages and limitations of the different noninvasive monitoring methods.
- Know the different technologies used in noninvasive monitoring.
- Correlate findings observed during noninvasive monitoring with the patient's changing physiology.

The modern paradigm of critical care medicine is not only to effectively treat the patient's underlying life-threatening illness but also to recognize, as early as possible, any potential complications that may occur because of the underlying disease or as a result of therapy. Indeed, the development of the modern coronary care unit in the early 1960s was born from the need to monitor the development of cardiac arrhythmia in patients who suffered acute myocardial infarction. Similarly, the impetus for the creation of the specialized respiratory care unit was also brought about by the need to care for patients who developed respiratory failure during polio epidemics.

Today, intensive care monitoring is widely practiced in most modern intensive care units (ICUs) across the country. In the context of ICU care, monitoring has been defined as making repeated or continuous observations or measurements of the physiologic functions, and the functions of the life support equipment, to guide management decisions, including when to make therapeutic interventions and to assess those interventions. Using this definition, intensive care monitoring can be as simple as frequent bedside assessment by an experienced clinician or the use of a noninvasive monitoring device such as pulse oximetry to assess the adequacy of oxygenation. Alternatively, ICU monitoring may use sophisticated medical technology that requires skilled physicians and health care workers to operate and maintain. The use of the pulmonary artery catheter in the ICU to continuously monitor hemodynamics and the use of an esophageal balloon to monitor auto-PEEP during mechanical ventilation are examples of invasive monitoring techniques. Regardless of the type of monitoring methods used in a particular clinical scenario, the success of any monitoring algorithm hinges on appropriate responses from physicians, nurses, and respiratory therapists. The type (invasive or noninvasive) and frequency (continuous inline or specified timed interval) of monitoring should be tailored to an individual patient's clinical condition. Thus, a patient in septic shock who requires multiple vasoactive drugs will often require invasive hemodynamic monitoring with pulmonary artery and peripheral artery indwelling catheters. In contrast, patients who are admitted to the ICU in status epilepticus often only require continuous electroencephalographic monitoring.

Invasive monitoring techniques are typified by the use of pulmonary and arterial catheters and invariably require a highly skilled physician, not only to obtain accurate physiologic measurements but also to troubleshoot problems. By its nature, invasive monitoring often contributes to pain and suffering and may potentially result in increased morbidity (infection, bleeding, pneumothorax), and even mortality. In contrast, noninvasive monitoring techniques are easier to use and maintain and are not associated with the complications inherent with invasive monitoring methods.

In this chapter, we discuss the noninvasive monitoring methods commonly used in ICUs throughout North America. Specifically, we discuss the different types of noninvasive methods used in respiratory and cardiac monitoring and also their advantages and disadvantages.

GOALS OF MONITORING

In general, the goal of intensive care monitoring is to decrease the morbidity and mortality resulting from life-threatening diseases or from complications that may arise during diagnostic and therapeutic interventions. Specifically, the goals of monitoring are to assess vital organ function, to detect early life-threatening complications, to determine the need for interventions such as mechanical ventilation or airway intubation, and to assess the effects of a particular therapeutic intervention. More important, monitoring should not cause undue pain and discomfort to the patient. Also, it should not be so cumbersome as to interfere with direct patient care.

The type of monitoring device or technique should be tailored to the particular disease process and to the need of individual patients. Thus, patients who are admitted to the ICU for gastrointestinal hemorrhage need frequent assessment of their vital signs. Patients who are admitted for an exacerbation of chronic obstructive lung disease may benefit from continuous monitoring of oxygen hemoglobin saturation in addition to routine vital signs. In certain situations, ICU monitoring is necessary in patients receiving therapy that may lead to fatal complications. For example, patients with stroke who are candidates for thrombolytic therapy require frequent neurologic monitoring in an ICU setting.

RESPIRATORY MONITORING

Bedside Assessment

An initial bedside assessment by an astute physician forms the foundation for subsequent respiratory monitoring in patients who are at risk for acute respiratory failure. In all circumstances, any measured physiologic variable obtained during routine ICU monitoring should be correlated with clinical findings. Occasionally, discrepancy between the measured physiologic variable as reported by the monitoring device and the clinical assessment may be encountered. In this situation, bedside clinical evaluation by the physician should always prevail. The old adage—treat the patient and not the laboratory abnormality—also applies in ICU monitoring.

Signs of acute respiratory distress:
- Tachypnea
- Inability to speak in sentences
- Use of accessory respiratory muscles
- Suprasternal, intercostal, subcostal retractions
- Tracheal tugging
- Dysynchronous movement of the thorax and abdomen

Acute respiratory distress is easy to recognize at the bedside. Clinically, impending respiratory failure is manifested by tachypnea, an inability to speak in complete sentences, and use of the accessory breathing muscles. Although tachypnea is a nonspecific sign that may result from fever, pain, anxiety, or metabolic acidosis, it is often one of the first signs of respiratory distress. An easy way to assess accessory muscle use is to palpate the sternocleidomastoid and feel for its contraction during each inspiration. Other signs such as alae nasi flaring, tracheal tugging, and intercostal and subcostal retractions also suggest an increased work of breathing. The onset of thoracoabdominal paradox during breathing in a patient in respiratory distress is a sign of respiratory muscle fatigue and usually signals the need for emergent ventilatory support. Similarly, mental obtundation suggests the presence of hypercapnia or of hypoxemia. Circumoral cyanosis usually indicates an oxygen hemoglobin saturation level below 80%.

Conditions associated with Cheyne–Stokes breathing:
- Congestive heart failure
- Stroke
- Narcotic overdose
- Intracranial hypertension
- High altitude

Breathing pattern may be an important clue to the etiology of respiratory failure, and also helps in the assessment of the level of brainstem function in comatose patients. Different breathing patterns include Cheyne–Stokes breathing, central neurogenic hyperventilation, apneustic breathing, chaotic breathing, and a Kussmaul breathing pattern. The most common recognizable abnormal breathing pattern is Cheyne–Stokes breathing.

Conditions associated with central neurogenic hyperventilation:
- Lower midbrain and upper pontine lesions
- Tentorial herniation

Apneustic breathing is commonly seen in brainstem stroke affecting the lower pons.

Biot, or chaotic breathing, is associated with lesions in the brainstem medulla.

Cheyne–Stokes breathing is characterized by a crescendo–decrescendo alteration in tidal volume that is interrupted by short periods of apnea, or hypopnea. This type of breathing pattern is commonly seen in patients with congestive heart failure, or in those with central nervous system diseases, such as stroke. It can also be seen in patients with increased intracranial pressure, with narcotic overdose, and when breathing at high altitudes. In central neurogenic hyperventilation, both the rate and depth of respiration are increased, akin to the breathing pattern observed in Kussmaul breathing. This type of breathing pattern is caused by lesions of the lower midbrain–upper pons and may also occur during tentorial herniation. Arterial blood gas examination in these patients shows profound respiratory alkalosis. Brainstem lesions occurring lower in the pons, as would be seen in acute basilar artery occlusion, lead to an apneustic breathing pattern. These patients have short and rapid respirations followed by periods of apnea at the end of each inspiration. Biot, or chaotic breathing, often suggests lesions in the medulla. This type of breathing pattern is device of any rhythmicity; each breath varies in both depth and rate, producing a breathing pattern that is devoid of any regularity. Kussmaul breathing is described as deep, regular, sighing respirations that result in an increased tidal volume. This type of breathing is most commonly seen in patients with acidemia, such as patients with diabetic ketoacidosis.

CASE STUDY: PART 1

A 55-year-old man was brought to the emergency room after being found unconscious on his living room floor by fire rescue personnel. The paramedics removed him from a room filled with thick smoke. He was spontaneously breathing with a palpable radial pulse and a blood pressure of 160/96 mmHg. On arrival to the emergency room, the patient was drowsy, intermittently agitated, and confused. He complained of mild dyspnea and vague anterior chest pain. He also complained of a severe headache, located mostly over both temporal areas. He was nauseated and vomited three times while in the ER. His past medical history was significant for hypertension and a "touch of asthma." He has a 25-pack-year history of smoking. On presentation, his vital signs were as follows: T = 98.6°F, P = 110 mm, BP = 156/88 mmHg, RR = 32 breaths/min, and SpO_2 = 100% while breathing on a 40% face mask. On physical exam, the patient had singed facial sideburns but without obvious signs of facial burns. Carbonaceous deposits were found in the nares, throat, and posterior pharynx. He appeared anxious and tachypneic but was not using the accessory muscles of respiration. His eyebrows and nasal hairs were singed. His lung exam revealed a few mild end-expiratory wheezes. Cardiac exam revealed regular tachycardia without any murmurs or gallops. The physical exam was otherwise completely unremarkable.

These different breathing patterns help justify the notion that breathing pattern manifests the underlying disease, the etiology of which needs to be elucidated to institute proper treatment.

Oxygenation

Pulse Oximetry

Noninvasive measurement of tissue oxygen saturation using an oximeter is based on the principle of differential light absorption characteristics of the different species of hemoglobin (oxyhemoglobin, deoxyhemoglobin, methemoglobin, carboxyhemoglobin, and sulfhemoglobin). Modern pulse oximetry uses two wavelengths of light, red (660 nm) and infrared (900–940 nm), to discriminate between oxyhemoglobin and deoxyhemoglobin. The absorption spectra for oxygenated and deoxygenated hemoglobins are shown in Figure 9-1. The reason oxygenated hemoglobin appears to be redder compared to deoxygenated blood is that oxygenated hemoglobin reflects red light better than other hemoglobin species. Earlier models of ear oximeters were large and cumbersome and required frequent calibration. Because the peripheral circulation contains a mixture of blood from arterial, venous, and capillary sources with different levels of oxygen saturation, the skin surface where the oximeter is applied has to be warmed or "arterialized" to increase arterial blood flow.

The widespread use of noninvasive measurements of oxyhemoglobin did not come about until the development of pulse oximetry. Pulse oximetry obviated the need for skin warming by assuming that the changes in light absorbance are mainly the result of the pulsatile flow of arterial blood. Oxygen saturation is calculated using an algorithm with a predetermined calibration curve stored in a microprocessor. The calibration curve is derived from healthy normal volunteers with oxygen saturation ranging from 70% to 100%. The accuracy of different pulse oximeters in measuring oxyhemoglobin saturation is excellent, with 95% confidence limits of 2%–4% when the oxygen saturation is above 70%. The accuracy of SaO_2 measurements substantially declines at lower oxyhemoglobin saturations; the error increases from ±4% at SaO_2 of 70% to as much as ±15% with SaO_2 levels below 50%. The accuracy of SaO_2 measurements at the lower range of SaO_2 values is further magnified by the presence of hypoperfusion states commonly encountered in ICU patients. If the heart rate

The accuracy of SaO_2 measurement by pulse oximetry is ±4% and becomes inaccurate with SaO_2 ≤60%.

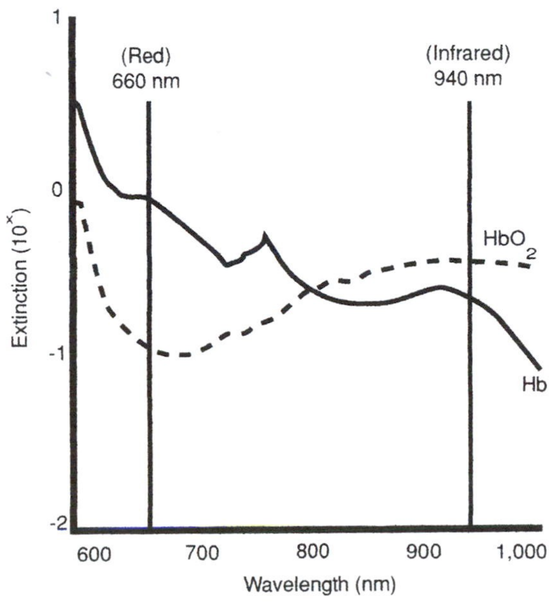

FIGURE 9-1

Modern pulse oximetry uses two wavelengths of light, red (660 nm) and infrared (940 nm), to differentiate oxyhemoglobin (HbO_2) from deoxyhemoglobin (Hb). (Adapted with permission from J Crit Illness 1989;4:23–31.)

FIGURE 9-2

The oxygen hemoglobin dissociation curve is sigmoidal. On the upper portion of the oxygen hemoglobin dissociation curve, a given oxygen hemoglobin saturation represents a wide range of PaO_2. (Adapted with permission from Am Rev Respir Dis 1988; 138:1625–1642.)

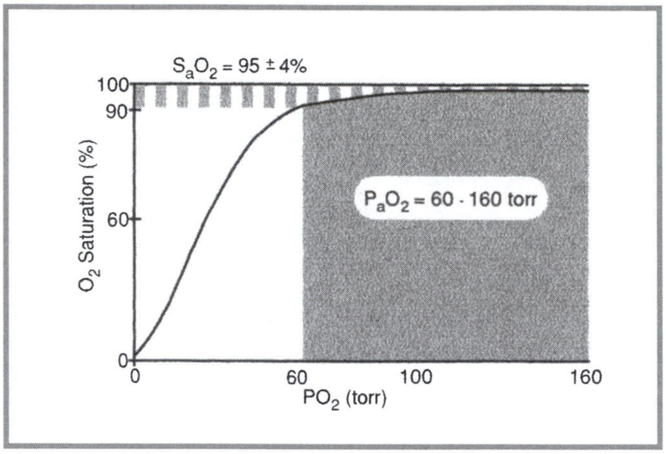

recorded by the pulse oximeter does not closely match the patient's true heart rate, the pulse oximeter reading is likely to be inaccurate.

Pulse oximetry measures only oxygenation function of the lung, not the adequacy of ventilation.

Although pulse oximetry is useful in different clinical situations requiring respiratory monitoring, it is not a substitute for arterial blood gas determination. Pulse oximetry does not provide any information on the adequacy of ventilation nor does it provide any information on the acid–base status of the patient. In addition, because of the sigmoidal shape of the oxygen hemoglobin dissociation curve, a given SaO_2 estimation by pulse oximetry represents a wide range of PaO_2 values (Figure 9-2). For example, an SaO_2 of 95%, assuming a measurement margin of error of $\pm 4\%$, represents PaO_2 values between 60 and 160 mmHg.

Both methemoglobinemia and carboxyhemoglobinemia result in false SaO_2 readings.

Other factors that may affect the accuracy of SaO_2 by pulse oximetry are listed in Table 9-1. Because pulse oximetry uses only two wavelengths, other forms of dyshemoglobinemia will not be detected by conventional pulse oximetry. For example, patients with methemoglobinemia (e.g., hemoglobin oxidized to its ferric state) may initially show a decrease in

TABLE 9-1

CAUSES OF INACCURATE PULSE OXIMETER READINGS OF OXYHEMOGLOBIN SATURATION

CONDITION	CAUSE	EFFECTS ON PULSE OXIMETER
Dyshemoglobinemia		
Carbon monoxide	Smoke inhalation	Falsely elevated
Methemoglobin	Local anesthetics (lidocaine, benzocaine), nitrates, sulfa drugs, EDTA	Initially decreased but falsely elevated at higher levels of methemoglobinemia
Dyes and pigments		
Methylene blue	Antidote for methemoglobinemia	Falsely low
Bilirubin	Hyperbilirubinemia from various causes	Inaccurate reading
Low perfusion	Hypothermia Hypovolemia Peripheral vascular disease Vasopressors	Inadequate pulse signal
Anemia	Bleeding, hemolysis	Inaccurate at hemoglobin < 5 g/dl
Increased venous pulsation	Right heart failure, tricuspid regurgitation	Any pulsatile flow is interpreted as arterial
External light source	Excessive light interference	Inaccurate reading

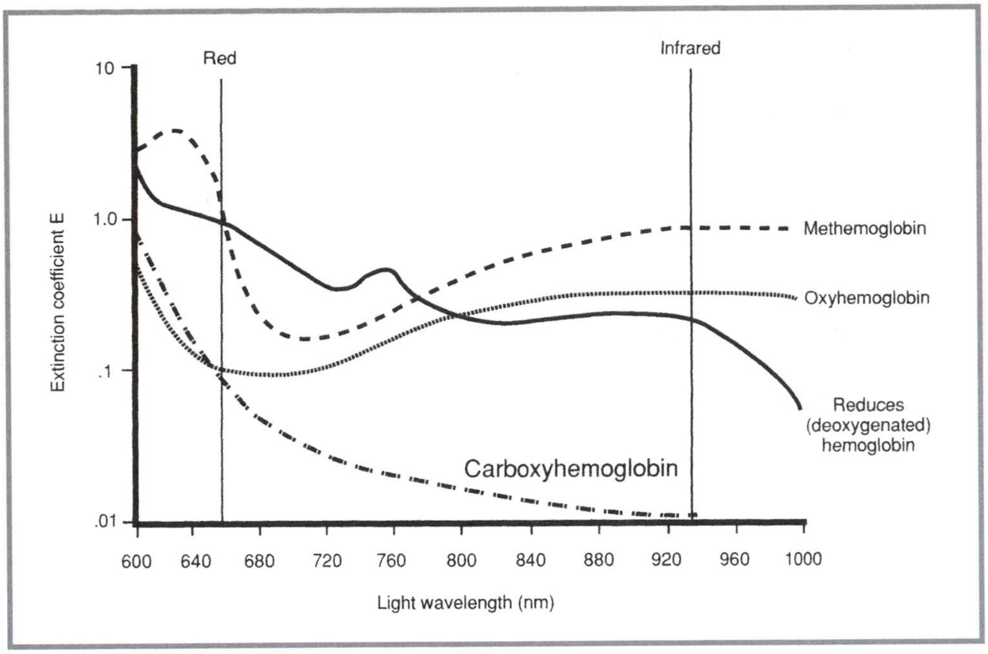

FIGURE 9-3

Different forms of dyshemoglobinemia, in particular methemoglobinemia and carboxyhemoglobin, mimic the light absorbance characteristics of oxyhemoglobin, resulting in false pulse oximetry reading of the true oxyhemoglobin saturation. (Adapted with permission from J Crit Illness 1988;3:103–107.)

pulse oximetry readings but plateau at 80%–85% even with increasing methemoglobin levels. This inconsistent $S\acute{a}O_2$ reading results from the absorbance characteristic of methemoglobin, which absorbs equally well at 660 nm (red) and 940 nm (infrared) (Figure 9-3). As methemoglobinemia worsens, both red and infrared absorption increase approaching an R (the ratio of pulsatile and baseline absorbance of red and infrared wavelengths) value of 1, which equates an SaO_2 of 85%. In contrast, methylene blue, which is used in the treatment of methemoglobinemia, leads to falsely low SaO_2 values. Similarly, carboxyhemoglobin, which mimics the light absorbance pattern of oxyhemoglobin, also results in falsely elevated oxyhemoglobin saturation determinations by pulse oximetry. If a dyshemoglobinemia is suspected, the SaO_2 should be measured directly in the blood utilizing a co-oximeter.

Hemoglobin F (fetal hemoglobin) behaves as does hemoglobin A (normal Hb) spectrophotometrically. Therefore, pulse oximetry can be accurately used in neonates and infants. The presence of hemoglobin S, the predominant Hb in sickle cell disease, can lead to inaccurate or inconsistent pulse oximetry readings. The abnormal geometry of the sickle cells alters the scatter of the light, thereby interfering with measurements made based on light absorption characteristics alone. Moreover, sickle cell disease shifts the oxygen–hemoglobin dissociation curve to the right, resulting in lower SaO_2 saturations for any given PaO_2 value. Finally, in sickle cell disease, significant hemolysis during painful crises can modestly increase carboxyhemoglobin concentration, thereby leading to falsely increased measurements of oxygen saturation.

> The oxygen–hemoglobin dissociation curve in sickle cell disease is shifted to the right, resulting in a lower SaO_2 for a given PaO_2.

Although pulse oximetry is widely used, not only in the ICU setting but also during intraoperative and perioperative situations and during outpatient procedures requiring conscious

CASE STUDY: PART 2

A portable chest x-ray of the patient was normal. An arterial blood gas sample was sent to the laboratory, with results as follows: pH = 7.43, $PaCO_2$ = 25 mmHg, PaO_2 = 225 mmHg, HCO_3 = 16 mEq/L, CoHb = 34%, and oxyhemoglobin saturation by co-oximeter = 82%. The patient was immediately given 100% supplemental oxygen via a nonrebreather mask. Six hours later, the patient was feeling much better and a repeat ABG revealed that the carboxyhemoglobin level decreased to less than 5%, with an improvement in oxyhemoglobin saturation as measured by co-oximeter.

sedation, such as bronchoscopy and colonoscopy, its effect on patient morbidity and mortality is unclear.

Transcutaneous Oxygen Measurement

Factors affecting $tcPO_2$ value:
- Skin thickness and capillary density
- Cutaneous metabolism
- Cardiac output

The measurement of transcutaneous PO_2 ($tcPO_2$) using a modified Clark electrode depends on the oxygen concentration gradient across the skin. It assumes minimal cutaneous metabolism. Local heat (to about 43°C) is applied to the electrode contact site to ensure adequate skin perfusion to produce a $tcPO_2$ approximating the PaO_2. The electrode site is changed every 4–6 h to prevent skin burn. In neonates or young infants, which have a thin epidermis and low metabolism for a given blood flow, the $tcPO_2$ closely approximates the PaO_2 value. Previous studies have shown that the oxygen tension gradient across the skin can be as low as 5%. In stable adult patients, the $tcPO_2$ is only approximately 80% of the simultaneously measured PaO_2 because adults have thicker skin with a decreased skin capillary density. The discrepancy between the measured PaO_2 and $tcPO_2$ is further magnified by changes in cardiac output and by skin perfusion abnormalities that are commonly encountered in critically ill patients (Figure 9-4).

Because of the limitations previously mentioned, $tcPO_2$ monitoring is mostly used in neonates and young infants to obviate the need for frequent arterial blood gas sampling. In these pediatric patients, the direction and percentage change in $tcPO_2$ correlates well with the PaO_2. In adult specialty care units, pulse oximetry has largely supplanted the use of PaO_2 measurement by arterial blood sampling. Because the $tcPO_2$ measurement in part depends on skin perfusion and thus reflects the adequacy of oxygen delivery, it has been used to monitor the results of vascular surgery in patients with peripheral vascular disease. The differences between transcutaneous and pulse oximetry are shown in Table 9-2.

Capnometry

Uses of capnometry in the ICU:
- Verify endotracheal tube placement
- Monitor ventilation adequacy
- Noninvasively estimate $PaCO_2$

Capnometry is the measurement of carbon dioxide concentration in respiratory gases. The measurement of carbon dioxide in expired respiratory gas was first used in the intraoperative setting to confirm endotracheal intubation and to aid in the quantitative assessment of ventilation during general anesthesia. Currently, capnometry in the ICU setting and in other emergent settings is used mainly to confirm endotracheal tube placement during intubation because of the inaccuracy of capnometry in the presence of significant intrinsic lung disease.

The capnometer is a device that quantitatively measures the amount of exhaled carbon dioxide; a capnograph has the added capability to display and track changes in end-tidal carbon dioxide over time. The principle of bedside capnometry is based on infrared spectroscopy, or calorimetry. Similar to pulse oximetry, capnometry utilizes the unique light absorption quality of carbon dioxide. In this case, carbon dioxide is measured in vitro by quantifying

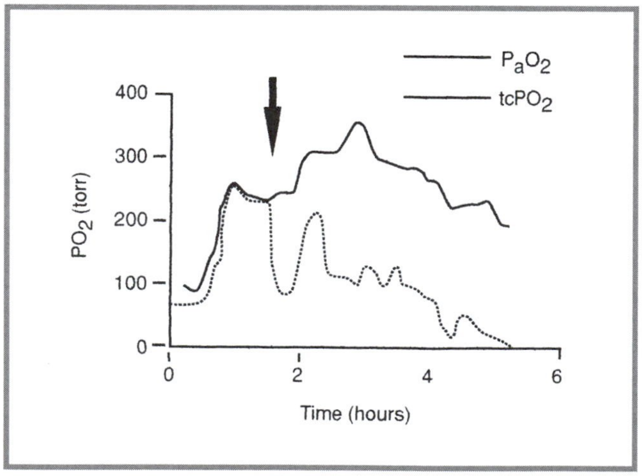

FIGURE 9-4

The accuracy of the transcutaneous oxygen measurement ($tcPO_2$) is decreased by the shock state, as shown in this patient, who developed low cardiac output. The arrow indicates the time of low cardiac output or onset of shock. (Adapted with permission from Crit Care Med 1981;9:706–709.)

TABLE 9-2

DIFFERENCES BETWEEN TRANSCUTANEOUS AND PULSE OXIMETRY

FACTOR	TRANSCUTANEOUS	PULSE OXIMETRY
Accuracy in adults	No	Yes
Detection of high PaO_2	Yes	No
Setup time	Minutes	Seconds
Time response	Minutes	Seconds
Measures pulse	No	Yes
Heated skin burns	Yes	No
Stability at one site	2–4 h	Yes
Motion artifact	Minimal	Yes
Sensitivity to perfusion	Yes	Yes

the absorption of infrared light at a wavelength of 4.3 μm as it passes through the sample gas. Because only carbon dioxide absorbs infrared light, the presence of oxygen, helium, or nitrogen in the expired gas does not interfere with its measurement. However, the presence of nitrous oxide may interfere with the capnometer reading because nitrous oxide also absorbs infrared light, resulting in an artifactual increase in the measured carbon dioxide concentration. In addition, nitrous oxide reduces the optical density of carbon dioxide, resulting in artificially low readings in less sophisticated capnometers.

Capnometers can be further categorized as mainstream or sidestream on the basis of the gas sampling method. The mainstream capnometer is attached inline to the endotracheal tube, resulting in rapid breath-by-breath gas analysis. The sensor used in the mainstream capnometer is typically heavy and bulky and therefore cumbersome to use. In contrast, the sidestream capnometer continuously withdraws gas from the breathing circuit into a gas sampling line. The gas sampling circuit, however, introduces a delay in overall carbon dioxide (CO_2) analyzer response time. The advantage of this system is that it can be used in an unintubated patient by holding the capnometer close to the patient's face.

In clinical practice, capnometry has three important uses: (1) to verify endotracheal tube placement, as previously mentioned, (2) to noninvasively estimate the arterial partial pressure of carbon dioxide ($PaCO_2$), and (3) to monitor the respiratory rate.

Confirmation of Endotracheal Tube Placement

Rapid confirmation of endotracheal tube position following intubation in patients with an unstable respiratory status is crucial. In most circumstances, tracheal intubation can be confirmed initially by an experienced physician by listening for equal breath sounds, visually inspecting for symmetric chest expansion with each assisted inspiration, and by observing a rising oxyhemoglobin saturation. However, none of these clinical methods is foolproof. The use of capnometry following intubation can further rapidly confirm successful tracheal intubation, especially in unstable patients or during a difficult airway intubation. Following airway intubation, a capnometer is connected to the tracheal tube. The colorimetric membrane inside the capnometer changes color when exposed to expired CO_2.

This method provides a rapid and accurate assessment of endotracheal tube placement within minutes. However, there are a few situations that may cause inaccuracy when using this technique. Normally, there is no appreciable amount of CO_2 in the gastrointestinal tract, but ingestion of carbonated beverages before intubation may result in high carbon dioxide readings; this is known as the "cola effect." In certain situations, cardiogenic shock and low flow states may lead to erroneous capnometer readings as a result of low exhaled carbon dioxide levels outside the range of the colorimetric assay.

Recent ingestion of carbonated drinks before intubation may lead to a high carbon dioxide reading.

Estimation of Arterial CO_2 with End-Tidal CO_2

In healthy individuals, the end-tidal carbon dioxide ($P_{ET}CO_2$) value is generally 1–3 mmHg lower compared to the arterial carbon dioxide level ($PaCO_2$). This difference between $P_{ET}CO_2$

The $P_{ET}CO_2$ is 1–3 mmHg lower than $PaCO_2$.

FIGURE 9-5

A–C. The relationship between end-tidal carbon dioxide ($P_{ET}CO_2$) and arterial carbon dioxide level ($PaCO_2$) is affected by the presence of ventilation perfusion inequalities. In normal individuals, $P_{ET}CO_2$ is usually 1–3 mmHg lower than simultaneously measured $PaCO_2$ **(A)**. The discrepancy between $P_{ET}CO_2$ and $PaCO_2$ becomes marked in the presence of deadspace **(B)** and shunt physiology **(C)**. (Adapted with permission from Airway Management. Philadelphia: Lippincott-Raven, 1996.)

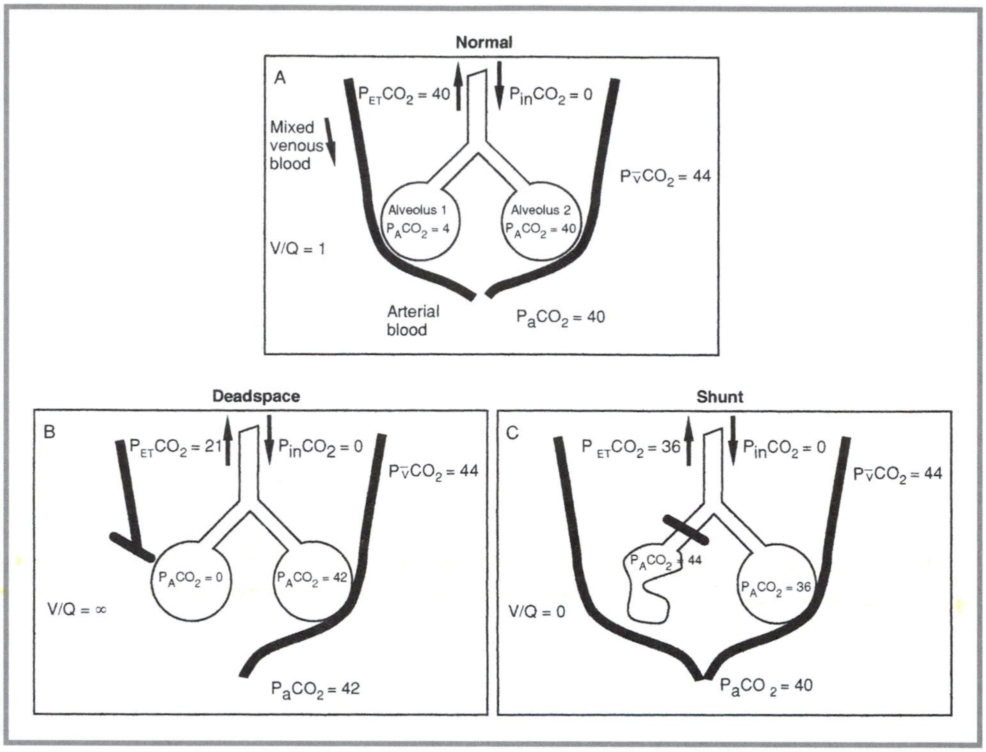

The accuracy of $P_{ET}CO_2$ in estimating $PaCO_2$ is affected by ventilation–perfusion inequality.

and $PaCO_2$ is mainly caused by minimal physiologic ventilation/perfusion imbalance found in the upper lobes because ventilation is greater than perfusion as a result of the gravitational effects influencing blood flow to more dependent lung regions. Thus, the measured $P_{ET}CO_2$ does not always reflect the $PaCO_2$, especially in the presence of ventilation/perfusion (V_A/Q) inequalities (Figure 9-5). When the V_A/Q ratio approaches 1.0, then $P_{ET}CO_2$ correlates well with $PaCO_2$. If the V_A/Q ratio is higher than 1.0, as in deadspace ventilation, then $P_{ET}CO_2$ will be lower than $PaCO_2$. An increase in deadspace ventilation is commonly seen in patients with acute pulmonary embolism. When the V_A/Q ratio is less than 1.0, then $P_{ET}CO_2$ will be lower than $PaCO_2$. A variety of clinical conditions are associated with changes in $P_{ET}CO_2$ (Table 9-3).

TABLE 9-3

CLINICAL CONDITIONS THAT MAY LEAD TO CHANGES IN END-TIDAL PCO_2

CONDITION	RESULT
Impaired central respiratory drive	Inadequate alveolar ventilation Apnea or hypopnea

Airway problems	Misplaced endotracheal tube
	  Bronchial intubation
	  Partial inadvertent extubation
	Presence of airflow obstruction
	  Bronchospasm
	  Mucous plug

Parenchymal disease	Massive pulmonary embolism Pneumothorax Aspiration Pneumonia Acute respiratory distress syndrome
Ventilator malfunction	Rebreathing of exhaled gas Ventilator circuit leak

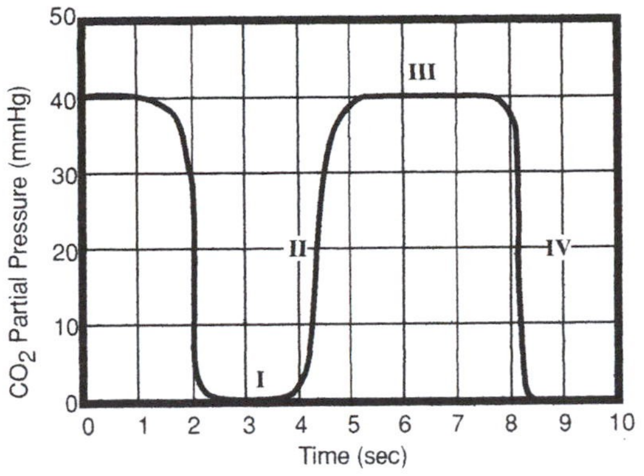

FIGURE 9-6

The four phases of a normal capnogram: *I*, inspiratory baseline; *II*, expiratory upstroke; *III*, expiratory plateau; *IV*, inspiratory downstroke. (Adapted with permission from Airway Management. Philadelphia: Lippincott-Raven, 1996.)

Interpretation of the Capnogram

A visual inspection of a capnogram may provide some clues to changes in the patient's ventilatory status. A normal capnograph has four phases: an inspiratory baseline (I), an expiratory upstroke (II), an expiratory plateau (III), and the inspiratory downstroke (IV) (Figure 9-6). The inspiratory baseline is normally at zero, indicating the absence of carbon dioxide in inhaled gas. Phase II or the expiratory upstroke corresponds with the beginning of expiration. The curve is normally steep due to the rapid emptying of gas from the anatomic deadspace followed immediately by mixed alveolar gas. The expiratory plateau, or phase III, results from good mixing of alveolar gas. $P_{ET}CO_2$ is measured at the end of the expiratory plateau phase. During the next respiratory cycle, the inspiration of fresh gas leads to a steep drop in CO_2 toward zero during phase IV. The cycle then repeats.

An abnormal capnograph suggests a change in the patient's condition, or malfunction of the breathing circuit such as an incompetent exhalation valve. An inspiratory baseline above zero suggests partial rebreathing of exhaled gas from breathing circuit malfunction. An upsloping expiratory plateau can be seen in patients with airflow obstruction resulting from poor mixing of alveolar gas. Similarly, ventilated patients with a partially obstructed endotracheal tube have capnograph readings showing a gradual rise in the expired CO_2, as opposed to the brisk increase that normally occurs during the expiratory phase. A dip in the

CASE STUDY: PART 3

The patient was admitted to the Burn Unit with a diagnosis of smoke inhalation injury and carbon monoxide poisoning. The next morning his nurse reported that Mr. Jones' pulse oximeter reading was 88% despite increasing his supplemental oxygen back to 50% FiO_2. His other vital signs were HR = 124/min (sinus tachycardia on the monitor), RR = 28 mm, BP = 100/60 mmHg, and T = 102°F. Physical exam revealed the patient to be in moderate respiratory distress, using his accessory muscles of respiration and complaining of shortness of breath. His jugular venous pressure was less than 6 cm. Lung exam revealed diffuse scattered bronchi with some bronchial breath sounds bilaterally. Heart exam was regular, tachycardic, and without murmurs or gallops. The remainder of his exam was normal. A stat portable chest x-ray showed diffuse bilateral fluffy infiltrates consistent with noncardiogenic pulmonary edema. An arterial blood gas showed pH = 7.47, $PaCO_2$ = 30 mmHg, PaO_2 = 60 mmHg, and HCO_3 = 20 mEq/l. Despite titrating the FiO_2 to 100%, the patient's SpO_2 remained at 88%, and he began to exhibit an abdominal paradoxical breathing pattern suggestive of incipient respiratory muscle fatigue. He was intubated and placed on mechanical ventilation. Proper placement of the ETT was confirmed with a colorimetric capnometer. His initial ventilator setting was assisted control with a rate of 14 breaths/min, V_T = 600 ml, FiO_2 = 100%, and PEEP = 5 cmH_2O. The positive end-expiratory pressure (PEEP) was titrated up to 12.5 cmH_2O and the FiO_2 was decreased to 60%. He was started on broad-spectrum IV antibiotics after all appropriate cultures were collected.

expiratory plateau phase, sometimes called curare clefts, is caused by small inspiratory efforts during expiration that could be due to hiccups, inadequate depth of anesthesia or muscle relaxation, or manipulation of the thoracoabdominal contents. Cardiac oscillations may be seen as sawtooth irregularities on the expiratory plateau.

Transcutaneous Carbon Dioxide Monitoring

Similar to transcutaneous oxygen tension measurement, carbon dioxide tensions can also be measured on the skin surface using either a Stowe–Severinghaus electrode or an infrared sensor. The Stowe–Severinghaus electrode is a small pH electrode that is covered by a bicarbonate buffer solution. The transcutaneous capnometer has a small (50-μl) collection chamber that analyzes CO_2 from the skin with an infrared sensor. The relative large gas collection chamber of the transcutaneous capnometer system compared to the volume of the bicarbonate buffer surrounding the pH electrode results in a slow response time of the infrared based system to changing CO_2 levels. The slow response time, however, can be improved by gentle skin abrasion to remove the epidermal stratum corneum layer or by heating the skin to 42°C to induce vasodilation. Because CO_2 solubility in tissue is temperature dependent, excessive skin heating or a poorly calibrated electrode results in spuriously high $tcPCO_2$ values. For every degree centigrade rise in temperature, the $tcPCO_2$ increases by 4.5%, resulting in an overestimation of $PaCO_2$ by a factor of 1.31–1.61 when skin heating is used.

Factors causing inaccurate $tcPCO_2$ measurement:
- Excessive skin heating
- Low cardiac output
- Thick skin

Because CO_2 has high tissue solubility severalfold higher than oxygen, the measured $tcPCO_2$ is affected less by tissue metabolism. However, the accuracy of $tcPCO_2$ degrades with low cardiac output states. In ICU and surgical patients with cardiac index >1.5 l/min, the $tcPCO_2$ is 23 $\pm$ 11 mmHg above the simultaneously measured $PaCO_2$ ($r = 0.8$). The difference in measured $PaCO_2$ and $tcPCO_2$ increases further with low cardiac output states. In studies of stable ICU patients using an infrared sensor, the measured $tcPCO_2$ showed excellent correlation with $PaCO_2$ with r values as high as 0.98; the mean difference between $tcPCO_2$ and $PaCO_2$ was 4–5 mmHg.

Despite the improving technology of $tcPCO_2$ measurement, it is not widely used in the ICU when compared to pulse oximetry because of its high cost, slow response time, the need to heat the skin to 43°C, and the need to frequently relocate the electrodes to prevent skin burn.

RESPIRATORY MECHANICS

The integrity of the respiratory pump can also be assessed at the bedside just as we are able to assess the gas exchange function of the lung. In the ICU setting, the clinical conditions that may benefit from frequent assessment of lung mechanics are those patients with acute or chronic airflow obstruction, patients with acute progressive neuromuscular disease, and patients who are being weaned from mechanical ventilation. In patients with acute asthma, a peak flowmeter is useful in following the response to treatment. Serial measurements of the forced expiratory volume in 1 s (FEV_1), and forced vital capacity (FVC) can be performed with a portable spirometer in the same patient group. FEV_1 is less dependent on patient effort and therefore may be more accurate in measuring airflow compared to the peak expiratory flow rate. Additionally, serial measurements of FVC are useful in timing the need for ventilatory support in patients with acute progressive neuromuscular diseases, such as the Guillain–Barré syndrome. Perhaps the most common indication for bedside spirometry in the ICU is the measurement of commonly used weaning parameters: tidal volume, FVC, maximum voluntary ventilation (MVV), negative inspiratory force (NIF), and the tidal volume/respiratory rate ratio. Finally, the pattern of breathing can be assessed by measuring changes in both rib cage and abdomen expansion during tidal breathing with elastic bands placed over the rib cage and abdomen that measure changes in electrical impedance (e.g., impedance plethysmography).

Serial FVC measurement is useful in timing the need for ventilatory support in patients with progressive neuromuscular weakness.

Commonly measured bedside respiratory mechanics in the ICU are FVC, TV, RR, MV, MVV, PEF, and NIF.

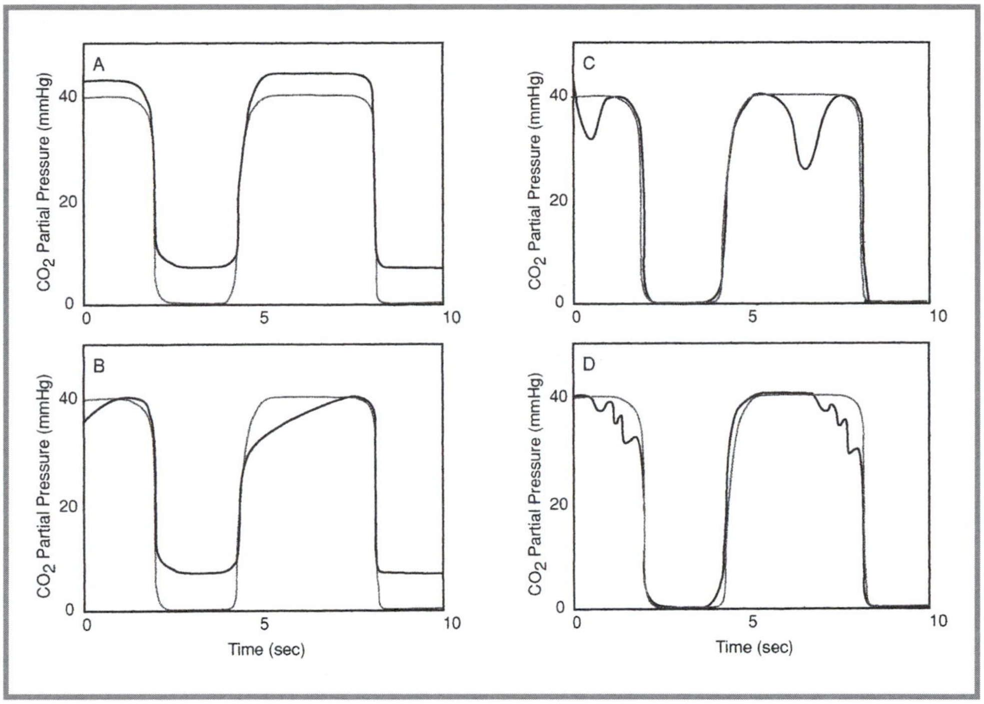

FIGURE 9-7

A–D. Changes in the shape of the phases of the capnogram may suggest the cause of ventilation abnormalities in a particular patient. An elevated baseline suggests elevated inspired carbon dioxide (CO_2) **(A)**. Sloping of the expiratory plateau is commonly seen in patients with chronic airflow obstruction **(B)**. A dip on the expiratory plateau indicates a superimposed breath during controlled ventilation **(C)**. A sawtooth pattern during periods of low expiratory flow is caused by cardiac oscillations **(D)**.

Bedside Spirometry

A portable flowmeter can be used in the ICU to assess the presence and severity of airflow obstruction and its response to therapy. Depending on the sophistication of the device being used, different expiratory flow and lung volume measurements can be performed to evaluate the overall respiratory status of critically ill patients. The commonly measured weaning parameters such as forced vital capacity (FVC), tidal volume (TV), respiratory frequency or rate (RR), minute volume (MV), maximum voluntary ventilation (MVV), peak expiratory flow (PEF), and negative inspiratory force (NIF) can be easily and repeatedly measured with a portable spirometer.

Two commonly used bedside spirometers are Wright's flowmeter and a pneumotachograph.

The two most commonly used flowmeter technologies are the Wright's respirometer and the pneumotachograph. The Wright's respirometer utilizes a rotating-vane technology that estimates flow based on the spinning rate of the turbine when exposed to gas flow (Figure 9-7). The volume of the expired gas is estimated from the velocity of the rotating turbine, which is directly proportional to the flow rate of the expired gas. The Wright's respirometer is small in size, light weight, simple to operate, and reasonably accurate except with very low flow rates (<3 l/min). The pneumotachnygraph estimates flow indirectly by measuring the differential pressure generated across the flow resistor placed in the gas stream. The pneumotachnygraph is more accurate in measuring flow and in detecting changing flow rates. The volume of the expired gas can also be measured indirectly by integrating flow. A modern pneumotachnygraph attached to a portable computer is shown in Figure 9-8.

Interpretation of Spirometry

Serial measurements of forced expiratory flow (FVC, FEV_1, and PEF) are useful to assess response to therapy and to detect early deterioration in a patient's clinical condition after intensive therapy for acute asthma exacerbation. In patients with neuromuscular dysfunction, serial measurements of forced vital capacity (FVC) are helpful in evaluating the need for partial or full ventilatory support. A decreasing FVC in patients with neuromuscular dysfunction usually suggests progressive respiratory weakness and is a harbinger of impending

In patients with progressive neuromuscular weakness, FVC $\leq$10 ml/kg is an indication for assisted ventilation.

FIGURE 9-8

An example of a modern portable spirometer using a pneumotach connected to a laptop computer.

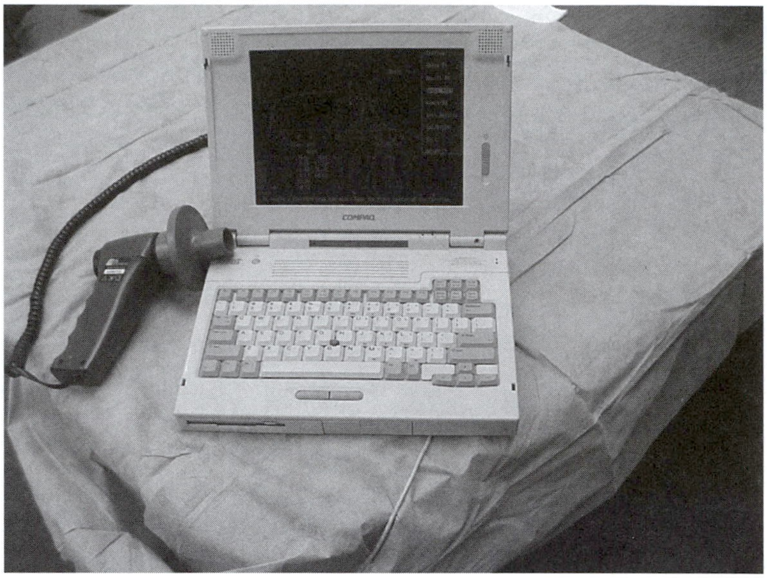

FVC ≤10 ml/kg is associated with impaired cough, retained secretions, and atelectasis.

Causes of high minute ventilation are intrinsic lung disease, pain, anxiety, fever, and central nervous system disorders.

An excessively high minute ventilation requirement may lead to respiratory muscle fatigue and acute respiratory failure.

Causes of low minute ventilation are hypothyroidism, oversedation, respiratory muscle dysfunction, and obesity hypoventilation syndrome.

Factors affecting peak flow measurements are volitional effort, respiratory muscle strength, recoil of the lung and chest wall, and airway resistance.

respiratory failure. At FVC less than 10 ml/kg, coughing becomes ineffective in clearing airway secretions, thereby increasing the risk for the development of atelectasis and pneumonia. Alternatively, the FVC can also be used as one of the criteria for the initiation of weaning trials and liberation from mechanical ventilation.

The minute ventilation is the amount of air that is inhaled and exhaled by an individual in 1 min. Therefore, minute ventilation is equal to the respiratory rate multiplied by tidal volume. Minute ventilation is composed of deadspace ventilation and alveolar ventilation. In healthy subjects, the normal minute ventilation is 5–6 l/min. Because minute ventilation is inversely proportional to $PaCO_2$, a high minute ventilation in the presence of hypercapnia suggests the presence of increased deadspace ventilation. Apart from intrinsic lung disease, a high minute ventilation may also result from pain, fever, or central nervous system disorders. An excessively high minute ventilation is not sustainable for prolonged periods of time, especially in critically ill patients. The majority of these patients often require ventilatory assistance if the cause of high minute ventilation cannot be easily reversed. For the same reason, a minute ventilation of less than 10 l is preferred in patients who are being weaned from mechanical ventilation. Conversely, a low minute ventilation may indicate decreased central respiratory drive as seen in conditions of oversedation, hypothyroidism, obesity hypoventilation syndrome, and respiratory muscle dysfunction. The ventilatory reserve of the respiratory system can be estimated by measuring the maximum minute ventilation, which is the maximum volume of gas that can be breathed over a specified period of time. Normal MVV values range from 50 to 250 l/min. The MVV is best interpreted in relationship to the resting minute ventilation. If a high minute ventilation is required to maintain a normal $PaCO_2$ in relation to the MVV (≥60%), the risk for the development of respiratory muscle fatigue increases during weaning trials.

A simple peak flowmeter can be used to measure airflow obstruction in highly motivated patients. It is a simple handheld device that is portable and easy to use. Serial measurements using the peak flowmeter gives more useful clinical information than a single absolute reading. Peak flow readings are affected by the volitional effort of the patient, the strength of the respiratory muscles, the recoil of the lungs and chest wall, and the degree of airway resistance. In patients with reversible airflow obstruction, the peak flow reading can be compared to their previously recorded personal best reading. Patients with chronic respiratory diseases such as asthma and chronic obstructive pulmonary disease (COPD), have their own optimal peak flows.

Serial measurement of respiratory muscle strength with a simple aneroid meter is important in patients with neuromuscular dysfunction. Maximum static mouth pressures, measured at the airway opening during a voluntary contraction against an occluded airway, are the most sensitive to assess respiratory muscle dysfunction in routine clinical practice. The extent of respiratory muscle weakness can be quantified by measuring the maximum inspiratory (PI_{max}) and expiratory pressures (PE_{max}) that can be generated by the respiratory muscles. It should be remembered that measurement of static mouth pressures is affected by the lung volume at which they are measured. Thus, PI_{max} is measured near residual volume where the inspiratory muscles are lengthened to their optimum precontraction length; PE_{max}, conversely, is measured near total lung capacity where expiratory muscles are lengthened to their optimum precontraction length. When respiratory muscle strength decreases to less than 30% of predicted, hypercapnic respiratory failure usually ensues.

PI_{max} is measured at residual volume; PE_{max} is measured at total lung capacity.

Inductive Plethysmography

Changes in breathing pattern herald the onset of respiratory muscle fatigue and ventilatory failure. In patients with respiratory muscle fatigue caused by either high resistive loads (e.g., patients with chronic airflow obstruction) or high elastic loads (e.g., morbidly obese patients), the breathing pattern is characterized as rapid and shallow. This rapid and shallow breathing pattern can be expressed as the ratio of tidal volume to respiratory rate, which is commonly referred to as the rapid shallow breathing index. In ventilator-dependent patients who are undergoing weaning trials, a rapid shallow breathing index less than 100 is highly predictive of weaning failure. Similarly, during breathing, thoracoabdominal rib cage paradox in the absence of upper airway obstruction also suggests respiratory muscle weakness or fatigue.

The breathing pattern in patients with ventilatory insufficiency can be followed qualitatively using inductive plethysmography. In inductive plethysmography, an elastic band that contains electrical wires or magnets is wrapped around the patient's rib cage and abdomen. The wires are then connected to an oscillator module. Changes in the compartmental volume of the rib cage or abdomen create proportional changes in the cross-sectional areas of the electrical inductance loops. This resultant change in volume displacement is compared to the calibration curve obtained from lung function data measured while performing spirometry. Using this technique, tidal volume can then be qualitatively estimated and followed serially during weaning trials.

Inductive plethysmography measures the qualitative compartment volume changes of the thorax in relation to the abdomen during inspiration and expiration.

CARDIAC MONITORING

Bedside Assessment

Cardiovascular monitoring is said to be the foundation of intensive care medicine. Cardiovascular dysfunction, either caused by primary cardiac disease or arising as complications from other organ dysfunctions, is frequently seen in patients admitted to the intensive care unit. A brief history and physical examination tailored to the patient's symptoms provide a cost-effective approach to the initial evaluation and monitoring of intensive care patients.

Acute circulatory shock or hypotension is a common clinical problem in the ICU. Occasionally, patients may not be able to provide any history because of respiratory distress, pain, or mental obtundation. The initial physical examination may provide the initial clue to the etiology of the shock state. For purposes of rapid assessment and therapy, acute circulatory shock can be broadly viewed as having hypovolemic, septic, cardiogenic, or obstructive causes. In both hypovolemic and cardiogenic shock, the pulse pressure is decreased by low stroke volume and high peripheral vascular resistance. The peripheral pulse volume is small and the skin is cool to the touch, with poor capillary refill. In patients with hypovolemic shock, the neck veins are flat even when the patient is in the supine position. The heart size is small and the lung fields are often clear to auscultation. In contrast, patients with cardiogenic shock present with an elevated jugular venous pulsation, bibasilar crackles on auscultation, cardiomegaly, and bipedal pitting edema. In addition, S3 or S4 gallops may be heard over the precordial region. In contrast to hypovolemic and cardiogenic shock, septic shock is characterized by a wide pulse pressure and a bounding pulse. The skin is often warm and

Types of circulatory shock are hypovolemic, septic, cardiogenic, and obstructive.

Causes of obstructive shock are valvular heart diseases, pericardial diseases, and restrictive cardiomyopathy.

CASE STUDY: PART 4

Reassessment of this patient's vital signs revealed that the automated blood pressure cuff was unable to record any blood pressure. His blood pressure could not be adequately ascertained manually with a bedside sphygmomanometer because of faint Korotkoff sounds. The systolic blood pressure on palpation was estimated at 80 mmHg, which was subsequently confirmed by a doppler-enhanced stethoscope; 1 l normal saline was rapidly infused and dopamine was initiated at 5 μg/kg/min. A radial arterial line was inserted for more accurate blood pressure monitoring.

flushed. The focus of infection may or may not be apparent on initial assessment. Common causes of obstructive circulatory shock include valvular heart disease such as aortic or mitral stenosis, constrictive pericarditis, cardiac tamponade, and restrictive cardiomyopathy.

Blood Pressure Monitoring

In the presence of shock, direct intraarterial blood pressure measurement is more accurate than noninvasive indirect blood pressure measurement.

Arterial blood pressure can be monitored either directly via an intraarterial catheter or indirectly using a traditional sphygmomanometer and a stethoscope. Although intraarterial blood pressure monitoring is more accurate, especially in the presence of shock, noninvasive blood pressure monitoring is easy to set up and not subject to the complications commonly associated with intravascular catheters such as pain, infection, bleeding, and thrombosis. Several indirect blood pressure monitoring techniques have been developed that even surpass the accuracy and convenience of the auscultory method.

Indirect Blood Pressure Measurement

In the indirect blood pressure monitoring method, a small cuff size falsely elevates blood pressure and a big cuff size results in falsely low blood pressure readings.

Although several techniques are currently available for the indirect measurement of blood pressure, the basic method remains the same: the application of external pressure via an appropriately sized cuff when flow is observed in the artery distal to the occlusion. It is important to note that what is actually detected is blood flow, not the intraarterial pressure itself. The accuracy of the blood pressure measurement is affected by the cuff size. An inadequate cuff size will result in a falsely elevated blood pressure reading. In contrast, an inordinately large cuff size will lead to a falsely low reading.

Manual Methods

Manual blood pressure measurement can be obtained by auscultatory, oscillation, or palpation methods. The auscultatory method of blood pressure measurement involves inflating a mercury or an aneroid sphygmomanometer cuff around an extremity and auscultating for the disappearance of blood flow in the distal artery. The resumption of blood flow when the cuff is released causes distinctive thumping sounds (Korotkoff sounds) due to vibrations of the artery under pressure. The level at which the Korotkoff sounds reappear, and the level at which these disappear or diminish in volume, are taken as the systolic and diastolic blood pressures, respectively. In most clinical conditions, the auscultatory method is more than adequate in estimating clinically relevant blood pressure readings. However, in shock states, the Korotkoff sounds becomes faint, making accurate readings difficult. In this circumstance, the oscillation or the palpation methods may help identify the systolic blood pressure in emergency situations. With the oscillation method, the resumption of blood flow as the cuff pressure is released is indicated by the pulsatile movement of the mercury column or the needle of the aneroid manometer, representing the systolic blood pressure. In the palpation method, the detection of the radial pulse as the cuff pressure is slowly released is the palpatory blood pressure. With either oscillation or palpation methods, the diastolic blood pressure cannot be measured. Overall, these noninvasive blood pressure techniques correlate poorly with the directly measured blood pressure value.

The oscillation or palpation methods are useful in rapidly estimating systolic blood pressure in the presence of shock.

CASE STUDY: PART 5

On the fourth hospital day, this patient was noted to have a heart rate of 171 beats/min. The rhythm appeared to be a narrow complex tachycardia on the patient's cardiac monitor. His blood pressure was 110/58 mmHg while receiving dopamine infused at 6 μg/kg/min. A 12-lead ECG showed a regular and narrow complex tachycardia with a consistent AV nodal reentrant tachycardia. Right carotid massage was attempted but without success. The patient was given 12 mg IV of adenosine with spontaneous conversion to sinus tachycardia at a rate of 110 beats/min. A stat electrolyte determination revealed a potassium of 3 mEq/l and a low normal serum magnesium level. A bedside echocardiogram revealed normal left ventricular function with an ejection fraction of 55%. His left atrial size was normal. He had no further recurrence of cardiac arrhythmia after adequate correction of his hypokalemia. The patient had a prolonged course in the ICU complicated by sepsis with multiorgan failure. On the seventh hospital day, he was weaned from dopamine, and his blood pressure remained stable. He was slowly weaned from the ventilator following a tracheostomy. He was subsequently transferred to the ventilator rehabilitation unit for further care.

Automated Methods

The automated indirect blood pressure measurement devices obviate the need to manually inflate and deflate the sphygnomanometer cuff. The automated blood pressure measurement is widely used in critical care units and offers the ability to repetitively measure the blood pressure with ease, convenience, and without the associated morbidity of intraarterial blood pressure monitoring. The most commonly used principles in automated blood pressure system include doppler flow, infrasound, oscillometry, volume clamp, and arterial tonometry. With the doppler flow system, the changes in the reflected echo signal in the distal artery during cuff inflation and deflation (doppler shift) are used to estimate blood pressure. In an uncompressed artery, the small amount of wall motion does change the frequency of the reflected signal. The first appearance of flow in the distal artery is the systolic pressure, and the disappearance of the doppler shift represents the diastolic blood pressure. In the infrasound system, a microphone is used to detect low-frequency sound waves associated with vibration of the arterial wall during cuff deflation. In the oscillometric method of blood pressure monitoring, oscillations of the arterial vessel wall due to pulsatile blood flow are detected by a sensor in the cuff. Systolic and diastolic blood pressure is estimated from the magnitude of the pressure fluctuation. The volume clamp technique is unique because a finger cuff applied over the proximal or middle phalanx is used instead of the arm cuff. The pressure on the finger cuff is regulated by a servo-control unit, strapped to the wrist, that keeps the artery at a constant size. The pressure needed to maintain the artery at a constant size is equal to the intraarterial pressure.

Overall, these automated blood pressure devices are adequate in frequent blood pressure monitoring, especially in patients who are essentially stable, or during transport when arterial lines cannot be easily used, or for burned patients in whom intraarterial blood pressure monitoring may lead to infections. The limitations of the automated indirect blood pressure measurement are similar to other noninvasive methods of blood pressure determination.

ELECTROCARDIOGRAPHIC MONITORING

Monitoring of cardiac rhythm using the principles of electrocardiography to detect life-threatening cardiac arrhythmia has been shown to improve prognosis in patients with acute myocardial infarction. The impact of routine cardiac rhythm monitoring in the ICU is unclear. However, because most patients who are admitted to the ICU are older, have multiple organ dysfunction, and have concomitant ischemic heart disease, continuous electrocardiographic monitoring should be used in all patients regardless of the admitting diagnosis. Common causes of cardiac arrhythmia in the ICU setting are shown in Table 9-4.

The ECG leads commonly selected are either for monitor display leads V_1 or lead II. The American Heart Association Task Force recommends using at least two and preferably three

> The preferred leads for monitoring myocardial ischemia are V_1, aVf, and V_5.

TABLE 9-4

COMMON CAUSES OF CARDIAC ARRHYTHMIA IN THE ICU

CONDITION	RESULT

Cardiac	Myocardial ischemia
	Myocardial infarction
	Congestive heart failure
	Sick sinus syndrome
	Atrioventricular bypass tract
	Postcardiac surgery arrhythmias
	Hypotension
	  Dehydration
	  Gastrointestinal bleeding
	  Sepsis

Noncardiac	

Metabolic	Electrolyte abnormalities
	  Hypokalemia
	  Hypomagnesemia
	High-catecholamine state
	  Pain
	  Sepsis
	Alcohol withdrawal syndrome
	Hyperthyroid state

Respiratory	Respiratory distress due to airflow obstruction or parenchyma lung disease Acute pulmonary embolism

Drugs	Vasopressors
	  Dopamine
	  Dobutamine
	  Epinephrine
	  Norepinephrine
	Theophylline
	Antiarrhythmic drugs

Lead V_5 is the most sensitive lead in detecting myocardial ischemia.

leads for patient monitoring. The use of multiple leads enhances recognition of abnormal ECG patterns and artifact detection. If the patient is at high risk for myocardial ischemia, a basic system using leads V_1, aVf, and V_5 is preferred for monitoring. Lead V_5 has been reported to have the greatest sensitivity for detecting myocardial ischemia. To enhance the recognition and interpretation of a wide QRS complex tachycardia, bipolar precordial leads, MCL1 and MCL6, are used to simulate leads V_1 and V_6, respectively.

Apart from choosing the optimal lead system, it is important to remember to clean the skin with alcohol and to remove the hair on the electrode site to decrease skin electrical resistance and to prevent artifacts. By properly following these techniques, the skin electrical resistance can be reduced from 200 to approximately 10 ohms in most patients. Other electro magnetic devices used in other monitoring systems can interfere with ECG monitoring. A common type of interference is caused by nearby 60-Hz power lines. This type of interference can be minimized by (1) using shielded electrodes and ensuring that the electrode cables are properly attached, (2) preparing the skin properly, (3) using an amplifier with common-mode rejection, and (4) using only monitors with built-in filtering systems.

Current continuous ECG monitoring system not only can detect cardiac arrhythmia but also can monitor ST segment morphology that may indicate ongoing myocardial ischemia. This added capability is important because (1) patients with coronary artery disease with ST segment changes may have no symptoms (silent myocardial ischemia), (2) patients with unstable angina with ischemic ST-T wave changes at rest or during pain have a poorer prognosis, and (3) patients in the ICU often are intubated or heavily sedated and may not be able to communicate their symptoms properly.

The modern ECG monitoring system includes analysis of the ST segment 60–80 mg after the J point.

In most ST segment monitoring systems, the computer analyzes ECG pattern and stores a normal QRS template. The computer algorithm used in the detection of ST segment changes compares the isoelectric points just before the QRS and the ST segment 60–80 ms after the

J point. The computer uses the stored QRS template to differentiate a normal QRS from an ectopic beat that makes the ST segment changes void. The use of a multiple lead system enhances the sensitivity and accuracy of ST segment monitoring.

Changes in the ST segment (e.g., elevation or depression) on the ECG monitoring leads need to be confirmed by a 12-lead ECG and interpreted in light of other clinical findings. In patients with known history of coronary artery disease, ST segment elevation or depression usually suggests ongoing myocardial injury or ischemia. Other causes of ST segment elevation include acute pericarditis, ventricular aneurysm, coronary artery spasm (Prinzmetal angina), change in body position, and benign early repolarization. In acute pericarditis, chest pain is worse when the patient leans forward, and a pericardial rub may be heard on cardiac auscultation. Moreover, ST segment elevation is often present diffusely on the ECG and is frequently accompanied by PR segment depression. In the presence of a ventricular aneurysm, the ST segment remains persistently elevated. These patients often have a history of prior anterior myocardial infarction. ST segment elevation in coronary artery spasm usually correlates with the patient's symptoms. It is important to remember that changes in body position can lead to artifactual ST segment elevation.

> Causes of ST segment elevation are acute myocardial infarction, acute pericarditis, ventricular aneurysm, coronary artery spasm, benign early repolarization, and a change in body position.

LIMITATION AND SIDE EFFECTS OF MONITORING

Although noninvasive monitoring in the ICU can alert the physicians, nurses, and respiratory therapists to potential life-threatening events, the limitations of the different ICU monitoring techniques must be remembered and applied in the right clinical setting. For example, pulse oximetry should not be used or relied on as a measure of adequate oxygenation in patients who are suspected of methemoglobin poisoning. It is incumbent on the health care practitioner to recognize artifactual as well as factitious data. A common cause of monitoring artifacts in the ICU is patient movement that causes dislodgement of the monitoring electrodes or probes. Electrical interference among different monitoring devices can also lead to artifactual results. This type of interference is commonly referred to as 60-Hz interference. Artifactual and factitious recordings may result in false alarms that may prompt less experienced health care providers to order unnecessary tests. In some studies, the incidence of false alarms generated by the multiple monitoring devices commonly used in the ICU can be as high as 50%–90%.

Apart from the measurement problems of the various monitoring devices, the alarms triggered by the different commonly used monitoring techniques contributes to noise pollution in the ICU environment, which may lead to sleep disruption in some patients. In one study, the noise level in a medium-sized ICU during the day and night exceeded the exposure threshold by the U.S. Environmental Protection Agency (>45 dB in 24 h).

Another emerging problem in ICU care is overreliance of health care givers on data from monitoring devices to the exclusion of the patient's physical examination. All too often work rounds in the ICU consist of discussion of the patient's monitoring data, rather than careful observation and physical examination of the patient. It is sometimes difficult to remember, amidst all the technologically advanced monitoring equipment in the ICU, that critically ill patients are more than the sum of their physiologic data.

SUMMARY

Noninvasive monitoring is widely used in the management of critically ill patients. It is safe, relatively easy to use, and is not associated with complications associated with invasive monitoring techniques. Its main use is to detect early changes in the patient's physiology so that appropriate interventions can be performed promptly. So long as the capabilities and limitations of the monitoring device are understood by physicians, nurses, and other health care workers, noninvasive monitoring is valuable in providing useful information and preventing complications.

REVIEW QUESTIONS

1. **A 12-year-old boy was rescued by a firefighter from a smoke-filled room of a burning 12-story apartment building. The following procedures are appropriate, except which of the following:**
   - **A.** A careful inspection of the upper airway passages to detect signs of inhalational injury.
   - **B.** A chest radiograph on admission to look for inhalation lung injury.
   - **C.** A 24-h hospital observation.
   - **D.** A normal oxygen hemoglobin saturation by pulse oximetry to exclude the presence of carbon monoxide poisoning.

2. **A 46-year-old bank executive was admitted to the neurointensive care unit for sudden onset of aphasia, right hemiparesis, and hypertension. Four hours after admission, the patient exhibited irregular breathing pattern. On examination, he was awake, alert, and could follow simple commands. He was afebrile and appeared anxious but comfortable. His breathing pattern was characterized by periods of tachypnea interrupted by apnea, especially during sleep. His oxygen hemoglobin saturation on 2 l/min of supplemental oxygen was 95%. The most likely explanation of his abnormal breathing pattern is which of the following:**
   - **A.** Cheyne–Stoke breathing is common following acute stroke and usually requires only low-flow supplemental oxygen.
   - **B.** Central neurogenic hyperventilation is commonly seen in patients with cephalocaudal brain herniation caused by compression of the pontine structures.
   - **C.** Biot breathing is a preterminal event caused by compression of the medulla.
   - **D.** Tachypnea in the setting of acute stroke could be a result of aspiration pneumonitis, of atelectasis caused by decreased phrenic nerve output to the diaphragm, or of compression of brainstem structures.

3. **The following statements about pulse oximetry are true except which of the following:**
   - **A.** Modern pulse oximetry uses two wavelength of light, red and infrared, to discriminate between oxygenated and deoxygenated blood.
   - **B.** Unlike transcutaneous oxygen measurement, pulse oximetry is not affected by low cardiac output state.
   - **C.** Different forms of dyshemoglobinemia can affect the accuracy of oxyhemoglobin measurement by pulse oximetry.
   - **D.** The accuracy of pulse oximetry degrades with oxygen saturation $\leq$65%.

4. **The following statements about capnometry and endotracheal tube placement are true except which of the following:**
   - **A.** Capnometry provides a rapid and accurate confirmation of a successful tracheal intubation in critically ill patients.
   - **B.** By looking at the end-tidal PCO_2 level, capnometry may also be able to discriminate right and left mainstem intubation.
   - **C.** Recent ingestion of carbonated drinks before attempted intubation may lead to positive CO_2 detection despite esophageal intubation.
   - **D.** Bedside proper endotracheal tube placement can also be assessed by listening for bilateral breath sounds, symmetric chest expansion, and absence of gastric sound following a positive inspiratory breath.

5. **ST segment elevation in the ICU may be seen in the following clinical scenario except which of the following:**
   - **A.** A 22-year-old man with cocaine overdose.
   - **B.** A 48-year-old executive presenting to the emergency room with chest discomfort and jaw pain radiating to the left arm.
   - **C.** A 70-year-old man with history of multiple anterior myocardial infarction and four-vessel coronary artery bypass surgery who now presents to the emergency room with symptoms and signs of congestive heart failure.
   - **D.** A 24-year-old man who complains of chest pain and shortness of breath 4 days after knee surgery.

ANSWERS

1. The answer is D. A normal oxygen hemoglobin saturation by pulse oximetry in patients with a history of smoke exposure does not exclude the presence of a significant carbon monoxide poisoning. Because the absorption characteristics of carboxyhemoglobin mimic the light absorbance pattern of oxyhemoglobin, a falsely elevated oxyhemoglobin saturation is invariably seen by pulse oximetry. The oxygen saturation should be measured directly in the blood samples by co-oximetry technique.
2. The answer is A. Cheyne–Stokes breathing is commonly seen in patients with stroke as well as in patients with congestive heart failure. In addition, it is also seen in neonates and at high altitudes in normal adults. It is easily recognized by a periodic crescendo–decrescendo breathing pattern associated with central apnea. Treatment usually requires supplemental oxygen or theophylline. Both central neurogenic hyperventilation and Biot breathing are caused by lesions located in the brainstem. Tachypnea due to aspiration of oropharyngeal contents usually occurs in patients with depressed mental status, poor gag reflex, fever, and an abnormal chest radiograph.
3. The answer is B. Pulse oximetry is unreliable in the low cardiac output state. Similarly, oxygen hemoglobin measurement by pulse oximetry becomes unreliable in the presence of dyshemoglobinemia, severe anemia, and severe hypoxemia.
4. The answer is B. Capnometry is increasingly used to confirm successful endotracheal intubation by the qualitative detection of expired CO_2. It will not differentiate an inadvertent bronchial intubation from tracheal intubation. Careful bedside examination for equal breath sounds and symmetric chest expansion, and listening for gastric sound on inspiration, are helpful in the detection of bronchial intubation. Capnometry may detect CO_2 release from carbonated drinks despite esophageal intubation.
5. The answer is D. In a small percentage of patients with acute pulmonary embolism, 12-lead electrocardiogram may show an S1-Q3-T3 pattern, that is, an S wave in lead I and Q-wave and T-wave

inversion in lead III. The cardiac toxicity of cocaine may be associated with either ST segment depression or elevation suggestive of myocardial ischemia or coronary vasospasm, respectively. Choice B is a classic presentation of acute myocardial infarction. Choice C is a patient with left ventricular aneurysm due to multiple episodes of myocardial infarction in the past. The typical 12-lead electrocardiographic finding is persistent ST segment elevation in the precordial leads.

SUGGESTED READING

Bowton DI, Scuderi PE, Harris L, Haponik EF. Pulse oximetry monitoring outside the intensive care unit: progress or problem? Ann Intern Med 1991;115:450–454.

Clark JS, Votteri B, Ariagno RL, Cheung P, Eichhorn JH, Fallat RJ, Lee SE, Newth CJL, Rotman H, Sue DY. Noninvasive assessment of blood gases. Am Rev Respir Dis 1992;145:220–232.

Clements FM, de Bruijn NP. Noninvasive cardiac monitoring. Crit Care Clin 4(3):435–445.

Curley FJ, Smyrnios NS. Routine monitoring of critically ill patients. In: Irwin RS, Cerra FB, Rippe JM (eds) Intensive Care Medicine, 4th Ed. Philadelphia: Lippincott-Raven, 1999.

Loeb RG, Santos WC. Monitoring ventilation. In: Hanowell LH, Waldron RJ (eds) Airway Management. Philadelphia: Lippincott-Raven, 1996.

Schnapp LM, Cohen NH. Pulse oximetry: uses and abuses. Chest 1990;98:1244–1250.

St. John RE, Thompson PD. Noninvasive respiratory monitoring. Crit Care Nurs Clin North Am 1999;11(4):423–435.

Tobin MJ. Respiratory monitoring in the intensive care unit. Am J Respir Dis 1988;138:1625–1642.

CHAPTER 10

GILBERT E. D'ALONZO AND DAVID FRIEDEL

Endoscopy in the Intensive Care Unit

CHAPTER OUTLINE

LEARNING OBJECTIVES

After studying this chapter, you should be able to do the following:

- Understand the indications for both respiratory and gastrointestinal endoscopy in critically ill patients.
- Describe the contraindications and potential complications that are associated with endoscopy and endosurgery.

During the past three decades, the technology of endoscopy has led to sophisticated optics and simple-to-use devices that are practical for use in critically ill patients. The upper airway, lung, and gastrointestinal passageways are accessible by endoscopy. In the intensive care unit, endoscopy is commonly performed for therapeutic reasons and for diagnostic purposes. This chapter reviews the indications, contraindications, techniques, and complications of laryngoscopy, bronchoscopy, and gastrointestinal endoscopy in critically ill patients.

LARYNGOSCOPY

The larynx can be examined directly with a laryngoscope or a bronchoscope. The traditional rigid laryngoscope is a lighted metal instrument that displaces the tongue and permits observation of the glottis, including the epiglottis and vocal cords. It consists of a handle containing batteries and a detachable blade, either straight (Miller) or curved (McIntosh), which comes in a variety of sizes, and a bulb to illuminate the tip of the blade. The straight blade bypasses and lifts the epiglottis, while the curved blade tip fits into the vallecula (Figure 10-1).

> The upper airway can be inspected by both rigid and flexible laryngoscopy techniques.

Fiberoptic laryngoscopy has enhanced the ease and comfort of visualizing the oronasopharynx and larynx. The flexible fiberscope, inserted via the nose, is considered the simplest method of visualizing the upper airway and an excellent way to monitor epiglottic swelling to evaluate the need to intubate or perform a tracheostomy. Rigid laryngoscopy should be performed for upper airway inspection, particularly in patients who are suspected of having upper airway obstruction (Table 10-1). The major indication for rigid laryngoscopy is endotracheal intubation.

> Rigid laryngoscopy facilitates endotracheal intubation.

Endotracheal intubation with a flexible fiberoptic laryngoscope or bronchoscope requires considerable experience. First, the larynx must be localized and the tip of the scope is ad-

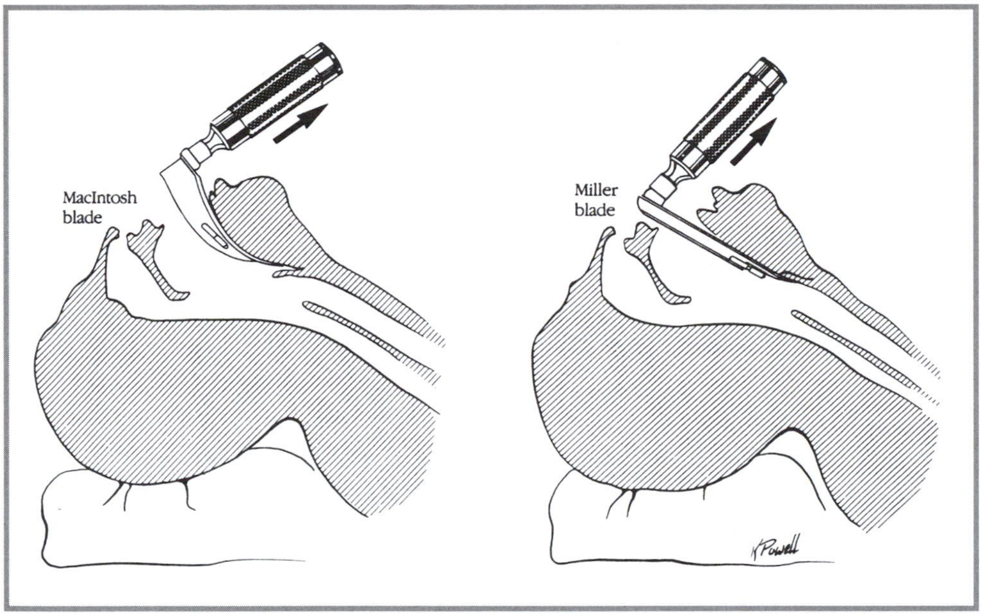

FIGURE 10-1

There are two basic types of laryngoscope blades, the MacIntosh (*left*) and the Miller (*right*) blades. The MacIntosh blade in curved and its use differs from that of the Miller blade. The MacIntosh blade tip is placed in the vallecula, and the handle of the laryngoscope is pulled forward at a 45° angle. This technique allows visualization of the epiglottis. With the Miller blade, which is straight, the tip is placed posterior to the epiglottis and, therefore, the epiglottis is pinned between the base of the tongue and the straight laryngoscope blade. The motion on the laryngoscope handle is the same as that used with the MacIntosh blade.

vanced into the trachea. Then the endotracheal tube is advanced over the scope into the trachea. Although the maneuver sounds simple, it can be very difficult. Visualization may be hampered by excessive secretions and tissue edema.

BRONCHOSCOPY

Bronchoscopy is the endoscopic examination of the larynx and tracheobronchial tree. In the intensive care unit, it is rarely performed using a rigid instrument but is often performed using a flexible bronchoscope. With the presence of bronchopulmonary disease in the intensive care unit and the use of mechanical ventilation with endotracheal tubes, bronchoscopy has become an essential tool in the management of these patients. Fiberoptic bronchoscopy is easily performed, is rarely associated with complications, and, with proper sedation, is very comfortable. It has surpassed rigid bronchoscopy as the instrument of choice for evaluating the tracheobronchial tree. Furthermore, as compared to rigid bronchoscopy, the flexible bronchoscope allows for more complete exploration of the airways, including access to

> Flexible fiberoptic bronchoscopy can be easily performed through an endotracheal tube while a patient is mechanically ventilated.

TABLE 10-1

CAUSES OF UPPER AIRWAY OBSTRUCTION

Trauma
Facial and neck injury
Laryngeal trauma and stenosis
Airway burn
Infection
Epiglotitis
Quinsey (acute tonsillitis)
Ludwig's angina (mouth floor abscess)
Retropharyngeal abscess
Endotracheal tube trauma
Foreign body
Tumor
Angioedema
Laryngospasm
Vocal cord paralysis
Postextubation stridor

the upper lobes, as compared to rigid bronchoscopy. The procedure can actually be performed at the bedside, with minimal technical assistance.

Flexible fiberoptic bronchoscopy allows the most complete inspection of the large airways.

Rigid bronchoscopy is most helpful in massive hemoptysis and the removal of a foreign body.

Despite the frequent use of flexible fiberoptic bronchoscopy, the rigid bronchoscope still has advantages in certain clinical situations, such as massive hemoptysis and the removal of large foreign bodies. Although laser surgery can be performed using a flexible fiberoptic bronchoscope, the rigid bronchoscope has distinct advantages for this intervention, as it does for certain dilation procedures of the tracheobronchial tree involving airway stricture and tumors, particularly the placement of airway stents. Nonetheless, flexible fiberoptic bronchoscopy can also be used for these procedures.

Diagnostic Indications

The diagnostic indications for bronchoscopy are numerous (Table 10-2). However, the most commonly encountered diagnostic indications in the ICU include the evaluation of hemoptysis, atelectasis, diffuse parenchymal disease, inspection of the airways following an inhalation injury or blunt trauma, assessment of the large airways following intubation, and for culturing airway secretions or washings, including bronchoalveolar lavage.

Bronchoscopy is often used to evaluate hemoptysis and to culture airway secretions and lung washings in critically ill patients.

Hemoptysis following intubation should always be evaluated by bronchoscopy.

Bronchoscopy is employed to identify the site of bleeding when a patient has hemoptysis. Because hemoptysis can be caused by a variety of tracheobronchial lesions, cardiovascular and hematologic conditions, and localized and diffuse parenchymal lung disorders, the clinician must decide when bronchoscopy is indicated in the patient with hemoptysis. For example, the patient who has hemoptysis as a complication of pulmonary embolism does not require bronchoscopy. On the other hand, a patient in respiratory failure with a localized lung infiltrate on chest x-ray and hemoptysis does require bronchoscopy to determine if there is an airway lesion, such as carcinoma, that is responsible for the clinical presentation. In patients who have been intubated, hemoptysis should always be evaluated to determine if tracheal damage has occurred at the time of or during intubation. It is the responsibility of the bronchoscopist to carefully inspect the airways and find the source of bleeding, when possible. The use of the fiberoptic bronchoscope allows the bronchoscopist to evaluate the areas to the segmental, and even subsegmental, bronchial level.

TABLE 10-2

INDICATIONS FOR BRONCHOSCOPY

DIAGNOSTIC INDICATIONS	THERAPEUTIC INDICATIONS
Acute inhalation injury	Airway stent placement
Assessment of intubation trauma	Bedside tracheostomy
Atelectasis	Brachytherapy for central airway neoplasms
Blunt chest trauma	Closure of bronchopleural fistula
Chest radiograph consistent with neoplasia	Endotracheal intubation
Cough	Excessive secretions and atelectasis
Cultures	Foreign bodies
Diaphragmatic paralysis	Hemoptysis
Diffuse parenchymal disease and/or bilateral hilar adenopathy	Laser resection for central airway neoplasms
Hemoptysis	Lung abscess
Laryngeal abnormalities	Preoperative assessment of resectability
Localized wheeze	Pulmonary alveolar proteinosis lavage
Lung abscess	
Metastatic disease with unknown primary	
Pleural effusion of unknown etiology	
Positive cytology and normal chest radiograph	
Recurrent laryngeal nerve paralysis	
Recurrent pneumonia	
Symptoms after resection surgery	
Unresolving infiltrate	

Not all chest x-ray abnormalities require diagnostic bronchoscopy. Intensive care patients with pneumonia may not require bronchoscopy unless they are immunocompromised and special cultures are necessary that can only be obtained with the use of a bronchoscope. However, certain chest x-ray abnormalities may indicate a need for diagnostic bronchoscopy (see Table 10-2). These abnormalities include atelectasis of a lung, lobe, or segment, enlarging or suspicious pulmonary parenchymal nodules, cavitated pulmonary lesions, and diffuse parenchymal processes that do not have an established diagnosis. Atelectasis often requires fiberoptic bronchoscopy to rule out endobronchial obstruction by carcinoma or a foreign body. However, most atelectasis is caused by mucous plugging of the airway. When atelectasis occurs in a critically ill patient who has had a normal chest x-ray on admission, mucous plugging is the most likely cause. In patients who are intubated, the position of the endotracheal tube may be responsible for the atelectasis, because the tube may have slipped down a mainstem bronchus, generally the right main stem, and obstructed the right upper lobe creating right upper lobe atelectasis. Additionally, the left lung may not have been aerated during this process, and complete left lung atelectasis may occur.

Lung atelectasis often necessitates bronchoscopy to rule out an endobronchial lesion, a foreign body, or mucous plugging.

Bronchoscopy can be helpful in the diagnosis of both bacterial and nonbacterial pulmonary infections in critically ill patients. Lung secretions can be obtained by bronchial washings, bronchoalveolar lavage, protected-catheter brushings, and, in select patients, transbronchial lung biopsy. Certain factors must be considered when choosing a certain bronchoscopy procedure in a critically ill patient with diffuse lung infiltrates: physician expertise, the patient's condition, and the potential for diagnostic success of a particular procedure in a select patient. Not only is physician expertise important, but the skill of the laboratory personnel in specimen processing and analysis is crucial, particularly cytopathologic and certain microbiologic issues.

Bronchoscopy can help diagnose a variety of pulmonary infections.

The two major bronchoscopic procedures used in the diagnosis of diffuse lung disease are bronchoalveolar lavage and transbronchial lung biopsy. Often the protected-brush catheter (Figure 10-2) is employed with bronchoalveolar lavage in the diagnosis of lung infection. Quantitative culturing using these techniques has improved the diagnosis of infection of the lung. Cultures obtained from the protected-brush catheter that provide 10^3 or more colony-forming units (CFU) per milliliter indicate active infection. This brush catheter technique is equivalent to needle aspiration biopsying of the lung in the identification of the etiology of bacterial pneumonia. The protected-brush catheter technique is limited by the fact that it only samples a very small area and that cultures obtained from this area may not alter the antibiotic therapy that is being used, because of the wider use of broad-spectrum antibiotics that treat most of the common bacterial infections. Bronchoalveolar lavage, performed through the flexible bronchoscope when wedged peripherally in an airway of the lung, allows for the recovery of both cellular and noncellular components of the lower respiratory tract. Bronchoalveolar lavage has been used to diagnose certain interstitial lung diseases, malignancies, and infections. However, bronchoalveolar lavage cannot be used to make a definitive diagnosis for most interstitial lung diseases. Bronchoalveolar lavage has been very successful in the diagnosis of *Pneumocystis carinii* pneumonia and other causes of diffuse pulmonary infiltrates in immunocompromised hosts. Its greatest efficacy is in a diagnosis of opportunistic infections, including *Pneumocystis carinii*, cytomegalovirus, a variety of fungi, and mycobacterium. The detection of hemosiderin-laden macrophages is helpful in the diagnosis of pulmonary hemorrhage. Occasionally, it can be helpful in the diagnosis of pulmonary malignancy, particularly those patients who have lymphangitic metastasis.

Protected-brush catheter and bronchoalveolar lavage techniques are useful in the diagnosis of pneumonia.

Bronchoalveolar lavage is the diagnostic procedural choice for *Pneumocystis carinii* pneumonia.

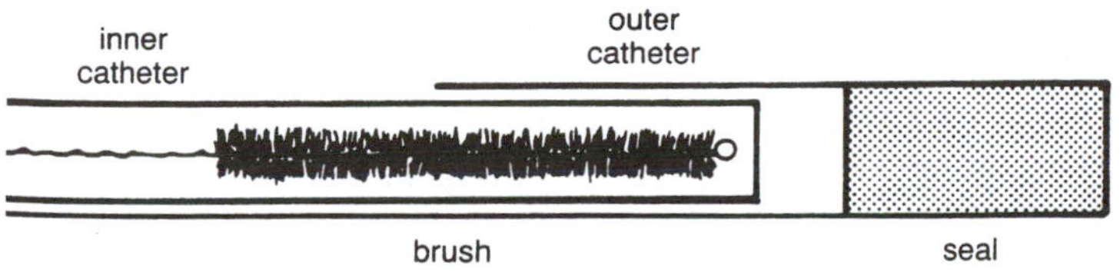

FIGURE 10-2

The plugged telescoping catheter brush is used to obtain selective samples from the lower airways and to keep the brush sterile until it is pushed out of the catheter at the time of culturing.

Critically ill patients who have sustained serious inhalation injuries or blunt chest trauma, or who are suspected of having intubation damage, require fiberoptic bronchoscopy for airway inspection. For patients who have sustained an inhalation injury, the presence of serious mucosal injury can be identified during fiberoptic bronchoscopy and a decision for prophylactic intubation can be better addressed. Likewise, fiberoptic bronchoscopy allows the trauma surgeon to evaluate the airways following blunt chest trauma to determine if the patient has sustained a fractured airway, particularly if atelectasis, pneumomediastinum, or pneumothorax is determined during the evaluation. Fiberoptic bronchoscopy can be used to determine whether laryngeal or tracheal complications have occurred during an intubation. If serious injury has occurred, then a tracheostomy should be considered. Fiberoptic bronchoscopy can easily be performed in patients who are intubated and have an endotracheal tube in place that is 7.5 mm or larger in internal diameter. Therefore, it is important for most of our adult patients to use an endotracheal tube at least 8 mm in internal diameter during intubation. A complete airway inspection can be done with a fiberoptic bronchoscope. With the endoscope inserted through the endotracheal tube, the balloon can be deflated and the tube withdrawn over the bronchoscope to look for subglottic damage. The tube can be carefully withdrawn up through the vocal cords over the fiberoptic bronchoscope for glottic and superglottic assessment. The presence of serious mucosal ulceration, necrosis, or edema indicates the need for a tracheostomy, which is done to avoid the serious consequences of tracheomalacia, tracheostenosis, and laryngostenosis.

Following blunt chest trauma, bronchoscopic inspection can determine airway fracture and laryngeal injury.

Therapeutic Indications

Airway secretion management can be facilitated by bronchoscopy in intubated patients.

The therapeutic uses of fiberoptic bronchoscopy (see Table 10-2) are as important as its diagnostic indications. Most bronchoscopies in the intensive care unit are performed for airway secretion management. It is common to perform bronchoscopy for both diagnostic and therapeutic reasons in patients who are intubated and are critically ill.

When aggressive pulmonary toilet, including physical therapy, incentive spirometry, and sustained maximum inspiration with cough, fails to clear the airways of excessive secretions or fails to reexpand significant lung atelectasis, then fiberoptic bronchoscopy should be considered. Retention of secretions and mucous plugging of the airways are common clinical complications in those patients with an altered level of consciousness and impaired cough, poor pulmonary function that often results from weakness, recurrent aspiration, ventilator dependence, or pain following thoracoabdominal surgery. Following thoracic surgery, blood clots often accumulate in the lung airways and induce atelectasis. Also, patients with airway mucosal injury are more likely to have serious secretion and mucous plugging problems. In all these situations, fiberoptic bronchoscopy may enhance pulmonary toilet and, in fact, may be lifesaving. For airway secretion management, it is better to use a flexible bronchoscope with large-channel suctioning capabilities. The airway secretions are often thick and tenacious and are generally aspirated with difficulty. In an intubated patient, the fiberoptic bronchoscope can be introduced and removed frequently to enhance secretion removal and maintain suction channel patency. Occasionally, the installation of acetylcysteine or pulmozyme through the bronchoscope may be necessary to help liquefy thick, tenacious inspissated mucus from the airways. The use of acetylcysteine may trigger bronchospasm, but patients who experience this complication generally respond to a bronchodilator nebulizer treatment. Pulmozyme is less likely to ellicit bronchospasm.

Bronchoscopy can remove retained secretions, mucous plugs, blood clots, and foreign bodies.

Fiberoptic bronchoscopy can be used to retrieve a foreign body lodged in an airway. Various techniques can be used either to grasp or net the object and to pull it out of the airway with the bronchoscope when it is withdrawn. Fiberoptic bronchoscopy is often used for endotracheal intubation. Essentially, the bronchoscope acts as an obturator for endotracheal intubation in patients for whom intubation is difficult, such as individuals with neck or head trauma or certain disease states such as ankylosing spondylitis. In individuals who have had laryngeal trauma or have vocal cord dysfunction, this technique can be particularly helpful. With the endotracheal tube over the bronchoscope, the bronchoscope is advanced either through the nose or orally to the vocal cords. After placing the endoscope through the cords,

Bronchoscopy can facilitate endo- or nasotracheal intubation.

the endotracheal tube can be slipped over the bronchoscope into the airway. This technique is also helpful in individuals with massive facial injuries.

Bronchoscopy helps locate the area of hemoptysis, and it can assist in tamponade.

Fiberoptic bronchoscopy can be used for the treatment of massive hemoptysis. Bronchial tamponade can be accomplished with a transbronchoscopic endobronchial balloon occlusion technique after the bronchoscope has been placed in an airway that is hemorrhaging. Bronchial tamponade can be used for either bronchial or pulmonary hemorrhage, as well as for refractory pneumothorax secondary to persistent air leaks following thoracotomy. Sometimes a bronchopleural fistula can develop between a bronchial tree and a pleural space. After chest tube placement, bronchoscopy can identify which airway is part of this phenomenon and then be used to distally occlude the bronchopleural fistula; however, this technique is not easy to do. A variety of materials have been injected through the bronchoscope to seal the fistula.

Airway stenting can open stenotic segments of large airways.

Central airway-obstructing lesions involving the larynx, trachea, or a major bronchus can be treated using a variety of bronchoscopic techniques including photoresection using laser technology or airway stenting. Airway stenting can be used in malignant or benign disease with severe airway narrowing from intrinsic or extrinsic processes. The trachea and main stem bronchi can be stented, but the technique is not suitable for lobar and distal bronchial stenosis. Many types of tracheobronchial stents are available, such as expandable metal wire (Figure 10-3), molded silicon stents, or a combination of these. After the area of stenosis

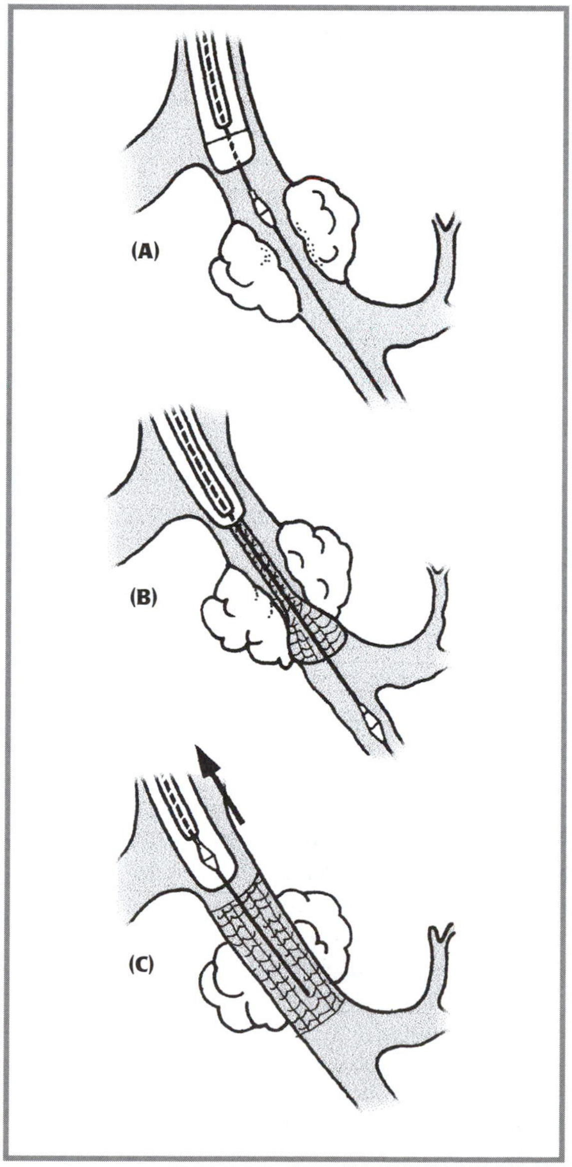

FIGURE 10-3A–C

Wire stent dilation of airway. **(A)** A guidewire is placed into the distal end of the delivery catheter. Under direct visualization with the bronchoscope, the catheter is threaded over the guidewire into the stricture. **(B)** The wire stent is expanded under fluoroscopic guidance to dilate the airway stricture. **(C)** The catheter and bronchoscope are withdrawn after the airway is dilated open.

has been identified and balloon dilatation has perhaps been used, then a stent is placed in that area and distended, expanding the airway lumen and relieving the critical stenosis. Complications can occur with balloon dilation and stenting, such as airway nupture, stent migration, increased mucosal secretions, and a granulomatous mucosal reaction.

Complications

Serious complications are rare with bronchoscopy.

When performed by a trained physician, flexible fiberoptic bronchoscopy has a very low morbidity and mortality incidence. Mortality does not exceed 0.1%, and overall complications should not exceed 10%. The complications may be related to the use of procedure premedications including sedatives or topical anesthetics, and vagal-mediated reactions or complications from the bronchoscopy itself or its related procedures. Absolute contraindications to performing bronchoscopy include an unstable cardiovascular status including life-threatening cardiac arrhythmias, severe hypoxemia that is likely to worsen during the procedure, and an inexperienced bronchoscopist and bronchoscopy team. It is important that the patient is cooperative, and if they are not, then sedation must be induced. Coagulation problems are not an absolute contraindication to bronchoscopy when a tracheobronchial inspection is needed or only bronchoalveolar lavage is to be performed. However, more invasive procedures including biopsy and needle aspiration techniques should not be performed until the coagulopathy has been corrected.

Premedication with sedatives may lead to respiratory depression, hypoventilation, hypotension, and syncope. Topical anesthetics can cause laryngospasm, bronchospasm, and, if given excessively, seizures. The bronchoscopy itself or its associated procedures such as brushing, biopsy, and bronchoalveolar lavage may also induce laryngospasm, bronchospasm, hypoxemia, and cardiac arrhythmias or cause fever, pneumothorax, and hemorrhage. Patients on mechanical ventilation who are receiving high positive end-expiratory pressure (PEEP) are at increased risk for barotrauma. Although fever is a relatively common complication, it is generally transient and not associated with sustained bacteremia. Perforation of the airway is exceedingly uncommon, but pneumothorax has been reported. Fortunately, tension pneumothorax is uncommon.

Procedure

Generally, before bronchoscopy, an anxiolytic, antisialagogue, and topical anesthetic are administered. Either the oral or nasal route can be used for flexible fiberoptic bronchoscopy. However, in the intensive care unit the procedure is generally done through the endotracheal tube while the patient is on the mechanical ventilator. This procedure is done with the use of a swivel adapter with a rubber diaphragm (Figure 10-4) through which the bronchoscope can be inserted safely without disconnecting the patient from the ventilator. The procedure should be done when the patient is as stable as possible. The risk for bronchospasm should be minimized. For critically ill patients, careful monitoring, including use of oximetry and electrocardiography, are necessary. The patient should not be allergic to the medications that are used.

When bronchoscopy is performed through an endotracheal tube, the tube should have a lumen at least 8 mm in internal diameter to ensure that the patient receives an adequate total volume and that excessive airway resistance and pressure do not develop. While the procedure is being done, the patient generally receives 100% oxygen to optimize the chances of keeping the arterial oxygen saturation greater than 90%. The procedure should be done as quickly as possible but without compromising thoroughness. It is best to perform the procedure in patients who have fasted or at least after the stomach has been emptied of its contents by gastric tube suctioning. In mechanically ventilated patients, after the procedure has been completed, it is best to return the ventilator settings to the preprocedure settings and to obtain a chest x-ray to look for a postprocedure pneumothorax. Although postbronchoscopy fever develops in approximately 15% of patients, it usually lasts less than 24 h and does not require antibiotic therapy. However, if the fever does last more than 24 h, then postprocedure pneumonia should be considered.

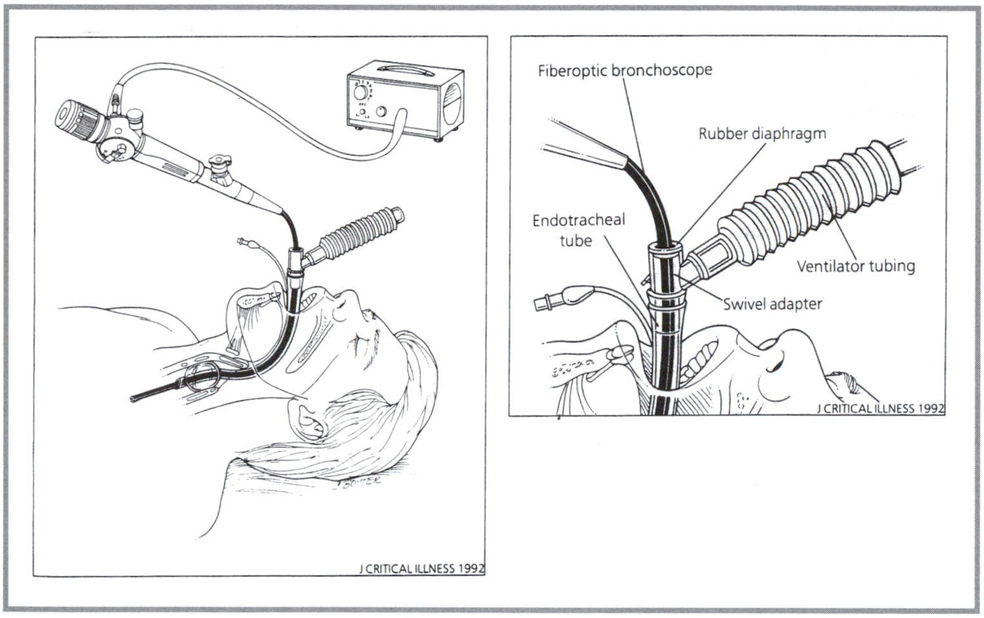

FIGURE 10-4

In an intubated, ventilated patient, a fiberoptic bronchoscope can be passed into the trachea via a swivel adapter, as shown at *left*. This adapter is equipped with taper joints that connect with the ventilator circuit manifold and the endotracheal tube (*right*). A rubber diaphragm on the adapter prevents loss of delivered oxygen, tidal volume, and, in some models, positive end-expiratory pressure.

GASTROINTESTINAL ENDOSCOPY

As compared to 25 years ago, current fiberoptic gastrointestinal endoscopes are highly flexible, slender, and capable of visualizing nearly 100% of the prejejunal upper gastrointestinal tract and colon using video technology. These procedures are commonly done on critically ill patients in the intensive care unit. Newer techniques allow even more of the small bowel to be visualized. This section reviews the indications, contraindications, and complications of gastrointestinal endoscopy in critically ill patients.

Indications

The indications for gastrointestinal endoscopy in the intensive care unit are found in Table 10-3. Gastrointestinal endoscopy should be delayed until the patient's cardiopulmonary status has been stabilized. Clinically insignificant gastrointestinal problems should not be evaluated by gastrointestinal endoscopy in seriously ill patients until they have been stabilized. However, sometimes critically ill patients require urgent gastrointestinal endoscopy. It is hard to separate therapeutic from diagnostic gastrointestinal endoscopy. Generally, in the intensive care unit, endoscopy of the gastrointestinal tract is performed for both therapeutic and diagnostic reasons.

GI endoscopy is done for both diagnostic and therapeutic reasons.

Upper gastrointestinal endoscopy is generally performed to evaluate serious gastrointestinal bleeding or the effects of caustic ingestion on the gastrointestinal tract or to remove

TABLE 10-3

INDICATIONS FOR GASTROINTESTINAL (GI) ENDOSCOPY

- Upper GI endoscopy
  - GI bleeding
  - Caustic ingestion
  - Foreign body ingestion
  - Feeding tube placement
- Endoscopic retrograde cholangiopancreatography
  - Severe gallstone pancreatitis
  - Severe cholangitis
- Lower GI endoscopy
  - GI bleeding
  - Acute adynamic ileus

Gastrointestinal endoscopy is commonly done for acute upper GI bleeding in critically ill patients.

a foreign body. Severe or recurrent gastrointestinal bleeding, in patients who are critically ill with cardiopulmonary diseases, increases the morbidity and mortality associated with these diseases. Endoscopy is performed with an intention to enhance hemostasis. Therefore, patients with a continuing need for blood product transfusions should be considered for urgent upper gastrointestinal endoscopy with the intent to stabilize bleeding. More elective endoscopy of the upper gastrointestinal tract is done in critically ill patients who require the placement of gastrostomy tubes for the administration of enteral nutrition. A percutaneous endoscopic gastrostomy (PEG) tube can be placed at the bedside with minimal sedation and local anesthesia.

A gastrostomy tube can be placed percutaneously by an endoscopic technique at the bedside.

Endoscopic retrograde cholangiopancreatoscopy (ERCP) occasionally is necessary in an ICU patient. ERCP would only be indicated in a patient who has severe gallstone pancreatitis or those with cholangitis unresponsive to medical therapy. ERCP combined with sphincterotomy and gallstone extraction reduces the complications that can occur in patients who have gallstone pancreatitis and cholangitis.

ERCP is indicated for the patient with cholangitis that is unresponsive to medical therapy.

Upper gastrointestinal hemorrhage usually prompts the use of endoscopy, but the role of lower endoscopy (colonoscopy) in severe lower gastrointestinal bleeding is less established. This lack is partially due to the technical difficulty of performing colonoscopy in the setting of acute bleeding where blood obscures the field, which lessens diagnostic accuracy and the therapeutic potential of colonoscopy. Colonoscopy is often performed in concert with technetium-labeled erythrocyte scanning and mesenteric angiography. Colonscopy can be diagnostic if the bleeding abates and the colon is purged of blood.

Low GI endoscopy is done to locate the site of large bowel bleeding and to decompress a markedly dilated colon.

Colonoscopy can be used to decompress a dilated colon in patients with acute adynamic ileus. Decompression of the bowel is indicated when the diameter of the right colon exceeds 12 cm because perforation can occur with this degree of severe distension. Endoscopic colonic decompression is especially indicated after an infusion of neostigmine, nasogastric tube suctioning, rectal tube drainage, and frequent body position changes do not lead to bowel decompression.

Complications

Major risks of colonoscopy are (1) biopsy bleeding and (2) bowel perforation.

Bleeding and perforation are the major risks of gastrointestinal endoscopy (Table 10-4). Bleeding can occur after biopsy, but most bleeding is minimal and self-limited. Perforation of the bowel lumen may result from direct pressure of the endoscope itself or the catheters and guidewires that are placed through the scope to complete certain procedures. With induced gastric distension during upper endoscopy, aspiration of stomach contents can occur. Finally, any of the medications used to sedate the patient can induce adverse reactions.

The best way to avoid serious procedural complications is to avoid the patient who has certain contraindications to the procedure (Table 10-5). Endoscopy and associated air insufflation of the bowel should be avoided in patients with known or suspected gastrointestinal perforation. Hemodynamic instability is a relative contraindication to endoscopy. A biopsy during endoscopy or a sphincterotomy during ERCP should not be done in patients who are coagulopathic. For many patients who are critically ill, sedation and endotracheal intubation are needed to safely facilitate the procedure.

Procedures

Upper gastrointestinal endoscopy should be done in stable patients. Obtunded patients should be intubated and placed on a mechanical ventilator before the procedure. Nasogastric lavage

TABLE 10-4

COMPLICATIONS OF GI ENDOSCOPY

Bleeding
Perforation of the gastrointestinal tract lumen by endoscope, catheters, or guidewires
Aspiration
Reaction to sedative medication

TABLE 10-5

CONTRAINDICATIONS TO GI ENDOSCOPY

Perforated viscus suspected/impending
Hemodynamic and respiratory gas exchange instability
Severe diverticulitis
Severe inflammatory bowel disease
Severe coagulopathy
Uncooperative patient
Unprotected airway in a confused or stuporous patient with acute upper GI bleeding

with a large-bore tube irrigation should be performed to empty the stomach of blood before the procedure. The endoscopy team should consist of an experienced endoscopist, a properly trained assistant, and a nurse skilled in monitoring patients who are under going endoscopy. When blood is to be removed from the stomach, a large operating channel endoscope should be employed.

A variety of procedures that can be used to localize the bleeding site and stabilize the bleeding area so that hemostasis can be achieved include laser photocoagulation, multipolar electrocoagulation, injection therapy, hemoclipping, and ligation. Laser photocoagulation is expensive and cumbersome. Injection therapy is simple and inexpensive, requiring only a needle catheter and various liquid media to induce hemostasis, including sclerosing agents and vasoconstrictors. Injection sclerotherapy is commonly used to treat bleeding esophageal varices but also can be used to control ulcer bleeds. However, the most commonly used methods are heater probe techniques, particularly electrocauterizing needle and injection therapy. A electrocauterizer delivers electrical current directly to the tissue inducing coagulation necrosis. In patients who have recurrent bleeding, one more attempt at endoscopic therapy is preferable to surgery.

Until recently, injection sclerotherapy was considered the endoscopic procedure of choice for variceal bleeding, but now endoscopic band ligation of varices is preferred. Sclerotherapy is performed by injecting a sclerosant chemical (ethanol, ethanolamine oleate, mecrylate) into and around the varix to induce thrombosis and fibrosis. Banding is performed to ligate the varix base and generally has fewer complications than sclerotherapy. Several complications of endoscopic coagulation and injection sclerotherapy can occur (Table 10-6).

Lower gastrointestinal endoscopy is employed in the intensive care unit in select patients in an attempt to localize the source of colonic bleeding. This procedure is difficult and often unsuccessful. The colon can hold a great deal of blood, making the procedure difficult to perform. Furthermore, it is difficult to prepare the colon properly for inspection in a patient who is critically ill. The same technical support is necessary for colonic inspection as is used during upper gastrointestinal endoscopy. Sedation and monitoring are similar. Decompression of the colon by endoscopy should not be first line therapy for a pseudoobstruction; it should only be used after all noninvasive measures have been employed and nasogastric tube

TABLE 10-6

COMPLICATIONS OF ENDOSCOPIC COAGULATION AND INJECTION SCLEROTHERAPY

- Esophageal complications
  - Ulceration
  - Stricture formation
  - Perforation (early or delayed)
  - Dysmotility
- Pulmonary complications
  - Pleural effusions and pleuritis
  - Pulmonary infiltrates
  - Aspiration
  - Mediastinitis
  - Adult respiratory distress syndrome
- Septic complications
  - Bacteremia
  - Sepsis
  - Subacute bacterial peritonitis

suctioning and rectal tube drainage have failed. Occasionally, the small bowel is suspected as the source of bleeding. This suspicion occurs after esophagogastroduodenoscopy and colonoscopy are found to be nondiagnositic. The small intestine can be evaluated by endoscopy using specially designed scopes and either an active or push technique or a passive method. Intraoperative endoscopy of the small bowel can be performed if these techniques are not available.

SUMMARY

Endoscopy has substantially broadened our diagnostic and therapeutic powers in the intensive care unit. Laryngoscopy, bronchoscopy and gastrointestinal endoscopy are rarely contraindicated and often simplify the care of patients who are seriously ill.

REVIEW QUESTIONS

1. **All the following statements are true concerning bronchoscopy, except:**
   A. Flexible bronchoscopy is commonly done in the ICU.
   B. Rigid bronchoscopy does not have any advantages over flexible bronchoscopy.
   C. Bronchoscopy is safely done often with minimal additional sedation in mechanical ventilated patients.
   D. The most common use of bronchoscopy in the ICU is for secretion management.

2. **The fiberoptic bronchoscopic is helpful in the ICU for all of the following conditions, except:**
   A. Location of bleeding
   B. Diagnosis of hospital-acquired pneumonia
   C. Removal of an airway mucous plug
   D. Diagnosis of inflammatory lung diseases

3. **All the following statements are true concerning gastrointestinal endoscopy in the ICU, except:**
   A. Nearly the entire GI tract can be evaluated.
   B. All GI problems should be considered for endoscopy evaluation.
   C. The most common cause for using endoscopy is bleeding.
   D. Bleeding and bowel perforation are the major risks of GI endoscopy.

ANSWERS

1. The answer is B. Massive hemoptysis, the removal of a foreign body, and the placement of an airway stent are often best approached with a rigid bronchoscope.
2. The answer is D. The bronchoscopic approach to the diagnosis of diffuse inflammatory noninfectious lung diseases is often unrewarding and is better approached by an open-lung biopsy, either by thoroscopy or thoracotomy.
3. The answer is B. Clinically insignificant GI problems should not be evaluated endoscopically. All patients who require endoscopy should be as stable as possible.

SUGGESTED READING

Anzueto A, Levine SM, Jenkinson SG. The technique of fiberoptic bronchoscopy. Diagnostic and therapeutic use in intubated, ventilated patients. J Crit Illness 1992;7:1657–1664.

Dellinger P, Bandi V. Fiberoptic bronchoscopy in the intensive care unit. Crit Care Clin 1992;8:755–772.

Hirschchowitz BI. Development and application of endoscopy. Gastroenterology 1993;104:337.

NIH Consensus Conference. Therapeutic endoscopy and bleeding ulcers. JAMA 1989;262:1369.

Shennib H, Baslaim G. Bronchoscopy in the intensive care unit. Chest Surg Clin N Am 1996;6:349–361.

Steer ML, Silen W. Diagnostic procedures in gastrointestinal hemorrhage. N Engl J Med 1983;309:646–650.

Van Dam J, Brugge WR. Endoscopy of the upper gastrointestinal tract. N Engl J Med 1999;341:1738–1748.

PHILLIP M. BOISELLE

Radiologic Imaging in the Critically Ill Patient

CHAPTER OUTLINE

LEARNING OBJECTIVES

After studying this chapter, you should be able to do the following:

- Know a systematic approach for interpreting ICU chest radiographs.
- Be aware of the common causes of increased lung opacification on ICU chest radiographs.
- Know the indications for obtaining thoracic CT scans, ultrasound exams, ventilation–perfusion scans, and pulmonary arteriography in ICU patients.
- Be aware of the radiographic signs of various abnormal thoracic air collections.
- Be familiar with the roles of various abdominal imaging procedures in the assessment of the ICU patient with suspected abdominal sepsis.
- Be aware of the relative merits of CT and MR imaging in the evaluation of the ICU patient with suspected neurologic abnormalities.

Radiology plays an important role in the care of the critically ill patient. The most commonly ordered imaging procedure is the portable chest radiograph, which is obtained on a daily basis for many critically ill patients. Other imaging procedures such as abdominal radiographs, computed tomography (CT), ultrasound (US), magnetic resonance (MR) imaging, ventilation–perfusion (VQ) imaging, and angiography are selectively ordered for specific indications. In this chapter, we review the fundamentals of radiologic imaging of the critically ill patient.

THORACIC IMAGING

Chest Radiography

Portable chest radiographs are the mainstay of radiologic imaging of the critically ill patient. Several studies have documented the value of this procedure in the critically ill patient population by showing that daily chest radiograph findings result in a change in patient management in up to two thirds of cases. Such alterations in management range from a change

Portable chest radiographs are the mainstay of radiologic imaging of critically ill patients.

In critically ill patients, daily chest radiographs result in a change in patient management in as many as two-thirds of cases.

in the position of a catheter or support device to a decision to institute specific therapy such as antibiotics or diuretics.

To maximize the utility of the portable chest radiograph in the ICU setting, it is important to optimize the quality of both the radiograph and its interpretation. A high-quality portable radiograph is the product of a number of important factors, including a well-trained technologist, up-to-date equipment, and a cooperative relationship between the the technologist, nursing staff, and respiratory therapist. Radiographic interpretation can be enhanced by daily rounds between the ICU clinical physicians and a thoracic radiologist who is specially trained in interpreting ICU radiographs. Such rounds promote optimal integration of the clinical history with the radiologic findings and ensure timely communication of radiographic findings.

Daily rounds with both the ICU team and a thoracic radiologist promote optimal integration of clinical data with radiographic findings and ensure timely communication of radiographic abnormalities.

In recent years, conventional portable radiographs have been replaced by digital portable radiographs in many hospitals. The most widely used digital system employs a storage phosphor cassette and an image processing system that converts an electronic image to a digital image. The final product of this process is a digital radiograph that can be displayed simultaneously at locations throughout the hospital by using a picture archiving and communications system (PACS). There are two main advantages of digital imaging over conventional radiography: (1) the ability to transmit an image simultaneously to the radiology department and to the ICU, and (2) the ability to electronically manipulate the image to produce more uniform consistency of exposure.

Digital radiography and picture archiving communications systems (PACS) allow for simultaneous transmission of radiographs to the radiology department and ICU.

Interpreting ICU Chest Radiographs

When interpreting radiographs of critically ill patients, it is important to have a systematic approach.

When interpreting ICU chest radiographs, it is important to have a systematic approach (Table 11-1). First, carefully evaluate the location of all catheters and support devices. Second, assess the cardiovascular status of the patient. Third, look for areas of abnormally increased lung opacification. Fourth, assess for pleural fluid. Finally, observe carefully for any abnormal air collections. In the following sections, we review the fundamentals of each of these steps.

Evaluating Catheters, Tubes, and Support Devices Several studies have shown that approximately one-half of ICU portable chest radiographs reveal unexpected findings. Such findings frequently relate to malpositioning of catheters, tubes, and cardiopulmonary support devices (Figure 11-1). Table 11-2 lists a variety of devices that are employed in the ICU setting, followed by their ideal positions and possible complications. The typical radiographic appearance of several of these devices is illustrated in Figure 11-2.

Assessing Cardiovascular Status The portable radiograph provides a noninvasive means for assessing the cardiovascular status of the critically ill patient. Important parameters include heart size, vascular pedicle width (see following), and pulmonary vascularity. When assessing these cardiovascular parameters on chest radiographs, it is extremely important to consider how the radiograph was obtained. For example, all ICU radiographs are performed portably using an anteroposterior technique, and most are obtained with the patient in the supine position. These technical factors result in magnification of the cardiac silhouette compared to its appearance on an upright, posteroanterior chest radiograph. Radiographs performed at shallow lung volumes (end-expiration) also result in accentuation of the heart size and pulmonary vascularity.

Important cardiovascular parameters to assess on chest radiographs include heart size, vascular pedicle width, and pulmonary vascularity.

TABLE 11-1

SYSTEMATIC APPROACH TO INTERPRETING ICU CHEST RADIOGRAPHS

1. Evaluate the locations of all catheters, tubes, and support devices.
2. Assess the cardiovascular status of the patient.
3. Look for areas of abnormally increased lung opacification.
4. Assess for pleural fluid.
5. Look carefully for abnormal air collections.

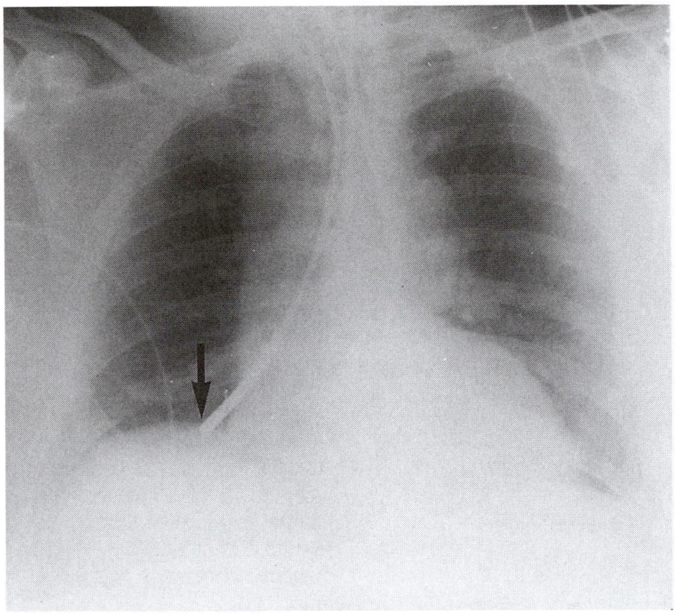

FIGURE 11-1

Portable supine chest radiograph reveals an unexpected finding: a feeding tube has been inadvertently passed into the airway, with its tip terminating in the right lower lobe (*arrow*). Note the expected midline position of a nasogastric tube within the esophagus.

HEART SIZE. The most common method of assessing the heart size on chest radiographs is the cardiothoracic ratio, which is obtained by dividing the widest transverse diameter of the heart by the widest transverse diameter of the thorax above the diaphragm. On a standard posteroanterior, erect chest radiograph, a cardiothoracic ratio of greater than 0.5 is considered abnormal. Because portable, supine radiographs magnify the cardiac silhouette, it has been suggested that a correction factor of −12.5% be applied to this equation for ICU radiographs.

VASCULAR PEDICLE. The vascular pedicle refers to a group of vascular structures that are located between the thoracic inlet and the top of the cardiac silhouette. The vessels that comprise the vascular pedicle include the right brachiocephalic vein, superior vena cava, and left subclavian artery. These distensible vessels increase in size in response to an increase in circulating blood volume (Figure 11-3).

It is important to keep in mind that the vascular pedicle width, similar to the cardiac silhouette, is dependent on technical factors. For example, it is magnified by portable technique and supine positioning, and it will artifactually increase with patient rotation. Because of the wide range of normal values (38 mm to 58 mm on an upright, posteroanterior chest radiograph), a comparison of vascular pedicle widths on serial radiographs of an individual patient is usually more useful than an absolute measurement.

PULMONARY VASCULARITY. The radiographic appearance of the pulmonary vascularity is dependent on the effect of gravity. In the erect position, gravity results in increased blood flow to the dependent, lower lobes of the lungs. Thus, in the erect position, the pulmonary vascular diameters are greater in the lower lobes than the upper lobes. In the supine position, however, gravitational changes result in an equalization of pulmonary blood flow to the upper and lower lobes. Thus, in the supine position, the caliber of the upper lobe and lower lobe vessels is similar.

> The radiographic appearance of the pulmonary vascularity is gravity dependent.

An increase in pulmonary vascularity can be detected on upright chest radiographs when the upper lobe pulmonary vessels appear similar (balanced blood flow pattern) or greater in size (cephalization or redistribution pulmonary blood flow pattern) than the lower lobe vessels. A balanced pattern is typically encountered in patients with hydrostatic edema from renal failure or volume overload, whereas a redistribution pattern is associated with congestive heart failure.

> A balanced pattern of pulmonary blood flow is associated with hydrostatic pulmonary edema from renal failure or fluid overload. A cephalized pattern is associated with hydrostatic pulmonary edema from congestive heart failure.

TABLE 11-2

LINES, TUBES, AND SUPPORT DEVICES

TUBE/LINE	IDEAL LOCATION	POSSIBLE COMPLICATIONS
Endotracheal tube	5–7 cm above carina	Malposition (15%) 1. Too low: endobronchial intubation and lung collapse 2. Too high: cord damage Overinflated cuff: tracheal stenosis Esophageal intubation Tracheal or laryngeal rupture Aspiration pneumonitis
Central venous catheter	Superior vena cava	Malposition (15%–40%) Pneumothorax (5%) Extrapleural hematoma Hemothorax Mediastinal hemorrhage Cardiac or vascular perforation Arrythmias (atrial placement) Catheter fragmentation Septic emboli Mycotic aneurysm
Swan–Ganz catheter	Central pulmonary arteries (within 2 cm of hilum)	Pneumothorax Malposition 1. Coiling in RA or RV may result in arrhythymias 2. Too distal location may result in pulmonary infarction, hemorrhage, infarction, or pulmonary artery pseudoaneurysm
Intraaortic balloon pump	Tip just below superior aortic knob contour	Malposition 1. If tip is too high, it may occlude left subclavian artery 2. If tip is too low, it may occlude abdominal or renal arteries Aortic dissection
Cardiac pacemaker	Right ventricular lead should project over the cardiac apex on PA view and lie anteriorly on lateral view	Pneumothorax Lead fracture Cardiac perforation
Automatic implantable cardiac defibrillator device (AICD)	Proximal lead, superior vena cava; distal lead, right ventricle; patch, left chest wall or pericardial space.	Fracture of lead Retraction of lead
Nasogastric tube	Side port and tip below left hemidiaphragm	Esophageal or gastric perforation Aspiration pneumonia Pneumothorax
Pleural drainage tubes	For pneumothorax, directed anteriorly and superiorly; for pleural effusion, posteriorly and inferiorly	Bleeding (laceration of vessel) Diaphragm perforation Lung contusion and laceration

SOURCE: Table partially adapted from Trotman-Dickenson B. Radiography in the critical care patient. In: McLoud TC (ed) Thoracic Radiology: The Requisites. St. Louis: Mosby, 1998:152

Because the upper and lower lobe vessels normally appear similar on supine radiographs, the recognition of increased pulmonary vascularity is more difficult on supine radiographs. Increased pulmonary blood flow can reliably be identified on ICU radiographs by comparing the caliber of the upper lobe vessels to the adjacent bronchi, both of which are normally seen end-on adjacent to the pulmonary hila. Normally, the artery and bronchus have a 1:1 size ratio. In the setting of increased pulmonary blood flow, the caliber of the artery will appear larger than the adjacent bronchus.

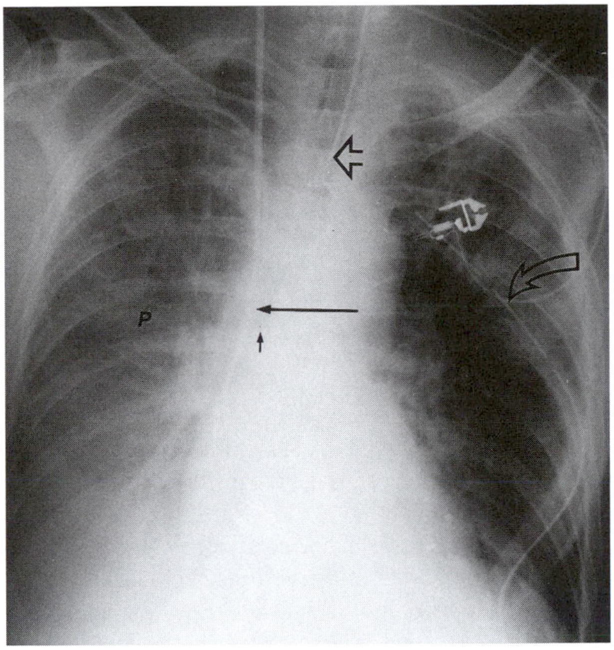

FIGURE 11-2

Portable supine chest radiograph demonstrates appropriate placement of endotracheal tube (tip 5 cm above carina; *straight open arrow*), central venous catheter (tip in superior vena cava; *long closed arrow*), Swan–Ganz catheter (tip in distal right main pulmonary artery; *short closed arrow*), and left-sided chest tube (*open curved arrow*). Also note diffuse haziness of the right hemithorax compared to the left side, corresponding to the presence of a layering right pleural effusion (*P*).

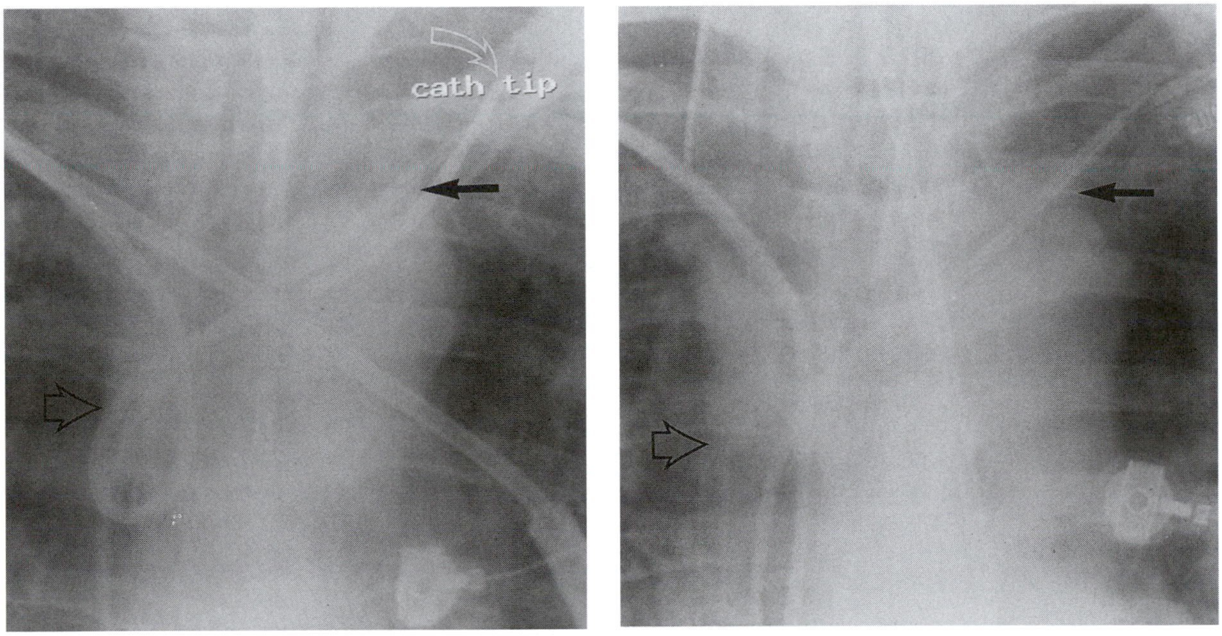

(A) **(B)**

FIGURE 11-3

(A) Coned-down image of the mediastinum reveals a normal vascular pedicle width of 46 mm. The pedicle is measured from where the right main bronchus crosses the superior vena cava (*open black arrow*) to a perpendicular dropped from where the left subclavian artery originates from the aorta (*closed black arrow*). Also note malpositioned right subclavian catheter, which has crossed over into the left subclavian vein (*open white arrow*, catheter tip). **(B)** Coned-down image of the mediastinum of same patient during an episode of fluid overload demonstrates interval widening of the vascular pedicle to a width of 65 mm (*arrows*). The right subclavian catheter has been successfully repositioned.

Common causes of lung opacification in the ICU setting include pulmonary edema, pneumonia, atelectasis, and aspiration.

Assessing Areas of Increased Lung Opacification There are a variety of causes of increased lung opacification, but only a few entities are commonly encountered in the ICU setting. These entities include pulmonary edema, pneumonia, atelectasis, and aspiration. The characteristic imaging features of these entities are reviewed in the following paragraphs.

There are two main forms of pulmonary edema: hydrostatic and increased capillary permeability edema.

PULMONARY EDEMA. Pulmonary edema is a common cause of diffuse parenchymal opacification in the ICU patient. It is important to try to differentiate hydrostatic pulmonary edema from increased capillary permeability edema. Several features can aid in this distinction (Table 11-3). Keep in mind, however, that this separation is not always possible on the basis of radiographic findings alone. Moreover, these forms of edema occasionally coexist in the same patient.

Hydrostatic pulmonary edema may occur secondary to congestive heart failure, renal failure, or fluid overload.

Hydrostatic pulmonary edema involves first the interstitial compartment of the lung, followed by the alveolar compartment.

Hydrostatic pulmonary edema. Hydrostatic pulmonary edema secondary to congestive heart failure or volume overload usually follows a typical course. Increased pulmonary vascularity is followed by the sequential development of fluid within the interstitial and alveolar compartments of the lung.

The interstitial compartment of the lung contains two major components: the peribronchovascular sheath and the interlobular septa. Fluid within the peribronchovascular sheath results in indistinctness of the pulmonary vessels and peribronchial cuffing. Fluid within the interlobular septa results in the presence of Kerley lines, a term that refers to linear opacities that are best visualized in the lung periphery (Figure 11-4). As interstitial edema progresses in severity, fluid may also accumulate within the subpleural space of the interlobar fissures; this is referred to as subpleural edema and results in thickening of the interlobar fissures on chest radiographs.

The next phase of pulmonary edema involves the extension of fluid into the alveolar spaces of the lung. Airspace involvement can be detected by identifying the presence of poorly defined lung opacities that coalesce to produce airspace consolidation. This term refers to the presence of confluent, cloudlike lung opacities. Airspace consolidation from hydrostatic pulmonary edema is usually bilateral and symmetric and often has a central, perihilar predominance (Figure 11-5). However, in some patients, alveolar pulmonary edema may be asymmetric or atypical in distribution. Although the appearance of pulmonary edema may vary among different patients, there is often a strikingly similar pattern in an individual patient from episode to episode. Thus, it may be helpful to compare the current radiograph to one obtained during a prior episode of pulmonary edema, particularly for patients who present with an asymmetric or atypical distribution.

Although the appearance of pulmonary edema may vary among different patients, there is often a strikingly similar pattern in an individual patient from episode to episode.

In addition to the features just described, patients with hydrostatic pulmonary edema frequently demonstrate an enlarged heart, an increased vascular pedicle width, and pleural effusions. Right-sided pleural effusions predominate in patients with congestive heart failure.

Hydrostatic pulmonary edema is frequently associated with cardiac enlargement, increased vascular pedicle width, and pleural effusions.

Increased capillary permeability pulmonary edema. Increased capillary permeability pulmonary edema is most closely associated with the acute respiratory distress syndrome (ARDS). This syndrome refers to a heterogeneous group of patients who develop acute respiratory failure, characterized by profound hypoxia, with associated diffuse lung opacification

TABLE 11-3

HYDROSTATIC VERSUS INCREASED CAPILLARY PERMEABILITY PULMONARY EDEMA: DISTINGUISHING RADIOGRAPHIC FEATURES

RADIOGRAPHIC FEATURE	HYDROSTATIC EDEMA	INCREASED PERMEABILITY EDEMA
Cardiomegaly	+	–
Widened vascular pedicle	+	–
Increased vascularity	+	–
Kerley lines	+	–
Peribronchial cuffing	+	–
Pleural effusion	+	–
Airspace consolidation	+	+

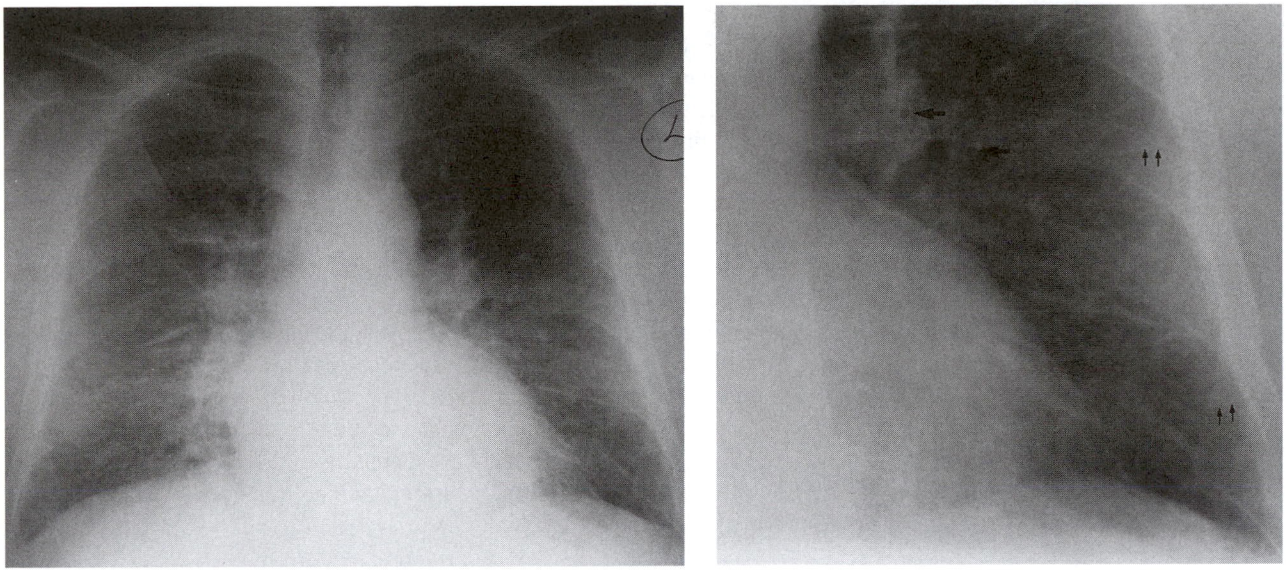

(A) (B)

FIGURE 11-4

(A) Frontal chest radiograph reveals typical features of interstitial pulmonary edema in a patient with congestive heart failure, manifested by peribronchial cuffing, indistinctness of the pulmonary vessels, and Kerley lines. Also note cephalization of the pulmonary vascularity and mild cardiomegaly. **(B)** The peribronchial cuffing (*single arrows*) and Kerley lines (*paired smaller arrows*) are seen in greater detail on the coned-down image of the left lung. (Reprinted with permission from Boiselle PM. Pulmonary vascular abnormalities. In: McLoud TC (ed) Thoracic Radiology: The Requisites. St. Louis: Mosby, 1998:403–419.)

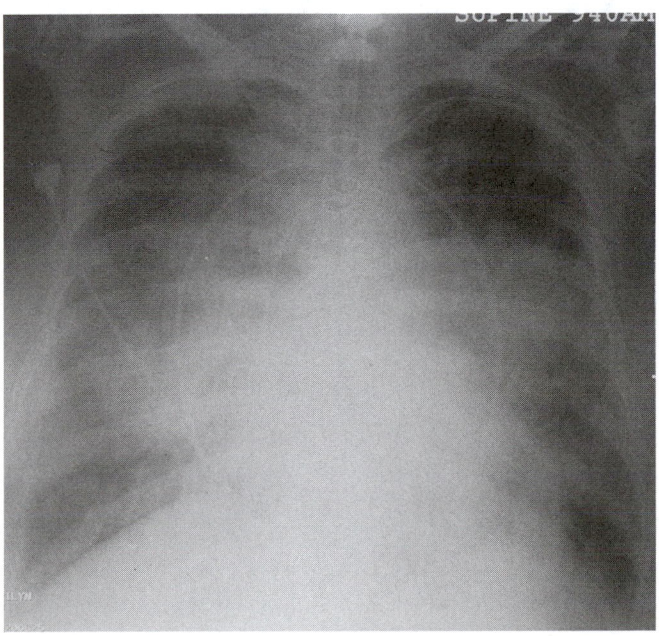

FIGURE 11-5

Portable supine chest radiograph of a patient with fluid overload demonstrates a bilateral pattern of alveolar consolidation with a central, perihilar distribution. Also note mild cardiomegaly and bilateral pleural effusions, right greater than left.

on chest radiography. There are a variety of risk factors for developing ARDS, including trauma, sepsis, severe pneumonia, circulatory shock, aspiration, inhaled toxins, and drug overdose.

Although both increased capillary permeability edema and hydrostatic edema are associated with alveolar consolidation, the pattern is frequently different. The former is usually patchy and somewhat peripheral in distribution, and the latter is usually confluent, central, and perihilar.

In contrast to patients with hydrostatic pulmonary edema, the heart size and vascular pedicle width are normal in patients with increased permeability pulmonary edema. Moreover, pleural effusions, Kerley lines, and peribronchial cuffing are not usually evident in patients with increased permeability pulmonary edema. Although both forms of pulmonary edema may be associated with diffuse airspace opacification, the distribution of lung opacities often differs between these entities. In patients with increased permeability pulmonary edema, the opacities are often patchy and somewhat peripheral in distribution, whereas in patients with hydrostatic pulmonary edema, lung opacities are often confluent, and they are usually central and perihilar in distribution. Finally, in comparison to hydrostatic pulmonary edema, lung opacities associated with ARDS are more often associated with air bronchograms.

Acute respiratory distress syndrome (ARDS) is frequently complicated by barotrauma, including subcutaneous emphysema, pneumothorax, pneumomediastinum, and pulmonary interstitial edema.

Because of decreased lung compliance and the need for prolonged mechanical ventilation, patients with ARDS frequently develop barotrauma, including subcutaneous emphysema, pneumothorax (Figure 11-6), pneumomediastinum, and pulmonary interstitial emphysema (see following). As ARDS progresses, areas of lung consolidation are replaced by areas of fibrosis and lung cyst formation.

PNEUMONIA. Pneumonia is a relatively common diagnosis in the ICU setting. For some patients, a severe pneumonia is the cause for admission to the ICU. For others, nosocomial pneumonia complicates another cause of respiratory failure such as ARDS.

When a focal area of alveolar consolidation develops in conjunction with the onset of fever and leukocytosis, a confident diagnosis of pneumonia can usually be rendered.

Because nosocomial pneumonia is associated with a high mortality rate, a prompt and accurate diagnosisis is extremely important. Unfortunately, however, nosocomial pneumonia is often difficult to diagnose both clinically and radiographically in the ICU setting. When a focal area of alveolar consolidation develops in conjunction with the onset of fever and leukocytosis, a diagnosis of pneumonia can usually be confidently rendered. In many cases, however, lung opacification from pneumonia may be difficult to distinguish from other causes, including pulmonary edema, atelectasis, and aspiration (Figure 11-7).

Diffuse bilateral pneumonia may occasionally be difficult to distinguish radiographically from asymmetric patterns of hydrostatic pulmonary edema. Findings that favor asymmetric pulmonary edema include a rapid onset of lung opacities, a change in distribution of opacities with changes in patient positioning, a rapid improvement in response to diuretic ther-

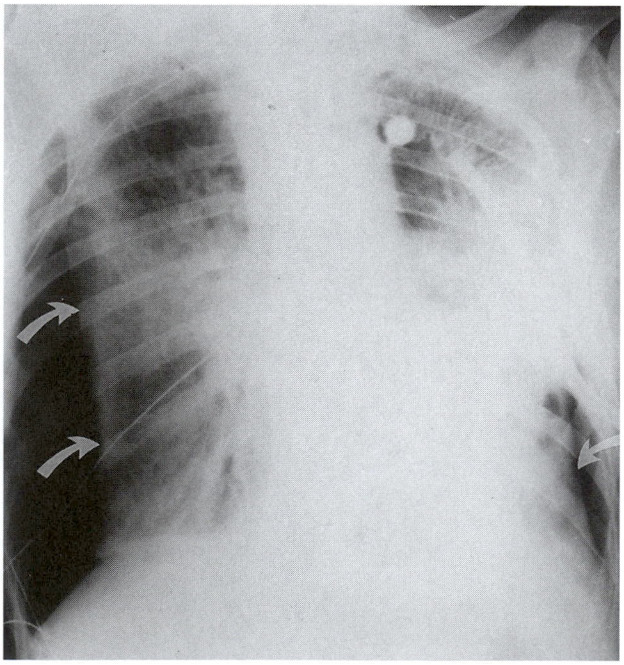

FIGURE 11-6

Portable supine chest radiograph of a patient with ARDS demonstrates diffuse bilateral alveolar opacities, with prominent air bronchograms in the right base. Note patchy areas of normally aerated lung that are spared by this process. The heart size cannot be assessed because the cardiac silhouette is obscured by adjacent areas of consolidation. Bilateral pneumothoraces are present (*arrows*), right greater than left.

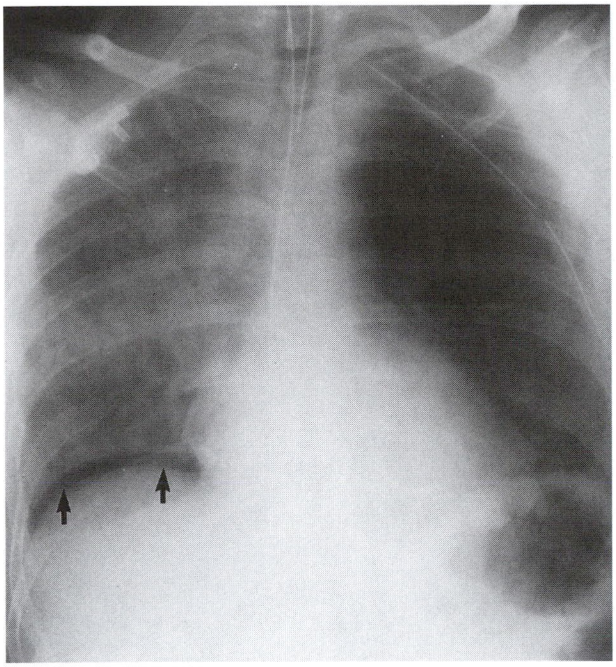

FIGURE 11-7

A portable supine chest radiograph reveals diffuse consolidation in the right lung, corresponding to diffuse pneumonia. The time course of development and the corresponding clinical features allowed accurate differentiation between pneumonia and other causes of alveolar consolidation such as aspiration. Despite the presence of right lower lobe consolidation, the right hemidiaphragm is sharply demarcated (*arrows*), indicative of a subpulmonic pneumothorax.

apy, and ancillary findings of congestive heart failure (e.g., enlarged heart, increased vascular pedicle width, and increased pulmonary vascularity).

ATELECTASIS. Atelectasis, which refers to areas of nonaerated lung, is a very common cause of lung opacification in the ICU setting. The degree of atelectasis may vary from minimal linear opacities, referred to as subsegmental or discoid atelectasis, to collapse of an entire lobe or lung (Figure 11-8). At these extremes of the spectrum, the radiographic diagnosis of atelectasis is relatively straightforward. However, degrees of atelectasis between these two extremes are often difficult to distinguish from pneumonia.

Atelectasis is most common in the lung bases, and the left lower lobe is very commonly affected following cardiac surgery. An important feature that favors atelectasis over pneumonia is the presence of associated volume loss, which may be manifested radiographically by displaced fissures, displaced hila, elevated hemidiaphragms, and shift of mediastinal structures. The time course may also be helpful in this distinction, as atelectasis typically develops and resolves more quickly than pneumonia.

An important feature that favors the diagnosis of atelectasis over pneumonia is the presence of volume loss.

When there is opacification of an entire hemithorax, the differential diagnosis includes complete atelectasis of a lung and a large pleural effusion. You can distinguish between these entities by assessing for mediastinal shift. If the mediastinal structures are shifted toward the side of opacification, the predominant abnormality is lung collapse, usually secondary to a mucous plug. On the other hand, if the mediastinum is shifted in the opposite direction, the predominant abnormality is a large pleural effusion, with associated passive atelectasis of the lung secondary to the effusion.

ASPIRATION. Aspiration is a common complication in the ICU setting. The radiographic appearance of aspiration depends on a number of factors, including the nature and volume of aspirated material and the position of the patient. For example, the aspiration of small amounts of water or blood may not result in clinical symptoms or detectable radiographic abnormalities. On the other hand, the aspiration of acidic gastric contents produces a chemical pneumonitis that resembles pulmonary edema, and the aspiration of food or oral pathogens frequently results in an aspiration pneumonia.

The radiographic appearance of aspiration is dependent on the nature and volume of aspirated material and the position of the patient.

A characteristic radiographic feature of aspiration is the presence of lung opacities in dependent portions of the lungs. If a patient aspirates in the upright position, the basal seg-

A characteristic radiographic feature of aspiration is the presence of lung opacities in a dependent distribution.

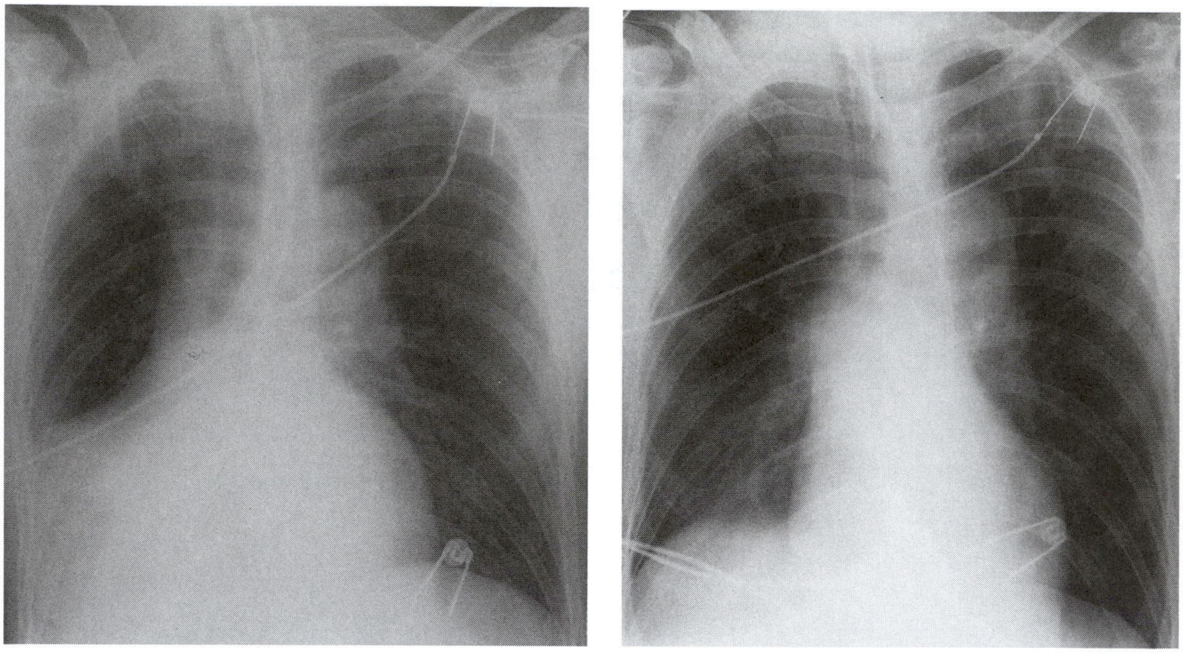

(A) (B)

FIGURE 11-8

(A) A portable supine chest radiograph demonstrates increased opacity in the right lower lung zone that obliterates the right heart border and right hemidiaphragm, corresponding to right middle and right lower lobe collapse. Note inferior displacement of the right hilum, indicative of volume loss. **(B)** A subsequent radiograph obtained several hours later demonstrates improved aeration of the right middle and lower lobes, with some remaining atelectasis at the right base medially. Note improved visualization of the right heart border and part of the right hemidiaphragm.

ments of the lower lobes are usually affected. In the supine position, the posterior segments of the upper lobes and the superior segments of the lower lobes are most often affected.

The time course can be helpful in distinguishing aspiration from other causes of lung opacification such as pneumonia. Aspiration typically has a rapid onset and it often clears rapidly, unless it is complicated by development of pneumonia or ARDS.

The radiographic appearance of a pleural effusion is dependent on the size of the effusion and the position of the patient.

Assessing for Pleural Fluid Pleural effusions are a relatively common finding on imaging studies of ICU patients and may occur secondary to a variety of conditions. The appearance of a pleural effusion on radiographs is dependent on the size of the effusion and the position of the patient.

On an upright radiograph, an effusion is manifested by blunting of the costophrenic sulcus, which results in a meniscus appearance. It requires approximately 200 ml fluid to produce this appearance on a frontal, upright radiograph. On supine radiographs, a unilateral, layering pleural effusion is manifested as a diffuse, hazy, increased opacity throughout the affected hemithorax (see Figure 11-2). Such an opacity does not usually obscure the pulmonary vessels. Moderate-sized effusions may result in a lateral or apical pleural opacity (apical cap) on supine radiographs.

Loculated pleural effusions suggest the presence of empyema or hemothorax.

Loculated pleural fluid collections suggest the presence of empyema or hemothorax. Hemothorax should also be considered when a large effusion develops rapidly and when an effusion develops following an invasive procedure such as catheter placement.

TABLE 11-4

ABNORMAL EXTRAALVEOLAR AIR COLLECTIONS

Subcutaneous emphysema
Pneumomediastinum
Pneumothorax
Pulmonary interstitial emphysema

Observing for Abnormal Air Collections Abnormal air collections in the thorax include subcutaneous emphysema, pneumothorax, pneumomediastinum, and pulmonary interstitial emphysema (Table 11-4). Such collections are often related to barotrauma from prolonged or high-pressure mechanical ventilation.

SUBCUTANEOUS EMPHYSEMA. The presence of air within the soft tissues of the chest wall is often one of the earliest signs of barotrauma. Subcutaneous emphysema is usually associated with pneumomediastinum and pneumothorax, which may be less apparent radiographically. Thus, the identification of subcutaneous emphysema should prompt a careful search for pneumothorax or pneumomediastinum.

The presence of subcutaneous emphysema is often one of the earliest signs of barotrauma.

Although it presents with a dramatic radiographic appearance, subcutaneous emphysema is a benign condition that resolves as pneumomediastinum and pneumothorax improve. It is important to recognize that extensive subcutaneous emphysema limits the diagnostic accuracy of the portable radiograph in the assessment of the pleura and lung parenchyma. CT of the thorax can be helpful for assessing for pneumothorax and lung parenchymal disease in such cases (Figure 11-9).

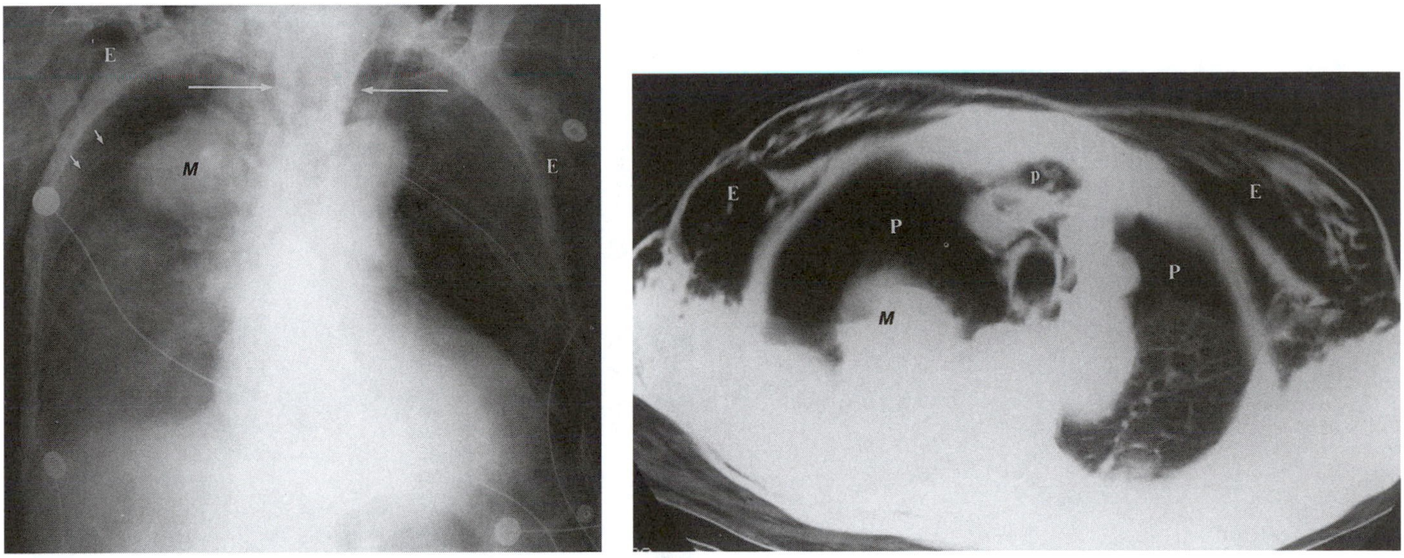

(A) (B)

FIGURE 11-9

(A) A portable supine chest radiograph demonstrates several abnormal air collections including subcutaneous emphysema (*E*), pneumomediastinum (*paired long arrows*), and right pneumothorax (*paired short arrows*). Also note the presence of a right upper lobe lung mass (*M*) and layering right pleural effusion. **(B)** CT confirms the presence of subcutaneous emphysema (*E*), pneumomediastinum (*p*), and right pneumothorax (*P*). CT also demonstrates a left pneumothorax (*P*), which was was obscured on the chest radiograph by extensive subcutaneous emphysema. *M*, mass.

TABLE 11-5

SIGNS OF PNEUMOTHORAX ON SUPINE RADIOGRAPHS

Anteromedial pneumothorax	
	Sharp outline of mediastinal vascular structures, heart border, and cardiophrenic angles
Subpulmonic pneumothorax	
	Hyperlucent upper quadrant of abdomen
	Deep costophrenic sulcus
	Sharp hemidiaphragm despite lung opacification in lower lobe
	Visualization of inferior surface of consolidated lung in lower lobe

Pneumothorax resulting from barotrauma is a life-threatening condition that requires prompt and accurate diagnosis.

In the supine position, air collects preferentially in the anteromedial and subpulmonic portions of the chest.

Only when a large amount of pleural air is present can an apicolateral pleural line be visualized on supine chest radiograph.

Flattening of the heart border and adjacent vascular structures is considered a relatively specific sign of tension pneumothorax.

When the diagnosis of pneumothorax is uncertain on the basis of a supine radiograph, additional views such as an upright or lateral decubitus radiograph may be helpful.

PNEUMOTHORAX. Pneumothorax resulting from barotrauma is a life-threatening condition that requires prompt and accurate diagnosis. A pneumothorax is usually readily identifiable on an upright chest radiograph as an apicolateral white line (the visceral pleural line) with an absence of vessels beyond it. However, a pneumothorax is much more difficult to detect on a supine radiograph. In the supine position, the apicolateral portion of the lung is no longer the most nondependent portion of the lung. Rather, air collects preferentially in the anteromedial and subpulmonic portions of the chest. Only when a very large volume of air is present in the pleural space will an apicolateral pleural line be visualized on a supine radiograph. The radiographic signs of pneumothorax on the supine radiograph (Table 11-5) are described in the following paragraphs.

Anteromedial pneumothorax is manifested by an unusually sharp outline of the mediastinal vascular structures, heart border, and cardiophrenic sulcus. A subpulmonic pneumothorax is manifested by a hyperlucent appearance of the upper quadrant of the abdomen, a deep costophrenic sulcus (Figure 11-10), a sharp hemidiaphragm despite lung opacification in the lower lobe (Figure 11-7), and visualization of the inferior surface of the consolidated lung.

Radiographic signs suggesting the presence of a tension pneumothorax include mediastinal shift, diaphragmatic inversion, and flattening of the heart border and adjacent vascular structures, such as the superior and inferior vena cava. Flattening of these structures is considered a relatively specific sign of tension pneumothorax, reflecting impairment of venous return to the right side of the heart.

When the diagnosis of pneumothorax is in uncertain on the basis of a supine radiograph, additional views such as an upright or decubitus radiograph may be helpful for confirmation. CT is the most sensitive method for detecting pneumothorax and may also help in guiding placement of chest tubes.

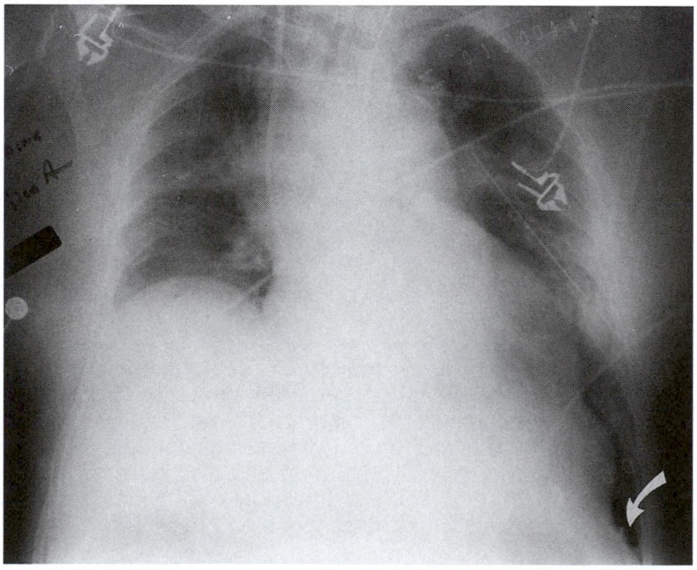

FIGURE 11-10

A supine portable chest radiograph demonstrates a deep left costophrenic sulcus (*curved arrow*), indicative of a subpulmonic pneumothorax. Note absence of a visible apicolateral visceral pleural line.

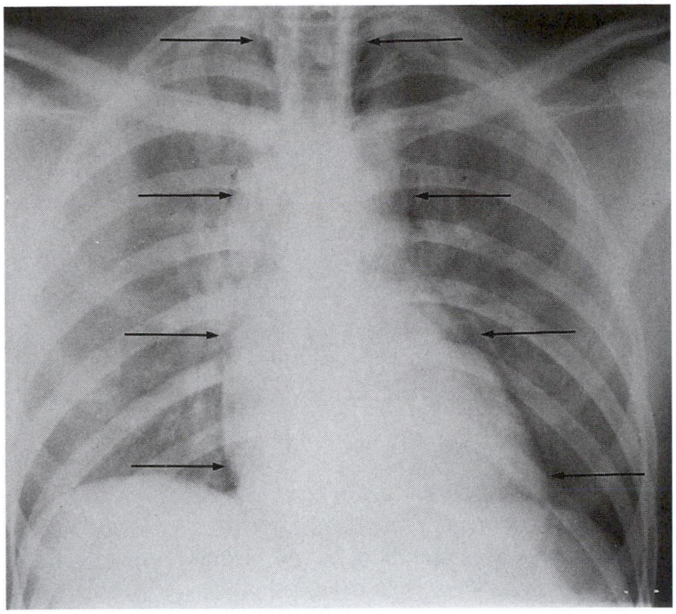

FIGURE 11-11

A supine portable chest radiograph reveals lucent streaks of air surrounding the mediastinal structures (*arrows*), consistent with pneumomediastinum.

PNEUMOMEDIASTINUM. Pneumomediastinum is usually a benign and self-limited condition. Although there are a variety of causes, the majority of cases that arise in the ICU setting are the result of barotrauma. It is important to recognize that pneumomediastinum frequently precedes the development of pneumothorax in patients with ARDS.

Pneumomediastinum frequently precedes the development of pneumothorax in patients with ARDS.

Pneumomediastinum manifests radiographically as lucent streaks of air that outline the mediastinal contours, elevate the mediastinal pleura, and frequently extend into the soft tissues of the neck (Figure 11-11). Thus, when you observe subcutaneous air in the neck, you should observe carefully for the presence of pneumomediastinum.

When you observe subcutaneous emphysema in the neck, you should carefully assess for the presence of pneumomediastinum.

PULMONARY INTERSTITIAL EMPHYSEMA. Pulmonary interstitial emphysema (PIE) is a form of barotrauma that occurs when the pressure in the airspaces of the lungs exceeds the tension in the adjacent perivascular connective tissues and interlobular septa. Rupture of alveoli results in dissection of air into the interstitium of the lung, producing interstitial emphysema.

Pulmonary interstitial emphysema occurs when the pressure in the airspaces of the lungs exceeds the tension in the adjacent perivascular connective tissue and interlobular septa.

The radiologic signs of PIE include small, mottled, and streaky lucencies, some of which radiate from the hilum to the lung periphery. These lucencies are best visualized when superimposed on diffuse consolidative changes, such as those related to ARDS. Small lung cysts may also develop, and the rupture of subpleural lung cysts may result in pneumothorax.

In patients with pulmonary interstitial emphysema, the rupture of small subpleural lung cysts may result in pneumothorax.

Thoracic CT

Although chest radiography is the mainstay of thoracic imaging of the ICU patient, it clearly has limitations in the detection and differentiation of various acute cardiopulmonary abnormalities. Thoracic CT is superior to radiography in the assessment of the pleura, lung parenchyma, mediastinum, and pulmonary vascularity. In certain clinical settings, the additional information provided by thoracic CT can aid in the diagnosis and management of the ICU patient (Table 11-6).

Pleura

The detection, localization, and characterization of pleural fluid collections is a common clinical indication for obtaining thoracic CT in the ICU setting. CT can help to distinguish simple, dependent effusions from complex, exudative effusions such empyema. An assessment of the Hounsfield units of the fluid can also aid in the diagnosis of a hemothorax.

The detection, localization, and characterization of pleural fluid collections is a common clinical indication for obtaining thoracic CT in the ICU setting.

TABLE 11-6

ROLE OF THORACIC CT IN THE ASSESSMENT OF THE ICU PATIENT

Pleura
- Detecting and characterizing pleural fluid collections
- Detecting pneumothoraces
- Guiding drainage procedures

Lung parenchyma
- Assessing ARDS patients with suspected pneumonia
- Identifying and characterizing complications of pneumonia

Mediastinum
- Assessing patients with mediastinal widening
- Evaluating mediastinal vascular disorders such as aortic dissection

Pulmonary vascularity
- Emerging role in the assessment for acute pulmonary embolus
- Evaluating complications of Swan–Ganz catheters such as pseudoaneurysm

As mentioned earlier in the discussion on abnormal air collections, CT is superior to radiography in the detection and localization of pneumothoraces. CT can also be used to guide the placement of drainage tubes for loculated pneumothoraces and pleural fluid collections.

Lung Parenchyma

The identification of alveolar consolidation in the nondependent portions of the lungs in patients with ARDS is suggestive of pneumonia.

CT may be helpful in the identification of nosocomial pneumonia in patients with diffuse lung disease such as ARDS. On CT scans, the parenchymal opacities from ARDS are usually dependent in distribution, with sparing of the anterior portions of the lungs. Thus, the identification of alveolar consolidation in nondependent portions of the lungs on CT scans of patients with ARDS is suggestive of pneumonia (Figure 11-12).

CT also aids in the assessment of complications of pneumonia, such as lung abscess, empyema, and bronchopleural fistula. Although lung abscess and empyema may appear similar radiographically, CT features usually allow an accurate distinction between these entities.

Mediastinum

CT can readily differentiate among various causes of mediastinal widening, including mediastinal hemorrhage, lymph node enlargement, and mediastinal lipomatosis.

CT can readily differentiate among various causes of mediastinal widening, such as mediastinal hemorrhage, lymph node enlargement, and mediastinal lipomatosis (Figure 11-13). CT can also be helpful in the diagnosis of postoperative mediastinitis.

With regard to mediastinal vascular structures, contrast-enhanced helical CT is an excellent method for assessing diseases of the thoracic aorta, such as aortic dissection and aortic

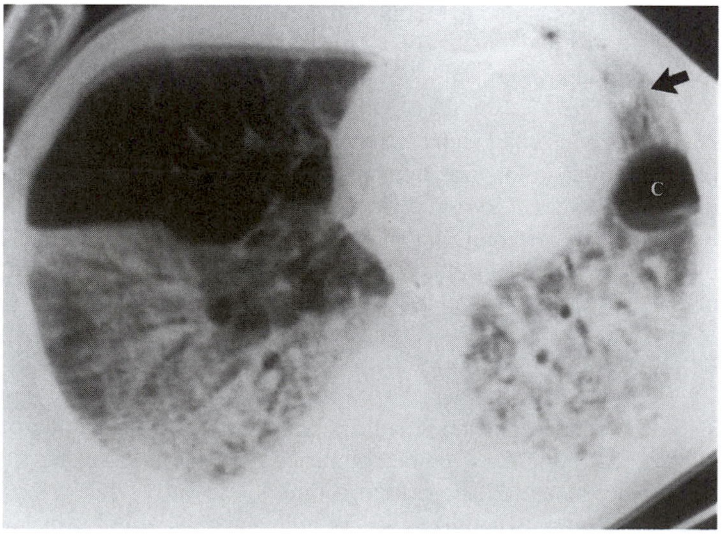

FIGURE 11-12

CT scan of a patient with acute respiratory distress syndrome (ARDS) demonstrates dependent distribution of lung opacities in the right lung, with sparing anteriorly. In the left lung, there is also lung opacification anteriorly (*arrow*), corresponding to a site of pneumonia within the lingula. Also note the presence of an adjacent lung cyst (*C*).

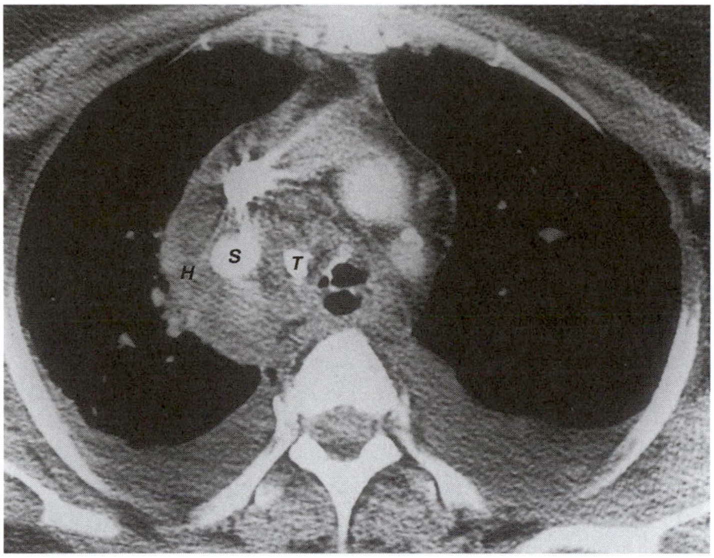

FIGURE 11-13

CT scan of a patient with mediastinal widening demonstrates high-attenuation opacity within the mediastinum, consistent with mediastinal hematoma (*H*). The hemorrhage occurred secondary to vascular perforation by a central venous catheter. Note that the catheter tip (*T*) is extravascular, located medial to the superior vena cava (*S*).

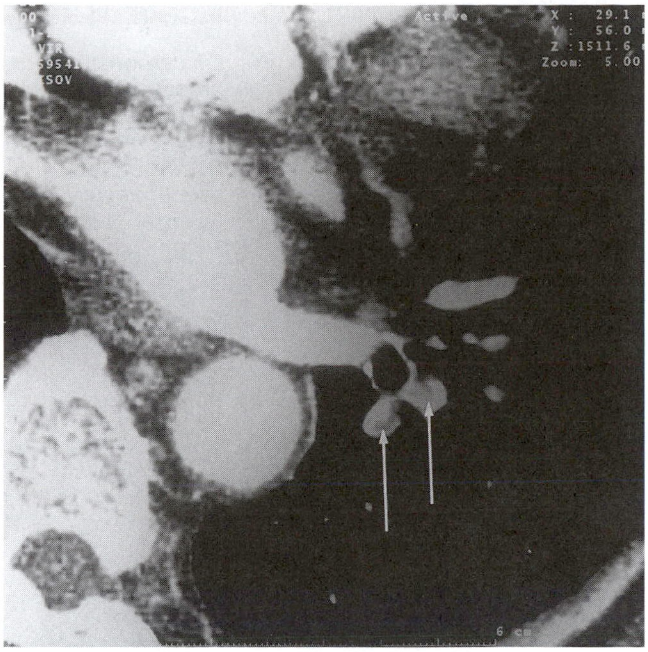

FIGURE 11-14

Coned-down image of the left lower lobe from a CT pulmonary angiogram demonstrates abnormal low-attenuation material within the posterior basal and lateral basal segmental arteries, consistent with acute, nonocclusive embolus.

aneurysm, as well as abnormalities of the superior vena cava such as superior vena cava obstruction.

Pulmonary Vascularity

In recent years, with the advent of spiral or helical technology, CT has been playing an increasingly prominent role in the diagnosis of pulmonary vascular disorders. For example, spiral CT has recently been advocated for the assessment of acute pulmonary embolism, particulary for patients with diffuse lung opacities on chest radiography. Such patients often have nondiagnostic ventilation–perfusion imaging studies. In several preliminary studies, spiral CT has been shown to have a relatively high sensitivity and specifity for the detection of central and segmental pulmonary emboli (Figure 11-14). Spiral CT scans obtained for assessing for pulmonary emboli should be performed using special protocols that optimize visualization of the pulmonary vascularity. It is important to recognize that a negative CT scan does not exclude the diagnosis of acute pulmonary embolus.

CT may also be helpful to detect iatrogenic pulmonary vascular complications, such as pulmonary artery pseudoaneurysms related to Swan–Ganz catheters (Figure 11-15).

Thoracic Ultrasound

The primary roles of thoracic ultrasound in the ICU setting are to assess for the presence of pleural fluid and to guide thoracentesis procedures. Advantages of ultrasound over CT include its portability, lower cost, and lack of ionizing radiation.

> The primary roles of thoracic ultrasound in the ICU setting are to assess for the presence of pleural fluid and to guide thoracentesis procedures.

Ventilation–Perfusion Imaging

The primary role of ventilation–perfusion imaging (VQ scan) in the ICU setting is to assess for the presence of acute pulmonary embolus. A VQ scan does not permit direct visualiza-

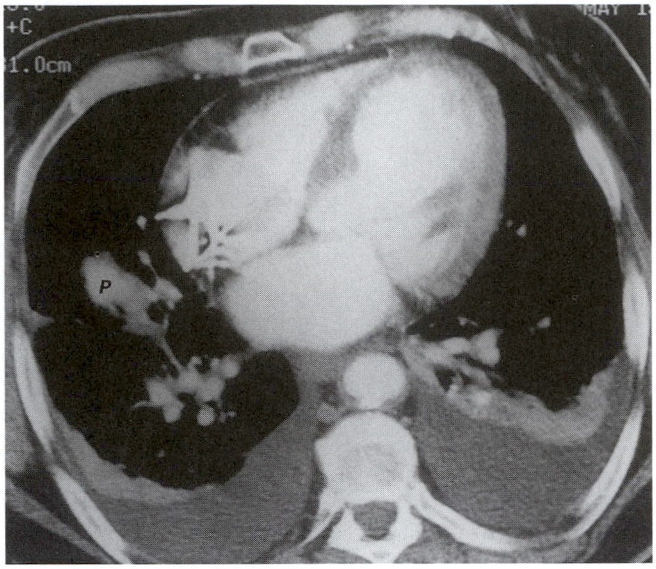

FIGURE 11-15

CT demonstrates aneurysmal dilatation (*P*) of the right middle lobe lateral segmental artery, corresponding to a pseudoaneurysm related to distal placement of a Swan–Ganz catheter.

Ventilation-perfusion imaging is a nuclear medicine study that uses indirect evidence (a ventilation–perfusion mismatch) to diagnose acute pulmonary embolism.

A normal VQ scan reliably excludes acute pulmonary embolus, and a high-probability VQ scan is sufficient evidence to treat a patient for acute pulmonary embolus.

Patients with a high clinical suspicion for acute pulmonary embolus and either a "low" or "intermediate" probability VQ scan should be evaluated with additional diagnostic studies such as pulmonary arteriography.

Pulmonary angiography is the most accurate imaging test for diagnosing acute pulmonary embolus.

tion of a pulmonary embolus. Rather, it relies on indirect evidence: a ventilation–perfusion mismatch. Although there are several interpretative schemes for diagnosing acute pulmonary embolus with VQ imaging, the most common criteria are those determined from the Prospective Investigation of Pulmonary Embolism Diagnosis (PIOPED) study. This study was a landmark prospective multiinstitutional investigation that assessed the value of the VQ scan in diagnosing acute pulmonary embolus, using pulmonary angiography as the gold standard. Using the PIOPED interpretative scheme, a VQ scan is categorized as normal, low probability, intermediate probability, or high probability for pulmonary embolus.

In general, a normal VQ scan reliably excludes the diagnosis of acute pulmonary embolus, and a high-probability VQ scan is considered sufficient evidence to treat a patient for acute pulmonary embolus. Unfortunately, however, the majority of VQ scan interpretations do not fall into these two categories. Because ICU patients frequently demonstrate pleural and parenchymal opacities on chest radiography, VQ scans are very often indeterminate for pulmonary embolus in this patient population. Based on their results, the PIOPED investigators recommended that patients with a high clinical suspicion for pulmonary embolus and either "low" or "intermediate" probability scans should be evaluated with additional diagnostic studies such as pulmonary angiography to exclude pulmonary embolus. Lower extremity doppler ultrasound may also be helpful in such a setting to exclude deep venous thrombosis, the source of most pulmonary emboli.

Pulmonary Arteriography

Pulmonary arteriography is presently considered the most accurate imaging test for diagnosing acute pulmonary embolus (Figure 11-16). It involves the percutaneous advancement of a catheter into the pulmonary arteries under fluoroscopic guidance, with subsequent injection of contrast media. The complication rate of the procedure is relatively low, estimated at 1%–5%. Complications include arrhythmias, cardiac arrest, cardiac perforation, and contrast reactions. The estimated mortality of the procedure is approximately 0.2%, increasing to approximately 2% in patients with severe pulmonary artery hypertension.

In addition to diagnosing acute pulmonary embolus, in certain clinical settings (such as a patient who is hemodynamically unstable from a massive pulmonary embolus), angiographers may also provide therapeutic intervention by administering lytic therapy.

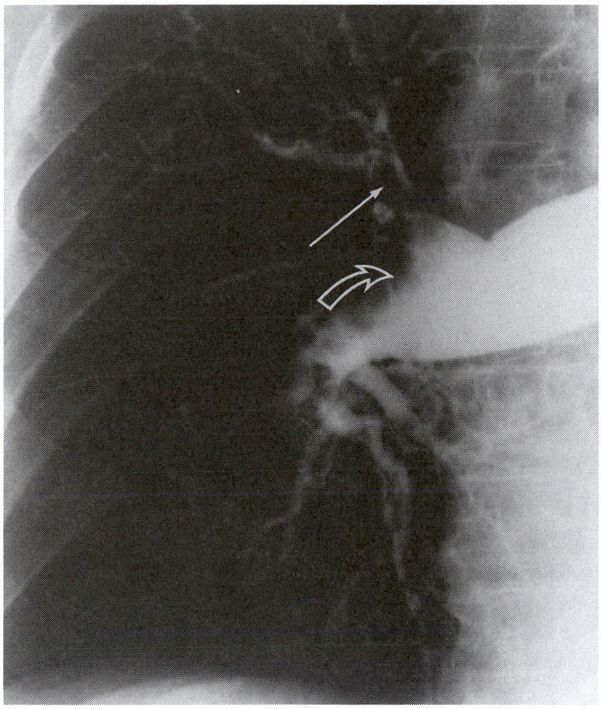

FIGURE 11-16

Pulmonary arteriogram demonstrates a large, central embolus in the distal right main pulmonary artery, manifested by a large filling defect (*curved arrow*) in the contrast column. Note additional nonocclusive thrombus within the truncus anterior, manifested as a filling defect (*curved arrow*) with peripheral contrast opacification.

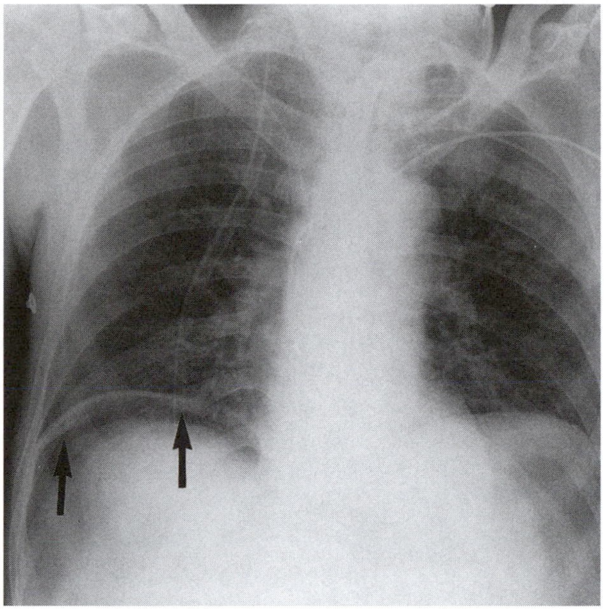

FIGURE 11-7

Upright portable chest radiograph demonstrates an abnormal crescenteric lucency (*arrows*) below the right hemidiaphragm, consistent with free intraperitoneal air.

EXTRATHORACIC IMAGING

Abdominal Imaging

One of the most important roles of abdominal imaging in the ICU patient is in the evaluation of the patient with sepsis of unknown origin. In the following paragraphs, we review the roles of various abominal imaging procedures in the assessment of the ICU patient with suspected abdominal sepsis.

Abdominal Radiography

One of the most ominous findings on abdominal radiographs of a septic patient is free intraperitoneal air, which is usually indicative of bowel perforation. Free intraperitoneal air can be quite difficult to detect on supine radiographs. Thus, an upright radiograph (Figure 11-17) or a lateral decubitus radiograph is recommended in the assessment of the patient with suspected free intraperitoneal air.

One of the most ominous findings on abdominal radiographs of a septic patient is free intraperitoneal air, which usually indicates bowel perforation.

An upright or right lateral decubitus radiograph is recommended in the assessment of the patient with suspected free intraperitoneal air.

Occasionally, abdominal radiography reveals other findings that point to the source of infection. Such findings may include bubbly, extraluminal lucencies, corresponding to an abdominal abscess; calcified gallstones; calcified renal stones; and a calcified appendicolith.

Outside the setting of suspected abdominal sepsis, abdominal radiographs play a frequent role in the assessment of accurate placement of nasogastric and feeding tubes and in the evaluation of patients with suspected bowel obstruction. In the patient with suspected obstruction, it is important to obtain a lateral decubitus or upright view (in addition to a supine radiograph) to allow assessment for fluid levels and free intraperitoneal air.

Abdominal Ultrasound

Abdominal ultrasound can be a valuable tool for assessing the abdomen and pelvis in critically ill patients. Because of its portability, ultrasound is ideally suited for the assessment of the critically ill patient, who may not be stable enough for transportation to the radiology department. In general, ultrasound provides excellent visualization of the liver, kidneys, gallbladder, spleen, pancreas, and female pelvis. However, it should be kept in mind that ultrasound is an operator-dependent modality. Careful attention to technical factors is important for optimal results, particularly when examinations are performed portably. Moreover, ultrasound is less successful at imaging obese patients, who are usually better imaged by CT.

> Ultrasound is less successful than CT at imaging obese patients.

> The best results with ultrasound are usually obtained when there is clinical suspicion for a specific abnormality such as suspected cholecystitis.

The best results are usually achieved when there is clinical suspicion for a specific abnormality such as suspected cholecystitis (Figure 11-18). Ultrasound fares less well than CT as a general screening examination for the patient with suspected abdominal sepsis of unknown origin, because abscesses may be obscured by overlying bowel gas on ultrasound examinations.

Ultrasound can occasionally be used at the bedside to guide drainage procedures. Its use is generally limited to situations in which fluid collections are well visualized with ultrasound and there is a bowel-free path to the fluid collection.

Abdominal CT

> CT is the most sensitive imaging modality for the detection of intraabdominal abscesses.

CT is the most sensitive imaging modality for the detection of intraabdominal abscesses. CT is also superior to ultrasound in its ability to guide drainage procedures. In contrast to ultrasound, however, CT is more expensive, it involves ionizing radiation exposure, and it requires that the patient travel to the radiology department.

> Whenever possible, it is important that abdominal CT be performed with oral and intravenous contrast.

Whenever possible, it is important that abdominal CT be performed with adequate oral and intravenous contrast to optimize sensitivity and specifity for diagnosing abscess collections (Figure 11-19).

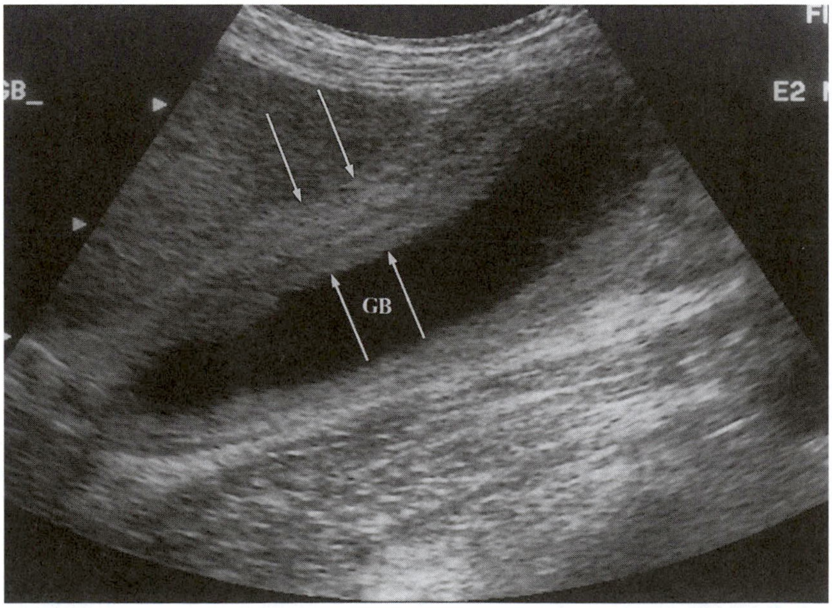

FIGURE 11-18

Right upper quadrant ultrasound of the gallbladder (*GB*) in a patient with acalculous cholecystitis demonstrates marked gallbladder wall thickening (*paired arrows* are on opposite sides of the gallbladder wall). (Case courtesy of Dr. Patrick O'Kane, Temple University.)

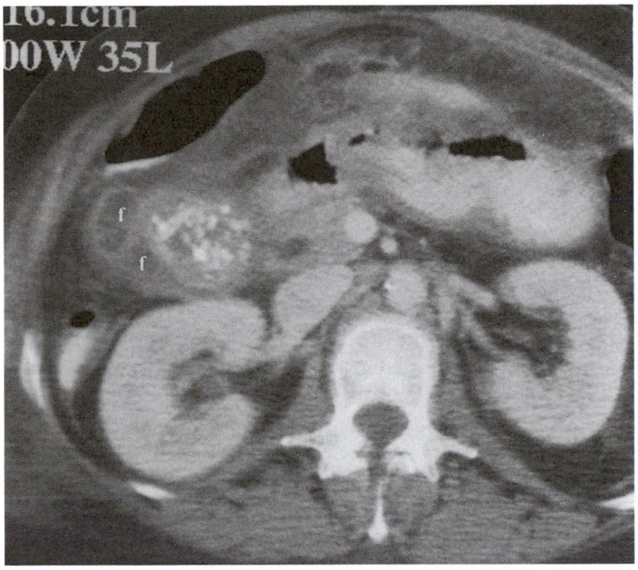

FIGURE 11-19

Abdominal contrast-enhanced CT image of a patient with gangrenous cholecystitis reveals numerous calcified gallstones and a pericholecystic fluid collection (*f*). (Case courtesy of Dr. Patrick O'Kane, Temple University.)

NEUROLOGIC IMAGING

In the evaluation of the critically ill patient, important roles of neurologic imaging include the assessment of intracranial hemorrhage, major cranial trauma, and acute stroke. CT is the preferred imaging modality for the assessment of suspected acute subarachnoid hemorrhage and in the evaluation of major cranial trauma. In these settings, a CT without intravenous contrast should be performed because both acute blood and intravenous contrast appear hyperdense (white).

CT is the preferred imaging modality for the assessment of intracranial trauma and nontraumatic intracranial hemorrhage.

CT can readily identify and distinguish among various sites of intracranial hemorrhage, including intraparenchymal hematoma, subdural hematoma, epidural hematoma, and subarachnoid hemorrhage (Figure 11-20). In the absence of trauma, subarachnoid hemorrhage

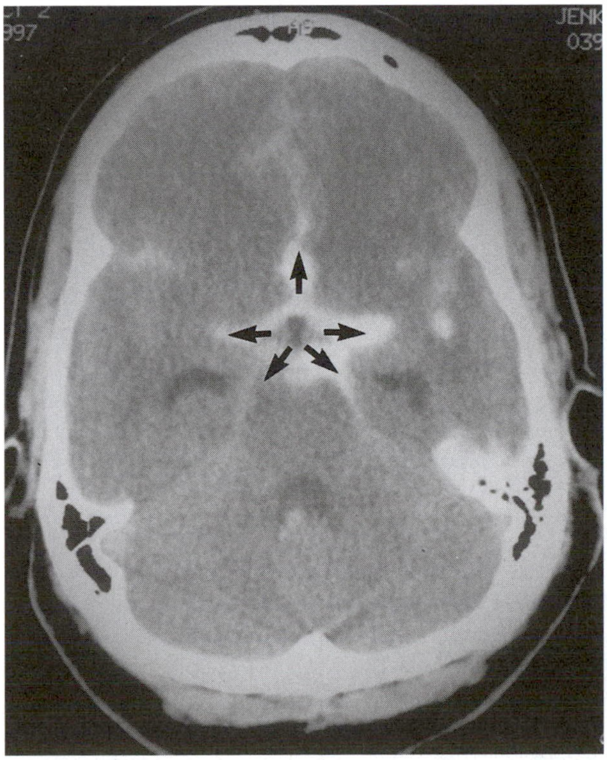

FIGURE 11-20

A noncontrast head CT near the base of the brain demonstrates the presence of a subarachnoid hemorrhage, manifested as a "star pattern" of increased density (*arrows*), corresponding to the presence of blood radiating from the suprasellar cistern into the sylvian fissures and the anterior interhemispheric fissure. (Case courtesy of Dr. Jeffrey Kochan, Temple University.)

is usually secondary to a ruptured aneurysm. Neuroangiography can be helpful for further assessment of the patient with subarachnoid hemorrhage, as it can aid in both the diagnosis and the treatment of a ruptured aneurysm.

It is important to recognize that CT may be normal within the first 24 h of an ischemic stroke.

With regard to a suspected acute stroke, it is important to recognize that CT may be normal in the setting of an acute ischemic stroke, particularly in the first 24 h. Early CT findings include a subtle loss of definition of the gray-white matter border and a loss of cortical definition. Another early CT sign of infarction is the presence of a hyperdense middle cerebral artery, which corresponds to either acute thrombus or calcified embolus lodged within the middle cerebral artery. Later CT findings (12–24 h) include an indistinct, low-density area within a vascular distribution, with associated mass effect. The latter becomes more pronounced more than 24 h following the stroke.

MR is more sensitive than CT for detecting acute ischemic strokes, and it is frequently positive in the first few hours.

MR is more sensitive than CT for detecting acute ischemic strokes, and it is frequently positive within the first few hours; this is because MR is extremely sensitive at detecting increased water (edema), which appears as bright signal intensity on T_2-weighted images. Despite the increased sensitivity of MR for detecting early ischemic infarction, CT can still be helpful in the acute assessment of a patient with suspected stroke by excluding an alternative cause of the patient's neurologic symptoms and by assessing for an acute hemorrhagic component of the stroke, which is usually readily apparent at CT. In the assessment of the ICU patient with suspected stroke, the decision to obtain CT or MR may vary according to local practice patterns and the relative availability of MR compared to CT. The stability of the patient is another factor to consider, as CT is the preferable modality for imaging the clinically unstable patient.

SUMMARY

Radiologic images are crucial tests in the evaluation of the critically ill patient. Imaging procedures and their interpretation as discussed in this chapter should provide the reader with the background to know when to appropriately order selected tests and how to interpret their results based on the fundamentals of radiologic imaging.

REVIEW QUESTIONS

1. **Which one of the following radiographic findings is present in both hydrostatic and increased permeability pulmonary edema?**
   A. Cardiomegaly
   B. Widened vascular pedicle
   C. Increased pulmonary vascularity
   D. Kerley lines
   E. Airspace consolidation

2. **Which one of the following causes of lung opacification is most closely associated with volume loss?**
   A. Pneumonia
   B. Pulmonary edema
   C. Atelectasis
   D. Aspiration

3. **Which one of the following is a radiographic sign of pneumomediastinum?**
   A. Hyperlucent upper quadrant of the abdomen
   B. Deep costophrenic sulcus
   C. Lucent streaks of air that outline the mediastinal contours
   D. Sharp hemidiaphragm despite lung opacification in lower lobe
   E. Visualization of inferior surface of consolidated lung in lower lobe

4. **Which one of the following is the most sensitive imaging modality for the detection of intraabdominal abscesses?**
   A. Abdominal CT scan
   B. Abdominal ultrasound
   C. Abdominal radiograph
   D. Abdominal MR exam

5. **With regard to neurologic imaging of the ICU patient, which one of the following is true?**
   A. MR is the preferred imaging modality in the evaluation of major cranial trauma.
   B. MR is more sensitive than CT for detecting acute ischemic strokes.
   C. CT with intravenous contrast is best for assessing patients with subarachnoid hemorrhage.
   D. MR is the preferable modality for imaging the clinically unstable patient.

ANSWERS

1. The answer is E. Both hydrostatic and increased permeability pulmonary edema are characterized by the presence of airspace consolidation. The other features listed (A–D) are typical of hydrostatic pulmonary edema, but they are not associated with increased permeability pulmonary edema.
2. The answer is C. Atelectasis, which refers to areas of nonaerated lung, is a very common cause of lung opacification in the ICU setting. An important feature that favors atelectasis over other causes of lung opacification such as pneumonia is the presence of associated volume loss. Radiographic signs of volume loss include displaced fissures, displaced hila, elevated hemidiaphragms, and shift of mediastinal structures.
3. The answer is C. Pneumomediastinum manifests radiographically as lucent streaks of air that outline the mediastinal contours, elevate the mediastinal pleura, and frequently extend into the soft tissues of the neck. The other listed features (A, B, D, E) are signs of a subpulmonic pneumothorax.
4. The answer is A. CT is the most sensitive imaging modality for the detection of intraabdominal abscesses. Whenever possible, it is important that abdominal CT be performed with adequate oral and intravenous contrast to optimize sensitivity and specificity for diagnosing abscess collections.
5. The answer is B. MR is more sensitive than CT for detecting acute ischemic strokes. MR is frequently positive within the first few hours of an acute ischemic stroke, because MR is extremely sensitive at detecting increased water (edema), which appears as bright signal intensity on T_2-weighted images.

SUGGESTED READING

Boiselle PM. Pulmonary vascular abnormalities. In: McLoud TC (ed) Thoracic Radiology: The Requisites. St. Louis: Mosby, 1998: 403–419.

Cascade PN, Meaney JB, Jamadar DA. Methods of cardiopulmonary support: a review for radiologists. Radiographics 1997;17:1141–1155.

Grossman RI, Yousem DM. Techniques in neuroimaging. In: Grossman RI, Yousem DM (eds) Neuroradiology: The Requisites. St. Louis: Mosby, 1994:1–23.

Grossman RI, Yousem DM. Vascular diseases of the brain. In: Grossman RI, Yousem DM (eds) Neuroradiology: The Requisites. St. Louis: Mosby, 1994:105–148.

Henschke CI, Yankelevitz DF, Wand A, Davis SD, Shiau M. Accuracy and efficacy of chest radiography in the intensive care unit. Radiol Clin North Am 1996;34:21–31.

McDowell RK, Dawson SL. Evaluation of the abdomen in sepsis of unknown origin. Radiol Clin North Am 1996;34(1):177–190.

MacMahon H, Giger M. Portable chest radiography techniques and teleradiology. Radiol Clin North Am 1996;34:1–20.

Miller WT. The radiologist in the intensive care unit setting. Semin Roentgenol 1997;27(2):86–88.

Miller WT. The chest radiograph in the intensive care unit. Semin Roentgenol 1997;27(2):89–101.

Miller WT Jr, Tino G, Friedburg JS. Thoracic CT in the intensive care unit: assessment of clinical usefulness. Radiology 1998;209:491–498.

Milne ENC, Massimo P. Pulmonary edema-cardiac and noncardiac. In: Putman CE (ed) Diagnostic Imaging of the Lung. New York: Dekker, 1990:253–336.

Thomason JWW, Ely EW, Chiles C, et al. Appraising pulmonary edema using supine chest roentgenograms in ventilated patients. Am J Respir Crit Care Med 1998;157:1600–1608.

Tocino I, Westcott JL. Barotrauma. Radiol Clin North Am 1996;34: 59–81.

Trotman-Dickenson B. Radiography in the critical care patient. In: McLoud TC (ed) Thoracic Radiology: The Requisites. St. Louis: Mosby, 1998:151–172.

Winer-Muram HT, Steiner RM, Gurney JW, et al. Ventilator-associated pneumonia in patients with adult respiratory distress syndrome: CT evaluation. Radiology 1998;208:193–199.

PART II

Pathophysiologic Disease States Encountered in the Critically Ill Patient

CHAPTER 12

GILBERT E. D'ALONZO, JOHN M. TRAVALINE,
AND MARIA ROSELYN LIM

Neurologic Illness and Critical Care

CHAPTER OUTLINE

LEARNING OBJECTIVES

After studying this chapter, you should be able to:

- Understand the various pathophysiologies of the most important neuromuscular conditions found in critically ill patients.
- Recognize the signs and symptoms of neurologic illness and describe the approach to their diagnosis.
- Discuss treatments used in a variety of severe neurologic and neuromuscular conditions.
- Appreciate the diversity of neurologic and neuromuscular diseases that can be identified in the intensive care unit.

ALTERED MENTAL STATUS

In a critically ill patient, an abnormal mental status has been associated with a higher mortality rate and a longer stay in the intensive care unit (ICU). Normally, patients should be aware of their surroundings and themselves and have an accurate perception of what they are experiencing. A patient should be able to process information into judgment and reasoning and store and retrieve information as memory. Orientation, judgment and reasoning, and memory constitute cognition. Therefore, disorders of awareness or mental status can be classified as problems with consciousness or cognition.

Cognition components:
Orientation
Judgment
Reasoning
Memory

Consciousness has two components: arousal or wakefulness and awareness or responsiveness. Obviously, awareness is not possible without arousal. There are various levels of consciousness (Table 12-1). A comatose patient is unable to be aroused or to be aware of their surroundings. Therefore, coma can be defined as a state of unarousible unresponsiveness. A vegetative state is a condition in which the patient is awake with sleep–wake cycles, spontaneous roving eye movements, and reflex activities at brainstem and spinal cord levels but neither is awake nor has purposeful behaviors. A vegetative state should not be confused with the locked-in syndrome. A patient with locked-in syndrome is awake and aware but is

Consciousness components:
Arousal or wakefulness
Awareness or responsiveness

Coma is a state of unarousable unresponsiveness.

TABLE 12-1

LEVELS OF CONSCIOUSNESS

Awake: aroused and aware
Somnolent: easily aroused and aware
Stuporous: aroused with difficulty, impaired awareness
Comatose: unarousable and unaware
Vegetative state: aroused but unaware

unable to generate any form of motor response to either verbal or noxious stimuli. The patient may be able to communicate with eye movements or blinking.

There are numerous reasons why a patient may have a depressed level of consciousness (Table 12-2). Many of these conditions can be classified as types of encephalopathies, such as infectious, ischemic, metabolic, or medication related. Often patients are admitted to an intensive care unit with an ischemic encephalopathy, whereas a septic encephalopathy generally develops after the patient has been in intensive care. Septic encephalopathy may be one part of a more widespread multiorgan injury process termed the systemic inflammatory response syndrome.

The systemic inflammatory response often includes encephalopathy.

The bedside evaluation of the unconscious patient is important to review. Ocular reflexes and mobility and the size and reactivity of the pupils are important features of this evaluation. The oculocephalic and oculovestibular reflexes are important determinants of the functional integrity of the brainstem. The oculocephalic reflex is elicited by briskly turning the patient's head from side to side. When the cerebral hemispheres are impaired but the brainstem is intact, the eyes deviate conjugately away from the direction of rotation. This eye movement resembles the fixed forward gaze of a doll's eyes, and for this reason it is called the doll's-eyes movement. When the lower brainstem is damaged or when the patient is awake, the eyes will follow the direction of head rotation. The oculovestibular reflex is elicited by injecting cold saline or tap water into the external auditory canal. In a normal awake person, it will cause nystagmus with the fast component away from the stimulated side. In a comatose patient, the fast component of the nystagmus is lost and the eyes are deviated toward the stimulus, usually for several minutes. Ocular movements may be altered in different ways. In comatose patients, spontaneous, roving, horizontal eye movements indicate that the midbrain and pontine tegmentum are intact. A persistent downward deviation of the eyes is seen in tectal compression by a thalamic hemorrhage and in anoxic and metabolic encephalopathies. Ocular bobbing, with downward deviation of the eyes and less rapid upward movement, occurs with lesions in the pons. Ocular dipping, characterized by slow downward deviations followed by rapid upward movement, may be observed with coma caused by anoxia and intoxication. There may be persistent conjugate deviation of the eyes to one side, away from the side of paralysis with a destructive cerebral lesion and toward the side of paralysis with a pontine lesion; seizure or "wrong-way" gaze paresis occurs with thalamic and brainstem lesions. The vestibuloocular reflexes are lost when the brainstem is damaged. It is important to remember that the maneuvers that elicit these reflexes must be temporized in patients with suspected injury to the cervical spine.

Oculocephalic and oculovestibular reflexes are determinants of the functional integrity of the brainstem.

Conditions that affect pupillary size and light reactivity are shown in Table 12-3. Dilated and unreactive pupils are generally a sign of cerebral injury. If the injury results from a mass lesion or cerebral edema with herniation, the pupillary abnormality will be unilateral; if the injury is more diffuse in character, the pupillary abnormality will be bilateral. Various medications, such as atropine, can affect pupillary size and ability to react to light.

Focal motor or sensory deficits in the extremities can be associated with a diffuse encephalopathy but may be a sign of a structural brain lesion. A patient may have semipur-

TABLE 12-2

POSSIBLE CAUSES OF DEPRESSED CONSCIOUSNESS AND DELIRIUM

Medications, drug intoxication	Hypoxic: ischemic encephalopathy
Sepsis, meningitis	Stroke, brain trauma, seizure
Acute metabolic or endocrine crisis	Fat or cholesterol embolization

TABLE 12-3

CONDITIONS THAT AFFECT PUPIL SIZE AND LIGHT REACTIVITY

- Constricted (1–2 mm diameter):
  - Reactive
    - Opiates
    - Pontine destruction/injury
    - Bilateral cortical lesions
  - Unreactive
    - Opiates
    - Ocular pilocarpine drops
- Midposition (5–7 mm diameter):
  - Reactive
    - Metabolic encephalopathy
    - Sedative-hypnotic therapy overdose
  - Unreactive
    - Barbiturates overdose
    - Glutethimide (unequal pupils)
    - Midbrain lesion
- Dilated (>7 mm diameter):
  - Reactive
    - Sympathomimetics
    - Atropine
  - Unreactive
    - Supratentorial injury or mass
    - Atropine (high dose)
    - Dopamine (high dose)
    - Scopolamine

poseful movement or no movement at all. In the absence of motor response to any stimulus, one should consider a locked-in-state, cervical trauma causing limb paralysis, or Guillain–Barré syndrome. Repetitive movements occurring on one side may represent seizure. The pattern of motor response or posturing stimulus may reveal the anatomic level of the altered mental state. Decerebrate posturing (extension at the elbows with internal rotation at the shoulders and forerarm together with lower extremity extension) correlates with brainstem disease or injury but may also be seen in metabolic states such as anoxic encephalopathy. A decorticate response (arm flexion at the elbow, adduction at the shoulder, and extension of the legs) signifies disease at the level of the cerebral hemispheres or compression of the thalamus, as well as metabolic depression of brain function.

Decerebrate posturing indicates brainstem injury.

Decorticate posturing suggests cerebral or thalamic disease.

The Glasgow Coma Scale

The Glasgow Coma Scale (Table 12-4) is used to gauge the severity of the level of consciousness depression. This coma scale is used for both nontraumatic and traumatic coma. Patients with higher scores are more likely to awaken. The Glasgow Coma Scale is determined by the ability of the patient to open their eyes, respond to verbal communication, and move to verbal and nonverbal stimuli. The predictive value of this scale, that is, the chance of a satisfactory neurologic recovery, can be found in Table 12-5. However, the value of this scale is enhanced if sufficient time has elapsed from the inciting event that induced coma to the time that the measurement was made.

Delirium

Delirium is the most common mental disorder in hospitalized patients, particularly elderly patients. Delirium can be defined as an abnormal mental status characterized by disorientation, irritability, fear, and, at times, hallucinations. Delirium can also be hypoactive, characterized by lethargy, particularly in an elderly patient. The essential feature of delirium is a global mental dysfunction marked by disturbance of consciousness. Delirium generally develops over a short time period, might actually fluctuate during the course of 24 h, especially at night, and is reversible. Dementia, on the other hand, evolves over a long period of time,

Delirium is the most common mental disorder in hospitalized patients.

Delirium can fluctuate whereas dementia does not.

TABLE 12-4

THE GLASGOW COMA SCALE

CRITERION	POINTS	
Eye opening:		
Spontaneous	4	
To speech	3	
To pain	2	
None	1	
		_____Points
Verbal communication:		
Oriented	5	
Confused conversation	4	
Inappropriate words	3	
Incomprehensible sounds	2	
None	1	
		_____Points
Motor response:		
Obeys commands	6	
Localizes to pain	5	
Withdraws to pain	4	
Abnormal flexion	3	
Abnormal extension	2	
None	1	
		_____Points
	Total Points[a]	_____

[a] Best score is 15 points; worst score is 3 points

usually with clear sensorium, but is characterized by progressive intellectual deterioration caused by a primary degenerative disease.

Delirium is the brain's complex reaction to metabolic, anoxic, toxic, and infectious insults. Clinicians have described delirium as acute brain failure, synonymous with cardiac angina. The differential diagnosis of delirium can be summarized by the mnemonic WHHHHIMP (Table 12-6). Numerous medications have been associated with delirium (Table 12-7). Also, a variety of medical conditions can cause delirium (Table 12-8).

The management of delirium should focus immediately on identifying the underlying cause and directing treatment as specifically as possible. When agitation is present, sedatives may be administered. However, one must be cautious in doing so. The amount of medication needed to suppress the agitation may dangerously affect vital function.

A benzodiazepine and thiamine are the treatment for alcohol withdrawal agitation.

Haloperidol can aggravate delirium tremens.

A delirious patient with extreme hypertension and papilledema will generally respond to antihypertensive medication. An alcoholic patient who is having withdrawal symptoms must immediately receive thiamine and a benzodiazepine. Postoperative delirium and the delirium of unidentified cause in a critically ill patient can be treated with haloperidol. Haloperidol should be avoided in alcohol-related delirium or delirium tremens because it can aggravate the delirium and actually lower seizure threshold. Cocaine-induced delirium is treated sim-

TABLE 12-5

PREDICTIVE VALUE OF THE GLASGOW COMA SCALE

	NEGATIVE PREDICTIVE VALUE POSTARREST		
PARAMETERS	**1 H (%)**	**24 H (%)**	**3 DAYS (%)**
No eye opening to pain	69	92	100
No motor response to pain	75	91	100
No response to verbal stimuli	67	75	94
Glasgow Coma Score ≤5	69	–	100

SOURCE: Data from Edgren E, et al. Assessment of neurologic prognosis in comatose survivors of cardiac arrest. Lancet 1994;343:1055–1059

TABLE 12-6

DIFFERENTIAL DIAGNOSIS OF DELIRIUM (WHHHHIMP)

Wernicke encephalopathy	Hypoxemic
Hypertension encephalopathy	Intracranial blood/sepsis
Hypoglycemia	Meningitis/encephalitis
Hypoperfusion of CNS	Poisons/medications

ilarly to delirium tremens. Benzodiazepines generally act quickly, whereas haloperidol is slow in its onset of effect. When delirium has abated, these medications should be tapered slowly over a 3- to 5-day period. A variety of ancillary measures are important in the treatment process, such as normalizing the patient's sleep–wake cycle, eliminating all nonessential medications, ensuring proper oxygenation, reducing environmental stimuli to a minimum, enhancing orientation influences to the patient's environment, and making sure that the patient, when appropriate, wears eyeglasses or a hearing aid.

TABLE 12-7

DRUGS THAT CAUSE DELIRIUM (REVERSIBLE DEMENTIA)

- Analgesics
  - Meperidine
  - Opiates
  - Pentazocine
  - Salicylates
- Antibiotics
  - Acyclovir, ganciclovir
  - Aminoglycosides
  - Amodiaquine
  - Amphotericin B
  - Cephalexin
  - Cephalosporins
  - Chloramphenicol
  - Chloroqine
  - Ethambutol
  - Gentamicin
  - Interferon
  - Sulfonamides
  - Tetracycline
  - Ticarcillin
  - Vancomycin
- Anticholinergics
  - Antihistamines (chlorpheniramine)
  - Antispasmodics
  - Atropine/homatropine
  - Belladonna alkaloids
  - Benztropine
  - Biperiden
  - Diphenhydramine
  - Phenothiazines (especially thioridazine)
  - Promethazine
  - Scopolamine
  - Tricyclic antidepressants (especially amitriptyline)
  - Trihexyphenidyl
- Anticonvulsants
  - Phenobarbital
  - Phenytoin
  - Valproic acid
- Antiflammatory drugs
  - Corticosteroids
  - Ibuprofen
  - Indomethacin
  - Naproxen
  - Phenylbutazone
  - Steroids
- Antineoplastic drugs
  - Aminogluthethimide
  - Asparaginase
  - Dacarbazine
  - 5-Fluorouracil
  - Hexamethylenamine
  - Methotrexate (high dose)
  - Tamoxifen
  - Vinblastine
  - Vincristine
- Antiparkinson drugs
  - Amantadine
  - Bromocriptine
  - Carbidopa
  - Levodopa
- Antituberculous drugs
  - Isoniazid
  - Rifampin
- Cardiac drugs
  - β-Blockers (propranolol)
  - Captopril
  - Clonidine
  - Digitalis
  - Disopyramide
  - Lidocaine
  - Mexiletine
  - Methyldopa
  - Procainamide
  - Quinidine
  - Tocainamide
- Drug withdrawal
  - Alcohol
  - Barbiturates
  - Benzodiazepines
- Sedative-Hypnotics
  - Barbiturates
  - Benzodiazepines
  - Glutethimide
- Sympathomimetics
  - Aminophylline
  - Amphetamines
  - Cocaine
  - Ephedrine
  - Epinephrine
  - Phenylephrine
  - Phenylpropanolamine
  - Theophylline
- Miscellaneous drugs
  - Baclofen
  - Bromides
  - Chlorpropamide
  - Cimetidine
  - Disulfiram
  - Ergotamines
  - Lithium
  - Metrizamide
  - Metronidazole
  - Phenelzine
  - Podophyllin (by absorption)
  - Procarbazine
  - Propylthiouracil
  - Quinacrine
  - Ranitidine
  - Timotol maleate (ophthalmic)

SOURCE: Wise MG, Brandt GT. Delirium. In: Hales RE, Yudofsky SC (Eds) Textbook of Neuropsychiatry, 2nd Ed. Washington, DC: American Psychiatric Press, 1992

TABLE 12-8

CAUSES OF DELIRIUM

CAUSE	EXAMPLES
Infectious processes	Encephalitis, meningitis, syphilis
Drug withdrawal	Alcohol, barbiturates, sedative-hypnotics, benzodiazepines
Acute metabolic disorders	Acidosis, alkalosis, electrolyte disturbance, hepatic failure, renal failure
Trauma	Heat stroke, postoperative severe burns, closed-head injury
Central nervous system pathology	Abscess, hemorrhage, normal pressure hydrocephalus, seizure, stroke, tumor, vasculitis
Hypoxia	Anemia, carbon monoxide poisoning, hypotension, pulmonary/cardiac failure
Vitamin deficiencies	B_{12}/niacin/thiamine; hypovitaminosis
Endocrinopathies	Hyperadrenocorticism or hypoadrenocorticism, hyperglycemia or hypoglycemia, parathyroidism
Acute vascular conditions	Hypertensive encephalopathy, shock
Toxins/drugs	Medications, pesticides, solvents
Heavy metal poisoning	Lead, manganese, mercury

Brain Death

Key diagnostic criteria for brain death:
- Coma
- Absent brainstem reflexes
- Apnea

Traditionally, the cessation of cardiopulmonary function defines death. With advancement in technology and the ability of medicine to sustain cardiopulmonary function, it soon became evident that cardiopulmonary function could be artificially maintained even in the absence of brain function. Severely ill patients with irreversible cessation of brain function, however, were recognized as being clinically dead. Guidelines to establish brain death criteria moved to the forefront by the early 1980s, and consensus regarding the determination of brain death appeared to be reached.

In the report of the Medical Consultant on the Diagnosis of Death to the President's Commission for the Study of Ethical Problems in Medicine and Biomedical and Behavioral Research, death is established when there is either irreversible cessation of circulatory and respiratory function or irreversible cessation of all functions of the entire brain, including the brainstem. The determination of brain death, moreover, is generally confirmed clinically by using the Harvard criteria as modified by the President's Commission for the Study of Ethical Problems in Medicine and Biomedical and Behavioral Research and guidelines for the determination of death.

The key diagnostic criteria for brain death are coma, absence of brainstem reflexes, and apnea. Specifically, the criteria require that the cause for coma is known and that there is at least sufficient evidence available to account for total loss of function. Typically, the history, physical examination, and imaging studies, most commonly computerized tomography (CT) of the brain, allow this determination. Physical examination and formal apnea testing are necessary to fulfill the requirements for the other criteria.

In addition to history, physical examination, and CT, electroencephalography (EEG) and cerebral blood flow studies are often useful in determining brain death. EEG is an important component of the original Harvard criteria for brain death and is almost always employed to help establish the diagnosis of brain death. In situations in which the cause of coma is clearly known, based on an anatomic imaging study of the brain, and other clinical criteria are met that confirm the absence of all brain function, however, an EEG may be unnecessary.

Cerebral blood flow studies include cerebral angiography, radionucleotide brain scanning, and transcranial doppler ultrasonography. These tools are sometimes employed in situations in which a diagnosis may be uncertain. Of these studies, cerebral angiography of the four main blood vessels supplying the brain provides the most complete information regarding brain blood flow. Radionucleotide brain scanning and transcranial doppler ultrasonography are limited by their inability to provide information about blood flow to the entire brain.

To declare brain death, the following must be evident:
- Core body temperature, 34°C
- Absence of drug intoxication, particularly with barbituates

A number of clinical conditions must be recognized as potentially incompatible with the diagnosis of brain death. For example, profound hypothermia with a core body temperature below 34°C, or drug intoxication, particularly with barbiturates, may mimic a condition otherwise indistinguishable from brain death. Similarly, decorticate or decerebrate posturing suggests intact reflexes and likewise is inconsistent with brain death. Spinal reflexes, however, may be present and generally are not tested as part of an examination for establishing brain death. Other clinical testing for establishing brain death includes examination of the pupils, which must be fixed to light, and the absence of corneal, oculocephalic, oculovestibular, and gag reflexes. Apnea must also be confirmed, and various guidelines have been established to ensure the presence of apnea. Most of these guidelines involve hyperoxia during a period of hypoventilation to allow arterial carbon dioxide to rise at least 15 mmHg to allow a potent stimulus to drive respiration. The maximum stimulus for breathing is an arterial carbon dioxide level greater than 60 mmHg.

SEIZURES

The intensivist often encounters a patient with seizure. A seizure can often be the initial indication of a serious central nervous system problem, and approximately 2% of the general population suffers from epilepsy. A patient who develops status epilepticus generally requires the care of a critical care specialist and a neurologist. Certain ICU patients are at high risk for seizures. A variety of medications used in the intensive care unit can predispose an individual to a seizure. Status epilepticus is associated with stroke, withdrawal from antiepileptic medication, alcohol withdrawal, anoxia, and a large variety of metabolic disorders. Systemic infection and central nervous system (CNS) infection, as well as trauma, can all cause seizure.

Seizures can be classified as partial or generalized.

Seizures can be classified as partial or generalized. A simple partial seizure starts focally in the cerebral cortex without invading other CNS structures. During the simple partial seizure, the patient is aware of what is happening. Partial seizures can become complex with impairment of consciousness. The initial clinical manifestation of a partial seizure depends on the function of the brain region involved in the seizure onset. Generalized seizures are accompanied by synchronous epileptiform activity in both hemispheres of the brain. If this diffuse seizure activity occurs from the onset, it is termed primary. A secondary generalized seizure begins as a partial seizure that eventually spreads throughout both cerebral hemispheres. These seizures may or may not involve tonic-clonic (grand mal) muscle contractions. Generalized seizures that do not involve prominent muscle contractions are called absence (petit mal) seizures.

Status epilepticus is defined as more than 10 min of continuous seizure or two or more sequential seizures without intervening consciousness.

Status epilepticus is defined as more than 10 min of continuous seizure activity or two or more sequential seizures without an intervening period of consciousness. This event is a medical emergency, and failure to treat in a timely and appropriate manner may result in serious medical and neurologic sequelae (including hyperthermia, acidosis, hypotension, hypoglycemia, and renal failure from myoglobinemia). During the attack, catecholamines are elevated and may trigger cardiac arrhythmia.

When an ICU patient seizes, it is important for the clinician to observe the event. Most patients stop seizing before medication can be administered and reach the brain. The postictal examination is also very valuable. Drugs are a major cause of ICU seizures, particularly in patients with substantial renal or hepatic dysfunction (Table 12-9). Withdrawal of medication or illicit drugs is also a frequent cause of seizure. The withdrawal of drugs such as ethanol and benzodiazepines may prompt convulsions 1–3 days later. Illicit drug screening can be helpful. Cocaine is a major cause of seizure. Electrolytes and serum osmolality should be measured. Hypocalcemia and hypomagnesemia are overstated causes of seizure in the adult patient. Evidence of cardiovascular disease or systemic infection must be sought. Imaging of the brain, either by CT or by MRI studies, should be performed in most ICU patients with new-onset seizure. Hypoglycemia and hyperglycemia can induce seizures. The EEG is a vital diagnostic tool for the seizure patient.

The administration of anticonvulsant therapy to an ICU patient depends on several factors. Provisional seizure etiology, estimation of recurrence, and the utility and limitations of anticonvulsant therapy must all be considered. For example, seizures during ethanol with-

TABLE 12-9

DRUG-RELATED SEIZURES IN THE ICU

Drug withdrawal	Pharmaceuticals
Barbiturates	Ciprofloxacin
Benzodiazepines	Imipenem
Opiates	Lidocaine
Drug intoxication	Penicillin
Drugs of abuse	Theophylline
Amphetamines	Tricyclics
Cocaine	
Phencyclidine	

drawal do not mandate chronic anticonvulsant therapy. The patient will need prophylaxis against delirium tremens, but the seizures themselves seldom require treatment. On the other hand, convulsions during barbiturate or benzodiazepine withdrawal should be treated with short-term lorazepam to prevent the development of status epilepticus. The ICU patient with structural CNS disease should start chronic anticonvulsant therapy. Phenytoin is frequently selected because of its ease of administration and lack of sedation. Because hypotension and arrhythmias may complicate the rapid administration of phenytoin, phenytoin is administered at a rate of less than 50 mg/min. Fosphenytoin, a phosphate ester prodrug of phenytoin, may be infused at a much faster rate, and it is dosed in phenytoin equivalents. Fosphenytoin is much less alkaline and causes less local infusion site irritation. The therapeutic range for phenytoin in the blood is 10–20 μg/ml. Failure to prevent seizures at a concentration of 25 μg/ml is an indication for the addition of phenobarbital. Patients with renal disease and hepatic disease may need careful dose adjustment of phenytoin by the measurement of free phenytoin blood levels. Hypersensitivity is a major adverse effect of phenytoin therapy. Fever, rash, and eosinophilia can occur. Paresthesia in the low back and groin is a unique side effect of fosphenytoin.

Treatment intensity for status epilepticus should reflect seizure risk in the individual patient and its etiology.

The intensity of treatment for status epilepticus should reflect the risk that a patient experiences from the episode and its etiology. During generalized convulsive status epilepticus, the patient is at risk for neurologic, cardiac, respiratory, hepatic, orthopedic, and renal problems. The seizure should be terminated as rapidly and as safely as possible. The basic aspects of airway and cardiovascular management should be employed. Rapid endotracheal intubation may be necessary. The use of near-immediate and short-acting benzodiazepine therapy in the form of lorazepam (0.1 mg/kg) or diazepam (0.2 mg/kg) may be initially considered. Diazepam can interrupt status epilepticus rapidly because of its high lipid solubility; it enters the brain rapidly but it redistributes widely and its toxic metabolites have long half-times. Lorazepam also has a rapid onset of action and a long duration of action in the CNS.

Midazolam has been shown to be effective in some patients who are refractory to other antiepileptic medications. In refractory status epilepticus, where lorazepam, phenytoin, and phenobarbital have been employed in conventional doses, three therapeutic interventions can be considered. High-dose barbituates, midazolam, and propofol (continuous infusion) have all been employed in the treatment of recalcitrant status epilepticus. General anesthesia with isoflurane may be required. These patients should have continuous EEG monitoring. It is valuable to have an expert in seizure disorder therapy at the bedside. It is important to treat the complications of status epilepticus. Rhabdomyolysis can be treated with hydration and diuresis and, if necessary, urinary alkalinization. Hyperthermia, which develops during the seizure, may persist and require external cooling. Cerebral edema, although rare, can occur and require hyperventilation and use of mannitol. Steroid therapy may also be helpful. Neurogenic pulmonary edema may occur, requiring mechanical ventilator support and diuresis.

Complications of status epilepticus:
- Hyperthermia
- Rhabdomyolysis and renal failure
- Cerebral edema
- Pulmonary edema and respiratory failure

STROKE

Most strokes are ischemic in nature. Strokes may be thrombotic, embolic, or lacunar.

Stroke is a common neurologic reason for hospital admission. Eighty percent of strokes are ischemic in character, with the remainder divided between intracerebral hemorrhage and subarachnoid hemorrhage. Abrupt neurologic deficit is the presentation hallmark of stroke.

TABLE 12-10

SYMPTOMS THAT ARE SELDOM THE RESULT OF CEREBROVASCULAR DISEASE

Vertigo alone	Tremor	Coma
Dysarthria alone	Tonic-clonic motor activity	Syncope
Dysphagia alone	Confusion	Incontinence
Diplopia alone	Memory loss	Tinnitus
Headache	Delirium	

Symptoms of unilateral weakness or sensory loss, speech/language impairment, visual disturbance, or impaired coordination are found. Confusion or lethargy occur less frequently.

Strokes may be thrombotic, embolic, lacunar, or hemorrhagic in character. Thrombotic strokes are generally caused by atherosclerotic stenosis or occlusion of a large vessel. Embolic strokes are generally associated with cardiac or carotid disease. Lacunar strokes are caused by intraparenchymal cerebral small vessel disease. The rupture of a conducting artery or intraparenchymal arterial is responsible for a hemorrhage stroke. Subarachnoid hemorrhage is often associated with leakage of blood from cerebral aneurysm and trauma. The medical intensivist most commonly encounters stroke patients in a setting of carotid artery disease or a cardiac disturbance, which is potentially embologenic.

There are numerous risk factors for stroke. Hypertension, diabetes, cardiac disease, age, gender, lipid disorders, excessive ethanol ingestion, cigarette smoking, an elevated hematocrit, asymptomatic carotid stenosis, and previous cerebrovascular disease should all be considered. About 30% of untreated patients with new-onset transient ischemic attack (TIA) will suffer a stroke within the next 2 years.

A prior transient ischemic attack is a major risk factor for subsequent stroke.

A CT scan of the brain is almost always indicated during the initial evaluation and critical care management of the stroke patient. Magnetic resonance imaging (MRI) is more sensitive but more difficult in terms of immediate access. Also, it is harder for the patient to lie still and remain calm during a MRI study. Transcranial doppler ultrasonography can be helpful, particularly when coupled to carotid duplex doppler testing. These studies can be performed at the bedside and provide a rapid assessment of abnormal cerebral blood flow. When added to CT of the brain scan results, these studies become even more valuable.

An acute localized neurologic problem almost always leads to the diagnosis of stroke. Stroke is by far the most common acute and focal brain disease. However, not all patients who present with neurologic impairment have stroke. There are a variety of neurological symptoms that are seldom the result of cerebrovascular disease (Table 12-10), and there are a variety of conditions which are frequently mistaken for stroke (Table 12-11). Epilepsy mimics stroke more often than other conditions. Drug intoxication and a variety of metabolic abnormalities can induce neurologic systems that can be mistaken for stroke. Brain tumors and abscesses, as well as subdural hematomas, may induce sudden neurologic impairment and also simulate a stroke.

Epilepsy frequently mimics stroke.

In evaluating a patient with cerebrovascular disease, it is crucial to determine whether the symptoms arise from the anterior cerebral circulation or the posterior circulation. Often the pathogenesis, diagnostic process, and therapy for stroke in these two vascular distribution regions are different. Impairment of blood flow through the carotid circulation causes a certain symptom complex (Table 12-12), whereas reduced blood flow through the vertebral-basilar circulation induces another symptom complex (Table 12-13). If a patient is aphasic or hemianopic, then the anterior cerebral circulation has likely been impaired. If the patient has cranial nerve dysfunction or serious brainstem neurologic impairment, then the posterior circulation has been seriously jeopardized. It is important to remember that more than 80% of all strokes involve the carotid circulation.

Hemorrhagic strokes are associated with hypertension and a poor prognosis and high mortality.

TABLE 12-11

CONDITIONS MOST FREQUENTLY MISTAKEN FOR STROKE

Seizures	Cerebral abscess	Hypoglycemia
Metabolic encephalopathy	Vertigo, Meniere disease	Encephalitis
Cerebral tumor	Peripheral neuropathy, Bell palsy	Migraine
Subdural hematoma	Multiple sclerosis	Psychogenic illness

TABLE 12-12

MOST COMMON SYMPTOMS OF CAROTID CIRCULATION ISCHEMIA

SYMPTOM	FREQUENCY (%)
Hemiparesis	65
Hemisensory loss	60
Monocular blindness	35
Facial numbness	30
Lower facial weakness	25
Aphasia	20
Headache	20
Dysarthria	15
Visual field loss	15

The clinical characteristics of the various types of strokes can be found in Table 12-14. Thrombotic strokes account for approximately 40% of all ischemic cerebrovascular disease whereas embolic strokes account for 30%. Atrial fibrillation or myocardial infarction are often associated with embolic strokes. Lacunar strokes constitute approximately 20% of all strokes and are associated with a reasonably good prognosis. Hemorrhagic strokes are often associated with hypertension and have a very poor prognosis and high mortality rate.

Brain CT scanning is an insensitive test for detecting an acute cerebral infarction.

Brain CT scanning is a sensitive test for detecting an intraparenchymal mass.

The typical laboratory investigation of stroke can be found in Table 12-15. The CT scan of the brain is very sensitive for detecting hemorrhage, tumor, and abscess, but it is not sensitive for detecting an acute cerebral infarction. This sensitivity is lowest within the first 24 h of the acute event. The MRI of the brain is more sensitive for cerebral infarction, particularly of the lacunar type.

Care of the stroke patient is largely supportive. In the absence of intracerebral hemorrhage, a common practice in the acute setting is to begin heparin, without an initial loading bolus, to maintain the partial thromboplastin time (PTT) at 1.5 fold normal. Thrombolytic and antithrombotic therapy has been clearly demonstrated to be efficacious in some patients with acute cerebral artery occlusions, although these drugs carry an elevated risk of brain hemorrhage. Therefore, heparin is usually started until an underlying etiology of stroke is defined; then choices concerning more aggressive therapy are pursued.

An intracerebral hemorrhage causes abrupt focal neurologic deficits resembling those of an ischemic stroke but also produces severe alterations in mental status including a decreased level of consciousness. Because the CT scan of the head is an extremely sensitive modality for detecting intraparenchymal hemorrhage, it is heavily relied upon in the early diagnostic process. An elevation in blood pressure often occurs. It has been recommended that blood pressure be below a mean arterial pressure of 130 mmHg in patients with hypertension. More aggressive neurosurgical management may also be necessary. Therapy focuses on reducing increased intracranial pressure by initially intubating and performing hyperventilation and then administering an osmotic diuretic agent such as mannitol or a loop diuretic such as furosemide. If more aggressive therapy is contemplated, such as high-dose barbituates, an intracranial pressure monitor should be inserted. Corticosteroid therapy has not shown ben-

TABLE 12-13

MOST COMMON SYMPTOMS OF VERTEBRAL-BASILAR CIRCULATION ISCHEMIA

SYMPTOM	FREQUENCY (%)
Ataxia	50
Crossed or hemisensory loss	30
Vertigo	30
Crossed or hemiparesis	25
Dysarthria/dysphagia	25
Syncope or light-headedness	25
Headache	20
Deafness or tinnitus	10
Diplopia	10

TABLE 12-14

CHARACTERISTICS OF DIFFERENT TYPES OF STROKES

TYPE OF STROKE	PERCENTAGE OF ALL STROKES	ONSET	PRECEDING TIAs (%)	SEIZURE AT ONSET (%)	COMA (%)	ATRIAL FIBRILLATION (%)	KNOWN CORONARY ARTERY DISEASE	MRI OR CT SCAN	OTHER FEATURES
Thrombotic	40	Stuttering, gradual	50	1	5	10	50	Ischemic infarction	Carotid bruit; stroke during sleep
Embolic	30	Sudden	10	10	1	35	35	Superficial (cortical) infarction	Underlying heart disease; peripheral emboli or strokes in different vascular territories
Lacunar	20	Gradual or sudden	30	0	0	5	35	Normal, or small, deep infarction	Pure motor or pure sensory stroke
Hemorrhagic	10	Sudden	5	10	25	5	10	Hyperdense mass	Nausea and vomiting; decreased mental status

TIAs, transient ischemic attacks.

TABLE 12-15

TYPICAL DIAGNOSTIC EVALUATION OF STROKE

DIAGNOSIS	METHOD
Anterior circulation ischemia	Carotid duplex, echocardiography, CT scan (MRI if lacunar)
Posterior circulation ischemia	Echocardiography, MRI (CT if unavailable), TCD, or MRA
The "unexpected stroke" (minimal risk factors or stroke in the young)	MRA (including cervical views) or conventional angiography echocardiography (TEE preferred), toxicology screen, prothrombotic workup

MRA, magnetic resonance angiography; TCD, transcranial doppler; TEE, transesophageal echocardiography

Subarachnoid hemorrhage often presents with severe headache but rarely with focal neurologic findings.

efit and is generally not recommended because of numerous potential complications. Neurogenic pulmonary edema may occur during any acute intracranial condition. Patients with subarachnoid hemorrhage seem particularly prone to neurogenic pulmonary edema. It is best to keep the pulmonary capillary wedge pressure close to normal in this setting.

Subarachnoid hemorrhage differs from other types of stroke in that it rarely causes focal neurologic findings. Severe headache, at times accompanied by collapse or loss of consciousness, occurs. Most spontaneous subarachnoid hemorrhages arise from ruptured berry aneurysms. Cerebral angiography is often performed acutely to identify the site of bleeding for the neurosurgeon. Key management issues for the intensivist include the maintenance of electrolyte and body fluid balances and blood pressure control by maintaining systolic blood pressure at about 150 mmHg until the aneurysm can be definitively treated. Calcium channel blocker therapy is used to prevent cerebral arterial vasospasm.

WEAKNESS

Three neuromuscular disorders that can produce severe and life-threatening neuromuscular weakness require review. Myasthenia gravis, Guillain–Barré syndrome, and critical illness polyneuropathy are all encountered in intensive care. These conditions have similarities and differences (Table 12-16).

Myasthenia Gravis

Myasthenia gravis is uncommon and characterized by intensifying weakness with repeated activity and intact deep tendon reflexes.

Myasthenia gravis is an autoimmune disease characterized by antibody-mediated destruction of postsynaptic acetylcholine receptors at neuromuscular junctions. It is an uncommon disease characterized by weakness that intensifies with repeated activity. The muscles of the eyelids and extraocular muscles are initially affected, followed by a generalized weakness. Proximal limb muscles are generally affected, and weakness of the diaphragm and thoracic muscles is common. Because of this, respiratory failure and eventual mechanical ventilator

TABLE 12-16

COMPARATIVE FEATURES OF THREE NEUROMUSCULAR DISORDERS

FEATURES	MYASTHENIA GRAVIS	GUILLAIN-BARRÉ SYNDROME	CRITICAL ILLNESS POLYNEUROPATHY
Ocular findings	Yes	No	No
Fluctuating weakness	Yes	No	NO
Bulbar weakness	Yes	Yes	No
Deep tendon reflexes	Intact	Depressed	Depressed
Autonomic instability	No	Yes	No
Nerve conduction	Normal	Abnormal	Abnormal

dependence can occur in a crisis fashion. There is no sensory loss in this disease, and deep tendon reflexes are generally preserved.

From a subclinical stage, myasthenia gravis can intensify to a crisis situation during a concurrent illness or surgery. This disease can accelerate when an individual is exposed to a variety of precipitating and aggravating medications, principally aminoglycosides, magnesium, and various antiarrhythmic agents such as lidocaine, quinidine, and procainamide.

When an anticholinesterase inhibitor such as edrophonium is administered, muscle strength returns, thus acting as a pharmacologic confirmatory test. Radioimmunoassay for acetylcholine receptor antibodies in the blood is positive in most patients with myasthenia gravis, confirming the diagnosis. Because thymic tumors and hyperthyroidism have been associated with myasthenia gravis, these conditions must be sought out and identified if present.

First-line therapy for myasthenia gravis is pyridostigmine, an anticholinesterase agent. The use of concomitant prednisone, azathioprine, or cyclosporine may be necessary, and with exacerbation, intravenous infusion of gammaglobulins or plasmapheresis to remove acetylcholine antibodies is often necessary for more immediate, but short-term, improvement. If a thymus tumor is identified, then surgical removal is indicated.

> First-line therapy for myasthenia gravis is pyridostigmine.

Guillain–Barré Syndrome

Guillain–Barré syndrome is an acute inflammatory demyelinating polyneuropathy. This condition is preceded by an acute infectious illness in the majority of cases. *Campylobacter jejuni* enteritis has recently been recognized as an important preliminary disease, often associated with severe neuropathy. Human immunodeficiency virus, cytomegalovirus, and Epstein–Barr virus with hepatitis or mononucleosis have been associated with Guillian–Barré syndrome. However, the exact etiology and mechanism of this disease remain unknown.

> *Campylobacter jejuni* enteritis is associated with the development of Guillain–Barré syndrome.

Symmetric limb weakness, often associated with paresthesias, which generally evolves over a few days to several weeks, is the clinical feature of this disease. Pain is common, as either bilateral sciatica or aching in large muscle groups. The development of weakness is clearly separated from the preceding acute illness. Nearly a quarter of patients develop respiratory failure and require mechanical ventilation. Autonomic dysfunctions are common but rarely persist for more than 1 or 2 weeks. Fortunately, nearly 85% of patients with Guillain–Barré syndrome recover, but residual neurologic deficits are common.

Progressive symmetric limb weakness with reduced and then absent reflexes following an acute infectious illness generally leads to the diagnosis of Guillain–Barré syndrome. At times, nerve conduction studies are necessary to confirm the diagnosis. Once Guillain–Barre syndrome has been diagnosed, early plasmapheresis or intravenous infusion of gamma globulins has proved to be beneficial. Mechanically assisted ventilation is sometimes warranted. In patients with oropharyngeal muscle involvement, aspiration precautions are needed.

> Plasmapheresis or IV immunoglobulin therapy can be used for severe Guillain–Barré syndrome.

Critical Illness Polyneuropathy

Multiorgan dysfunction or failure is often found in patients in the intensive care unit, often associated with sepsis. As part of this condition, the peripheral nervous system can be affected. A diffuse peripheral neuropathy called critical illness polyneuropathy is the result of this peripheral nervous system dysfunctional state.

> Critical illness polyneuropathy is a combined motor and sensory polyneuropathy without autonomic and bulbar weakness.

Critical illness polyneuropathy is a combined motor and sensory polyneuropathy. Although most patients with this condition have very mild peripheral nerve dysfunction, some patients develop severe limb and truncal weakness. The more severely affected patients require mechanical ventilation. At times, the condition is identified after the patient has been intubated and placed on the mechanical ventilator. Often the acute situation that created multiorgan failure has resolved, and the patient is left with diffuse muscle weakness requiring mechanical ventilation. Because this condition occurs in the intensive care unit, many of the patients have received neuromuscular blocking agents. Unlike Guillain–Barré syndrome, autonomic dysfunction and bulbar weakness are uncommon. Nerve conduction studies or electromyography may be necessary to confirm axonal degeneration. There is no specific treatment for this condition but fortunately it resolves in most patients.

NERVOUS SYSTEM INFECTIONS

Meningitis

Suspected meningitis should be treated immediately. Often there is delay in the performance of a diagnostic lumbar puncture. Some clinicians prefer to have a CT of the brain performed before doing the lumbar puncture; however, generally patients who are alert and have normal fundi and neurologic examination can undergo lumbar puncture without scanning. The possibility of the patient in that setting herniating after lumbar puncture is extremely small. Cefotaxime or ceftriaxone should be used for empiric therapy. Vancomycin can be added until spinal fluid culture and sensitivities are available, particularly where pneumococcal resistance to third-generation cephalosporins has emerged. Chloramphenicol is often recommended for penicillin-allergic patients.

Blood cultures should be obtained before antibiotics are administered. If listeriosis is suspected, then ampicillin or sulfa-trimethoprim, an acceptable alternative, should be added until an organism is isolated or blood and spinal fluid cultures have been negative for at least 3 days. Imipenem should be avoided in central nervous system infections because it is epileptogenic. The use of systemic corticosteroid therapy in adult meningitis remains controversial. Increased intracranial pressure, hyponatremia, and cerebral venous thrombosis are all complications of severe meningitis. Additionally, seizures may occur and are initially managed with benzodiazepines and phenytoin.

Encephalitis

The most common and important cause of fatal sporadic encephalitis in the United States is herpes simplex virus. When encephalitis is suspected, acyclovir is begun as a workup proceeds. The most sensitive test for herpetic encephalitis is demonstration of viral DNA in the cerebrospinal fluid by polymerase chain reaction (PCR) amplification, followed by an MRI with gadolinium and electroencephalography. A brain biopsy should be avoided unless absolutely necessary. Generally, a brain biopsy is reserved for those patients who do not respond to empiric therapy or those in whom the workup raises a question as to the diagnosis. Seizures, increased intracranial pressure, and cerebral edema are common complications of encephalitis.

Brain Abscess

Empiric therapy for suspected brain abscess should include a third-generation cephalosporin, vancomycin, and metronidazole. If *Listeria* is suspected, then the addition of ampicillin or sulfa-trimethoprim should be considered. Neurosurgery may be indicated for most patients with brain abscess for drainage and biopsy reasons. A high-grade astrocytoma can mimic a brain abscess. Increased intracranial pressure is often associated with brain abscess and can be additionally improved with neurosurgery.

FEBRILE MUSCLE RIGIDITY SYNDROMES

Neuroleptic Malignant Syndrome

Neuroleptic malignant syndrome is associated with nearly every mixed dopamine secretion agent and neuroleptic agent.

Neuroleptic malignant syndrome can be treated with bromocriptine and dantrolene after the inciting medication has been stopped.

The neuroleptic malignant syndrome occurs in a very small number of patients who have received medications such as haloperidol, thioxanthine, or fluphenazine. The syndrome has been associated with almost every mixed dopamine-serotonin agent and neuroleptic agent. The condition can be lethal.

Neuroleptic malignant syndrome appears to be generated from central dopaminergic blockade. Often this syndrome develops a short time after the initiation of neuroleptic treatment or an increase in dosage. Fever, rigidity, tremor, obtundation, and autonomic dysfunction, including diaphoresis, hypotension, and tachycardia, develop. Pulmonary edema can

TABLE 12-17

DIFFERENTIAL DIAGNOSIS OF RHABDOMYOLYSIS IN ASSOCIATION WITH ACUTE CENTRAL NERVOUS SYSTEM DYSFUNCTION

- Myofiber metabolic exhaustion
  - Seizures
  - Delirium
  - Tetanus
  - Strychnine intoxication
  - Extremes of environmental temperature
  - Malignant hyperthermia
  - Neuroleptic malignant syndrome
  - Diabetic ketoacidosis
- Infectious myositides
  - Influenza
  - HIV
  - Toxic shock
  - Clostridial myonecrosis *(Clostridium perfringens bacteremia)*
- Toxins and abused drugs
  - Alcohol
  - Cocaine and other CNS stimulants
  - LSD
  - Narcotics
  - Phencyclidine
  - Envenomations (wasps, bees, spiders, snakes, etc.)
- Medications
  - Salicylate overdose
  - Theophylline
  - Lithium
- Fluid and electrolyte disturbances
  - Hyperosmolar states
  - Hypoosmolar states
  - Severe hypophosphatemia
- Trauma

occur. Rhabdomyolysis related to sustained muscular contraction, immobility, and volume depletion can occur. The differential diagnosis of rhabdomyolysis and acute central nervous system dysfunction is extensive (Table 12-17). Disseminated intravascular coagulation, thrombocytopenia, and deep venous thrombosis with pulmonary embolism have all been reported.

Neuroleptic malignant syndrome should be treated supportively, but suspected inciting medications should be withdrawn. Aggressive hydration is mandatory. The administration of a dopaminergic agonist, such as bromocriptine, and the direct muscle relaxant dantrolene may be helpful.

Malignant Hyperthermia

Malignant hyperthermia is often familial in an autosomal dominant disorder pattern, but many cases are sporadic and typically follow exposure to an anesthetic agent. Most human cases are associated with a defect on chromosome 19. The sustained muscle contraction associated with malignant hyperthermia causes excessive oxygen consumption with its eventual heat production. Known triggering agents of malignant hyperthermia are listed in Table 12-18. As this syndrome intensifies, there is a rapid rise in temperature, metabolic acidosis, hypoxemia, and cardiac arrhythmias. The combination of rhabdomyolysis and acidosis results in hyperkalemia. The syndrome can actually develop during surgery or can follow after several hours. Often, the patient who develops malignant hyperthermia has a family history of anesthetic complication. The condition can often be diagnosed by muscle biopsy, and it can be treated by termination of the triggering agent and the use of dantrolene.

> Malignant hyperthemia is an autosomal disorder associated with a chromosome defect.

> Dantrolene can improve malignant hyperthermia.

TABLE 12-18

TRIGGERING AGENTS FOR MALIGNANT HYPERTHERMIA

Recognized agents	
Inhalational anesthetics	
	Desflurane
	Enflurane
	Halothane (most common)
	Sevoflurane
Depolarizing NMJ blockers	
	Decamethonium
	Succinylcholine (most common)
Possible agents	
	Calcium
	Catecholamines
	Ketamine
	Monoamine oxidase inhibitors
	Phenothiazines
"Safe" agents	
	Barbiturates
	Beta-blockers
	Benzodiazepines
	Local anesthetics
	Nitrous oxide
	Nondepolarizing NMJ blockers
	Propofol

Lethal Catatonia

Lethal catatonia is indistinguishable from neuroleptic malignant syndrome. Lethal catatonia can begin with extreme psychotic excitement that leads to fever, exhaustion, and death. Severe muscle rigidity is generally not part of this syndrome. Lethal catatonia may require neuroleptic treatment, although electroconvulsive therapy is more commonly used. The underlying pathophysiology of lethal catatonia remains unknown.

Serotonin Syndrome

When receiving a serotonergic agent or a monoamine oxidase inhibitor, which also raises extracellular serotonin concentrations, the patient is at risk for developing the serotonin syndrome. Like neuroleptic malignant syndrome, serotonin syndrome involves muscle rigidity and high fever. Autonomic instability can occur. Generally the intensity of serotonin syndrome is less than that of neuroleptic malignant syndrome. Treatment for this condition is supportive after recognizing and removing the offending agent.

SUMMARY

Numerous neurologic issues and problems are found in critically ill patients. Consultation with a neurologist or neurosurgeon is often necessary, but the intensivist must be able to recognize the conditions and initiate treatment appropriately.

REVIEW QUESTIONS

1. **All the following statements are true concerning delirium except:**
   - **A.** The most common mental disorder in hospitalized patients
   - **B.** Never characterized by lethargy
   - **C.** Cognition changes
   - **D.** Fluctuates during the course of day
   - **E.** Caused by many types of medicine

2. **Delirium tremens should not be treated with:**
   - **A.** Haloperidol
   - **B.** Diazepam
   - **C.** Lorazepam
   - **D.** Ethyl alcohol
   - **E.** Thiamine

3. **What type of stroke is associated with cardiac or carotid disease?**
   - **A.** Thrombotic
   - **B.** Lacunar
   - **C.** Hemorrhagic
   - **D.** Embolic

4. **Which condition is rarely associated with focal neurologic deficit?**
   - **A.** TIA
   - **B.** Ischemic stroke
   - **C.** Intracerebral hemorrhage
   - **D.** Grand mal seizure
   - **E.** Subarachnoid hemorrhage

5. **Each of the following clinical features can be used to distinguish myasthenia gravis from Guillain–Barré syndrome except:**
   - **A.** Deep tendon reflexes
   - **B.** Ocular finding
   - **C.** Bulbar weakness
   - **D.** Autonomic instability
   - **E.** Fluctuating weakness

ANSWERS

1. The answer is B. In fact, delirium in an elderly patient can present with lethargy and the clinical course can be hypoactive in character.
2. The answer is A, B. Benzodiazepines, such as diazepam and lorazepam, are primary therapies for alcohol withdrawal, often in combination with thiamine and multivitamins. Ethyl alcohol is an alternative therapy, but haloperidol should be avoided. Haloperidol can actually aggravate the delirium, and it can lower seizure threshold.
3. The answer is D. Embolic strokes are associated with atrial fibrillation and artherosclerosis of the carotid artery.
4. The answer is E. Subarachnoid hemorrhage differs from other types of stroke because it rarely causes neurologic deficits but does cause headache and syncope.
5. The answer is C. Myasthenia gravis and Guillain–Barré syndrome both can be associated with bulbar weakness. Ocular findings and fluctuating weakness with intact deep tendon reflexes are found in patients with myasthenia gravis. Patients with Guillain–Barré syndrome generally have progressive weakness, absent deep tendon reflexes, and autonomic constability, especially with advanced disease. A nerve conduction test may be necessary to distinguish between these two diseases. Patients with myasthenia gravis have normal nerve conduction but nerve conduction is abnormal in patients who have Guillain-Barré syndrome.

SUGGESTED READING

A definition of irreversible coma. Report of the Ad Hoc Committee on the Harvard Medical School to examine the definition of brain death. JAMA 1968;205:337–340.

Bleck TP, Smith MC, Pierre-Louis JC, et al. Neurologic complications of critical medical illnesses. Crit Care Med 1993;21:98–103.

Epilepsy Foundations of America. Treatment of convulsive status epilepticus: recommendations of the Epilepsy Foundation of America's Working Group on Status Epilepticus. JAMA 1993;270: 854–859.

Guidelines for the determination of death. Report of the Medical Consultants on the diagnosis of death to the President's Commission for the Study of Ethical Problems in Medicine and Biomedical and Behavioral Research. JAMA 1981;246:2184–2186.

Guze BH, Baxter LR. Neuroleptic malignant syndrome. N Engl J Med 1985;313:163–166.

Kam PC, Chang GW. Selective serotonin reuptake inhibitors. Pharmacology and clinical implications in anaesthesia and critical care medicine. Anaesthesia 1997;52:982–988.

Kelly BJ, Matthay MA. Prevalence and severity of neurologic dysfunction in critically ill patients. Chest 1993;104:1818–1824.

Mosewich RK, So EL. A clinical approach to the classification of seizures and epileptic syndromes. Mayo Clin Proc 1996;71:405–414.

Plum F, Posner JB. The diagnosis of stupor and coma. Philadelphia: Davis, 1980.

Quagliarello V, Scheld WM. Treatment of bacterial meningitis. N Engl J Med 1997;336:708–716.

Ropper AH. Guillain-Barre syndrome. N Engl J Med 1992;326:1130–1136.

Wijdicks EFM, Scott JP. Stroke in the medical intensive-care unit. Mayo Clin Proc 1998;73:642–646.

Zochodne W, Bolton CF, Wells GA, et al. Critical illness polyneuropathy: a complication of sepsis and multiple organ failure. Brain 1987;110:819–842.

CHAPTER 13

GERARD J. CRINER

Respiratory Failure

CHAPTER OUTLINE

LEARNING OBJECTIVES

After studying this chapter, you should be able to:

- Define respiratory failure.
- Classify respiratory failure as hypoxemic or hypercapnic.
- Recognize the signs and symptoms of respiratory failure.
- Define the alveolar gas equation and apply it to the evaluation of respiratory failure.
- Recognize the changes in blood gases that accompany respiratory failure.
- Know the major treatment strategies for respiratory failure.

DEFINITION OF RESPIRATORY FAILURE

Respiratory failure affects all ages and varies markedly in presentation.

Despite the varied causes of respiratory failure, the pathophysiologic mechanisms and approach to the evaluation, diagnosis, and treatment are similar.

Respiratory failure is one of the most common and important entities treated by the critical care practitioner. Respiratory failure affects patients of all ages and can vary markedly in presentation. Episodes of respiratory failure may present as an acute crisis in a previously normal host (e.g., the patient sustains a flail chest after a motor vehicle accident), or as an acute exacerbation of a chronic disorder (an exacerbation of chronic obstructive pulmonary disease [COPD]). Although the causes of respiratory failure are diverse, the pathophysiologic mechanisms and the approach to the evaluation, diagnosis, and treatment of respiratory failure are similar.

This chapter provides an organized overview of respiratory failure by (1) defining respiratory failure; (2) reviewing the pathophysiologic mechanisms responsible for its develop-

CASE STUDY: PART 1

A 70-year-old woman with a known history of mild chronic obstructive pulmonary disease (COPD) developed worsening shortness of breath during the past several days, following an upper respiratory tract infection. During the past 4 days, the patient complained of purulent nasal discharge, postnasal drip, cough, and fever. Recently, these symptoms had been complicated by the expectoration of thick, yellow mucus and increased shortness of breath. Her chronic airways obstruction had been well maintained by regular administration of inhaled beta-agonists and anticholinergic bronchodilators, use of supplemental oxygen at 1 l/min continuously, and intermittent courses of systemic steroids.

Today, the patient's breathlessness was worse upon awakening and had increased in severity through the day. She failed to respond to several bronchodilator treatments, and on examination was found to have marked increased work of breathing, heralded by the use of accessory muscles of the neck, a respiratory rate of 38 breaths/min, and evidence of paradoxical inward motion of the upper abdomen during inspiration. She was transported from the outpatient pulmonary clinic to the emergency room for further evaluation and treatment.

ment, and (3) providing indications for the evaluation, diagnosis, and treatment of respiratory failure.

In general terms, respiration defines the process whereby gas exchange occurs between an organism and its surrounding environment. Specifically, the respiratory system supplies the body with adequate oxygen for aerobic metabolism while simultaneously removing its major metabolic waste product, carbon dioxide. Respiration is achieved through three distinct processes: (1) ventilation, the process by which ambient air is delivered to the alveoli where it is exposed to blood; (2) diffusion, the movement of oxygen and carbon dioxide in opposite directions across the alveolar air sac and capillary walls; and (3) circulation, the process whereby oxygen is carried from the site of gas exchange, in the lung, to the cells of the body where active aerobic metabolism occurs.

To accomplish the task of respiration as defined here, the respiratory system must function as a pump for effective ventilation and also as an area of gas exchange (Figure 13-1). Failure of the respiratory system to perform optimally, either in its role as a pump or as an area of gas exchange, results in an elevation of carbon dioxide in the blood (i.e., hypercapnia), or a reduction in blood oxygen (i.e., hypoxemia). Both parameters are considered indices of respiratory system failure. Therefore, respiratory failure is defined as impaired gas exchange, that is, hypoxemia with or without hypercapnia.

Respiration defines the processes by which gas exchange occurs between an organism and its environment.

The function of the respiratory system is to supply the body's organ with adequate oxygen and to remove its metabolic waste product, carbon dioxide.

Respiration is accomplished by three distinct processes: ventilation, diffusion, and circulation.

The respiratory system acts both as a pump and as an area of gas exchange.

Respiratory failure defines the inability to maintain normal gas exchange: hypoxemia with or without hypercapnia.

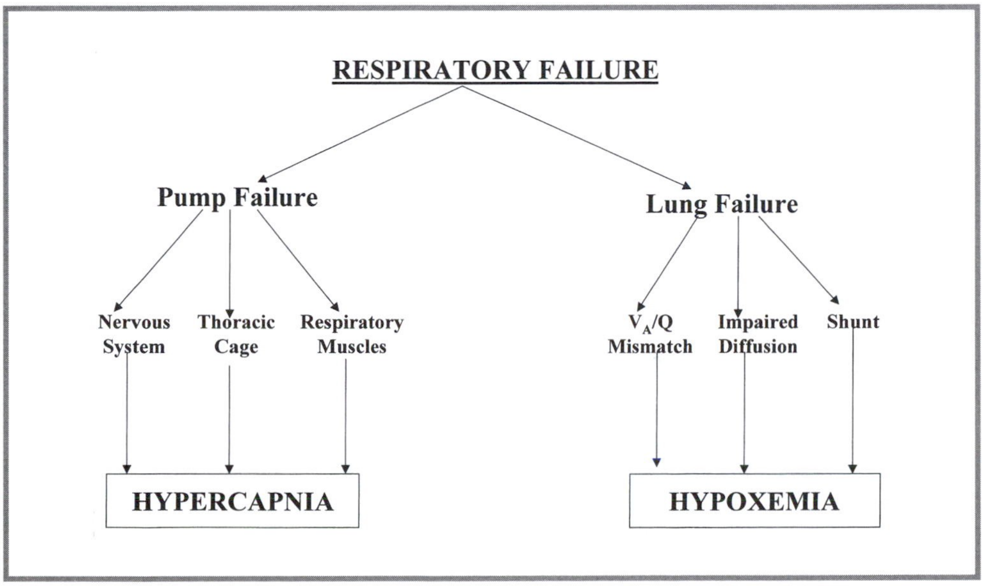

FIGURE 13-1

Characterization of respiratory failure as hypercapnic (i.e., pump failure) and hypoxemic (i.e., lung failure) subtypes. Pump failure results in hypercapnia; lung failure results in hypoxemia.

FIGURE 13-2

Anatomic components of the respiratory system. Optimum and integrated function are vital to maintaining normal respiration. Disruption in function of any component can have serious implications for normal respiration and can precipitate the development of respiratory failure.

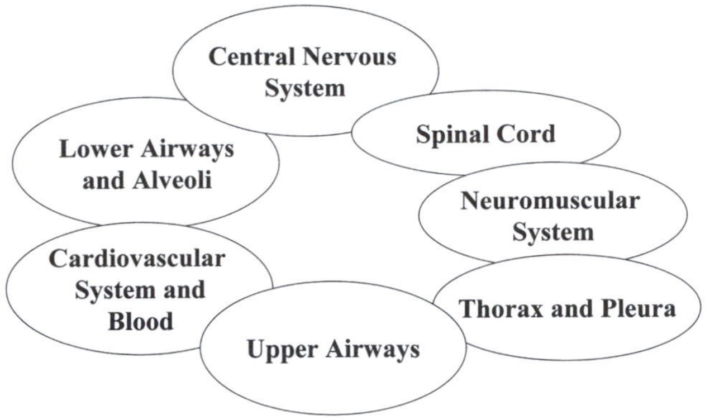

Characterization of the process causing respiratory failure as hypercapnic or hypoxemic serves as a tool to determine the cause and choose the most appropriate treatment.

Although it is helpful to characterize respiratory failure into the primary disorder that results in either pump or lung failure, it is important to recognize that patients who present with hypoxemic respiratory failure may also develop impaired pump function. However, characterization of the primary process causing respiratory failure into hypercapnic and hypoxemic subtypes remains useful as a tool to guide the clinician in determining the underlying etiology and choosing the most efficient and successful methods of treatment.

Pump failure indicates impairment in the respiratory system acting as a bellows.

Pump failure indicates conditions that impair the bellows function of respiration. Even if a patient has normal lung function, a decrease in central respiratory drive, impaired peripheral nerve transmission to contract the respiratory muscles, or severe weakness of the respiratory muscles may result in inability to exhale carbon dioxide and, if severe enough, may cause arterial hypoxemia. Similarly, conditions that severely impair chest wall integrity, such as flail chest or kyphosoliosis, may negatively impact the task of ventilation. On the other hand, lung failure occurs in conditions where the neuromuscular and chest wall apparatus functions normally but the lung parenchyma is severely impaired by the underlying disease process. In this scenario, abnormalities that affect the lung at the level of the alveolus, airway, lung interstitium, or pulmonary vasculature may result in the development of severe arterial hypoxemia.

Severe arterial hypoxemia results from processes that affect the lung at the levels of the alveolus, airway, interstitium, or pulmonary vasculature.

Although the function of the respiratory system can be easily subdivided into its pump and gas exchange functional components, the anatomic components that constitute the respiratory system are greater in number and more diverse in nature. Overall, the respiratory system is divided into seven distinct anatomic components: (1) the central nervous system; (2) the peripheral nervous system, including the spinal cord; (3) the neuromuscular system, including the myoneural junction and respiratory muscles; (4) the thorax and pleura; (5) the upper airways; (6) the cardiovascular system, including the red blood cells and hemoglobin,

Respiration is dependent on optimum and integrated function of several discrete anatomic units.

CASE STUDY: PART 2

On presentation to the emergency room, the patient was found to be in severe respiratory distress. She appeared to be lethargic, could not speak in complete sentences, secondary to dyspnea, and was unable to follow simple commands. On examination, her respiratory rate was 40 breaths/min. She had obvious contractions of the sternocleidomastoid and salenus muscles of the neck; paradoxical inward motion of the upper abdomen was more pronounced, as was flaring of the ala nasi. The patient was promptly intubated with an endotracheal tube and placed on mechanical ventilation. While inspiring 100% oxygen on ventilator settings at a respiratory rate of 10 breaths/min and tidal volume of 500 ml, an arterial blood gas showed PaO_2 was 110, $PaCO_2$ was 38, and pH was 7.44. A chest x-ray showed evidence of diffuse alveolar infiltrates with slight hyperinflation.

After intubation, rectal temperature was recorded at 101°F, respiratory rate was 12 breaths/min, blood pressure was 128/72 mmHg, and heart rate was 114 beats/min. Chest examination showed diffuse end-expiratory wheezes with bilateral rhonchi and end-inspiratory crackles and bronchial breath sounds. The rest of the physical examination was within normal limits.

TABLE 13-1

CLASSIFICATION OF DISEASES THAT CAUSE RESPIRATORY FAILURE INTO PUMP (I.E., HYPERCAPNIC) OR LUNG FAILURE (I.E., HYPOXEMIC) SUBTYPES

PUMP FAILURE	LUNG FAILURE
Central nervous system	Asthma
Drug overdose	Chronic obstructive pulmonary disease
Stroke	Bronchitis
Head Trauma	Pneumonia
Spinal cord, neuromuscular disease	Pulmonary embolism
Myasthenia gravis	Acute respiratory distress syndrome
Guillain–Barré	Alveolar hemorrhage
Polio	Cardiac
Polymyositis	Pulmonary edema
Neuromuscular blocking agents	Valvular abnormalities
Critical illness polyneuromyopathy	
Chest wall	
Kyphoscoliosis	
Burn eschar	
Flail chest	
Upper airways	
Glottic stenosis	
Paradoxical vocal cord dysfunction	
Laryngospasm	

which carry oxygen and carbon dioxide; and (7) the lower airways, including the alveoli. Normal respiration is dependent on the optimum and integrated action of all these vital links, and malfunction of one or several of these components can lead to respiratory failure (Figure 13-2). As one may expect, because of all the different components required for optimum respiration, the disease processes that can precipitate respiratory failure are great in number and diverse in nature.

A useful way to characterize the many different diseases causing respiratory failure is to separate disorders that cause pump failure from those which cause lung failure.

A method helpful in characterizing the many different disease processes that precipitate respiratory failure is, once again, to separate disorders primarily causing pump failure from those that precipitate lung failure. Table 13-1 lists the pathophysiologic processes that cause primarily pump versus lung failure. In addition to classifying respiratory failure into its pump and lung failure subtypes, it is important to further subdivide respiratory failure into acute and chronic presentations (Table 13-2). In acute presentations of either hypoxemic or hypercapnic respiratory failure, the disease process occurs within minutes to hours, whereas in chronic conditions respiratory failure ensues over several days or longer. Patients who present with acute episodes of respiratory failure, whether hypercapnic or hypoxemic in nature, usually present with obvious and severe symptoms and physical exam findings because patients having acute episodes of respiratory failure lack full development of compensatory mechanisms that attenuate the negative sequelae of hypercapnia or hypoxemia.

Respiratory failure must be classified not only into hypercapnia and hypoxemic subtypes but also into acute and chronic presentations.

In an acute episode of respiratory failure, compensatory mechanisms do not have time to develop; therefore, symptoms and physical exam abnormalities are more severe.

In cases of chronic hypoxemia, patients develop secondary polycythemia, and the severe manifestations of hypoxemia are somewhat attenuated by increased blood oxygen content. In cases of chronic hypercapnic respiratory failure, renal conservation of bicarbonate buffers chronic elevations in carbon dioxide levels, and the resultant pH is higher. In addition to clinical history taking, measurement of blood pH can aid in distinguishing acute from chronic presentations of hypercapnic respiratory failure (see Table 13-2).

Secondary polycythemia and bicarbonate elevation are two examples of compensatory mechanisms attenuating chronic hypoxemia and acidemia, respectively.

TABLE 13-2

CLASSIFICATION OF RESPIRATORY FAILURE INTO ACUTE AND CHRONIC PRESENTATIONS

PREDOMINANT TYPE	HYPERCAPNIC	HYPOXEMIC
Acute		
Time course	Minutes to hours	Minutes to hours
Compensatory changes	None	None
Chronic		
Time Course	Days to minutes	Days to minutes
Compensatory Changes	↑ HCO_3 ↑ pH	↑ Hemoglobin, Hematocrit

PATHOPHYSIOLOGY OF RESPIRATORY FAILURE

Six different pathophysiologic processes can lead to severe derangements in gas exchange and respiratory failure. However, reduction in inspired partial pressure of oxygen and increased venous admixture are less common causes.

The mechanisms of normal gas exchange are extensively reviewed in other textbooks and are not discussed here. This discussion focuses only on abnormalities that result in disturbed gas exchange, which leads to hypoxemic and/or hypercapnic respiratory failure. Although there are six different pathophysiologic processes that can lead to severe derangements in gas exchange and episodes of respiratory failure, not all of them are commonly encountered clinically. Reductions in the inspired partial pressure of oxygen and venous admixture are less common mechanisms for the development of respiratory failure.

When increased venous admixture leads to hypoxemia, patient management centers around cardiac dysfunction.

Reductions in inspired oxygen concentration may be encountered in patient populations residing at high altitude or patients exposed to reductions in ambient oxygen in commercial aircraft, which are pressurized to simulate altitudes as high as 10,000 feet and provide ambient concentrations of oxygen as low as 100 mmHg. Increased venous admixtures leading to hypoxemic respiratory failure arise in conditions where cardiac output is significantly reduced or oxygen consumption is extremely high. Under these conditions, pulmonary venous oxygen is significantly reduced and, as a consequence, arterial oxygenation is severely impaired. In clinical scenarios where increased venous admixture leads to hypoxemia, patient management and prognosis center around cardiac dysfunction. This topic is extensively covered in Chapters 14, 23, and 36.

Diffusion abnormalities are rarely the sole cause of respiratory failure.

The transfer of oxygen and carbon dioxide across the alveolar capillary membrane is accomplished by the process of diffusion, a process that depends on the physical characteristics of the membrane, including its thickness, area, and diffusibility, and the solubility of the gases diffusing across it. However, from a clinical standpoint, impaired diffusion is a minor contributor to arterial hypoxemia and plays only a minor role in gas exchange imbalance in patients with acute respiratory failure. Even in patients with severe lung disease with markedly reduced diffusion, ventilation–perfusion imbalance and intrapulmonary shunting appear to be far more important determinants of arterial oxygenation.

The most important pathophysiologic mechanisms impairing gas exchange include intrapulmonary shunt, mismatched pulmonary blood flow and ventilation, and decreased alveolar ventilation.

The three most important abnormalities resulting in disturbances in gas exchange that lead to respiratory failure are ventilation–perfusion inequality, intrapulmonary shunt, and hypoventilation.

Ventilation–Perfusion Inequality

Ventilation–perfusion mismatch is the most frequent contributor to clinically important oxygen desaturation.

Ventilation–perfusion imbalance exists even in the normal lung, depending on region, but remains fairly tightly regulated when assessing normal lung aggregate function.

Ventilation–perfusion (V_A/Q) mismatch is the most frequent contributor to clinically important oxygen desaturation. Ideally, each alveolar capillary exchange unit would have perfect matching of ventilation and perfusion, such that optimum gas exchange occurs across each alveolar unit. Realistically, however, the lungs do not act as multiples of identical and ideal gas exchange units, but rather as millions of units that are perfused in parallel and ventilated both in parallel and in series, resulting in some degree of V_A/Q imbalance even in healthy individuals. In normal individuals, there is a spectrum of V_A/Q ratios that range from relatively underventilated units to those lung units which are ventilated but not perfused. In normal lungs, V_A/Q may range from 0.6 to 3.0, with the distribution usually centered around a V_A/Q of approximately 1. The distribution of ventilation varies with common events, such as changes in body posture, lung volumes, and age. Increasing age produces a gradual increase in the degree of the V_A/Q inequality. However, despite this range of ventilation–perfusion imbalance in a normal lung, ventilation–perfusion balance on the whole remains a fairly tightly controlled process. In the setting of disease, however, the distribution of V_A/Q may become markedly abnormal, and lower and higher V_A/Q units predominate and may contribute to the development of respiratory failure.

Figure 13-3 shows examples of ventilation–perfusion imbalances that occur in different disease states. In patients with obstructive or restrictive ventilatory diseases, decreased ventilation may result from structural or functional abnormalities of the airway and can lead to decreased V_A/Q units (Figure 13-3B). On the other hand, lung units with increased V_A/Q ratios can develop in disorders that lead to overventilation of lung units, conditions such as emphysema, for example, in which patients have airspace enlargement as a result of the de-

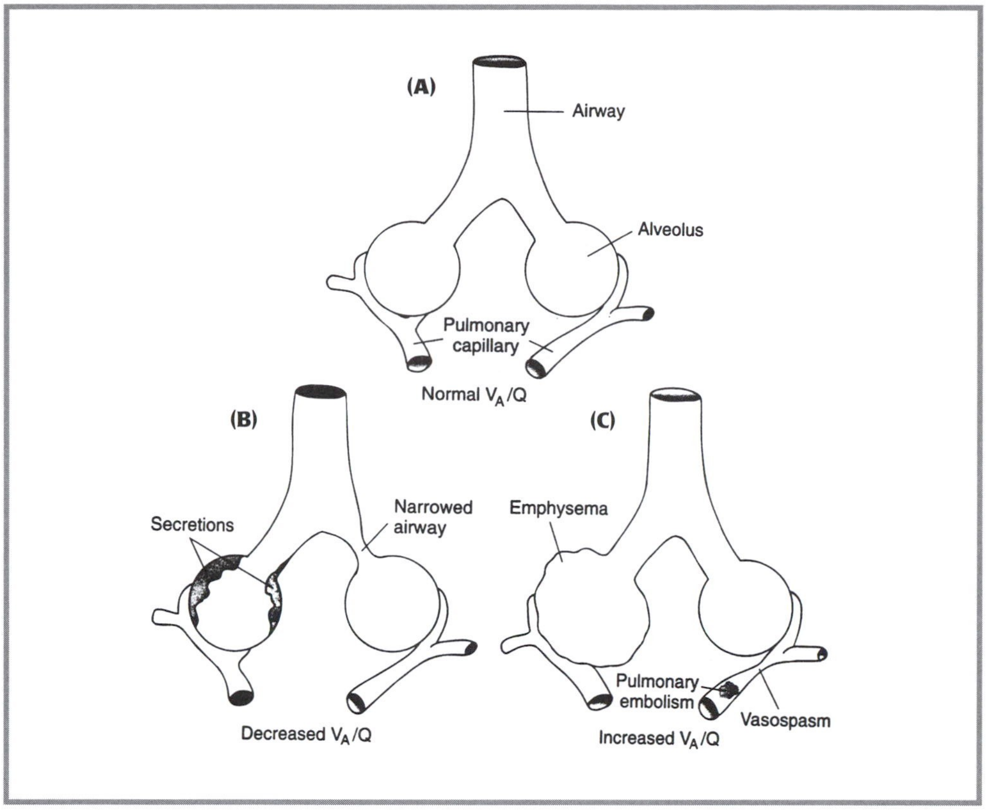

FIGURE 13-3

Examples of ventilation–perfusion imbalance. **(A)** Normal idealized alveolar capillary unit. **(B)** Examples of decreased ventilation–perfusion units as a result of secretions in the airway or airway bronchoconstriction. **(C)** Examples of increased ventilation–perfusion units due to the development of emphysema or decreased pulmonary blood flow secondary to pulmonary embolism or pulmonary artery vasospasm.

struction of the alveolar sac distal to the terminal bronchiole. Moreover, the development of pulmonary vascular underperfusion, as observed in cases of pulmonary embolism or pulmonary vasospasm, may cause high V_A/Q ratios (Figure 13-3C). Reflex mechanisms are present in the lung to minimize the effect of V_A/Q inequality, thus avoiding the detrimental effects of impaired gas exchange. One mechanism is hypoxic vasoconstriction, whereby a fall in V_A/Q leads to the development of alveolar hypoxia, which in turn causes vasoconstriction of the perfusing arteriole. This effect is beneficial for pulmonary gas exchange because it decreases the denominator of the V_A/Q relationship, thereby partially correcting regional V_A/Q imbalance and improving arterial hypoxemia. Hypoxic vasoconstriction appears to operate over a range of alveolar PO_2 values between 30 and 150 mmHg. The mechanism by which alveolar hypoxia sends the message to trigger regional vasoconstriction is unknown, but it may involve the release of humoral messengers.

Hypoxic vasoconstriction is a reflex mechanism that tends to minimize the effects of V_A/Q inequality to avoid the detrimental effects of impaired gas exchange.

Hypoxic vasoconstriction operates at alveolar PO_2 from 30 to 150 mmHg.

Many factors, however, can significantly interfere with hypoxic vasoconstriction, including certain drugs, such as calcium channel blockers and beta agonists, or diseases such as those causing elevations in left atrial pressure or lower respiratory tract infection. In addition, although hypoxic vasoconstriction may be helpful in improving arterial hypoxemia, a progression in vasoconstrictor effect can lead to the development of secondary pulmonary hypertension and, eventually, right heart failure.

Hypoxic vasoconstriction, if unabated, can lead to the development of secondary pulmonary hypertension and right heart failure.

The development of V_A/Q abnormalities can have a dramatic affect on gas exchange and interfere with the transfer of both oxygen and carbon dioxide. The oxygen and carbon dioxide content of end-capillary gas for each of the two gases depends on the gas pressure in the alveolus and their respective hemoglobin dissociation curves. One may expect, therefore, that V_A/Q inequality would result in both hypoxemia and hypercapnia; however, most of the clinical derangement observed following mild V_A/Q inequality is attributable to the development of profound hypoxemia rather than hypercapnia. In fact, most patients with mild V_A/Q inequality have normal $PaCO_2$ levels or are hypocapnic. Hypoxemia with normocapnia as a result of V_A/Q inequality appears to be best explained by the differences in the shapes of the oxyhemoglobin and carbon dioxide hemoglobin dissociation curves (Figure 13-4). An

Hypercapnia is not seen in mild V_A/Q imbalance, secondary to the linear relationship of the partial pressure of CO_2 and carbon dioxide hemoglobin dissociation curves.

FIGURE 13-4

Oxygen and carbon dioxide contents versus the partial pressures of carbon dioxide and oxygen. An increase in oxygen partial pressure above a certain level (60 mmHg) does not result in increased in oxygen content of the blood. However, a linear relationship is seen between the partial pressure of carbon dioxide and carbon dioxide blood content. (Adapted from Dantsker MD, David R. Pulmonary gas exchange: In: Bone R, (ed) Pulmonary and Critical Care Medicine. St. Louis: Mosby, 1997.)

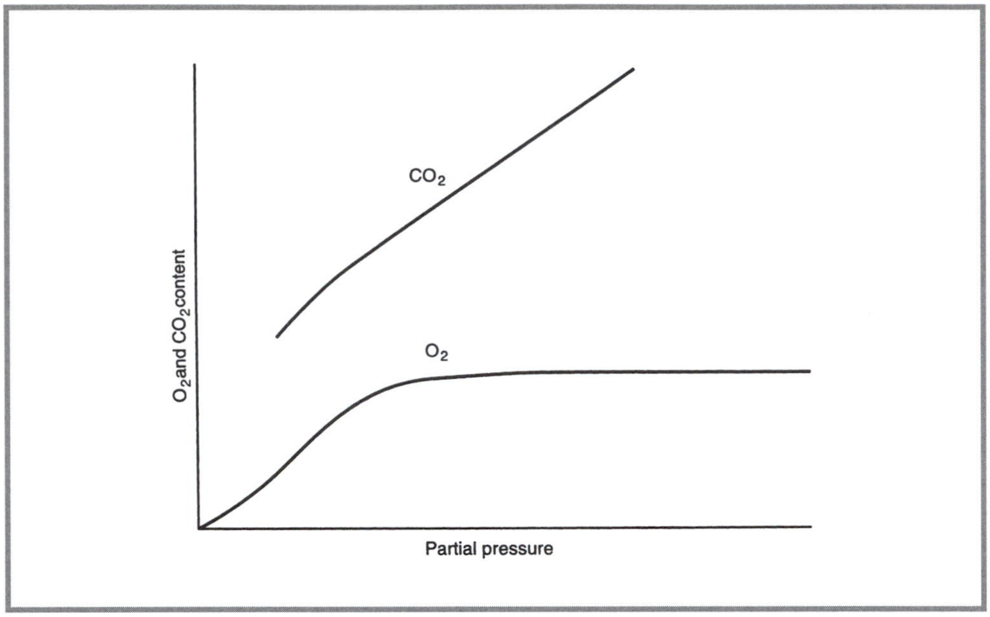

increase in $PaCO_2$ is sensed by chemoreceptors and stimulates increased ventilation, predominantly to lung units already ventilated. However, because of the nonlinear portion of the oxyhemoglobin curve, increased PaO_2 does not result in an increase in blood oxygen content. In contrast, because of the linear relationship of carbon dioxide content with the partial pressure of carbon dioxide, an increased minute ventilation results in a decrease in the partial pressure of carbon dioxide and consequently a lower carbon dioxide content. In essence, in the presence of V_A/Q inequality, an increased minute ventilation prevents CO_2 retention but cannot influence the development of hypoxemia.

V_A/Q inquality causing hypoxemia is relatively responsive to the inspiration of supplemental oxygen.

Hypoxemia as a result of ventilation–perfusion imbalances responds in a variable way to increases in the concentration of inspired oxygen. This fact helps to distinguish ventilation–perfusion imbalance from intrapulmonary shunt as the primary cause of hypoxemia. As shown in Figure 13-5, disease processes associated with mild ventilation–perfusion imbalance show an increase in arterial PaO_2 in response to increasing concentrations of inspired oxygen that is relatively linear and may even approximate the normal condition. With moderate or more severe ventilation–perfusion imbalances, however, higher concentrations of oxygen are required to demonstrate an increase in arterial PaO_2. It is important to note that even with severe ventilation–perfusion imbalances, high concentrations of supplemental oxygen may result in substantial increases in arterial PaO_2.

Intrapulmonary shunt indicates that lung units are being perfused but not ventilated.

Intrapulmonary shunt represents lung units that are perfused but receive no ventilation. Although intrapulmonary shunt can be considered an extreme case of V_A/Q inequality, intrapulmonary shunt results from a different category of clinical disorders that require different forms of therapy. Because of this, intrapulmonary shunt should be considered as an entity distinct from ventilation–perfusion imbalance. Under normal conditions, 1%–3% of mixed venous blood flows directly from the systemic circulation through the bronchial and thebesian blood vessels. Clinical disorders causing hypoxemic respiratory failure may be found in diseases associated with shunt physiology resulting from either cardiac or pulmonary diseases.

Disorders causing hypoxemic respiratory failure, secondary to shunt physiology, occur in cardiac or pulmonary diseases.

The intracardiac shunts include right to left intraatrial or intraventricular blood transit.

Examples of intracardiac shunts include atrial and ventricular septal defects, especially in conditions in which pulmonary hypertension is present. When pressure becomes high enough in the pulmonary vascular circuit, right to left intracardiac shunt occurs and profound hypoxemia may develop. In cases of intrapulmonary shunt, mixed venous blood passes through the capillary walls of alveoli that are collapsed (i.e., atelectatic) or filled with fluid (i.e., congestive heart failure) or inflammatory debris (i.e., pneumonia) and are thus nonventilated (see Figure 13-5A).

Intrapulmonary shunts are caused by alveoli that are collapsed, filled with fluid or inflammatory debris, and not ventilated.

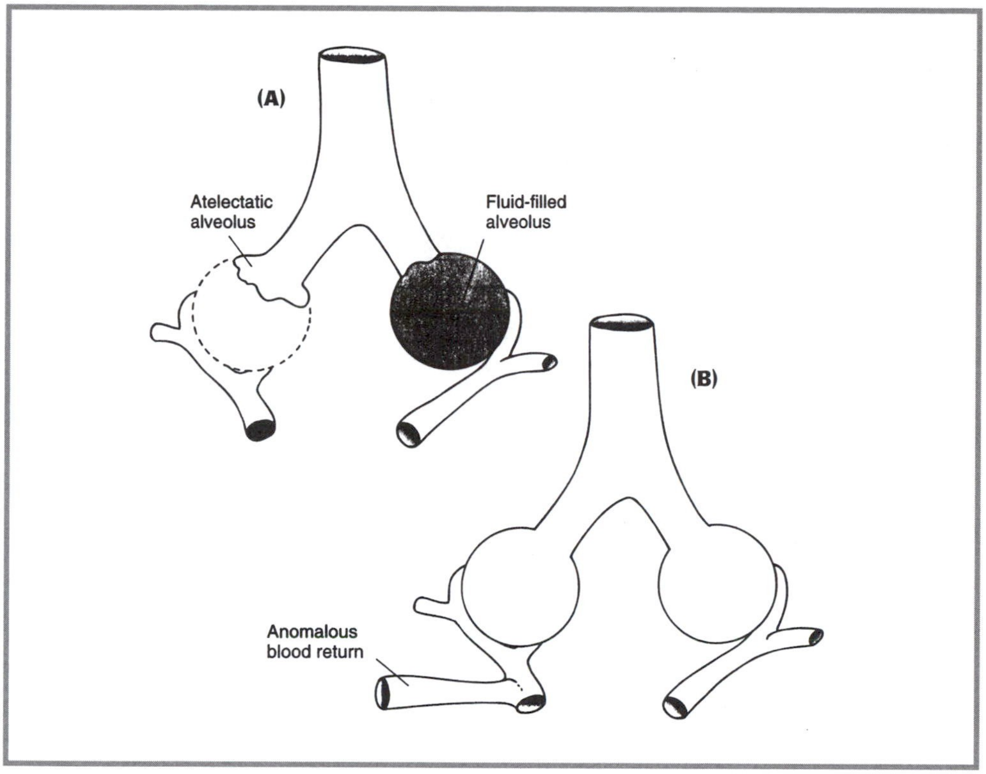

FIGURE 13-5

Examples of intrapulmonary shunt. **(A)** Collapsed and fluid-filled alveoli are examples of intrapulmonary shunt. **(B)** Anomalous blood return of mixed venous blood bypasses the alveolus and thereby contributes to the development of intrapulmonary shunt.

As shown in Figure 13-6B, intrapulmonary shunts 30% or greater are remarkably resistant to the inspiration of high inspired oxygen concentrations. Even breathing 100% oxygen has minimal impact on increasing arterial PaO_2 in patients with severe shunts. In fact, use of 100% oxygen can serve as a clinical tool to help distinguish intrapulmonary shunt from V_A/Q inequality as the underlying major pathophysiologic mechanism responsible for hypoxemia in patients with elevated alveolar–arterial (A-a) oxygen gradients. In contrast to patients with severe shunts, patients with elevated A-a gradients resulting from V_A/Q inequality exhibit substantial increases in PaO_2 when breathing high levels of inspired oxygen. When testing for the presence of intrapulmonary shunt, it is important to remember to administer

Intrapulmonary shunts greater than 30% cause hypoxemia that is relatively refractory to the inspiration of supplemental oxygen.

When testing for intrapulmonary shunt, it is important to remember to administer 95%–100% inspired oxygen.

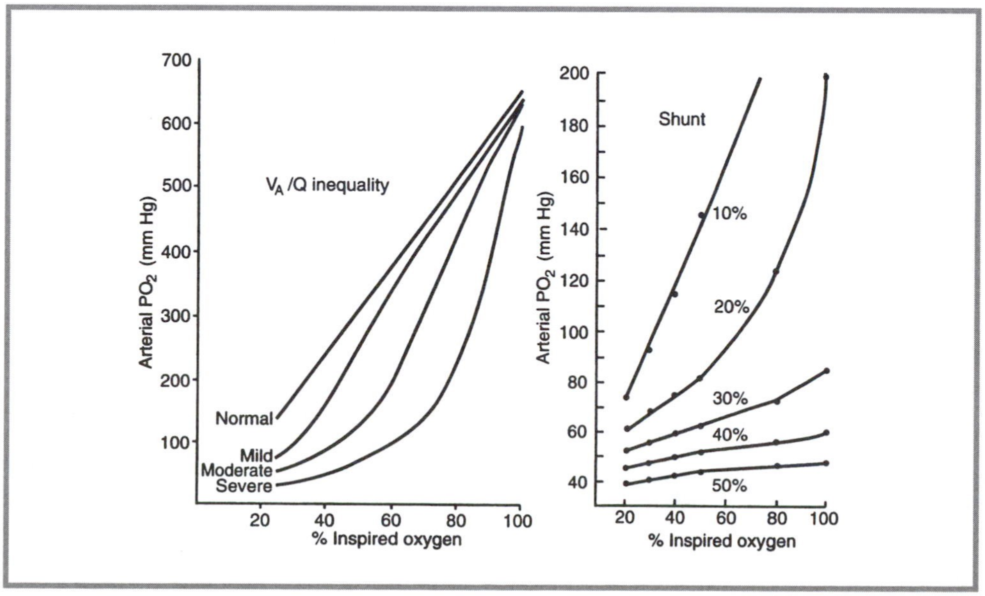

FIGURE 13-6

Differing responses of ventilation–perfusion inequality or intrapulmonary shunt to increases in inspired oxygen. **(A)** Ventilation–perfusion inequality under mild to severe circumstances. Even in the presence of severe ventilation–perfusion imbalance, high levels of supplemental oxygen have a profound effect on increasing arterial PaO_2. **(B)** In contrast, intrapulmonary shunts of 30% or greater are relatively refractory to supplemental oxygen increasing arterial PaO_2. (Adapted from Dantzker MD, David R. Pulmonary gas exchange. In: Bone R (ed) Pulmonary and Critical Care Medicine. St. Louis: Mosby, 1997.)

95%–100% inspired oxygen because severe V_A/Q inequalities may result in levels of hypoxemia similar to shunt until 100% oxygen is administered (Figure 13-6a).

To test for the percentage of intrapulmonary shunt present, the patient should be administered 100% supplemental oxygen for 15 min, until all the alveoli can be presumed to be filled with pure oxygen. The percentage of shunt can then be calculated by the following formula:

$$Q_S/Q_T = (Cc'O_2 - C_aO_2)/(C_C'O_2 - C_{\overline{V}}O_2) \times 100$$

In this equation, C denotes content, and c, a, and v denote end-capillary, arterial, and mixed venous blood, respectively. When making these calculations, it is assumed that end-capillary and calculated alveolar oxygen tensions are equivalent.

The treatment of intrapulmonary shunt requires methods that increase lung volume with either CPAP, PEEP, or mechanical ventilation.

Because of the refractoriness of moderate to severe shunts to respond with an increase in arterial oxygen to inspiring higher concentrations of supplemental oxygen, the application of positive pressure to the airway in the form of continuous positive airway pressure (CPAP) or positive end-expiratory pressure (PEEP) is considered. A full discussion of the treatment of refractory oxygenation is given in Chapters 2, 22, and 37.

Hypoventilation

$PaCO_2$ is directly related to VCO_2 production and inversely directed to alveolar ventilation.

To avoid the development of respiratory acidosis, the carbon dioxide produced each day as an end product of aerobic metabolism (approximately 17,000 mEq of acid) must be exhaled. To achieve balance between the production and elimination of carbon dioxide, the central nervous system and carotid body chemoreceptors must be able to adjust ventilation over a broad range of carbon dioxide production. Hypoventilation, therefore, can be defined as an inadequate delivery of fresh alveolar gas required to maintain a normal $PaCO_2$.

Carbon dioxide must be eliminated from the body at a rate equal to that at which it is produced.

The relationship between alveolar ventilation (V_A), carbon dioxide production (VCO_2), and the partial pressure of carbon dioxide in the blood ($PaCO_2$) can be described using a modification of the Fick principle of mass balance that quantitates VCO_2 as the product of V_A and the fractional concentration of carbon dioxide in the alveolar gas. Under steady-state conditions, with elimination of carbon dioxide from the body at a rate equal to the rate at which it is produced, the relationship between $PaCO_2$, VCO_2, and V_A is:

$$PaCO_2 = \frac{VCO_2K}{V_A}$$

V_E is the total expired ventilation measured during 1 min.

Deadspace ventilation (V_D) is that portion of minute ventilation that insufflates the conducting airways and does not precipitate directly in gas exchange.

Alveolar ventilation (V_A) is equal to the total expired minute ventilation minus deadspace ventilation.

In this condition, K is a constant that equals 0.863. This constant is required because VCO_2 is expressed at standard temperature and pressure dry (STPD), whereas alveolar ventilation is expressed at body temperature, ambient pressure, and saturation conditions (BTPS). Within the normal lung, V_A is a fixed proportion of overall expired minute ventilation (V_E). V_E is the total expired ventilation, usually measured over a 1-min collection period. V_E has two components, ventilation that contributes to the elimination of CO_2, termed alveolar ventilation (V_A), and ventilation which does not contribute to the elimination of CO_2, termed deadspace ventilation (V_D). Deadspace ventilation (V_D) is the portion of minute ventilation that insufflates the conducting airways and does not participate directly in gas exchange. V_D therefore approximates the volume of the conducting airways. However, in disease states that result in conditions of higher physiologic deadspace (e.g., exacerbation of COPD), if the patient does not mount a corresponding proportional increase in V_E, alveolar ventilation will decrease.

Alveolar ventilation (V_A) can be expressed as total expired minute ventilation minus deadspace ventilation ($V_A = V_E - V_D$). If one rewrites the equation provided earlier and substitutes $V_E - V_D$ for V_A, the relationship between $PaCO_2$, VCO_2, and V_A becomes:

$$PaCO_2 = \frac{K(VCO_2)}{V_E - V_D}$$

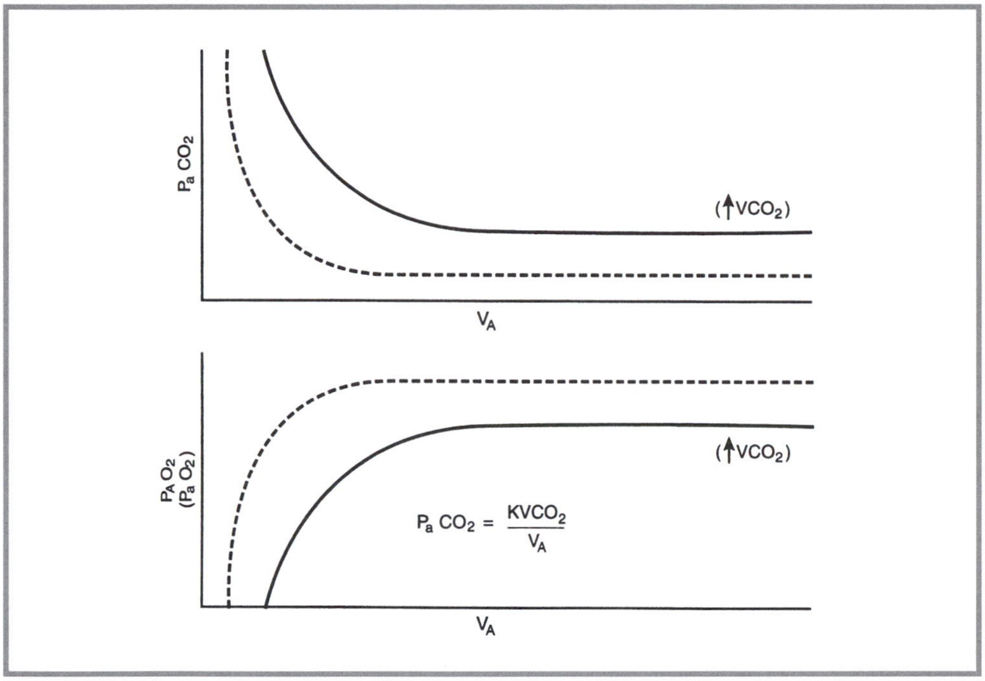

FIGURE 13-7

Relationships of $PaCO_2$, P_AO_2, and PaO_2 to alveolar ventilation (V_A). As V_A increases, $PaCO_2$ decreases. As CO_2 production (VCO_2) increases, the relationship shifts upward and to the right. In contrast, with an increase in V_A, alveolar oxygen (P_AO_2) and consequently arterial oxygen (PaO_2) increase. (Adapted from Dantzker MD, David R. Pulmonary gas exchange. In: Bone R (ed) Pulmonary and Critical Care Medicine. St. Louis: Mosby, 1997.)

Therefore, states of alveolar hypoventilation are those in which minute ventilation (V_E) is reduced or deadspace ventilation (V_D) is high. Either or both of these mechanisms will result in decreased alveolar ventilation. Alveolar ventilation that is inadequate to compensate for the increased metabolic production of VCO_2 results in a rise in $PaCO_2$.

Alveolar ventilation inadequate to compensate for increased metabolic production of VCO_2 results in a rising $PaCO_2$.

Hypoventilation may also indirectly reduce the partial pressure of oxygen in the blood (PaO_2) by reducing alveolar oxygen tension (P_AO_2). As illustrated in Figure 13-7, a fall in alveolar ventilation or a rise in carbon dioxide production greater than the increase in alveolar ventilation results in an increase in $PaCO_2$, a decrease in alveolar PO_2, and a consequent decrease in PaO_2. In this latter case, because all the parameters used in calculating the alveolar PO_2 change simultaneously, the alveolar–arterial (A-a) oxygen gradient remains normal.

When alveolar hypoventilation occurs, the A-a gradient remains normal.

It is important to differentiate between hypoxemia caused by alveolar hypoventilation and hypoxemia caused by ventilation–perfusion imbalance or intrapulmonary shunt because the disease processes and their treatments differ markedly. Determination of the alveolar gas equation, which is discussed later in this chapter (see Arterial Blood Analysis) is extremely useful in determining whether hypoxemia is caused by hypoventilation, as opposed to hypoxemia caused by conditions attributable to V_A/Q inequality, or intrapulmonary shunt. Although hypoxemia regardless of pathophysiologic mechanism may be treated by the inspiration of enriched oxygen, in most cases hypoventilation must be treated with an augmentation of ventilation to avoid progressive respiratory acidosis.

It is important to differentiate hypoxemia that results from alveolar hypoventilation from V_A/Q inequality or intrapulmonary shunt because the treatments are different.

Hypoventilation in most cases must be treated by augmentation of ventilation.

DIAGNOSIS OF RESPIRATORY FAILURE

History

The diagnosis of respiratory failure begins with a high clinical suspicion on the part of the practitioner, coupled with the clinical manifestations and symptoms of severe gas exchange imbalance. Hypoxemia and hypercapnia are the major precipitating disturbances that elicit abnormalities found on history and physical examination in patients presenting in respiratory failure (Table 13-3). However, the severity and acuity of the inciting event causing respiratory failure, and the patient's underlying condition, are important influences on the severity of the patient's symptoms and their requirement for prompt evaluation and treat-

Hypoxemia and hypercapnia precipitate disturbances that elicit abnormalities on history and physical exam in patients presenting in respiratory failure.

TABLE 13-3

SYMPTOMS OF RESPIRATORY FAILURE

Impaired gas exchange: neurologic symptoms
Headache
Visual disturbances
Anxiety
Confusion
Memory loss
Hallucinations
Loss of consciousness
Asterixis (hypercapnia)
Weakness
Decreased functional performance
Specific organ symptoms
Pulmonary
Cough
Chest pains
Sputum production
Stridor
Dyspnea (resting vs. exertional)
Cardiac
Orthopnea
Peripheral edema
Chest pain
Other
Fever
Abdominal pain
Anemia
Bleeding

ment. In patients who represent with catastrophic disorders or have severe underlying diseases with already compromised respiratory reserve, respiratory failure may develop acutely. Examples of these types of patients include those who suffer an intracranial hemorrhage, pneumothorax, or acute tracheobronchitis with underlying COPD. In circumstances where respiratory failure is chronic in nature, symptoms and clinical manifestations present insidiously over weeks to months after compensatory mechanisms fail to further attenuate the progression of hypoxemia and hypercapnia. Examples include chronic respiratory failure developing in patients with slowly progressive neurologic diseases, such as myotonic dystrophy or chronic spinal muscle atrophy.

> Most patients who present in respiratory failure complain of dyspnea.

Most patients who present with respiratory failure complain of dyspnea. Dyspnea appears first with exertion and later, with progression of the disease, is present even at rest. Hoarseness, cough, sputum production, and chest pain are not symptoms of respiratory failure per se but are clues that a primary pulmonary process may be the trigger for the development of respiratory failure. As the condition precipitating respiratory failure progresses and severe gas exchange imbalances appear (i.e., hypoxemia with or without hypercapnia), neurologic manifestations predominate (headache, visual disturbances, confusion, memory loss, anxiety, seizures, or, in extreme cases, loss of consciousness).

> As gas exchange imbalances worsen, neurologic manifestations predominate.

Physical Examination

> Physical examination of patients in respiratory failure begins with a quick, but thorough, general assessment.

> The initial priority is to triage patients who present with severe forms of respiratory failure from those with less severe forms.

Physical examination in patients presenting in respiratory failure begins with a quick but thorough general assessment (Table 13-4). The initial priority on the part of the clinician should be to characterize those patients who are presenting with severe manifestations of respiratory failure who may need prompt assessment for airway control, oxygenation, and ventilation. In those patients who present with more severe presentations of respiratory failure, a decrease in mental alertness, more severe breathlessness, and evidence of an elevated respiratory workload are present. Hypoxemia and hypercapnia both can contribute to neurologic manifestations, which in their most severe form result in a decrease in cognitive function that ranges from anxiety to coma. Patients who have severe airways obstruction are unable to speak in complete sentences, signifying a FEV_1 of 1 l or less. A respiratory rate

TABLE 13-4

PHYSICAL EXAMINATION IN RESPIRATORY FAILURE

- General findings
  - Mental alertness
  - Ability to speak in complete sentences
  - Respiratory rate >35 breaths/min
  - Heart rate > or < 20 beats from normal
  - Pulsus paradoxus present?
  - Elevated work of breathing?
    - Using accessory muscles
    - Rib cage or abdominal paradox
- Specific organ dysfunction
  - Pulmonary
    - Stridor
    - Wheezes
    - Rhonchi
    - Crackles
  - Cardiac
    - Tachycardia, Bradycardia
    - Hypertension, Hypotension
    - Crackles
    - New murmurs
  - Renal
    - Anuria
  - Gastrointestinal
    - Distended
    - Pain to palpation
    - Decreased bowel sounds

greater than 35 breaths/min, heart rate 20–30 beats/mm greater or lesser than normal, and the presence of pulse paradoxus (e.g., a 15- to 20-mmHg decrease in systolic pressure during inspiration) are all manifestations of an increased ventilatory workload.

Parameters that show metabolic instability, or show severe respiratory distress, signify more severe episodes of respiratory failure.

An elevated work of breathing may also be indicated by the pattern of breathing exhibited by the patient. The use of accessory muscles of the neck (palpable or visual contraction of the sternocleidomastoid muscles, flaring of the ala nasi), tensing of the abdominal muscles, or paradoxical movements of the rib cage and abdominal compartments are indications of respiratory distress. Paradoxical rib cage or abdominal motions during inspiration (e.g., rib cage and abdominal compartments move in opposite directions, rather than similar outward movements) signify the development of a ventilatory workload that is higher than ventilatory capacity or the development of underlying respiratory muscle dysfunction such as respiratory muscle fatigue or respiratory muscle weakness.

A change in breathing pattern is helpful in indicating the severity of the episode of respiratory failure.

The presence of specific abnormalities on physical examination related to isolated organ dysfunction may indicate the primary underlying process contributing to the development of respiratory failure (see Figure 13-4). The presence of abnormal ausculatory sounds of the upper airway (stridor) or lower airways (wheezes, rhonchi, or rales) may indicate a primary underlying pulmonary process (i.e., exacerbation of airflow obstruction, pneumonia, or interstitial lung disease). Similarly, the presence of cardiac, renal, or gastrointestinal abnormalities on physical examination may indicate those organs as the source of the patient's severe illness. Although these findings may indicate the severity of or in some cases provide clues to the etiology of respiratory failure, in most cases the clinical history and physical examination of patients who present with respiratory failure are fairly nonspecific, and identification of the cause of respiratory failure requires laboratory testing.

Extrapulmonary abnormalities on physical examination may identify the cause of respiratory failure.

Because physical and historical symptoms are nonspecific in diagnosing all aspects of respiratory failure, laboratory testing is necessary.

USE OF LABORATORY TESTS IN THE DIAGNOSIS

Laboratory testing for respiratory failure encompasses four major areas: (1) arterial blood gas analysis; (2) measurement of respiratory mechanics; (3) chest imaging; and (4) general laboratory testing (Table 13-5). A brief description of the most important features of each of these tests as they pertain to the management of respiratory failure follows.

Laboratory testing for respiratory failure includes arterial blood gas analysis, measurement of respiratory mechanics, chest imaging, and general laboratory testing.

TABLE 13-5

LABORATORY TESTING IN RESPIRATORY FAILURE

Arterial blood gas
PaO_2
$PaCO_2$
pH
Chest imaging
Chest x-ray
CT scan
Ultrasound
Ventilation–perfusion scan
Respiratory mechanics
Spirometry (FVC, FEV_1, peak flow)
Respiratory muscle pressures
MIP (maximum inspiratory pressure)
MEP (maximum expiratory pressure)
MVV (maximum voluntary ventilation)
Other tests
Hemoglobin, hematocrit
Electrolytes, blood urea nitrogen, creatinine
Creatinine phosphokinase, aldolase
EKG, echocardiogram
Swan–Ganz catheter
Electromyography (EMG)
Nerve conduction study

Arterial Blood Gas Analysis

An arterial blood gas provides an indication of the duration and severity of the episode of respiratory failure. It measures PaO_2, $PaCO_2$, and pH.

Analysis of arterial blood gas is the single most important laboratory test that can classify the subtype of respiratory failure. This test indicates the duration and severity of the episode of respiratory failure. Analysis of the arterial blood gas provides information on the presence and magnitude of three distinct abnormalities: hypoxemia (reduction of partial pressure of oxygen in the blood), hypercapnia ($PaCO_2 > 45$ mmHg), and arterial pH.

Hypoxemia

Oxygenation failure is defined as $PaO_2 < 60$ mmHg while inspiring oxygen concentrations $\geq 40\%$.

Hypoxemia is a reduction in the partial pressure of oxygen in the blood. The normal resting PaO_2 ranges from 75 to 80 mmHg. A PaO_2 below 60 mmHg is considered the lower limit of safety, because lower values represent displacement to the steep slope of the oxyhemoglobin dissociation curve. At PaO_2 values less than 60 mmHg, even small declines in the partial pressure of oxygen result in much more substantial decreases in arterial oxygen content (see Figure 13-4). In cases of respiratory failure, oxygenation failure is usually defined as a PaO_2 less than 60 mmHg while inspiring oxygen concentrations of 40% or greater.

As previous discussed, the mechanisms by which clinically significant reductions in PaO_2 occur include right-to-left intracardiac shunts, intrapulmonary shunts, ventilation–perfusion imbalance, and alveolar hypoventilation. Hypoxemia caused by alveolar hypoventilation is characterized by a normal alveolar–arterial oxygen difference ($P_AO_2 - PaO_2$), a feature that distinguishes hypoxemia associated with hypoventilation from hypoxemia caused by shunt or ventilation–perfusion imbalance. The alveolar arterial oxygen gradient can be calculated by using the alveolar gas equation to estimate alveolar oxygen (P_AO_2) and measuring the arterial oxygen blood tension during arterial blood gas analysis (PaO_2).

Water vapor pressure observed at 100% saturation is 47 mmHg.

As fresh gas is inspired at atmospheric pressure, the gas is warmed and humidified. The concentration of inspired oxygen (P_IO_2) depends on the barometric pressure (P_B). At sea level, P_B is 760 mmHg, or 1 atm. $P_IO_2 = F_IO_2$ (P_B − water vapor pressure), where P_IO_2 is the partial pressure of oxygen in the central airways, F_IO_2 is the concentration of inspired oxygen, and P_B represents barometric pressure at sea level (760 mmHg). Water vapor pressure exerted at 100% saturation is 47 mmHg, the condition that exists in the lower airways at one atmosphere (1 atm).

Measurement of alveolar gas exchange is important because the gradient between P_AO_2 and measured PaO_2 serves as an index of the efficiency of gas exchange by the lung. The amount of oxygen at the alveolar level (P_AO_2) can be calculated by the simplified alveolar gas equation:

The A-a gradient serves as an index of the efficiency of gas exchange by the lung.

$$P_AO_2 = \frac{P_IO_2 - PaCO_2}{R}$$

The alveolar–arterial oxygen gradient is normally 10–20 mmHg in the normal patient, but increases with age and the percent of inspired oxygen and is also affected by body posture.

An example calculation of the alveolar–arterial oxygen gradient is provided for a representative patient:

$$\text{Alveolar–arterial (A-a) oxygen gradient} = \frac{P_IO_2 - PaCO_2}{R} - PaO_2$$

R equals the respiratory exchange ratio (R = 0.8), which is determined by metabolic events ($R = VCO_2/\dot{V}O_2$). $P_IO_2 = F_IO_2$ (P_B − 47 mmHg), and PaO_2 and $PaCO_2$ are measured by the arterial blood gas.

R is determined by metabolic events: $VCO_2/\dot{V}O_2$.

If the patient breaths room air oxygen ($F_IO_2 = 0.21$) at sea level (P_B = 1 atm = 760 mmHg), water vapor pressure is 47 mmHg and P_IO_2 becomes 150.

$$\begin{aligned} PIO_2 &= FIO_2\,(760 - \text{water vapor}) \\ &= 0.21\,(760 - 47) \\ &= 150 \end{aligned}$$

If arterial blood gas measures $PaCO_2$ of 56 mmHg and PaO_2 of 70 mmHg, the alveolar–arterial oxygen gradient becomes 10. Mild hypoxemia in this case is a result of hypoventilation, not intrapulmonary or cardiac shunting or ventilation–perfusion imbalance.

$$\begin{aligned} \text{Alveolar–arterial (A-a) oxygen gradient} &= P_IO_2 - \frac{PaCO_2}{R} - PaO_2 \\ &= 150 - \frac{80}{0.8} - 40 \\ &= 10 \end{aligned}$$

Hypercapnia

Hypercapnia is an elevation in arterial carbon dioxide tension ($PaCO_2$) greater than the upper limit of 45 mmHg. Hypercapnia is commonly present in chronic cases of respiratory failure resulting from neuromuscular disease, thoracic cage abnormalities, or chronic obstructive pulmonary disease (COPD). Hypercapnia that presents in acute situations (i.e., status asthmaticus or sepsis) usually represents acute respiratory failure and has more ominous implications. In most cases, hypercapnia results from the presence of hypoventilation, and is not caused by V_A/Q imbalance, because of the linear relationship of the partial pressure of carbon dioxide with CO_2 content (see Figure 13-4). However, in extreme cases of ventilation–perfusion imbalance, hypercapnia may develop.

Hypercapnia is $PaCO_2 \geq 45$ mmHg.

Hypercapnia usually results from hypoventilation, not V_A/Q imbalance.

Arterial pH

The relationship described by the Henderson–Hasselbach equation between $PaCO_2$ and plasma bicarbonate dictates the arterial pH.

The Henderson–Hasselbach equation defines the relationship between $PaCO_2$, pH, and plasma bicarbonate.

$$\text{Henderson–Hasselbach Equation: pH} = 6.1 + \log \frac{[HCO_3]}{PaCO_2 \times 0.0301}$$

FIGURE 13-8

Effects of acute and chronic variation in $PaCO_2$ on plasma bicarbonate and pH. The line connecting points *C* and *A* represents the effect of an acute change in $PaCO_2$ to a value above or below 40 mmHg. A more chronic rise in $PaCO_2$ that allows renal compensation to occur shows a shift in this relationship to the line connecting points *D* and *B*. During the chronic rise in $PaCO_2$, identified by the line connecting points *D* and *B*, renal conservation of bicarbonate attenuates the decline in pH induced by a rise in arterial carbon dioxide. (Reproduced with permission from Murray JF. The Normal Lung. Philadelphia: Saunders, 1997:224.)

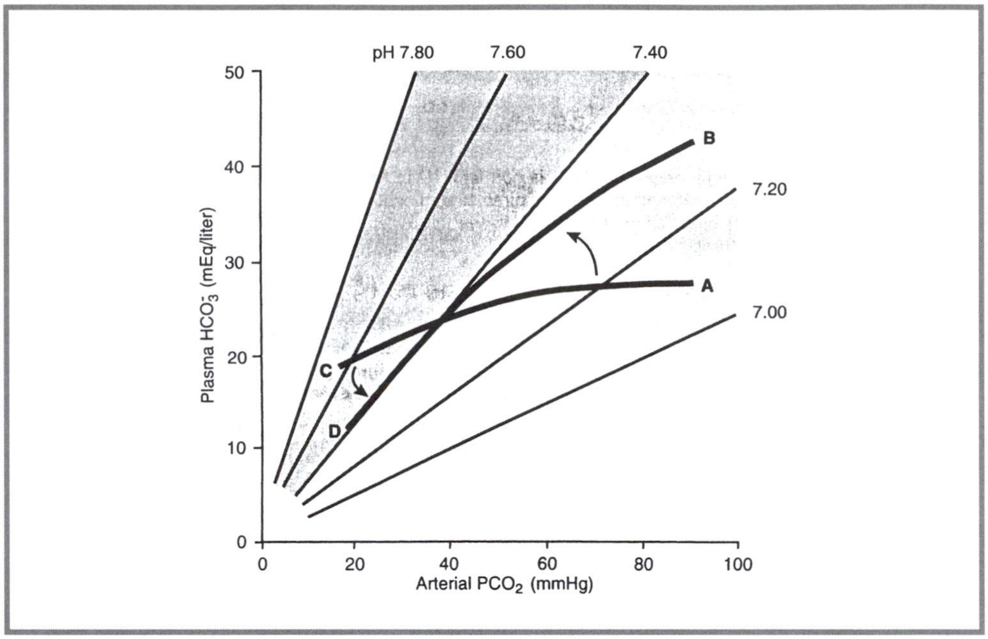

By using the arterial blood gas to measure arterial pH and $PaCO_2$, the Henderson–Hasselbach equation can be used to calculate the bicarbonate level. Only small to negligible increases in plasma bicarbonate accompany acute increases in $PaCO_2$ that occur over hours. Over a period of several days to weeks, however, the renal conservation of bicarbonate results in increased bicarbonate levels. A higher serum bicarbonate attenuates the decline in pH that would otherwise occur because of an increased partial pressure of carbon dioxide. As a result, reductions in pH are less severe in situations in which carbon dioxide is chronic, in contrast to conditions associated with acute elevations in CO_2. Examples of acute and chronic $PaCO_2$ elevation in regards to the impact of plasma bicarbonate and pH levels are shown in Figure 13-8.

Measurement of Respiratory Mechanics

Measurement of respiratory mechanics might not only help to grade the severity of the abnormality provoking respiratory failure but also can provide causative insight.

Respiratory mechanics measured at the bedside in patients with respiratory failure include spirometry and measurement of respiratory muscle pressures.

Although the measurement of respiratory mechanics is limited in critically ill patients, in certain circumstances measurement of respiratory mechanics might help not only to grade the severity of the abnormality causing respiratory failure but also to provide some insight into the mechanism. In most cases, measurement of bedside spirometry or respiratory muscles pressures are the only respiratory mechanics tests applicable for evaluating patients presenting in respiratory failure.

A vital capacity <10 ml/kg of body weight indicates significant dysfunction of the respiratory system.

Measurements of vital capacity (VC), forced expiratory volume in 1 s (FEV_1), and peak expiratory flow rate (PEFR) are the most common parameters used in patient assessment. VC is the maximum volume of air exhaled after a maximal inspiration; it provides an indication of the patient's maximum ventilatory capacity. VC is influenced by optimum functioning of the central and peripheral nervous systems, the elastic properties of the lung and the chest wall, and airway caliber. It cannot be used to assess specific abnormalities of the individual components of the respiratory system but helps to provide a simple global estimate of respiratory system function. In most patients, the minimal acceptable VC before respiratory failure develops is approximately 10–15 ml/kg of body weight. Lower values usually signal significant respiratory muscle pump dysfunction and predict imminent need for ventilatory assistance. However, as with any other laboratory tool used in the assessment of respiratory failure, the results of this test must be used only in the context of an individual patient's clinical scenario.

FEV_1 is that portion of the forced VC measured during the first 1 s of expiration and is another method to measure the severity of airflow obstruction. FEV_1 values less than 25% of predicted are usually associated with increases in $PaCO_2$. Measurement of the peak expiratory flow rate (PEFR) is the maximum point on the forced expiratory limb of the flow volume curve and provides information similar to the FEV_1. Both FEV_1 and PEFR can be used to serially assess the patient's response to bronchodilator therapy.

Both FEV_1 and PEFR are used to diagnose airflow obstruction and assess the response to treatment.

Measurements of respiratory muscle pressures may be helpful in identifying the cause and also the severity of muscle weakness contributing to respiratory failure. Maximum inspiratory and expiratory mouth pressures are global assessments of inspiratory and expiratory muscle strength, respectively. Measurement of respiratory muscle pressures must be performed under conditions of maximum effort at a known lung volume. Because lung volume affects the precontraction length of the respiratory muscles, maximum inspiratory pressure must be recorded at or near residual volume and expiratory muscle pressure must be recorded at or near total lung capacity. When measured under the conditions addressed here, the precontraction length of the inspiratory and expiratory muscles is optimized, and maximum muscle contraction results in a more accurate measurement of muscle strength. However, controlling for lung volume and ensuring maximum patient effort is problematic when measurements are conducted at the bedside in critically ill patients. To obtain meaningful results of respiratory muscle testing, methods must be used that optimize patient and operator performance and simultaneously minimize the impact of lung volume on measured values.

Respiratory muscle pressures may help to identify the cause of respiratory failure by examining the degree of respiratory muscle strength.

Measurement of respiratory muscle pressures depends on patient effort, operator technique, and the lung volumes at which the pressures are measured.

CHEST IMAGING

Chapter 11 reviews radiologic imaging in the critically ill patient in detail. This section only discusses chest imaging as it relates to the evaluation of respiratory failure. In selected patients, chest imaging can provide important information as to the cause of respiratory failure. The imaging test most commonly used for evaluating respiratory failure is the chest x-ray; however, in some circumstances chest computed tomography (CT) and ventilation–perfusion lung scanning may also be valuable.

Common chest imaging in the evaluation of respiratory failure includes the portable chest x-ray and occasionally chest CT and ventilation–perfusion lung scanning.

The chest x-ray may be important in demonstrating the severity of the chest wall abnormality that contributes to the development of respiratory failure. The chest x-ray can identify patients who present in respiratory failure due to severe kyphosiolosis or flail chest. In patients with severe kyphoscoliosis, the amount of thoracic spine deviation on chest x-ray can be quantitated and used to predict the onset of hypercapnic respiratory failure. Other abnormalities seen on chest x-ray that may indicate the presence and magnitude of underlying disease contributing to respiratory failure include the presence and extent of severe COPD, pneumonia, diffuse infiltrates, or pulmonary edema. Chest x-ray findings may suggest the cause and magnitude of the primary pulmonary process that is contributing to the presence of respiratory failure. A chest x-ray may also be helpful in assessing the patient's response to therapy.

In comparison to the chest x-ray, the chest CT is a more sensitive and specific imaging tool in differentiating pleural from parenchymal abnormalities. The chest CT may also be more specific in characterizing the pattern of lung involvement by the underlying disease process. The use of intravenous contrast during chest CT imaging may also help to identify pulmonary vascular abnormalities (e.g., pulmonary embolism, arteriovenous malformation) and their potential role in the pathogenesis of respiratory failure.

In patients who suffer predominantly from unexplained hypoxemic respiratory failure, lung ventilation–perfusion scanning may be helpful in assessing individual lung region participation in ventilation and perfusion. Specific patterns of ventilation–perfusion abnormalities can be considered diagnostic of pulmonary thromboembolism and aid in the diagnosis of pulmonary embolism as a cause for respiratory failure. If lung ventilation–perfusion scanning is nondiagnostic, pulmonary angiography or spiral CT with contrast may help rule in or rule out pulmonary embolism.

Ventilation–perfusion lung scanning may be important in the diagnosis of pulmonary embolism as the cause of respiratory failure.

CASE STUDY: PART 3

The patient was admitted to the intensive care unit and maintained on mechanical ventilation in the assist control node. She remained on 100% oxygen with increasing levels of positive end-expiratory pressure (PEEP) to decrease intrapulmonary shunt and to improve oxygenation by increasing end-expiratory lung volume. After 12 cmH_2O PEEP was applied with an FIO_2 of 100%, her PaO_2 increased to 220 mmHg. F_IO_2 was decreased to 60% to maintain an SaO_2 at 94%. The patient continued to aggressively receive bronchodilator agents to alleviate bronchospasm and was given general sedation and intermittent neuromuscular blocking agents to facilitate patient–ventilator synchrony and to decrease patient effort.

Sputum Gram stain showed a marked increase in the number of white blood cells and gram-negative cocci. The patient was administered cefepime at 1 g twice daily and placed on prophylactic therapy for gastritis and deep venous thrombosis. She was started on enteral feeding via a nasogastric feeding tube.

Other Laboratory Tests

Laboratory tests helpful in diagnosing problems contributing to respiratory failure include hemoglobin, hematocrit, electrolytes, bicarbonate level, anion gap, and concentration of electrolytes, including calcium, magnesium, potassium, and phosphate.

In selected patients, assessment of neuromuscular and cardiovascular status is important.

In some patients, nonpulmonary tests may help provide clues to the cause or the temporal nature of the disorder precipitating respiratory failure. The presence of secondary polycythemia indicates the presence of chronic hypoxemia. Metabolic testing can show electrolyte abnormalities that may explain respiratory pump dysfunction (e.g., hypocalemia, hypokalemia, hypomagnesemia, and hypophosphotemia all impair skeletal muscle contractility) and also related metabolic abnormalities, such as metabolic acidosis or alkalosis, which have major implications for respiratory workload, cardiopulmonary function, and the oxyhemoglobin dissociation curve. In some patients, cardiac ischemia and cardiac dysfunction may contribute to respiratory failure, and assessment with electrocardiography, echocardiogram, or even, at the bedside, right heart catheterization (e.g., Swan–Ganz catheter) may be indicated. Finally, measurements of creatine phosphokinase or aldolase, or electromyography, or tests for nerve conduction may be important to determine whether systemic neurologic diseases are causing respiratory pump failure.

TREATMENT OF RESPIRATORY FAILURE

As is true for identifying the cause of respiratory failure, treatment of respiratory failure is based on characterizing the underlying process as to whether it impairs the respiratory system primarily in its pump capacity (i.e., hypercapnia) or as an area of gas exchange (i.e., hypoxemia). Therefore, organizing diagnostic testing and treatment for respiratory failure is best done after it has been first characterized as hypoxemic, hypercapnic respiratory failure, or as hypoxemic, nonhypercapnic respiratory failure. Figure 13-9 outlines the approach of respiratory failure based on pump or lung failure as predominant causes. More specific guidelines for oxygenating the patient (Chapter 2), the use of mechanical ventilation (Chapters 34 and 35), and providing hemodynamic support (Chapters 37 and 38) are provided in specific chapters. This section briefly outlines treatment as it relates to the patient who presents in respiratory failure.

Oxygenation

Oxygen should always be used as the initial treatment for hypoxemic respiratory failure.

Many devices may be able to provide supplemental oxygen to patients in respiratory failure; nasal prongs are comfortable, but inefficient.

Regardless of etiology, the initial approach to the treatment of patients with respiratory failure is to identify those who need supplemental oxygen. Oxygen is frequently necessary for patients who present with hypoxemia or with conditions known to predispose to hypoxemia. Most of the initial morbidity and mortality found in patients who present in respiratory failure results from untreated hypoxemia.

Various types of external oxygen delivery devices are now available to provide variable concentrations of inspired oxygen. The choice of a particular device depends on (1) the magnitude of supplemental oxygen required by the patient to achieve effective oxygenation;

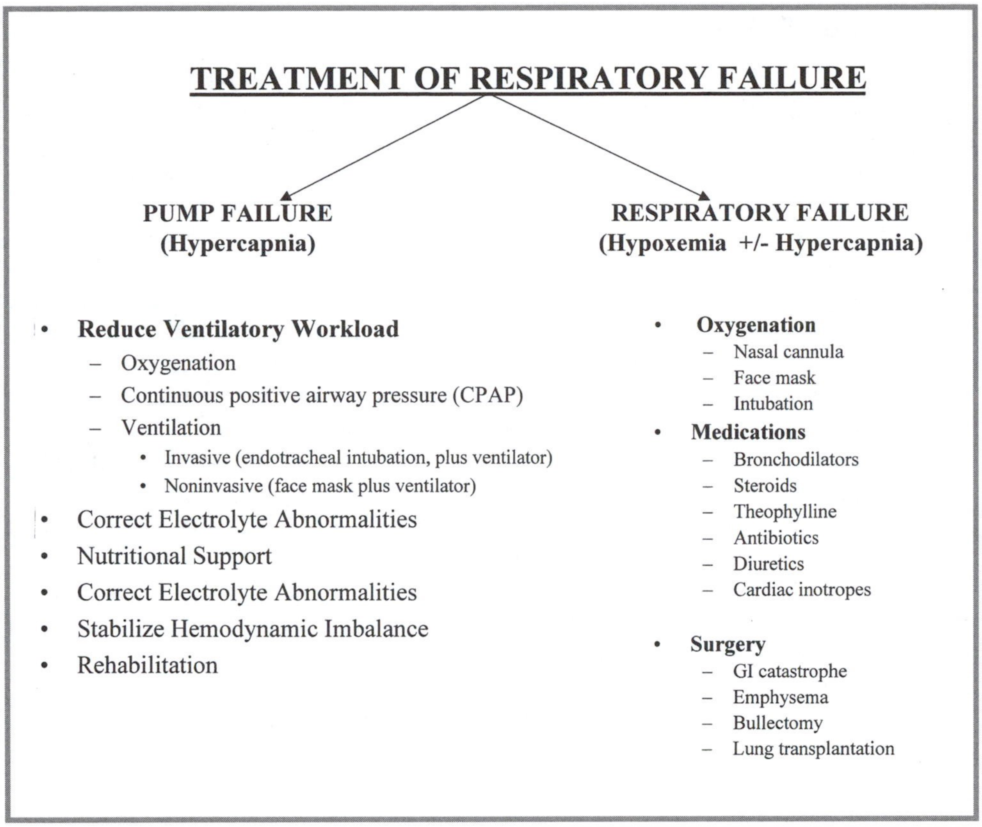

TREATMENT OF RESPIRATORY FAILURE
PUMP FAILURE
(Hypercapnia)
RESPIRATORY FAILURE
(Hypoxemia +/- Hypercapnia)
• Reduce Ventilatory Workload
– Oxygenation
– Continuous positive airway pressure (CPAP)
– Ventilation
• Invasive (endotracheal intubation, plus ventilator)
• Noninvasive (face mask plus ventilator)
• Correct Electrolyte Abnormalities
• Nutritional Support
• Correct Electrolyte Abnormalities
• Stabilize Hemodynamic Imbalance
• Rehabilitation
• Oxygenation
– Nasal cannula
– Face mask
– Intubation
• Medications
– Bronchodilators
– Steroids
– Theophylline
– Antibiotics
– Diuretics
– Cardiac inotropes
• Surgery
– GI catastrophe
– Emphysema
– Bullectomy
– Lung transplantation

FIGURE 13-9

Treatment of respiratory failure organized into pump (hypercapnic) and lung (hypoxemia with, or without, hypercapnic) respiratory failure.

(2) the need for precise control of supplemental oxygen to avoid excessive oxygenation and the development of hypercapnia; (3) whether airway control is needed to suction the patient for excessive secretions; and (4) whether other techniques are needed to increase oxygen by increasing lung volume (externally applying positive pressure to the airway by continuous positive airway pressure (CPAP) or positive end-expiratory pressure (PEEP).

Delivering supplemental oxygen using nasal prongs is the simplest and most comfortable method. However, despite its comfort, this apparatus cannot be used to provide high levels of oxygen. Moreover, it does not provide enriched oxygen in an extremely precise manner, because room air is entrained when patients mouthbreathe or during high levels of spontaneous ventilation. Face mask devices (outlined in Chapter 2) fit more tightly and have nonrebreathing valves that, coupled with an inspiratory reservoir of oxygen, provide higher and more precise concentrations of supplemental oxygen. Using these types of face masks, inspired oxygen concentration may reach 80%–95%. In addition, these devices can accommodate the use of valves to allow titrating external levels of PEEP to simultaneously increase lung volume and therefore decrease intrapulmonary shunt and improve oxygenation. Moreover, delivery of oxygen by means of a face mask with a venturi device, a calibrated inline device, can provide high flows of oxygen in a more precise manner and avoid the effect of room air entrainment on decreasing the amount of inspired oxygen.

Masks are more cumbersome but more efficient in increasing supplemental oxygen concentration.

A venturi delivery device allows more precise prescription of supplemental inspired oxygen.

Medications

The use of medications in treatment of respiratory failure depends on the underlying disorder. In patients who present with an exacerbation of airway obstruction, bronchodilators, corticosteroids, theophylline preparations, and antibiotics are required. In patients who present with pulmonary edema due to volume overload, or with cardiac dysfunction, diuretics are in order. In patients who have more pronounced cardiac dysfunction, the selected use of cardiac inotropes may be required.

Supportive Therapy

Acid–base or electrolyte disturbances may compromise respiratory pump function and contribute to an elevated ventilatory workload. Hypocalemia, hypomagnesemia, hypokalemia, and hypophosphotemia all have been identified as conditions that lead to skeletal muscle weakness and, specifically, respiratory skeletal muscle weakness. Correction of these abnormalities can markedly improve ventilatory muscle strength and increase respiratory reserve. Additionally, regardless of etiology, metabolic acidosis increases ventilatory workload and its presence should be identified and appropriately treated. For example, diabetic ketoacidosis responds to fluid, electrolyte management, and administration of insulin. In other cases, severe metabolic acidosis that causes respiratory compromise and leads to respiratory failure may be best treated by hemodialysis. The use of ancillary testing and physical examination must appropriately diagnose the cause of metabolic acidosis because effective treatment is required before the episode of respiratory failure will resolve.

Besides identification of electrolyte metabolic disturbances, nutritional support and, in some cases, reconditioning are important in restoring respiratory pump function and reversing the presence of respiratory failure. Undernutrition, found in at least 40% of hospitalized COPD patients, has major implications on decreasing respiratory muscle mass and affecting respiratory muscle fiber type composition. Renutrition increases respiratory muscle mass and restores ventilatory muscle endurance, an important beneficial physiologic effect that results in an improvement in respiratory pump function. Moreover, rehabilitation of patients who present in a deconditioned state because of the underlying disease, or with disuse atrophy after a critical illness, is similarly important in restoring respiratory pump function.

Reducing Ventilatory Workload

In some patients, the methods described here are inadequate for reducing ventilatory workload so as to permit spontaneous ventilation. In these cases, ventilatory workload far exceeds ventilatory capacity, and the patient's spontaneous effort must be augmented with mechanical ventilation. Mechanical ventilation is required until the condition causing the higher workload resolves or the patient's ventilatory capacity increases.

Invasive or noninvasive mechanical ventilation is used to augment spontaneous ventilation.

Augmentation of the patient's spontaneous breathing effort can be achieved by either invasive or noninvasive forms of mechanical ventilation. In noninvasive mechanical ventilation, a nasal or nasal oral face mask is used to augment the patient's spontaneous efforts without the use of an artificial airway. In the case of invasive ventilation, an artificial conduit is inserted in the patient's airway, either an endotracheal tube or a subglottically placed tracheotomy tube. In both cases, the ventilator can be manipulated to adjust the amount of applied ventilation, the pattern of breathing, the inspiratory flow rate, and the concentration of inspired oxygenation. Details on the specific use of noninvasive mechanical ventilation are provided in Chapter 35 and the use of invasive mechanical ventilation is discussed in Chapter 34.

Invasive ventilation is the method most frequently used to augment a patient's spontaneous respiratory effort. When using invasive ventilation, airway intubation is considered to be mandatory for the patient's therapy so as to (1) provide airway protection; (2) serve as a conduit for suctioning patients with excessive mouth or lower respiratory tract secretions; (3) achieve higher inspired oxygen concentrations than are possible with a face mask; and (4) apply positive pressure via the ventilator to increase lung volume to treat refractory hypoxemia.

As outlined in Chapter 1, endotracheal intubation may be accomplished by either nasal or oral translaryngeal intubation. Oral intubation uses a larger endotracheal tube and is easier to perform under emergent conditions because the vocal cords are visualized by the use of a fiberoptic endoscope or a laryngoscope. In addition, nosocomial sinusitis is less likely to develop in patients who have oral, in contrast to nasal, intubation. However, in the long term, the oral intubation route is uncomfortable for patients, securing of the endotracheal tube is less stable, and providing optimal oral hygiene is difficult. Nasal intubation is easier to perform in the spontaneously breathing patient, is anchored to the patient's face less obtrusively, and therefore facilitates patient comfort. However, nasal intubation is not without complications. Nasal intubation for longer than 5–7 days is associated with a higher incidence of nosocomial sinusitis and nosocomial pneumonia; also, because of its smaller size, the nasal tube has higher resistance than larger, orally placed tubes. These latter factors may be important in patients who require intubation for treatment of respiratory failure for more than several days, or have a primary increase in airways resistance due to asthma or COPD as a cause of respiratory failure. In both these examples, nasal intubation may hinder the weaning process and lead to more complications. Although no general guidelines can be given for all patients, patients who require a longer intubation for respiratory failure, on balance, probably benefit more from oral versus nasal intubation. If the weaning process continues further, a tracheotomy to provide longer-term positive pressure ventilation should be considered.

Mechanical ventilators are intended to stabilize gas exchange imbalances until the primary process resolves, not necessarily to achieve normal gas exchange parameters of pH, PaO_2, or $PaCO_2$. In some patients, normal values of gas exchange cannot be easily obtained without significant complications arising because of mechanical ventilation. For example, if maintaining a normal $PaCO_2$ or pH predisposes the patient to unacceptably high airway pressures or lung volumes, and results in hypotension or ventilator-induced lung injury, the perceived benefit from achieving normal gas exchange is lost. The goal of ventilation must be readjusted to one that stabilizes the patient's gas exchange imbalance without further subjecting patients to undue complications from the mechanical ventilation process itself. More details on choosing the appropriate form of ventilation and ventilator settings and identifying the complications of mechanical ventilation are provided in Chapters 34 and 35.

> The goal of mechanical ventilation is to stabilize gas exchange disturbance. Obtaining normal values for $PaCO_2$ and PaO_2 is not the primary objective.

Other Therapy

In some patients, surgery may have a limited but occasionally important role in the treatment of respiratory failure. Patients who present with an intraabdominal catastrophe from a ruptured viscus, vascular accident, or severe gastrointestinal bleeding may be required to undergo surgery to treat the underlying problem contributing to respiratory failure. These cases are mainly patients who present with acute manifestations of respiratory failure and usually require surgical intervention during the initial phases of their treatment for respiratory failure.

> Surgery has a limited, but occasionally important, role in the treatment of respiratory failure.

On the other hand, selected patients with severe, advanced lung disease with chronic forms of respiratory failure may be candidates for surgical treatment of respiratory failure per se. In these cases, stabilization of the chest wall in patients who suffer from flail chest, decortication of fibrotic pleura trapping the lung after a preceding pleural space inflammatory process, and resection of large bulla that compromise otherwise viable lung tissue in patients with advanced COPD are some indications for surgery as treatment for chronic respiratory failure. In the past 10 years, single-lung, double-lung, and heart-lung transplantation have

CASE STUDY: PART 4

The patient continued to improve with the use of bronchodilators, antibiotics, and supportive care measures. Subsequent chest x-rays showed significant clearance of pulmonary infiltrates, the patient was able to be lowered to an inspired oxygen concentration of 40%, and PEEP was discontinued. While performing a spontaneous breathing trial via a 40% T-piece setup, the patient demonstrated satisfactory hemodynamic parameters, and respiratory variables, and was extubated. Following extubation, the patient continued to exhibit severe weakness of the lower extremities, secondary to the prior use of high steroids and intermittent use of neuromuscular blocking agents. The patient was transferred to an intermediate care unit where she received whole-body rehabilitation, respiratory toilet, continuation of bronchodilator therapy, and completion of an antibiotic course. As the patient improved, swallowing function was evaluated, and the patient was restored to normal eating. The tracheotomy tube was downsized and eventually the patient was decannulated. The patient was discharged successfully from the hospital to home. The final diagnosis for this patient was mild chronic obstructive lung disease with the development of multilobar *Pseudomonas* pneumonia and respiratory failure.

also been used to treat some patients with advanced lung diseases causing respiratory failure. In these cases, respiratory failure is most likely the result of end-stage COPD, interstitial lung disease, cystic fibrosis, or pulmonary hypertension. However, this therapy, to optimize survival, is relegated to those patients who present with chronic forms of respiratory failure that do not require intensive care unit hospitalization or the use of invasive ventilation.

SUMMARY

The approach to the patient who presents in respiratory failure includes a systematic effort to identify the cause of respiratory failure and categorize it as a pump or lung failure subtype, using clinical history, physical examination, and selected laboratory tests. Treatment options are also organized on the basis of whether pump or lung failure is the predominant cause of respiratory failure and are implemented in a logical fashion to treat the underlying disorder, correct derangements in gas exchange, and reduce ventilatory workload.

REVIEW QUESTIONS

1. **An example of a disorder that primarily causes respiratory system pump failure is multilobar pneumonia. This statement is:**
   A. True
   B. False

2. **A 30-year-old woman presents to the emergency room 1 h after injecting heroin and is found to have an oxygen saturation of 82% by pulse oximetry. An arterial blood gas taken while the patient breathes room air oxygen shows PaO_2 is 55 mmHg, $PaCO_2$ is 48 mmHg, and pH is 7.32. The patient is placed on a 100% face mask; 1 h later, oxygen saturation by pulse oximetry is 88%–90%. The most likely cause of hypoxemia in this patient is:**
   A. Ventilation–perfusion mismatch
   B. Intracardiac shunting
   C. Intrapulmonary shunting
   D. Alveolar hypoventilation

3. **The most important and initial laboratory test to perform in assessment of respiratory failure is:**
   A. Chest x-ray
   B. Serum magnesium
   C. Ventilation-perfusion lung scan
   D. Hemoglobin level
   E. Arterial blood gas

4. **One of the first therapies to consider in a patient presenting in respiratory failure is:**
   A. Mechanical ventilation
   B. Surgical intervention
   C. Antibiotics
   D. Bronchodilators
   E. Supplemental oxygen

5. **A 28-year-old man presents with a change in mental status over the past 4 days. He has a known diagnosis of chronic spinal muscle atrophy and is followed in neurology clinic. Over the last several days to weeks, the patient's family has noted an increase in morning headaches, the development of hypersomnolence, and increased forgetfulness. An arterial blood gas while the patient is breathing room air oxygen shows PaO_2 is 40 mmHg, $PaCO_2$ is 80 mmHg, and pH is 7.29. The most likely cause of hypoxemia in this patient is:**
   A. Ventilation–perfusion imbalance
   B. Intracardiac shunting
   C. Intrapulmonary shunting
   D. Alveolar hypoventilation

ANSWERS

1. The answer is B. False. Multilobar pneumonia is an example of lung failure wherein hypoxemia results when the alveolus becomes filled with inflammatory debris and fluid; this results in hypoxemic respiratory failure as a result of intrapulmonary shunting and ventilation–perfusion imbalance. Diseases in which respiratory failure is caused by pump failure include disorders that affect the cerebral and peripheral nervous system, chest wall, upper airways, and respiratory muscles.

2. The answer is C. Intrapulmonary shunting. Although this patient presented with a disorder that could lead to alveolar hypoventilation, namely heroin overdose, the patient's blood gas does not show profound hypoventilation. By using the alveolar gas equation, the patient's A-a gradient was found to be 35. The patient demonstrated refractoriness to improving her oxygenation by use of a high concentration of inspired oxygen. Hypoxemia in this patient's cause is associated with an elevated A-a gradient, which is re-

fractory to a high concentration of inspired oxygen; this would most likely be a result of intrapulmonary or intracardiac shunting. In this case, without prior cardiac history, and in light of a known condition that can lead to pulmonary aspiration of gastric contents or heroin-induced cardiogenic edema, a pulmonary disease such as multilobar pneumonia, aspiration pneumonia, or acute respiratory distress syndrome, leading to intrapulmonary shunting, is the most likely diagnosis.

3. The answer is E. The arterial blood gas. The arterial blood gas analysis allows one to measure three important components in determining the cause, the severity, and finally the chronicity of the disturbance causing respiratory failure. With a blood gas, one measures PaO_2, $PaCO_2$, and pH. One can also calculate the alveolar–arterial oxygen gradient to determine whether a reduction in PaO_2 is secondary to hypoventilation vs intrapulmonary, intracardiac shunt, or ventilation–perfusion imbalance.
4. The answer is E. Supplemental oxygen. In most patients who present in respiratory failure, hypoxemia is present. In fact, in almost all cases of respiratory failure, hypoxemia is the most important derangement in gas exchange. If untreated, hypoxemia can contribute to the development of stroke, myocardial dysfunction, or some other manifestation of severe organ dysfunction. Therefore, oxygen is the first therapy to contemplate in the patient who presents in respiratory failure. In patients who present with pump dysfunction, the use of devices to augment spontaneous ventilation are required, that is, mechanical ventilation in the form of noninvasive or invasive modalities. Similarly, bronchodilators and antibiotics have a role as adjunctive therapy when patients present with bronchospasm or infection. However, oxygen is the first therapy to consider because hypoxemia is the major disturbance in patients who present with respiratory failure, which has substantial morbidity and mortality.
5. The answer is D. Alveolar hypoventilation. In the patient breathing room air at sea level, the P_IO_2 is 150. Subtracting from this value, the $PaCO_2/R$ (assuming $R = 0.8$) and then subtracting PaO_2 of 40 mmHg measured from an arterial blood gas, the alveolar–arterial oxygen gradient is 10. An A-a gradient of 10 suggests that the lung is normal and the patient's hypoxemia is a result of respiratory pump failure, or hypoventilation. The pH is greater than expected if this was due to an acute condition causing respiratory failure, suggesting that this is an acute-on-chronic presentation of respiratory failure, or a compensated chronic respiratory acidosis. Features from the patient's history documenting a decline in mental function over several days to a week, the development of hypersomnolence, and an early morning headache all suggest an insidious onset of progressive hypercapnia.

SUGGESTED READING

Dantzker MD, David R. Pulmonary gas exchange. In: Bone R (ed) Pulmonary and Critical Care Medicine. Mosby: St. Louis, 1997: [Part B] 1–13.

Grippi MA. Respiratory failure: an overview. In: Fishman AP (ed) Fishman's Pulmonary Diseases and Disorder. New York: McGraw-Hill, 1998:2525–2535.

Irwin RS, Pratter MR. A physiologic approach to managing respiratory failure. In: Rippe JN, Irwin RS, Fink NP, Cerra FB (eds) Intensive Care Medicine. Boston: Little, Brown, 1996:581–586.

CHAPTER 14

PAUL MATHER AND GILBERT E. D'ALONZO

Heart Failure

CHAPTER OUTLINE

LEARNING OBJECTIVES

After studying this chapter, you should be able to:

- Define congestive heart failure.
- Classify the epidemiology of congestive heart failure.
- Understand the morbidity and mortality statistics of congestive heart failure.
- Recognize the signs and symptoms of congestive heart failure.
- Know the major treatment algorithms of congestive heart failure.
- Understand the pharmacology and pathophysiology behind the treatment regimens.
- Understand the limitations of the treatment regimens.

CONGESTIVE HEART FAILURE

Congestive heart failure (CHF) is a major health problem in the United States with a prevalence that has been increasing and a mortality rate that remains high, even as adverse outcomes from other forms of cardiovascular disease have declined. In a critically ill patient, cardiac failure is an ominous sign that requires prompt recognition and aggressive management. Cardiac failure can be acute or more subtle in character, even as a chronic disease process. Heart failure can involve the right heart or left heart, or it can be biventricular in character, and it can occur during diastole or systole. Diastolic left ventricular failure can be very difficult to recognize and diagnose. The degree of valvular dysfunction associated with cardiac failure can vary even in an individual patient, depending on the status of ventricular function and the intravascular volume of the patient.

More than 4 million people in the United States have CHF, and about 400,000 new cases are diagnosed each year. Heart failure is responsible for nearly 1 million hospitalizations an-

CASE STUDY: PART 1

The patient was a 52-year-old man who was admitted to the coronary care unit after presenting in the emergency room with crushing substernal chest pain accompanied by pulmonary edema. This 52-year-old African-American man had a history of hypertension and coronary artery disease and had several acute myocardial infarctions in the preceding decade. He also had a history of tobacco abuse and hypercholesterolemia. During the past 2 years, he had three admissions to the hospital for acute pulmonary edema and angina. He presented to the emergency room with crushing substernal chest pain accompanied by pulmonary edema, and he required intubation and mechanical ventilatory support with intraaortic balloon counterpulsation. His wife stated that he awoke at 2:00 A.M. that morning with complaints of chest pain and severe shortness of breath.

His family history was significant for coronary artery disease: myocardial infarction in his father at age 55 and in two brothers in their sixth decade. His current medications included a beta-blocker for hypertension and an HMG-CoA reductase inhibitor for cholesterol control. He was intermittently compliant with both medications.

His physical findings were as follows:

- Age: 52 years
- Sex: Male
- Race: African-American
- Height: 5 ft, 10 in.
- Weight: 225 lb
- BP: 100/70 mmHg
- Pulse: 120 bpm
- Funduscopy: Diffuse arteriolar narrowing
- Lungs: Clear to auscultation and percussion
- Cardiac exam: Tachycardia with an S4 and the sounds of an intraaortic balloon counterpulsation; jugular venous distension (JVD) to 12 cm; diminished pulses in the lower extremities.
- Edema: Trace pitting edema

nually. For each decade above the age of 45 years, the incidence of heart failure more than doubles. The prevalence of heart failure is similar for males and females. Males before the age of 64 years have the highest prevalence, but after 65 years of age the difference between males and females is insignificant.

Congestive heart failure (CHF) rates are increasing as the U.S. population ages.

Patients with hypertension and a prior history of myocardial infarction have the highest incidence of CHF. It has been postulated that the steady increase in the number of patients with heart failure is directly linked to the decreasing mortality rates of coronary artery disease, myocardial infarction, and stroke. With improved management of these underlying problems, patients are surviving long enough to develop CHF.

The number of deaths from CHF has increased fourfold over the past 20 years. As for most diseases, the mortality rate increases with age and is higher in men than in women. Racially, it is higher at all ages in African-Americans than Caucasians. Hispanics and Asians appear to have a lower incidence of heart failure. Sudden death occurs in nearly 40% of patients with chronic heart failure.

Sudden death occurs in ~40% of chronic CHF patients.

Prognostically, patients with CHF are in a difficult situation. Half will die within 5 years of diagnosis, and for patients with advanced heart failure, the 1-year survival is approximately 30%. On the brighter side, there has been an improvement in death rates during the first year after diagnosis, with a decrease from approximately 50% to 10% for some categories. Mortality quickly increases when the left ventricular ejection fraction declines below 20%; this is usually found in patients who have poor functional performance. A functional class assessment by the New York Heart Association (NYHA) criteria of class IV is known to have a mortality of 50% at 1 year. A simple and prognostically relevant exercise test, the 6-min walk test, has been used to predict poor survival. Patients with heart failure who are allowed to walk at a self-pace for 6 min and who cannot travel more than 300 m have been shown to have a poor prognosis. Finally, certain hemodynamic abnormalities have been associated with a poor prognosis in patients with heart failure. A cardiac index of less than 2.25 $l/min/m^2$, a pulmonary arterial occlusion pressure of greater than 25 mmHg, and a right atrial pressure greater than 10 mmHg are all indicators of poor survival.

NYHA function class IV has a 1-year mortality ≥50%.

Definitions

Heart failure can be acute or chronic in character. In fact, acute heart failure can occur in individuals with chronic heart failure. The heart failure could be biventricular in nature or

CHF is mainly systolic in nature but can be a manifestation of diastolic disease.

TABLE 14-1

ETIOLOGIES OF DIASTOLIC DYSFUNCTION

Abnormal relaxation
Ischemia
Ventricular hypertrophy from hypertension
Increased stiffness
Infiltrative disorders such as amyloidosis
Extrinsic compression
Pulmonary hypertension
Pericardial diseases
Positive-pressure mechanical ventilation

could involve mainly the left or right heart. Generally, cardiac failure is systolic in character, but in certain individuals, diastolic heart failure is the predominant feature.

In approximately 40% of patients with newly diagnosed heart failure, systolic function is normal. The problem in these patients is a decrease in left ventricular distensibility, a condition referred to as diastolic dysfunction or heart failure. Diastolic dysfunction refers to the inability of the left ventricle to accept blood at a low ventricular pressure, with an associated delay in chamber filling. In a compensatory fashion, left atrial pressure increases, and this condition can lead to pulmonary congestion and, with more progressive disease, even systemic congestion. Systemic congestion can actually occur in the absence of an abnormality in systolic function of the left ventricle. There are numerous etiologies responsible for diastolic dysfunction (Table 14-1) but the common causes include ventricular hypertrophy myocardial ischemia, pericardial disease, and positive-pressure mechanical ventilation. Most patients are elderly with ischemic heart disease and recurrent pulmonary edema despite normal left ventricular systolic function. These patients generally have a long-standing history of systemic hypertension. Finally, patients with renal insufficiency and mitral regurgitation are even more likely to develop pulmonary edema when they have diastolic dysfunction.

Most patients with CHF in the United States are elderly with ischemic disease.

Etiologies

At present, the major causes of heart failure in the United States include ischemic heart disease, idiopathic or viral cardiomyopathy, and hypertensive heart disease. Many other disease processes can have an impact on the heart and cause cardiomyopathy. Regardless of the cause, the three major mechanisms for systolic dysfunction are loss of viable ventricular muscle, a primary abnormality of cardiac muscle, or a serious mechanical abnormality of the muscle, valves, or path of blood flow through the heart (Table 14-2). Determining the cause of heart failure in each patient is crucial to identifying potentially reversible causes, such as correcting a valvular abnormality surgically or aggressively treating systemic hypertension. Although some patients may have relentless disease progression with no precipitating cause, many others have a definite triggering event. Before patients can be labeled as having idiopathic cardiomyopathy or nonischemic cardiomyopathy, they must be evaluated for subtle endocrine abnormalities, a variety of metabolic diseases, and certain connective tissue disorders.

Determining the cause of CHF is crucial to identifying potentially reversible causes.

Metabolic and endocrinologic abnormalities must be excluded for a diagnosis of idiopathic CM.

Potentially reversible causes of cardiomyopathy include alcohol-induced disease, viral infection, noninfectious myocarditis, nutritional deficiencies such as thiamine deficiency or beri beri, and ischemic heart disease.

Chronic heart failure can take an acute course due to a variety of influences. Dietary indiscretion, especially sodium and alcohol intake, and inappropriate changes in medical therapy are the most common reasons for stable patients to decompensate suddenly. Other precipitating causes include new arrhythmias, specifically atrial fibrillation, metabolic abnormalities such as ketoacidosis, electrolyte imbalance, uremia, and pulmonary embolism.

TABLE 14-2

MECHANISMS OF SYSTOLIC DYSFUNCTION

Loss of viable ventricular muscle
Coronary artery disease
Infectious and/or inflammatory damage
Traumatic damage
Acquired cardiomyopathies (i.e., postpartum, obesity)
Primary abnormality of cardiac muscle
Infiltrative disorders
Glycogen storage disorders
Muscular dystrophies
Metabolic damage
Neoplastic disorders
Fibroelastic disorders
Genetic disorders (i.e., hypertrophic cardiomyopathies, hereditary dilated)
Mechanical abnormalities
Valvular
Congenital malformations

DIAGNOSIS

Patients with systolic heart failure show persistence of various signs and symptoms. When these signs and symptoms occur despite maximum medical therapy, we call this form of heart failure refractory. Dyspnea that occurs during or following moderate exertion results from the development of anaerobic metabolism and its consequent metabolic factors such as lactic acidosis, which activates respiratory drive to eliminate carbon dioxide as a buffering effect. In contrast, the dyspnea that occurs at rest in patients with refractory heart failure results from elevated atrial and intrapulmonary vascular pressure.

Lactic acidosis can activate the respiratory drive.

Dyspnea at rest is caused by elevations in atrial and intrapulmonary vascular pressure.

Orthopnea, often accompanied by anorexia and gastrointestinal distress, is related to systemic venous congestion. Systemic venous congestion can be suspected if jugular venous

CASE STUDY: PART 2

The laboratory results were as follows.

- Chest x-ray: intraaortic balloon pump in the appropriate position.
- Mild cephalization and an enlarged cardiac silhouette with a large left pleural effusion. The left atrium (directly under the bifurcation of the carina) was enlarged, as was the right ventricle.
- Echocardiogram: severe left ventricular dysfunction with an ejection fraction of 10%–15%; anterior, apical, and septal dyskinesia with an aneurysm. Normal right ventricular function with mild mitral regurgitation, no aortic regurgitation, and an enlarged left ventricular diastolic dimension. No pericardial effusion.
- Electrocardiogram: sinus tachycardia with a complete left bundle branch block and left axis deviation.
- Cardiac catheterization: normal main left coronary artery; 100% proximal occlusion of the left anterior descending coronary artery with right to left collaterals. Significant occlusions of the right and left circumflex coronary arteries, and extremely poor distal targets, which were considered to be unsuitable for surgical or noninterventional treatment. Right heart hemodynamics were as follows: right atrial (RA) pressure, 14 mmHg; pulmonary artery (PA) pressure, 52/29 mmHg (mean, 37 mmHg); pulmonary capillary wedge pressure, 28 mmHg; cardiac index, 1.90 l/min/m^2; and systemic vascular resistance (SVR), 1550 dynes/s/cm^5.

The impression is that of a 52-year-old man with multiple coronary risk factors and a prior history of myocardial infarctions. The patient presented with acute angina and pulmonary edema. He has developed a severe dilated cardiomyopathy from an ischemic origin. He continues to have myocardial infarctions as a result of poor coronary artery perfusion. He has nonrevascularized lesions and is in acute cardiogenic shock. His renal insufficiency is most likely caused by long-standing hypertension and a low cardiac index, which has led to diminution of the glomerular filtration rate. He may also have renal arteriopathy because of multiple areas of vascular disease, as noted in the decrease of his peripheral pulses when the intraaortic balloon pump was placed. The signs and symptoms of CHF in this patient indicate that acute ischemia has exacerbated an underlying ischemic cardiomyopathy.

Only an occasional patient has lung crackles.

distension is noted. Peripheral edema is present in only a minority of patients with heart failure. Only an occasional patient has lung crackles on physical examination of the chest. Patients with anorexia and early satiety often have abdominal discomfort and evidence of liver engorgement on palpation. Tenderness on palpation of the right upper quadrant of the abdomen, but not hepatomegaly, is often found on examination.

Cheyne–Stokes respiration has been associated with a low cardiac output states.

In the presence of a sinus heart rhythm, the proportional blood pressure measurement is an important physical finding in patients with advanced heart failure. An arterial pulse pressure of less than 25% of the systolic pressure has been shown to be an indicator of a severely reduced cardiac index, generally less than 2 $l/min/m^2$. Finally, patients with severe left ventricular dysfunction can experience disrupted sleep because of either sleep apnea or periodic breathing. Periodic breathing during sleep, or Cheyne–Stokes respiration, has been associated with a low cardiac output state.

The earliest sign of ventricular dysfunction is dyspnea on exertion.

With decompensated CHF, peripheral vasoconstriction occurs.

The earliest sign of ventricular dysfunction is dyspnea at rest and during exertion. As already mentioned, an elevated jugular venous pressure and hepatojugular reflux or a positive abdominojugular test is associated with an increase in pulmonary capillary wedge pressure. At this stage, the stroke volume of the heart is maintained because the left ventricle is still preload responsive. The next stage is a substantial decrease in left ventricular stroke volume with an increase in heart rate. Tachycardia helps compensate for the reduction in stroke volume, so that the cardiac output remains unchanged. At this stage, the dyspnea, especially during exertion, worsens, but there is still no evidence of peripheral edema. The final stage of heart failure is characterized by a decrease in cardiac output, marking the transition from compensated to decompensated heart failure. With decompensation, peripheral vasoconstriction occurs, which eventually causes further reduction in cardiac output and peripheral blood flow (Figure 14-1).

Cardiac filling pressures do not distinguish systolic versus diastolic pressure.

Routine hemodynamic measurements cannot distinguish diastolic from systolic heart failure. The decrease in stroke volume occurs in both systolic and diastolic failure. In systolic failure, the end-diastolic left ventricular volume is elevated at a high diastolic pressure whereas in diastolic, failure the end-diastolic volume at a comparable end-diastolic pressure is much lower. Therefore, monitoring cardiac filling pressures as an index of ventricular preload does not allow a distinction between systolic and diastolic heart failure.

The end-diastolic volume is the best measure for identifying systolic and diastolic heart failure. End-diastolic volume (EDV) can be derived by the relationship between stroke volume (SV) and the ejection fraction (EF): EDV = SV/EF. The EF of the left ventricle can be measured noninvasively by radionuclide or echocardiographic techniques. The stroke volume can be determined by right heart catheterization.

Right heart failure is prevalent in the intensive care unit, especially in patients who are ventilator dependent. The relationship between central venous pressure (CVP) and pulmonary

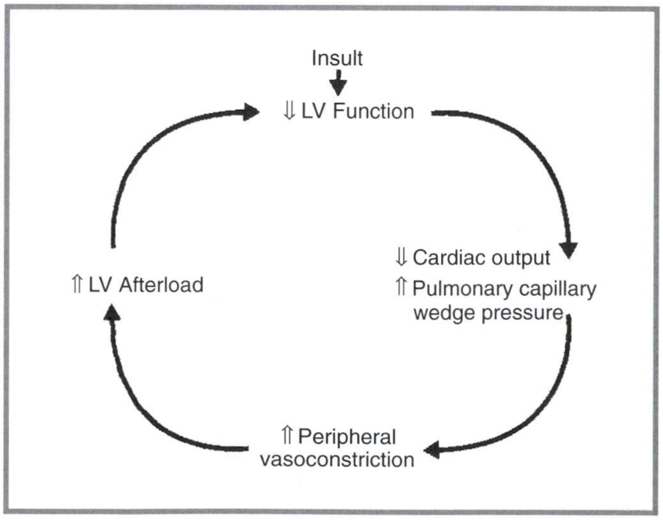

FIGURE 14-1

Pathophysiology of congestive heart failure. *LV*, left ventricular.

TABLE 14-3

NEW YORK HEART ASSOCIATION FUNCTIONAL CLASSIFICATION OF HEART FAILURE

Class I:	No limitations. Activities of daily living do not cause undue fatigue, malaise, dyspnea, or symptomatic palpitations.
Class II:	Mild limitations. Ordinary physical activity causes profound fatigue, dyspnea, and or anginal symptoms. The patient is generally asymptomatic at rest.
Class III:	Severe limitations. Minimal activity causes significant symptoms; however, at rest, the patient is usually relatively asymptomatic.
Class IV:	Any physical activity will cause severe symptoms and discomfort. Symptoms of congestive heart failure are present even at rest.

SOURCE: Adapted from the Criteria Committee, New York Heart Association, Inc. Diseases of the Heart and Blood Vessels. Nomenclature and Criteria for Diagnosis, 6th Ed. Boston: Little, Brown, 1964:114

capillary wedge pressure (PCWP) can be useful in identifying patients with right heart failure. In patients with a CVP that is greater than 15 mmHg and a CVP that equals PCWP or a CVP greater than PCWP, right heart failure should be considered. However, about one-third of patients with acute right heart failure do not satisfy these criteria because of the insensitivity of CVP. An increase in CVP is seen only in the later stages of right heart failure.

If the central venous pressure (CVP) ≥ pulmonary capillary wedge pressure (PCWP), then right heart failure should be considered.

Another problem with measuring cardiac filling pressures to identify right heart failure is the interaction between the right and left sides of the heart, so-called ventricular interdependence. Because the ventricles share the same septum, an enlargement of the right ventricle pushes the septum toward the left side, compromising left ventricular chamber size and influencing pressure and function. This relationship can confuse the interpretation of ventricular filling pressures to the point that hemodynamic changes in right heart failure appear as pericardial tamponade. Finally, echocardiography can be useful at the bedside for determining right from left heart failure. Typically, right heart failure is associated with an increase in right ventricular chamber size and paradoxical motion of the interventricular septum. These findings must be interpreted according to the clinical situation.

Echocardiography at the bedside can be useful to assess right ventricular (RV) and left ventricular (LV) function.

Heart failure can take months to years to develop. Patients commonly present with symptoms of exercise intolerance and dyspnea. Heart failure can also occur in asymptomatic patients with left ventricular dysfunction. Identification of these patients with no or minimal symptoms, with the aim of preventing the development of overt heart failure, is an important diagnostic and therapeutic challenge. Currently, functional classification of heart failure is based on the New York Heart Association (NYHA) classification system (Table 14-3). NYHA I patients have no symptoms, but their physiology is consistent with left ventricular or right ventricular dysfunction, whereas NYHA IV patients have serious symptoms at rest.

Identification of asymptomatic LV dysfunction is a diagnostic and therapeutic challenge.

PATHOPHYSIOLOGY

Heart failure is a clinical syndrome that results from the complex interaction between an initial myocardial insult and reactive, compensatory processes. During the natural course of heart failure development, patients progress from a clinically silent state in which the heart muscle undergoes changes in cellular function to preserve cardiac output and to normalize ventricular wall stress (e.g., by hypertrophy) to overt symptoms resulting from ventricular decompensation. Clinically, heart failure is classified as systolic or diastolic or both and can occur in the left or right ventricle or be biventricular. This definition can be extended to include chronic or acute decompensation. Understanding the pathophysiology of heart failure is vital to the management of this disease. Ventricular hypertrophy and remodeling occur in response to pressure-overloaded conditions, volume-overloaded conditions, or tissue injury and infarction. The role of the hypertrophic process is to preserve stroke volume and cardiac output. Pressure-overloaded conditions stimulate cardiac hypertrophy. In this type, there is lateral expansion of the myocytes through addition of myofibril units in parallel. In contrast, volume-overloaded conditions stimulate ventricular cavity enlargement without a change in wall thickness. This enlargement occurs through replication of sarcomeres in series. Myocardial infarction leads to ventricular dilation because the infarcted segment ex-

CHF is characterized as systolic, diastolic, or biventricular.

Hypertrophy and remodeling are ventricular responses to pressure overload conditions.

Volume overload stimulates LV cavity dilatation.

pands or stretches. The dilation involves loss of myocytes and disruption of the normal architecture of the ventricular wall. Within the surviving myocytes, abnormal stretching increases tension in each cell and promotes hypertrophy. The dilation of the infarcted segment increases pressure on the noninfarcted myocardium and stimulates hypertrophy.

Chronic systolic dysfunction is the most common type of CHF.

Chronic systolic or low-output heart failure is the most common type of heart failure. Systolic failure is the condition that results when the weakened, dilated heart is unable to eject an adequate stroke volume. The syndrome of systolic heart failure begins with a period of adaptive cardiac myocyte remodeling that involves changes in both wall geometry and cavity size. Left untreated, the systolic dysfunction will continue until compensatory mechanisms can no longer sustain circulatory function. The volume-overloaded ventricle will eventually decompensate. Contractility continues to decline, and ventricular filling pressure rises. The resulting greater oxygen demand on surviving cells promotes further cell loss. This continuous loss of cells disrupts the normal architecture of the ventricular wall, and the shape of the ventricle changes from elliptic to globular; hence, cardiomegaly develops, which is characteristic of end-stage CHF.

Wall geometry and cavity size change as the ventricle decompensates.

Loss of ventricular compliance impairs relaxation.

Diastolic heart failure results when the heart cannot fill effectively during diastole. It is most common when there is a loss of ventricular compliance that impairs relaxation, as can occur with left ventricular hypertrophy, coronary artery disease, and normal aging. The characteristic hemodynamic disturbance in diastolic dysfunction is higher ventricular filling pressures at the same volume. With this pathology, symptoms of pulmonary venous congestion develop in the absence of systolic dysfunction. If a hemodynamic evaluation, perhaps by echocardiography, shows that systolic function of the left ventricle is preserved and there is a reduced degree of diastolic filling, then therapy should be directed at improving diastolic ventricular function.

A characteristic hemodynamic disturbance in diastolic dysfunction (DD) is higher ventricular filling pressures at the same volume.

Three mechanisms are involved in the pathophysiology of diastolic heart failure (Table 14-4). These mechanisms often operate concomitantly, and all of them elevate the pressure–volume relationship of ventricular filling, in other words, decrease ventricular compliance. The first mechanism is impaired, slowed, or incomplete ventricular wall relaxation. During early diastolic filling, left atrial pressure can exceed left ventricular pressure and pulmonary congestion symptoms can develop. Another mechanism increases the stiffness of the ventricle during both early and late diastole as a result of increased left ventricular thickness and decreased internal chamber dimensions; it can be caused by an infiltrative disease process such as amyloidosis or by wall hypertrophy, which is seen in chronic, poorly controlled systemic hypertension. The final mechanism, high concentrations of ventricular wall collagen, generally occurs in conjunction with myocardial infarction where excess collagen is deposited in the injured segment; this change can affect each myocardial unit, causing increased stiffness, and can affect diastolic pressure as a whole. The left ventricular hypertrophy associated with diastolic failure results from pressure overload, which stimulates concentric hypertrophy. As myocytes expand through addition of myofibril units in parallel, fibrous tissue is laid down to maintain structural integrity. In most cases, myocytes in a concentrically hypertrophied human heart contract normally, whereas the laying down of fibrous tissue impairs contractile efficacy. Active fibrosis isolates the individual muscle cells, destroying the ventricular structure and leading to diastolic stiffness. Hence, the loss of contractility that is considered the hallmark of heart failure is not the instigating mechanism in diastolic failure but rather the consequence of the initial insult.

Pressure overload causes LV hypertrophy.

Fibrous tissue impairs myocyte contraction.

Loss of contractility occurs as a result of an insult in diastolic CHF.

Coronary artery disease (CAD) is the most common cause of systolic CHF.

Coronary artery disease (CAD) is the most common cause of systolic heart failure, but it is frequently associated with diastolic dysfunction as well. Diastolic function deteriorates

TABLE 14-4

PATHOPHYSIOLOGY OF DIASTOLIC DYSFUNCTION

Impaired ventricular wall relaxation
Increased ventricular stiffness
Increased collagen deposition in the ventricular walls

with normal aging. Both loss of myocytes and increased fibrosis have been described. Apoptosis or programmed cell death may be one factor contributing to the loss of myocytes, or hypertrophy itself may accelerate the cellular death process. Aging is also associated with collagen remodeling following myocyte necrosis. Some of this remodeling consists of fibrosis that replaces lost myocardium, but the predominant change occurs in the interstitium, where deposition of collagen occurs around myocytes, isolating individual muscle cells.

The depression of contractile function that occurs in heart failure and is associated with myocardial remodeling is the result of certain changes in biochemical and molecular function and gene expression. Myocardial remodeling includes both structural and functional reorganization of cardiac cells. Various mechanisms appear to be involved in the development of hampered contractility, including alterations in the excitation–contraction coupling process, neurohumoral changes, and various actions of certain growth factors. Disruption in the mechanisms for handling calcium ion distribution within cardiac cells has been found in patients with heart failure.

Myocardial remodeling includes both structural and functional reorganization of cardiac cells.

A number of neurohumoral alterations are present in heart failure. Even before patients become symptomatic, there is a reflex increase in neurohumoral activity in response to the decreased cardiac output. Initially, activation of the sympathetic nervous system results in an increase in heart rate and myocardial contractility, which leads to enhanced cardiac output. Also, there is an increase in sympathetic vascular tone that maintains peripheral vascular resistance and perfusion pressure gradients to systemic organ beds. However, this intensified cardiac functioning places an increased demand for myocardial oxygen on the already weakened myocardial cells.

In heart failure, there is an increase in sympathetic vascular tone that maintains peripheral vascular resistance and perfusion pressure gradients to systemic organ beds.

As heart failure progresses, the heart is exposed to increasing levels of catecholamines that are toxic to the failing organ. Catecholamines have been shown to stimulate protein synthesis and enhance collagen deposition and myocardial fibrosis, leading to ventricular hypertrophy and remodeling. High doses of norepinephrine also can cause myocarditis, myocardial necrosis, and cardiomyopathy, and selective downward regulation of beta-1 receptor density occurs in response to this high adrenergic drive. The decrease of beta-1 receptors appears to be proportionate to the amount of ventricular dysfunction. Plasma levels of norepinephrine have prognostic importance. Elevated plasma norepinephrine is an important predictor of mortality in heart failure patients. Catecholamines, especially in the presence of myocardial ischemia, cause serious arrhythmias, a frequent mode of sudden death in heart failure patients. Also, norepinephrine increases arterial vasoconstriction, thus enhancing afterload on the failing left ventricle.

As heart failure progresses, the heart is exposed to increasing catecholamines that are toxic to the failing organ.

Plasma levels of norepinephrine have prognostic importance.

The renin-angiotensin-aldosterone system is activated in heart failure. The immediate response to a decrease in heart function and a reduction in blood pressure is a decrease in stretch stimulation of baroreceptors in the carotid and aortic sinuses. This change reduces the number of nerve impulses sent to regulatory centers in the CNS, resulting in a reflex increase in sympathetic outflow and a decrease in vagal stimulation to the heart and vasculature. The cumulative effect is to return blood pressure toward its previous level through increased heart rate and contractility and vasoconstriction of arterials. Underlying these rapid events is a slowly developing series of neurohumoral alterations that are also promoted by the decrease in cardiac output and blood pressure. These alterations include increases in plasma renin activity, promoting sodium and water retention, and increases in arginine vasopressin, aldosterone, and endothelin, which induce vasoconstriction. Because the responsiveness to atrial natruretic peptide is blunted, peripheral dilation, diuresis, and natruresis are attenuated, and a vasoconstrictive and volume-overloaded environment ensures.

The renin-angiotensin-aldosterone system is activated in heart failure.

The abnormal neurohumoral cascade includes increases in plasma renin activity, promoting sodium and water retention and increases in arginine vasopressin, aldosterone, and endothelin, which induce vasoconstriction.

The systemic reflexes of vasoconstriction, fluid retention, and increase in heart rate generally maintain blood pressure at the expense of cardiac output. Accordingly, most patients with chronic heart failure are not hypotensive. However, the impaired heart must continue to work under excessive loading conditions. Continuous ejection of blood into this vasoconstricted vascular system, coupled with compensatory excess fluid volume in the circulatory system, increases myocardial oxygen consumption, contributes to myocardial ischemia, and produces an unstable cardiac cellular environment that increases the likelihood of lethal arrhythmias. All these factors act together to accelerate the deterioration of overloaded myocardial cells.

Systemic reflexes generally maintain blood pressure at the expense of cardiac output.

Increased myocardial oxygen consumption is ongoing in heart failure.

CASE STUDY: PART 3

Treatment and Follow-Up. The patient was continued on his intraaortic balloon counterpulsation and was started on intravenous nitroglycerin. He was also given an intravenous pressor (dobutamine) to increase his cardiac output. Intravenous dobutamine and intravenous nitroglycerin allowed weaning the patient from his intraaortic balloon counterpulsation. He was given oral angiotensin-converting enzyme (ACE) inhibitors, digoxin, and diuretics, which were used to wean him from his intravenous pressor support. His right heart hemodynamics improved significantly with this medical regimen.

The rationale for the choice for intravenous dobutamine was to improve the patient's hemodynamics by increasing his cardiac index with a positive inotropic agent. The oral ACE inhibitors, digoxin, and diuretics were used to decrease his peripheral resistance and also increase his cardiac index. Once the burden of the acute ischemic event was overcome, the patient's CHF symptoms were stabilized with oral medication.

The patient was successfully weaned from the intravenous dobutamine and stabilized on his oral regimen. Because his coronary artery disease was considered to be inoperable, he was placed on a rigorous outpatient heart failure therapy program with close monitoring. He and his family had received intensive education regarding the signs, symptoms, and treatment of CHF while he was in the hospital. He was also strongly urged to cease alcohol and tobacco abuse and was given a plan for doing so. This patient would be considered for possible intervention with an orthotopic heart transplant in the future if necessary.

The decrease in contractility characteristic of heart failure can be viewed as a series of adaptive and maladaptive processes in response to an initiating pathologic event.

The decrease in contractility characteristic of heart failure can be viewed as a series of adaptive and maladaptive processes in response to an initiating pathologic event. After an initial insult from any number of causes, the heart adapts to various metabolic and structural changes. These changes, which result from a series of biochemical, biophysical, and molecular events that are set into motion by myocardial injury, can continue for months to years and keep the patient nearly symptom free.

PHARMACOLOGIC MANAGEMENT STRATEGIES

Systolic Left Ventricular Failure

Managing heart failure should involve the maintenance of cardiac output with a secondary goal of decreasing venous capillary pressure and edema formation.

The optimal PCWP is the pressure that augments cardiac output without inducing clinically relevant pulmonary edema.

Managing heart failure should involve the maintenance of cardiac output with a secondary goal of decreasing venous capillary pressure and edema formation. Left heart failure can be either systolic or diastolic in nature. The approach to left ventricular systolic failure generally focuses on optimizing PCWP and then on systemic arterial pressure. The correction of an inadequate filling pressure is imperative in the management of systolic left ventricular heart failure. The optimal PCWP is the pressure that augments cardiac output without inducing clinically relevant pulmonary edema. This pressure can be best demonstrated by reviewing ventricular function curves for the normal and failing left ventricle. As PCWP increases, cardiac index increases, but there is a balance between intravascular volume or left ventricular filling pressure and the formation of lung edema. The optimal PCWP or ventricular filling pressure must be determined on an individual basis. When the colloid osmotic pressure (COP) of the blood is normal (20–25 mmHg), the optimal PCWP ranges between 18 and 20 mmHg. If the COP is lower, then the optimal PCWP is lower. Higher pressures, in a low colloid osmotic pressure state, will induce pulmonary edema.

Once the optimal PCWP is determined, attention must be directed to optimizing systemic arterial blood pressure. Vasoconstrictor medications may be needed to optimize arterial blood pressure. Certain medications, such as dopamine, may be necessary to improve a low systemic arterial blood pressure; other medications, such as nitroprusside or nitroglycerin, may be necessary to reduce a high systemic arterial pressure. Medication such as dobutamine is used to enhance inotropic function of the myocardium and to increase cardiac output without significantly altering systemic arterial vascular resistance. Medication such as milrinone is used to increase cardiac output and lower afterload. All these medications are used to optimize cardiac index.

If a high left ventricular filling pressure or PCWP cannot be safely reduced with diuretic therapy, therapies such as dobutamine and milrinone can be used if the cardiac output is low.

Nitroglycerin or nitroprusside can be used if the cardiac output is normal. The use of a diuretic alone, such as furosemide, often causes a decrease in cardiac output in patients who have high left ventricular filling pressures or PCWP with a normal cardiac output, which again emphasizes the importance of intravascular volume as a partial determinant of cardiac output.

The optimal treatment for diastolic heart failure remains unknown. In diastolic heart failure, the systolic function of the left heart is normal and is unresponsive to changes in afterload. Therefore, diuretic therapy should be avoided. Medications that relax myocardial tissue are likely to be most helpful; these are called lusitropic agents. Medications such as calcium channel blockers and angiotensin-coverting enzyme (ACE) inhibitors and receptor blockers may have lusitropic actions.

The optimal treatment for diastolic dysfunction is unknown.

Lusitropic agents are most likely to be useful in diastolic dysfunction.

Diastolic dysfunction can be related to abnormalities of ventricular muscle relaxation or abnormalities of a relaxed ventricle. Hypertrophic states caused by aortic stenosis, systemic hypertension, and hypertrophic cardiomyopathy; ischemic states caused by unstable angina and myocardial infarction; and cardiomyopathic states caused by diabetes mellitus are all associated with abnormalities of dynamic relaxation. Abnormalities of a relaxed ventricle include atrial fibrillation with a decreased ventricular filling time, mitral stenosis with a reduced ventricular filling capacity, and increased myocardial stiffness caused by infiltrative diseases such as amyloidosis or endomyocardial fibrosis. Also, one must consider in the differential diagnosis a variety of extrinsic abnormalities relating to pericardial constriction and tamponade and the interventricular interaction of an overloaded right ventricle or right ventricular infarction. Compared to systolic heart failure, diastolic heart failure appears to be less morbid.

There are no large clinical trials to help us understand how to treat diastolic dysfunction. Lowering the systemic arterial blood pressure by treating essential hypertension, including systolic hypertension, lowers left ventricular filling pressures and helps reduce dyspnea. Maintaining a sinus heart rhythm at a low rate is important. When patients with diastolic dysfunction develop rapid atrial fibrillation, especially in the presence of mitral regurgitation, they experience a major increase of symptoms and sometimes cardiovascular collapse and pulmonary edema. Diuretic therapy is often required. Finally, ACE inhibitors, angiotensin I receptor blockers, beta-blockers, nitrates, and calcium channel blockers have all been used with some success.

Treatment of Systolic Heart Failure

Preload and Afterload Reduction

Patients with chronic heart failure often achieve their best cardiac output when their left ventricular filling pressures are close to normal. Lower filling pressures are likely to improve subendocardial perfusion and reduce ventricular wall stress. Actually, lower left ventricular filling pressures may occur without a significant change in left ventricular volume, suggesting that there was a beneficial influence on right ventricular distension and right atrial distension and a consequent decrease in coronary sinus pressures, resulting in improved myocardial venous drainage and left ventricular compliance. Even more so, a higher stroke volume from the left ventricle might occur because of a forward redistribution of regurgitant flow. The redistribution of regurgitant flow occurs in the right and left ventricle by reducing mitral and tricuspid regurgitant stroke volumes. Pulmonary arterial wedge pressures less than 16 mmHg have been associated with a significantly lower 1-year mortality in patients with advanced systolic heart failure.

Pulmonary arterial wedge pressures less then 16 mmHg have been associated with a significantly lower 1-year mortality in patients with advanced systolic heart failure.

Preload reduction is likely indicated in patients with dilated cardiomyopathy, provided they have reasonable renal function. Diuretics are commonly used to reduce preload. Diuretics reduce circulatory volume, thereby decreasing end-diastolic volume and myocardial oxygen consumption, which reduces ventricular wall tension.

Afterload reduction is indicated for nearly every patient with heart failure. Angiotensin-converting enzyme inhibitors (ACE inhibitors) are the primary class of medications prescribed to reduce afterload. ACE inhibitors vasodilate and reduce circulatory fluid volume.

ACE I inhibitors are the drugs of choice in CHF.

FIGURE 14-2

Starling curves show ventricular end-diastolic volume plotted on the *x*-axis and stroke volume (ventricular performance) plotted on the *y*-axis. *Increase* means an increased contractile state; *decrease* means a decreased contractile state. The *normal curve* is shown for comparison.

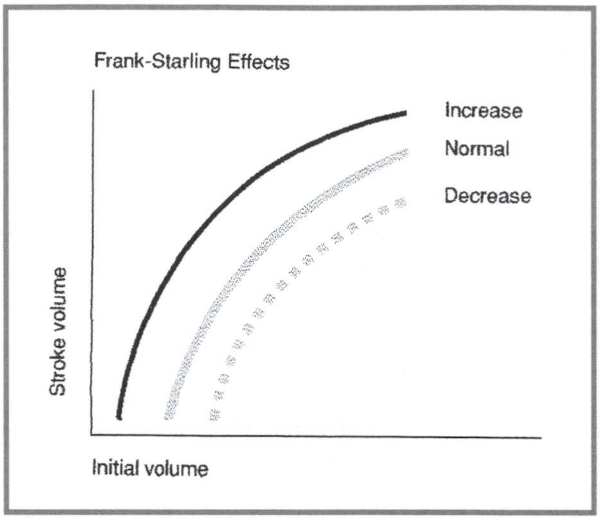

ACE inhibitors vasodilate and reduce circulatory fluid volume.

The resulting decrease in systemic vascular resistance allows better ventricular emptying, which, along with the decrease in circulatory fluid volume, shifts the pressure–volume curve to the left (Figure 14-2). Other medications can reduce systemic vascular resistance and thereby decrease left ventricular afterload.

Inotropic Therapy

The improvement in cardiac performance produced by inotropic therapy allows end-systolic pressure and volume to decrease.

End-stage heart failure often requires the use of more potent inotropic agents to support the failing heart.

Inotropic therapy can benefit patients with heart failure. Digoxin, an historically important medication, increases myocardial contractility without significantly increasing myocardial oxygen consumption. The resulting augmentation of stroke volume stimulates the arterial baroreceptors, which, in turn, decreases sympathetic outflow to the peripheral vasculature. The improvement in cardiac performance produced by inotropic therapy allows end-systolic pressure and volume to decrease, thus shifting the pressure–volume curve to the left. End-stage heart failure often requires the use of more potent inotropic agents to support the failing heart. Beta-adrenergic agonists such as dobutamine and phosphodiesterase inhibitors such as milrinone should be considered.

Combination Therapy

Interrupt the conditions that contribute to myocardial deterioration when treating heart failure.

Combination therapy increases the ejection fraction, reduces LV end-diastolic diameter, and contributes to an improved cardiac performance.

The ideal management strategy for patients with heart failure, particularly when it has progressed beyond the compensatory stage, is to interrupt the conditions that contribute to myocardial deterioration. An elevated preload, an elevated afterload, and a reduced contractility must all be addressed. Diuretics, ACE inhibitors, and digoxin are often used in combination to gain a synergistic benefit of the combined individual actions, namely, volume reduction, decreased peripheral resistance, and increased myocardial contractility. The pressure–volume curve often shifts substantially to the left. Combination therapy increases the ejection fraction, reduces left ventricular end-diastolic diameter, and contributes to a substantially improved cardiac performance and reduced myocardial oxygen consumption.

PHARMACOLOGY OF HEART FAILURE

The cocktail of therapies is often led by the ACE inhibitors in combination with digoxin and a diuretic.

All therapies would fail if they were not supported by important dietary restrictions and exercise regimens.

The pharmacology of heart failure consists of a myriad of treatments, often administered concurrently. The cocktail of therapies is often led by the ACE inhibitors in combination with digoxin and a diuretic. More recently, beta-blockers have been added to this therapy. When treating heart failure, multiple issues must be addressed to maintain patient stability. All these therapies would fail if they were not supported by important dietary restrictions and exercise regimens. The multidisciplinary approach coupled with close follow-up care is essential to assuring a reasonable quality of life for the patient with heart failure.

Diuretics

Diuretics, considered a mainstay of therapy for heart failure, are used to decrease hypervolemia, which helps reduce body edema including pulmonary congestion. Many diuretics could be considered, and they vary according to their site of pharmacologic activity, effects on fluid and electrolyte balance, and adverse reactions. The choice of the appropriate diuretic and its dosage requires careful consideration of individual patient factors. Loop diuretics decrease sodium reabsorption by interfering with the sodium chloride/potassium chloride cotransport system located on the apical membrane of the ascending limb (thick segment) of Henle's loop. Thiazides decrease sodium reabsorption by inhibiting the same cotransport system located on the apical membrane of the early portion of the distal convolution. Potassium-sparing diuretics decrease sodium reabsorption in the late portion of the distal convolution and in the collecting tubule. Diuresis with diuretic therapy can cause renin release. Increased renin blood level stimulates the release of aldosterone, which in turn enhances sodium reabsorption. Therefore, diuretics when used in large doses may paradoxically contribute to the reaccumulation of fluid and actually exacerbate heart failure.

Loop diuretics decrease sodium reabsorption by interfering with the sodium chloride/potassium chloride cotransport system located on the apical membrane of the ascending limb (thick segment) of Henle's loop.

Diuresis with diuretic therapy can cause renin release.

Common adverse effects from diuretics include hypotension, weakness, sexual dysfunction, and a variety of metabolic and electrolyte changes such as hypokalemia, hypomagnesemia, hypercalcemia, hyperglycemia, hypercholesterolemia, hypertriglyceridemia, and hyperuricemia. Tolerance can develop with the consistent use of certain diuretics. Tolerance to loop diuretics may be managed by more frequent dosing, continuous intravenous dosing, or coadministration of a thiazide diuretic coupled with more stringent dietary sodium restriction. Diuretic resistance arising from a decline in cardiac function should be managed by optimizing vasodilator therapy and ensuring patient compliance with the prescribed medical regimen.

Tolerance can develop with the consistent use of certain diuretics.

Glycosides

The role of digoxin and other cardiac glycosides in heart failure remains a subject of ongoing debate and controversy. Proponents believe that the use of digoxin and its mild positive inotropic effects help prevent worsening of congestive heart failure and improve the symptoms of this low cardiac index state. However, opponents maintain that exposure to the continuous positive inotropism of digoxin may actually hasten myocardial cell demise.

Exposure to the continuous positive inotropism of digoxin may actually hasten myocardial cell demise.

Digoxin is generally recommended for patients with more severe forms of heart failure who have a dilated left ventricle and a moderate to severely diminished ejection fraction. Studies have demonstrated that digoxin substantially reduces the risk of congestive heart failure exacerbation, but it does not improve exercise tolerance. The effect of digoxin on survival remains unclear.

The effect of digoxin on survival remains unclear.

The principal mechanisms of action of digoxin and other cardiac glycosides are not completely understood and are probably very complex. Involvement of cardiac muscle directly and of the cardiac autonomic nervous system indirectly results in a positive inotropic action, specifically an increase in the force in velocity of myocardial systolic contraction and a decrease in conduction velocity through the atrioventricular node. In the failing heart, digoxin increases cardiac output and decreases end-diastolic pressure. The magnitude of the positive inotropic effect depends on contraction frequency; the rate of onset is dependent on serum concentration of ions, particularly potassium, sodium, and magnesium.

The factors affecting digitalis pharmacokinetics include serum electrolyte abnormalities, drug interactions affecting gastrointestinal absorption, drug interactions with other cardiovascular agents, and thyroid disease, renal dysfunction, autonomic nervous system tone, and respiratory disease. Hypokalemia, hypomagnesemia, and hypercalcemia potentiate the effects of digoxin, thus producing digitalis toxicity.

Many factors affect digitalis pharmokinetics.

Angiotensin-Converting Enzyme Inhibitors

Angiotensin-converting enzyme (ACE) inhibitors have emerged as important agents in the treatment of heart failure. Despite growing evidence from a variety of important clinical trials that they improve symptoms, increase exercise capacity, and improve survival, ACE in-

ACE inhibitors are underused in treating CHF.

hibitors are underused in treating congestive heart failure. Furthermore, when ACE inhibitors are used, the dosages are often inadequate.

ACE inhibitors increase cardiac index and stroke volume and decrease systemic and pulmonary vascular resistance.

ACE inhibitors may slow the progression of heart failure.

ACE inhibitors, when used in patients with congestive heart failure, increase cardiac index and stroke volume and decrease systemic and pulmonary vascular resistance. Tachyphylaxis does not occur. Improved myocardial compliance with diminished or reversed left ventricular hypertrophy, and, most importantly, improved survival have been reported with the regular use of ACE inhibitor therapy. ACE inhibitors may slow the progression of disease, delaying the onset of overt heart failure in patients with asymptomatic left ventricular dysfunction.

ACE inhibitors decrease the formation of angiotensin II.

Pharmacodynamically, ACE inhibitors decrease the formation of angiotensin II with a resultant decrease in vasoconstriction and decrease in aldosterone secretion, leading to decreased sodium and water reabsorption, attenuation of sympathetic activity, and increased bradykinin levels. ACE inhibitors reduce arteriolar constriction, thus decreasing total peripheral resistance. Cardiac output and stroke volume improve in patients with heart failure and PCWP, and left atrial and ventricular filling volumes both decrease. ACE inhibitors block the conversion of angiotensin I to angiotensin II, a potent vasoconstrictor that also fosters the secretion of aldosterone from the adrenal cortex. Reduction in plasma levels of angiotensin II decreases blood pressure, reduces salt and water reabsorption in renal tubules, and increases plasma renin activity via a negative feedback.

Bradykinin appears to participate in the beneficial effects of these ACE inhibitors by stimulating the production of cGMP, nitric oxide, and prostaglandins.

ACE inhibition reduces presynaptic release of norepinephrine.

ACE inhibitors reduce the local accumulation of bradykinin. Bradykinin appears to participate in some of the beneficial effects of these drugs by stimulating the production of cyclic guanosine monophosphate (cGMP), nitric oxide, and prostaglandins. ACE inhibitors attenuate the abnormally high levels of sympathetic nervous system activity found in congestive heart failure. This attenuation may result from improved hemodynamics as well as direct inhibition of angiotensin II-mediated control of peripheral nervous system activity. Angiotensin II can stimulate sympathetic activity. ACE inhibition reduces presynaptic release of norepinephrine. ACE inhibitors decrease the amount of circulating angiotensin II, which results in less angiotensin I receptor activation on vascular and smooth muscle membranes as well as sympathetic postganglionic terminals, which attenuates sympathetic activity.

Adverse effects associated with ACE inhibitors include hypotension, renal dysfunction, hyperkalemia, cough, and angioedema.

A persistent, dry cough occurs in as many as 20% of patients treated with ACE inhibitors.

Angiotensin II type 1 (ATI) receptor blockers can be used as substitutes or concomitantly with ACE I inhibitors.

ACE inhibitors increase circulating levels of bradykinin because kinase, which degrades bradykinin, is identical to the angiotensin-converting enzyme. Bradykinin is a potent vasodilator, but the importance of bradykinin-related effects to the hemodynamics of ACE inhibitors remains unknown. However, bradykinin has been implicated in the genesis of cough and angioedema associated with the entire class of ACE inhibitors. Other significant adverse effects associated with ACE inhibitors include hypotension, renal dysfunction, and hyperkalemia. Patients at the greatest risk for renal dysfunction are those who are volume depleted or salt depleted, or both, from aggressive diuretic therapy and individuals with bilateral renal artery stenosis. Increases in serum potassium may occur from decreased aldosterone levels induced by ACE inhibitors. Finally, a persistent, dry cough occurs as many as 20% of patients treated with ACE inhibitors. This cough can substantially affect quality of life. The cough does not respond to conventional antitussive preparations or antiasthmatic preparations, and the ACE inhibitor must be discontinued to eliminate the coughing.

There are now angiotensin II type 1 (AT1) receptor antagonists. The AT1 receptor blockade provides an alternative for heart failure patients who are intolerant of ACE inhibitors because of the adverse effects of angioedema or cough. Clinical trials assessing the efficacy and safety of these receptor antagonists in heart failure have shown improvement in symptoms and exercise capacity similar to that seen with ACE inhibitors.

Direct Vasodilators

Other direct vasodilators are an effective alternative therapy for patients who have heart failure and cannot tolerate ACE inhibitors. Hydralazine and isosorbide dinitrate, in combination, can be considered a definitive alternative therapeutic approach. This combination therapy improves symptoms and the prognosis of chronic heart failure. Direct vasodilators can also be used as second-line therapy in combination with ACE inhibitors.

The rationale for the use of vasodilators in the therapy of heart failure is based on the concept that, in the context of a high-afterload state coupled with a high-preload state, peripheral arterial vasodilation improves cardiac output. As already mentioned, in some patients a decrease in preload volume may also improve cardiac output, depending on the position of the patient on the Frank–Starling curve of ventricular function. Direct vasodilators relax vascular smooth muscle and induce vasodilatation. Vasodilators may have a predominant effect on the arterial or venous circulation. An arterial vasodilator such as hydralazine can improve cardiac output with little change in end-diastolic left ventricular pressure. Nitrates, used primarily as venous dilating agents, decrease preload with little change in systemic arterial resistance. Balance vasodilation, with equal action on vascular capacitance and resistance, can be a desirable effect in heart failure treatment. Often, the combination of a predominantly arterial vasodilator and a strong venodilating agent improves forward flow while decreasing filling pressure and improving congestive symptoms.

A decrease in preload volume may also improve cardiac output.

Hydralazine can improve cardiac output with little change in end-diastolic LV pressure.

Nitrates decrease preload with little change in systemic arterial resistance.

Problems with vasodilators, in general, derive from the induction of symptomatic arterial hypotension, especially in the setting of intravascular volume depletion. Patients who use chronic vasodilator therapy should be assessed frequently and carefully for orthostatic changes in pulse and blood pressure as well as a deterioration in renal function.

Inotropic Support

The principal use of intravenous inotropic support is for the patient with advanced heart failure, generally decompensated, with evidence of a reduction in systemic blood pressure and cardiac output that threatens vital end-organ perfusion. These patients are generally either end-stage CHF patients or individuals with severe CHF that has been unresponsive to conventional therapy. Intravenous inotropic support can often temporarily improve ventricular performance and achieve clinical stabilization. The choice of a particular parenteral inotropic agent for an individual patient generally depends on the experience of the clinician and the target actions of the drug that has been selected.

Intravenous inotropic support can often temporarily improve ventricular performance and achieve clinical stabilization.

The two most commonly used parenteral inotropic agents are the sympathomimetic amine dobuttamine and the phosphodiesterase inhibitor milrinone. Both beta-adrenergic stimulation and phosphodiesterase inhibition share a final common pathway in leading to an increase in intracellular cyclic AMP. Cyclic AMP increases the intracellular concentration of calcium via subsequent phosphorylation of several proteins. These actions enhance myocardial contractility and improve diastolic relaxation.

The two most commonly used parenteral inotropic agents are the sympathomimetic amine dobutamine and the phosphodiesterase inhibitor milrinone.

Treatment with intravenous inotropic agents is usually done in the hospital setting, either in the intensive care unit or a special cardiac unit where intravenous therapy can be used. The patients are carefully monitored and the medication is titrated, generally with a right heart catheter in place and a continuous electrocardiogram. Blood pressure monitoring is done on a frequent basis. Daily monitoring of urine output, serum electrolytes, and renal function is advisable.

Dobutamine is a synthetic catecholamine. It has a predominant beta-1 agonist effect and produces increased cardiac contractility and reduced aortic impedance, thereby augmenting stroke volume and cardiac output while decreasing left ventricular filling pressure. The reason why dobutamine enhances clinical improvement, including a reduction in symptoms and an increase in exercise performance, remains an enigma. An improvement in myocardial energetics may occur with a course of dobutamine therapy. A major limitation in the use of dobutamine is the potential for a progressive loss of beta-1 receptor responsiveness to this agonist, or so-called desensitization, necessitating the use of this drug in an intermittent infusion fashion. As with any parenterally administered medication, dobutamine may cause problems at the injection site, particularly if infiltration occurs. Often, this medication is given via a central line catheter. Other problems with dobutatmine use reflect its positive inotropic and chronotropic effects, that is, an increased heart rate, blood pressure, and ventricular ectopy, all of which are dose related. Hypotension may also occur suddenly with the use of this medication, and thus continuous electrocardiogram and blood pressure monitoring are advisable.

A major limitation in the use of dobutamine is a progressive loss of beta-1 receptor responsiveness.

Dobutamine has chronotropic effects that can induce arrhythmias.

Milrinone is a selective inhibitor of phosphodiesterase isoenzyme in the myocardium and vascular smooth muscle. The inhibition of phosphodiesterase reduces the degradation of cyclic AMP, which is associated with an increase in intracellular calcium, which in turn in-

Milrinone is a selective inhibitor of phosphodiesterase isoenzyme in the myocardium and vascular smooth muscle.

Degradation of cAMP increases intracellular calcium concentrations and myocardial contractility.

creases myocardial contraction force. Also, the decrease in cyclic AMP breakdown results in increased phosphorylation of contractile proteins and relaxation and vascular smooth muscle. Thus, milrinone, similar to dobutamine, exerts positive inotropic as well as vasodilatory effects. The vasodilatory properties of milrinone are more likely than dobutamine to cause hypotension, particularly in patients with underlying renal insufficiency. The hypotension induced by milrinone can be dangerous because the average elimination half-life of milrinone is nearly 2 h in patients with substantial heart failure. Finally, milrinone has shown an ability to reduce pulmonary hypertension because of its potent vasodilatory action.

Milrinone is more likely than dobutamine to cause hypotension.

Calcium Channel Blockers

Calcium channel blocker therapy is avoided in CHF because of negative inotropic effects.

Calcium channel blocker therapy has historically been avoided in congestive heart failure because of negative inotropic effects. However, newer therapies are reported to have less pronounced cardiodepressant effects than the earlier generation drugs. Calcium channel blockers may prove useful in some patients with heart failure because they are effective vasodilators, thereby reducing systemic vascular resistance. They also decrease myocardial oxygen demand in the ischemic heart. However, calcium channel blockers as a class tend to worsen symptoms, and may even increase mortality in CHF patients with systolic ventricular dysfunction, including patients with CHF caused by ischemic disease. Calcium channel blockers may have value in treating heart failure caused by diastolic left ventricular dysfunction, such as heart failure resulting from hypertensive or idiopathic hypertrophic cardiomyopathies.

Calcium channel blockers inhibit the transmembrane influx of calcium into vascular smooth muscle and cardiac muscle.

Calcium channel blockers inhibit the transmembrane influx of calcium into vascular smooth muscle and cardiac muscle. The contractile mechanism of cardiac muscle relies on the movement of extracellular calcium ions in the cardiac muscle cells through specific ion channels.

New-generation dihydropyridine drugs, such as amlodipine, do have a role in the treatment of CHF.

The most significant adverse effects related to calcium channel blocker therapy is hypotension, lightheadedness, bradycardia, palpitations, and peripheral edema. The only class of calcium channel blockers used in the treatment of heart failure are the dihydropyridine drugs such as amlodipine, because other classes of calcium channel blockers induce a negative inotropic effect.

Beta-Blocker Therapy

Beta-adrenergic blocking agents have had an erratic history in the treatment of heart failure. Early studies demonstrated a trend toward prolongation of survival in dilated cardiomyopathy with the use of a beta-blocker. There is likely a subset of patients, those with dilated cardiomyopathy and impaired systolic function, who benefit from the use of a beta-blocker therapy, such as metoprolol. Later, it was found that beta-blocker therapy could be cautiously used in some patients with CHF caused by ischemic cardiomyopathy. Beta-blocker therapy was used at low doses with very slow and gradual upward titration. Metoprolol improves myocardial performance and energetics in patients with dilated cardiomyopathy.

At present, several beta-blockers, including carvedilol and metoprolol, have shown survival benefit, reduced progression of heart failure, and improvement in functional performance. Beta-blockers have been shown to be particularly helpful in patients who are already taking digoxin, a diuretic, and an ACE inhibitor. Bucindolol is another beta-blocker that may have benefit in the management of heart failure. The ultimate mechanisms of beta-blocker effects in CHF are unknown but probably lead beyond the beta receptor and into the ensuing cascade of effects down to the cellular membrane milieu.

Sympathetic neurotransmitters can cause heart cell death and impair cardiac cell function.

The physiologic rationale for beta-blocker therapy in the treatment of chronic heart failure involves several mechanisms related to the adverse effects of chronic sympathetic stimulation of the heart. Sympathetic neurotransmitters can cause heart cell death and impair cardiac cell function, thereby reducing contractility. Increased activity of the sympathetic nervous system can lead to downregulation of beta-1 receptors on the myocardial cell surface. Antagonism of the sympathetic nervous system with beta-blocker therapy can improve the metabolic and hemodynamic status of the failing heart. In heart failure, the compensatory increase in sympathetic nerve activity compromises cardiac function. The resulting chronic elevation of norepinephrine produces a change in intracellular activity that "downregulates" beta-1 receptors so that there are fewer receptors available for activation. This downregulation of beta receptors further impairs cardiac cell function and decreases myocardial contractility. When a beta receptor antagonist is used, many of these effects are blocked, resulting in an increase in beta receptor function and upregulation of beta-1 receptors. Beta blockage combined with the upregulation of beta-1 receptors may improve overall cardiac function in the presence of compensatory sympathetic stimulation, as occurs in heart failure.

Downregulation of beta receptors further impairs cardiac cell function and decreases myocardial contractility.

Beta-blocker therapy, as a class, can be associated with numerous adverse effects. Congestive heart failure symptoms may initially be exacerbated by the negative inotropic effect of the beta-blocker therapy, but over time a crucial benefit may actually occur. The use of beta-blocker therapy is typically limited to patients with less severe heart failure, although new studies may shed further light on patients with class IV NYHA CHF. Beta-blocker therapy is avoided in patients with potential for bronchospasm, including patients with asthma and other chronic obstructive pulmonary diseases. In the elderly, a beta-blocker may increase fatigue and reduce mental acuity. Obviously, beta-blocker therapy can precipitate chronic CHF and induce serious hypotension. Various types of cardiac arrhythmias can develop while patients are on beta-blocker therapy, including AV nodal conduction problems and even more serious heart block. In the diabetic, blunting of the epinephrine effect may impair the ability of the patient to perceive the onset of a hypoglycemic attack.

In the elderly, a beta-blocker may increase fatigue and reduce mental acuity.

MECHANICAL SUPPORT

Intraaortic Balloon Pump

Intraaortic balloon counterpulsation can provide mechanic circulatory support in patients with severe left ventricular dysfunction. The intraaortic balloon pump (IABP) induces diastolic augmentation of blood pressure with systolic afterload reduction, and it is the most common assist device used today. A balloon tip catheter is inserted through the femoral artery, up the aorta, and positioned just beyond the origin of the left subclavian artery. The balloon can be inflated during diastole, accelerating blood to the periphery of the body, and it deflates during systole, reducing end-diastolic pressure, thereby reducing left ventricular afterload and promoting stroke volume. During diastole, when the balloon is inflated, coronary perfusion also increases.

The intraaortic balloon pump (IABP) induces diastolic augmentation of blood pressure with systolic afterload reduction.

IABP is contraindicated in patients with substantial aortic regurgitation or aortic dissection.

IABP is generally used before and after coronary artery bypass surgery and cardiac transplantation, during acute myocardial infarction with cardiogenic shock, and during acute mitral insufficiency. Most frequently, it is used immediately postoperatively following cardiopulmonary bypass surgery. IABP is contraindicated in patients with substantial aortic regurgitation or aortic dissection. The procedure is complicated by leg ischemia and infection. Finally, weaning from intraaortic counterpulsation can be difficult, but in most patients it occurs within a 24-h period.

Ventricular Assist Devices

A ventricular assist device (VAD) (Figure 14-3) is a pump that is implanted into the body and can either support the right ventricle (RVAD), the left ventricle (LVAD), or both ventricles (BiVAD). The pump enhances total systemic arterial blood flow and is generally used in patients with severe or end-stage cardiac disease with a life expectancy of less than 1 year; it is often used as a bridge to heart transplantation. LVAD is generally employed in patients who are dependent on vasopressor therapy, with hemodynamics that are poorly supported with such pressors: these hemodynamics include high PCWP, low mean systemic arterial pressure, and low cardiac index, generally less than 2 $l/min/m^2$.

VADs are not used in patients who have noncorrectable bleeding disorders, bone marrow suppression, or severe immune suppression. Bleeding, systemic embolization, and infection

Bleeding, systemic embolization, and infection are the most frequent complications of ventricular assist devices (VADs).

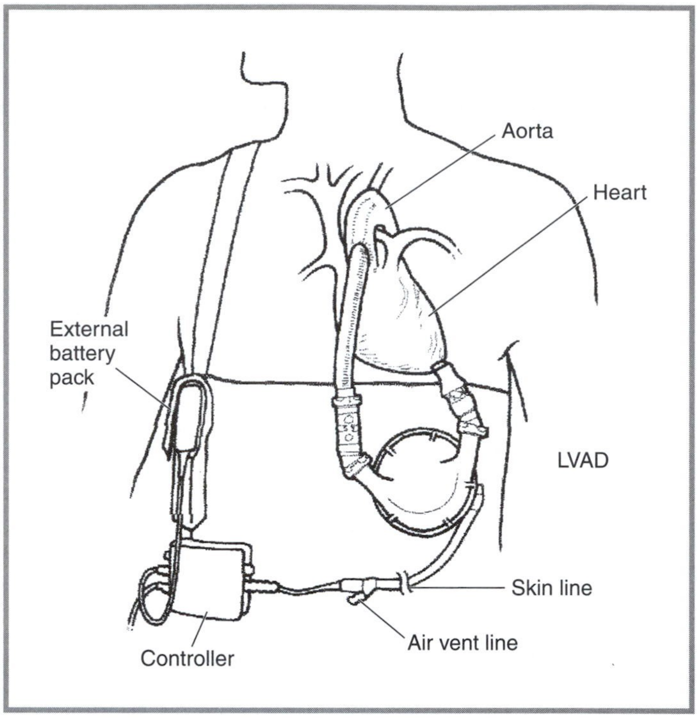

FIGURE 14-3

A left ventricular assist device (VAD). The outflow cannula is in the LV apex and the return (inflow) cannula is in the proximal ascending aorta.

are the most frequent complications. However, thromboembolic complications have been kept to a minimum because the device often undergoes vascular surface changes, namely endothelialization of the pumping chamber.

HEART TRANSPLANTATION

Donor availability remains the rate-limiting step for heart transplantation.

Despite aggressive medical management, many patients with end-stage heart failure may require heart transplantation. The mortality rate for NYHA classification IV heart failure remains 30%–40% per year. For patients whose disease progresses rapidly despite optimal treatment or whose 1-year life expectancy is far less than the survival probability for transplant patients, cardiac transplantation may be a viable option. However, donor availability remains the rate-limiting step for heart transplantation for patients with advanced heart failure.

CASE STUDY: PART 4

This patient had several systemic complications of his acute coronary event. He had pulmonary edema requiring mechanical ventilatory support, and he required intraaortic counterpulsation to increase coronary artery perfusion and to provide afterload reduction. His physical examination findings were consistent with long-standing hypertension and vascular disease, including diffuse arteriolar narrowing and poor peripheral pulses. His habitus was that of an obese patient having multiple coronary risk factors including tobacco and alcohol use.

The patient had signs and symptoms of CHF that were acute in presentation but probably chronic in origin from an underlying ischemic cardiomyopathy due to his multiple infarctions. His echocardiogram showed an aneurysmal left ventricular apex, which suggested a previous old myocardial infarction, and his new event showed a minimal spillage of creatinine, phosphokinase, and isoenzymes, suggestive of a small area of ischemia.

However, in the context of severely decompensated and diminished ventricular performance and function, as in this patient, these small ischemic events can precipitate acute pulmonary edema and cardiogenic shock. This patient required intravenous inotropic support and mechanical ventilation with mechanical counterpulsation to try to augment his cardiac performance. With the use of oral ACE inhibitors and medical management, he could be weaned from his mechanical support.

The patient's clinical evidence suggests that his renal insufficiency is probably multifactorial, deriving from a vascular etiology, a hypertensive etiology, and a low cardiac output state.

SUMMARY

Our increased understanding of the pathophysiology of heart failure has led to better treatment strategies and prolonged survival. However, more effective and earlier recognition of disease is still needed, and the challenge for the futures rests in preventing the disease from occurring or progressing to its morbid state. For now, proper therapy includes not only the correct combination of medications but also proper diet, fluid intake, and exercise, which can often prevent repeated hospitalizations for heart failure patients.

REVIEW QUESTIONS

1. **Which of the following cardiovascular disease entities has increased in prevalence over the last decade?**
   A. Coronary artery disease
   B. Hypertension
   C. Valvular heart disease (including mitral valve prolapse)
   D. Congestive heart failure

2. **NYHA class III–IV patients have a 1-year survival rate of:**
   A. 10%–20%
   B. 80%–90%
   C. 30%–50%
   D. 60%–70%

3. **Which of the following factors are important in the regulation of the stroke volume?**
   A. Venous return
   B. Systemic vascular resistance
   C. Concentration of extracellular calcium
   D. All of these
   E. A and C only

4. **The cardiac remodeling that occurs during chronic failure is part of the compensatory response to preserve cardiac output and to normalize ventricular wall stress.**
   A. True
   B. False

5. **"Higher ventricular filling pressures at the same volume" best describes the hemodynamic disturbance found during:**
   A. Congestive heart failure
   B. Right ventricular failure
   C. Systolic heart failure
   D. Diastolic heart failure
   E. Biventricular failure

ANSWERS

1. The answer is D. Heart failure is the only major cardiovascular condition in the United States for which the incidence and prevalence have steadily increased. Approximately 4.8 million American suffer from heart failure, and about 400,000 new cases are discovered each year. This steady increase in the number of patients with heart failure is directly linked to the decreasing mortality rates of coronary heart disease, myocardial infarction, and stroke. The improved management of these underlying problems has resulted in patients surviving long enough to develop a weakened heart and subsequent heart failure.
2. The answer is C. The outlook for patients with congestive heart failure (CHF) remains poor. Half will die within 5 years of diagnosis, and for patients with severe heart failure, 1-year survival is only 30%–50%.
3. The answer is D. Stroke and volume is the amount of blood ejected with each heart beat. All the factors listed are important in regulating stroke volume. Stroke volume depends on (1) the end-diastolic volume, which is dependent on venous return; (2) the load against which the heart must contract, which is dependent on the systemic vascular resistance; and (3) the level of cardiac contractility, which is determined by the concentration of intracellular calcium that attaches to troponin C. In cardiac muscle, the amount of calcium released from internal stores to attach to troponin C is related to calcium entry from outside the cell, which is related in part to the extracellular concentration.
4. The answer is A. Cardiac remodeling is an extremely important part of the initial response to myocardial injury. Remodeling is associated with several changes in cardiac geometry, including ventricular hypertrophy. Compensatory ventricular hypertrophy results in an increase in the number of myofilaments (which helps to maintain stroke volume and thus cardiac output) and an increase in myocardial wall thickness (which decreases ventricular wall stress, thereby reducing myocardial oxygen consumption).
5. The answer is D. Diastolic heart failure is associated with inability of the ventricle to fill adequately during diastole. In diastolic heart failure, filling pressure becomes disproportionately elevated in relation to small changes in diastolic volume. This situation occurs with loss of ventricular compliance. Diastolic heart failure can lead to congestive heart failure, with the development of pulmonary or systemic edema (or both). Right ventricular failure can result from diastolic failure, but it can also occur because of systolic failure, in which the characteristic ventricular dysfunction is inadequate emptying during systole rather than improper filling during diastole. Diastolic as well as systolic failure can occur in both ventricles (i.e., be biventricular).

SUGGESTED READING

ACC/AHA Task Force Report. Guidelines for the evaluation and management of heart failure. J Am Coll Cardiol 1995;26:1376–1398.

Cohn JN, Archibald DG, Ziesche S, et al. Effect of vasodilator therapy on mortality in chronic congestive heart failure: results of a Veterans Administration Cooperative Study (CONSENSUS). N Engl J Med 1986;314:1547–1552.

Dracup K, Walden JA, Stevenson LW, Brecht ML. Quality of life in patients with advanced heart failure. J Heart Lung Transplant 1992;11:273–279.

Gillum RF. Epidemiology of heart failure in the United States. Am Heart J 1993;126:1042–1047.

Packer M. The neurohormonal hypothesis: a theory to explain the mechanism of disease progression in heart failure. J Am Coll Cardiol 1992;20:248–254.

Pfeffer MA, Braunwald E, Moyè LA, et al. (and the SAVE Investigators). Effect of captopril on mortality and morbidity in patients with left ventricular dysfunction after myocardial infarction. Results of the Survival and Ventricular Enlargement Trial. N Engl J Med 1992;327:669–677.

Stevenson WG, Stevenson LW, Middlekauff HR, et al. Improving survival for patients with advanced heart failure: a study of 737 consecutive patients. J Am Coll Cardiol 1995;26:1417–1423.

Tresch DD, McGough MF. Heart failure with normal systolic function. A common disorder in older people. J Am Geriatr Soc 1995;43:1035–1042.

CHAPTER 15

ROBERT SANGRIGOLI AND HENRY H. HSIA

Cardiac Arrhythmias

CHAPTER OUTLINE

LEARNING OBJECTIVES

After studying this chapter, you should be able to:

- Understand the fundamental properties of excitability and refractoriness and, in particular, understand the timing of these events during the action potential of a cardiac cell.
- Know basic conduction system anatomy.
- Develop a basic understanding of arrhythmia mechanisms, with particular attention to reentry, which is responsible for most clinically relevant arrhythmias.
- Develop a systematic approach to the diagnosis and treatment of common bradycardic and tachycardic rhythms.
- Understand the impact, evaluation, and treatment options of arrhythmias occurring during several common clinical syndromes (long QT syndrome, sudden cardiac death, and acute myocardial infarction).

This chapter provides an overview of basic cellular electrophysiology, conduction system anatomy, and mechanisms of common cardiac arrhythmias. A discussion follows on the clinical recognition of common arrhythmias, based primarily on ECG characteristics and arrhythmia response to noninvasive maneuvers. The clinical characteristics, diagnostic features, and treatment options of specific arrhythmias are discussed. The last section provides an overview of specific arrhythmia syndromes.

CELLULAR ELECTROPHYSIOLOGY

Understanding the fundamental electrical properties of the cardiac cell allows a greater understanding of the basic mechanisms of arrhythmia initiation, maintenance, and termination. Cardiac electrical activity is determined by the cellular transmembrane potential, the voltage difference between the intracellular and extracellular environments. This potential difference is created by an electrochemical gradient that is maintained by the selectively permeable cardiac cell membrane. Within this membrane specialized proteins act as channels or pumps that allow passage of certain ions. These channels are voltage sensitive and are selective for a particular ion (Na^+, K^+, or Ca^{2+}). In the resting state, the intracellular compartment is polarized to a negative potential relative to the extracellular space. Most normal cardiac cells are polarized to approximately −90 mV. Changes in cell membrane potential are caused by the flow of charged ions (Na^+, K^+, Ca^{2+}) across the membrane. The relatively high extracellular sodium and calcium concentrations provide the driving force for

> Cardiac electrical activities are determined by the cellular transmembrane potential, the voltage difference between the intracellular and extracellular environments. The action potential is expressed as the curve of voltage change over time during depolarization and repolarization of the cardiac cell: it consists of five phases.

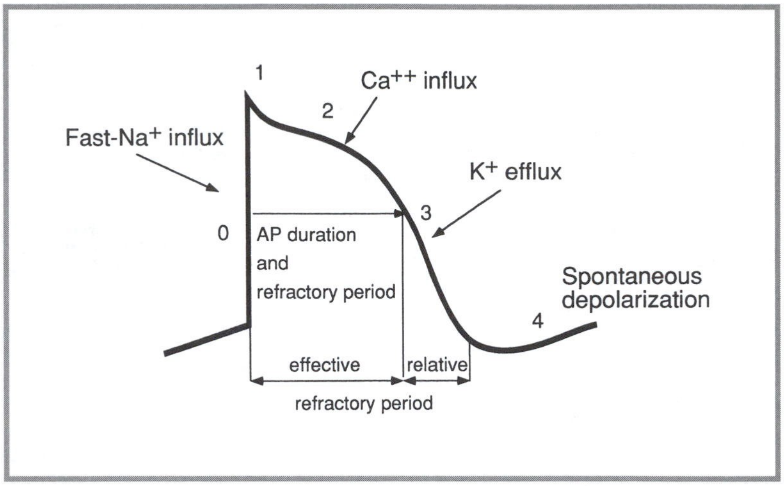

FIGURE 15-1

Cardiac action potential. The rapid upstroke represents cellular depolarization, referred to as phase 0. Repolarization is divided into three phases: phase 1 represents early and rapid repolarization, phase 2 is known as the plateau phase, and phase 3 represents the final, rapid repolarization of the cell. Phase 4 is the period from the end of repolarization until another AP is generated. Also depicted are the effective (absolute) and relative refractory periods. *AP*, action potential.

positive currents into the cell when the channels are opened; this depolarizes the cell membrane. Potassium has a higher intracellular concentration and carries current outward, repolarizing the cell membrane. An action potential (AP) is created when a sufficiently strong stimulus activates opening of enough sodium channels to raise the resting membrane potential to threshold (about −70 mV), which activates the remainder of the sodium channels, fully depolarizing the cell.

Cardiac cell action potential: during phases 0, 1, and 2 the cells are inexcitable. During phase 3, cells gradually recover excitability; during phase 4, the cell is fully excitable.

The action potential (AP) is expressed as the curve of voltage change over time during depolarization and repolarization of the cardiac cell. It consists of five phases (Figure 15-1). The rapid upstroke, referred to as phase 0, results from a rapid inward sodium current causing cell membrane depolarization. The slope of phase 0 determines the conduction velocity of the AP. Phase 1 represents early and rapid repolarization caused by inactivation of the inward sodium current and activation of a transient outward potassium current. The cell at this stage is inexcitable or refractory. Phase 1 repolarization is terminated by the plateau phase of the AP. During this plateau phase, phase 2, a slow inward calcium current is activated, but membrane conductance to all ions is low and cells are unresponsive to stimuli regardless of strength. The cell is said to be in its absolute refractory period. Phase 3 represents the final rapid repolarization of the cell, caused by inactivation of the slow inward calcium current and activation of outward potassium current. During phase 3, cells gradually recover their ability to respond to stimuli; that is, they recover "excitability." A sufficiently strong stimulus applied near the end of phase 3 may encounter enough recovered sodium channels to allow depolarization to threshold and generate a new action potential; this is known as the relative refractory period of the cell. Still later in phase 3, essentially all sodium channels are readily available. The cell is once again fully excitable, and stimuli will generate a normal AP. Phase 4 represents the period from the end of repolarization until another action potential is generated. It is a period of electrical quiescence when the cell is said to be at its resting membrane potential. Although most cardiac fibers require a stimulus sufficient to move the resting membrane potential to threshold to produce a depolarization, some specialized cardiac cells display spontaneous phase 4 depolarization. These cells, which are said to possess the property of automaticity, include the sinoatrial (SA) node, parts of the atria, the atrioventricular (AV) junctional region, and the His–Purkinje system.

CONDUCTION SYSTEM ANATOMY

Figure 15-2 shows the basic anatomy of the cardiac conduction system. Under normal conditions the pacemaker function of the heart is in the sinoatrial (SA) node, which is located epicardially in the high lateral right atrium near the entrance of the superior vena cava. The blood supply for the SA node is from the right coronary artery (RCA) in 60% of cases and

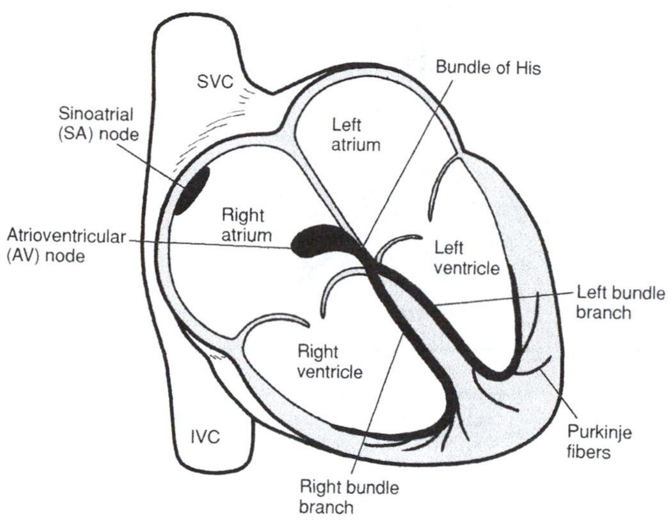

FIGURE 15-2

Anatomy of the conduction system. *SVC*, superior vena cava; *IVC*, Inferior vena cava.

from the left circumflex artery in 40% of cases. Once an impulse exits the SA node, it traverses the atrium until it reaches the atrioventricular (AV) node which lies at the base of the right interatrial septum. The electrophysiologic properties of the AV node provide delay in atrioventricular conduction under normal circumstances. Blood supply for the AV node is from the RCA in 90% of cases; this may explain the frequent occurrence of AV nodal conduction disturbances during inferior myocardial infarctions. Parallel bands of Purkinje fibers emerge from the AV node to form the bundle of His. The His bundle then branches into left and right bundle branches that course over the left and right sides of the interventricular septum. Conduction is especially rapid through the His–Purkinje system (HPS). The His bundle and the right bundle branch have dual blood supply from the RCA and left anterior descending (LAD) coronary artery. The left bundle branch divides into two fascicles. The blood supply to the anterior fascicle is from the LAD, and the posterior fascicle has dual blood supply from the LAD and the RCA. Consequently, the development of left posterior hemiblock after myocardial infarction is a poor prognostic sign, indicating compromise of two major circulations. In addition to the normal conduction pathway (atria → AV node → HPS → ventricles), some individuals have accessory pathways that bypass the normal route. These pathways have major clinical importance when involved in reciprocating tachycardias such as the Wolff–Parkinson–White syndrome.

The SA and AV nodes are significantly influenced by autonomic tone. Vagal tonic effects dominate during normal resting conditions. Vagal influence depresses automaticity of the sinus node and prolongs AV nodal conduction and refractoriness; it is responsible for the rapid modulation of heart rate and AV conduction. Sympathetic influence increases sinus node automaticity, accelerates AV nodal conduction, and shortens AV nodal refractoriness; it is responsible for sustained acceleration of pacemaker activity (chronotropic) and enhanced conduction (dromotropic) responses.

The sinoatrial (SA) and atrioventricular (AV) nodes are significantly influenced by autonomic tone.

Electrophysiologic properties of the AV node result in a delay in atrioventricular conduction.

Vagal tonic forces dominate during normal resting conditions.

MECHANISMS OF ARRHYTHMIAS

The mechanisms responsible for cardiac arrhythmias are typically divided into abnormalities of impulse formation such as abnormal automaticity and triggered activity and abnormalities of impulse conduction such as reentry or heart block. This section provides an overview of these mechanisms, with a particular focus on reentry. Understanding the concept of reentry is critical to understanding how most arrhythmias are initiated and maintained

Mechanisms responsible for cardiac arrhythmias are typically divided into abnormalities of impulse formation and impulse conduction.

FIGURE 15-3

Reentry. The cardiac impulse encounters a transient, unidirectional conduction block in one limb (*right*) of the circuit (*1*). The impulse travels down an alternative limb (*left*) in the circuit (*2*). There is a critical degree of conduction slowing (*shaded area*) that allows the area of prior unidirectional block to recover excitability and the impulse to reenter the circuit (*3*).

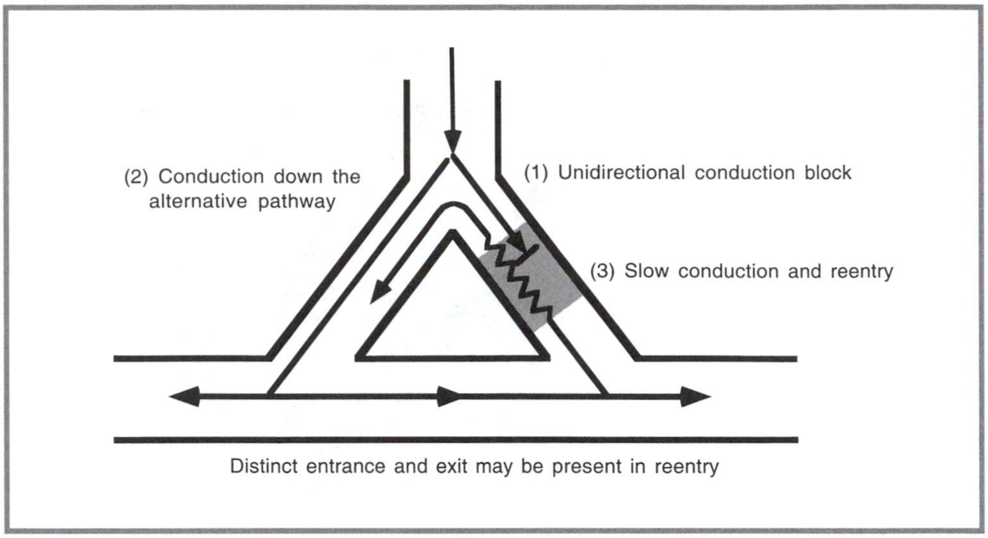

and why antiarrhythmic drugs may work (antiarrhythmic drug therapy is discussed in detail in Chapter 37).

Automaticity occurs when cardiac cells undergo spontaneous diastolic (phase 4) depolarization and form action potentials at an abnormally fast rate. Clinical arrhythmias believed to be caused by abnormal automaticity include paroxysmal sinus tachycardia, some causes of atrial tachycardia, accelerated junctional tachycardias, and rare cases of ventricular tachycardia.

Arrhythmias caused by triggered activity are initiated by "afterdepolarizations," which are abnormal depolarizing oscillations in cell membrane voltage triggered by one or more preceding action potentials. Triggered depolarizations may occur before the cell membrane has completely repolarized, called an early afterdepolarization (EAD), or after full recovery of the cell, called a delayed afterdepolarization (DAD). EADs may be responsible for reperfusion arrhythmias and polymorphic ventricular tachycardia of torsades de pointes associated with the long Q-T syndrome. DADs can be induced by digitalis excess and exposure to catecholamines and thus may be responsible for certain digitalis toxic arrhythmias as well as catecholamine dependent atrial and ventricular tachycardias.

> Reentry is responsible for most clinical tachycardias.

> Basic to all forms of reentry are (1) multiple limbs in a circuit, (2) unidirectional conduction block in one limb, and (3) slow conduction via an alternative pathway.

Reentry is responsible for most clinical tachycardias. In the presence of multiple anatomically or functionally defined pathways, impulses may reexcite areas that were just activated and have now recovered from the initial depolarization. This phenomenon is known as reentry. Basic to all forms of reentry are (1) multiple anatomic or functional pathways in a circuit, (2) unidirectional conduction block in one limb of the circuit, and (3) slow conduction down the alternative pathway, slow enough that the tissue proximal to the area of unidirectional block recovers excitability and allows the impulse to reenter the circuit Figure 15-3. It is important that all these conditions be present to initiate and maintain the reentrant circuit. Reentry may be the result of (1) a microreentrant circuit, as found in ischemic ventricular tachycardia, (2) a macroreentrant circuit that encompasses larger areas of the heart, as in bypass tract-mediated tachycardias, or (3) multiple reentrant circuits (wavelets), as found in atrial and ventricular fibrillation.

> Determining the underlying mechanisms of a particular arrhythmia requires review of the patient's history and attention to morphologic characteristics of the arrhythmia, particularly its mode of initiation or termination and response to certain cardiac maneuvers and drugs.

CLINICAL RECOGNITION OF CARDIAC ARRHYTHMIAS

Accurate diagnosis of the arrhythmia allows prompt and appropriate treatment, which may center primarily on the arrhythmia or on the underlying cause. At the bedside it is often difficult to determine the underlying mechanism of a particular arrhythmia. A careful review of the patient's history, as well as close attention to the morphologic characteristics of the arrhythmia, its mode of initiation or termination, and its response to certain maneuvers and drugs, however, often provide enough information for a reasonably accurate diagnosis.

Information gathered from a review of the patient's history may provide important diagnostic clues. For instance, in patients with known history of prior myocardial infarction, a wide complex tachycardia is far more likely to be ventricular than supraventricular in origin. The physician should also be aware of circumstances that immediately preceded or coexist with the arrhythmia such as angina, myocardial infarction, hypoxia, metabolic abnormalities, and the use of ionotropic or antiarrhythmic medications. These conditions may trigger arrhythmias and may be the primary target for arrhythmia intervention.

Heart rate and the regularity of an arrhythmia are often the first signs to be noticed. Although these signs may sometimes assist in the differentiation of arrhythmias, there is considerable overlap. Determining the presence and morphology of P waves and their relationship to the QRS complexes, as well as assessing the QRS morphology, is of paramount importance in diagnosing an arrhythmia. No single lead can provide enough information to make the correct diagnosis. Therefore, multiple simultaneous leads must be examined and a 12-lead ECG obtained whenever possible. These tracings should always be compared to a sinus rhythm tracing if available.

Determining the presence and morphology of P waves and their relationship to the QRS complexes and assessing the QRS morphology is of paramount importance.

Multiple simultaneous leads must be examined and a 12-lead EKG obtained whenever possible.

The mechanism responsible for certain arrhythmias may occasionally be determined from the mode of initiation and termination of the arrhythmia or from its response to atrial and ventricular premature beats. Automatic arrhythmias are initiated spontaneously or following a "late" premature beat and often exhibit a "warm-up" phenomenon. The ECG appearance of the first beat of an automatic tachycardia is usually identical to the rest of the beats of the tachycardia. A reentrant arrhythmia is frequently initiated by a "early" premature beat followed by a pause. This pattern corresponds to a premature stimulus, unidirectional block with slow conduction, and then reentry. The ECG appearance of the first beat of a reentrant tachycardia may not be identical to the rest. Automatic arrhythmias are not terminated by overdrive pacing and may be incessant. Reentrant arrhythmias can usually be terminated by overdrive pacing or introduction of properly timed premature extra stimuli. The mode of initiation and termination of triggered activity in clinical human arrhythmias has not been well studied.

Noninvasive cardiac maneuvers, often greatly underutilized, may provide important diagnostic information. The Valsalva maneuver and application of carotid sinus pressure (CSP) result in increased vagal tone. This slows the rate of sinus nodal discharge, slows AV nodal conduction and prolongs refractoriness producing AV nodal block. Clinically, this often results in abrupt termination of AV node-dependent tachycardias. Tachycardias, especially narrow-QRS supraventricular tachycardias (SVT), can be divided into AV node-dependent and AV node-independent tachycardias. AV node-dependent tachycardia includes the AV node as a critical part of the circuit. Interruption of conduction through the AV node terminates these reentrant arrhythmias. The prototypes of AV node-dependent arrhythmias include AV nodal reentry (AVNRT) and AV reciprocating tachycardia (AVRT) utilizing a bypass tract. AV node-independent tachycardias, such as sinus or atrial tachycardias, may slow in response to the increased vagal tone, but the tachycardia quickly resumes as the vagal maneuver is terminated. Ventricular tachycardia (VT) shows no response to vagal maneuvers. Heart rate during atrial fibrillation (AF), atrial flutter (AFL), and atrial tachycardia (AT) will often slow in response to an increased degree of AV block, allowing the underlying atrial activity to be seen and thus establishing the diagnosis. The Valsalva maneuver should generally be avoided in patients with ischemic heart disease because of the accompanying fall in coronary blood flow. The carotid arteries should be carefully auscultated, so that pressure is not applied to patients with carotid bruits indicative of carotid artery disease. Induced gagging (suctioning via an endotracheal tube) also causes intense vagal stimulation. These maneuvers are potentially dangerous, because they may result in prolonged AV block, asystole, and even death. Appropriate precautions include continuous ECG monitoring, intravenous access, and easy availability of a code cart.

Noninvasive (vagal) cardiac maneuvers may provide important diagnostic information.

The Valsalva maneuver should be avoided in patients with ischemic heart disease because of the accompanying fall in coronary blood flow.

The response of supraventricular tachycardias to specific drugs may be diagnostic. Adenosine is a short-acting potent endogenous nucleoside that slows conduction through the AV

Adenosine is a short-acting endogenous nucleoside that slows conduction through the AV node.

node. If the arrhythmia is AV node dependent, 6–12 mg IV adenosine restores sinus rhythm in the majority of cases. If the tachycardia is atrial fibrillation, adenosine will slow the ventricular response, but only rarely does the arrhythmia convert into sinus rhythm. If the rhythm is atrial flutter or atrial tachycardia, adenosine will slow the ventricular response and allow the underlying flutter or P waves to be recognized. Verapamil also has a potent negative dromotropic effect on the AV node. However, verapamil has a longer duration of action and may cause significant vasodilatation and hypotension, making IV adenosine the drug of choice. In general, verapamil should not be used if the rhythm is a wide complex tachycardia. With either drug, asystole has rarely been observed; thus, the capability for temporary pacing should be available whenever these drugs are administered.

ARRHYTHMIA DIAGNOSIS

> Characterize the rhythm as slow or fast.
> Assess the AV relationship.
> Assess the morphologic characteristics.
> Assess response to maneuvers of drugs.

There are many approaches to arrhythmia diagnosis, but the simplest and most clinically relevant approach is to first categorize the rhythm as slow or fast, then fine tune arrhythmia differentiation according to its regularity, AV relationship, morphologic characteristics, and response to maneuvers or drugs. Characterization of every arrhythmia is beyond the scope of this text, which discusses only the more common, clinically relevant arrhythmias.

Bradycardias

Sinus Bradycardia

> Sinus bradycardia is defined as a sinus rate <60 beats/min in the adult.

Sinus bradycardia (SB) in the adult is defined as a sinus rate less than 60 bpm. In the general population, this rhythm is normal in the majority of cases, often reflecting good cardiovascular condition or periods of enhanced vagal tone such as sleep. In the ICU setting, however, this is often a distinctly abnormal rhythm. Causes include drugs with a negative chronotropic effect (beta-blockers, calcium channel blockers, amiodarone), parasympathomimetic drugs, myocardial infarction (especially inferior), hypothermia, gram-negative sepsis, hypothyroidism, and CNS disorders. Therapy is primarily directed at the underlying cause. Symptomatic patients require treatment with IV atropine, isoproterenol infusion, or temporary pacing.

Sinus Node Dysfunction

> Sick sinus syndrome is frequently intermittent and mostly common found in the elderly.

Sinus node dysfunction (SND), also called sick sinus syndrome, is frequently intermittent and is most commonly found in the elderly. SND describes a group of disorders of sinus node function including "inappropriate" SB, sinus arrest, and sinoatrial (SA) exit block. SND accounts for more than half of all permanent pacemaker implantations in the United States. SND is often caused by idiopathic degeneration of the sinus node, hypertension, ischemia, infiltrative or inflammatory diseases, or the normal aging process.

> Manifestations of SND include sinus bradycardia, sinoatrial (SA) arrest, tachy-brady syndrome, and brady-tachy syndrome.

> Tachy-brady syndrome is the most common cause of cause of symptomatic sinus node dysfunction and is associated with syncope.

Inappropriate sinus bradycardia refers to a primary rhythm disorder (depressed automaticity) in which the bradycardia is persistent, inappropriate for the physiologic condition of the patient, and unexplained by other factors such as medication effect. When marked sinus bradycardia (heart rate < 50 beats/min) occurs, symptoms of fatigue and weakness predominate. Prolonged sinus pauses (>3 s) caused by failure of sinus node impulse formation (sinus arrest) or block of conduction of the sinus impulse to the surrounding atrial tissue (sinus exit block) may result in paroxysmal dizziness, presyncope, or syncope (Figure 15-4). Other manifestations of SND include the tachy-brady syndrome in which a supraventricular tachycardia, most often atrial fibrillation or flutter, bombards the sinus node, suppressing its function. When the tachycardia ceases, the sinus node may be abnormally slow to recover and need several seconds to resume its function. If there is an inadequate escape rhythm, dizziness and even syncope may result. The tachy-brady syndrome is the most common cause of symptomatic SND and is associated with the highest incidence of syncope. Tachycardia may also follow bradycardia—the brady-tachy syndrome. Atrial fibrillation, for instance, may develop in the presence of bradycardia or pauses.

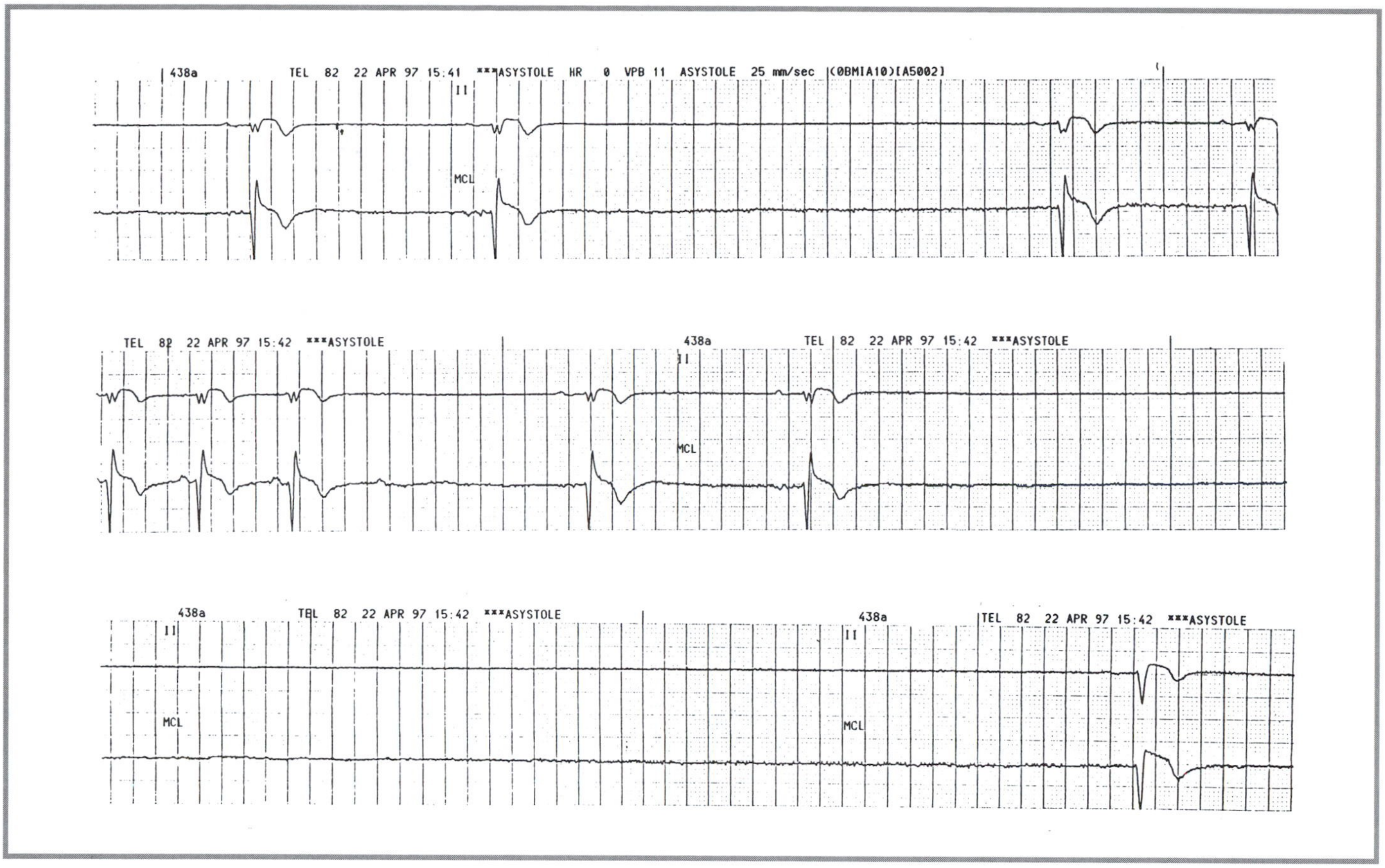

FIGURE 15-4

Sinus node dysfunction. Continuous telemetry recording shows sinus pause greater than 13 s duration and failure of an adequate escape rhythm.

Asymptomatic patients require no immediate treatment. Symptomatic bradycardia may be treated with atropine, isoproterenol, or temporary pacing. In the long term, these patients often require permanent pacemakers.

AV Block (Heart Block)

Abnormalities of the AV conduction system include (1) prolonged AV conduction (first-degree AV delay), (2) intermittent AV conduction (second-degree AV block), and (3) no AV conduction (third-degree AV block). Causes of abnormal AV conduction include degeneration of the conduction system, ischemic heart disease, drug effect (beta-blockers, calcium channel blockers, digitalis, antiarrhythmic drugs), recent cardiac surgery, and infiltrative diseases of the heart. Lesser degrees of AV block can be seen in normal individuals with heightened vagal tone, especially during sleep.

Abnormal AV conduction: (1) prolonged AV conduction; (2) intermittent AV conduction; (3) no AV conduction.

First-degree AV delay is defined as a P-R interval greater then 0.2 s. P-R interval prolongation may be caused delay in impulse conduction in the atria, AV node, or HPS. A narrow QRS complex and a P-R interval that exceeds 0.26 s strongly suggest delay in the AV node. Asymptomatic patients require no further evaluation or treatment.

Second-degree AV block (AVB) occurs when some atrial impulses fail to reach the ventricles. Type I (Wenckebach) second-degree AVB is characterized by progressive lengthening of the P-R interval until block of the atrial impulse develops resulting in dropping out of a QRS complex Figure 15-5. Type I second-degree AVB may infrequently progress to complete heart block. Type II second-degree AVB occurs when AV conduction intermittently fails without a preceding change in P-R intervals Figure 15-6, which is most often caused

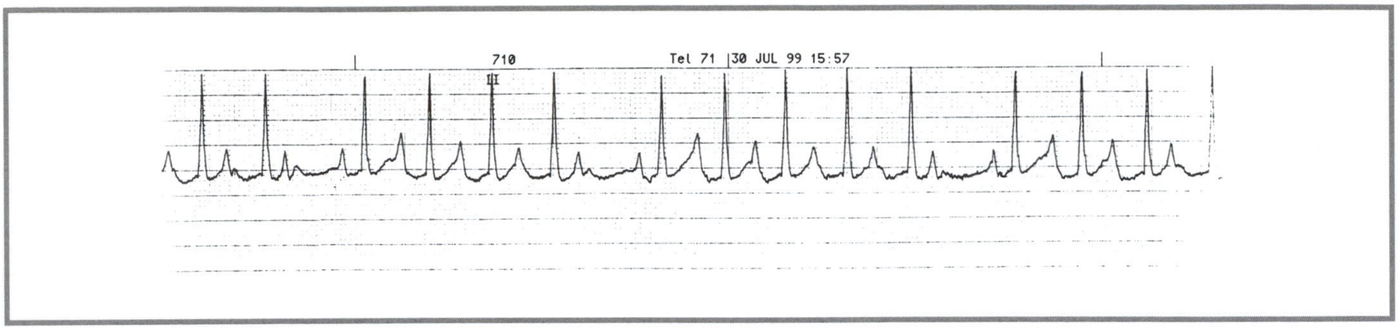

FIGURE 15-5

Type I (Wenckebach) second-degree heart block with sinus tachycardia at approximately 125 beats/min. Note progressive lengthening of the PR interval until a QRS complex is "dropped." The conduction ratio is 5:4; that is, there are five P waves for four QRS complexes in the Wenckebach cycle.

by disease within the HPS. Narrow QRS complexes during the conducted beats suggest the block is within the His bundle, whereas a wide QRS complex during conducted beats suggests a block below the His bundle (infra His) and is associated with a high risk of progressing to complete heart block.

Third-degree AV block, also known as complete heart block (CHB), occurs when there is complete failure of conduction between the atria and the ventricles (Figure 15-7). CHB is most commonly found in the later decades of life, with 80% of cases presenting after the age of 50. The site of AV conduction block may be suggested by the width of the escape rhythm (Table 15-1). If the escape rhythm has a narrow QRS complex and occurs at a rate of 40–55 beats/min, block within the AV node is likely. If the QRS is wide and the rate is less than 40 beats/min, block usually is distal to the His bundle, although considerable overlap is seen. The response of AV conduction to various maneuvers or drugs may also assist in differentiating the site of block (Table 15-2). If exercise, atropine, or isoproterenol improve AV conduction, the site of block is likely to be the AV node. However, if conduction worsens, the site of block is probably below the AV node. If vagal maneuvers, such as carotid sinus pressure, worsen AV conduction, the site of block is likely the AV node. Improvement in AV conduction after vagal maneuvers suggests infranodal block.

Management of patients with AV block (AVB) is usually straightforward. Asymptomatic first-degree AVB and type I second-degree AVB require no specific treatment. Type II second-degree AVB and third-degree AVB associated with active transient problems usually resolve spontaneously as the underlying problem improves. Such patients may be observed

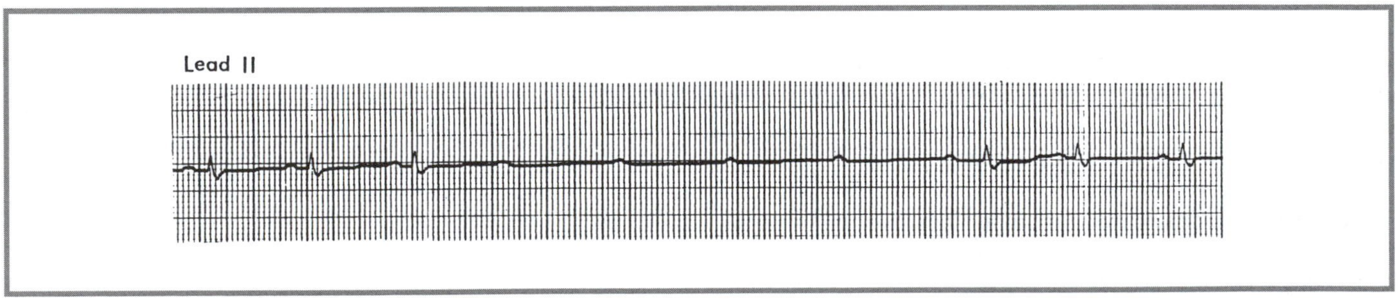

FIGURE 15-6

Type II second-degree heart block with abrupt loss of AV conduction (P waves not followed by QRS complexes) without a preceding change in the PR interval; this is also an example of high-grade AV block.

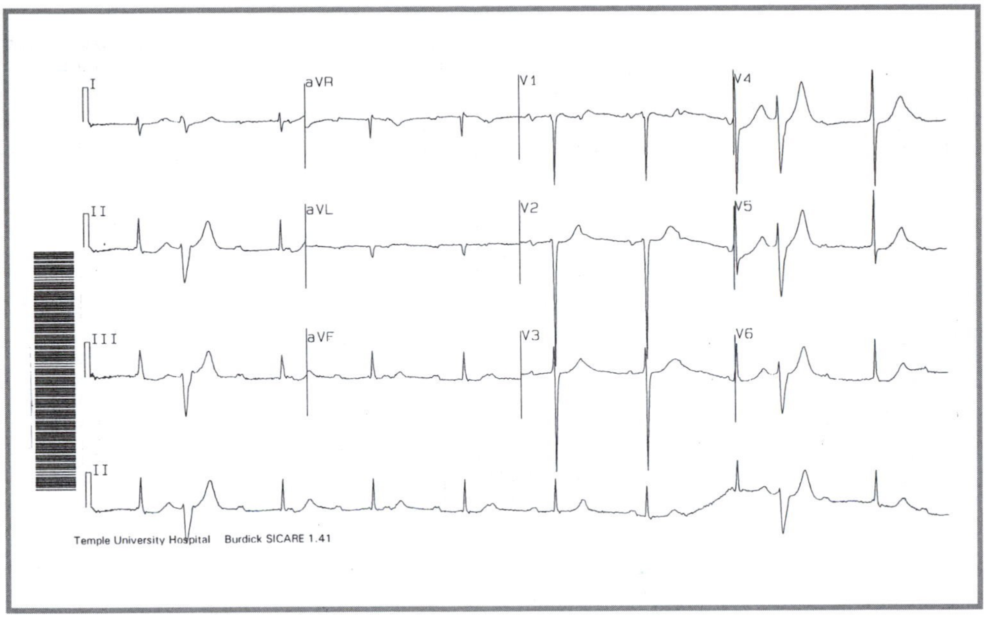

FIGURE 15-7

Third-degree heart block shows sinus tachycardia with occasional ventricular premature depolarizations (VPDs) and complete heart block with a junctional escape rhythm (narrow QRS complexes) at approximately 55 beats/min. Note that the P waves march through the tracing without any association to the QRS complexes.

carefully without immediate intervention if a hemodynamically stable, narrow QRS rhythm is present. Symptomatic patients and patients with a wide QRS complex and slow rhythm require immediate transvenous pacing. If the level of block is at the AV node, IV atropine and isoproterenol infusion may be useful. Transvenous pacing may be required if the site of block is below the AV. Atropine should not be used in the setting of acute myocardial infarction (see Acute Myocardial Infarction, later in this chapter).

Escape Rhythms

The AV node or the ventricles may take over the role of dominant pacemaker in cases of sinus node dysfunction or heart block. The AV node (AVN) normally escapes at an inherent rate of 40–60 beats/min (idiojunctional rhythm), and the ventricle normally escapes at less than 40 beats/min (idioventricular rhythm). The ECG is characterized by lack of P waves preceding each QRS. The QRS is normally narrow in the case of junctional escape and wide in the case of ventricular escape. Retrograde conduction to the atria may occur with either rhythm. Treatment is directed at the underlying cause. Atropine, isopreterenol, or cardiac pacing may be used to treat symptomatic bradycardia. Antiarrhythmics are never indicated to treat escape rhythms.

TABLE 15-1

AV CONDUCTION ABNORMALITIES

ECG	SITE OF BLOCK
First-degree heart block	AVN>>HPS
Second-degree heart block	
Type I: normal QRS	AVN>>>HPS
Type I: wide QRS	AVN>HPS
Type II: normal QRS	HPS>AVN
Type II: wide QRS	HPS>>>AVN
2:1: normal QRS	AVN = HPS
2:1: wide QRS	HPS>>AVN
Third-degree heart block	
Normal QRS	HPS = AVN
Wide QRS	HPS>>AVN

AV, atrioventricular; AVN, atrioventricular node; HPS, His–Purkinje system

TABLE 15-2

SITE OF CONDUCTION DEFECT

	AV NODE	INFRANODAL
QRS	Narrow	Wide
PR interval	>0.26	0.26
Wenckebach pattern	Yes	No
Exercise	Improve	Worsen
Atropine	Improve	Worsen
Carotid sinus message	Worsen	Improve (?)
Isoproterenol	Improve	????

Tachycardias

Sinus Tachycardia

Sinus tachycardia (ST) in the adult is defined as a sinus rate greater than 100 beats/min.

Sinus tachycardia (ST) in the adult is defined as a sinus rate greater than 100 beats/min. The maximal rate is age dependent but typically does not exceed 150–180 beats/min. The age-related maximum physiologic heart rate can be approximated at about 220 beats/min minus age. Sinus tachycardia is probably the most commonly encountered arrhythmia in the ICU setting. In the majority of cases it is an appropriate response to an underlying stimulus such as pain, fever, or hypotension in the setting of vagal withdrawal and adrenergic stimulation. It is critical to determine and direct therapy at the underlying cause and not simply treat the tachycardia. Rarely, "inappropriate" sinus tachycardia is observed, which is a primary rhythm disorder caused by enhanced automaticity or reentry within the sinus node.

Multifocal Atrial Tachycardia

MAT is usually seen in the setting of severe pulmonary disease.

MAT often precedes a development of atrial fibrillation.

The treatment of MAT is directed toward improving the underlying pulmonary status.

Multifocal atrial tachycardia (MAT) describes a rhythm in which multiple foci within the atria fire and conduct to the ventricles, producing an irregularly irregular rhythm at a rate exceeding 100 beats/min with at least three different P wave morphologies and varying P-R intervals (Figure 15-8). MAT is usually seen in the setting of severe pulmonary disease; it may precede the development of atrial fibrillation. Treatment is directed at improving the underlying pulmonary status. If slowing of the ventricular rate is desired, verapamil may be of some benefit. Beta-blockers are generally avoided because of the risk of bronchospasm. Digitalis should be avoided as it is unlikely to be of any benefit and exposes the patient to the risk of toxicity. This arrhythmia is termed wandering atrial pacemaker (WAP) when the heart rate is less than 100 beats/min. Treatment is unnecessary unless symptomatic bradycardia occurs.

Atrial Fibrillation and Atrial Flutter

Atrial fibrillation (AF) is the most frequently encountered arrhythmia. The prevalence increases with advancing age.

Atrial fibrillation (AF) is the most frequently encountered arrhythmia. The prevalence of AF increases with advancing age, occurring in more than 10% of the elderly population. AF usually develops in patients with structural heart disease, such as mitral valvular disease, thyrotoxicosis, myocarditis, pericarditis, cardiomyopathy, hypertension, or pulmonary disease or

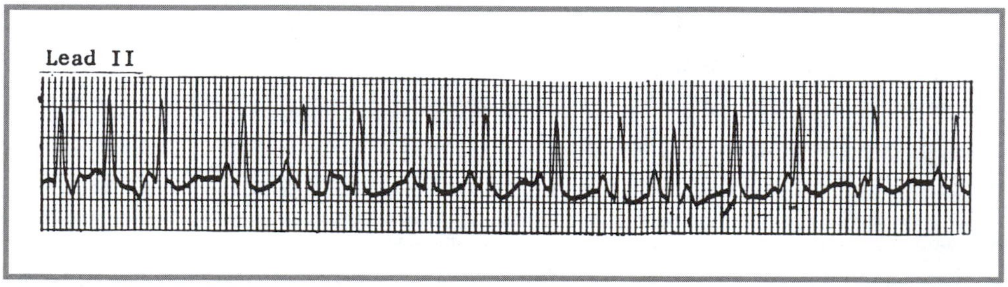

FIGURE 15-8

Multifocal atrial tachycardia (MAT). Note the irregularly irregular rhythm with varying P-wave morphologies and varying PR intervals.

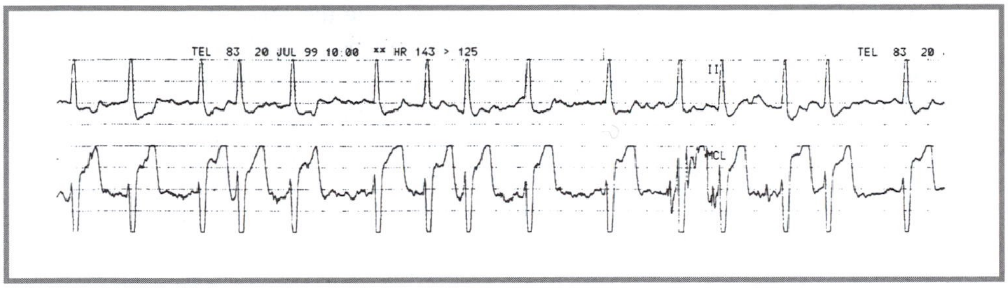

FIGURE 15-9

Atrial fibrillation. Note the irregularly irregular rhythm with coarse and rapid baseline undulations. No distinct P wave is evident.

early after open heart surgery and in association with the Wolf–Parkinson–White (WPW) syndrome. Most commonly, AF is caused by multiple random wavelets of reentry circulating within a critical mass of atrial tissue. Less often, AF appears to have a focal origin, usually in one of the pulmonary veins. Atrial fibrillatory activity, called f waves, may appear on the ECG as coarse or fine irregular baseline undulations at a rate of 350–600 beats/min (Figure 15-9). The refractory period and conductivity of the AV node determine the ventricular rate. Very fast and very slow ventricular rate response may appear regular at first glance. If left untreated, the ventricular rate response generally ranges from 130 to 200 beats/min, but can be accelerated with thyrotoxicosis, fever, sympathetic stimulation, or in the presence of a bypass tract. The QRS complexes are narrow unless aberration occurs. Aberration is a common finding after a long–short cycle (Ashman's phenomenon). More recently, electrophysiologic remodeling of the atria has been demonstrated in both animal models and humans with persistent atrial fibrillation. AF itself induces physiologic and anatomic changes (atrial dilatation, myofibrillary disarray and fibrosis, and shortening of the atrial refractory period) that reinforce the likelihood that fibrillation will persist. This finding underscores the importance of early intervention.

Atrial flutter (AFL) typically occurs in patients with structural heart disease. It may also be seen in the setting of acute pulmonary embolus, hyperthyroidism, pericarditis, and repaired congenital heart disease and in the early days following open heart surgery. Typical (type 1) atrial flutter originates from a macroreentrant circuit within the right atrium in which the impulse travels counterclockwise down the right atrial free wall and up the intraatrial septum. The ECG characteristically shows negative sawtooth flutter waves in the inferior leads (I, II, and aVF) and sharply peaked flutter waves in lead V1 (Figure 15-10). In the absence of a drug effect, the atrial rate ranges from 250 to 350 beats/min. Atypical (type 2) atrial flutter may originate from reentry within either the right or left atrium, occurring at a rate of 350–450 beats/min, and does not have the typical negative flutter waves in the inferior leads. Untreated, the AV conduction in typical (type 1) atrial flutter is normally 2:1, giving a regular ventricular rate at approximately 150 beats/min. The diagnosis of AFL should always be suspected when a narrow QRS tachycardia at 150 beats/min is seen. Higher-degree blocks or variable AV block often occur. If the AV conduction ratio varies, the ventricular rhythm will be irregular. Accentuating AV block by applying vagal maneuvers or using pharmacologic blockade may aid in the diagnosis because flutter waves often become better visualized with a slower ventricular rate. AFL tends to be unstable, reverting to sinus rhythm or degenerating into atrial fibrillation.

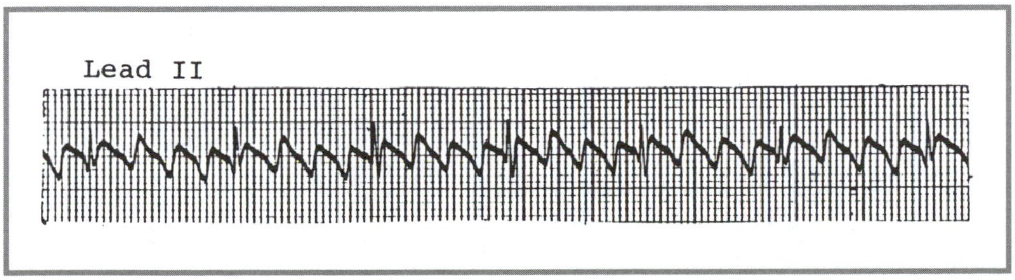

FIGURE 15-10

Atrial flutter with 4:1 atrioventricular (AV) conduction. Note the negative, sawtooth flutter waves in lead II. The atrial flutter rate is approximately 300 beats/min.

In unstable patients with atrial fibrillation or flutter, emergent cardioversion is needed.

In stable patients with flutter or fibrillation, the goals of treatment are to (1) control ventricular rate, (2) restore sinus rhythm, and (3) prevent thrombobolic complications.

A bradycardic ventricular response during AF or AFL, in the absence of drugs, suggests disease of the AV nodal conduction system and may be associated with sinus node dysfunction. In such cases, conversion to sinus rhythm may be complicated by prolonged bradycardia requiring temporary pacing. Unstable patients require emergent synchronized direct current (DC) cardioversion. In stable patients, the goals of treatment are to (1) control the ventricular rate, (2) restore and maintain sinus rhythm, and (3) prevent thromboembolic complications. AV nodal blocking agents (beta-blockers and calcium channel blockers) should be used preferentially for the acute control of the ventricular rate, whereas digitalis should be reserved for rate control in chronic AF. Digitalis should be avoided in AFL because it tends to be ineffective at controlling the ventricular rate during AFL and, if used, exposes the patient to unnecessary toxic risk.

Pharmacologic conversion may be achieved using the Vaughan Williams class 1 or class 3 agents. If class 1A agents (quinidine, procainamide, and disopyramide) are used, pretreatment with AV nodal blocking drugs is recommended to avoid accelerating the tachycardia (refer to Chapter 39 on antiarrhythmic agents), which is more likely to occur with AFL than AF. Additionally, typical AFL may be terminated by right atrial overdrive pacing whereas atypical AFL and AF are refractory to pacing. Synchronized DC cardioversion may be attempted instead of pharmacologic treatment and can be reserved for drug-refractory cases. Antiarrhythmic drug therapy may be necessary for successful electrical cardioversion or to maintain sinus rhythm after cardioversion. In patients with refractory AF or AFL and an uncontrollable ventricular response, radiofrequency (RF) catheter modification of the AV node or ablation of the AV junction followed by permanent pacemaker insertion can be very effective.

Patients with repetitive paroxysmal or sustained AF or AFL of greater than 48–72 h duration should be anticoagulated to reduce the risk of thromboembolic complications unless specific contraindications are present. In these patients, effective anticoagulation for 3–4 weeks before and 3–4 weeks after pharmacologic or electrical cardioversion is recommended. Anticoagulation before cardioversion may not be necessary if a transesophageal echocardiography excludes the presence of left atrial thrombi. Lone AF describes AF occurring in young (<60 years old) individuals with structurally normal hearts. These patients are at lower risk for thromboembolic complications and may therefore be safely treated with aspirin alone.

Paroxysmal Supraventricular Tachycardias

Paroxysmal supraventricular tachycardias (PSVT) include narrow QRS complex tachycardias caused by AV nodal reentry (AVNRT), orthodromic AV reciprocating tachycardia (AVRT) utilizing an AV bypass tract, and atrial tachycardias (AT) that may arise near the sinus node or other regions of the atria. Table 15-3 shows the relative incidence of the various forms of supraventricular tachycardias. In general, these arrhythmias are reentrant in nature, have abrupt onset and termination, and range in rate from 150 to 230 beats/min. A P wave is constantly related to a narrow QRS unless aberrant conduction produces a wide QRS.

AVNRT can occur at any age and is usually unrelated to structural heart disease. The rate is variable but usually ranges from 180 to 200 beats/min. AVNRT is caused by reentry within the AV node along two functionally distinct pathways. These dual AV nodal pathways consist of a fast-conducting (beta) pathway that generally has a longer refractory period and a

TABLE 15-3

SUPRAVENTRICULAR TACHYCARDIAS

AVNRT (50%–60%)	
Typical	95%
Atypical	5%
AV Reentrant Tachycardia (30%)	
Fast BPT	90%
Slow BPT	10%
Atrial Tachycardia (10%)	
Sinoatrial reentrant tachycardia	10%
Automatic atrial tachycardia	90%

AVNRT, atrioventricular nodal reentry

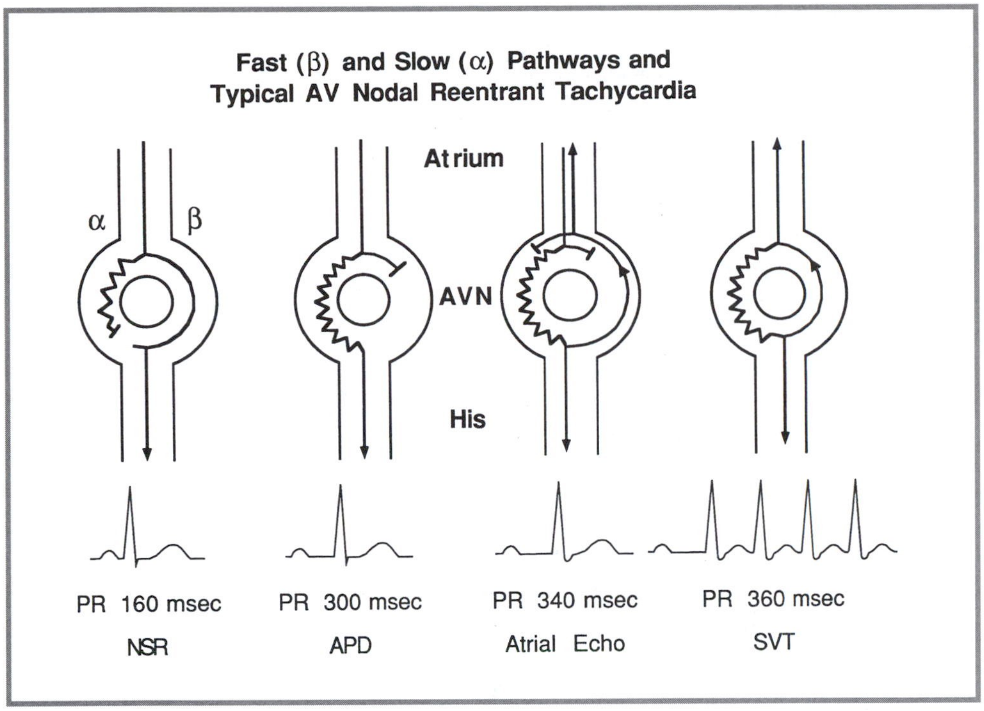

FIGURE 15-11

Dual AV nodal pathways. The AV node (*AVN*) is schematically divided into dual AV nodal pathways that consist of a slowly conducting α-pathway and a rapidly conducting β-pathway. The refractory period of the β-pathway is usually longer than the α-pathway. During normal sinus rhythm (NSR), the impulse preferentially conducts over the β-pathway. Progressively premature atrial depolarizations (APD) block in the β-pathway and travel down the slowly conducting α-pathway, resulting in a prolonged PR interval. When a critical degree of slow conduction within the circuit is present (PR interval reaches 340 ms), a single atrial echo results (single reentrant beat). Further slowing in the circuit results in sustained reentry.

slower-conducting (alpha) pathway which has a shorter refractory period (Figure 15-11). Anterograde conduction normally occurs down the fast pathway during sinus rhythm, but an atrial premature beat (APB) may find the fast pathway refractory and travel down the alternative slow pathway. If conduction in the alpha-pathway is sufficiently slow, the fast limb will recover excitability and reentry may occur. During this common (slow–fast) form of AVNRT, retrograde conduction over the fast beta-pathway depolarizes the atria at almost the same time that the impulse reaches and depolarizes the ventricles. Thus, the P wave is inscribed within the QRS complex and is invisible on the surface ECG. Occasionally, the P wave may be seen in the terminal portion of the QRS. Figure 15-12 illustrates the P/QRS

A P wave buried within the QRS suggests typical AV nodal reentry (AVNRT).

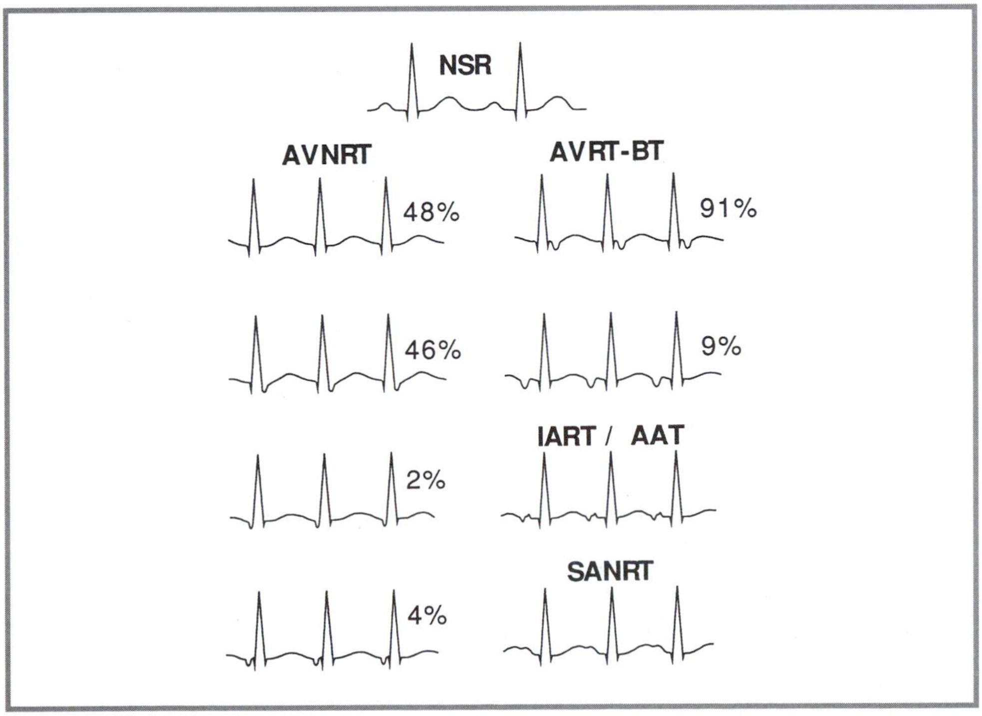

FIGURE 15-12

P/QRS relationship in SVT. The P/QRS relationships are illustrated for normal sinus rhythm (*NSR*), AV nodal reentry tachycardias (*AVNRT*), AV reentry tachycardias using retrogradely conducting AV bypass tracts (*AVRT-BT*), intraatrial reentry (*IART*), automatic atrial tachycardias (*AAT*), and sinoatrial nodal reentry tachycardia (*SANRT*). The *numbers* represent relative incidences of these arrhythmias.

RP > PR is consistent with atypical AVNRT and AVRT using a slow accessory pathway.

relationship in SVT. The uncommon (fast–slow) form of AVNRT occurs when anterograde conduction occurs over the fast beta-pathway and retrograde conduction to the atria occurs over the slow alpha-pathway. In this situation, atrial depolarization occurs late after ventricular depolarization and the P wave is inscribed after the QRS, producing a long R-P and a short P-R interval.

AVRT utilizing an AV bypass tract as the retrograde limb and the normal AV conducting system as the anterograde limb (orthodromic AVRT) is the second most common form of PSVT. During orthodromic AVRT, the atria are activated after the impulse traverses the ventricles and the retrograde limb of bypass tract. The P wave therefore must follow the QRS, producing an R-P interval that is shorter than the P-R interval. In 10% of orthodromic AVRTs, the AV bypass tract conducts slowly, producing a long R-P and short P-R interval. The differential diagnosis of a long RP tachycardia includes the uncommon form of AVNRT, orthodromic AVRT utilizing a slowly conducting or sick bypass tract, and atrial tachycardia.

RP < PR suggests AV reciprocating tachycardia (AVRT) using a fast accessory pathway.

Atrial tachycardias (AT) are more commonly associated with structural heart disease. The paroxysmal forms of atrial tachycardias are caused by reentry within the sinus node or, more commonly, within other regions of the atria. The incessant forms of AT are more likely the result of abnormal automaticity. Atrial tachycardias may demonstrate 1:1 conduction or variable ratios of AV block. During atrial tachycardias, the P waves may be seen anywhere among the QRS complexes. Sinus node reentry tachycardia (SNRT) and intraatrial reentry tachycardia (IART) are generally slower than other forms of PSVT, with an average rate of 130–140 beats/min. In SNRT, the P wave is very similar or identical to the sinus rhythm P wave whereas the P wave of IART is frequently bizarre and different.

The P wave during atrial tachycardia (AT) may be anywhere.

Automatic atrial tachycardia is caused by enhanced automaticity rather than reentry and may be commonly associated with underlying structural heart disease. This tachycardia can also be seen in the setting of cor pulmonale, digitalis toxicity, hypokalemia, amphetamine ingestion, acute alcohol ingestion, and hypoxia. Unlike reentrant rhythms, automatic atrial tachycardias cannot be initiated or terminated by a premature beat. This arrhythmia typically appears to warm-up on its initiation, increasing its rate for the first several beats; the atrial rate typically ranges from 150 to 200 beats/min. Digitalis increases automaticity within the atria and slows conduction in the AV node; thus, when AV block occurs in the setting of atrial tachycardias, digitalis toxicity should be suspected.

Table 15-4 outlines a stepwise approach of differentiation of narrow complex tachycardias. First, one must decide if atrial activity is clearly evident on the surface ECG. Second, is AV block present (spontaneous or induced via vagal maneuvers)? Because orthodromic AVRT requires both atrial and ventricular components in a circuit, the presence of AV block during a persistent tachycardia excludes this diagnosis. AV block during AVNRT is extremely unlikely, although rarely observed. The presence of AV block during a regular tachycardia strongly favors the diagnosis of atrial tachycardia. Third, is QRS alternans present? Alternation of the amplitude of the QRS complexes (>1 mm in height) seen at least 5 s after initiation of the tachycardia favors the diagnosis of orthodromic AVRT, especially when the heart rate is less than 200 beats/min during tachycardia. Fourth, the location of the P wave (P-R relationship) may aid in the differentiation of AVNRT from orthodromic AVRT. A P wave buried within the QRS, and therefore not visible on the surface electrogram, is consistent with the typical form of AVNRT. An R-P interval that is less than the P-R interval is seen during orthodromic AVRT utilizing a fast-conducting retrograde accessory pathway. An

TABLE 15-4

STEPWISE APPROACH TO DIFFERENTIATE NARROW COMPLEX TACHYCARDIAS

1. Is atrial activity present?
2. Is heart block present?
3. Is there QRS alternans? (SVT duration longer than 10 s)
4. P-wave location: RP vs. PR
5. P-wave morphology/axis: superior–inferior, left–right
6. Mode of initiation, termination, and influence of BBB on the SVT

BBB, bundle branch block; SVT, supraventricular tachycardia

R-P interval longer than the P-R interval is usually observed during the atypical form of AVNRT and during orthodromic AVRT utilizing a slowly conducting retrograde accessory pathway. The location of the P wave is variable during atrial tachycardias. A variable R-P relationship during a tachycardia suggests a lack of temporal dependence of the QRS with the subsequent P waves and favors the diagnosis of atrial tachycardia.

Fifth, the P-wave axis can further fine-tune the differentiation of narrow QRS tachycardias. A P-wave axis indicating superior to inferior activation (positive P-wave deflection in leads II, III, and aVF) is found during atrial tachycardia. A P wave axis indicating inferior to superior activation (negative P wave deflection in leads II, III, and aVF) is usually observed during AVNRT or orthodromic AVRT. The direction of atrial activation in the horizontal plane may be right to left or left to right during atrial tachycardia or orthodromic AVRT, depending on the location (right atrium or left atrium) of the atrial focus or the accessory pathway. Finally, the mode of initiation and termination of the SVT also provides diagnostic information. An atrial premature beat can initiate or terminate atrial tachycardia, AVNRT, or orthodromic AVRT. A ventricular premature beat should have no effect on atrial tachycardia and is unlikely to affect AVNRT (small reentrant circuit within the AV node). However, ventricular premature beats can commonly initiate and terminate orthodromic AVRT.

Treatment is guided by the hemodynamic response to the PSVT. Unstable patients require prompt electrical cardioversion. Relatively low energies (approximately 50 J) are usually sufficient to restore sinus rhythm. In stable patients, noninvasive vagal maneuvers are the first therapy of choice, as this often terminates arrhythmias that utilize the AV node as part of the reentrant circuit (AVNRT and AVRT) and may also slow and terminate SNRT. If vagal maneuvers fail, pharmacologic blockade of the AV node with IV adenosine should be attempted. Conduction block at the AV node will not terminate atrial tachycardia, but it may slow the ventricular response and allow confirmation of the diagnosis. Persistence of SVT in the presence of AV block excludes AVRT and makes AVNRT very unlikely. If these maneuvers fail to restore sinus rhythm, electrical cardioversion can be attempted. If antiarrhythmic medications are required, class 1 and class 3 drugs are most useful. Automatic atrial tachycardia is notoriously difficult to treat, often even resistant to electrical cardioversion. If possible, therapy must be directed at the underlying cause. If digitalis toxicity is implicated, digitalis must be discontinued and hypokalemia corrected. Radiofrequency catheter ablation may be required in management of drug-refractory SVTs.

Ventricular Tachycardia and Ventricular Fibrillation

Most ventricular tachycardia (VT) originates from reentry within the ventricular myocardium, which occurs most frequently within the subendocardial layer and less frequently from the epicardial layer. VT most often occurs in the setting of structural heart disease. In fact, more than 90% of patients presenting with sustained VT have underlying coronary artery disease (CAD). VT can also occur in patients with nonischemic cardiomyopathies, congenital and valvular heart diseases, drug toxicity, metabolic disorders, hypoxia, long Q-T syndrome, and, less commonly, in structurally normal hearts. Electrocardiographically, VT appears as a run of ventricular premature complexes (VPBs, wide QRS complexes) and is defined as three consecutive VPBs at a rate in excess of 100 beats/min. This rhythm most often is regular, but irregularity may occur, particularly during nonsustained episodes. Ventricular activation independent of atrial activity (VA dissociation) is the hallmark of VT. However, the atria may be activated retrogradely by the ventricles (VA association) in up to 50% of cases. Thus, the presence of VA association does not exclude VT. If the tachycardia lasts less than 30 s and is self-terminated, it is termed nonsustained VT (NSVT). If the tachycardia lasts more than 30 s or requires intervention for hemodynamic deterioration, it is termed sustained VT. Monomorphic VT has a single stable morphology (Figure 15-13), whereas polymorphic VT (Figure 15-14) has multiple QRS morphologies and irregular QRS patterns. The rate of polymorphic VT is often faster than 200 beats/min and frequently degenerates into VF. Sustained monomorphic VT most commonly occurs in patients with healed myocardial infarction or myocardial scar and is caused by reentry. Multiple morphologies are possible depending on the site of origin and the direction of the reentry circuit.

Ventricular-tachycardia (VT) most often occurs in setting of structural heart disease, particularly coronary artery disease.

FIGURE 15-13

Monomorphic ventricular tachycardia (VT) at approximately 300 beats/min (ventricular flutter). The QRS complexes all have the same morphology.

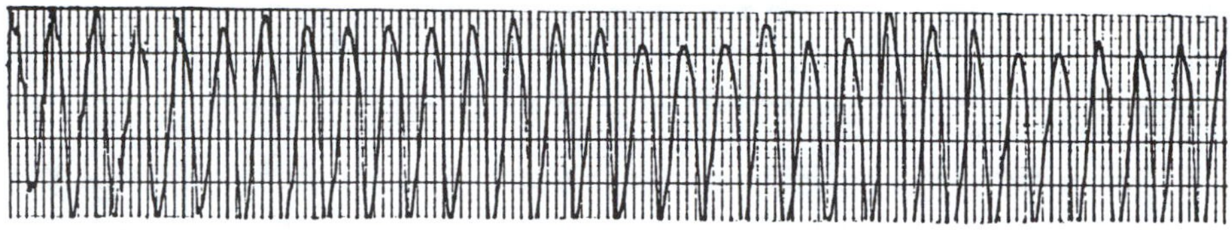

Other less common forms of VTs include bundle branch reentry (BBR), VT from the right ventricular outflow tract (RVOT), and fascicular VT. BBR VT typically occurs in patients with ventricular dysfunction caused by dilated, nonischemic cardiomyopathy. The circuit of reentry consists of the right and left bundle branches and intervening ventricular myocardium. One bundle branch serves as the anterograde limb and the other as the retrograde limb. The ECG morphology is typically that of the left bundle branch block (LBBB) pattern. Radiofrequency catheter ablation of the right bundle branch is very effective in curing BBR VT.

As its name implies, RVOT VT originates in the right ventricular outflow tract. It is generally associated with structurally normal hearts in young patients and should be suspected whenever a left bundle branch morphology of VT with an inferior axis is observed. RVOT VT may be exercise induced and thus is termed catecholamine sensitive and tends to respond to beta-blocker therapy. Fascicular VT describes an idiopathic form of reentrant VT that generally originates from the inferior left ventricular septum producing a QRS pattern of right bundle branch block with left axis deviation. The mechanism is postulated to be reentry involving the Purkinje network or various fascicles. This form of VT is also frequently observed in young people with structurally normal hearts and usually responds to verapamil, thus being termed verapamil-sensitive VT. Radiofrequency catheter ablation is an effective therapeutic option for treatment of both RVOT VT or fascicular VT and is associated with a good success rate.

Ventricular fibrillation (VF) is characterized by extremely rapid (>300 beats/min) erratic ventricular depolarizations, often giving the appearance of an undulating baseline (Figure 15-15). VF is a self-sustaining rhythm based on multiple wavelets of random reentry within a critical mass of myocardium. VF usually follows another arrhythmia such as sustained monomorphic or polymorphic VT; it also may occur during acute myocardial ischemia, metabolic derangement, or drug toxicity. Immediate hemodynamic collapse ensues, and death quickly follows. Because the defibrillation efficacy has been negatively correlated to the duration of VF, emergent DC defibrillation is essential to terminate the lethal arrhythmia. The ability of VT to cause hemodynamic decline is related to the tachycardia rate, abnormal ventricular contraction, and the underlying cardiovascular condition of the patient. Hemodynamically poorly tolerated wide complex tachycardias (WCT), regardless of cause, require prompt DC cardioversion. Sustained VT that does not cause hemodynamic compromise may

Wide complex tachycardia, regardless of cause, is poorly tolerated hemodynamically and requires prompt DC cardioversion.

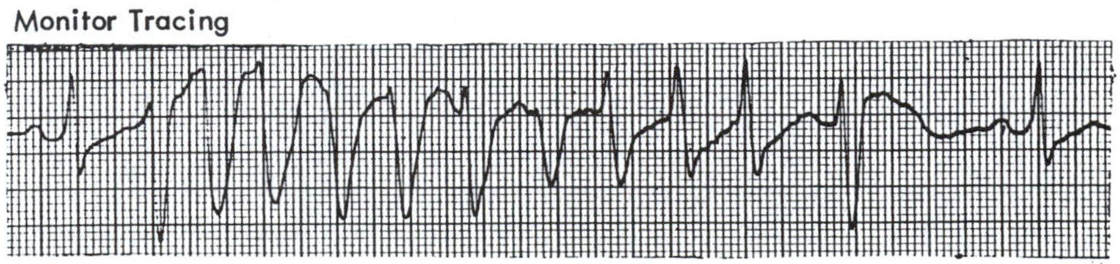

FIGURE 15-14

Polymorphic VT. A brief run of nonsustained ventricular tachycardia. The QRS complexes have multiple morphologies.

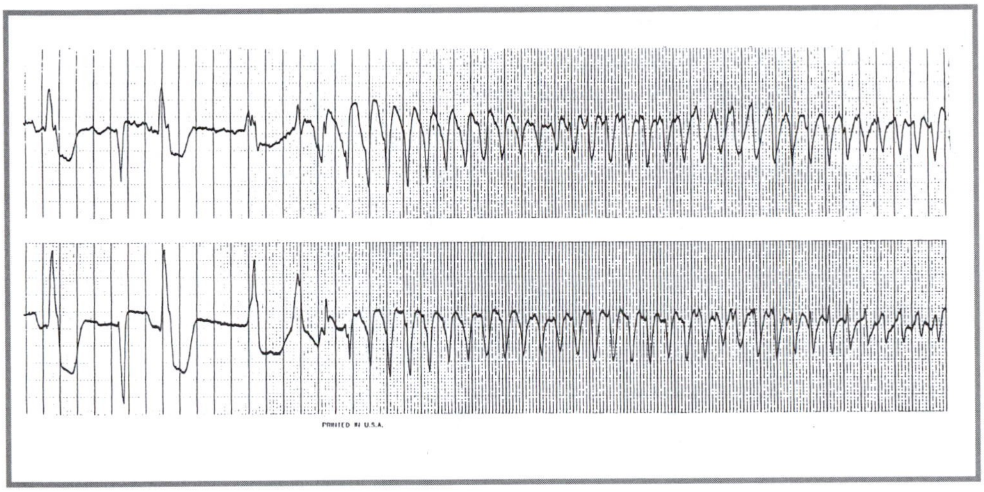

FIGURE 15-15

Ventricular fibrillation develops after a premature ventricular depolarization with R-on-T phenomenon.

be treated with a variety of pharmacologic agents including IV lidocaine, procainamide, and amiodarone. Lidocaine, however, is often ineffective outside the setting of acute cardiac ischemia. Because beta-blockers have been shown to raise the VF threshold and antagonize the catecholamines that trigger arrhythmia recurrences, they may be effective at preventing the recurrence of VT or VF.

Preexcitation

Preexcitation refers to activation/excitation of the ventricle by the atrial impulse earlier than would have occurred if the impulse had traveled exclusively down the normal AV conducting system. Preexcitation of the ventricles may occur via one of several anatomic connections, known as accessory pathways (AP), between the atria and ventricles (atrioventricular, the Kent bundle), the atria and His–Purkinje system (atriofascicular), the AV node and His–Purkinje system (nodofascicular), the AV node and ventricles (nodoventricular), and between the His–Purkinje system and the ventricles (fasciculoventricular). The latter four forms of accessory pathways or bypass tracts are collectively called Mahaim fibers.

The Wolf–Parkinson–White (WPW) syndrome is the classic form of preexcitation, caused by the abnormal presence of an accessory pathway or pathways (bundle of Kent) between the atria and the ventricles. The prevalence of WPW syndrome is estimated at between 0.1% and 0.4%; it is congenital. The classic ECG findings include (1) a short P-R interval (<0.12 s), (2) a wide QRS complex (>0.12 s) with slurring of the initial upstroke of the QRS (delta wave), and (3) abnormal repolarization (T waves). The delta wave represents a fusion of impulse conduction over the accessory pathway(s) as well as the normal AV conducting system (Figure 15-16). The degree of preexcitation (the width of the delta wave) is dependent on the relative contribution of the accessory pathway versus conduction via the normal AV node and the His–Purkinje system in producing ventricular depolarization. A larger contribution by the accessory pathway results in a wider delta wave. This syndrome has been associated with other forms of congenital heart disease such as Ebstein's anomaly and atrial septal defect, as well as mitral valve prolapse.

The clinical significance of the WPW syndrome relates primarily to the high frequency of associated arrhythmias. Orthodromic AVRT is the most prevalent arrhythmia associated with the WPW syndrome (see AVRT). The second most common, but often more dangerous, arrhythmia is atrial fibrillation. During atrial fibrillation, rapid atrial impulses may conduct over the accessory pathway and result in vary rapid ventricular rate response (up to 300 beats/min); this can precipitate significant hemodynamic decline (Figure 15-17), and degeneration into ventricular fibrillation may also occur. Electrocardiographically, atrial fibrillation in the WPW syndrome is characterized by a rapid, irregular, wide complex tachycardia that occasionally shows a normal (narrow) QRS complex because of intermittent conduction over the normal AV conducting system. Antidromic AVRT accounts for less

Orthodromic AVRT is the most common arrhythmia associated with the WPW syndrome.

The second most common, but dangerous, arrhythmia is fibrillation.

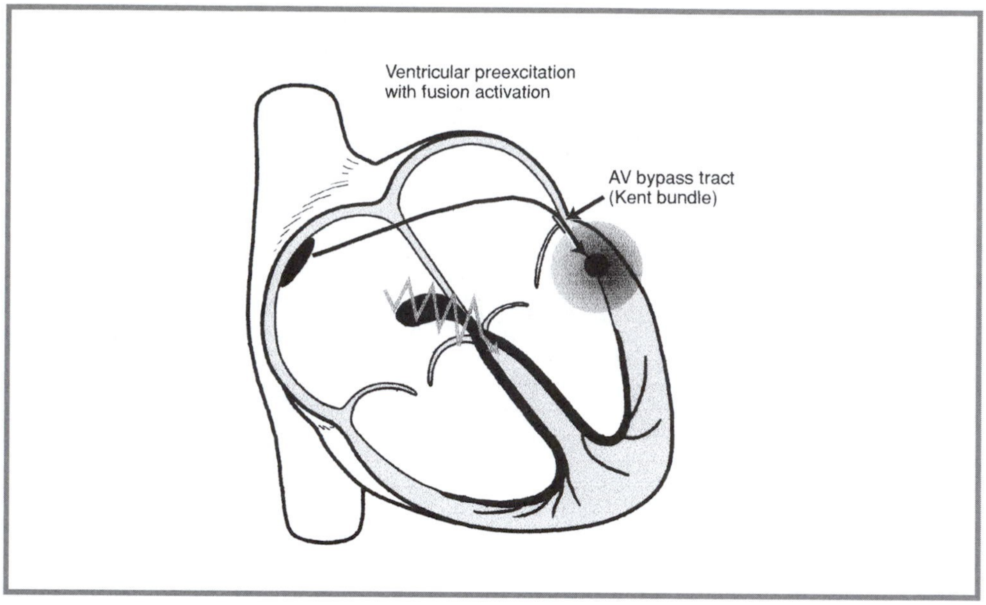

FIGURE 15-16

The Wolf–Parkinson–White (WPW) syndrome. The activation of the ventricles occurs over both the normal AV node–His–Purkinje system and an AV bypass tract. Anterograde conduction over the bypass tract preexcites the ventricular myocardium.

than 5% of cases in which the accessory pathway is the anterograde limb and the AV node–His–Purkinje system is the retrograde limb of the reentrant circuit. Ventricular activation in antidromic AVRT occurs exclusively over the bypass tract and is characteristically marked by bizarre, wide, complex tachycardia that may be indistinguishable from VT. Atrial flutter occurs rarely, but can be a significant problem if 1:1 conduction over the accessory pathway results.

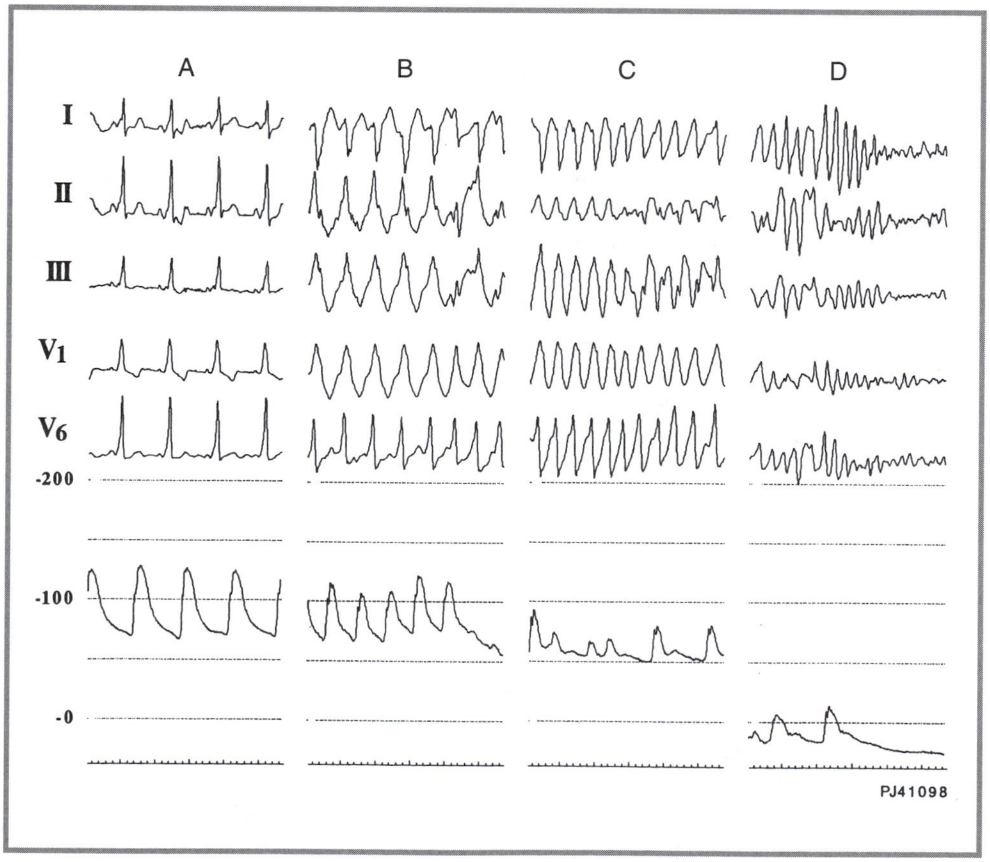

FIGURE 15-17

Surface electrogram (leads *I, II, III, V1,* and *V6*) and arterial blood pressure recordings from a patient with WPW syndrome. Note the short PR interval and slurred upstroke of the QRS complex (delta wave) during normal sinus rhythm in (*A*). The tracings in (*B*) were recorded early after the onset of atrial fibrillation while those in (*C*) were taken later in the course of atrial fibrillation during rapid AV conduction over the accessory pathway. Finally, the rhythm degenerates into ventricular fibrillation with hemodynamic collapse, (*D*).

Therapeutic options are determined by the hemodynamic state of the patient and the type of arrhythmia encountered. The unstable patient requires prompt DC cardioversion. A regular narrow complex tachycardia in a patient known to have WPW can be assumed to be orthodromic AVRT. AV nodal blockade via vagal maneuvers or IV adenosine often terminates this arrhythmia. IV procainamide or DC cardioversion should be considered in resistant cases. In patients with AF and WPW, IV procainamide or DC cardioversion is the treatment of choice. Digoxin, verapamil, and lidocaine must not be used in the emergent treatment of AF in patients with known or suspected WPW because these agents can facilitate conduction over the accessory pathway and accelerate the tachycardia. Any patient suspected of having WPW syndrome should receive a cardiology/electrophysiology consultation.

Differentiating Wide Complex Tachycardias

A differential diagnosis of WCT includes (1) VT, (2) SVT with functional bundle branch block, (3) SVT with preexisting bundle branch block, (4) SVT with ventricular preexcitation, and (5) SVT with ventricular preexcitation.

The differential diagnosis of wide QRS complex tachycardia (WCT) includes (1) VT, (2) SVT with functional bundle branch block (BBB) or aberrant conduction, (3) SVT with preexisting, fixed BBB or aberrant conduction, and (4) SVT with ventricular preexcitation. The last category includes SVTs with innocent bystander bypass tract and antidromic tachycardia. In wide complex SVTs with an innocent bystander bypass tract, the bypass tract does not participate in the SVT mechanism. These preexcited SVTs may be difficult to distinguish from VT. To differentiate supraventricular from ventricular WCTs, heart rate and hemodynamic response are usually nondiagnostic. Known history of coronary artery disease or other structural heart disease favors VT, although SVT can also occur in this population. Certain ECG features may be used to distinguish VT from wide complex SVT.

Table 15-5 outlines a stepwise approach to the differentiation of WCT. First and foremost, the AV (P-R) relationship must be defined. The presence of VA dissociation, fusion beats, and captured beats strongly favor the diagnosis of VT. Unfortunately, these findings occur infrequently and are often difficult to recognize on the surface ECG or the telemetry tracings. Vagal maneuvers, such as CSP (carotid sinus pressure), may induce AV dissociation and make the diagnosis of SVT. Second, the QRS width should be carefully measured. By convention, QRS complexes that are predominately positive in lead V1 are designated as right bundle branch block (RBBB) morphology and QRS complexes that are predominantly negative in lead V1 are designated as left bundle branch block morphology (LBBB). In the absence of antiarrhythmic drugs that slow myocardial conduction, a QRS width greater than 0.14 s with a RBBB morphology and a QRS width greater than 0.16 s with a LBBB morphology favor VT. Third, the QRS axis may offer additional diagnostic clues. During a WCT, a RBBB morphology with a superior axis (negative QRS in leads II, II, and aVF) favors VT, whereas a LBBB morphology with a right-axis deviation (QRS axis +90° to +210°) favors VT. Fourth, certain morphologic characteristics are extremely valuable in determining the origin of WCT. The absence of an RS complex in all precordial leads is highly specific for VT. In addition, when an RS complex is present in any precordial lead, an RS interval of 100 ms is also highly suggestive of VT.

Brugada et al. incorporated these findings with prior morphologic criteria developed by Wellens and Kindwall to construct a simple stepwise algorithm for the differential diagnosis of wide complex tachycardias (Figure 15-18). Table 15-6 and Figure 15-19 outline the differentiating configurational characteristics of RBBB and LBBB pattern wide complex tachycardias. During WCT with RBBB pattern QRS, a monophasic or biphasic QRS complex in lead V1 and an R:S less than 1 in lead V6 favor the diagnosis of VT. A triphasic QRS complex in leads V1 or V6 favor SVT. During a WCT with LBBB pattern QRS, a R wave

TABLE 15-5

STEPWISE APPROACH TO DIFFERENTIATE WIDE COMPLEX TACHYCARDIAS

1. What is the relationship of atrial and ventricular events?
2. What is the width of the QRS complex?
3. What is the axis of the QRS complex?
4. What are the morphologic features of the QRS complex?

FIGURE 15-18

Differential diagnosis of wide QRS complex tachycardia. (From Brugada et al. Circulation 1991;83:1649.)

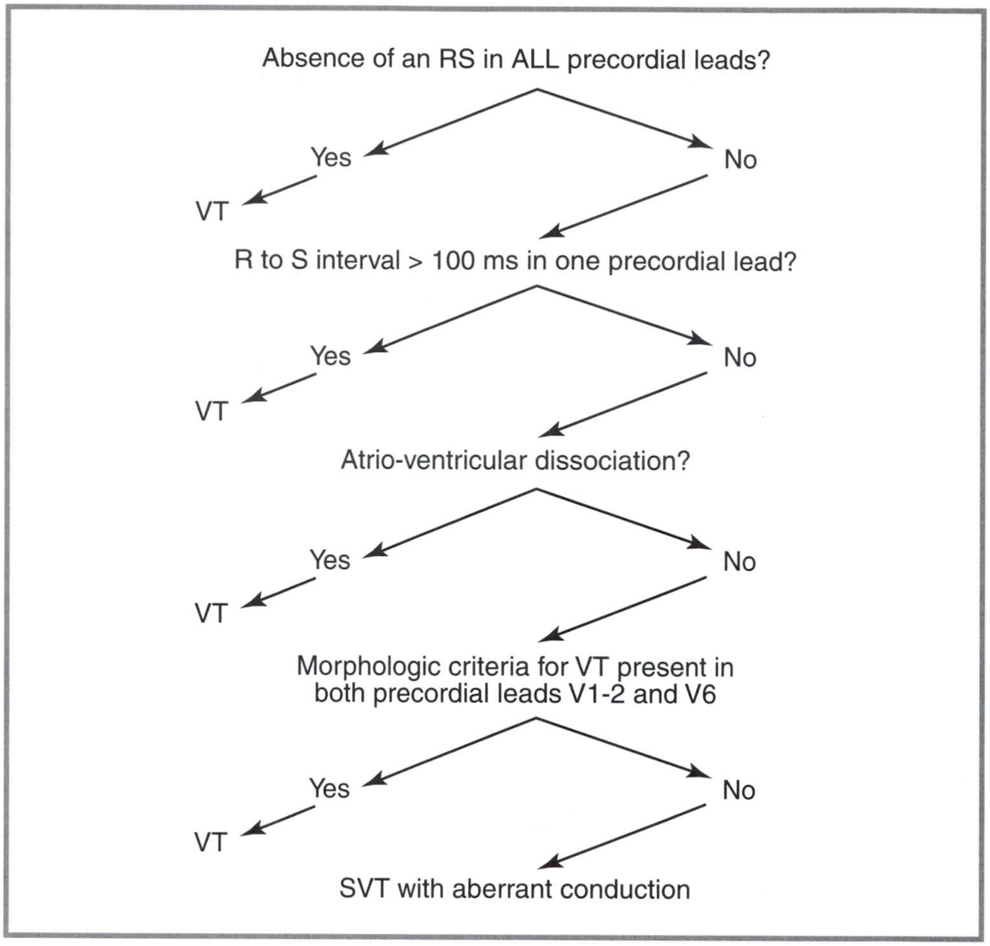

greater than 30 ms in duration in leads V1 or V2, an interval greater than 30 ms from the onset of the QRS to the S nadir, and notching of the downstroke of the S wave favor the diagnosis of VT. In lead, V6, the presence of a Q wave favors VT. The sensitivity of the four consecutive steps was 99% and the specificity was 97%. An additional feature that is characteristic of VT is a QRS width during the tachycardia that is narrower than the QRS width during sinus rhythm, because it is highly unlikely that aberrant conduction during a tachycardia will result in a narrower QRS.

Therapeutically, a wide complex tachycardia associated with hemodynamic decline is always treated with prompt DC cardioversion. In hemodynamically stable patients in whom the diagnosis remains unclear, IV adenosine may be used as a diagnostic agent. If the arrhythmia is supraventricular, adenosine often terminates the tachycardia or makes the diagnosis apparent by causing transient AV block and unmasking atrial activity. Adenosine usually has no effect on VT, except for RVOT VT.

TABLE 15-6

DIFFERENTIATION OF RBBB AND LBBB PATTERN WIDE COMPLEX TACHYCARDIAS

When V_1 is mainly upright ("RBBB" pattern):
In V_1: Monophasic or biphasic pattern (R, qR, QR, RS) suggests VT
In V_6: R to S ratio less than 1 (R/S<1) suggests VT
When V_1 is mainly negative ("LBBB" pattern):
In V_{1-2}: broad R wave (>30 ms duration)
Slurred or notched downslope to S suggests VT
>60 ms from the R to the nadir of S wave suggests VT
In V_6: R < S, any significant Q wave suggests VT
R > S and large monophasic R waves suggest SVT

RBBB, right bundle branch block; LBBB, left bundle branch block

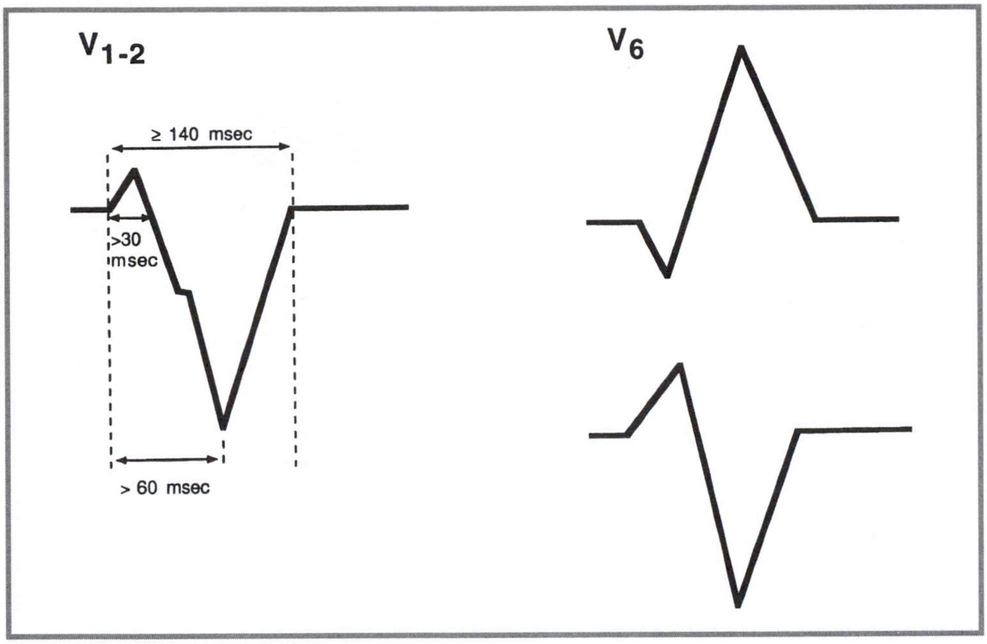

FIGURE 15-19

Morphologic characteristics of left bundle branch block (LBBB) pattern ventricular tachycardia (VT). *Left*: QRS configuration of a LBBB pattern VT in leads *V1* and *V2*. Note the broad R wave (>30 ms duration), slurred/notched downstroke of the S wave, and >60 ms duration from the beginning of the R wave to the S nadir. *Right*: typical QRS configurations of LBBB pattern VT in lead *V6*. Note the significant Q-wave and the R-wave amplitude, which is less than the S-wave amplitude (R/S ratio < 1).

SPECIAL CONSIDERATIONS

The Long QT Syndrome

The upper limit of normal for the duration of the QT interval corrected for the heart rate (QTc) is generally accepted as 0.44 s (Figure 15-20). Prolongation of the QT interval is due to abnormalities of cardiac repolarization. These abnormalities allow the formation of early depolarization- (EAD-) related triggered activity and possibly reentry that may be responsible for the development of polymorphic VT. Torsade de pointes (TdP, twisting of the points) is defined as polymorphic VT associated with prolonged QT intervals. It is characterized by QRS complexes with oscillating axis of positive and negative deflections giving the appearance of twisting along the isoelectric line (Figure 15-21). The long QT syndrome (LQTS) occurs in congenital or acquired forms.

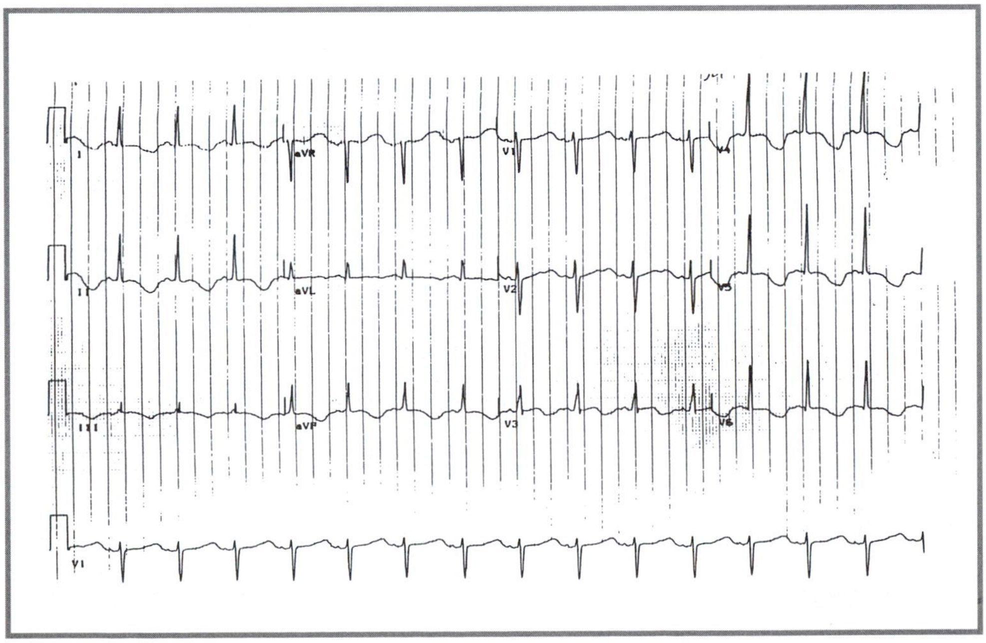

FIGURE 15-20

QT interval prolongation. Note the markedly prolonged QT interval of 540 ms. The corrected QT interval (QTc.) is 657 ms.

FIGURE 15-21

Torsades de pointes. Note the presence of complete heart block and bradycardia. Torsades de pointes was initiated by a R-on-T event with prolonged QT intervals.

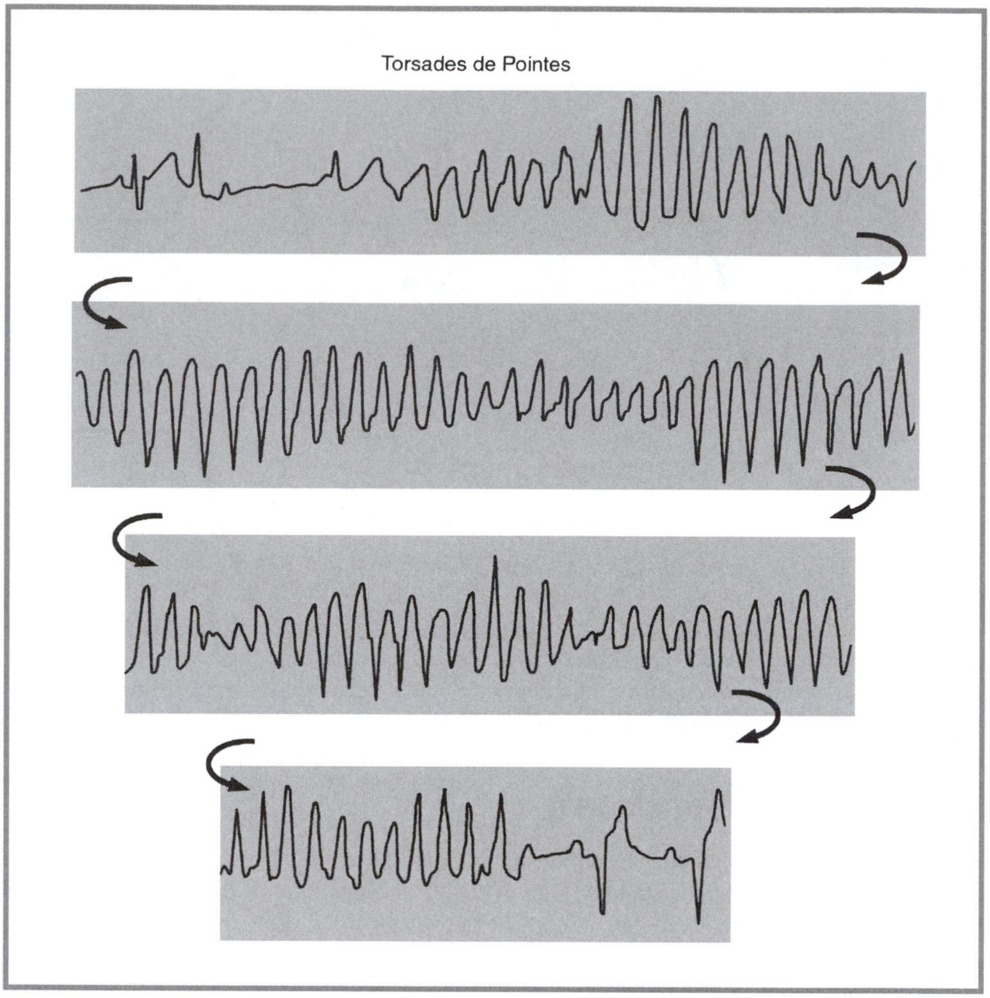

Patients with congenital LQTS typically present with syncope or cardiac arrest, and there is often a family history of sudden death.

Three types of congenital LQTS have been identified: (1) an autosomal recessive type (Jervell and Lange–Nielsen) associated with congenital deafness, (2) an autosomal dominant type (Romano–Ward) not associated with deafness, and (3) a sporadic type. Patients with congenital LQTS typically present with recurrent syncope or cardiac arrest, and often there is a family history of sudden death. This syndrome is responsible for approximately 4000 cases of sudden cardiac death in children and young adults each year in the United States. The acquired form is characteristically associated with bradycardic pauses and prominent late diastolic U waves. Clinically, it occurs in association with certain antiarrhythmic drugs (particularly class I-A and class III agents), electrolyte disturbances (primarily hypokalemia), bradycardia, psychoactive drugs, and macrolide antibiotics. Other miscellaneous drugs that have been linked to QT prolongation and TdP include terfenadine, probucol, papaverine, ketanserin, cocaine, and bepridil. Table 15-7 lists drugs commonly associated with QT interval prolongation.

Treatment for sustained tachyarrhythmias associated with the LQTS is immediate cardioversion. Magnesium sulfate administered intravenously has been shown to suppress polymorphic VT in this setting. Electrolyte imbalances must be corrected, and any potential offending drug must be discontinued. Attempts to shorten repolarization (shorten the QT interval) by increasing the heart rate with atropine, isoproterenol infusion, or temporary overdrive pacing may also be effective. Because the risk of sudden death is relatively high even in asymptomatic patients with congenital LQTS, prophylactic treatment with beta-blockers is often recommended. Other forms of chronic treatment include cervicothoracic sympathectomy, permanent pacing, and placement of an implantable cardioverter-defibrillator.

TABLE 15-7

DRUGS REPORTED TO CAUSE QT INTERVAL PROLONGATION AND TORSADE DE POINTES

TYPE	EXAMPLES
Antiarrhythmics	Class IA and III
Antifungal	Fluconazole, itraconazole, ketoconazole
Antihistamine	Astemazole, diphenhydramine, terfenadine
Antibiotics	Erythromycin, TMP-sulfa
Antimalarial/antiprotozoal	Chloroquine, mefloquine, pentamidine, quinine
Gastrointestinal	Cisapride
Psychiatric	Haloperidol, lithium phenothiazine, tricyclic antidepressants
Other	Amantidine, chloral hydrate, indapamide, probucol, tacrolimus, vasopressin papaverine, cocaine, bepridil

Sudden Cardiac Death

Sudden cardiac death (SCD) is defined as an unexpected death from a cardiac cause within a short period of time (<1 h) after the onset of symptoms. It is responsible for as many as 500,000 deaths annually in the United States (Table 15-8). Most patients have underlying coronary artery disease (CAD) (>80%), but only 20%–25% of patients have evidence of acute myocardial infarction at presentation. Other risk factors of sudden cardiac death include a previous history of SCD, left ventricular dysfunction (particularly if associated with coronary artery disease and nonsustained ventricular tachyarrhythmia), hypertrophic obstructive cardiomyopathy, syncope associated with ventricular arrhythmias, early postinfarction ventricular arrhythmias (VT or VF occurring 3 days to 2 months after an myocardial infarction), survival of myocardial infarction with frequent or complex ventricular ectopy, NYHA class III–IV heart failure, and the long Q-T syndrome. Myocardial ischemia, metabolic abnormalities, drug toxicity, and abnormalities of the autonomic nervous system (sympathetic overactivity and/or parasympathetic underactivity) may trigger life-threatening arrhythmias in patients with the appropriate underlying substrate. VT or VF are responsible for the majority of cases in which a cause can be identified. AV block, asystole, and mechanical failure may also cause SCD in the remainder of patients.

Survivors of SCD should be evaluated for reversible causes such as myocardial ischemia, acute infarction, severe metabolic abnormalities, and drug toxicity. Coronary angiography is recommended to define the presence and the extent of coronary artery disease. An echocardiogram is performed to assess ventricular function and structural abnormalities. Electrophysiologists should be available for consultation. If no reversible cause is found, an implantable cardioverter-defibrillator (ICD) is recommended because of the high risk for recurrence. Early observational reports and recent prospective, randomized trials have uniformly documented the benefit of ICD therapy in reduction of SCD, both in survivors of cardiac arrest (secondary prevention) and in high-risk patients for future arrhythmic event (primary prevention). If an ICD implantation is not an option, alternative drug treatment with amiodarone is indicated.

Survivors of sudden cardiac death should be evaluated for reversible causes to define the underlying structural abnormalities and arrhythmia substrate.

TABLE 15-8

SUDDEN CARDIAC DEATH

400,000–500,000 sudden deaths per year in the United States
50% of all cardiovascular deaths
80% of patients die out of hospital
50% of out-of-hospital cardiac arrest survivors die in hospital:
- 60% from CNS deficits
- 30% from CHF
- 10% from arrhythmia

Acute Myocardial Infarction

> As many as 30% of acute myocardial infarction (MI) patients have AV conduction disturbances.

Arrhythmias and conduction defects occur frequently in the setting of an acute myocardial infarction (AMI). It is important to distinguish benign from potentially life-threatening arrhythmias. Sinus tachycardia is usually an appropriate physiologic response during an AMI and is therefore the most commonly seen arrhythmia. In hemodynamically stable patients, judicial use of beta-blockers is recommended. Sinus bradycardia is also not an uncommon occurrence, particularly in the first few hours of an inferior wall infarction. AV conduction disturbances occur in up to 30% of patients with AMI. Those disturbances occurring with inferior wall infarction are caused by heightened vagal tone on the AV node (Bezold–Jarisch reflex) or RCA or AV nodal artery hypoperfusion resulting in AV nodal ischemia. Temporary pacing is indicated for symptomatic patients; however, permanent pacing is rarely necessary as these conduction disturbances are typically transient and associated with a benign clinical course. AV block associated with anterior wall infarction usually results from LAD occlusion with subsequent infranodal, His bundle necrosis. In this instance, the conduction disturbance tends to be permanent, necessitating permanent pacing if high-grade AV block develops. Overall, complete heart block develops in 5%–8% of patients with AMI and is associated with increased mortality regardless of the location of infarction.

> Approximately 10%–20% of acute MI patients develop an atrial arrhythmia.

> VT or VF occurs in less than 5% of patients with acute MI.

Symptomatic bradycardia should be treated with temporary transvenous pacing. The use of atropine should be avoided in AMI. The increasing sinus automaticity and tachycardia rate response can precipitate a worsening of ischemia and the development of ventricular arrhythmia. Approximately 10%–20% of patients develop an atrial arrhythmia, mostly atrial fibrillation or flutter, within 24 h of an AMI. These arrhythmias are also often transient although they are associated with a worse prognosis. In postinfarction patients, ventricular ectopy and nonsustained ventricular tachycardia occur frequently, but sustained episodes of VT or VF occur in less than 5% of cases. VT or VF occurring early in the periinfarction period (within 48 h of an AMI) is often transient and usually requires only short-term antiarrhythmic drug therapy. Sustained VT occurring after 48 h postinfarction is associated with increased mortality and recurrent arrhythmia. Therefore, complete electrophysiologic evaluation with aggressive antiarrhythmic drug therapy is warranted.

Implantation of an ICD may be necessary in high-risk patients. The incidence of VF is highest within the first 4 h of an acute myocardial infarction and may occur in up to 5% of patients. Immediate defibrillation followed by intravenous antiarrhythmic drug treatment is indicated. Accelerated idioventricular rhythm can also occur, either as an escape mechanism or as an abnormal ectopic focus that often follows reperfusion or thrombolytic therapy. Prophylactic use of antiarrhythmic agents (except beta-blockers and possibly amiodarone) is not indicated. The American College of Cardiology and the American Heart Association (ACC/AHA) Guidelines on acute myocardial infarction do not recommend antiarrhythmic therapy for isolated ventricular ectopy, couplets, accelerated idioventricular rhythm, or nonsustained ventricular tachycardia.

SUMMARY

Arrhythmia diagnosis may often appear to be an imposing task. However, a fundamental understanding of cellular electrophysiology, conduction system anatomy, the mechanisms of arrhythmogenesis, and the clinical scenarios common to a particular arrhythmia coupled with a systematic analysis of rhythm disturbances often leads the clinician to the correct diagnosis. The importance of a systematic approach to arrhythmia diagnosis cannot be overemphasized. Once a diagnosis is reached with reasonable certainty, therapeutic interventions can be attempted. This chapter has centered mostly on arrhythmia diagnosis with only a brief overview of therapeutic interventions. A more detailed discussion of antiarrhythmic medications and implantable cardioverter-defibrillators is presented elsewhere in this text.

REVIEW QUESTIONS

1. **Which of the following statements regarding arrhythmia management is/are true?**
   - **A.** Automatic arrhythmias occur when cells undergo spontaneous diastolic (phase 4) depolarizations and form action potentials.
   - **B.** Arrhythmias caused by triggered activity are initiated by after-depolarizations.
   - **C.** Multiple anatomic or functionally defined pathways are required for reentry to occur.
   - **D.** Unidirectional conduction block is required for reentry to occur.
   - **E.** All of the above.

2. **Interruption of conduction through the AV node terminates AV nodal-dependent tachycardias. AV nodal-dependent tachycardias include which of the following?**
   - **A.** Atrial tachycardias
   - **B.** Orthodromic AV reentry tachycardias utilizing a bypass tract
   - **C.** Atrial flutter
   - **D.** AV nodal reentry tachycardia
   - **E.** B and D
   - **F.** A and C

3. **Which of the following is/are true regarding differentiation of the site of AV conduction block?**
   - **A.** Narrow QRS complex escape rhythm greater than 40 beats/min usually indicates block within or above the level of the AV node.
   - **B.** A wide QRS complex escape rhythm greater than 40 beats/min usually indicates block within the AV node.
   - **C.** If exercise, atropine, or isoproterenol administration improve AV conduction, the site of block is likely at the AV node.
   - **D.** If vagal maneuvers, such as carotid sinus pressure, improve AV conduction, the site of block is likely at the AV node.
   - **E.** A and C.
   - **F.** B and D.

4. **The differential diagnosis of long R-P tachycardias includes which of the following?**
   - **A.** The uncommon (fast–slow) form of AV nodal reentry tachycardia
   - **B.** Atrial tachycardia
   - **C.** Orthodromic AV reentry tachycardia utilizing a slowly conducting bypass tract
   - **D.** Orthodromic AV reentry tachycardia utilizing a fast-conducting bypass tract
   - **E.** A and C
   - **F.** A, B, and C

5. **In the absence of antiarrhythmic drugs that slow myocardial conduction, which of the following excludes the diagnosis of ventricular tachycardia?**
   - **A.** Monophasic or biphasic QRS complex in lead V1 and an R:S <1 in lead V6 during an RBBB pattern wide complex tachycardia (WCT).
   - **B.** R wave >30 ms, >60 ms from the onset of the QRS to the S nadir, and notching of the downstroke of the S wave in anterior precordial leads (V1 or V2) leads during a WCT.
   - **C.** AV association.
   - **D.** AV dissociation with fusion beats or capture beats.
   - **E.** None of the above.

ANSWERS

1. The answer is E: All of the above. Automatic and triggered arrhythmias account for a minority of arrhythmias. Arrhythmias due to automaticity are caused by phase 4 diastolic depolarization of cellular membrane potentials that reach the threshold and generate abnormal action potentials. Arrhythmias associated with triggered activity are caused by cellular membrane potential oscillation that forms afterdepolarizations. Reentry is responsible for most clinically relevant tachyarrhythmias. Prerequisites of reentry include (1) an initiating event, most likely a premature beat that results in unidirectional block; (2) multiple anatomic or functional pathways; and (3) sufficiently slow conduction down the alternative pathway so that the tissue proximal to the block recovers excitability and allows the impulse to reenter the circuit.
2. The answer is E: B and D. AV nodal-dependent SVTs utilize the AV node as a critical path in the arrhythmia circuit. These arrhythmias include AVNRT, which is a reentrant circuit within the AV nodal region utilizing the dual AV nodal pathway physiology (fast and slow pathways), and orthodromic AVNRT, which is a macroreentrant circuit utilizing anterograde conduction through the AV node and retrograde conduction through bypass tract(s). The mechanism responsible for the initiation and maintenance of AV nodal-independent SVTs reside above the AV node, and interruption of conduction at the AV node does not terminate these arrhythmias but may slow the ventricular response.
3. The answer is E: A and C. The site of AV block may be suggested by the width of the escape rhythm (see Table 15-1). A narrow QRS complex rhythm at a rate of 40–55 beats/min suggests a junctional escape rhythm and therefore the site of block is within the AV node, proximal to the AV junction. A wide QRS rhythm at a rate less than 40 beats/min suggests infranodal block. The response of AV conduction to various maneuvers or drugs may also localize the site of the block (see Table 15-2). Sympathetic stimulation or parasympathetic withdrawal (exercise, atropine, or isoproterenol) improves AV nodal conduction. These maneuvers may worsen infranodal conduction block by enhancing proximal AV nodal impulse propagation and thus stress the distal His–Purkinje system. If vagal maneuvers worsen AV conduction, the site of block is likely within the AV node, whereas an improvement in conduction suggests block below the AV node.
4. The answer is F: A, B and C. The P-wave location is variable during atrial tachycardias, but usually with a shorter PR than RP intervals. The uncommon form of AVNRT utilizes anterograde conduction down the fast AV nodal pathway (short PR) and retrograde conduction up the slow AV nodal pathway (long RP). Dur-

ing the common forms of orthodromic AVRT, the retrograde conduction up the bypass tract is sufficiently fast that the result is a shorter RP than PR. A long RP is seen during the uncommon forms of orthodromic AVRT. The retrograde limb of the reentrant circuit is a slowly conducting bypass tract with a longer RP than PR.

5. The answer is E: None of the above. The differential diagnosis of a WCT includes (1) VT, (2) SVT with functional aberrant conduction, (3) SVT with preexisting "fixed" aberrant conduction, and (4) SVT with ventricular preexcitation. Certain electrocardiographic morphologic criteria can be useful in distinguishing VT from wide complex SVT (see Tables 15-5, 15-6; Figures 15-18, 15-19). The presence of a monophasic or biphasic QRS complex in lead V1 and an R:S <1 in lead V6 suggests VT during an RBBB pattern WCT. A broad R wave (>30 ms), with a slow and inhomogeneous ventricular conduction (R-to-S >60 ms with notching on the downstroke of the S wave) suggests VT during a LBBB pattern WCT. Although VA dissociation is a hallmark of VT, AV association may be observed in up to 50% of VTs.

SUGGESTED READING

Brugada P, Brugada J, Mont L, et al. A new approach to the differential diagnosis of a regular tachycardia with a wide QRS complex. Circulation 1991;83:1649–1659.

El-Sherif N, Turitto G. The long QT syndrome and Torsade de Pointes. PACE 1999;22(Pt I):91–110.

Josephson ME. Clinical Cardiac Electrophysiology: Techniques and Interpretations, 2nd Ed. Philadelphia: Lea & Febiger, 1993.

Josephson ME, Wellens HJJ. Differential diagnosis of supraventricular tachycardia. Cardiol Clin 1990;8(3):411–442.

Kindwall EK, Brown J, Josephson ME. Electrocardiographic criteria for ventricular tachycardia in wide complex left bundle branch block morphology tachycardias. Am J Cardiol 1988;61:1279–1283.

Marriot HJL. Practical Electrocardiography, 8th Ed. Philadelphia: Williams & Wilkins, 1988.

Wellens HJ, Bar FW, Liek I. The value of the electrocardiogram in the differential diagnosis of a tachycardia with a widened QRS Complex. Am J Med 1978;64:27–33.

CHAPTER 16

GILBERT E. D'ALONZO AND DAVID FRIEDEL

Gastrointestinal Hemorrhage

CHAPTER OUTLINE

LEARNING OBJECTIVES

After studying this chapter, you should be able to:

- Discuss the differential diagnosis of acute gastrointestinal bleeding.
- Describe the diagnostic and therapeutic maneuvers necessary to identify the cause and control of gastrointestinal hemorrhage in the ICU.
- Understand the role of endoscopy, surgery, and tube placement in upper and lower GI bleeding.
- Appreciate the complications of stress ulceration and how it occurs in the critically ill patient.

ACUTE GASTROINTESTINAL HEMORRHAGE

Acute gastrointestinal hemorrhage is a common emergency that either necessitates admission to an intensive care unit or complicates the course of the ICU patient initially hospitalized for other reasons. Mortality associated with gastrointestinal hemorrhage is significant and has remained about 10% since World War II. Mortality has not changed despite technologic advances, perhaps due to increased patient age and the presence of comorbid disease. The upper gastrointestinal tract is the site of origin for most acute gastrointestinal bleeding, but the lower small intestine and the colon can often be the source of such bleeding. This chapter reviews the evaluation and management of the ICU patient with gastrointestinal bleeding, including differential diagnosis, diagnostic modalities, and treatment options.

DIFFERENTIAL DIAGNOSIS

Gastrointestinal hemorrhage occurs in 15%–35% of patients admitted to the ICU for reasons other than GI bleeding (Table 16-1). A wide variety of conditions may cause upper gastrointestinal hemorrhage. The most common potential etiologies are ulcers (peptic, stress), gastritis (drug- or alcohol-related), varices (esophageal, gastric), or a Mallory–Weiss tear. Bleeding related to peptic ulceration or varices can be obvious on admission or can manifest later in the hospitalization. Stress ulceration occurs after admission and relates to acute illness (pneumonia, trauma, burns) or systemic disease. Less common causes of upper gastrointestinal hemorrhage include esophagitis, malignancy, and angiodysplasia. Occasionally, the source of gastrointestinal bleeding (upper or lower) remains unknown despite an ex-

Upper and lower gastrointestinal (GI) lesions are the cause of bleeding in the critically ill.

CASE STUDY: PART 1

A 43-year-old lawyer with a known history of cigarette smoking developed shortness of breath, cough productive of discolored sputum, and fever. Despite taking appropriate oral antibiotics as an outpatient, his respiratory condition deteriorated. He was admitted to the intensive care unit (ICU) after evaluation in the emergency department with a respiratory rate of 42 breaths/min, blood pressure of 80/40 mmHg, heart rate of 140 beats/min, and a temperature of 102.9°F. He was stuporous and complaining of left-sided chest pain.

On subsequent examination he had diffuse left lung crackles. He was emergently intubated and placed on assist-control mechanical ventilation. Intravenous antibiotic therapy was initiated, and a diagnosis of severe community-acquired pneumonia is made. Within 48 h, his condition began to improve. Tachypnea and mental status improved, and his blood pressure and heart rate were now 110/80 mmHg and 100 beats/min, respectively. On the fifth hospital day his blood pressure dropped dramatically to 70/40 mmHg and his heart rate increased to 132 beats/min. His mental status remained stable and he had no additional complaints. He denied abdominal discomfort. His chest pain had actually improved, and he claimed that his breathing was more comfortable. There were no ischemic changes on his electrocardiogram, and his arterial blood gases had substantially improved since admission to the hospital.

On physical examination, his mental status had improved. He had fewer crackles and better breath sounds in his left chest, and his right chest was normal on auscultation. The cardiac examination, with the exception of tachycardia, was normal. An abdominal examination revealed mild epigastric tenderness on deep palpation and he had hyperactive bowel sounds. Rectal examination revealed melanotic stool.

haustive diagnostic evaluation. Bleeding from an obscure origin in an ICU patient with multisystem disease significantly increases mortality.

> Stress ulcers are common but preventable shallow mucosal lesions that occur in critically ill patients.

Stress ulcerations are erosions or small ulcers in the gastroduodenal mucosa that develop acutely in critically ill patients who experience serious physiologic instability. These ulcerations occur chiefly in the gastric fundus but may also occur at the level of the pylorus and duodenum. These lesions are generally small, shallow mucosal erosions without serious submucosal penetration. Many of these ulcers do not progress to bleeding. They are usually multiple and begin to appear within 24 h of admission to the ICU. However, over time they become larger, deeper, and in fact may bleed by 72 h after admission. Histologically, they have minimal acute inflammatory cell infiltration. Although stress ulceration is frequently found in critically ill patients, these patients are generally asymptomatic. Abdominal pain is rarely reported. Gastroduodenal perforation only rarely occurs. Hematemesis and frank melena are unusual, but trace positive blood in the stool frequently occurs. Fortunately, stress ulceration has become much less common with the widespread use of pharmacologic prophylaxis, early enteral nutrition, and greater attention to reestablishment of systemic perfusion and oxygenation.

TABLE 16-1

CAUSES OF UPPER GASTROINTESTINAL HEMORRHAGE

- Common (75%–90%)
  - Peptic ulcer (gastric, duodenal)
  - Stress ulcer
  - Gastritis (nonsteroidal antiinflammatory drugs, alcohol)
  - Esophageal varices
  - Mallory–Weiss tear
- Less common (10%–15%)
  - Esophagitis
  - Malignancy
  - Anastomotic ulcer
- Rare
  - Angiodysplasia
  - Mucocutaneous syndromes (Osler–Weber–Rendu disease, Peutz–Jeghers disease, Ehlers–Danlos disease)
  - Polyps
  - Hemobilia
  - Aortoenteric fistula
  - Dieulafoy's lesion

Gastric or duodenal peptic ulceration is responsible for up to 50% of the episodes of acute upper gastrointestinal hemorrhage. Most patients have abdominal pain or dyspepsia; only a small percentage of patients are asymptomatic. Patients with peptic ulceration often have hematemesis and melena. The epigastric pain associated with peptic ulceration is often nocturnal and relieved by food, antacids, or histamine blockers. Esophageal varices are a manifestation of portal hypertension caused by cirrhosis. The bleeding associated with esophageal varices is usually abrupt and severe. There is a high mortality risk with bleeding esophageal varices, ranging from 40% to 70% during the first episode of bleeding. It is important to realize that a patient with known esophageal varices frequently has upper gastrointestinal bleeding from sites other than the varices. This bleeding may emanate from a peptic ulcer, a Mallory–Weiss tear, or portal gastropathy (gastric wall edema related to portal hypertension).

Peptic ulcer disease is the most common cause of GI bleeding and is associated with melena and hematochezia.

Varices are thin, bulbous venous channels that are enlarged and engorged when blood is pathologically shunted from the systemic to the portal circulation because of the loss of functioning liver cells in cirrhosis. Large collateral channels or varices are invariably present at the gastroesophageal junction in patients with portal hypertension, and bleeding occurs with increased intravariceal pressure. The onset of bleeding tends to be abrupt, painless, and massive and generally follows vomiting. Bleeding risk depends on variceal size and hepatic venous pressure and the severity of the underlying liver disease. These patients often have soluble clotting factor disorders and thrombocytopenia. Variceal bleeding recurs in nearly 50% of patients, and two-thirds of patients die within 12 months of the initial hemorrhagic episode.

Variceal bleeding is associated with portal hypertension secondary to cirrhosis.

A Mallory–Weiss tear occurs at the esophagastric junction and is an often unappreciated cause of severe upper gastrointestinal bleeding in an ICU patient. It is more common in patients with active alcoholism, and classically such patients have antecedent retching of gastric contents before developing hematemesis. Patients with prior aortic graft surgery may develop torrential upper gastrointestinal bleeding from an aortoenteric fistula. These patients classically have a "herald bleed" of a lesser magnitude hours to days before this.

Previous vomiting is an important clue to distal esophageal tearing.

Patients with lower gastrointestinal hemorrhage, distal to the second portion of the duodenum (ligament of Treitz), usually present with hematochezia or bright red blood coming from the rectum. Causes of lower gastrointestinal hemorrhage are found in Table 16-2. Rapid lower gastrointestinal hemorrhage is usually caused by diverticular disease or angiodysplasia. Cutaneous or mucous membrane arteriovenous malformations may signal the presence of Osler–Weber–Rendu (OWR) syndrome. A variety of conditions are associated with slower hemorrhage including inflammatory and ischemic bowel diseases, radiation-induced colitis, polyps, hemorrhoids, and neoplasm. In contrast to upper gastrointestinal bleeding, which is almost always rapidly and accurately diagnosed, lower gastrointestinal bleeding remains undiagnosed in 10%–15% of patients.

Lower GI bleeding is associated with hematochezia.

Two major causes of hematochezia are diverticulosis and angiodysplasia.

Bleeding from colonic diverticuli and angiomata are the two most common causes of lower gastrointestinal bleeding. Diverticuli are most frequent in the sigmoid colon, but torrential diverticular bleeding is usually from the right side. Bleeding can be mild or massive. Massive bleeding can be associated with hemodynamic instability including orthostatic hypotension. Fortunately, most diverticular bleeding ceases spontaneously. Angiodysplasic lesions are vascular abnormalities that can range from 3 to 15 mm. These lesions could be found throughout the gastrointestinal tract, but there is a particular predilection for the stomach, ileum, and right colon. They become more common with age, and there is an associa-

TABLE 16-2

CAUSES OF LOWER GASTROINTESTINAL HEMORRHAGE

Diverticulosis
Angiodysplasia
Polyps
Hemorrhoid
Inflammatory disease
Ischemic colitis
Radiation-induced colitis
Malignancy

CASE STUDY: PART 2

The presence of melena and hypotension with tachycardia signaled that severe gastrointestinal hemorrhage was occurring. The priority at this time was to stabilize the patient by repleting his intravascular volume and avoiding the consequences of irreversible shock. Hypotension and tachycardia existed. There also was no evidence of significant abdominal pain. There also was no evidence of mental confusion, agitation, diaphoresis, skin mottling, or cold extremities. The patient was resuscitated with intravenous volume replacement, initially using normal saline solution, then following up with packed red blood cell transfusions. The hemoglobin and hematocrit initially returned at 8.0 g and 27%, respectively. The coagulation profile was normal. Fresh-frozen plasma transfusion was not necessary. Because the rectal bleeding had a melanotic appearance, a nasogastric tube was inserted, and gastric suctioning followed by normal saline lavage was performed. With the placement of the nasogastric tube and suctioning, it was determined that the patient had serious ongoing gastric hemorrhage. Gastric lavage using room temperature normal saline was employed to clear the stomach of blood, and an upper gastrointestinal endoscopy was performed once the patient was hemodynamically stable. A histamine-2 receptor antagonist was administered intravenously. Careful attention was paid to the urine output, and intravenous fluids were adjusted to maintain urination at least 50 ml/h.

tion with OWR syndrome, chronic renal insufficiency and aortic stenosis. Bleeding manifestations of angiodysplasia are similar to diverticular bleeding in that bleeding can be inconsequential or massive and life-threatening, with most bleeds stopping spontaneously. Angiodysplasia appears as flat furry-like lesions during endoscopy. Dieulafoy's lesion is a vascular abnormality of the bowel mucosa, more specifically, a small-caliber artery abnormally close to the mucosa that can bleed briskly with minimal mucosal effacement. Dieulafoy's lesions are typically located in the proximal stomach but can be present anywhere in the gastrointestinal tract; they can be difficult to identify at endoscopy because of their small and innocuous appearance.

> Angiodysplasia is common to the right colon and ileum.

Patients with larger colorectal cancers tend to bleed intermittently. Frank hematochezia is more common in advanced and distal lesions. Iron deficiency anemia is a common presentation. Bleeding from internal and external hemorrhoids can occasionally be massive. Such bleeding is more common in patients with poor hemostasis, including those with cirrhosis. Colitis associated with inflammatory bowel disease, bowel ischemia, or induced by radiation has been associated with subacute and massive gastrointestinal hemorrhage. Radiation colitis follows abdominal radiotherapy for malignancy when the total radiation dose has exceeded 4000 rads. Ischemic colitis generally occurs in patients older than 50 years who have evidence of arterial vascular disease elsewhere. Ulcerative colitis and Crohn's disease, from time to time, can be associated with serious gastrointestinal hemorrhage.

> Hemorrhoids can be the cause of serious GI bleeding, especially in the patient with cirrhosis.

> Ischemic colitis occurs in older patients with arterial insufficiency.

TREATMENT OF ACUTE GASTROINTESTINAL HEMORRHAGE

Examination of vomitus or aspirated gastric content and the appearance of the stool can help localize the site of bleeding. Hematemesis indicates an upper gastrointestinal bleed. "Coffee grounds" gastric aspirate through an appropriately placed nasogastric tube also signifies an upper gastrointestinal bleed.

> Upper GI bleeding is usually distinguished from lower tract bleeds by the history and physical exam.

A nasogastric tube is usually inserted to determine whether the bleeding is in the upper or lower gastrointestinal tract. Generally speaking, the presence of blood in the gastric aspirate indicates upper gastrointestinal bleeding and the absence of blood, especially if bile is aspirated, suggests a lower gastrointestinal source. However, nearly 15% of patients with upper gastrointestinal bleeding have negative gastric aspirates. These false-negative cases occasionally occur in duodenal bleeds. Sometimes massive upper gastrointestinal bleeding can produce hematochezia, or bright red rectal bleeding, but this type of hemorrhage generally originates from a lower site. Melena, or black tarry stools, results from blood digestion by acid and bacteria and signifies upper gastrointestinal blood loss. Maroon-colored stools generally signify right colonic bleeding, whereas bleeding from the left colon results in bright

> Some patients with upper GI bleeding have gastric tube aspirates negative for blood.

TABLE 16-3

INDICATORS OF MAJOR BLOOD LOSS

Resting tachycardia (>100 beats/min)
Orthostasis (pulse increase >20 beats/min, systolic BP decrease >20 mmHg, diastolic BP decrease >10 mmHg)
Acidosis
Azotemia (BUN ≥40 mg/dl without prior renal disease)
Transfusion requirements >1 unit packed red blood cells q 8 h (or 6 units total)
Hematochezia from upper GI source
Failure to clear bright red blood from gastric lavage
Continued bleeding or rebleeding during endoscopy

red blood coming from the rectum. Distal colonic bleeding is suggested by a mixture of formed stool with blood.

Estimation and replacement of blood loss is perhaps the most important aspect of therapy. Intravascular hypovolemia must be quickly corrected to prevent permanent end-organ damage. It is important not to underestimate the amount of blood lost. An estimation of blood loss depends on an assessment of the vital signs, the hemoglobin and hematocrit, and on the degree of clinical experience of the physician who is caring for the patient. Indicators of major blood loss are found in Table 16-3. Severe hemorrhage is generally defined as a blood loss of greater than 1 l. The acute physiologic response to hypovolemia includes orthostatic changes in blood pressure and pulse, vasoconstriction, and end-organ dysfunction (Table 16-4). In acute blood loss, the hemoglobin and hematocrit may drop slowly until crystalloid fluid replacement begins; then a precipitous fall may be seen. Chronic blood loss usually is associated with stable hemodynamics, appropriate end-organ function, and anemia with the retention of hypotonic fluid. The clinical picture associated with gastrointestinal bleeding can often be clouded by medication, the status of the cardiopulmonary system, and kidney and neurologic impairment.

Acute blood loss causes changes in pulse and arterial pressure while chronic bleeding is associated with stable hemodynamics.

Abdominal pain generally implies a mucosal lesion and suggests a peptic ulcer. Vomiting before the onset of bleeding suggests an esophageal tear, commonly called a Mallory–Weiss tear. Previous bleeding from a known source usually means that that same source is bleeding again. When bleeding was previously unidentified and it occurs again, then there is a high likelihood of angiodysplasia. The stigmata of chronic liver disease might be an important clue for the diagnosis of esophageal varices. A patient with known diverticular disease is always at risk for lower gastrointestinal hemorrhage.

Aggressive fluid resuscitation of patients with acute and subacute gastrointestinal bleeding is extremely important and cannot be overemphasized. After appropriate intravenous access has been established, generally using two large-bore (14- to 16-gauge) peripheral intravenous catheters, then fluid and blood replacement should be initiated. The maximum infusion rate for intravenous fluids is determined by the diameter of the catheter and not the size of the vein that is cannulated. Because the major pathophysiologic defect in hemorrhage is intravascular fluid depletion, the best initial therapy is fluid replacement, not vasopressor infusion therapy. The most convenient fluid to use is isotonic crystalloid solutions until blood replacement is available. Colloid therapies offer little advantage over crystalloids, except that

Aggressive fluid resuscitation and correction of coagulopathy during acute GI bleeding are essential.

TABLE 16-4

CLASSIFICATION OF HEMORRHAGE

CLASS	CLINICAL SIGNS	VOLUME LOSS (%)
I	Tachycardia	15
II	Orthostatic hypotension	20–25
III	Supine hypotension, oliguria	30–40
IV	Obtundation, cardiovascular collapse	>40

SOURCE: Committee on Trauma, American College of Surgeons. Early Care of the Injured Patient, 3rd Ed. Philadelphia: Saunders, 1982

TABLE 16-5

MEDICATIONS USED IN THE EMPIRIC TREATMENT OF UPPER GASTROINTENSTIAL HEMORRHAGE

Drugs that raise gastric pH
Histamine-2 receptor antagonists
Antacids
Drugs that induce splanchnic vasoconstriction
Vasopressin
Somatostatin
Octreotide
Drugs that correct coagulopathy
Vitamin K
Fresh-frozen plasma

a small volume of colloid is required to produce a similar degree of intravascular volume expansion. However, colloid therapies are expensive and have allergic potential. Whole blood therapy is rarely used, but specific components, such as packed red blood cells and plasma, are often employed. Patients with blood loss greater than 500 ml, hypotension, or end-organ dysfunction should be admitted to the ICU. The older patient who has preexisting cardiopulmonary, liver, or renal disease should also be considered earlier rather than later for intensive care treatment. Any patient who has a gastrointestinal hemorrhage with a coagulopathy should be treated in the ICU. There is ongoing debate as to the optimum target hemoglobin that should be achieved and maintained, but for most patients it seems to be 8–10 g/dl. It is most important to optimize tissue oxygenation rather than correct an anemia to a certain level. During resuscitation, the patient should be evaluated for underlying organ dysfunction. Lactic acidosis, renal failure, bowel ischemia, myocardial injury, cerebral ischemia, and limb ischemia may all complicate hemorrhage.

Pharmacologic intervention is then initiated (Table 16-5). Generally, medication that raises gastric pH such as a histamine-2 receptor (H2R) antagonist or an antacid is initiated. A H2R blocker intravenously is preferred because endoscopy is likely to be done. Other medications could be considered, such as vasopressin and somatostatin or its long-acting form, octreotide. The gastrointestinal effect of vasopressin is its ability to contract vascular smooth muscle, thereby reducing splanchnic blood flow. Portal venous flow and pressure and total hepatic flow are reduced, which could be advantageous in patients with variceal bleed. However, the value of vasopressin in peptic and stress ulceration remains questionable. Similarly, somatostatin and octreotide are used in esophageal variceal bleed and not in peptic ulceration or stress ulceration hemorrhage. Somatostatin and octreotide lower portal venous and presumably esophageal venous blood flow in patients with portal hypertension. Propranolol decreases portal blood flow and pressure, and when used chronically, it reduces rebleeding risk, but it should not be used during acute bleeding because of compensatory cardiovascular blockade. Ice water lavage has no hemostatic value. Correcting coagulopathy is essential and is done with fresh-frozen plasma and vitamin K. Sometimes platelet transfusion may be necessary. Stopping medications that induce coagulopathy, such as warfarin and heparin, is essential. Reversing coagulopathy and volume replacement are the only medical interventions that can be done for a lower gastrointestinal hemorrhage.

ENDOSCOPY FOR DIAGNOSIS AND TREATMENT

With the possible exception of varices and ulcers containing visible bleeding vessels, most GI bleeding ceases spontaneously.

Upper endoscopy is a rapid, safe, precise method to diagnose the source and cause of upper GI bleeding.

No form of empiric medical therapy has been shown to definitively improve the outcome of upper gastrointestinal hemorrhage. Most patients stop bleeding spontaneously. Nonetheless, because of its safety, ease of administration, and the possibility of efficacy, patients are generally administered an H2R intravenously at the time of admission to the ICU. Endoscopy is the procedure of choice for diagnosing the cause of upper gastrointestinal hemorrhage; it also has strong therapeutic value. Rarely, endoscopic intervention should be considered for patients who have acute gastrointestinal hemorrhage and present with shock or serious hemodynamic instability, a hemoglobin less than 8 g/dl, coagulopathy, bright red nasogastric tube aspiration after the initial resuscitation, or onset of bleeding while in the hospital. Patients who are older and who have serious concomitant disease should also be considered for early endoscopy. Upper endoscopy or esophagogastroduodenoscopy (EGD) can identify a source of bleeding in 80%–90% of patients. This high diagnostic yield drops when the procedure is delayed beyond 24 h after presentation. It has a particular value in the early diagnosis of gastric erosions including stress ulceration, peptic ulceration, angiodysplasia, and Mallory–Weiss tears of the esophagus. Certain endoscopic findings suggest an increased risk for rebleeding (Table 16-6). Upper endoscopy has the added, important advantage of therapeutically delivering thermal or injection therapy that can control hemorrhage. Even when a specific diagnosis cannot be made by endoscopy, it often localizes the area of bleeding, which is helpful to the surgeon or interventional radiologist who will subsequently treat the patient. EGD has some limitations. During the procedure, rapid bleeding can obscure the view and sedation can influence ventilation. In an uncooperative patient, viseral perforation can occur.

Upper endoscopy often provides useful prognostic information concerning risk of rebleeding.

When the endoscope is used therapeutically, it is called endotherapy. Endotherapy has been used primarily in the treatment of upper gastrointestinal bleeding. Endotherapy for hemostasis is indicated for patients at high risk for persistent or recurrent upper gastrointestinal hemorrhage (Table 16-6) and death. The prognostic criteria listed in Table 16-6 can be helpful in selecting this therapeutic subgroup. If there is endoscopic evidence of ongoing bleeding or a nonbleeding visible vessel, then endotherapy should be performed. Rates of hemostasis for the first endoscopy exceed 90%, and recurrent bleeding is often controlled with a second procedure. The modalities commonly used are thermal therapy (heater probe coagulation, electrocoagulation, laser), injection therapy (ethanol, epinephrine, hypertonic saline, other sclerosing solutions), hemoclipping, and ligation. These therapies can decrease the incidence of further bleeding, shorten the hospital stay, decrease the need for transfusions, and reduce the need for emergent surgery.

When lower gastrointestinal bleeding is suspected, sigmoidoscopy and colonoscopy may be helpful if the bleeding has nearly stopped and the bowel has been sufficiently cleansed. As a bedside procedure in the ICU, colonoscopy helps determine the state of bleeding in about one-half of patients. Even when the exact cause of bleeding cannot be determined, these procedures help localize the area of bleeding, which again is important for the surgeon or interventional radiologist. A radionuclide bleeding scan using technetium-99m-labeled red blood cells offers a reasonable noninvasive early diagnostic approach for patients suspected of having gastrointestinal bleeding below the second portion of the duodenum, an area that is difficult to reach by upper endoscopy. To be helpful, a minimal degree of bleeding must be occurring as the scan is performed. This procedure helps identify the area in which the bleeding is occurring. Finally, one of the most attractive features of radionuclide scanning is the complete absence of morbidity and the ability to perform repeat studies at reasonable intervals to determine if bleeding has reinitiated.

If the bowel can be cleansed, colonoscopy usually provides an etiologic diagnosis for lower GI bleeding.

Mesenteric arteriography is sometimes helpful. Again, ongoing bleeding is necessary. It is generally indicated when endoscopy is not available or it fails, there is a contraindication to endoscopy such as esophageal perforation, or there is a suspected lesion amenable to an-

Briskly bleeding lower GI lesions can be found by arteriography or by tagged red blood cell nuclear scanning.

TABLE 16-6

ENDOSCOPIC FEATURES SUGGESTIVE OF INCREASED RISK OF REBLEEDING

Peptic ulcer
- Arterial spurting of blood (Dieulafoy's lesion)
- Visible vessel at the ulcer base
- Clot at the ulcer base
- An elevated red dot
- Gastric or giant (>2 cm) duodenal ulcer

Esophageal varices
- Erosions, ulcerations, or craters
- Erythema over varices
- Varices on varices

Stress ulcers
- Numerous deep mucosal lesions

giography-directed interventional therapy. Serious complications that can occur with this intervention include catheter-related arterial trauma, contrast allergy, and renal failure.

The interventional radiologist can be very helpful in the management of serious upper and lower gastrointestinal hemorrhage, both diagnostically and therapeutically. With arteriography, the radiotherapist can infuse intraarterial vasopressin to control a variety of bleeding lesions found in the esophagus, stomach, duodenum, and colon. Material embolization can also be very effective at reducing recurrent hemorrhage. Either a delivered dose of gel foam or a metal coil inserted into a terminal vessel can result in localized thrombosis and cessation of hemorrhage. This so-called angiotherapy may be first-line treatment for lower gastrointestinal hemorrhage associated with diverticula and angiodysplasia. The use of angiotherapy for bleeding stress or peptic ulceration is generally reserved for those patients who fail endotherapy.

NONENDOSCOPIC MANAGEMENT OF ESOPHAGEAL BLEEDING

Esophageal variceal hemorrhage is the most serious complication of portal vein hypertension, which is secondary to cirrhosis, and it carries a high mortality. The principal treatment to control variceal hemorrhage is fiberoptic endoscopy with either band ligation or sclerotherapy. However, for certain patients who fail either procedure, balloon tamponade of the esophagus can be lifesaving. A Sengstaken–Blakemore or Minnesota (Figures 16-1 and 16-2) tube is indicated in certain patients with a diagnosis of esophageal variceal hemorrhage in which sclerotherapy is either technically impossible or has failed or is not readily available. Before the placement of one of these esophageal tubes, it is best to have a confirmed diagnosis of esophageal varices by endoscopy. Balloon compression for a variceal bleed should not be done in patients with recent esophageal surgery, esophageal stricture disease, or a large hiatal hernia. When the procedure is done, it is essential to have appropriate airway control. Endotracheal intubation is necessary in patients who are hemodynamically unstable or encephalopathic. Also, sedatives are necessary to provide comfort for patients who have an esophageal balloon in place. Therefore, endotracheal intubation is generally necessary.

Esophageal balloon tamponade techniques can be used when endoscopy ligation and sclerotherapy fail to stop variceal bleeding.

As mentioned, a diagnostic endoscopic procedure should be done to verify the diagnosis of bleeding esophageal varices; at the same time, this procedure should also decompress the stomach of air and blood to reduce the risk of aspiration of gastric contents into the lungs

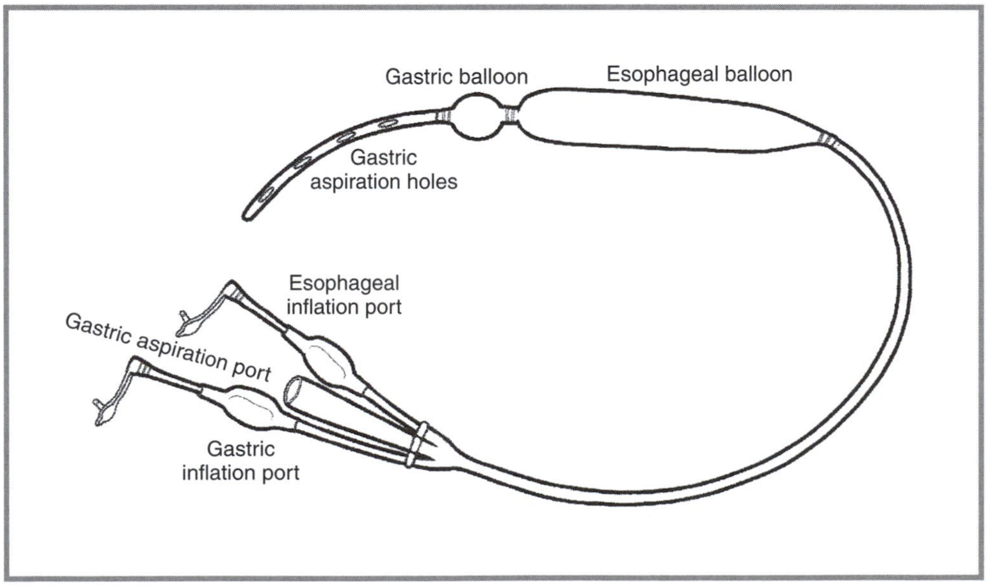

FIGURE 16-1

Sengstaken–Blakemore tube.

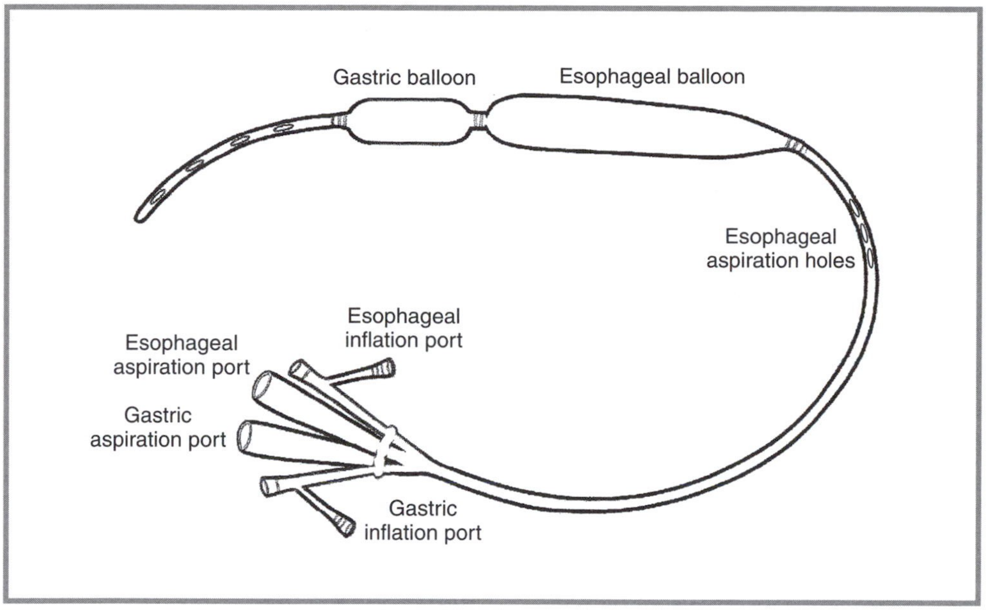

FIGURE 16-2

Minnesota tube.

during esophageal balloon placement. Before placement of one of the esophageal balloon catheters, all balloons should be inflated and checked for leaks and all tube lumens should be patent. The difference between a Minnesota tube and a Sengstaken–Blakemore tube is the presence of a fourth tube lumen in the Minnesota tube, the esophageal aspiration channel with port, which allows for intermittent suctioning above the esophageal balloon (see Figure 16-2). When a standard Sengstaken–Blakemore tube is used, a standard surgical suction catheter must be tied to the Sengstaken–Blakemore tube so that the tip of this suction catheter is just above the esophageal balloon to facilitate upper esophageal and hypopharyngeal suctioning. With the balloons completely deflated, the tube should be generously lubricated with lidocaine jelly. The tube can then be inserted either through the nose or the mouth, but because most patients have a serious coagulopathy, most tubes are placed through the mouth. The tube is then passed into the stomach, and, after verification by auscultation, the gastric balloon is inflated and brought up against the esophageal gastric sphincter. Furthermore, verification of gastric balloon placement is done by abdominal x-ray. With the balloon below the diaphragm, more air can be added to the gastric balloon; this in itself often leads to hemostasis. Volumes as high as 450 ml can be placed in the gastric balloon to accomplish this. At times extreme traction must be applied to the catheter to enhance hemorrhagic control. If the bleeding continues, then the esophageal balloon can be inflated as high as 45 mmHg of mercury using a bedside manometer for pressure control. The tube is then in place (Figure 16-3).

Both the Sengstaken–Blakemore and Minnesota tubes have instructions that must be carefully followed. Balloon volume, catheter traction, and fixation guidelines must be carefully performed. The gastric lumen is placed to intermittent suction. The esophageal lumen or catheter above the esophageal balloon must be placed to low intermittent suction. The tautness, position, and inflation of the gastric balloon should be checked hourly by experienced personnel. The tubes should be left in place at least 24 h, and perhaps up to 48 h if clinically necessary. The esophageal balloon must be deflated for 30 min every 8 h. Positioning of the tubes and its balloons should be checked roentgenographically at least daily. After hemorrhage control, the esophageal balloon is deflated first, followed by the gastric balloon, which is left inflated for an additional 24 h before deflation. If no further bleeding occurs, then the entire tube is removed.

Band ligation for variceal hemorrhage control is considered first-line treatment, followed by sclerotherapy. Balloon tamponade techniques are an important alternative therapeutic option, especially when band ligation and sclerotherapy work. These therapies should be coupled with appropriate pharmacologic therapy such as the use of vasopressin or somatostatin.

FIGURE 16-3

The Sengstaken–Blakemore triple lumen tube. Some newer tubes (Minnesota) have a fourth lumen to permit aspiration of blood or secretions from the esophagus. If a conventional triple lumen tube is employed, an additional sump tube should be passed alongside the Sengstaken–Blakemore tube and positioned in the midesophagus.

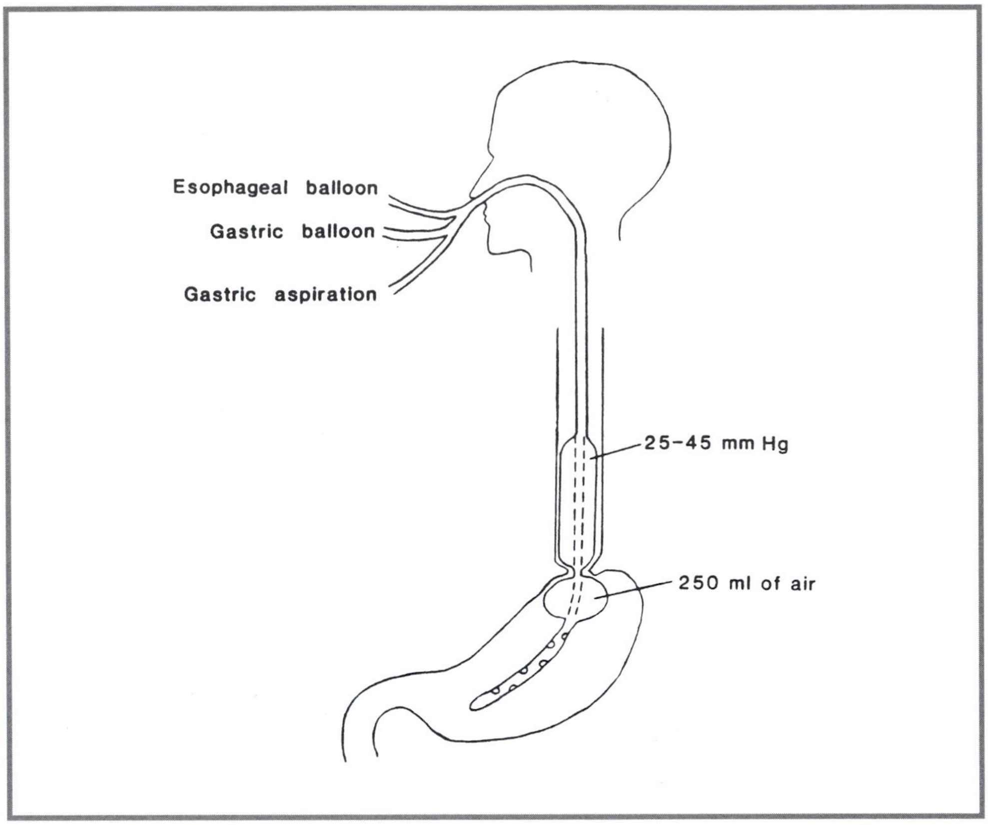

Aspiration pneumonia is the most serious complication associated with esophageal balloon tamponade. Laryngeal obstruction and suffocation can occur with balloon migration. Esophageal perforation and mucosal ulceration at the gastroesophageal junction also can occur. Percutaneously placed hepatic shunts can be lifesaving for those patients with variceal bleeding who are poor surgical candidates. Transjugular intrahepatic portal–systemic shunting (TIPSS) is an interventional radiologic procedure in which a fistula is created between hepatic vein and portal vein. This technique is done by an invasive radiotherapist and requires passing a catheter, under fluoroscopic guidance, through the internal jugular vein to the level of the hepatic vein. A needle is subsequently passed through the hepatic vein until a branch of the portal vein is cannulated. This tract is then dilated, and a metallic expandable stent is placed in the liver to create a shunt between the portal and hepatic veins. The TIPSS procedure can control variceal bleeding. This procedure is generally done to avoid emergent surgery. For patients with severe, recurrent, or persistent bleeding, surgical treatment becomes necessary.

Transjugular intrahepatic portal–systemic shunting (TIPSS) can reduce recurrent esophageal variceal bleeding and help the cirrhotic patient awaiting surgery.

SURGERY

Surgical consultation should be requested in the early stages of GI bleeding resuscitation and evaluation.

Surgical consultation should be obtained in the early stages of resuscitation and evaluation especially if the patient continues to bleed or more than a total of six units of packed red blood cells have been administered. Furthermore, if endoscopic risk factors suggest high morbidity and mortality, or an increase risk of rebleeding (see Table 16-6), surgical consultation is mandatory. There are no rigid indications for surgery. Indications for surgery are based on the overall assessment of the patient and inability to maintain hemodynamic stability. These patients usually have failed appropriate medical, including endoscopic, therapies. For the patient with massive overwhelming hemorrhage, surgery is part of the resuscitative process, which is carried out immediately by moving the patient from the intensive care unit to the surgical suite. The surgical procedure performed depends on the lo-

CASE STUDY: PART 3

Endoscopy was performed on our patient who had serious upper gastrointestinal bleeding. Multiple stress ulcerations of the gastric fundus were found, several of which were bleeding actively. Surgical intervention was avoided by endotherapy. A heater probe thermal coagulation technique via the endoscope was utilized to control the active bleeding ulcers. Following endoscopy, the patient was maintained on an H2R antagonist intravenously. His pneumonia continued to improve with general supportive measures and intravenous antibiotic therapy, and he was weaned from mechanical ventilation and extubated. The patient was discharged from the hospital 11 days after admission.

cation of hemorrhage and the stability of the patient. The surgeon usually opts for "oversewing" of a distal gastric or duodenal ulcer that bleeds continuously and necessitates a quick operation. A vagotomy and pyloroplasty would lessen the chance for ulcer recurrence. A more stable patient with a bleeding ulcer would typically undergo a Billroth procedure with a selective vagotomy and antrectomy. Rarely, a total gastrectomy is performed for severe hemorrhagic gastritis.

Surgery is considered for patients who have severe rebleeding associated with angiodysplasia or diverticulosis and for those patients who have serious lower gastrointestinal bleeding of undetermined organ. If the site of bleeding is known, then the involved colonic segment can be removed. Blind resection of colon is performed in patients with active bleeding of undetermined colonic origin; this may include a total colectomy or, possibly, a left hemicolectomy because of the predominance of diverticulosis in the left colon in the elderly.

Unremitting or recurrent variceal bleeding may require surgical intervention. Surgically created portal–hepatic shunts or portal–systemic shunts have the advantage of being the most reliable means to control acute variceal bleeding and prevent recurrent bleeding. The main limitation to emergent surgical intervention in the acutely bleeding cirrhotic patient is a high incidence of mortality. Finally, liver transplantation is the only therapy that treats both the underlying liver disease and portal hypertension. Liver transplantation is considered for patients with variceal bleeding and who have advanced liver disease that is refractory to all other therapy.

SUMMARY

The successful management of acute gastrointestinal hemorrhage demands a highly organized and multidisciplinary diagnostic and treatment approach. The intensivist must quickly involve the gastroenterologist and, when necessary, the invasive radiotherapist and surgeon in the diagnostic and treatment process. The intensivist must quickly identify that bleeding is present and with the help of the gastroenterologist determine the site of bleeding. During this diagnostic process, the magnitude of bleeding must be assessed and aggressive resuscitation must occur. The urgency of these processes depends heavily on the severity of the hemorrhage and its etiology. The therapeutic resources that are available must play an important part in this treatment equation. The availability of endoscopic therapy and interventional radiology has diminished the frequency of surgical intervention for upper gastrointestinal hemorrhage. However, surgical intervention is usually necessary for unremitting lower gastrointestinal bleeding.

For our patient who had stress ulceration as the cause of severe upper gastrointestinal hemorrhage, it was extremely important to initiate prophylactic therapy at the time of hospitalization. The prevalence of stress ulceration seems to be decreasing because of the prophylactic use of H2R antagonist therapy and, more recently, the use of proton pump inhibitor therapy. Critically ill patients in the ICU (especially those with burns and acute neurologic events) are at great risk for stress ulceration and should be treated aggressively with stress ulceration prophylaxis.

REVIEW QUESTIONS

1. **All the following are common causes of gastrointestinal bleeding except:**
   A. Gastric ulcer
   B. Esophagitis
   C. Gastritis
   D. Diverticulosis

2. **Peptic ulcer disease is least likely to be associated with:**
   A. Melena
   B. Pain
   C. Hematochezia
   D. Hematemesis

3. **The most important therapeutic intervention during urgent resuscitation of acute GI bleeding is:**
   A. Intravascular volume expansion
   B. Vasopressor therapy
   C. Correct coagulopathy
   D. Endotherapy

4. **The immediate treatment of choice for bleeding esophageal varices is:**
   A. Liver transplantation
   B. TIPSS procedure
   C. Esophageal balloon tamponade
   D. Endoscopy with band ligation

ANSWERS

1. The answer is B. Esophagitis is common in the critically ill patient and in patients in general, but it is rarely a cause of bleeding.
2. The answer is C. Hematochezia is bright red rectal bleeding, a sign of lower GI bleeding that is generally caused by hemorrhoids or diverticulosis.
3. The answer is A. Intravascular hypovolemia must be quickly corrected to prevent end-organ damage with volume expansion. While blood is being readied, crystalloid or colloid fluids should be administered through two large-bore peripheral intravenous lines.
4. The answer is D. Cirrhosis and hepatic insufficiency are best treated by liver transplantation, but acute variceal bleeding is most immediately controlled by endotherapy. Band ligation and sclerotherapy control approximately 25% of variceal bleeds.

SUGGESTED READING

Beckman JW, Tedesco FJ. Acute lower GI bleeding: the differential diagnosis. J Crit Illness 1986;1:56–64.

Beckman JW, Tedesco FJ. Acute management of lower GI bleeding. J Crit Illness 1986;1:14–20.

Gostout CJ, Wang KK, Ahlquist DA. Acute gastrointestinal bleeding: experience of a specialized management team. J Clin Gastroenterol 1992;14:260–267.

Gottlieb JE, Menasha PI, Cruz E. Gastrointestinal complications in critically ill patients: the intensivist's overview. Am J Gastroenterol 1986;81:227.

Grace ND. Diagnosis and treatment of gastrointestinal bleeding secondary to portal hypertension. Am J Gastroenterol 1997;92:1081–1091.

Lau JYW, Sung JJY, Lam YH, et al. Endoscopic retreatment compared with surgery in patients with recurrent bleeding after initial endoscope control of bleeding ulcers. N Engl J Med 1999;340:751–756.

NEH Consensus Conference. Therapeutic endoscopy and bleeding ulcers. JAMA 1989;262:1369.

Rankin RA. Acute upper gastrointestinal bleeding: therapy and prophylaxis. Prog Crit Care Med 1985;2:167–174.

Richter JM, Christensen MR, Kaplan LM, et al. Effectiveness of current technology in the diagnosis and management of lower gastrointestinal hemorrhage. Gastrointest Endosc 1994;41:93–98.

Schaffer J. Acute gastrointestinal bleeding. Med Clin N Am 1986;70:1055.

Schuster DP. Stress ulcer prophylaxis: in whom? with what? Crit Care Med 1993;21:4.

Van Dam J, Brugge WR. Endoscopy of upper gastrointestinal tract. N Engl J Med 1999;341:1738–1748.

Zuckerman GR, Cort D, Shuman RB. Stress ulcer syndrome. J Intens Care Med 1988;3:21.

CHAPTER 17

WISSAM CHATILA

Hepatic Failure

CHAPTER OUTLINE

LEARNING OBJECTIVES

After studying this chapter, you should be able to:

- Recognize patients presenting in fulminant hepatic failure.
- Identify different etiologies of fulminant hepatic failure.
- Understand the pathophysiology underlying various organ and system dysfunctions in fulminant hepatic failure.

Acute hepatic failure, also called fulminant hepatic failure (FHF), is an uncommon liver disorder characterized by an acute onset of severe hepatic dysfunction resulting in jaundice, encephalopathy, and coagulopathy that frequently progresses to cause cerebral edema, multiorgan failure, and eventually death. More than two decades ago, before the advent of liver transplantation, mortality from FHF approached 80%. Currently, liver transplantation is offered as salvage therapy for select patients with FHF, resulting in 1-year survival rates of 40%–80%. Despite the encouraging results from liver transplantation, patients suffering from hepatic failure are among the most difficult patients to manage while awaiting for liver donation, and, unfortunately, many succumb to their disease before receiving a liver. Patients with cirrhosis frequently present to the intensive care unit in hepatic failure; however, they differ from FHF in regard to pathophysiology, management, and prognosis. This chapter is limited to the discussion of patients with FHF.

Fulminant hepatic failure (FHF):
- Occurs in patients without previous history of liver disease.
- Is defined as development of encephalopathy within 12 weeks of the onset of hepatic symptoms.
- Is associated with a mortality rate up to 80% in patients who do not receive liver transplantation.

DEFINITIONS AND ETIOLOGY

Fulminant hepatic failure has been defined as the development of hepatic encephalopathy within 8 weeks of the onset of acute liver disease in a previously healthy person. Many patients, however, have a very rapid deterioration of liver function whereas others have a much slower progression of their disease (up to 12 weeks). Recently, several authors have suggested redefining the syndrome of FHF into three categories depending on the time interval between the onset of jaundice and encephalopathy: hyperacute (0–7 days), acute (1–4 weeks), and subacute (4–12 weeks). The timing of onset of encephalopathy and the etiology of liver

TABLE 17-1

CAUSES OF FULMINANT HEPATIC FAILURE

Viral hepatitis
Hepatitis A (HAV), hepatitis B (HBV), hepatitis C (HCV), hepatitis E (HEV)
Herpes simplex virus (HSV)
Epstein–Barr virus (EBV)
Drug toxicity
Acetaminophen
Antimicrobials (tetracycline, ampicillin-clavulanate, trovafloxacin, isoniazid)
Antiepileptics (valproate, phenytoin)
Anesthetic (halothane)
Antihyperglycemic (troglidazone)
Antidepressants (tricyclic antidepressants, monoamine oxidase inhibitors)
Others: loratadine, pemoline, antabuse, cyclophosphamide, lovastatin
Toxins
Mushrooms (*Amanita phalloides*)
Organic solvents
Ethanol
Herbal remedies (ginseng, chaparral, pennyroyal oil, teucrium polium)
Bacterial toxins (cyanobacteria, *Bacillus cereus*)
Circulatory impairment
Ischemia (hepatic vascular occlusion, shock)
Septic shock
Cardiac failure
Heat stroke
Pregnancy induced
Acute fatty liver of pregnancy
Eclampsia
Malignant infiltration
Hematologic (leukemia, lymphoma)
Liver metastasis
Metabolic
Wilson disease
Galactosemia
Hereditary tyrosinemia
Miscellaneous
Autoimmune hepatitis
Budd–Chiari syndrome
Malaria
Tuberculosis
Coxiella burnettii
Reye syndrome

Viral hepatitis and idiosyncratic drug reactions are the most common causes of FHF.

failure have major impacts on prognosis; the shorter the presentation, the better the outcome. Hepatic failure occurs as a result of severe liver injury from either hepatocellular necrosis or microvesicular steatosis. Viral hepatitis and hepatotoxic drugs, inducing hepatocellular necrosis, are the most common causes of FHF, but there is a great geographic variation in regard to the etiology of FHF. Hepatitis B virus is the most common virus causing FHF (25%–75% of all viral hepatitis). Acetaminophen toxicity is frequently encountered in the United States and the United Kingdom but is less frequent in some parts of Europe. In 15%–20% of patients, the etiology of FHF remains indeterminate despite an exhaustive workup (Table 17-1).

CLINICAL FEATURES

Development of encephalopathy is required to diagnose FHF. Hepatic encephalopathy (HE) masks the onset of cerebral edema.

The hallmark of FHF is the development of hepatic encephalopathy (HE) in the setting of acute and severe liver injury. The severity of encephalopathy, which manifests as neuropsychiatric dysfunction, has been stratified into four stages (Table 17-2). Unlike HE of decompensated cirrhosis, HE of FHF responds poorly to therapy and often masks the development

TABLE 17-2

STAGES OF HEPATIC ENCEPHALOPATHY

STAGE	MENTAL STATE
Stage 1	Impaired intellect, affect, and psychomotor function, euphoria, untidiness, arousable and coherent
Stage 2	Increased drowsiness, inappropriate behavior, lack of sphincter control, arousable and conversant
Stage 3	Very drowsy and sleeps most of the time, may become agitated and aggressive, incoherent speech, arousable
Stage 4	Comatose, may or may not respond to painful stimuli

SOURCE: Modified from Shakil et al. (1999)

of cerebral edema, a catastrophic complication of FHF. Cerebral edema is characterized by systemic hypertension, hyperventilation, increased muscle tone, decorticate or decerebrate posturing, abnormal pupillary reflexes, and eventually altered brainstem reflexes in the event of uncal or cerebellar herniation. Unfortunately, it is not uncommon for cerebral edema to develop in the absence of significant physical findings. Moreover, FHF usually affects all organ function, resulting in cardiovascular instability, hypoxemic respiratory failure, renal insufficiency, coagulopathy, severe malnutrition, and life-threatening infections. Therefore, in addition to the signs of HE and jaundice, patients with FHF have fetor hepaticus and present with tachycardia, tachypnea, hypotension, and hypoxemia. The aforementioned signs may also be related to sepsis or gastrointestinal hemorrhage, which are common complications of FHF. Laboratory abnormalities vary according to the etiology of the hepatic failure, but it is the severity of HE rather than specific test results that distinguishes FHF from severe active hepatitis. Common laboratory findings in FHF include elevation in liver function tests (e.g., aminotransferases and alkaline phosphatase), abnormal coagulation profile, and increase in ammonia level.

Fulminant hepatic failure is associated with high cardiac output shock and multiorgan dysfunction.

PATHOPHYSIOLOGY OF LIVER FAILURE

Hepatic Encephalopathy and Cerebral Edema

The neural depression and generalized slowing seen on electroencephalography (EEG) associated with HE are thought to be mediated through increased inhibitory neurotransmitters such as ammonia and γ-aminobutyric acid A (GABA). It is unclear whether cerebral edema represents the end stage of the spectrum of HE or if it constitutes a separate complication. Cerebral edema occurs mostly in stages 3 and 4 of HE and is a major cause of death in FHF. Three mechanisms may be involved in the pathogenesis of cerebral edema: (1) increase in the cerebral interstitial fluid; (2) increase in fluid transfer across the blood–brain barrier; and (3) cellular edema. The progression of cerebral edema is accelerated by volume overload and a hypooncotic state and leads to a significant increase in intracranial pressure (ICP). Multiple interventions (such as tracheal suctioning, tactile stimulation, and hemodialysis) and other factors (hypertension and agitation) accentuate the rise in ICP, hence exacerbating the brain injury.

Cerebral edema:
- Develops in patients with advanced HE (stage 3 or stage 4).
- Leads to brain death if unrecognized and untreated.

Renal Impairment

Renal insufficiency (serum creatinine >2 mg/dl) in FHF can result from hepatorenal syndrome, acute tubular necrosis (ATN), or intravascular volume depletion, all manifested by oliguria (<300 ml/24 h) and water retention. Renal insufficiency has been reported to occur in 30%–84% of the cases of FHF, some of which progress to end-stage renal failure requiring hemodialysis. The hepatorenal syndrome is a functional renal impairment resulting from an intense renal arterial vasoconstriction caused by a hormonal imbalance (there is an increase in renin and aldosterone versus a reduction in prostaglandin). ATN also may result from the same toxic substances that precipitated FHF (e.g., acetaminophen) or from iatrogenic factors introduced in the ICU (hypotension, nephrotoxic drugs, or contrast agents). Typically in hepatorenal syndrome, the urine sodium (UNa) is less than 10 mEq/l and the urine sediment is unremarkable. By contrast, in ATN the urine shows the presence of cellular casts and UNa is greater than 40 mEq/l.

Circulatory Impairment

The hemodynamic changes in FHF are comparable to those of sepsis and are consistent with high cardiac output shock, a state characterized by systemic vasodilatation, high cardiac output, hypotension, and impaired tissue oxygen uptake. Some patients experience a reduction in their cardiac output and heart rate (relative bradycardia), both of which exacerbate the presence of hypotension. Of note, one should be careful to detect infections and hemorrhages, commonly encountered in patients with FHF, that can contribute to hypotension and further blur the clinical picture. It has been suggested that this state of systemic vasodilatation is centrally mediated or mediated via circulating endotoxin, increased inflammatory mediators (tumor necrosis factor, interleukin-6), and unregulated production of nitric oxide (NO). Systolic hypertension in a patient with stage 3 or 4 encephalopathy may indicate the development of increased ICP.

Respiratory Failure

Hypoxemia is extremely common in FHF. Noncardiogenic pulmonary edema (pulmonary artery occlusion pressure <18 mmHg) accounts for almost one-third of cases with hypoxemia, but the true incidence of pulmonary edema also varies with the nature of the inciting event. Other causes of hypoxemia include aspiration of gastric contents in encephalopathic patients, nosocomial pneumonia, intrapulmonary hemorrhage, and pulmonary vascular dilatation. Hypoxemia is multifactorial in the majority of patients with FHF. In addition to hypoxemia, a respiratory alkalosis may be observed, except in cases of advanced cerebral edema that results in respiratory depression.

Coagulopathy

The liver is involved in the synthesis of numerous coagulation factors (other than factor VIII) and some of the inhibitors of fibrinolysis. In FHF, the abnormal prothrombin time found in all patients confirms the loss of liver synthetic function and is used as an indicator for the severity of hepatic injury. A high prothrombin time reflects more impaired hepatic synthetic function and more severe liver injury. Moreover, thrombocytopenia (<100,000/ml) and platelet dysfunction have been demonstrated in FHF. A low-grade disseminated intravascular coagulation (DIC), increased peripheral consumption, and fibrinolysis may coexist with impaired hepatic synthetic function, further exaggerating the risk of major hemorrhage (gastrointestinal and intrapulmonary).

Infections

Infectious complications in FHF are very common and occur early in the course of the disease.

Infectious complications occur early in the course of FHF in up to 80% of patients. Patients with FHF are predisposed to multiple infections and sepsis because of their compromised immune function (related to complement and opsonin deficiency and impaired neutrophil function) and the use of invasive ICU instrumentation. Bacterial as well as fungal infections have been reported. Isolated organisms include *Staphylococcus aureus*, *Streptococcus* species, gram-negative lactose fermenters, and *Candida* species, causing catheter-related infections or respiratory and urinary tract infections. Worsening liver function and hemodynamic status may indicate a superimposed infection, even in the absence of fever and leukocytosis, and should prompt a sepsis workup with initiation of broad-spectrum antimicrobial coverage. Several authors advocate obtaining daily surveillance cultures while others initiate systemic antimicrobial prophylactic throughout the course of FHF.

Metabolic Disturbances

The liver is the site of glycogen stores, gluconeogenesis, and lactate metabolism. In the presence of severe hepatic necrosis, and despite the hypercatabolic state of patients with FHF, the liver is rendered ineffective as a source of glucose. Therefore, it is common to observe that such patients have high glucose requirements (continuous intravenous 10% dextrose is usually administered to prevent hypoglycemia). Moreover, severe lactic acidosis may complicate the metabolic acidosis associated with renal failure.

PROGNOSIS OF LIVER FAILURE

The prognosis in FHF is related to the etiology and the severity of the liver injury. The highest survival rates have been reported in acetaminophen toxicity and hepatitis A infections. In contrast to the 80% mortality rate reported in patients without liver transplantation, other reports have documented 39%–67% survival in patients with FHF with supportive therapy alone. To allocate donated livers to the most appropriate patients early in the course of the FHF, liver transplant centers have identified certain criteria that have been associated with worse outcome. The King's College Hospital Criteria are the most widely applied prognostic criteria. Patients are divided into acetaminophen and nonacetaminophen hepatic injury (Table 17-3). In addition, persistent deterioration of HE and coagulopathy despite aggressive supportive therapy also indicate a poor prognosis. Refractory increases in ICP, factor V, factor VIII/factor V ratio, liver histology, hepatic volumetry (by CT scanning), arterial ketone body ratio, and plasma Gc protein have been proposed to have prognostic significance; however, some variables require further validation, and others are more difficult to obtain (e.g., liver biopsy or CT scans).

MONITORING AND MANAGEMENT

Currently, available measures or antidotes that are used to minimize hepatic injury are limited to specific types of liver failure (e.g., *N*-acetylcysteine for acetaminophen, Silymarin or penicillin G for *Amanita* mushroom poisoning; charcoal hemoperfusion to reduce circulating toxins). Unfortunately, there have been no breakthroughs in pharmacologic approaches to reverse existing hepatic injury. Because of the scarcity of available organs for donation, many nonpharmacologic approaches for liver replacement are under investigation (hepatocyte transplantation, bioartificial liver support, extracorporeal liver perfusion, and xenotransplantation). Until the efficacy and safety of nontraditional approaches are established, the management of patients in FHF consists of aggressive supportive care along with the

TABLE 17-3

CRITERIA FOR POOR SURVIVAL AND SELECTION FOR LIVER TRANSPLANT

ACETAMINOPHEN TOXICITY	NONACETAMINOPHEN TOXICITY
pH <7.30, irrespective of grade of encephalopathy Or Stage 3 or 4 encephalopathy with • PT >100 s (INR >6.7) • Serum creatinine >3.4 mg/dl	PT >100 s (INR >6.7), irrespective of grade of encephalopathy Or Any 3 of the following variables: • Age <10 or >40 years • Unfavorable etiology: non-A, non-B hepatitis, drug reactions • Jaundice >7 days before onset of encephalopathy • PT >50 s (INR >4) • Serum bilirubin >17.5 mg/dl

PT, prothrombin time; INR, international normalized ratio
SOURCE: Modified from O'Grady et al. (1989)

recognition and treatment of complications while awaiting liver transplantation or until spontaneous liver function recovery occurs.

There is no specific treatment to reverse the hepatic injury in FHF. The only effective therapeutic intervention is liver transplant. Early transfer to a liver transplant center for patients with progressive disease is recommended.

Aggressive central and cerebral hemodynamic monitoring is required to guide the therapy for complications.

Because of multiorgan involvement, frequent complications, and rapid deterioration in patients with FHF, optimal supportive care cannot be delivered without appropriate monitoring performed by medical and surgical teams familiar with management of such patients. Therefore, acknowledging that the only effective therapy is liver transplantation, patients whose disease is progressive should be transferred to a transplant center. Hemodynamically unstable patients require arterial and pulmonary arterial cannulation to titrate fluid resuscitation and vasopressor support. Monitoring of cerebral hemodynamics (ICP, cerebral perfusion pressure, cerebral blood flow, and cerebral oxygen consumption) is not universally accepted for all patients with FHF, but some transplant centers strongly advocate its early use in patients with advanced encephalopathy because this allows early identification and treatment to minimize risks of significant brain injury. On the other hand, ICP monitoring is essential for diagnosis as well as for guiding therapy in patients with deteriorating neurologic status who are suspected to have intracranial hypertension. Computed brain tomography (head CT) has not been shown to be useful in the diagnosis and management of cerebral edema.

The management of patients with cerebral edema, always rendered while monitoring cerebral hemodynamics, consists of acute hyperventilation in the early phases of the cerebral edema. With progression of cerebral edema and reduction of cerebral blood flow, hyperventilation becomes ineffective; osmotic diuresis administered in boluses becomes the mainstay of management and has been shown to be effective in reducing ICP. Mannitol (1 g/kg) is usually given as needed (so long as serum osmolarity remains less than 320 mOsm/l) to maintain an ICP less than 30 mmHg or a cerebral perfusion greater than 40 mmHg. Additional supportive management to prevent deterioration of ICP includes early intubation, avoiding stimulation, treatment of fever, and sedation for agitation. Some liver transplant centers also induce a state of hypothermia and barbiturate coma and treat all patients with *N*-acetylcysteine, which has been shown to improve oxygen transport and consumption even in nonacetaminophen FHF.

Mechanical ventilation is recommended as encephalopathy progresses to protect the patient from overt or covert aspiration and to optimize alveolar recruitment in the presence of pulmonary edema. Fluid resuscitation and vasopressors are essential to maintain adequate tissue perfusion pressure and to minimize organ dysfunction. Patients with FHF seem to respond better to epinephrine or norepinephrine as compared to dopamine and dobutamine. Low-dose dopamine (2–4 μg/kg/h) and loop diuretics (e.g., furosemide) are almost always given in the face of deteriorating renal function. The effectiveness of such interventions to salvage the kidneys has not been demonstrated; it is more important to ensure that patients have adequate intravascular filling pressures. Frequently, patients ultimately require renal replacement therapy (hemodialysis or continuous venovenous hemodiafiltration). Frequent blood draws are done to assess and to treat electrolyte abnormalities, hypoglycemia, bleeding, and coagulopathy. Several centers advocate the use of systemic prophylactic antibiotics early in the course of FHF. Antimicrobial coverage should be directed against all organisms listed earlier.

SUMMARY

Patients with severe liver dysfunction are extremely difficult to manage because of the nature of multiorgan involvement during the course of their illness. However, successful outcome is possible with aggressive monitoring and management in tertiary care transplant centers. Early recognition of FHF allows expedited transfer of high-risk patients to specialized centers where sophisticated supportive therapy is instituted while patients await their only curative therapy, liver transplantation. Any blunders in delivering appropriate and meticulous care to these patients, such as failure to recognize infections and cerebral edema, are life-threatening and often result in a dismal outcome.

REVIEW QUESTIONS

1. **In fulminant hepatic failure:**
   - **A.** The slower the progression the better the outcome.
   - **B.** Liver failure caused by drug toxicity has the worst prognosis.
   - **C.** The most common viral etiology is hepatitis B virus.
   - **D.** Patients always need liver transplant because of the associated high mortality.

2. **The signs of cerebral edema:**
   - **A.** Include hypotension, hyperventilation, and worsening mental status
   - **B.** Should prompt insertion of intracranial pressure monitoring before initiating therapy
   - **C.** Can be exacerbated by stimulation of the patient such as during tracheal suctioning
   - **D.** Occur most commonly in stage 2 hepatic encephalopathy

Questions 3 and 4 refer to the following:
A 32-year-woman, previously healthy, was admitted to a small community hospital because of acetaminophen overdose after a suicide attempt. In the emergency room, she was alert and oriented, in no distress, and without complaints. Her laboratory results revealed toxic acetaminophen levels, AST 4509, ALT 5745, INR 5.2, direct bilirubin 13 mg/dl, pH 7.35, PaO_2 112 mmHg, and serum creatinine 3.0 mg/dl. The patient was started on intravenous hydration, fresh-frozen plasma, and *N*-acetylcysteine, and transferred to the four-bed intensive care unit. On the second day, she became lethargic, but still appropriate when aroused, and her laboratory studies showed lower acetaminophen levels, AST 4202, ALT 4897, direct bilirubin 15 mg/dl, INR 5.2, pH 7.30, PaO_2 99 mmHg, and serum creatinine 3.2 mg/dl. The closest tertiary care center, where liver transplant can be offered, is approximately 5 h away by ambulance.

3. **Based on the current history and present illness, the next step in the patient's management should be:**
   - **A.** Stop transfusion of fresh-frozen plasma but continue *N*-acetylcysteine
   - **B.** Transfer to the tertiary care center
   - **C.** Perform a liver biopsy
   - **D.** Obtain blood cultures and start broad-spectrum antibiotics

4. **Over the next day, the patient became comatose, without any focal neurologic deficit; her systolic blood pressure dropped to 80 mmHg, requiring aggressive intravenous fluid resuscitation and dopamine; and her laboratory studies were essentially unchanged compared with the previous day. The next step in her management should be:**
   - **A.** Transfer to the tertiary care center
   - **B.** Obtain a head CT scan to exclude cerebral edema
   - **C.** Intubate and initiate hyperventilation to treat cerebral edema
   - **D.** Transfuse with packed red blood cells, investigate for possible blood loss, and treat with broad-spectrum antibiotics

ANSWERS

1. The answer is C. Among the viral infections, hepatitis B is the most common cause of fulminant hepatic failure. A more rapid progression of liver failure portends a better prognosis compared to slower deterioration, and acetaminophen overdose has a high likelihood of spontaneous recovery. Although a high percentage of patients may need liver transplant to salvage them, some have spontaneous recovery; prognostic factors help differentiate which patients need liver transplantation most.
2. The answer is C. Hypertension, rather than hypotension, is one of the signs of cerebral edema, which occurs mostly in stage 3 or 4 hepatic encephalopathy. Once suspected, intracranial monitoring is recommended but should not delay initiation of therapy; patients who sustain prolonged increase in intracranial pressure have the worst prognosis.
3. The answer is B. Patient is not improving and actually is showing evidence of progression to stage 2 hepatic encephalopathy, despite conservative and supportive therapy. The best plan of action is to transfer her, while she is stable, to the transplant center where aggressive monitoring and therapy can be offered should she continue to deteriorate. Until she is transferred, supportive therapy should continue, including fresh-frozen plasma because of significant coagulopathy. A liver biopsy is a high-risk procedure, and current data to support such practice are limited.
4. The answer is D. If the patient was not transferred to a transplant center, she should be stabilized before taking a 5-h trip. First, the reason for her hypotension should be identified and treated. The patient has progressed to stage 4 hepatic encephalopathy, and causes of hypotension include major hemorrhage and sepsis; hypotension is not among the early signs of cerebral edema. Therefore, treatment with antibiotics and transfusion should be started. Although intubation is recommended in comatosed patients for airway protection, hyperventilation is not advised unless cerebral edema is suspected.

SUGGESTED READING

Lewis TH, Schmidt GA. Acute and chronic hepatic disease. In: Principles of Critical Care, 2nd Ed. New York: McGraw-Hill, 1998.

O'Grady JG, Alexander GJ, Hayllar KM, et al. Early indicators of prognosis in fulminant hepatic failure. Gastroenterology 1989;97:439.

O'Grady JG, Schalm SW, Williams R. Acute liver failure: redefining the syndromes. Lancet 1993;342:273.

Shakil AO, Mazariegos GV, Kramer DJ. Fulminant hepatic failure. Surg Clin North Am 1999;79(1):77.

CHAPTER 18

Michael S. Lagnese and David E. Ciccolella

Pathophysiology of the Sepsis Syndromes

CHAPTER OUTLINE

LEARNING OBJECTIVES

After studying this chapter, you should be able to:

- Name the different sepsis syndromes.
- Understand how dysfunction of the host immune system contributes to development of the sepsis syndromes.
- Identify the hemodynamic and oxygen utilization abnormalities observed in septic patients.
- Recognize the clinical presentation and progression of the sepsis syndromes.
- Describe the intensive care unit management of the sepsis syndromes.

SEPSIS SYNDROMES DEFINED

Invasion of the body by microorganisms alters homeostasis and can cause sepsis.

Sepsis results when invasion of the body by microorganisms (including bacteria, fungi, viruses, and parasites) causes alterations in the normal homeostatic balance maintained by the human host in health. Patients with sepsis or septic shock may present with a constellation of variable symptoms and signs including fever or low body temperature, tachypnea, tachycardia, low blood pressure, low urine output, mental status changes, and multiple laboratory abnormalities such as high white blood cell counts, hyperglycemia, and hypoxemia. The number and severity of these clinical manifestations represent a spectrum of clinical conditions, which may progress along a disease continuum from sepsis to more severe sepsis and septic shock. The frequency of these clinical conditions is rising as a result of changing population risk factors, and the mortality rate for severe sepsis and septic shock has remained high, ranging between 40% and 60%.

CASE STUDY: PART 1

A 50-year-old man presented to the emergency department with a 4-day history of high fevers, chills, left-sided pleuritic pain, and productive cough with thick yellow sputum. He also had a small amount of blood-tinged sputum the day before presentation. He reported that 4 days ago he felt unusually fatigued and had a sore throat. By the next day, he had developed fevers to 103.5°F, taken orally, and associated chills. His fever persisted, and anorexia and nausea and vomiting developed 1 day before presentation. His past medical history was significant for noninsulin-dependent diabetes mellitus and hypertension (usual BP, 130/85), both controlled with medications. He had a 30-pack-year smoking history and drank alcohol rarely. He had worked as a bus driver for many years.

Some of the risk factors for development of sepsis include diseases such as diabetes mellitus, acquired immunodeficiency syndrome, liver failure, kidney failure, and cancer, being among the very old or very young, and the use of invasive technology from urinary and vascular catheterization to cardiac mechanical-assist devices.

To standardize the terms used in describing the sepsis syndromes, the definitions used here were recommended in the American College of Chest Physicians/Society of Critical Care Medicine consensus statement of 1992. Systemic inflammatory response syndrome (SIRS) is present when two or more of the following are present: (1) leukocytosis, white blood count (WBC) > 12,000, or leukopenia, WBC < 4,000 or significant band forms (>10%); (2) hyperthermia (>38°C) or hypothermia (<36°C); (3) hypocapnia (P_aCO_2 <32 mmHg) or respiratory rate >20 breaths/min; (4) heart rate >90 beats/min. The presence of infection is not required for the diagnosis of SIRS because it can be caused by noninfectious diseases such as trauma, pancreatitis, tissue ischemia, and hypovolemic shock. Sepsis is present when the systemic inflammatory response syndrome is caused by infection. Severe sepsis is sepsis associated with organ hypoperfusion, dysfunction, or hypotension. Examples of these hypoperfusion and perfusion abnormalities are oliguria, mental status alterations, or lactic acidosis. Septic shock is a subset of sepsis that is associated with hypotension refractory to adequate fluid resuscitation and signs of organ hypoperfusion and dysfunction. The term sepsis with hypotension has been used to describe sepsis states that are responsive to intravenous fluid resuscitation. Finally, bacteremia refers to the presence

Systemic inflammatory response syndrome (SIRS) can result from both infectious and noninfectious insults.

SIRS caused by infection is sepsis.

Severe sepsis with low blood pressure is referred to as septic shock.

CASE STUDY: PART 2

On physical exam, the patient appeared lethargic but was easily aroused. He was in moderate respiratory distress and was just able to complete sentences without pausing to catch his breath. There was prominent use of accessory respiratory muscles. His rectal temperature was 104.5°F, heart rate was 118, respiratory rate was 28, blood pressure was 98/60 mmHg, and O_2 saturation by pulse oximetry was 92% while the patient was breathing through a nonrebreather facemask with a FiO_2 of 1.0. His skin was cool and moist. The only other significant findings on physical examination were inspiratory crackles and some wheezing over the left lower lung field on auscultation. Except for these findings, the cardiovascular, abdominal, and neurologic examination results were normal.

During the initial evaluation and treatment in the Emergency Department, laboratory studies were obtained. Arterial blood gas revealed hypoxemia, despite high supplemental oxygen, and a mixed acid–base disorder with hypocapnia and metabolic acidosis. The electrolytes showed a sodium of 142 mmol/l and an elevated anion gap. Serum glucose was elevated at 180 mg/dl. Creatinine and blood urea nitrogen were 1.4 mg/dl and 36 mg/dl, respectively. The complete blood cell count showed a white blood cell count of 22,800 cells/mm^3 with increased band forms, a hematocrit of 42%, and a platelet count of 200,000 cells/mm^3. Sputum Gram stain showed no epithelial cells, many gram-positive diplococci, and many white blood cells, some containing intracellular bacteria. The chest x-ray showed a dense left lower lobe consolidation with a very small pleural effusion. The cardiac silhouette appeared normal.

The patient continued to receive bronchodilators, supplemental oxygen, and intravenous fluids and also started on broad-spectrum intravenous antibiotics, third-generation cephalosporin and macrolide. The patient was admitted to the intensive care unit (ICU) with a diagnosis of community-acquired pneumonia with sepsis and respiratory distress.

In sepsis or septic shock, infection may occur in a variety of sites but lung, abdomen, and urinary tract appear to be the most common. However, a definite site of infection cannot be found in a significant proportion of patients.

of bacteria in the blood, proven either by growth on blood culture or by visible microorganisms in the blood on Gram staining.

The clinical manifestations of sepsis result from the interaction between the defenses of the human body and the microbial infection. Through a complex cascade of cellular and humoral defenses, the human immunologic system provides the means by which infection is attenuated and eliminated. Although it is usually carefully contained and regulated, the immune system has great potential to become harmfully uncontrolled, as occurs with the sepsis syndromes. This chapter presents an overview of the pathophysiologic processes responsible for sepsis and sepsis-related syndromes.

PATHOPHYSIOLOGY

Cellular and Inflammatory Mediators

Both locally active and circulating mediators play a role in coordinated immune function.

Normally protective cellular mediators released during sepsis can also cause tissue damage if not attenuated.

Many of the clinical signs seen in sepsis are manifestations of systemic host protection.

The host defense system involves the interaction of a variety of cells and humoral systems. As part of the host immune reaction, a series of both local and systemic soluble factors are released. Their primary coordinated function is to identify, limit, and eliminate the infecting organism and its products from the body. Analysis of bronchoalveolar lavage fluid has demonstrated that a large number of biologically active molecules can be found in the alveoli of patients with sepsis. These molecules are collectively referred to as mediators, and they play an important role in the development of sepsis. Many of these inflammatory mediators have been identified and their function characterized (Table 18-1), but many more likely exist and remain unknown. A fundamental concept in sepsis pathophysiology is that the cellular mediators and hormones released can be just as harmful to normal human tissue as they are to the invading organism. For this reason, the defense cascade usually is under tight homeostatic control that limits the extent of damage. Many of the systemic effects of the circulating immunologic mediators produce clinical changes that play a role in resolving infection.

Cellular Elements

The stimulated macrophage is the initiator of much of the immunologic cascade.

To understand the abnormalities encountered in the sepsis syndromes, it is important to first review some of the basic mechanisms involved in normal immune function following microbial invasion. The tissue mononuclear phagocyte (also known as a macrophage) is the primary cell that initiates much of the local and systemic immune response (Figure 18-1). These

TABLE 18-1

SELECTED INFLAMMATORY MEDIATORS AND THEIR FUNCTIONS

MEDIATOR	SELECTED FUNCTIONS
Tumor necrosis factor-α (TNF-α)	Stimulates polymorphonuclear neutrophils (PMN) Increases vascular permeability Stimulates IL-1, IL-6, IL-8, IL-9 Stimulates PAF Stimulates cyclooxygenase production
Platelet-activating factor (PAF)	Stimulates platelet degranulation Attracts eosinophils Stimulates neutrophil activity
Interferon-γ	Stimulates macrophage protein synthesis Stimulates monocyte maturation
Interleukin-1	Stimulates mononuclear phagocyte function Stimulates IL-2 Stimulates fibroblast and endothelial proliferation
Interleukin-2	Stimulates T-lymphocyte production and activity
Interleukin-5	Stimulates eosinophil production and activity
Interleukin-6	Stimulates B-lymphocyte production and activity Decreases TNF production

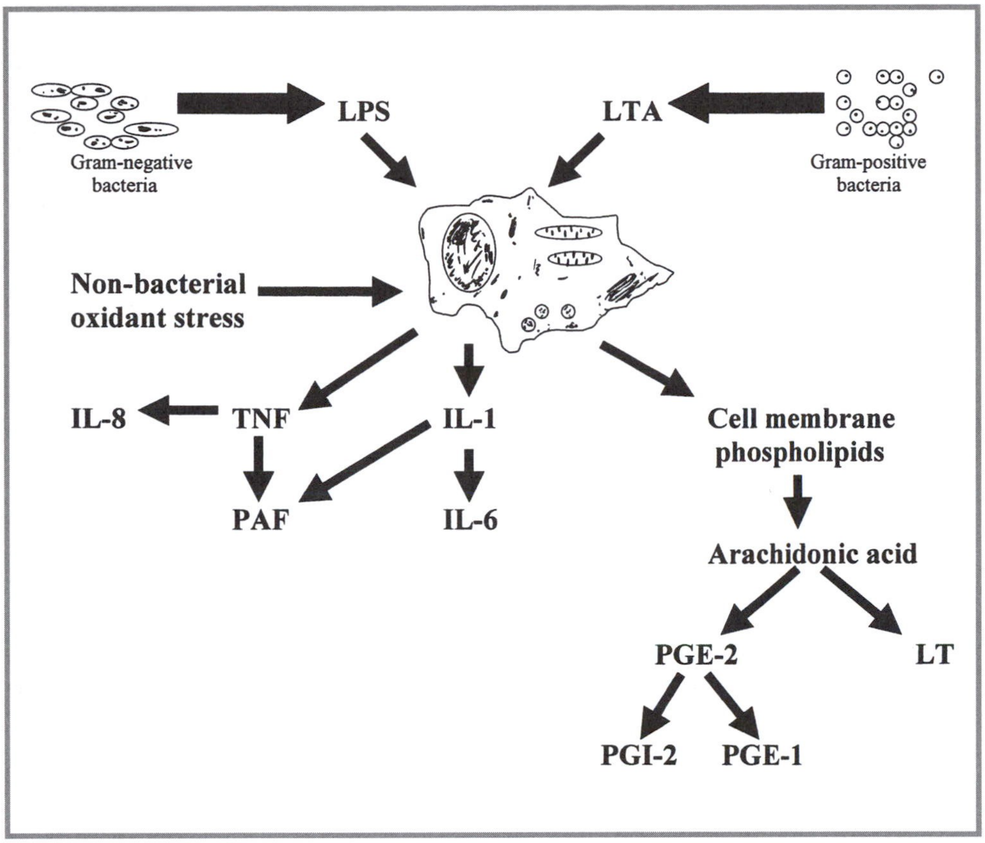

FIGURE 18-1

Schematic diagram of interactions of several common macrophage stimuli and potential subsequent macrophage activity. *LPS*, lipopolysaccharide; *LTA*, lipoteichoic acid; *TNF*, tumor necrosis factor; *PAF*, platelet–activating factor; *IL*, interleukin; *LT*, leukotriene; *PG*, prostaglandin.

cells can be found in most body tissues and secretions, and in many organ systems, these cells have highly specialized organ-specific subpopulations. Specific microbial antigens act as a stimulus to the mononuclear phagocyte and cause them to release a variety of humoral factors that in turn act on various other tissues and organ systems. These antigens generally are microbial proteins and have variable ability to activate the host immune system.

Recognition of bacterial antigens by the host macrophage initiates the immune response.

One of the most important of these microbial antigens is lipopolysaccharide (LPS), otherwise known as gram-negative endotoxin. Lipopolysaccharide is a large, complex cell membrane component necessary for bacterial growth and survival. The host receptor protein that recognizes and interacts with LPS is called CD14. CD14 is primarily found on the cell membrane of the macrophage. Binding of LPS to host macrophage CD14 initiates the production and release of many of the elements involved in the immune cascade. Several soluble forms of CD14 have also been identified and have been shown to bind with LPS. These circulating LPS–CD14 compounds are able to activate the immune response and initiate the sepsis syndromes independent of primary macrophage involvement. The LPS–CD14 interaction is complex and is incompletely understood; specifically, there appear to be several proteins that have the ability to alter the binding properties of these two compounds at the molecular level. The liver produces a protein called lipopolysaccharide-binding protein (LBP) that binds to circulating LPS and facilitates the LPS–CD14 interaction.

Lipopolysaccharide (LPS) is a bacterial cell wall constituent that interacts with the macrophage membrane protein CD 14.

Circulating CD14 can also bind with LPS and trigger the immunologic response.

Cytokines

Macrophages and other inflammatory cells produce cytokines, which are large molecules that have the ability to modulate the function and secretory response of other host cells by interacting with specific cell membrane receptors. The cytokine–cell membrane interaction results in altered cell gene expression and, ultimately, altered cellular function. These effects take place at the local cellular level causing, among other things, chemotaxis, which results in the migration of more phagocytic cells to the areas of infection. A systemic effect also occurs with many cytokines acting as hormones and circulating to areas distant from the site

Cytokines induce and alter target cell secretory function. They are released from inflammatory cells.

TABLE 18-2

CLINICAL EFFECTS OF TNF-α, IL-1, AND IL-6

MEDIATOR	CLINICAL EFFECTS	SOURCE
Tumor necrosis factor-α	Hypotension Fever Cachexia Capillary leak syndrome Capillary thrombosis	Polymorphonuclear lymphocytes Mononuclear phagocytes
Interleukin-1	Hypotension Fever Skeletal muscle breakdown	Endothelial cells T lymphocytes B lymphocytes Mononuclear phagocytes
Interleukin-6	Fever	Endothelial cells T lymphocytes B lymphocytes Mononuclear phagocytes

Cytokines released from host immune cells have both local and systemic effects, resulting in many of the clinical signs of sepsis and septic shock.

Tumor necrosis factor (TNF), a cytokine, causes local tissue destruction and tissue edema and promotes intravascular coagulation.

Interleukin-1 (IL-1) causes fever, stimulates muscle breakdown, and attracts and stimulates host immune cells.

of secretion. It is this systemic release of dozens of inflammatory cytokines that is responsible for the clinical features of sepsis.

Many cytokines have been well characterized in terms of their structure and specific function, but many others have yet to be fully defined (Table 18-2). Tumor necrosis factor (TNF) is one of the most important cytokines; it has both local and systemic effects. In the immediate area of infection, TNF can cause direct damage to endothelial cells. Upon systemic release, it causes intravascular coagulation leading to tissue ischemia, gross increase in capillary permeability leading to tissue edema, and fever. It is also a potent stimulator of other cytokines and other mediators of inflammation, including cyclooxygenase species and several molecules in a class of cytokines known as the interleukins (IL), including interleukin-1 (IL-1). IL-1 causes fever through its stimulatory effects on the preoptic nucleus of the hypothalamus, which is why it is also referred to as the endogenous pyrogen. It is also the primary mediator of skeletal muscle catabolism observed in severe sepsis. IL-1 release from the macrophage also occurs independent of TNF stimulation, as when the phagocytic cells are stimulated by LPS. IL-1 also stimulates neutrophil and lymphocyte activity, causing production and release of cellular products and cellular replication and migration. Many other cytokines (including many other interleukins) are released by the macrophage on microbial stimulation (see Table 18-1).

Platelet-Activating Factor and Leukotrienes

Arachidonic acid is a substrate for production of many other inflammatory mediators and regulatory hormones and is itself liberated from the macrophage cell membrane.

Platelet-activating factor (PAF) has both local and systemic effects, including platelet chemotaxis and bronchoconstriction, and contributes to hypotension as seen in septic shock.

The stimulated macrophage also releases membrane phospholipids that are converted to arachidonic acid. Arachidonic acid, in turn, is the biochemical substrate for conversion to various other mediators of inflammation by cyclooxygenases and lipoxygenases. These end products are mediators of many cellular processes, including alteration in vascular permeability and immune cell chemotaxis. Among the more important of these membrane phospholipid derivatives are platelet-activating factor (PAF) and leukotriene B_4. PAF is secreted by many host cells in response to interaction with LPS and has a number of local cellular effects, including stimulation of other immune mediators and initiation of platelet chemotaxis. It also plays a role in stimulating further release of other mediators of inflammation, including TNF, and IL-1. Clinically, PAF causes pulmonary hypertension, bronchoconstriction, and profound systemic hypotension and is likely a key factor in the development and progression of septic shock, which, as already mentioned, is characterized by profound and refractory systemic hypotension. Leukotriene B_4 (LTB_4) is biosynthesized from membrane-derived arachidonic acid in the lipoxygenase pathway. LTB_4, a potent chemotactic factor for neutrophils, promotes vascular fluid leakage at the capillary, contributing to tissue edema and, ultimately, to gas exchange abnormalities in the lung.

Nitric Oxide and Oxygen Radicals

As hypotensive shock progresses during sepsis, so does tissue hypoxia and subsequent ischemic injury. A major goal of therapy for septic shock has been improvement and maintenance of the tissue oxygen supply. However, if adequate amounts of oxygen can be restored, several species of reactive oxygen radicals are produced as a result of normal cellular respiration. Under physiologic conditions, an adequate supply of local defense antioxidants is present to absorb the chemical reactivity of these potentially harmful oxygen radials. When previously ischemic tissue is reoxygenated, oxygen radical release overwhelms any antioxidant defense species available. Endogenously produced nitric oxide (NO) is the substrate for production of the highly reactive free radical peroxynitrite, which is involved in microbial destruction. However, like other elements in the inflammatory cascade, peroxynitrite has also been shown to cause direct tissue damage when present in substantial amounts. This process is referred to as NO-induced reperfusion injury and can affect any tissue.

Improvement in tissue oxygen delivery is a major goal of therapy for septic shock.

NO is produced endogenously and is converted to highly reactive free radicals that are involved in microbial destruction.

NO can also induce direct tissue damage if homeostatic control is not maintained.

Again, the entire defense cascade is necessarily under careful autoregulation and homeostatic control. The many redundant inflammatory cascade pathways underscore the complexity of both the inflammatory response itself and the regulatory pathways that initiate and control it. Because of the harmful cellular effects that the activated system can have on normal tissue were it to go unchecked, various regulatory pathways have evolved. Most of these regulatory mechanisms involve modulation of either the cytokine receptor function or number or cytokine production itself. To a variable extent, all the sepsis syndromes involve at least some initial dysfunction of these normal control mechanisms. Furthermore, as sepsis progresses, these control mechanisms become increasingly dysfunctional and perpetuate the disease state.

Dysfunction of the regulation of the immune cascade is a fundamental observation seen in all the sepsis syndromes.

Oxygen Consumption and Delivery

An attempt has been made recently to include the concept of deranged oxygen metabolism in the definition of sepsis and in the description of septic patients. This trend underscores the importance of oxygen delivery and oxygen consumption in the septic state. A more complete description of oxygen metabolism in critically ill patients can be found elsewhere in this volume. Here, we explain some basic and specific relationships as they pertain specifically to the sepsis syndromes.

Dysfunctional oxygen metabolism is common in the sepsis syndromes.

Systemic oxygen delivery (DO_2) is defined as the product of cardiac output and arterial oxygen content, or, more simply:

$$DO_2 = Q \times CaO_2 \qquad (18\text{-}1)$$

where Q is cardiac output and CaO_2 is the arterial oxygen content. Systemic oxygen consumption ($\dot{V}O_2$) is defined as the product of the cardiac output and the difference between the arterial and venous oxygen contents, or

$$\dot{V}O_2 = Q \times (CaO_2 - C\bar{v}O_2) \qquad (18\text{-}2)$$

where $C\bar{v}O_2$ is the mixed venous oxygen content. In the healthy state, the relationship between DO_2 and $\dot{V}O_2$ is a biphasic one (Figure 18-2), in which the normally perfused organs are able to maintain a constant $\dot{V}O_2$ independent of the delivered oxygen (DO_2). This effect is primarily accomplished by altering the percentage of oxygen that is extracted from the capillaries. In other words, as DO_2 decreases, the oxygen extraction ratio (O_2ER) increases. The result is physiologic maintenance of $\dot{V}O_2$, referred to as physiologic independence of $\dot{V}O_2$ on DO_2. Below a certain critical DO_2, however, cellular metabolism reaches a point of maximal oxygen extraction and $\dot{V}O_2$ can no longer be maintained; this point is referred to as DO_{2crit}. Oxygen consumption below the DO_{2crit} is linearly related to the DO_2 (see Figure 18-2).

Normally, the rate of oxygen uptake from the tissues is constant despite variable oxygen delivery.

The application of these basic physiologic concepts to the septic state is more controversial and has been the topic of numerous studies. Early studies suggested that, in the septic state, cellular metabolism was altered in such a way that DO_{2crit} was increased, resulting in

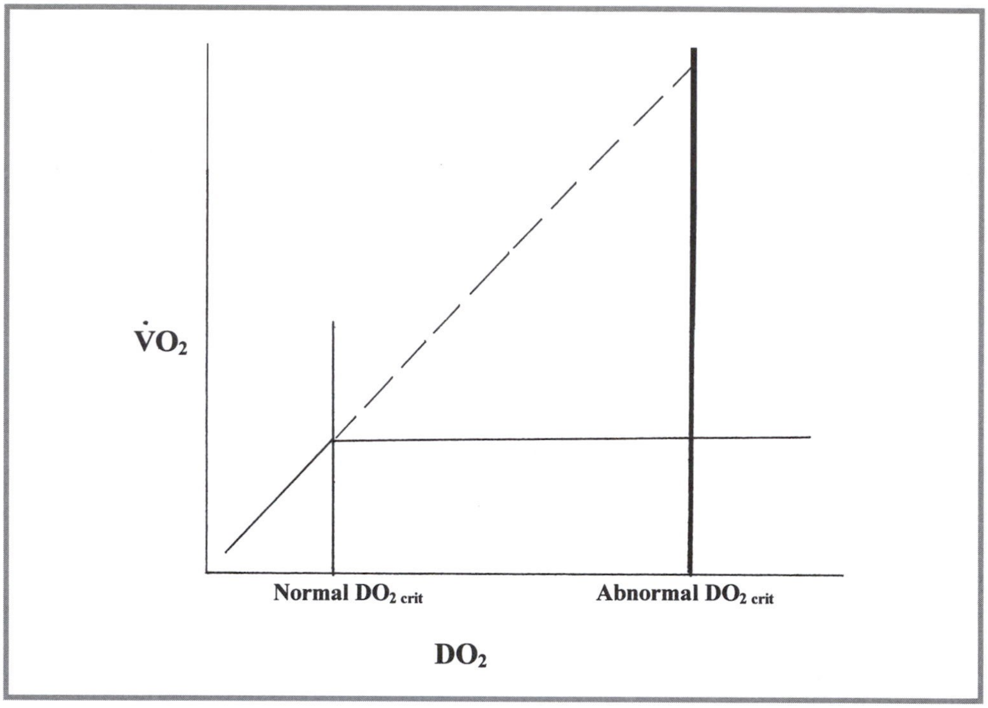

FIGURE 18-2

In the healthy state, there is physiologic independence of $\dot{V}O_2$ on DO_2 beyond the DO_{2crit} (*solid line*), primarily because of the alteration of the cellular extraction ratio as DO_2 varies. It had been postulated that, in the septic patient, the DO_{2crit} could be greatly increased and the oxygen extraction ratio could be unable to compensate for significant changes in DO_2; this is thought to result in a supposed physiologic dependence of $\dot{V}O_2$ on DO_2 (*broken line*).

Initial research suggested that the septic state was characterized by pathologic dependence of oxygen uptake on oxygen delivery.

Recent studies have shown that there likely is no pathologic dependence of oxygen uptake on oxygen delivery in the septic state.

Cellular and organ oxygen demand is increased in hypermetabolic states such as sepsis.

a pathologic dependence of $\dot{V}O_2$ on DO_2. A progressive, linear decline in oxygen consumption was thought to be directly related to lower systemic oxygen delivery. It was postulated that occult tissue hypoxia resulted and that this, in turn, was a possible explanation for the development of SIRS and multiple organ dysfunction (MODS). At least a dozen studies in both septic and nonseptic patients have presented evidence for this theory of impaired oxygen delivery–consumption metabolism. However, closer examination of the data has since pointed out several mathematical and statistical errors common to many of these studies that flaw the original conclusions.

To date, there is no clear evidence that a pathologic dependence of $\dot{V}O_2$ on DO_2 exists in septic patients. On the other hand, there is general acceptance that sepsis does alter oxygen metabolism significantly at both the cellular and organ system levels and that this disturbance plays a role in the development of more severe manifestations of the disease, such as SIRS and MODS. Specifically, it has been shown that in hypermetabolic states such as sepsis, cellular oxygen demand is increased, resulting in a net increase in tissue and organ oxygen demand. This demand and subsequent consumption may outpace the ability of the cardiorespiratory system to compensate at the cellular and organ levels. Although invasive monitoring and testing and bedside diagnosis allow for such systemic manifestations of this oxygen derangement to be identified, there is currently no reliable way to identify it at the cellular level. Given the current data available, it is reasonable to direct efforts at diagnosing sepsis in terms of the cellular mechanisms affected.

CASE STUDY: PART 3

Soon after admission to the ICU, the patient developed signs of septic shock and respiratory failure. He became mildly confused and more lethargic, systolic blood pressure decreased to 75 mmHg and respirations were labored. His urine output had decreased as well. He was intubated and ventilated and rapidly given further intravenous fluids and vasoactive drugs for circulatory support. Placement of a pulmonary artery catheter revealed a pulmonary capillary wedge pressure (PCWP) of 12 cmH_2O, a high cardiac output of 10 l/min, and a calculated systemic vascular resistance (SVR) of 700. The pulmonary artery catheter was used to further optimize his hemodynamic status.

CLINICAL ASPECTS

Clinically, there is much overlap among the sepsis syndromes. For this reason, it is important to be able to recognize the broad, cardinal manifestations of sepsis. The clinical progression of the patient with sepsis can be acute and rapidly fatal, and early consideration of the diagnosis and institution of appropriate therapy are essential. Multiple organ systems are usually involved with variable acute dysfunction of each. In fact, in late-phase severe septic shock with multiple organ dysfunction syndrome, it is rare to find an organ system that is spared.

Sepsis must be considered early in the differential diagnosis because it can be rapidly progressive and fatal.

Cardiovascular Effects

The cardiovascular effects present the most immediate and life-threatening danger to the patient with sepsis. The most prominent cardiovascular effect is arterial and venous bed dilation. Several mechanisms are responsible for this, including phospholipase-mediated release of endothelial prostaglandins and leukotrienes. An initial physiologic response to this is increased cardiovascular sympathetic tone resulting in early tachycardia, increased pulse pressure and warm, red skin as peripheral capillary beds dilate. Hypotension resulting from decreased systemic vascular resistance and decreased intravascular volume is a hallmark of septic shock and is usually seen later in the course of sepsis. Pale, cool skin at this stage reflects the underlying tissue hypoperfusion. Also, as released prostaglandins and leukotrienes each increase vascular permeability, large molecular weight proteins move more readily into the extravascular space, resulting in decreased total blood volume. Additionally, other cytokines inhibit tissue cells from releasing fluid into the extracellular matrix. This altered fluid balance results in a net loss of intravascular volume, contributing to inadequate tissue perfusion. Tumor necrosis factor (TNF) is another well-known mediator of increased vascular permeability in the sepsis syndromes. A third mechanism responsible for impaired cardiovascular function is decreased cardiac contractility.

Cardiovascular collapse is responsible for many of the common signs and symptoms observed in the septic patient.

Cytokine-mediated alterations in vascular permeability and vasoactivity result in many of the clinical cardiovascular signs of sepsis.

Decreased cardiac inotropy contributes to hemodynamic failure during sepsis.

Hemodynamic Changes and Pulmonary Artery Monitoring

Because the clinical minute-to-minute assessment of cardiovascular and hemodynamic function can be extremely challenging, pulmonary artery monitoring has become an important adjunct in the management of the septic patient. Because treatment of sepsis is supportive only, continuous monitoring of multiple systems, such as the respiratory, cardiovascular, metabolic, and central nervous systems, is crucial. The pulmonary artery (PA) catheter allows comprehensive monitoring of the hemodynamic function of the body at the bedside. Here we examine the hemodynamic profile specific to the septic state. Details of PA catheter insertion and function are given elsewhere in this volume.

Hemodynamically, the sepsis syndromes actually progress through a series of different phases. Early sepsis is characterized by a hyperdynamic cardiovascular pattern. The vascular system is diffusely dilated as a result of the systemic effects of the various circulating catecholamines. Reflexive tachycardia usually ensues, and this can be one of the earliest signs of systemic infection. Pulmonary arterial monitoring usually reflects this: the systemic vascular resistance (SVR) and pulmonary capillary wedge pressure (PCWP) are decreased, reflecting low cardiac filling pressures. Cardiac output, however, is usually elevated as the heart rate reflexively increases. Increased cardiac contractility generally is not a feature of early sepsis. Although several catecholamines function to increase contractility, a net decrease in systolic and diastolic function is characteristic. As the septic process progresses, hemodynamic compensations begin to fail. Cardiac output appears to normalize as cardiovascular function deteriorates. The PCWP begins to increase as well. The SVR also tends toward normal as the process progresses. As further systemic collapse continues, the late septic hemodynamic profile becomes similar to that seen in cardiogenic shock.

The pulmonary artery (PA) catheter allows continuous bedside assessment of many hemodynamic parameters.

Sepsis has a specific pattern of hemodynamic derangement as measured by the PA catheter.

Early sepsis is characterized by increased cardiac output and decreased systemic vascular resistance.

Early in the septic state, cardiac filling pressures are depressed but cardiac output is elevated.

Late sepsis is characterized by deteriorating cardiovascular function.

Respiratory Changes

Tachypnea is the most common respiratory finding in early sepsis.

Hypercapnia generally is not observed in septic patients.

In early sepsis, tachypnea is a common finding. Although incompletely understood, the mechanism may be partly explained by cytokine stimulation of respiratory centers in the brainstem. Significant alveolar hyperventilation can occur in this setting, especially if preexisting pulmonary reserve is already low. Hypercapnia, however, is generally not a feature of early sepsis. Likewise, usually only modest, if any, hypoxemia is present in sepsis unless there is significant underlying pulmonary disease. However, in more advanced sepsis, as more organ systems become involved, the lungs themselves may be primarily affected with severe, refractory hypoxemia being a manifestation. Primarily as the result of abnormal alteration in the pulmonary vasculature endothelial membrane permeability, extravasation of fluid occurs, resulting in the acute respiratory distress syndrome (ARDS).

Renal Effects

Decreased urine output in the septic patient dramatically worsens prognosis.

An early goal of volume resuscitation in sepsis is maintenance of urine output.

Renal dysfunction may occur as the functional intravascular volume decreases and normal compensatory mechanisms fail to maintain adequate organ perfusion. The renal vascular supply has an integrated humoral autoregulatory mechanism that allows the glomeruli to maintain perfusion adequate to produce urine over a wide range of varying volume states. However, as even these compensations fail, renal blood flow decreases. Prerenal oliguria results, and eventually anuric renal failure can occur. In early sepsis, volume expanders such as crystalloid and colloid solutions usually can improve renal blood flow and increase urine output. This effect is important prognostically because increased urine output generally has been associated with a more favorable outcome.

Neurologic Effects

Some degree of neurologic dysfunction is almost always observed in septic patients.

Cytokines and other mediators of the host immune response probably contribute to the CNS dysfunction observed in septic patients.

The central nervous system (CNS) is almost always affected in sepsis. Alteration in the patient's thermoregulatory function is common. Hyperthermia reflects macrophage release of IL-1 and TNF. Hypothermia is also a common sign, usually seen in chronically ill or elderly patients. The most common CNS effects usually are varying degrees of mental status change, which can range from mild confusion to complete obtundation and even coma. Mental status poorly correlates with the degree of sepsis, and even mild early disease can present with profound alterations in higher neurologic function. The pathophysiology of CNS dysfunction in the sepsis syndromes is unclear; however, the multiple systemic immune products released from the macrophage probably play a key role. Also, low circulating blood volume in more severe cases can result in decreased cerebral perfusion, contributing to the toxic encephalopathy seen.

Hematologic Effects

Altered production and function of white cells, red cells, and platelets is common in septic patients.

Anemia in septic patients is caused by both hematopoietic suppression and hemodilution following aggressive volume resuscitation.

All three hematologic cell lines can be affected in the sepsis syndromes. Cytokine-mediated release of immature polymorphonuclear neutrophils (PMNs) is reflected in the leukocyte differential as a left shift. Unless there is underlying bone marrow pathology that would otherwise result in a decrease in liberated white blood cells, most patients demonstrate such a shift. Patients with normal bone marrow who fail to mount such a response have a poor prognosis.

Anemia is also seen in most sepsis patients, usually as a result of early massive volume resuscitation with consequent hemodilution. There is also suppression of normal hematopoiesis caused by both endogenous and exogenous mediators that are released as a result of the systemic inflammatory response.

Circulating platelets are particularly sensitive, both quantitatively and qualitatively, to local and systemic infection. Mild to moderate thrombocytopenia is evident in less severe sepsis, but intractable disease and septic shock are the usual setting for more profound and clinically significant decrease in the peripheral platelet count.

Disseminated intravascular coagulation (DIC) is a syndrome of variable severity that can be associated with sepsis. It is characterized by intravascular thrombosis with resultant tissue ischemia, abnormal bleeding, and accelerated breakdown of fibrinogen.

DIC is commonly observed in sepsis syndromes.

Gastrointestinal, Endocrinologic, and Metabolic Processes

In addition to the multiple roles of IL-1 already discussed, IL-1 and TNF also have influence on several metabolic and hepatic processes that are often quite prominent in the septic patient. However, fulminate hepatic failure is usually not a common feature of sepsis. When it occurs, the so-called shock liver is more often associated with low circulating flow states and resultant decreased organ perfusion, as seen in septic shock. Less well understood factors contributing to liver failure in sepsis are the direct effects of the various inflammatory mediators released as part of the systemic inflammatory response.

Liver failure is usually not a feature of sepsis syndromes.

Loss of gross muscle mass has been shown to begin very early in the course of sepsis, primarily as a result of increased muscle protein catabolism mediated by IL-1 and cachectin.

Muscle mass loss is mainly a result of the catabolic effects of IL-1 and cachectin.

Blood glucose metabolism is altered in sepsis. Hyperglycemia is common and has been attributed to increased levels and activity of endogenous glucocorticoids and catecholamines. Heightened glucagon activity and production also impair glucose metabolism and contribute to clinical hyperglycemia.

The syndrome of inappropriate antidiuretic hormone secretion (SIADH) is a common feature in critical illness, including sepsis, especially when the underlying etiology of the sepsis is bacterial lower respiratory tract infections. The result can be hyponatremia as a result of the impaired renal water excretion.

Syndrome of inappropriate antidiuretic hormone secretion (SIADH) is particularly common when sepsis is caused by infection of the lower respiratory tract.

Multiple Organ Dysfunction Syndrome

As systemic infection progresses and affects a particular organ system, basic function of the organ will begin to fail. Maintenance of homeostatic stability requires coordination of multiple organ systems and subsystems for survival. Disruption of the primary functions of more than one organ system as related to sepsis is referred to as the multiple organ dysfunction syndrome (MODS). This syndrome usually reflects uncontrolled and advanced disease and can develop rapidly. The prognosis for patients at this endstage of disease is extremely poor and has not improved in recent years, despite advances in the knowledge base of the pathogenesis of sepsis and the introduction of evolving and novel treatments.

When more than one organ system is affected by sepsis, multiple organ dysfunction syndrome (MODS) is present.

MODS portends a poor prognosis for recovery.

THERAPY

There is currently no specific therapy for sepsis or septic shock. Initial management of these syndromes is supportive and should focus on treatment of any actually identified or suspected infections with appropriate antimicrobials and on maintenance of hemodynamic sta-

CASE STUDY: PART 4

In our previous evaluation of the patient, a rapid and profound deterioration was seen in his respiratory and cardiovascular status. The patient developed respiratory failure despite maximum therapy and was intubated and placed on mechanical ventilation. At the same time, the patient was rapidly given more intravenous fluids with minimal improvement in his arterial blood pressure. He was started on a dopamine drip but despite increasing dose titration there was only a small improvement in circulatory support. Initiation of a norepinephrine drip significantly improved the shock state and the dopamine was tapered; his BP increased to 92/50 mmHg. Measurements obtained by the pulmonary artery catheter revealed a hyperdynamic shock state. The pulmonary artery catheter was used to further optimize his cardiovascular hemodynamics. His sputum and blood cultures revealed gram-positive diplococci later identified as Streptococcus pneumoniae, and antibiotic therapy was simplified accordingly.

There is no specific cure for sepsis at present.

bility. However, more recent data suggests that administration of activated protein C may reduce mortality in patients with severe sepsis, but may be associated with an increased risk for bleeding. Initially, broad empiric antimicrobial therapy allows coverage for most possible causative infections. As sepsis progresses, and systemic involvement becomes more evident, therapy is directed more toward hemodynamic and organ system support. Furthermore, definitive antimicrobial therapy can be instituted as infectious sources are identified.

Antimicrobial Therapy

Early, empiric use of intravenous antibiotics is mandatory as part of the initial therapy of sepsis.

Antimicrobial therapy is imperative in the initial management of sepsis, even when no obvious source of infection can be identified. Therefore, the patient presenting with clinical signs and symptoms of sepsis poses challenges in terms of selection of an optimal antimicrobial regimen. When the source of infection is unknown, the initial antimicrobial choice is necessarily empiric. Other times, there may be clinical findings or patient complaints that suggest a potential source of infection, allowing a more focused regimen. However, even when a source is suspected or known, broad initial coverage is still indicated in addition to directed antimicrobial coverage. Studies have shown wide variation in terms of benefit to be gained from specific combinations of empiric antimicrobials and the timing of administration of directed antimicrobials when a source of infection is identified. Nonetheless, early, broad antimicrobial therapy is essential to successful management of sepsis.

Selection of antibiotics should be guided by a logical assessment of the potentially infecting organisms.

In general, severe infections of unknown source as seen in the sepsis syndromes require empiric broad-spectrum antibiotic coverage. Several regimens have been suggested, all with common features. Initial therapy should be directed toward gram-positive cocci, aerobic bacilli, and usually anaerobes as well. Bactericidal drugs are preferred to those that are bacteriostatic. A cephalosporin with good gram-positive coverage, such as cefazolin, combined with an aminoglycoside such as gentamicin is a reasonable regimen when there is no clear source of underlying infection. Many clinicians also include anaerobic coverage with either clindamycin or metronidazole to this empiric regimen. Other cephalosporins such as ceftriaxone, cefotaxime, or ceftizoxime can also be considered in place of cefazolin. Augmented antipseudomonal beta-lactamase-susceptible penicillins such as ticarcillin/clavulanate or piperacillin/tazobactam or other beta-lactams such as imipenem have also been used as single agent alternatives. If serious beta-lactam allergy is present, a fluoroquinolone such as ciprofloxacin can be used in combination with either clindamycin or metronidazole.

Bactericidal antibiotics are generally preferred in the treatment of the septic patient.

Directed antibiotic therapy should be added to the initial regimen if a particular invading organism is suspected, based on the history and physical exam.

Certain clinical situations necessitate modification of the chosen antibiotic regimen.

At times, clinical clues may suggest a possible source of infection. In these circumstances, antimicrobials can be added to the foregoing regimens. For example, if there is any suspicion that methicillin-resistant *Stapholococcus aureus* (MRSA) is the causative organism, vancomycin should be added. Such might be that case if the patient has an indwelling venous catheter that appears red, edematous, or has a purulent discharge. Likewise, if there is a recent history of surgery and the surgical wound appears to be infected, treatment for MRSA should be added as part of the regimen. When there is a suspected intraabdominal or pelvic infection, anaerobic and gram-negative coverage is necessary. Clindamycin or metronidazole should definitely be added in these situations.

Patients with chronic obstructive pulmonary disease (COPD) have an increased risk of developing resistant gram-negative lower respiratory infections.

Patients with underlying respiratory disease, such as chronic obstructive pulmonary disease (COPD), are predisposed to developing lower respiratory tract infections caused by gram-negative organisms such as *Hemophilus influenzae* and *Moraxella catarrhalis*. Pneumonia caused by these organisms can result in sepsis and should be treated with either a second- or third-generation cephalosporin instead of cefazolin if suspected.

When meningitis is suspected, high-dose ampicillin, a third-generation cephalosporin plus vancomycin should be included in the empiric antibiotic management.

Patients who have been confined to a hospital or other long-term care facility for more than 72 h are typically colonized with antimicrobial-resistant gram-negative bacteria and MRSA. When they develop sepsis syndromes, initial antibiotic regimens should reflect these modifying circumstances by including coverage with vancomycin or extended-spectrum beta-lactams, such as imipenem, or fluoroquinolones, such as ciprofloxacin. Patients who are neutropenic following therapy for malignant disease represent a well-defined, specific subpopulation who have been documented to benefit from early semiempiric antibiotic therapy directed toward aerobic gram-positive cocci (*Streptococcus*, *Staphylococcus*, *Enterococcus*, and *Corynebacterium*) and toward certain gram-negative organisms (*Escherichia coli*, *Pseudomonas*, *Klebsiella*).

Regardless of the initial broad antibiotic therapy chosen, the regimen should be tailored as microbiologic culture and sensitivity data become available. Surgical or percutaneous drainage of any localized, potentially infected fluid collections should always be performed promptly in addition to antimicrobial therapy.

Definitive surgical drainage and debridement of any suspected infected fluid or tissue is imperative.

Supportive Therapy

Although there is no known specific therapy for the sepsis syndromes, vital organ support is essential and requires the level of care and continuous monitoring that only the intensive care unit environment can provide. Because septic shock is defined, in part, by systemic hypotension that is refractory to volume resuscitation, vasoactive pressors are frequently used to support hemodynamic and cardiac function. Patients who are supported hemodynamically earlier have better outcomes than patients for whom the same therapy is delayed.

Intensive care unit monitoring and full vital organ system support of the septic patient is the standard of care.

Initial pressor support of blood pressure should be with intravenous dopamine, which has dose-dependent alpha- and beta-agonist properties. Once injected, dopamine is systemically converted to norepinephrine, which is the primary active metabolite. Because this enzyme-mediated conversion may be dysfunctional in the septic patient, treatment with intravenous norepinephrine should be instituted in a patient who continues to have hypotension despite treatment with dopamine. Intravascular volume should be supported with either crystalloid or colloid solutions concurrently with pressor therapy unless there is a history of severe decompensated left ventricular dysfunction. In such cases, dobutamine, with its dose-dependent beta-2 agonist and cardiac inotropic effects, is preferred over dopamine. Epinephrine can be added when these other pressors have failed to adequately support the patient hemodynamically. Catecholamine vasopressor-induced tachycardia is common, especially in patients who have either underlying intrinsic cardiac disease or who are not adequately intravascularly resuscitated. In these situations, phenylephrine, an alpha-1 agonist can be used for hemodynamic support.

Initial vasoactive pressor support, when needed, should be instituted with dopamine as the first-line pressor.

If hypotension is initially refractory to dopamine, norepinephrine should be administered.

Volume resuscitation should be administered concurrently with pressor therapy.

SUMMARY

Mortality of patients suffering from severe sepsis remains excessive despite advances in our knowledge of the pathophysiology of the disease and novel therapies. This problem primarily reflects the fact that there still remains no specific treatment for sepsis and thus management is primarily supportive. Because hemodynamic collapse represents the fulminant stage of this illness, supportive interventions are directed mainly toward maintenance of cardiovascular, respiratory, and hemodynamic integrity. However, many patients with sepsis often already have preexisting and sometimes multisystem disease, and are unable to sustain the derangements imposed by systemic infection, even with aggressive and intensive systemic support. Important concepts that the clinician must consider are early consideration of occult infection in the differential diagnosis and the rapid identification of the offending organism, if possible. If a source of infection is found, primary treatment must include both

CASE STUDY: PART 5

After continued antibiotics directed toward *Streptococcus pneumoniae* and supportive treatment, the patient's vital signs, including blood pressure, gradually improved. His mental status, cardiovascular hemodynamics, and urine output improved over the next 2 days. His pulmonary artery catheter was removed. Over the next 10 days, his pneumonia improved and he was weaned from mechanical ventilator support. He was later evaluated as an outpatient and was found, as expected, to have chronic obstructive pulmonary disease (COPD).

surgical and medical interventions because delay in either approach can be catastrophic. If a source cannot be identified, empiric antibiotic therapy is the rule. In any case, the process may continue unattenuated despite all direct and supportive therapy, even when such therapy is guided by invasive hemodynamic monitoring. With new data and novel therapies being investigated at a vigorous pace, the management of sepsis is sure to evolve rapidly, and clinicians will likewise need to advance their own understanding of the clinical aspects of the disease on the basis of the pathophysiologic mechanisms outlined here.

REVIEW QUESTIONS

I. *Multiple Choice Questions*

1. Which one of the following is NOT one of the criteria required for diagnosis of the systemic inflammatory response syndrome (SIRS), as established by the American College of Chest Physicians/Society of Critical Care Medicine?

A. Tachycardia greater than 90 beats/min
B. Elevated white blood cell count
C. Low white blood cell count
D. Peripheral edema
E. Low P_aCO_2 on arterial blood gas analysis

2. Which one of the following statements is FALSE?

A. Sepsis is diagnosed when SIRS is found to have an infectious etiology.
B. At least two blood culture samples need to be positive for bacterial growth for the systemic inflammatory response syndrome to be present.
C. Hypotension is NOT the main criteria required for a diagnosis of septic shock to be made.
D. Septic shock is associated with signs of organ hypoperfusion and dysfunction.
E. A P_aCO_2 of 22 torr on arterial blood gas analysis would be one of the criteria needed for SIRS to be diagnosed.

3. All the following are true concerning inflammatory mediators released during sepsis syndromes except:

A. They are tightly regulated during sepsis and therefore pose no threat to normal host tissue.
B. Their release from the macrophage results in both local and systemic immune responses.
C. Bacterial lipopolysaccharide (LPS) is recognized by the host immune system and can result in activation of the immune response.
D. Interleukin-1 (IL-1) can mediate fever in the host through its activity in the hypothalamus.
E. Tumor necrosis factor (TNF) is a potent stimulator of several interleukins and can also cause local tissue destruction directly.

4. Which one of the following statements is false?

A. Systemic release of tumor necrosis factor (TNF) has been shown to have a stimulatory effect on host intravascular coagulation.
B. Both tumor necrosis factor and interleukin-1 (IL-1) can cause fever in the host.
C. Interleukin-1 release from the macrophage does not occur unless first stimulated by tumor necrosis factor (TNF).
D. Arachidonic acid release from the host cell membrane is a common feature of the sepsis syndromes.
E. Interleukin-1 (IL-1) is a potent stimulator of phagocytes and lymphocytes.

II. *True/False Questions*

5. Interleukin-1 release from the macrophage occurs after stimulation by tumor necrosis factor (TNF) and also after stimulation by gram-negative cell membrane lipopolysaccharide (LPS).

6. Platelet-activating factor (PAF) causes platelet degranulation and pulmonary hypertension but has no effect on platelet chemotaxis.

7. Peroxynitrite is produced from endogenously liberated nitric oxide and has been shown to cause direct host tissue damage.

8. In the healthy state, the relationship between oxygen uptake and oxygen delivery is biphasic, with tissue metabolism able to maintain a constant oxygen uptake over a variable degree of oxygen delivery.

9. In the septic state, occult tissue ischemia has been shown to be caused by a pathologic dependence of oxygen uptake on oxygen delivery, thus inciting the acute respiratory distress syndrome (ARDS).

10. Antibiotics are an essential element of early treatment of the critically ill septic patient.

ANSWERS

1. The answer is D. The American College of Chest Physicians and the Society of Critical Care Medicine have jointly established consensus criteria, which should be applied when considering the diagnosis of systemic inflammatory response syndrome in a patient, as an attempt to standardize diagnostic, therapeutic, and investigational efforts. By these criteria, SIRS is present when at least two of the following findings are present: (1) leukocytosis or leukopenia; (2) hyperthermia or hypothermia; (3) hypocapnia or tachypnea $>$ 20 breaths/min; or (4) tachycardia $>$ 90 beats/min. Peripheral edema is not one of the established criteria required to define the presence of SIRS.
2. The answer is B. Consensus definitions have been established for sepsis and the sepsis syndromes. By these definitions, if SIRS is caused by infection, sepsis is present. Although infection is a common cause of SIRS, noninfectious causes are recognized as well; therefore, bacteremia is not required for the diagnosis to be made. Although the diagnosis of septic shock has previously focused on relative or absolute hypotension, this finding has recently been deemphasized in favor of the more conceptual theory of relative or absolute tissue ischemia, reflected clinically as gross organ dysfunction. Hypocapnia is one of the established criteria that may define SIRS in combination with other consensus criteria.
3. The answer is A. Mediators involved in the inflammatory response are subject to complex and integrated control under homeostatic conditions. Because they function to influence host cells both locally and systemically, any abnormal propagation or acceleration of the immune response has systemwide potential to alter gross host function and result in the clinical syndrome of SIRS, with sepsis being SIRS caused by infection. Many stimulants of the immune cascade are recognized, both exogenous and endogenous. Bacterial LPS is a common exogenous macromolecule that results in mediator release and activation of the immune cascade. Endogenous stimulants, such as IL-1 and TNF, cause effects on host hypothalamic thermal regulation and activation of other mediators, respectively. Additionally, TNF has been shown to cause biochemical tissue damage directly. A fundamental concept in sepsis physiology is that abnormal proliferation of the normally activated immune response results in ultimate host damage.
4. The answer is C. Mediators such as TNF and IL-1 that are released on activation and propagation of the immune cascade work to influence or modify the activity of host cells and organ systems distant to the site of their secretion. TNF has many effects on host cells. For example, TNF is a potent stimulator of the coagulation cascade, which can manifest clinically as a syndrome of disseminated intravascular coagulation (DIC), involving inappropriate activation of the blood coagulation factors in the vascular pool. The result is formation of capillary microthrombi that can cause tissue ischemia or infarction. TNF also plays a role in mediation of IL-1 release. Macrophage stimulation by TNF will elicit IL-1 production and secretion but it is not required. Cell membrane phospholipid liberation and subsequent bioconversion by increased phospholipase activity can be caused by both IL-1 and TNF in sepsis. The result is an increase in the arachidonic acid pool, making the precursor metabolite available for further inflammatory mediator generation. One of the first descriptions of IL-1 described its efficiency as a phagocytic and lymphoid cell stimulator.
5. The answer is True. There are many potential stimulators of IL-1 release, including both endogenous mediators such as TNF and exogenous mediators such as the gram-negative bacterial cell membrane constituent LPS.
6. The answer is False. PAF, like most other inflammatory mediators released during sepsis, has systemic effects, such as pulmonary hypertension, as well as local effects on platelets, including chemoactivation and chemoattraction.
7. The answer is True. Peroxynitrate, an oxygen species free radical, has been shown to cause profound tissue damage local to its release. Basic sepsis physiology describes both an increase in the liberation of these free radicals and attenuated host clearance mechanisms.
8. The answer is True. By adjusting the fraction of oxygen extracted from perfused blood at the cellular level, normal host tissues are able to maintain a constant intracellular supply of oxygen needed to support the metabolic demands of respiration; this is referred to as physiologic independence of oxygen uptake on oxygen delivery.
9. The answer is False. Since first postulated and following intense investigation and academic debate, this theory of oxygen dysmetabolism, known as physiologic dependence of oxygen uptake on oxygen delivery, has largely been abandoned. The exact nature of the oxygen metabolism disturbance observed in sepsis remains to be fully described.
10. The answer is True. There is no cure for sepsis, which is defined as SIRS caused by infection. Therapeutic intervention is largely supportive and is organ- or system-targeted. Although the infecting organism responsible is rarely identified initially, and is relatively infrequently identified at all, early empiric antibiotic coverage is mandatory. Broad coverage is preferable, with directed antibiotic therapy added if clinically indicated.

SUGGESTED READING

Light RB. Sepsis syndrome. In: Hall JB, Schmidt GA, Wood LDH (eds) Sepsis Syndrome in Principles of Critical Care. New York: McGraw-Hill, 1992:645–655.

Marik PE, Varon J. The hemodynamic derangements in sepsis. Implications for treatment strategies. Chest 1998;114:854–860.

Schlichtig R. Oxygen delivery and consumption in critical illness. In: Civetta JM, Taylor RW, Kirby RR (eds) Oxygen Delivery and Consumption in Critical Illness in Critical Care, 3rd ed. Baltimore: Williams & Wilkins, 1997:337–342.

Wheeler AP, Bernard GR. Treating patients with severe sepsis. N Engl J Med 1999;340:207–214.

Zimmerman JL, Taylor RW. Sepsis and septic shock. In: Civetta JM, Taylor RW, Kirby RR (eds) Sepsis and Septic Shock in Critical Care, 3rd ed. Baltimore: Williams & Wilkins, 1997:405–412.

CHAPTER 19

UBALDO J. MARTIN AND GERALD M. O'BRIEN

Acute Renal Failure

CHAPTER OUTLINE

LEARNING OBJECTIVES

After studying this chapter, you should be able to:

- Understand the basic pathophysiology of renal failure.
- Recognize factors that are associated with the development or worsening of acute renal failure.
- Elicit a concise, pertinent history and conduct a targeted physical exam in patients with acute renal disease.
- Interpret urinary sediment and urinary index results.
- Formulate a differential diagnosis of acute renal failure based upon history, physical findings, and laboratory data.
- Recognize the attributes and limitations of current and potential treatment modalities in acute renal failure.

Despite advances in critical care, improvements in supportive therapy, and the advent of hemodialysis almost 25 years ago, acute renal failure continues to be a highly prevalent cause of morbidity and mortality in the hospital setting. In hospitalized patients, acute renal failure has been associated with a marked increment in mortality. The following chapter reviews acute renal failure in the critically ill patient; specifically, its pathophysiologic mechanisms, methods of diagnosis, and treatment plan.

DEFINITIONS

Acute renal failure (ARF) is usually diagnosed by observing a rise in blood urea nitrogen (BUN) and plasma creatinine and a decrement in urine production. Interestingly, there is a great disparity in terms and definitions among different studies. Commonly used definitions of ARF include an increment in serum creatinine of 0.5 mg/dl greater than baseline value, an increase in serum creatinine 50% greater than baseline value, a 50% reduction in calculated creatinine clearance, or a decrement in renal function that requires dialysis. However, these definitions are not without problems.

Creatinine is a suboptimal indicator of renal function during ARF. Patients with ARF frequently are edematous; this condition results in a dilution of creatinine and may obscure the recognition of ARF. As glomerular filtration rate (GFR) decreases, tubular excretion of creatinine tends to increase; hence, creatinine clearance overestimates GFR by as much as 50%–100% once true GFR falls below 15 ml/min. In addition, large decrements in GFR that occur acutely are manifested by small increments in creatinine.

Serum creatinine is a poor indicator of renal function during acute renal failure.

ARF is classified as oliguric when urinary output is less than 400 ml/24 h or nonoliguric when urinary output is more than 400 ml/24 h. Anuria is defined as urinary output of less than 100 ml/24 h. ARF can also be classified according to the anatomic location where it originates, namely, prerenal, postrenal, or intrinsic renal failure.

Acute renal failure (ARF) can be classified anatomically or functionally by the amount of urine produced during 24 h.

EPIDEMIOLOGY

Incidence

The annual incidence of azotemia in the United States is about 275,000 cases yearly. Considering that about 40% of patients with azotemia have ARF, the incidence of ARF can be estimated to be approximately 115,000 cases per year. The frequency of ARF varies, depending on clinical setting. ARF occurs in approximately 1% of patients on admission to the hospital; 2%–5% of patients develop ARF during hospitalization, and perhaps 15% of patients develop ARF after cardiopulmonary bypass. The prevalence of ARF in the intensive care unit (ICU) is very high; approximately 16% of ICU patients with ARF require long-term dialysis.

Risk Factors

Patients with preexisting renal insufficiency are at high risk of developing ARF from radiocontrast agents, aminoglycosides, atheroembolism, and following cardiovascular surgery. Patients with both renal insufficiency and diabetes mellitus are particularly susceptible to radiocontrast agents. Other notable risk factors are hypotension, septic shock, old age, and hyperbilirubinemia.

Mortality

The mortality of ARF during WW II was about 91%, 68% during the Korean War, and 67% during the Vietnam War. Most modern studies have shown a modest improvement in mortality, possibly related to the advent of hemodialysis about 25 years ago and more successful supportive measures in the ICU. Mortality in ARF correlates with the number and severity of other comorbidities present. In the absence of other comorbidities, mortality due to ARF is 7%–23%. In the ICU setting, mortality in patients with ARF increases and ranges from 50% to 70%. ARF is far from being a simple bystander or a marker for severity of other comorbid conditions. In one study, 16,000 relatively healthy patients who were exposed to radiocontrast agents were followed for development of ARF; 189 patients eventually developed ARF. When age matched, patients who developed ARF were five times more likely to die. Because these were relatively healthy patients with minimal comorbidities, this study emphasizes the role of ARF as an independent risk factor for mortality.

The presence of acute renal failure in a seriously ill patient increases the risk of dying.

PATHOPHYSIOLOGY

The pathophysiology of ARF is complex, and our understanding remains limited. Acute tubular necrosis (ATN) is the clinical term used to designate ischemic acute renal failure and some forms of acute toxic injury to the kidney. The terms are frequently interchanged. ATN adequately identifies the anatomic site where lesions occur, but necrosis is not always the dominant pathologic characteristic. The pathogenesis of ARF is thought to be related to poor perfusion of the kidney cell, causing specific cellular changes or direct cellular damage due to toxins. In most cases the relative contribution of poor renal perfusions states versus direct renal epithelial damage is unclear. In certain entities, such as acute exposure to cyclosporine or the hepatorenal syndrome, renal arteriolar vasoconstriction is the predominant feature. In contrast, in patients exposed to aminoglycosides, direct renal epithelial injury is likely to be more important than alterations in blood flow to the kidney.

The pathophysiology of acute renal failure is a complex interaction of vascular, cellular, and immunologic events that propagates inflammation.

Local changes to the kidney vasculature and cells may be extremely important in the genesis and persistence of ARF. Several theories have been postulated, but it has become increasingly clear that one single paradigm cannot entirely explain the underlying mechanisms in ARF. Instead, ARF is a complex interaction of vascular, cellular, and immunologic alterations that ultimately leads to renal failure.

Vascular Alterations

The vascular injury theory states that systemic or local vasoactive substances may cause intrarenal ischemia, thereby injuring the renal tubular epithelium and altering the production of local vasodilatory factors. An imbalance between nitric oxide (vasodilator) and endothelin (vasoconstrictor) may alter renal blood flow, especially at the medullary level. There also seems to be a decreased response to vasoactive substances, such as prostaglandins and other vasodilators, leading to further tissue ischemia.

Cellular Injury

Renal cells possess an actin cytoskeleton, a protein matrix that maintains the integrity of the cell structure. This actin skeleton also allows the renal tubular cells to maintain a determined polarity. Cell polarity is essential for normal tubular function and regulation of the net movement of electrolytes, ions, and water.

Marked structural changes can be recognized in the renal epithelial cells during acute renal ischemia. The actin cytoskeleton is disrupted. These alterations in cell structure may not be lethal to the cell but can impair the cell's ability to maintain its polarity, resulting in abnormal tubular function. Alterations in sodium and fluid transport can be caused by structural alterations in the sodium pump.

Ischemia also causes alterations in renal tubular cell tight junctions, thereby impairing cell-to-cell integrity. The renal tubular cells also become detached from their matrix. Ischemia and toxins particularly damage a group of proteins known as integrins that are responsible for maintaining the adhesive qualities of the cells. After losing their polarity, as a result of integrin and tight junction alterations, renal tubular cells slough into the tubule lumen. Sloughed cells contribute to cast formation in the tubules, creating increased intraluminal pressure and a reduction in GFR (Figure 19-1). In summary, the cellular theory postulates that the decrement in GFR seen in ARF is likely caused by structural abnormalities in the tubular cells, resulting in altered ion, electrolyte, and water movement, and by tubular lumen obstruction with sloughed cells and tubular debris.

Inflammatory and Immune Alterations

There are several instances whereby ischemia and toxins are not able to explain the development of ARF/ATN. Local immune and inflammatory events, alterations in cell-to-cell interaction, and the release of substances into the local renal environment may play an important role in ischemic- and nonischemic-mediated ARF. The kidney produces several inflamma-

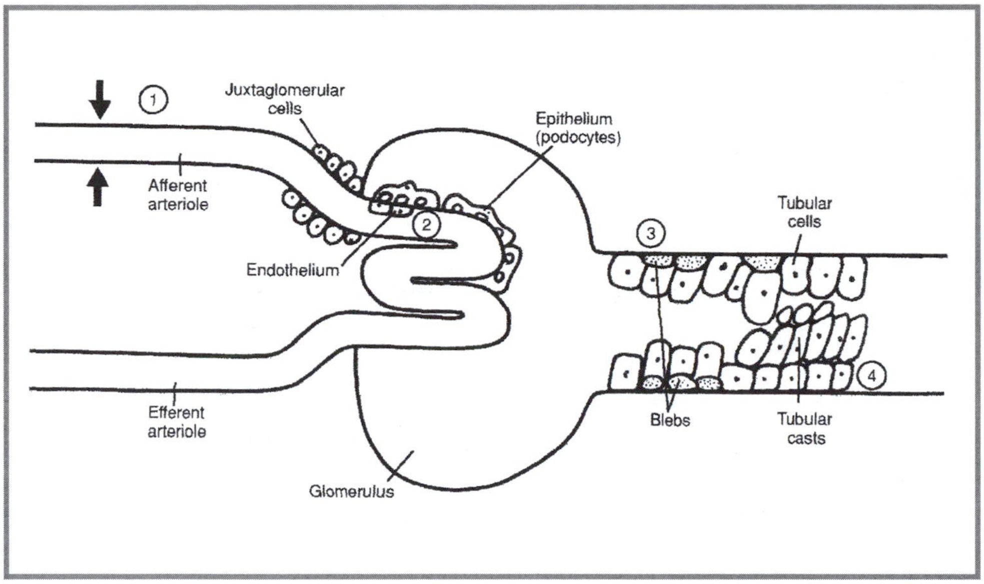

FIGURE 19-1

According to the cellular theory, the decrease in glomerular filtration rate (GFR) seen in acute renal failure (ARF) results from structural changes in the renal epithelial cells during acute renal ischemia. (*1*) Systemic and local vasoactive substances cause ischemia, decreased nitric oxide, and increased endothelin. (*2*) Ischemia affects endothelial cells, causing a decrease in local vasodilator substances. (*3*) Blebs form, possibly secondary to ischemia; there is loss of integrins and sloughing of tubular cells. (*4*) Tubular casts form, intraluminal pressure increases, and GFR further decreases.

tory mediators in response to systemic (sepsis, ischemia, etc.) and local stimuli, such as tumor necrosis factor-α (TNF-α) and interleukin (IL)-1, IL-8, and macrophage chemoattractant protein-1 (MCP-1). The kidney also synthesizes molecules that are potentially cytotoxic to the tubular cells, including superoxide and nitric oxide. These soluble inflammatory mediators recruit and activate neutrophils, the most important mediators in the inflammatory phenomenon. Cytokines and complement activation products also upregulate adhesion molecules, such as intercellular adhesion molecule-1 (ICAM-1). ICAM-1 is located on endothelial cells and promotes adherence and immobilization of activated neutrophils. After adhering to the endothelium, neutrophils release reactive oxygen species and proteases and other enzymes. The inflammatory process is amplified, and further increment in the expression of adhesion molecules and recruitment of neutrophils occurs. The increased number of recruited neutrophils plugs small vessels, impedes the passage of red blood cells, and increases ischemic damage (Figure 19-2).

In vitro studies have shown that administration of monoclonal antibodies directed against ICAM molecules protects against renal failure, possibly reducing the interaction between neutrophils and the endothelium. Studies in humans have shown that certain hemodialysis membranes that activate complement and neutrophils prolong the course and severity of renal failure. These studies further substantiate the critical role of neutrophils and adhesion molecules in the pathogenesis of ARF.

DIAGNOSIS

The diagnosis of ARF, especially in the intensive care unit, requires a careful, stepwise approach. Figure 19-3 depicts such an approach, the different components of which are discussed in the following sections.

History and Physical Examination

The history and physical examination can provide important clues to the etiology of renal failure.

The patient's history and physical evaluation can often yield important clues toward the diagnosis of ARF. A detailed history should include questions regarding exposure to nephrotoxic agents, history of sinus problems, pulmonary hemorrhage to consider pulmonary–renal syndromes, fever or purpura suggesting vasculitis, presence of bone pain in the elderly to suggest multiple myeloma, history of trauma (pigment nephropathy), and recent radiocontrast exposure (i.e., cardiac angiography). Physical examination may reveal signs of volume depletion such as tachycardia and hypotension, raising the question of prerenal etiology for

FIGURE 19-2

Ischemia and toxins may not always be directly responsible for the development of acute renal failure/acute tubular necrosis (ARF/ATN). The kidney produces several inflammatory mediators in response to systemic and local stimuli. The inflammatory phenomenon is probably responsible for the genesis and perpetuation of ARF in a multitude of situations: (*1*) ischemic or toxic injury to the kidney; (*2*) release of inflammatory mediators, interleukin-8 (IL-8), tumor necrosis (TNF)-α, chemoattractant protein, and oxygen radicals; (*3*) damage of cells by toxic oxygen radicals and nitric oxide; (*4*) inflammatory mediators recruit cells, especially neutrophils, that interact with ICAM molecules; (*5*) neutrophils release proteases and elastases, augmentation of the inflammatory process occurs, and direct damage to the interstitium and tubular cells results; and (*6*) neutrophils clump inside vessels, causing ischemia and further injury.

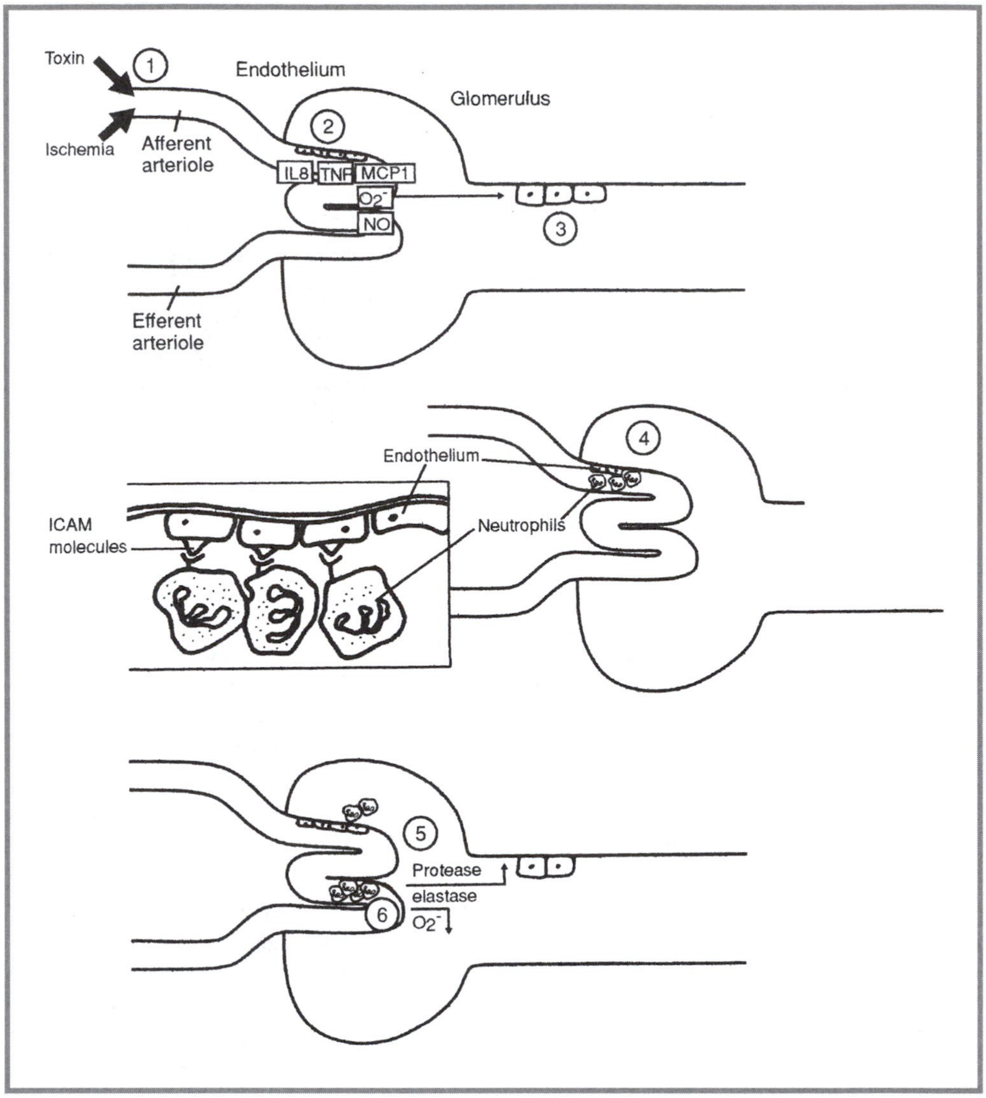

ARF. A rash can accompany allergic interstitial nephritis. Livedo reticularis can be seen in patients with atheroembolic renal failure and signs of embolism to the legs. Rhabdomyolysis should be suggested by signs of ischemia to the limbs and evidence of muscle compartmental syndrome associated with trauma or vascular occlusion.

Urine Analysis

White blood cell casts are found in the urine sediment of patients with interstitial nephritis, and red blood cell casts are found in glomerulonephritis.

Analysis of urine indexes and sediment is an important part of the diagnostic evaluation of patients with ARF. The analysis of sediment, when casts are present, is particularly helpful. Pigmented granular casts are seen in ischemic and toxic acute renal failure; white cell casts are typical of interstitial nephritis, and red cell casts are seen in glomerulonephritis. The finding of hemepositive urine, in the absence of red cells, suggests myoglobinuria or hemoglobinuria. Eosinophils can be seen in the sediment of patients with allergic interstitial nephritis, but they may also be present in patients with atheroembolism and pyelonephritis. The detection of eosinophils in urine is improved by using staining methods such as the Hansel stain.

Urine electrolyte indexes are useful, especially in patients with oliguria. Their usefulness decreases during the use of diuretics. Parameters that are commonly measured are urine-specific gravity, urine osmolality, urinary concentration of sodium (Na), and urinary con-

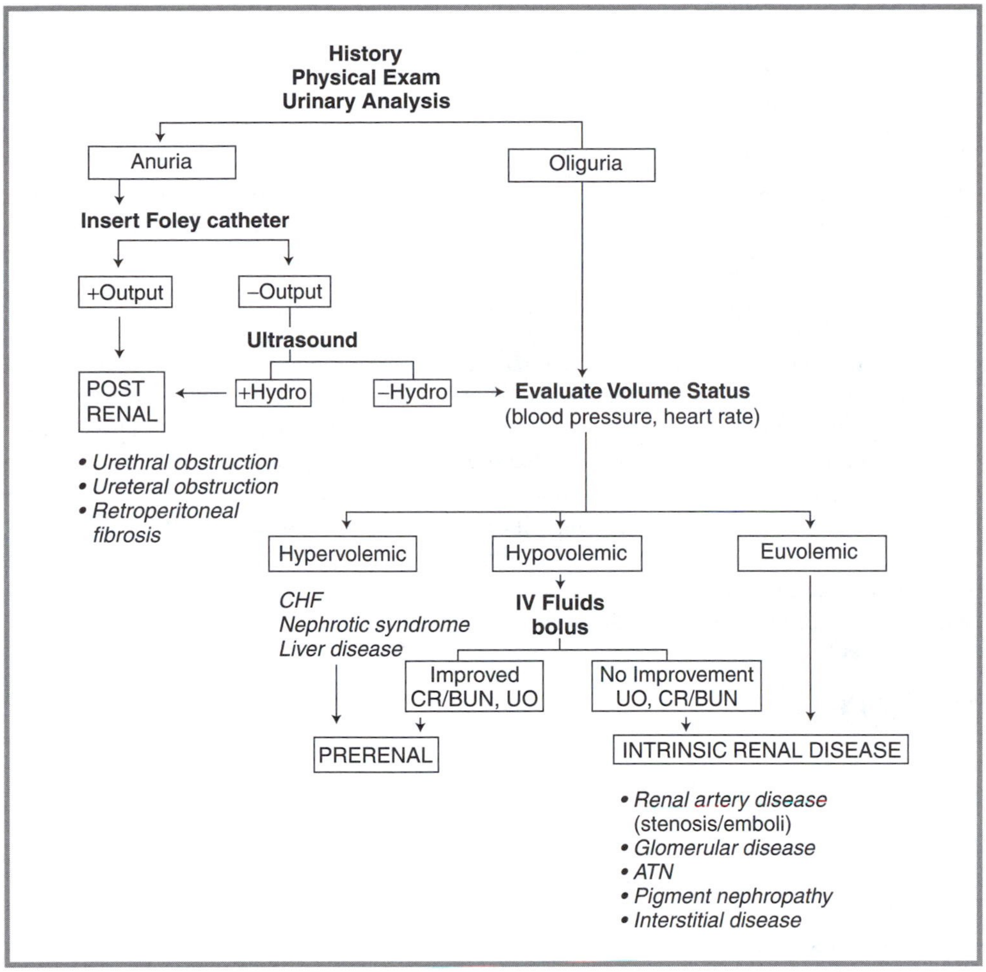

FIGURE 19-3

Algorithm for the diagnosis of ARF.

centration of creatinine. From these parameters, fractional excretion of sodium (FENa) can be calculated as follows:

$$\text{FENa} = \frac{\text{urine Na concentration/plasma Na concentration}}{\text{urine creatinine concentration/plasma creatinine concentration}}$$

Table 19-1 shows urinary indexes for different conditions.

Blood Tests

In addition to measurement of serum creatinine and blood urea nitrogen (BUN), other laboratory tests may aid in the differential diagnosis of ARF. Elevated calcium and uric acid are seen in tumor lysis syndrome, which can complicate patients with leukemia or lymphoma

TABLE 19-1

URINARY INDICES IN PATIENTS WITH ACUTE RENAL FAILURE

	PRERENAL	ATN	AGN	OBSTRUCTION
Urine Osm	>500	<350	300–500	300–500
Urine Na	<20	>40	<40	>40
FE Na	<1	>1	<1	>1

ATN, acute tubular necrosis; AGN, acute glomerulonephritis; Osm, osmolarity; FE Na, fractional excretion of sodium

TABLE 19-2

ANTIBODIES IN RENAL DISEASE

DISEASE	ANTIBODY	TARGETED PROTEIN
Wegener's	c-ANCA	Granulocyte serine protease
Polyarteritis nodosa	p-ANCA	Granulocyte myeloperoxidase
Goodpasture's syndrome	Anti-GBM	Alpha-3 chain of type IV collagen

c-ANCA, cytoplasmic antineutrophil cytoplasmic antibodies; p-ANCA, perinuclear staining antineutrophil cytoplasmic antibodies; anti-GBM, antiglomerular basement membrane antibodies

receiving chemotherapy. Serum creatine kinase is high in patients with rhabdomyolysis, and multiple myeloma can be suspected with an abnormal serum protein electrophoresis. Blood eosinophilia can be found in patients with allergic interstitial nephritis. Antiglomerular basement membrane antibodies may confirm the presence of Goodpasture's syndrome, and perinuclear antineutrophil cytoplasmic antibodies (p-ANCA) are associated with polyarteritis nodosa syndromes, whereas cytoplasmic antineutrophil cytoplasmic (c-ANCA) antibodies are found in patients with Wegener's granulomatosis (Table 19-2). The presence of an osmolar gap, which is the difference between measured and calculated osmolarity, may suggest the presence of a low molecular weight nephrotoxin such as ethylene glycol.

ETIOLOGY

Postrenal Azotemia

Urinary tract obstruction should be considered in patients with poor urine output and previous pelvis surgery radiation or a history of prostate disease.

ARF occurs when both urinary outflow tracts are obstructed, or a single tract obstruction occurs in a patient with a single functional kidney (Table 19-3). Patients with acute urinary tract obstruction may present with abdominal pain, flank pain, nausea, and vomiting. The diagnosis should be considered in patients with previous pelvic, gynecologic, or abdominal surgery, and in patients with a history of prostate carcinoma or prior radiation to the region. Patients can present with anuria, which is suggestive of complete obstruction.

Bladder catheterization is sufficient to diagnose urethral obstruction. Documentation of hydronephrosis with ultrasound is both sensitive and specific. It is important to remember that

CASE STUDY: PART 1

Mr. J.P. is a 64-year-old patient with a past medical history significant for hypertension, coronary artery disease, ischemic cardiomiopathy with an ejection fraction of 25%, benign prostatic hypertrophy, chronic cigarette smoking (1 pack/day for 35 years), and chronic obstructive pulmonary disease (COPD). He was admitted to the hospital with a 1-week history of cough productive of discolored sputum, fever, chills, and progressively worsening shortness of breath. He denied chest pain and denied leg swelling or other signs of heart failure. His vital signs upon admission were oral temperature, 39.1°C; respiratory rate, 24 beats/min; heart rate, 116 beats/min; blood pressure, 100/55 mmHg; and oxygen saturation, 91% on room air by pulse oxymetry.

On examination he was sitting in bed in mild respiratory distress. His neck had an easily seen jugular venous pulse. His heart was regular with a soft ejection murmur along the left sternal border. His lung examination was remarkable for crackles in the right base and diffuse wheezing. The abdomen was slightly tender to palpation over the suprapubic region. Extremities showed mild edema but no clubbing or cyanosis. Rectal examination evidenced a large prostate.

His laboratory work showed a white blood cell count of 16,000 with a left-shift hemoglobin of 14 g/dl. Creatinine was 1.6 mg/dl and BUN was 44 mg/dl; potassium, bicarbonate, calcium, phosphorus, and magnesium were normal; creatine kinase was 125 mg/dl. A chest radiograph showed a right lower lobe consolidation consistent with pneumonia.

Our patient was admitted with a diagnosis of community-acquired pneumonia and was started on cefotaxime. During the first 12 h in the hospital, his urinary output was found to total 10 ml; he also complained of worsening suprapubic pain. A Foley catheter was placed with difficulty, and 2,500 ml of urine was obtained. On hospital day 2, the patient's serum creatinine improved to 1.3 mg/dl and BUN decreased to 31 mg/dl.

TABLE 19-3

CAUSES OF POSTRENAL AZOTEMIA

- Extrarenal obstruction
  - Urethral occlusion or stricture
  - Neoplasm
    - Bladder
    - Pelvic
    - Prostate
    - Retroperitoneum
  - Benign prostatic hyperplasia
  - Calculi
  - Pus
  - Blood clots
  - Papillary necrosis
  - Trauma
  - Retroperitoneal fibrosis
- Intrarenal obstruction by crystals
- Bladder rupture
- Neurogenic bladder

in ARF hydronephrosis may not be present initially. If ultrasonographic results are equivocal or further pathology needs to be delineated, computed tomography (CT) could be helpful.

Urinary obstruction is most commonly caused by prostatic hypertrophy, prostatic cancer, cervical carcinoma, or retroperitoneal disorders; it frequently occurs in the outpatient setting. Postrenal ARF can be a manifestation of neurogenic bladder. Other less common causes include intraluminal disorders such as papillary necrosis, bilateral renal calculi, bladder carcinoma, and fungal disease or extraluminal conditions such as retroperitoneal fibrosis or colorectal carcinoma. Intratubular obstruction can be caused by crystaluria due to uric acid, calcium oxalate, acyclovir, sulfa drugs, methotrexate, and multiple myeloma.

Urate Nephropathy

Urate nephropathy is caused by the deposition of urate crystals in the tubules. It is seen most often in patients with lymphoproliferative disorders and hematologic malignancies, although it has also been described to occur with solid tumors. Hyperuricemia occurs spontaneously with tumor cell lysis; more often, it is the consequence of chemotherapy or radiotherapy. ARF is usually associated with release of other ions from neoplastic cells, resulting in hyperphosphatemia and hyperkalemia. Prevention is accomplished by administering allopurinol before chemotherapy, by volume repletion, and by keeping the urinary pH above 7.0. Serum electrolytes are followed carefully. Patients with ARF frequently require dialysis, but in general the prognosis is good.

Severe polyuria as a result of postobstructive diuresis can ensue after relief of urinary obstruction, possibly because of high plasma osmolality and increased tubular absorption of sodium and water. Physiologic diuresis should be distinguished from the pathologic state marked by volume depletion, hypotension, and worsening azotemia. It is important to diagnose postobstructive causes of ARF expeditiously because recovery of renal function is in-

CASE STUDY: PART 2

On the second hospital day and after relief of postrenal obstruction, the patient developed a brisk spontaneous diuresis. His blood pressure dropped to 85/45 mmHg and he became tachycardic. Because of poor intravenous access, a central line was placed and the patient was given 3 l normal saline over several hours. Subsequently, the patient developed acute shortness of breath and chest pain. Chest radiography was consistent with pulmonary edema. The patient responded to aggressive diuresis with intravenous furosemide and topical nitrates. On hospital day 3, his creatinine increased to 1.9 mg/dl.

versely related to the duration of the obstruction. Long-term treatment options include ureteral stenting and percutaneous nephrostomy.

Prerenal Azotemia

Prerenal azotemia is secondary to volume depletion or poor renal perfusion.

Prerenal azotemia can be found in both volume-depleted and volume-overloaded patients; it results from poor perfusion to the kidneys. Poor perfusion can be caused by decreased intravascular volume (as in dehydration), poor forward flow (as in heart failure), or vascular obstruction generating poor perfusion (renal artery stenosis). The most common cause of prerenal azotemia is volume depletion. Causes include vomiting, diarrhea, nasogastric suction, and protracted hemorrhage. Elderly patients are particularly susceptible to prerenal disease as a result of their predisposition to hypovolemia and the increased prevalence of renal vascular disease. Prerenal states are usually reversible if the underlying cause is quickly corrected.

Certain drugs have been associated with prerenal azotemia. The combination of angiotensin convertase inhibitors (ACEI) and diuretics can induce prerenal azotemia, particularly in patients with renal vascular disease. ACEI decrease resistance in the efferent arterioles with a concomitant decrement in GFR. Nonsteroidal antiinflammatory agents (NSAIDs) inhibit vasodilatation of afferent arterioles, thereby decreasing GFR and renal flow. Cyclosporin (especially intravenous administration) can cause vasoconstriction and induce a prerenal state. Among hospitalized patients, prerenal azotemia is usually caused by cardiac dysfunction, liver failure, septic shock, and accumulation of fluid in body cavities (such as the peritoneum).

Acute Tubular Necrosis

Acute tubular necrosis (ATN) is the most common cause of acute renal failure.

Acute tubular necrosis (ATN) is the most common form of intrinsic ARF. It is usually associated with ischemia or nephrotoxic agents (Table 19-4). The pathogenesis of ATN is unclear but disorders of ATP, calcium metabolism, tubular polarity, generation of free radicals, and proteases have all been implicated. The pathology of ATN involves tubulointerstitial injury, but the glomerulus is spared. This injury causes tubular epithelial cells to slough into the lumen of the tubules and creates obstruction, which reduces the net filtration rate across the glomerular capillaries. These events result in decreased GFR. ATN typically presents with an oliguric phase, associated with worsening serum creatinine, azotemia, and a progressive decrement in GFR. This oliguric phase can be followed by a diuretic phase, marked by the presence of electrolyte abnormalities and volume depletion. Some patients never develop a decrement in urinary output; this is termed nonoliguric ATN. Patients with nonoliguric ATN have a better prognosis than patients with oliguric renal failure, the latter have a greater likelihood of requiring hemodialysis and a significantly higher mortality. In the past, the use of diuretics and osmotic agents has been advocated to revert oliguric failure. However, evidence that patients who convert from an oliguric to a nonoliguric state after a pharmacologic intervention have an improvement in their prognosis is under current investigation.

CASE STUDY: PART 3

On hospital day 5, the patient had a rise in temperature to 39.2°C; blood cultures were obtained. On day 6 methicillin-sensitive *Staphylococcus aureus* was detected. He was started on nafcillin. On day 7, the patient developed chest pain with electrocardiographic changes consistent with ischemia. He underwent cardiac angiography, evidencing a subtotal occlusion of the left anterior descending coronary artery. A coronary artery stent was placed; 2 days later his creatinine was found to be 2.4, and it continued to increase over the next several days.

TABLE 19-4

CAUSES OF ACUTE TUBULAR NECROSIS

- Postischemic
  - Sepsis
  - Circulatory shock
- Pigment induced
  - Hemolysis-hemoglobin
  - Rhabdomyolysis-myoglobin
- Toxin induced
  - Antibiotics
  - Cyclosporin
  - Radiocontrast agents
  - Organic solvents
  - Heavy metals
- Pyelonephritis
- Eclampsia

Drug-Related Nephrotoxicity

Previous renal disease, volume depletion, and old age predispose the patient to drug-induced nephropathy.

Aminoglycosides are a common cause of hospital-acquired ARF. Patients who are elderly, volume depleted, or have preexisting renal disease are at higher risk. Other risk factors for toxicity from aminoglycosides include preexisting liver disease, shock, female gender, and high peak and trough levels.

Tubular cells and cells in the pars recta are predominantly affected. Tubular abnormalities are usually seen in the early phases of renal injury; they are marked by glycosuria, aminoaciduria, and proteinuria. Electrolyte abnormalities such as potassium and magnesium wasting can be seen, and polyuria and nephrogenic diabetes insipidus may be present. Nephrotoxicity caused by aminoglycoside administration usually results in nonoliguric renal failure. It can be seen at any time 1–2 weeks after starting treatment, although the time to onset of renal dysfunction may be shortened in patients with predisposing factors. Treatment is supportive with discontinuation of the drug. Recovery of renal function is slow, usually 4–6 weeks. In some patients, especially those with previous renal disease, recovery of renal function is incomplete; this is possibly related to residual interstitial fibrosis. Penicillins, cephalosporins, and quinolones have also been associated with acute renal failure, but they are usually associated with interstitial nephritis.

Amphotericin B is a polyene antifungal agent that interacts with membrane sterols, causing cell membrane disruption and an increment in cell wall permeability. Lesions have been noted in several different places in the nephron, such as the tubules and the medulla. The nephrotoxic effect of amphotericin is initially manifested as a loss of urine concentration, distal renal tubular acidosis, hypokalemia, and hypomagnesemia. Most patients receiving amphotericin experience a rise in serum creatinine. ARF due to amphotericin B is usually nonoliguric, slowly progressing, and dose related. Renal function usually returns to baseline after a short interruption of the drug or a reduction in the administered dose. The most important risk factor for development of nephrotoxicity due to amphotericin is volume and salt depletion; therefore, prevention of toxicity includes volume and sodium repletion. Newer formulations of amphotericin, such as lipid complex formulations and liposome-encapsulated amphotericin B, are less likely to cause renal dysfunction and may be an option in patients with previous renal disease.

Acyclovir can induce ATN in 10%–30% of patients treated. Nephrotoxicity becomes evident 24–48 h after treatment is initiated. Acyclovir crystals precipitate in the distal tubules and cause intratubular obstruction. Treatment consists of volume repletion and discontinuation of the drug.

Cyclosporine and tacrolimus are agents commonly used to provide immunosuppression in patients with solid organ and bone marrow transplantation. These agents are associated with vasoconstriction causing nonoliguric ARF and have also been implicated in the development of thrombotic microangiopathy (thrombi deposition in small vessels) in the kidney.

Cisplatin is a chemotherapeutic agent, frequently used in the treatment of ovary, testicular, and lung cancer; it can cause damage to the proximal and distal tubules. Initially, it causes polyuria with preserved GFR. Reduction in GFR and nephrogenic diabetes insipidus can be seen after 3–4 days of treatment. Recovery of renal function usually is seen 2–4 weeks after discontinuation of the drug.

Contrast Nephropathy

The overall risk for contrast nephropathy for ARF is low in the general population, but the risk increases up to 30% in patients with previous renal disease or diabetes mellitus. The pathogenesis of contrast-induced nephropathy is possibly related to a reduction in renal medullary blood flow. An increment in creatinine can be seen as early as 24 h after the procedure with radiocontrast material. Only a small percentage of the patients develop oliguric renal failure. Serum creatinine tends to return to baseline in 10–14 days. Hydration with half-normal saline solution should be used as prophylaxis in high-risk patients. The appropriate dose seems to be 1 ml/kg/min for 12 h before and after the procedure. Hypotonic solutions provide less volume expansion than isotonic solutions, but they have been shown to increase prostaglandin excretion; this, in turn, has been associated with improved medullary blood flow. Nonionic contrast agents are an option for reducing toxicity in patients who are at high risk. The use of nonionic contrast agents is not indicated in patients at low risk for contrast-induced nephropathy.

Pigment Nephropathy

Rhabdomyolysis (RML) has been described in a variety of settings, including crush injuries, strenuous exercise, peripheral arterial embolism, alcoholism, cocaine use, protracted seizures, heat-induced disorders, and viral infections. In this disorder, creatine released from the muscles is eventually transformed to creatinine, resulting in disproportionately high levels of serum creatinine. Pigmenturia, hyperkalemia, hyperphosphatemia, and elevation of lactate dehydrogenase and creatine kinase characterize RML.

The development of ARF in patients with RML has been attributed to various mechanisms, including (a) the direct toxic effects of myoglobin or its by-products, such as ferrihemate, (b) disseminated intravascular coagulation, (c) obstruction of renal tubules with myoglobin or uric acid crystals, and (d) renal ischemia caused by release of vasoconstrictor substances. The risk of developing ARF is not uniform among patients who present with RML.

Clinical factors that increase the risk of developing RML include liver dysfunction, hypotension, seizures, severe muscle damage (manifested by high muscle enzyme levels), disseminated intravascular coagulation, and dehydration. In a series of 200 patients with traumatic RML, patients who received intensive IV fluid therapy within 12 h of trauma were less likely to develop ARF than patients who received therapy after 12 h (2.5% vs. 25%). It has been recommended that patients with crush injuries immediately receive IV fluids on the accident scene and then in the hospital to achieve a urinary output of 200–300 ml/h. It is apparent that early volume resuscitation and intensive IV fluid administration may reduce the incidence of ARF. The use of solutions containing bicarbonate has been recommended to maintain a urinary pH greater than 6.5. Maintaining an alkaline urinary pH may reduce the conversion of myoglobin to ferrihemate, an iron compound that can cause vasoconstriction and local production of toxic oxygen radicals. An alkaline urinary pH may also prevent the precipitation of uric acid crystals in the tubules.

Atheroembolic Disease

Atheroembolic disease causing ARF occurs mainly in the elderly, usually heavy smokers. It is more likely to occur in patients with atheromatous disease who undergo procedures such as cardiac angiography, intraaortic balloon placement, and vascular surgery. Atheroembolic disease has been reported to occur spontaneously and, rarely, after the institution of anticoagulation. Clinical manifestations are a consequence of cholesterol crystal migration and atheromatous debris in the circulation. ARF may ensue; it is frequently associated with visual disturbances and with cerebral and intestinal ischemia. Physical examination can reveal the presence of refractive plaques in the retinal arteries (Hollenhorst bodies), rash, petechiae, livedo reticularis, and bluish discoloration of the toes. Eosinophilia, eosinophiluria, and hypocomplementemia can be seen; these features can also be associated with acute interstitial nephritis, vasculitis, allergic reactions, and some of the entities causing rapidly progressive glomerulonephritis. Definitive diagnosis can be made by muscle, skin, or renal biopsy showing characteristic biconcave crystals. The course of renal failure in these cases is highly variable, but renal dysfunction usually occurs 3–8 weeks after the initial insult. No treatment has been shown to be effective in these cases, and therapeutic measures are usually aimed at removing anticoagulation and preparing the patient for hemodialysis.

Acute Interstitial Nephritis

The first cases of acute interstitial nephritis (AIN) were described in patients with diphteria and scarlet fever. Among patients with ARF of undetermined origin, 11% have AIN by biopsy. Today, AIN is most often caused by medications. Other causes of AIN are shown in Table 19-5.

Clinical manifestations include fever, rash, and eosinophilia. This triad suggests AIN, but its absence does not rule out the disorder, because the triad is only present in 10%–40% of patients. Renal impairment manifests 5–25 days after initial exposure. Recovery of renal function after discontinuation of the offending drug is frequent. Patients who develop AIN after exposure to NSAIDs tend to have worse RF and only a partial recovery of renal function. There is only limited evidence in the literature to support the use of steroids in patients with medication-induced AIN.

> Fever, rash, and blood eosinophilia can signal the presence of acute interstitial nephritis (AIN).

Glomerulonephritis and Other Intrinsic Renal Diseases

Glomerulonephritis (GN) can present as acute or subacute renal failure. Rapid diagnosis using serologic markers is important to institute treatment rapidly. Immunosuppressive therapy, plasma exchange, or both can reduce morbidity and eventual progression to end-stage renal failure.

Wegener's granulomatosis is an idiopathic disorder characterized by the presence of granulomatous vasculitis in the kidney and upper and lower respiratory tract. Diagnosis can be made by serologic detection of c-ANCA or biopsy. Standard therapy for Wegener's consists of a combination of cyclophosphamide (2 mg/kg) and prednisone (1 mg/kg). This regimen achieved remission in 75%–91% of patients. The role for plasma exchange is less clear.

Anti-GBM-mediated disease is an entity characterized by the deposition of antibodies directed toward the glomerular basement membrane (GBM). These antibodies can also be seen

TABLE 19-5

CAUSES OF INTERSTITIAL NEPHRITIS

Infectious
Immunologic diseases
Hypercalcemia
Idiopathic
Drugs
Penicillins
Cephalosporins
Nonsteroidal antiinflammatory medications
Diuretics
Allopurinol
Cimetidine

in the alveolar basement membrane. The syndrome usually presents as rapidly progressive glomerulonephritis (RPGN). Renal biopsy shows proliferative GN with crescent formation. It can present with or without hemoptysis; smokers are more likely to present with hemoptysis. Therapy for anti-GBM-mediated GN consists of early administration of immunosuppressive drugs and plasmapheresis.

The combination of acute renal failure, fever, thrombocytopenia, and microangiopathic anemia should raise the suspicion of hemolytic uremic syndrome/thrombotic thrombocytopenic purpura (HUS/TTP).

Patients with HUS/TTP have a normal coagulation profile.

Hemolytic uremic syndrome (HUS) and thrombotic thrombocytopenic purpura (TTP) are two closely linked entities associated with ARF, hemolytic microangiopathic anemia, and thrombocytopenia. TTP is also associated with fever and central nervous system abnormalities. Prothrombin time (PT) and activated partial thromboplastin time (PTT) are normal in these entities. HUS and TTP likely represent different spectra of the same disease. Other manifestations of the disease include neutrophilic leukocytosis, bowel perforation, and normal coagulation profile. Treatment consists of supportive therapy and plasmapheresis.

MEDICAL MANAGEMENT OF ACUTE RENAL FAILURE

The treatment of ARF is aimed at treating the underlying disorder(s) or mechanism(s) that precipitated it. Patients with prerenal failure should be treated with aggressive fluid resuscitation if they are volume depleted, with inotropes and afterload reduction if poor forward flow or low cardiac output is suspected (heart failure, cardiomyopathy, etc.), or by relief of renal artery stenosis via percutaneous angioplasty or renal artery bypass surgery.

In patients with postrenal failure, prompt relief of the obstruction is key for preservation of renal function. Depending on the site and nature of the obstruction, several therapeutic modalities are available. Surgery may be helpful for patients with benign prostate hyperplasia or confined carcinoma. A suprapubic catheter can be placed in cases of urethral stricture. Urethral strictures can be dilated, and a stent can be deployed to maintain lumen patency. Percutaneous nephrostomy catheters provide relief for patients who have extensive peritoneal disease or numerous calculi or who are poor surgical candidates. Treatment for ATN is one of the most challenging areas in critical care. In the remainder of this section we discuss old and new approaches to the treatment of ATN, as well as some experimental therapeutic options.

Diuretics and Mannitol

Furosemide is loop diuretic and a vasodilator. It works on the thick ascending limb of the nephron and increases flow, possibly allowing removal of casts and decreasing toxins such as myoglobin or hemoglobin. Furosemide may convert oliguric renal failure to nonoliguric renal failure. Patients who convert from an oliguric to a nonoliguric state are able to tolerate more liberal fluid intake and total parenteral nutrition.

Furosemide and mannitol can aggravate radiocontrast-induced nephropathy.

Mannitol is a diuretic that also appears to be able to scavenge free radicals. It has been used in organ preservation solutions for renal transplant, where it appears to be beneficial. It also may be useful when given very early in the course of rhabdomyolysis. Other than these selected cases, its role in prevention or treatment of ARF has not been proven. Both furosemide and mannitol can aggravate radiocontrast-induced nephropathy.

Dopamine

Dopamine is a selective renal vasodilator that can induce natriuresis and an increase in GFR and urinary output. The dopamine dose at which mainly dopaminergic receptors are activated is 0.5 μ/kg/min to 2.5 μg/kg/min. Clinical studies have failed to show the utility of dopamine to either prevent or treat ARF. Dopamine does not improve survival or delay dialysis. In individual cases, however, dopamine may increase urinary output or enhance the renal response to diuretics.

EXPERIMENTAL TREATMENT OPTIONS

Atrial Natriuretic Peptide

Atrial natriuretic peptide (ANP) vasodilates the afferent arteriole and constricts the efferent arteriole, thereby increasing GFR. It also inhibits tubular absorption of sodium. The net result of these actions is an increase in urinary output. In preliminary studies, ANP appeared to increase GFR and decrease the need for dialysis. In a randomized, placebo-controlled trial, ANP improved dialysis-free survival in a subgroup of patients who converted from oliguric to nonoliguric renal failure. This effect was not seen in patients who presented with nonoliguric renal failure. A subsequent randomized trial of oliguric patients with ARF was discontinued prematurely when an interim analysis found no difference between the placebo-treated and the ANP-treated group.

Insulin-Like Growth Factor

Insulin-like growth factor (IGF-1) is secreted in large amounts by the developing kidney where it induces cell proliferation and differentiation. IGF may have a role in renal cell repair and preventing injury following renal transplant, and it may preserve GFR in patients following renal vascular surgery.

RENAL REPLACEMENT THERAPY

Dialysis is required in 80% of the patients with oliguric renal failure and 30% of patients with nonoliguric renal failure. In the setting of ARF, patients who undergo hemodialysis have a significant improvement in morbidity and mortality over patients who do not receive this therapeutic modality. Hemodialysis carries important risks. Bleeding from the access site, hemorrhage, and infection are a few of the complications that can be seen. Hypotension and arrhythmias can be induced by changes in compartment volumes and electrolyte disturbances.

Dialysis improves morbidity and mortality in patients with acute renal failure.

There is a risk that dialysis actually prolongs or worsens ARF, likely the result of hypotension causing worsening ischemia or the activation of an inflammatory reaction by the blood–dialyzer interface. Dialysis with biocompatible membranes shortens the course of ARF in nonoliguric patients, decreases hospital stay, and improves survival. Dialysis with biocompatible membranes results in less complement activation, better survival from sepsis, and fewer dialysis sessions. In terms of the amount or dose of dialysis, new studies show that dialysis with biocompatible dialyzers on a daily basis improves mortality as compared to alternate day dialysis (21% vs. 47%). Renal replacement therapy and dialysis are discussed further in Chapter 20.

SUMMARY

Acute renal failure (ARF) is frequently seen in the ICU setting and carries a high morbidity and mortality. In most cases, early diagnosis results in an improved prognosis. A stepwise diagnostic approach to ARF (see Figure 19-3) in the critically ill patient that includes a detailed history and physical examination, along with urine analysis and serum tests, should help in determining the etiology of ARF and instituting the appropriate therapy.

REVIEW QUESTIONS

1. **Regarding hemolytic uremic syndrome/thrombotic thrombocytopenic purpura (HUS/TTP), all the following are correct except:**
   - **A.** Treatment consists of supportive therapy and plasmapheresis.
   - **B.** They are associated with thrombocytopenia.
   - **C.** Patients can present with neutrophilic leukocytosis.
   - **D.** Prothrombin time (PT) and partial thromboplastin time (PTT) are usually abnormal.
   - **E.** TTP is associated with central nervous disease abnormalities.

2. **A 32-year-old American traveler has spent the past 2 weeks in Guatemala City; he had eaten in the local market to reduce his expenses. Over the past 2 days he has experienced low-grade fever, mild abdominal pain, and explosive diarrhea, about 7–10 episodes per day. Upon admission to a local hospital, his oral mucosa appeared dry and his skin showed decreased turgor. His blood pressure was 86/45 and his heart rate 120; serum creatinine was 2.3 mg/dl and blood urea nitrogen 62 mg/dl. Analysis of his urine electrolyte indexes is likely to reveal:**
   - **A.** Urine osmolarity of 200, urine sodium >40, fractional excretion of sodium >1
   - **B.** Urine osmolarity of 600, urine sodium <20, fractional excretion of sodium <1
   - **C.** Urine osmolarity of 500, urine sodium >40, fractional excretion of sodium >1
   - **D.** Urine osmolarity of 300, urine sodium = 30, fractional excretion of sodium <1

3. **The following conditions are associated with postrenal azotemia, except:**
   - **A.** Uric acid crystaluria
   - **B.** Retroperitoneal fibrosis
   - **C.** Neurogenic bladder
   - **D.** Atheroembolic disease
   - **E.** Prostate carcinoma

4. **Regarding the pathophysiology of acute renal failure, all of the following are correct, except:**
   - **A.** Ischemia can cause imbalance between local vasoactive substances.
   - **B.** Inflammatory mediators such as tumor necrosis factor and interleukin-8 are elevated in acute renal failure.
   - **C.** Cytotoxic substances such as superoxide are locally produced and may induce cell damage.
   - **D.** Intercellular adhesion molecule-1 (ICAM-1), located in the renal endothelium, promotes adhesion of neutrophils.
   - **E.** Macrophages are the most important mediators in the inflammatory process that occurs in acute renal failure.

5. **A 50-year-old patient with a history of sinus infection develops acute renal failure; he is thought to have Wegener's granulomatosis. Diagnosis can be confirmed with:**
   - **A.** Serologic detection of p-ANCA
   - **B.** Serologic detection of c-ANCA
   - **C.** Serologic detection of lupus anticoagulant
   - **D.** Renal biopsy
   - **E.** B and D are correct

ANSWERS

1. The answer is D. An abnormal coagulation profile associated with renal failure and thrombocytopenia can be seen in patients with sepsis and diffuse intravascular coagulopathy. Patients with renal failure due to systemic lupus erythematosus can present with thrombocytopenia and an elevated partial thromboplastin time. An abnormal coagulation profile is not characteristic of HUS/TTP and should raise the suspicion of a different etiology for renal failure. Thrombocytopenia and neutrophilic leukocytosis are seen in HUS/TTP. Plasmapheresis is the most effective therapeutic option.
2. The answer is B. The patient in this case is suffering from traveler's diarrhea. The profuse diarrhea has resulted in hypovolemia. The clinic manifestations of hypovolemia are low blood pressure, tachycardia, dry mucous membranes, and decreased urinary output; this results in a prerenal state marked by elevated serum creatinine and blood urea nitrogen. The set that better depicts a prerenal state is B (see Table 19-1); set A is consistent with acute tubular necrosis, set C is consistent with prostrenal obstruction, and set D is consistent with acute glomerulonephritis.
3. The answer is D. All these conditions are associated with postrenal azotemia, except for atheroembolic disease. Atheroembolic disease, which can occur after instrumentation of the aorta, after vascular surgery, or rarely spontaneously, causes intrarenal disease.
4. The answer is E. Neutrophils are the most important mediators of the inflammatory reaction in acute renal failure. They may interact via intercellular adhesion molecules located in the endothelium. Dialysis membranes that activate neutrophils have been associated with poorer outcomes in acute renal failure, further emphasizing the pivotal role of neutrophils in this disease.
5. The answer is E. The diagnosis of Wegener's granulomatosis can be established with a renal biopsy showing granulomatous vasculitis or serologic detection of c-ANCA. p-ANCA can be seen in polyarteritis nodosa and other autoimmune diseases. Lupus anticoagulant is the name for several antibodies that have been associated with alterations in platelet number and hypercoagulable states, not renal failure.

SUGGESTED READING

Briglia A, Paganini E. Acute renal failure in the intensive care unit: therapy overview, patient risk stratification, complications of renal replacement and special circumstances. Clin Chest Med 1999;20: 347–366.

Gesualdo L. Acute renal failure in critically ill patients. Intens Care Med 1999;25:1188–1190.

Kribben A, Edelstein GL. Pathophysiology of acute renal failure. J Nephrol 1999;12(Suppl 2):S142–S151.

Meyer MM. Renal replacement therapies. Crit Care Med 2000;16: 29–58.

Wagener O, Lieske J. Molecular and cell biology of acute renal failure: new therapeutic strategies. New Horizons 1995;3:634–649.

CHAPTER 20

Ronald Rubin

Bleeding Diathesis

CHAPTER OUTLINE

LEARNING OBJECTIVES

After studying this chapter, you should be able to:

- Know the history, physical examination, and laboratory tests useful in assessing the bleeding patient.
- Be aware of the disorders of vascular and tissue components and platelet dysfunction as they relate to bleeding diathesis.
- Evaluate patients with disorders of platelet immune destruction.
- Diagnose hereditary and acquired coagulation disorders found in ICU patients.

BLEEDING DYSCRASIAS

Normal hemostasis requires an intact interrelating mechanism composed of vascular and tissue components, platelets, and coagulation proteins. Deficiency or disease of any of these components may cause either spontaneous or trauma-related hemorrhage. The intensive care setting, by definition, involves a population that is characterized by multiorgan failure, polypharmacy, and multiple wounds of both accidental or iatrogenic variety. Such pathophysiology significantly stresses even an initially normal hemostatic mechanism. It is not surprising, then, that bleeding is a frequent complication encountered in the intensive care setting. A thorough history, physical findings as well as a broad battery of laboratory tests, often serves to differentiate the different bleeding dyscrasias.

A thorough history, physical findings as well as a broad battery of laboratory tests, often serves to differentiate the bleeding dyscrasias.

History

A carefully taken history provides clues to the pathogenesis of bleeding dyscrasias. Immediate bleeding in mucocutaneous areas (nose, mouth, bladder, skin) suggests vascular or platelet abnormality, whereas delayed deep tissue bleeding such as internal hematoma formation suggests coagulation protein deficiency. Genetic transmission of bleeding disorders, such as the hemophilias and von Willebrand's disease, also can be elicited by history, as will the ingestion of drugs (e.g., warfarin, aspirin, nonsteroidal antiinflammatory drugs [NSAIDs]), which can profoundly affect hemostasis. Similarly, a history of no hemostatic difficulties during past hospitalizations or surgeries or during the time period before arrival in the intensive care unit (ICU) suggests that any bleeding dyscrasia is an acquired one, and investigation of recent events and medications often yields an etiology.

Physical Findings

A thorough examination often yields clues to the underlying derangement in hemostatic pathophysiology resulting in a bleeding diathesis. Mucocutaneous petechiae and purpura suggest platelet disorders whereas spreading hematomas suggest coagulopathy.

Mucocutaneous petechiae or purpura suggests platelet disorders; spreading hematomas suggest coagulopathy.

Laboratory Testing

Laboratory tests are vital to the evaluation of bleeding disorders. Because single tests rarely provide conclusive results, various batteries of tests have been developed. The coagulation cascade is shown in Figure 20-1. The interpretation of common tests of hemostasis and blood coagulation is shown in Table 20-1, with the diagnosis of common bleeding disorders based on commonly used tests. These studies provide a basis upon which a proper differential diagnosis and reasonable attempts at therapy can then be formulated.

DISORDERS OF VASCULAR TISSUE COMPONENTS

On occasion, bleeding may result from pathology involving the vessel area itself, with secondary leakage of blood. When the skin is a dominant target area, as with vasculitic disease, these disorders have palpable skin lesions as their hallmark. Testing performed on patients with these bleeding disorders shows normal coagulation testing and platelet counts and, occasionally, increased bleeding times. A history of exposure to drug allergens or the presence of an infection by appropriate pathogens is very important in arriving at a diagnosis. When clarification of this mechanism is deemed vital to alterations in therapy, skin biopsy and culture are indicated.

Autoimmune Purpura

Autoimmune (allergic) purpura is a prototype lesion, also known by its eponym, Henoch–Schönlein purpura. It is a vasculitis of small vessels with associated IgG deposits caused by

Autoimmune purpura is a vasculitis of small vessels with associated IgG deposits.

FIGURE 20-1

The blood coagulation cascade has two pathways, intrinsic and extrinsic, involving multiple factors. The integrity of the intrinsic pathway is tested by a partial thromboplastin time (PTT) assay and the extrinsic pathway measuring prothrombin time (PT).

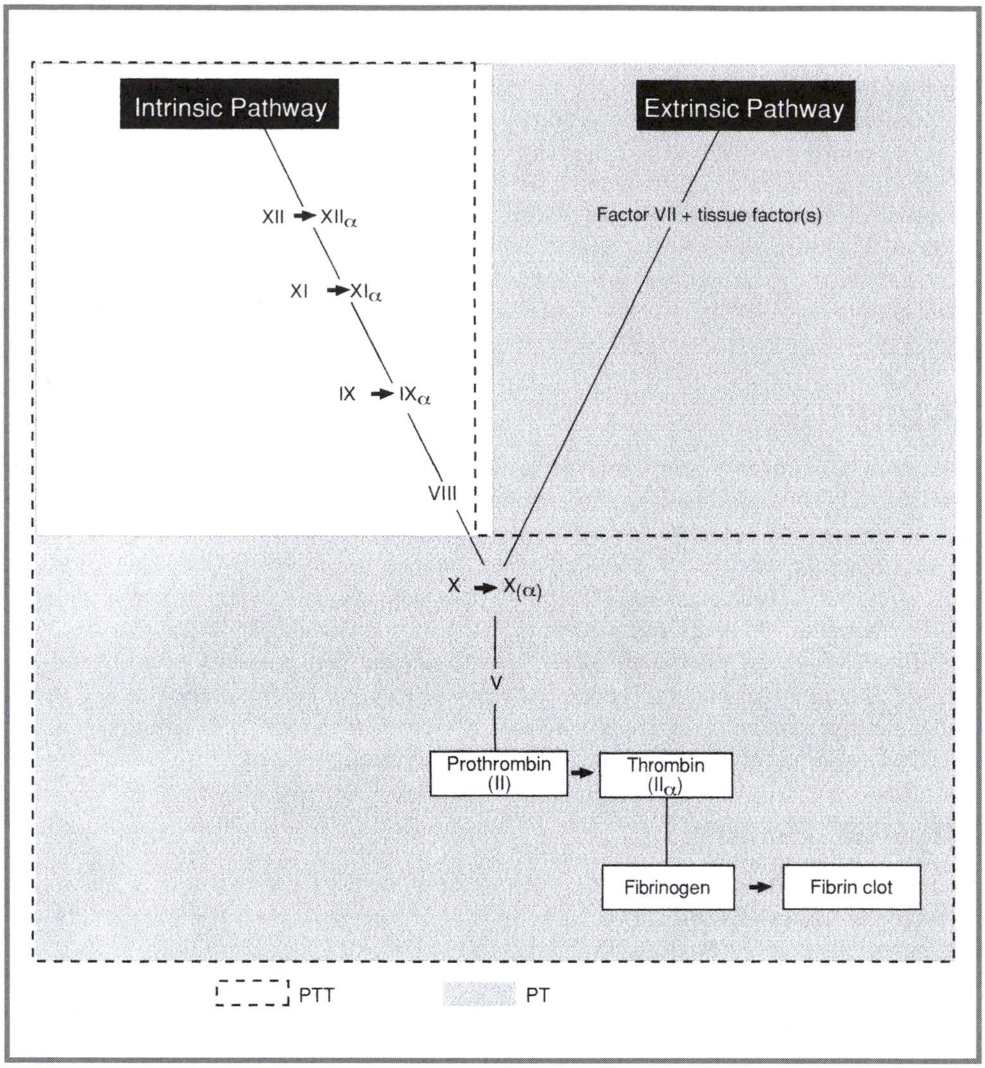

TABLE 20-1

COMMONLY USED TESTS OF HEMOSTASIS AND ASSOCIATED DIAGNOSES

TEST	NORMAL RANGE	IMPORTANT ASSOCIATED CONDITIONS
Essential screening tests		
Platelet count	150,000–450,000/μl	Thrombocytopenias
Template bleeding time	2.0–7.5 min	Thrombocytopenias Vascular disorders (scurvy) von Willebrand's disease Platelet dysfunction
Partial thromboplastin time (PTT)	25–40 s	Intrinsic factor protein deficiencies Anticoagulant overdose
Prothrombin time (PT)	12–17 s	Liver disease Warfarin overdose Vitamin K Deficiency
Secondary tests		
Fibrinogen assay	150–400 mg/dl	Severe liver disease Fibrinolytic drugs Disseminated intravascular coagulation (DIC)
Fibrinogen/fibrin digest product assays and D-dimer assays	–	Fibrinolytic agents DIC

allergy, most classically to infectious agents such as streptococci and to drugs such as penicillin. Palpable, symmetric, often pruritic lesions are most commonly seen on the extremities. Lesions can occur in the bowel, causing gastrointestinal bleeding, in the kidney, causing hematuria, and in joints, causing clinical arthritis. Biopsy reveals perivascular inflammatory lesions with leakage of plasma and blood into the skin, mucosa, and serosa. Therapy requires recognition, cessation of the offending agent, or treatment of the infection causing the reaction. Recognition is important because this is a vascular lesion and not a true coagulopathy or platelet defect, and therapies along those lines should not be used. The prognosis is good, except that 5%–10% of patients can develop chronic glomerulonephritis.

Infectious Purpura

These conditions can also cause formation of a palpable purpuric lesion that is often also painful. These lesions may be symmetric and in classical distributions, as with *Rickettsia* infections, or be quite random, as with bacterial infections such as endocarditis. The lesions are caused by actual endothelial damage by the infectious agent (*Rickettsia*) or by embolic occlusion of the microvasculature (endocarditis). Biopsy and culture of lesions can be particularly helpful in these patients, because such procedures demonstrate that the lesions are not primarily coagulopathic or platelet related, and in addition can actually demonstrate and identify a specific infection.

Structural Malformations

A variety of structural malformations are associated with friability of vessels with a resulting hemorrhagic tendency.

A variety of structural malformations are associated with friability of blood vessels with resulting hemorrhagic tendencies.

Scurvy

Scurvy is caused by vitamin C deficiency, which impairs collagen synthesis in vessel walls. These vessels are thus friable because of lack of collagen support; they rupture very easily and, once ruptured, do not vasoconstrict and thus allow excess bleeding. Classical sites are perifollicular petechiae, gum bleeding, and periosteal hemorrhages. This syndrome is most frequently seen today in severe alcoholics who are malnourished. Laboratory study of such patients usually reveals a prolonged bleeding time. Scurvy patients respond well to vitamin C at 1 g/day.

Scurvy patients respond well to vitamin C.

Steroid Purpura

Steroid therapy also results in impaired collagen synthesis, involving particularly the dermal layer of the skin. These patients manifest a vascular fragility and increased skin bleeding that can often mimic a true platelet quantitative or qualitative problem.

Steroid therapy causes vascular fragility and increased skin bleeding that often mimics a true platelet dysfunction.

Miscellaneous Conditions

Paraproteinemias, including cryoglobulinemias and amyloidosis, are associated with skin bleeding and prolonged bleeding times.

Surgical Bleeding

Profuse bleeding from a single area of the body, in the absence of any abnormality of platelet or coagulation testing, is not an infrequent situation in the ICU. When no other obvious or subtle lesion involving the vasculature, platelets, or coagulation proteins is found, one must consider the possibility of inadequate surgical hemostasis or the damage to a vessel severe enough to require exploration and ligature, rather than hemostasis therapy. Classic and common examples include tearing of a vein when placing a central catheter, tearing of an artery during cardiac catheterization, or profound bleeding from a chest tube related to sur-

Profuse bleeding in a single area of the body in the absence of an abnormality of platelet or coagulation testing is frequently observed in the ICU.

gical hemostasis after thoracotomy and cardiac surgery. This problem is discussed later with specific common bleeding situations and entities.

DISORDERS OF PLATELETS

Platelet Structure and Function

Platelets are small cells composed of granules critical to proper platelet function. When platelets aggregate, fibrinogen serves as the adhesive molecule cofactor.

Platelets are small (2–3 μm) cells that circulate in the blood. They do not possess a nucleus but do have mitochondria and other organelles that are critical to proper platelet function. Most important are the systems of granules evident using the electron microscope (see Figures 20-2 and 20-3). Three granule types are identified: (1) dense granules that contain ATP, ADP, serotonin, and calcium; (2) alpha granules that contain many proteins, including trace amounts of plasma proteins (albumin, fibrinogen, von Willebrand's factor [vWF]) and platelet-specific proteins (beta-thromboglobulin, platelet-derived growth factor); and (3) lysosomal granules. All these proteins are released as part of the platelet release reaction.

Platelet Physiology During Coagulation

A series of events occurs when platelets are stimulated in vivo. The usual physiologic stimulants are exposure of the platelet membrane to damaged endothelium and exposure of platelets to biologically active substances such as thrombin, which is present in the area of a thrombosis. When these events happen, the platelets first undergo a shape change that is mediated by membrane changes. The oblong disks become stellate forms with pseudopod-like structures, these coincide with the phenomenon of platelet adhesion, wherein the adhesion molecule platelets, with von Willebrand factor (vWF) as a cofactor, adhere to vascular endothelium exposed by injury. The platelet receptor in this reaction is GPIb. The next reaction is clumping of platelets to each other, or platelet aggregation, in which platelets adhere to each other with fibrinogen serving as the adhesive molecule cofactor. The platelet membrane complex receptor IIb–IIIa is required for this step. Also at this time, the platelets begin to secrete and release the substances contained in their granules. When sufficient release has occurred, the release reaction is irreversible with total degranulation of platelet granule substances, loss of distinct membranes, and formation of a platelet syncytial mass that is, in essence, the primary hemostatic plug. These reactions are summarized in Figure 20-4.

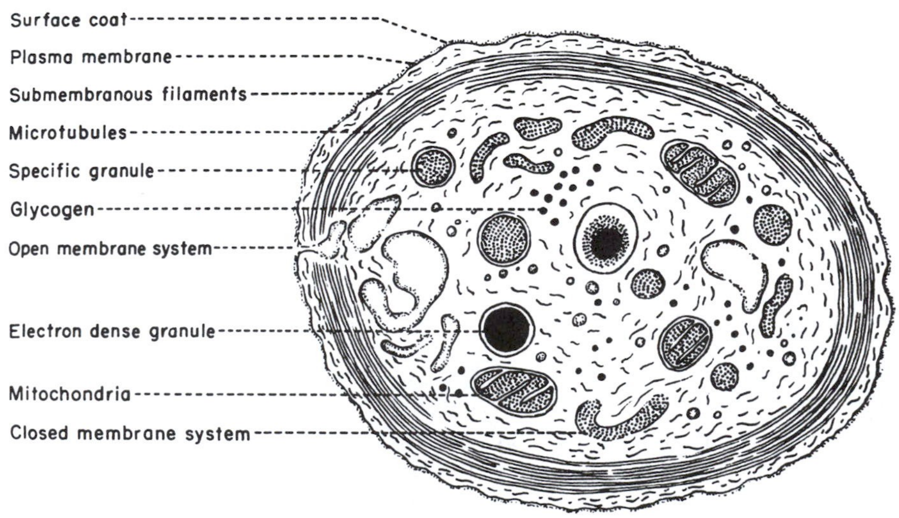

FIGURE 20-2

Diagram of an intact platelet shows numerous organelles but no nucleus.

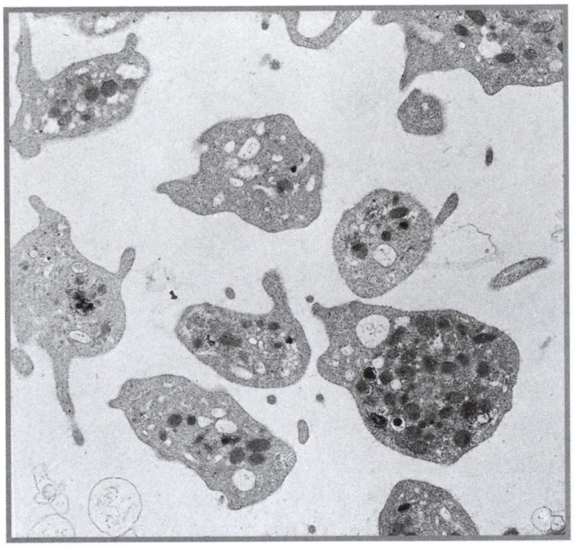

FIGURE 20-3

Electron photomicrograph of numerous intact platelets.

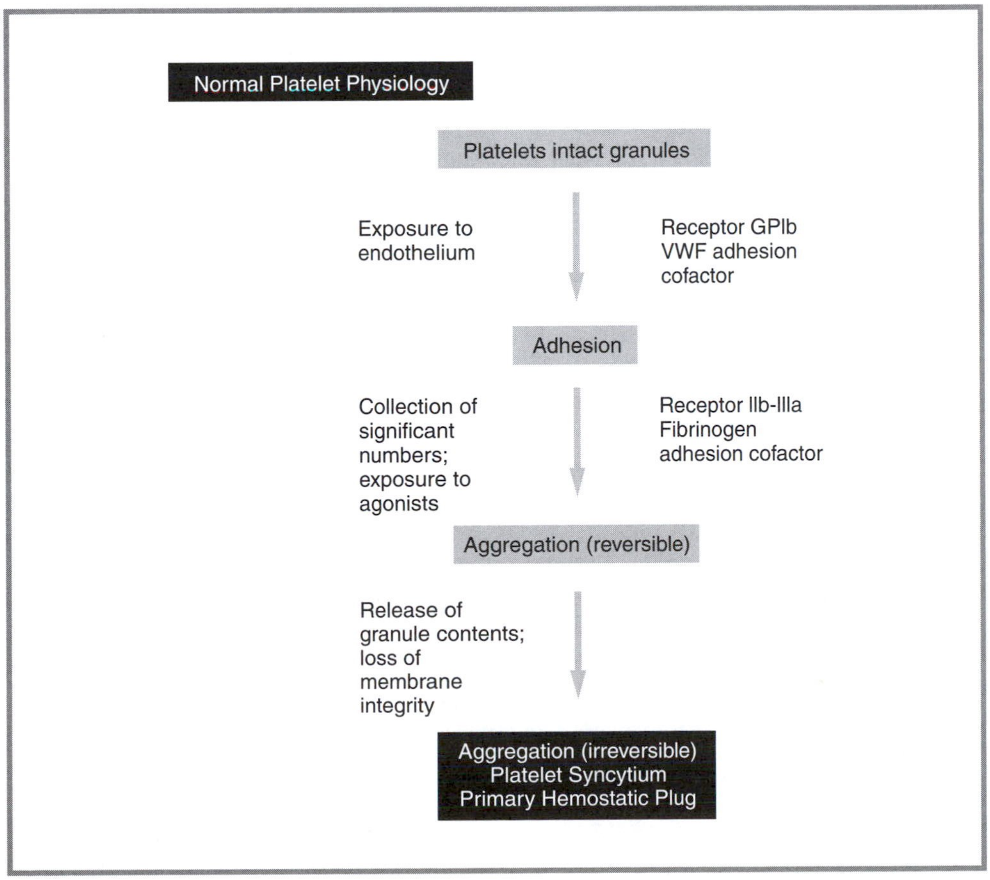

FIGURE 20-4

When an intact platelet membrane is exposed to damaged endothelium, a series of events leads to the formation of a primary hemostatic plug.

TESTS OF PLATELET FUNCTION

The two major tests of platelet integrity as a component of normal hemostasis are platelet counts and the template bleeding time of platelet function.

Platelet Counts

Normal platelet count ranges between 150,000 and 400,000 cells/mm^3.

The normal range of platelet counts is between 150,000 and 400,000 cells/mm^3. Platelets can be counted easily and accurately using current Coulter technology. A series of clinically significant platelet counts has been recognized (Table 20-2).

Bleeding Time

A normal bleeding time requires a platelet number of at least 50,000 cells/mm^3.

In this test, a small iatrogenic wound is made on the patient's arm under standardized conditions and the time for hemostasis in minutes is measured; normal time is 2–7 min. The bleeding time tests platelet function but also requires normal vascular tissue and can indeed be abnormal because of vascular diseases such as scurvy. In addition, a normal bleeding time requires a platelet number of at least 50,000/mm^3 and, in fact, can be prolonged whenever a platelet count is less than 100,000/mm^3. Thus, a Coulter platelet count should be performed before ordering a bleeding time. If the number is less than 100,000/mm^3, the test cannot discriminate between thrombocytopenia and abnormality caused by platelet function and should be deferred. Only when there is a normal platelet count and a bleeding time then reveals prolongation can a defect in platelet function be deduced.

Specific Tests of Platelet Function

A variety of tests are available to directly test platelet function, including platelet aggregometry, in which various known platelet agonists such as ATP and thrombin are added to platelet-rich plasma and the extent of aggregation is measured, and platelet secretion assays wherein known platelet granule contents are measured in plasma after the platelets have been induced to aggregate and degranulate. The latter is the assay most commonly used in the entity of heparin-induced thrombocytopenia (see following section). It should be noted that, unlike the platelet count and bleeding time, special coagulation laboratory facilities and technical knowledge and expertise are required for these tests. Further, they are labor intensive and have a slow turnaround time by ICU standards. Thus, they are often done "after the fact" in bleeding situations and have rather limited utility in the acute setting of bleeding.

QUANTITATIVE PLATELET DISORDERS

Thrombocytopenia

Thrombocytopenia is the most common disorder of hemostasis.

Thrombocytopenia is by far the most common disorder of hemostasis. The condition is suspected when the classical immediate and mucocutaneous bleeding pattern of platelet bleed-

TABLE 20-2

CLINICALLY SIGNIFICANT PLATELET COUNTS

PLATELET COUNT (MM^3)	CLINICAL SIGNIFICANCE
>100,000	Normal hemostasis and testing Tolerate trauma and surgery
100,000–50,000	Bleeding time affected Risk of hemorrhage with trauma/surgery
50,000–20,000	Bleeding time prolonged Bleeding expected with trauma/surgery Signs of skin bleeding on exam
20,000–10,000	More serious (GI, GU) spontaneous bleeding
<10,000	Life-threatening hemorrhage, such as CNS

ing is encountered in a patient and is confirmed by the easily measured Coulter platelet count. Finding a lowered platelet count is only the initial step in such patients, however. The more important diagnosis is why the thrombocytopenia is occurring; this can be classified very effectively by identifying the mechanisms that resulted in thrombocytopenia.

Decreased Production

In all these conditions, some factor has resulted in decreased production of platelets in the marrow. Examples includes marrow failure (i.e., aplastic anemia), that is, marrow invasion and replacement by tumor, leukemia, or fibrosis, and marrow injury, as with drugs such as benzene, chemotherapy, alcohol, and infectious agents.

Abnormal Distribution

In humans, approximately 75% of the total body platelets circulate while the remaining 25% are sequestered in the normal spleen. These platelets are alive and normal but are not immediately available in the circulation (in contrast, in dogs and cats these platelets can be immediately mobilized when needed). In the presence of pathologically enlarged spleens as with chronic leukemias, lymphomas, and cirrhosis of liver with portal hypertension, the ratio of circulating to sequestered platelets can invert with a resulting thrombocytopenia that is clinically significant from a hemostatic view. Such spleens should be readily apparent on physical exam or routine imaging studies.

> Seventy-five percent of the total body platelets circulate; the remaining 25% are sequestered in the normal spleen.

Increased Platelet Destruction

Increased platelet destruction is the most common pathophysiology for thrombocytopenia. In these conditions, platelets are utilized, consumed, or destroyed in the circulation faster than even a normal marrow, with its ability to become hyperplastic by roughly a factor of six, can compensate. Again, a convenient and effective classification schema can be structured on the basis of whether the enhanced destruction is immune- or nonimmune mediated (Table 20-3).

> Increased platelet destruction is the most common pathophysiologic mechanism for thrombocytopenia.

THROMBOCYTOPENIA CAUSED BY PLATELET IMMUNE DESTRUCTION

The forms of thrombocytopenia that are caused by platelet immune destruction have, as a common mechanism, the accelerated destruction of platelets mediated by an antiplatelet antibody. There is almost always a brisk marrow response, although this may take up to 7 days to manifest (see following section). A marrow exam reveals either normal or increased numbers of megakaryocytes.

TABLE 20-3

DISORDERS CAUSED BY PLATELET DESTRUCTION

- Immune disorders
  - Idiopathic (ITP)
  - Drug induced: quinidine, pronestyl, heparin
  - Infections: HIV infection, sepsis-related thrombocytopenia
  - Autoimmune disorders: Systemic lupus erythematosus (SLE)
- Nonimmune disorders
  - Thrombotic thrombocytopenia purpura (TTP)
  - Disseminated intravascular coagulation (DIC): septicemias, massive trauma, obstetric emergencies
  - Dilutional: massive trauma, prolonged surgeries, CABG
  - Microangiopathy: malignant hypertension, cardiac valve dysfunction

Autoimmune Thrombocytopenia

Autoimmune thrombocytopenia (ITP) is the most common form of thrombocytopenia and the most common serious bleeding disorder.

The diagnosis of ITP is based on finding isolated thrombocytopenia, a peripheral smear that shows no evidence of other hematologic abnormality, and an appropriate history and physical examination.

Autoimmune thrombocytopenia (ITP) is the most common form of thrombocytopenia and is also the most common serious bleeding disorder. One must note that most patients will be known to be ITP patients before ICU situations, and the coincident occurrence of symptomatic ITP with another serious condition requiring ICU intervention should be an uncommon event. The American Society of Hematology has recently published a clinical pathway and paradigm for ITP diagnosis and therapy. The diagnosis of ITP is based on the finding of an essentially isolated thrombocytopenia, examination of a peripheral smear without evidence for other hematologic abnormality, and an appropriate history and physical examination. Thus, other causes of thrombocytopenia should be excluded, such as drugs (e.g., quinidine, procainamide, and heparin), other immune diseases (e.g., systemic lupus erythematosus, SLE), and other hematologic diseases such as leukemia or lymphoma. Abnormalities such as the presence of splenomegaly, profound changes in other blood counts, and other abnormal forms on smear strongly suggest another diagnosis. The presence of HIV-positive status or the presence of antiretroviral drugs also excludes the diagnosis of idiopathic, classic ITP, although HIV patients commonly manifest an immune-mediated thrombocytopenia, especially very early in their natural history. The presentation of ITP can be explosive, with profound, life-threatening thrombocytopenia ($<5,000/mm^3$ range) causing profuse mucocutaneous bleeding with melena and oral blood blisters being the reason for presentation to the ICU setting. More subtle, lesser degrees of thrombocytopenia in the range of 30,000–50,000 cells/mm^3 complicating a surgical situation or some other serious medical condition may also require therapy for bleeding.

Therapy

The various, very effective treatments for ITP require judgment depending on the overall clinical situation, the platelet counts, and the bleeding symptoms. An important principle is the excellent functional status of ITP patient platelets. Because of rapid turnover and short half-life, the platelets are young and retain much of their metabolic capacity, such as membrane integrity and granule content. This condition translates into enhanced functional physiology, such that these patients can perform hemostatically at much lower platelet counts than normal patients. Therapy is thus usually considered for patients with platelet counts less than 20,000–30,000/mm^3 and for those less than 50,000/mm^3 who are at risk for bleeding from surgery, peptic ulcer disease, or related situations. If a patient with ITP is already bleeding in a worrisome fashion, higher counts may be preferred in the ICU setting. Therapies are all designed to slow either antibody synthesis or reticuloendothelial destruction or both. A course of high-dose steroids (1 mg/kg) remains the basic therapy. Frequently, a response can be seen within several days. If immediate responses are deemed necessary, reticuloendothelial system (RES) blockade methods are used that include either intravenous immunoglobulins or anti-RhD immunoglobulin, frequently resulting (e.g., 80%) in rises in platelet counts within 24–48 h and sustained elevations for 2–3 weeks. This method can be a very effective emergent maneuver in an acute ICU setting. In extremely dangerous and urgent settings, such as intracranial hemorrhage in an active, thrombocytopenic ICU patient, emergency splenectomy must be considered. The prognosis overall, however, is quite good, with a 5-year mortality rate of about 3%–4% from intercurrent bleeding events.

In extremely dangerous and urgent settings, emergency splenectomy must be considered for ITP.

Drug-Immune Purpura

In drug-immune purpuras, a drug usually acts as a hapten, creating a neoantigen with either plasma proteins or the platelet membrane. An antibody is then formed that is capable of reacting with the neoantigen and causing innocent bystander immune complex or complement-mediated platelet destruction. The classic and still most common medicine causing this condition is quinidine/quinine. Other common drug etiologies include procainamide, sulfa, high doses of penicillins as seen with endocarditis therapies, and phenytoin. These thrombocytopenias are often explosive and acute, to less than 10,000/mm^3 with mucosal bleeding.

They can be caused by a single dose of drug in sensitive patients. Fortunately, platelets recover quickly, usually within 48 h after the drug is stopped. There is anecdotal evidence that the immune maneuvers discussed earlier (IVIg and anti-Rho D) also have some efficacy in this setting, but when a drug is suspected, the medicine must be stopped. Any immune therapies are merely adjunctive.

Heparin-Induced Thrombocytopenia

Heparin-induced thrombocytopenia (HIT) is a special case of drug-related immune thrombocytopenia. Because of the ubiquitous use of heparin in the general hospital and ICU settings, HIT has now become the most common drug-related thrombocytopenia. In patients using full-dose intravenous porcine heparin, an incidence of 2%–3% can be expected. Lower rates occur for prophylaxis, flush, and other heparin regimens, but the denominator of these is so large that cases will still be seen. The other special aspect of HIT is the unique immune mechanism. In this syndrome, heparin elicits a platelet-active antibody that specifically interacts with the IIb-IIIa receptor and is biologically active. In the presence of heparin, this antibody elicits platelet membrane activation similar to that occurring after exposure to a vascular wound. These activated platelets thus aggregate and cause thrombocytopenia.

Heparin-induced thrombocytopenia is the most common drug-associated thrombocytopenia.

If vascular pathology is present, particularly as in coronary artery procedures and peripheral vascular surgery cases, platelet thrombi with life- and limb-threatening thrombosis of arteries and veins ensues, with mortality rates in this subgroup ranging from 20% to 50%. The syndrome usually occurs within 5–10 days of heparin exposure, although in patients with prior heparin exposure 24–48 h may suffice. Due to the potential morbidity and mortality of the lesion, heparin must be stopped in any suspected case, particularly now that an alternative anticoagulant, hirudin derived from genetically engineered leech salivary glands, is now available. Laboratory testing for HIT remains very problematic. There is a serotonin release assay, but the test has many problems: (1) false negatives as high as 30%–40%, (2) the requirement for technical skill, and (3) prolonged turnaround time. An ELISA assay is being developed but is not yet routinely available. Thus, HIT remains a clinical diagnosis and, in the urgent setting, unexplained thrombocytopenia in patients on heparin is an indication for stopping the drug.

Other Immune-Mediated Thrombocytopenias

Infectious immune thrombocytopenias result when either cross-reactive antibodies or nonspecific immune reactions result in platelet destruction. In HIV infection, two mechanisms have been found: immune complex formation with typical innocent bystander-type pathophysiology and the more common true cross-reactive antiplatelet antibody resulting from shared antigens between the HIV virus and the platelet IIb-IIIa receptor. This immune thrombocytopenia responds to classical ITP therapy as well as to antiretroviral therapy against the HIV virus. Other infectious thrombocytopenias include septic thrombocytopenia, a usually moderate (50,000–90,000/mm^3) thrombocytopenia associated with sepsis physiology and positive blood cultures. The precise role of circulating immune complexes and inflammatory cytokines remains unclear. This thrombocytopenia responds in time to therapy of the underlying sepsis.

Infectious immune thrombocytopenia results when cross-reactive antibodies cause platelet destruction.

NONIMMUNE DESTRUCTIVE THROMBOCYTOPENIAS

Nonimmune destructive thrombocytopenias are caused by abnormalities in the circulation that result in some type of enhanced usage or destruction of otherwise intrinsically normal platelets. Such usage or destruction is more rapid than marrow production. If a marrow exam is performed, the hyperplasia will be evident and manifest as at least normal and usually increased numbers of megakaryocytes. There are three main causes; each occurs frequently in the critical care setting.

Thrombotic Thrombocytopenic Purpura

Thrombotic thrombocytopenic purpura (TTP) is defined by a pentad of findings.

Thrombotic thrombocytopenic purpura (TTP) is an important syndrome that has been long recognized and classically is defined by a pentad of findings: (1) thrombocytopenia, (2) microangiopathic hemolytic anemia, (3) renal failure or dysfunction with hematuria, (4) fever, and (5) neurologic manifestations such as seizures. We now recognize that the full-blown syndrome is a rather late development and that the nonblood findings are the result of the more basic, primary hematologic pathophysiology. The current etiology is thought to be an abnormality of endothelial cells caused by a variety of lesions such as drugs (e.g., cyclosporine), toxins (e.g., enterotoxic *E. coli* 157), viruses, and autoantibodies (that probably account for the idiopathic cases) such that they release an abnormal, unprocessed factor VIII molecule, which is a super platelet aggregant rather than the normal platelet adhesion cofactor seen in normals. This molecule results in hyperaggregation of platelets in the microcirculation. Associated sequelae are then microangiopathic hemolytic anemia, fevers, neurologic signs, and renal failure. The latter likely result from microthrombi in cerebral and glomerular microvasculature.

The diagnosis must be suspected in patients who manifest either microangiopathic hemolysis or thrombocytopenia. Blood changes almost always precede any other indication, and a complex ICU patient whose mental, renal, and febrile status is being attributed to TTP almost always has quite diagnostic changes on peripheral smear, which is the initial line of diagnosis. Biopsy material (e.g., kidney, skin) will reveal characteristic hyaline material in the subendothelial areas of small vessels. Studies of factor VIII in the coagulation laboratory will frequently show the abnormally large multimers of unprocessed factor VIII typical of this disease. Plasma-based maneuvers have become the mainstay of therapy in TTP and have within a decade or so changed the prognosis from $>90\%$ mortality to $>80\%$ remission rates. The preferred therapy is plasmapheresis for at least 7 days, followed by cautious weaning from plasmapheresis in responders. In urgent situations (off-hours), the infusion of plasma is a good temporizing measure pending plasma exchange. These plasma maneuvers have been shown to remove the abnormal VIII multimers as well as provide a metalloprotease in increased amounts that can cleave the VIII to less noxious fragments in the patient's circulation. A similar pathophysiologic picture is encountered in the eclampsia of pregnancy and in the vasculitis syndromes of SLE and other collagen vascular diseases.

The preferred therapy for TTP is plasmapheresis.

Disseminated Intravascular Coagulation

The basic abnormal pathophysiology in disseminated intravascular coagulation (DIC) is an abnormal presence of thrombin in the systemic circulation.

In disseminated intravascular coagulation (DIC), the basic abnormal pathophysiology is the presence of thrombin in the systemic circulation. The thrombin can be generated by a variety of mechanisms but results in abnormal fibrin deposition in the microcirculation. This fibrin mesh acts as a sieve through which the blood will flow. As this occurs, once again a microangiopathy ensues and platelets are consumed. The key here is to be aware of the variety of mechanisms that can precipitate this process, because the therapy is indirect and involves addressing that trigger mechanism (see full discussion of DIC later in this chapter).

Dilutional Thrombocytopenia

Dilutional thrombocytopenia occurs if the patient is transfused with large volumes of blood products devoid of functioning platelets.

Dilutional thrombocytopenia disorders are most frequently iatrogenic. The disorders occur when patients have a loss of blood/platelets or very abnormal, large, yet volumetrically correct usage of blood components outside of their ability to produce clotting factors or platelets and in excess of the replacements given. This is the situation in massive transfusions and in cardiac bypass surgery when there are large blood losses either intraoperatively or in the bypass circulation. In vivo, this situation results in an acute depletion of platelets. If the platelets are not replaced, as in the case with many blood recirculation devices, this acute thrombocytopenia will register in vivo and initiate first the formation of thrombopoietin and then a hyperplasia of megakaryocytes. However, this process takes about 5–7 days, such that there will be an immediate, often significant, thrombocytopenia postoperatively and in the early days after surgery. This finding is usually well recognized but can be confirmed by a relatively normal presurgery platelet count, a prolonged procedure, and the use of large amounts of transfused blood that is platelet poor. If the postoperative thrombocytopenia, usually in the 30,000–60,000/mm^3 platelet count range, is homoeostatically inadequate for the critically ill patient, therapy is transfusion of platelets pending marrow response, which is expected in 5–7 days.

Other related thrombocytopenias caused by nonimmune destruction include abnormally functioning prosthetic valves and malignant hypertension, both of which are also examples of angiopathy, this time a local variety in a specific circulation. Both disorders show a microangiopathic smear. Correction of the blood pressure ameliorates the malignant hypertension, whereas valve angiopathy is almost always a sign of dysfunction or infection that requires repair or replacement of the malfunctioning valve.

Abnormally functioning prosthetic valves and malignant hypertension are also associated with nonimmune destruction of platelets.

In all these entities, the basic pathology is platelet destruction in excess of marrow ability to compensate for the losses. In theory, transfused platelets will suffer the same fate and are therefore expected to be of limited efficacy. Correction of the primary abnormal lesions, as discussed with each entity, is the main goal of therapy. Nonetheless, in difficult situations, when a patient is bleeding and has a dangerously low platelet count, platelet transfusions may be considered. TTP is one exception because transfused platelets have been shown to worsen the situation in some cases. In the other entities, assuming that therapy based on the primary insult has been put into place, platelet transfusion should not be withheld.

QUALITATIVE PLATELET DISORDERS

Qualitative platelet disorders share common abnormalities in platelet function (i.e., adhesion, aggregation; see preceding section). Platelet counts are usually within normal limits but the bleeding time, a test of intrinsic platelet function when platelet count is normal, is prolonged. Although characterized by the typical mucocutaneous and immediate-type bleeding pattern found with platelet disorders, the severity and clinical features vary more than seen with the thrombocytopenias. These disorders may be acquired or congenital, but for this chapter, which is concerned with intensive care medicine, the acquired type is discussed at more length. Acquired platelet disorders are more common, in any setting, than congenital forms, and even more so in the setting of critical care. The prototype congenital disorder of platelet function is von Willebrand's disease (vWD). Recall that the large portion of factor VIII, or von Willebrand factor (vWF), is a required cofactor for adhesion of platelets to the subendothelium. vWD is a clinical disease caused by the absence, or at least lowered levels, of vWF on a genetic basis, such that the amount is inadequate to support normal platelet adhesion, with resultant platelet-type bleeding diathesis. A variety of forms of vWD exist, some being caused by abnormally low amounts of vWF and others by an abnormally functioning vWF. Unlike the classical hemophilias, which are sex-linked recessive and thus found in males, vWD in almost all its forms is genetically transmitted autosomally and thus is seen in both males and females. Clues to its presence are platelet-type bleeding in the presence of a normal platelet count, a prolonged bleeding time, and, frequently, a prolonged PTT resulting from a general lowering of the coagulant function of factor VIII with the platelet tropism function of that molecule.

The prototype congenital disorder platelet qualitative function is von Willebrand's.

Laboratory confirmation is readily available in cases once the diagnosis is suspected and consists of specific platelet function abnormalities (normal aggregometry, excepting nonreaction with ristocitin as the agonist), the finding of a lowered level of the factor VIII molecular complex, and testing of factor VIII multimers for abnormalities of amounts, molecular mixtures, and function. Most cases are moderate to mild and respond to 1-desamino-8-D-arginine vasopressin (DDAVP), which elicits increased factor VIII secretion from endothelial cells and is usually adequate to raise levels at least to effectively hemostatic levels if not to normal. In more severe cases in which the VIII and vWF levels are profoundly low, this maneuver is not adequate to raise levels to hemostatic values and transfusion of vWF-containing blood products is required. Such products include fresh-frozen plasma, or more effectively, concentrates such as cryoprecipitates and related products that have been pre-

Most cases of von Willebrand's disease are mild and respond to the use of DDAVP.

TABLE 20-4

DISORDERS OF PLATELET FUNCTION

DISORDER	PATHOGENESIS	THERAPY
Aspirin	Permanent acetylation of platelet membrane interferes with production of agonist thromboxane	Remove ASA Recovery may require 3–7 days
Other NSAIDs	Reversible inhibition of platelet agonist and membrane metabolism	Remove agent Fully reversible with clearance of NSAIDs
Uremia	Toxic molecules deaggregate platelet adhesive cofactor vWF	Dialysis, DDAVP Cryoprecipitates
Exposure to foreign surfaces (cardiac bypass)	Degranulation and metabolic fatigue of platelet membrane	Reversible within hours of removal from apparatus

pared by methods which enrich the amounts of factor VIII-vWF in relation to their volume, an important consideration in many critical care patients.

ACQUIRED DISORDERS OF PLATELET FUNCTION

A broad variety of conditions can and do cause platelet dysfunction (Table 20-4). The proposed mechanism, clinical setting, and treatment principles of these disorders share the findings of platelet-type bleeding diathesis: prolonged bleeding times in the presence of essentially normal (or at least $>100,000/\mu l$) platelet counts and theoretical or actual demonstration in-vitro platelet testing of lesions interfering with the normal and required platelet physiology (i.e., adhesion, aggregation, secretion of granule contents). Therapy involves reversing, if possible, the causative lesion (i.e., discontinuation of aspirin or NSAIDs; dialysis to remove toxic molecules that are deaggregating vWF). Transfusion of normal platelets may be required to temporize bleeding in patients whose platelets are dysfunctional. However, if the causative lesion is not properly addressed, such as stopping drugs or dialysis for uremia, the transfused platelets will quickly experience the same lesions, and become hypofunctional, and hemostasis will not be effectively attained.

DISORDERS OF THE COAGULATION SYSTEM

The third component of normal hemostasis physiology is the coagulation protein system (see the coagulation cascade in Figure 20-1). This series of proteins acts as a biologic amplifier system wherein proteases and cofactors are generated with the ultimate product being a powerful serine protease, thrombin, which cleaves a soluble plasma protein, fibrinogen, which then polymerizes into insoluble fibrin, the basic meshwork of a thrombus. Table 20-5 lists and describes the proteins of the coagulation system, which are quite arbitrarily named according to their discovery sequence. The table also lists the coagulation disorders associated with hereditary deficiency in these proteins.

Coagulation disorders are usually classified as being hereditary or acquired.

Coagulation disorders are usually classified as being hereditary or acquired. The hereditary types result from gene mutations that render the corresponding proteins either qualitatively or quantitatively deficient. The acquired types are almost always complex disorders in which the pathophysiology is so deranged that multiple deficiencies or defects in the normal hemostatic pathways ensue.

TABLE 20-5

PROTEINS OF THE COAGULATION SYSTEM AND THEIR DISORDERS

FACTOR	BIOCHEMISTRY	BIOSYNTHESIS	BIOLOGIC HALF-LIFE (H)	SERUM	ADSORBED PLASMA	FUNCTION	HEREDITARY CONDITION
Fibrinogen	Multimeric glycoprotein; three paired peptide chains; MW 340,000	Liver	72–120	Absent	Unchanged	Precursor of fibrin and common pathway	–
Prothrombin	Monomeric glycoprotein; MW 69,000	Liver: vitamin K-dependent	67–106	Absent	Absent	Proenzyme, precursor of thrombin, and common pathway	–
Factor V	Multimeric glycoprotein; MW 200,000–400,000	Liver	12–36	Absent	Unchanged	Cofactor and common pathway	–
Factor VII	Monomeric glycoprotein; MW 63,000	Liver: vitamin K-dependent	4–6	Increased	Absent	Proenzyme and extrinsic pathway	Rare, but seen; requires ≥20% activity for adequate hemostasis; FFP source
Factor VIII_{VWF} complex	Multimeric glycoprotein; MW ~1,200,000; functionally heterogeneous subunits	–	–	Absent	Unchanged	Cofactor, intrinsic pathway, and platelet adhesion	von Willebrand's disease; autosomal inheritance; treated with DDAVP, cryoprecipitate
Factor VIII C	Monomeric glycoprotein; MW 267,000	Unknown	10–14	Absent	Unchanged	Cofactor, intrinsic pathway and "carrier" molecule for VIIIC	Hemophilia A; sex-linked inheritance; severe delayed bleeding with surgery; requires ≥50% levels for surgery hemostasis
Factor IX	Monomeric glycoprotein; MW 55,000	Liver: vitamin K-dependent	18–40	Increased	Absent	Proenzyme and intrinsic pathway	Hemophilia B; sex-linked inheritance
Factor X	Two-chain glycoprotein; MW 55,000	Liver: vitamin K-dependent	24–60	Unchanged	Absent	Proenzyme and common pathway	–
Factor XI	Two-chain glycoprotein; MW 160,000	Liver	48–84	Unchanged	Slightly decreased	Proenzyme and intrinsic pathway	Common in Ashkenazic Jews; autosomal inheritance; variable bleeding risk
Factor XII	Monomeric glycoprotein; MW 80,000	Unknown	52–60	Unchanged	Unchanged	Proenzyme and intrinsic pathway	–
Prekallikrein	Monomeric γ-globulin; MW 88,000	Liver	Unknown	Unchanged	–	Proenzyme, kinin system, and intrinsic pathway	–
Factor XIII	Multimeric glycoprotein; two paired peptide chains; MW 320,000	Megakaryocytes, liver	72–168	Decreased	Unchanged	Proenzyme and common pathway	Fibrin-stabilizing protein; wound-healing problems in newborns

HMW, high molecular weight; MW, molecular weight

SOURCE: Adapted with permission from Lee GR, et al. Wintrobe's Clinical Hematology, 9th Ed. Philadelphia: Lea & Febiger, 1993:1309

COAGULATION TESTING IN COAGULATION SYSTEM DISORDERS

Coagulation testing and proper interpretations are vital in the diagnosis and therapy of bleeding.

The prothrombin time (PT) test examines the extrinsic pathway of clotting.

The partial thromboplastin time (PTT) tests the intrinsic pathway.

Coagulation testing and proper interpretations are vital in the diagnosis and therapy of bleeding. A relatively easy initial strategy is to perform a prothrombin time (PT) and partial thromboplastin time (PTT). In PT, a tissue factor (usually brain extract) is added to plasma to quickly activate factor VII, which then fires down the common pathway of coagulation (factors C, V, thrombin, and fibrinogen). This portion of the coagulation cascade is referred to as the extrinsic pathway. The PTT test introduces surface-active substances, such as kaolin, to the plasma; this reaction activates factors XII and XI and proceeds, more slowly than with the PT, to activate factors VIII and IX, which then fire down the common pathway. This portion of the coagulation cascade is referred to as the intrinsic pathway. These tests are excellent screens because if either one is normal then the common pathway must be intact and any prolongation found can be isolated to the extrinsic or intrinsic wings of the pathway, allowing relatively simple diagnosis corroboration by specific factor assays. Almost all the congenital diseases (i.e., the hemophilias) have this mechanism and result from a single gene defect causing a single protein deficiency. On the other hand, when both the PT and PTT are abnormal, this finding usually suggests an acquired and complex disorder with multiple defects in the coagulation pathways being simultaneously present. In addition to being able to provide such a bleeding abnormality with a classification and name, proper utilization of this coagulation testing schema and diagnosis allows proper therapy. The only blood product containing all the coagulation factors is fresh-frozen plasma (FFP). If one tried to treat all lesions this way, volume considerations would prevent efficacy and cause morbidity and even mortality. Thus, excellent specialized plasma derivatives have evolved that are rich in specific proteins or groups of proteins (i.e., cryoprecipitates for fibrinogen, factors VIII and V) and are much more volumetrically appropriate and factor enriched. However, to use these correctly, one must know where the deficiencies are and what factors are needed: thus, accurate diagnosis is needed before using definitive treatment. Refer again to Figure 20-1, which shows the extrinsic and intrinsic coagulation protein pathways with tests for each, that is, the prothrombin time (PT) for the extrinsic pathway and the partial thromboplastin time (PTT) for the intrinsic pathway.

HEREDITARY COAGULATION DISORDERS

The prototype example of hereditary coagulation disease is hemophilia A, the most common hereditary deficiency.

Encountering an occult hereditary coagulation disorder in the critical care setting should be an unusual event. These conditions in their milder forms may not cause any spontaneous bleeding symptoms or history, yet may result in morbid hemorrhage with severe hemostatic stress (i.e., surgery). The author diagnosed mild forms of hemophilia A and B four times during a 2-year experience in the Army. The prototype example of hereditary coagulation disease is hemophilia A, which is discussed in some detail here; other less common hereditary coagulation diseases are summarized in Table 20-5.

Hemophilia A

Hemophilia A, the most common hereditary deficiency, results from a genetic defect in the factor VIII gene that causes deficient amounts (or, less commonly, deficient functioning) of factor VIII. Many different genetic defects have been described, ranging from deletion of the gene with essentially no factor VIII protein in the circulation to more subtle single base mutations that result in intact antigenic amounts but hypofunctional factor VIII. The former defect tends to result in severe variants whereas the latter results in milder forms. However, there is no mild hemophilia with trauma or surgery. All affected patients will bleed severely in such instances. Clinical severity aspects and levels of factor in hemophilia are correlated and summarized in Table 20-6. It should be noted that hemophilia A and its variants can now be diagnosed by genetic mapping. All hemophilia A subtypes as well as hemophilia B sub-

TABLE 20-6

CLINICAL AND LABORATORY SEVERITY IN HEMOPHILIA

FACTOR LEVEL	CLINICAL SEVERITY	MANIFESTATIONS
<1% (0–1 μm/ml)	Severe	Spontaneous hemorrhages Morbid arthropathy
2%–5% (2–5 μm/ml)	Moderate	Spontaneous hemorrhage, including joints, but infrequent
>5%	Mild	No spontaneous bleeds, but life-threatening hemorrhage with trauma or surgery

types are transmitted on the X chromosome and display sex-linked heredity with male subjects and female carriers. Factor IX, or hemophilia B, has similar genetics. The other hereditary disorders most often display autosomal recessive heredity.

Clinical Features

Hemophilia, like most of the other coagulation protein diseases, results in a bleeding pattern somewhat different from platelet disorders. The bleeding may not be immediate, but rather delayed. Thus the trauma physician or surgeon may not detect any undue bleeding initially, but later in the recovery room or ICU, hematoma formation or body cavity bleeding ensues. Joint bleeding or hemarthrosis is the diagnostic hallmark of these conditions, but for critical care specialists it will be the bleeding with surgery or trauma that is problematic. It cannot be overemphasized that all hemophiliacs, whether defined as mild or not by factor analysis and degree of spontaneous bleeding, will display a severe and potentially life-threatening hemorrhagic diathesis with major trauma or surgery. Diagnosis in most cases comes with the patient, for example, a young male with severe hemorrhage at surgery and a sex-linked positive family history, although fully one-third of cases arise de novo genetically. Conversely, in any male, particularly with a positive past history of stress-related hemorrhage, who displays unexpected delayed, deep tissue bleeding with trauma or surgery, the presence of a variant of hemophilia should be suspected. Both hemophilia A and B show marked prolongation of the PTT with normal PT, thus localizing the lesion to the intrinsic arm of coagulation. The PTT corrects with addition of normal plasma, thus indicating deficiency of a protein. Analysis of specific intrinsic pathway coagulation factors then isolates with precision which factor, VIII or IX, is deficient. The time required for such testing in a coagulation laboratory is quite reasonable, no more than several hours being required for factor levels.

Bleeding in hemophilia is not immediate but rather delayed.

Management

Management of all the hereditary disorders of coagulation is predicated on several issues: (1) the required level of factor needed for hemostasis, (2) the distribution space of the clotting factor, (3) the plasma half-life of the factor, and (4) the time needed for firm hemostasis for the particular event involved. Table 20-7 presents these facts and therapeutic principles for the more common hereditary bleeding disorders. It should be emphasized that this is a quite specialized aspect of coagulation medicine, and consultation with physicians experienced with the care of such patients is highly recommended.

ACQUIRED COAGULATION DISORDERS

The acquired coagulopathies are more commonly seen in the critical care setting because they often are the result of other organ failures and therapeutic side effects so frequently encountered in this difficult population. These disorders are characterized by multiple and mixed deficiencies, involving not only different parts of the coagulation cascade but often other as-

Acquired coagulation disorders are commonly seen in the ICU and are characterized by multiple and mixed deficiencies of the coagulation cascade, as well as platelet dysfunction.

TABLE 20-7

BASIC PRINCIPLES OF COAGULATION FACTOR REPLACEMENT

CONDITION (FACTOR DEFICIENCY)	PHARMACOLOGY	CLINICAL ASPECTS
Hemophilia A (VIII)	$T_{1/2}$ 8–12 h 90% plasma compartment No loading dose	Surgery usually requires 5–7 days Activity ≥50%
Hemophilia B (IX)	$T_{1/2}$ 24 h 50% plasma compartment Requires loading dose	Identical
Fibrinogen	$T_{1/2}$ 3–4 days > 50% plasma compartment	Levels ≥100 mg% needed for hemostasis
Factor VII	$T_{1/2}$ 6–8 h 50% plasma compartment	Activity ≥25% required for hemostasis

pects of hemostasis such as the platelet count and bleeding time as well. These disorders manifest a diffuse effect on coagulation tests, prolonging many of them and crossing the extrinsic–intrinsic–common pathway boundaries. Clinical acumen as to which entities complicate specific conditions (i.e., liver disease, anticoagulant misadventures, and disseminated intravascular coagulopathy with sepsis) and the ability to properly perform and interpret a more complex and comprehensive array of coagulation tests are needed to accurately diagnose and to provide effective therapy for these conditions.

COAGULOPATHY ASSOCIATED WITH CARDIOPULMONARY BYPASS AND MASSIVE TRANSFUSIONS

Coagulopathy associated with cardiopulmonary bypass and massive transfusions is complex and involves several different factors.

A patient with prolonged surgery and large transfusion requirements often is deficient in clotting proteins and platelets.

A very common and at times clinically significant coagulopathy is observed in the setting of cardiopulmonary bypass and in the setting of prolonged surgery with use of massive transfusions and cell-saver techniques. Bleeding incidence in these settings has been estimated to be in the 2%–5% range. The pathogenesis is complex but basically involves several key elements. First, the use of massive amounts of transfused blood results in a dilution of coagulation proteins and platelets. The stability of these components in banked blood is quite poor, and within days the amounts in a stored unit are minimal. Because the red cell storage time is 35 days, much banked blood given for hemoglobin support in the OR is essentially devoid of platelets and coagulation factors. Cell-saver technology also is designed for RBC salvage, and the material reinfused in the OR is once again essentially devoid of platelets and clotting proteins. Thus, a patient with prolonged surgery and large transfusion requirements often is deficient in clotting proteins and platelets. If the pump team or anesthesia team fails to note this and to adequately supplement the transfused material with FFP and platelets, hemostatic function deteriorates and a bleeding diathesis manifests. This condition is a complex bleeding diathesis associated with surgical bleeding (i.e., chest tube) as well as diffuse bleeding at other sites. As one should surmise from the pathophysiology, multiple aspects of hemostasis and the attendant coagulation tests are abnormal. Thus, there is thrombocytopenia as well as prolonged PT and PTT in lab testing. The diagnosis should be suspected when a hemostatically normal patient manifests bleeding diathesis and diffuse laboratory abnormalities intraoperatively or postoperatively in association with cardiopulmonary bypass or other extensive surgery requiring large amounts of transfused blood. When this diagnosis is suspected, "resuscitation" with blood and blood products, FFP, platelets, and, if significantly hypofibrinogenemic, cryoprecipitates will stop the bleeding. Over time, normal synthesis replaces the deficiency and the situation normalizes. However, this may take days to occur and ongoing blood bank support may be needed in the first postoperative days.

A special situation is cardiopulmonary bypass, where in addition to the dilution discussed above, an acquired transient platelet dysfunction (in addition to the dilutive thrombocytopenia) occurs. This disorder has been shown to result from a qualitative platelet defect related to activation of platelets with release of granule contents elicited by the hypothermia, exposure to synthetic surfaces of the bypass circuitry, and exposure of platelets to the oxygenator, all of which occur during surgery in these patients. Immediately postoperatively, these platelets are hypofunctional and patients display prolonged bleeding times even with normal platelet counts. If postoperative bleeding is associated with this lesion, platelet transfusions will temporize the situation while normal endogenous platelet function is being restored.

A special situation in cardiopulmonary bypass is an acquired transient platelet dysfunction.

COMPLICATIONS OF ANTICOAGULANTS

Another acquired, iatrogenic bleeding diathesis in critical care medicine is complications related to anticoagulants. The most common anticoagulants involve heparins and warfarin. Less common are problems related to newer agents such as plasminogen activator and hirudin.

Heparin

Heparin is a commonly used polysaccharide anticoagulant that, via an allosteric interaction with plasma antithrombin III, potently inactivates thrombin and thus inhibits the coagulation protein cascade from forming a fibrin thrombus. When excessive heparin is in place, or when a patient with therapeutic levels of heparin is bleeding from a pathologic or iatrogenic lesion, serious and life-threatening hemorrhage will result until the effect of heparin is reversed. The diagnosis is entertained when a patient on heparin has abnormal bleeding. Heparin overdose is defined as a PTT in excess of 2–2.5 times control. The coagulation laboratory will perform a mixing study to confirm that the PTT is caused by heparin inhibition rather than factor depletion due to dilution or decreased synthesis. Protamine sulfate is a heparin antidote in these instances and can reverse the heparin effect within minutes. A reasonable initial dose is 1 mg/kg. Some authorities use an empiric lesser dose of 50 mg; this is effective in most patients and utilizes less protamine, which has its own intrinsic anticoagulant effect.

Warfarin

Warfarin is a commonly used oral anticoagulant that, via competitive antagonism of vitamin K, interferes with the gamma carboxylation of clotting proteins II, VII, IX, and X. The functional levels of these proteins is thus titrated lower with an anticoagulant effect. If excessive doses are used, the lowering of clotting proteins becomes excessive and a situation very similar to hereditary coagulation factor deficiency results. This complication can result in spontaneous bleeding, bleeding from surgery or trauma, or bleeding from pathologic sites such as gastric erosions. The patient usually will have a history of warfarin use and demonstrate an excessively prolonged PT International Normalization Ratio (INR in excess of 3.0). Because many coagulation factors are involved, the PTT is also prolonged. Laboratory testing shows correction with mixing, and factor analysis shows concordant lowering of factors II, VII, IX, and X. Treatment depends on clinical severity and requires judgment. In uncontrolled situations, the factors must be replaced quickly, and this is done by giving FFP. In less urgent situations, if the liver synthetic function is intact, vitamin K acts as an antidote. Doses vary between 1 and 10 mg depending on the clinical situation. The medicine should be given IV (after a small test dose for allergy) because intramuscular hematomas may result in this setting if intramuscular (IM) injections are used. Response usually occurs within 12 h, but ongoing vitamin K may be needed because the half-life of warfarin exceeds that of vitamin K.

PLASMINOGEN ACTIVATORS AND HIRUDIN

Plasminogen activators actually lyse already formed fibrin thrombus. Bleeding from these drugs is usually transient as the half-life of tissue plasminogen activator (tPA) is measured in minutes. However, a more sustained coagulopathy can result from the lysis of fibrinogen and other coagulation factors by the tPA. In such instances, the PT and PTT are usually prolonged and in addition there is a profound hypofibrinogenemia. Such patients benefit from replacement of factors, particularly fibrinogen in the form of transfusions of cryoprecipitates. Hirudins are new anticoagulants derived from genetically engineered leech salivary extracts. Hirudins are used as anticoagulants in cases of HIT (see full discussion of HIT earlier in this chapter); they are direct thrombin inhibitors. Problems with their use are renal excretion such that significant dose reductions must be made with decreases in glomerular filtration rate and the absence of a known antidote. Thus, bleeding problems with these agents are very problematic with the only therapy available being support until the drug half-life effects disappear (measured in hours with normal renal function).

VITAMIN K DEPLETION

A frequent coagulopathy encountered in the ICU is vitamin K depletion.

A coagulopathy frequently encountered in the ICU is vitamin K depletion. As already discussed, this fat-soluble vitamin is required for posttranslational gamma-carboxylation of the vitamin K-dependent clotting proteins II, VII, IX, and X. This step results in the formation of a carboxyl-rich group whose negative domain is required for adsorption of the proteins and hence for function. Vitamin K has two sources in humans: dietary, from green leafy vegetables, and endogenously, from vitamin K made by colonic flora that is subsequently absorbed. The common manifestation of deficiency occur in the patient not ingesting anything by mouth for reasons of surgery or other morbid conditions who also is being treated with broad-spectrum antibiotics, which obliterate normal bowel flora and thus impair the endogenous source of vitamin K. The condition presents itself most often as a gradual prolongation of, first, the PT (because the shortest half-life for the vitamin K family is factor VII, a protein of the extrinsic pathway and therefore PT), and later, in extreme cases, of the PTT. Diagnosis is suspected by the coincident findings of poor oral intake and broad-spectrum antibiotics and confirmed by demonstrating correction of the PT in laboratory mixing studies with lowered vitamin K family clotting proteins on assay. These patients respond quickly to parenteral vitamin K, and supplements can be placed into their nutrition, either enterally or parenterally, to prevent recurrence.

Vitamin K depletion most commonly occurs in patients that are not ingesting anything by mouth and are being treated with broad-spectrum antibiotics.

LIVER DISEASE

The coagulopathy of liver disease is one of the most frequent bleeding diatheses seen in the ICU.

The coagulopathy of liver disease is one of the most frequent bleeding dyscrasias in critical care medicine. Review of Figure 20-1 and Table 20-5 reveals the ubiquitous extent of hepatic synthesis of coagulation proteins in all pathways, suggesting that derangements in liver function should result in a variety of disturbances of clotting function. The major defect is deficiency of synthesis of clotting factors. Newer data have revealed that there is a hierarchy of resistance to disease in factor synthesis. Thus, the earliest, least specific, and least prognostic change is defects in the gamma-carboxylation pathways already discussed. The very same factors II, VII, IX, and X are depressed, again with the PT laboratory test being affected first because of the short half-life of VII. As liver disease worsens, the ability to properly synthesize fibrinogen is affected next, with the finding of hypofibrinogenemia and even dysfibrinogenemia (an abnormal fibrinogen molecule). These findings suggest more serious clinical liver disease (i.e., Childs' class B or C) and a worse prognosis. Finally, in the most serious and advanced situations, the usually resistant factor V synthetic mechanism fails, with lowering of that factor. This finding is an ominous prognostic sign, both for acute survival and for reversibility. Many hepatologists now use factor V levels as a trigger for candidacy for liver transplantation.

Many hepatologists now use factor V levels as a trigger for liver transplantation.

Coagulation profiling is now acquiring an important role in the management of liver patients. On routine testing, prolonged PT and PTT result from the diffuse lowering of many factors. Further testing of fibrinogen specific factor levels, especially VII and V, can reveal a more complete prognostic picture with therapeutic value as well (i.e., need for transplantation). Management of bleeding patients is extremely difficult and problematic, and this is among the most difficult bleeding diatheses to treat. Initial attempts involve replacing the extensive array of deficient factors with FFP (plus cryoprecipitates for profoundly hypofibrinogenemic patients <100 g%) as the standard of care. However, as the half-life of the factors is short, especially VII, this therapy has fleeting or negligible benefit. The volumes involved become prohibitive and bleeding in these cases carries a high mortality. Virally safe, effective concentrates of vitamin K complex proteins are now under examination and would be a beneficial alternative if proven efficacious in this group of patients.

In addition to the coagulopathy, other events in liver failure significantly add to bleeding diathesis and morbidity. As portal hypertension increases, there is enlargement of the spleen with a degree of hypersplenism, sequestration of platelets, and thrombocytopenia. The degree is usually moderate in the 50,000–100,000 range, but enough to contribute to serious hemorrhage in these cases, especially because platelet transfusions will be similarly sequestered and less efficacious than in normals. Portal hypertension raises the venous pressures in the abdominal wall, as well as in the portal circulation, further increasing the tendency to bleed with surgery or from comorbid gastrointestinal lesions such as the varices or erosions so frequent in these patients.

As portal hypertension increases in patients with liver disease, splenic enlargement promotes further sequestration of platelets and thrombocytopenia.

DISSEMINATED INTRAVASCULAR COAGULATION

Disseminated intravascular coagulation (DIC) is, along with hepatic coagulopathy, one of the most frequently encountered bleeding diatheses in critical care medicine. DIC is the end result of an intermediary syndrome that has as its basis the abnormal generation and presence of the serine protease thrombin in the systemic general circulation, usually in the microcirculation. In fact, DIC can result from any disease process that activates either the intrinsic pathway (i.e., infections, gram-negative sepsis) or the extrinsic pathway (i.e., introduction of tissue factors via obstetric complications, carcinomatosis, massive trauma). Figure 20-5 presents an overview of these pathophysiologic models with the clotting pathways. Once either of these pathways is activated, the common pathway fires, with the diffuse, systemic production of thrombin and fibrin formation. This process in due time therefore depletes the plasma of its clotting moieties, which are consumed in this process. Paradoxically, this microvascular consumptive storm then causes a profound bleeding diathesis.

The clinical features of DIC are quite heterogeneous and depend on the levels and balance of diffuse microclotting and clotting factor depletion. Three arbitrary patterns are described. (1) In acute hemorrhagic DIC (e.g., abruption of placenta), the coagulopathy overwhelms the microthrombus aspect of the syndrome; these cases demonstrate the most profound derangement of coagulation testing and clinically bleed. (2) In laboratory DIC (common in infections), the process is less explosive such that there is sufficient factor depletion for laboratory findings to become manifest but not so severe as to result in serious bleeding; in the author's experience, this is the most common situation. (3) In subacute and chronic forms of DIC, most typical of malignancy, the microthrombosis aspect dominates and even evolves into grossly evident thrombi (e.g., Trousseau's syndrome). Laboratory evaluation, as is typical of the acquired coagulopathy states, utilizes a battery of tests that demonstrate the presence of consumption of clotting proteins and platelets by the process and the presence of microvascular clotting. For the former, PT is measured as a surrogate for the clotting cascade proteins, the fibrinogen and platelets. For the latter, the presence of fibrin clots is deduced by measuring their physiologic digestion products, fibrinogen degradation products and/or D-dimers. Until a valid assay for thrombin levels is available, which would be a more specific test of this condition, we continue to use this classical battery (Table 20-8).

The clinical features of DIC are heterogenous and depends on levels and balance of diffuse microclotting and clotting factor depletion.

Management of DIC is difficult and controversial. A variety of schemas have been proposed. All authorities agree, however, that the keystone of therapy is removal of the initiat-

Management of DIC is difficult and controversial.

FIGURE 20-5

Numerous clinical conditions have been associated with the development of disseminated intravascular coagulation (DIC).

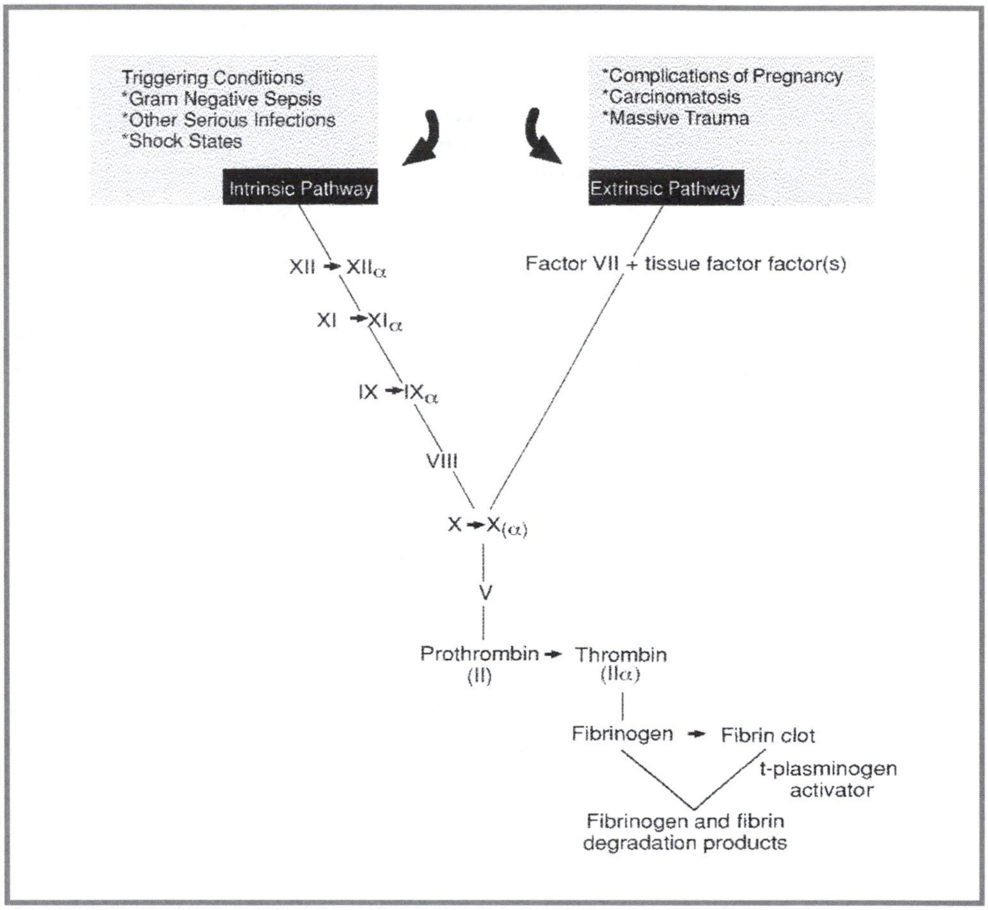

ing process. Regardless of what else is done, this maneuver is primary and no amount of other treatment will be effective if the trigger process is not addressed. Thus, surgery to drain an abscess must not wait for correction of the DIC lab abnormalities. Conversely, draining the abscess will indeed reverse and correct the abnormalities. Sometimes the removal of the trigger is relatively easy, as with evacuating the uterus, draining an infection, or giving antibiotics. Other situations, such as carcinomatosis or refractory hypoperfusion and shock, are much more problematic. Supportive therapy may be needed in coagulopathic patients with severe depletion of clotting moieties and uncontrolled hemorrhage. Blood products should not be withheld from these patients, especially if maneuvers targeting the trigger process are in place or at least attempted. A broad mixture of coagulation support is used: plasma, platelets, and cryoprecipitates depending on the degree and specifics of the laboratory abnormalities encountered. When an overt thrombosis such as acral gangrene is present, the microcirculatory thrombosis may require the judicious use of heparin as well. Fortunately,

TABLE 20-8

LABORATORY DIAGNOSIS OF DISSEMINATED INTRAVASCULAR COAGULATION (DIC)[a]

LABORATORY TEST	NORMAL	MEAN VALUES IN DIC (%)[b]
Platelets	150–400,000/μl	52 (93)
Prothrombin time (PT)	11–14 s	18 (90)
Fibrinogen	150–400 mg/dl	137 (71)
Fibrin degradation products/D-dimers	–	High titer (92)

[a] Clinical diagnosis of DIC required at least three tests abnormal
[b] %, percentage of cases with autopsy-confirmed DIC in author's trial who manifested an abnormal value

many patients have only laboratory manifestations with little clinical bleeding. In these cases, reversal of the initiating process is the only therapy required. It must be mentioned that the presence of DIC in a critical care patient is an ominous prognostic. In the author's series, a 1-month mortality of 66% was associated with the presence of DIC regardless of mechanism.

DIC is a serious disease. A 1-month mortality of 66% has been reported, regardless of mechanism.

SUMMARY

Bleeding diathesis are common problems facing the ICU practitioner in caring for critically and complexly ill patients. Fundamentals of a good history and physical examination along with appropriate laboratory testing enable the critical care practitioner to approach the patient with a logical differential diagnosis and appropriate treatment plan.

REVIEW QUESTIONS

1. **A purpuric skin rash found on a patient who is using prednisone on a daily basis is likely caused by:**
   A. Infection
   B. Steroid therapy
   C. Allergy to antibiotic
   D. Amyloidosis
   E. Vitamin C deficiency

2. **In a patient with thrombocytopenia, an increased number of megakaryocyte in a bone marrow assay may indicate:**
   A. Tumor invasion of the bone marrow
   B. Acute bleeding event
   C. Splenic sequestration of platelets
   D. Toxic effect of alcohol
   E. Autoimmune platelet destruction

3. **All the following statements concerning heparin-induced thrombocytopenia (HIT) are correct, except:**
   A. The serotonin release assay is valuable in diagnosing HIT.
   B. HIT is the most common drug related thrombocytopenia.
   C. HIT has a unique immune mechanism.
   D. Life- and limb-threatening thrombosis can occur.
   E. When HIT is suspected, heparin should be immediately stopped.

4. **What is the most common hereditary coagulation deficiency?**
   A. von Willebrand's disease
   B. Hemophilia A
   C. Hemophilia B
   D. Antithrombin III deficiency
   E. Protein S deficiency

5. **All the following statements concerning disseminated intravascular coagulopathy (DIC) are correct, except:**
   A. DIC and hepatic coagulopathy are the most common bleeding diathesis in the medical ICU.
   B. Initially, diffuse microthrombosis with depletion of clotting factors, then profound bleeding occurs.
   C. A microthrombosis clinical state can dominate.
   D. Management is well defined and straightforward.
   E. Blood tests for fibrinogen degradation products and D-dimer are almost always elevated.

ANSWERS

1. The answer is B. All the responses are associated with purpura. Patients who are administered daily systemic corticosteroid therapy commonly have areas of purpura because steroids impair collagen synthesis in the dermal layer of skin, leading to vascular fragility and skin bleeding. Infection and a variety of antibiotics can cause purpura, and patients who use daily prednisone are often at risk for infection, but the steroid therapy itself presents the greatest risk for purpura development.
2. The answer is E. The most common pathophysiology for thrombocytopenia is increased platelet destruction, particularly autoimmune-mediated disease. With increased platelet destruction, bone marrow megakaryocytes increase in number. Bone marrow megokaryocytes do not change with platelet splenic sequestration, and they decrease when the bone marrow is replaced by tumor or suppressed by alcohol.
3. The answer is A. The serotonin release assay is not very helpful. This assay has a high false-negative rate and prolonged turnaround time. Because HIT involves activated platelets that aggregate, as soon as thrombocytopenia is recognized heparin should be discontinued. HIT remains a clinical diagnosis.
4. The answer is B. Hemophilia A is caused by a genetic defect in the factor VIII gene, causing a decrease in functional factor VIII, and is the most common hereditary coagulation disorder. Both type A and B hemophilia are transmitted on the X-chromosome and display sex-linked hereditary with male subjects and female carriers.

5. The answer is D. Management of DIC is difficult, undefined, and controversial. However, all agree that treating the underlying causal factor(s) is most important, such as surgically removing the abscess, treating shock, and administering antibiotics. Supportive therapy may include the use of blood products in patients with uncontrolled bleeding or the use of heparin for gangrene.

SUGGESTED READING

Addonizio VP. Platelet function in cardiopulmonary bypass and artificial organs. Hem Oncol Clin North Am 1990;4:31–51.

Alving BM, Krishnamurti C. Recognition and management of heparin-induced thrombocytopenia (HIT) and thrombosis. Semin Thromb Hemost 1997;23:569–575.

Furie B, Limentani S, Rosenfeld CG. A practical guide to the evaluation and treatment of hemophilia. Blood 1994;84:3–9.

Furlan M, Rodolfo R, Galbusera M, Remuzzi G, et al. Von Willebrand factor-cleaving protease in thrombotic thrombocytopenic purpura and hemolytic-uremic syndrome. N Engl J Med 1998;339:1578–1584.

George JN, Shattil SJ. The clinical importance of acquired abnormalities of platelet function. N Engl J Med 1994;331:1207–1211.

George JN, Woolf SH, Raskob GE, Wasser JS, et al. Idiopathic thrombocytopenic purpura: a practice guideline developed by explicit methods for the American Society of Hematology. Blood 1996; 88:3–40.

George JN, Raskob GE, Shah SR, Rizvi MA. Drug-induced thrombocytopenia: a systemic review of published case reports. Ann Intern Med 1998;129:886–890.

Mammen E. Coagulation defects in liver disease. Med Clin North Am 1994;78:544–545.

Penner JA. Managing the hemorrhagic complications of heparin administration. Hematol Oncol Clin North Am 1993;7:1281–1289.

Rubin RN, Colman RW. Disseminated intravascular coagulation: approach to treatment. Drugs 1992;44:963–971.

Wandt H, Frank M, Ehninger G, Schneider C et al. Safety and cost-effectiveness of a 10 × 10/L trigger for prophylactic platelet transfusions compared with the traditional 20 × 10/L trigger: a prospective comparative trial in 105 patients with acute myeloid leukemia. Blood 1998;91:3601–3606.

Woodman RC, Harker LA. Bleeding complications associated with cardiopulmonary bypass. Blood 1990;76:1680–1697.

CHAPTER 21

JOSEPH I. BOULLATA AND FRANCIS C. CORDOVA

Nutrition Assessment and Nutrition Support in Intensive Care Unit Patients

CHAPTER OUTLINE

LEARNING OBJECTIVES

After studying this chapter, you should be able to:

- Describe the neurohormonal changes on the body during stress and its effect on fuel utilization by the body.
- Describe the indications for nutrition support in a critically ill patient.
- Explain the timing, route, and administration of nutrition support in the critically ill.
- List dosing parameters for macronutrients and micronutrients delivered enterally or parenterally to critically ill patients.
- Describe the monitoring parameters used to assess therapeutic effect and adverse effects of nutrition support.

Malnutrition in the hospital setting remains largely underrecognized by health care workers despite increasing awareness of the value of nutrition in clinical practice. The incidence of malnutrition in hospitalized patients has remained the same over the past 20 years (40%–50%) despite progress in clinical nutrition. More importantly, studies show that many patients lose weight during their hospital stay.

The problem of malnutrition in critically ill hospitalized patients, particularly those who are undernourished, is magnified severalfold because of the profound metabolic alterations associated with critical illnesses, regardless of the type of the initial body insult (e.g., trauma, burn, surgery, or sepsis). Apart from the hypermetabolic state contributing to undernutrition after injury, critically ill medical patients admitted to the intensive care unit (ICU) often have chronic, lingering illnesses, including acquired immunodeficiency syndrome, malignancy, chronic obstructive pulmonary disease, congestive heart failure, and hepatic and renal diseases, that often further contribute to the problem of their undernutrition. In essence, undernutrition is common in the ICU patient because of preexisting malnutrition compounded by the hypermetabolic response of injury. Also, critically ill patients have in common a state of restricted food intake following admission to the ICU.

Undernutrition is common in hospitalized patients, especially in the ICU setting.

Among the numerous therapeutic interventions made in the intensive care unit, provision of nutrition support is common. Regardless of subspecialty, the intensivist should understand the altered metabolism that may occur in the critically ill patient and the role for nutrition support in this population. Critically ill patients often require specialized nutrition support, delivered enterally and/or parenterally, not as a substitute for food so much as to provide needed substrate for a metabolism altered by their illness.

Critically ill patients often require enteral or parenteral nutrition or both.

In this chapter we describe the pathophysiology and clinical assessment of malnutrition and the approach to nutrition support in all critically ill adult patients. Where appropriate, information relevant to a subgroup of critically ill patients is included.

DEFINITIONS

Nutritional status is an expression of the degree to which an individual's nutritional needs are being met based on body composition and function. Poor nutritional status, or malnutrition, refers to any imbalance between nutrient intake and requirements (from starvation to obesity). Disease states obviously influence clinical outcome, but nutritional status is also a comorbid factor.

Undernutrition refers to a state of food intake inadequate to meet the daily nutrient requirements of the body. Starvation is the extreme example of the undernourished state, which can result from insufficient nutrient intake, malabsorption, or increased metabolic requirements due to disease or injury. Undernutrition can be defined as a body weight less than 90% of predicted ideal weight or a body mass index (body weight/height^2) less than 18.4 kg/m^2. Undernutrition is also said to exist with an unintentional weight loss of at least 10% that occurs over the preceding 3–6 months. The opposite extreme of nutritional imbalance is obesity, defined as a body weight above 130% of predicted ideal weight, or a body mass index greater than 30 kg/m^2. Individuals over 110% of ideal weight, or with body mass index greater than 25 kg/m^2, are considered preobese or overweight. It is important to realize that undernutrition should be viewed not only as a decrease in body weight but also as an alteration in body composition in response to a perturbation in physiologic function. Various screening tools, devices, and nutritional indices have been developed to further define malnutrition. Clearly, there is no single best parameter to define undernutrition in every clinical situation, especially in the ICU. The actual body weight remains an objective, easy, and reproducible measure of undernutrition and is an important initial screening tool of nutritional status in the ICU. Different measures of nutritional health, such as midarm muscle circumference, tricep skin fold thickness, serum albumin, prealbumin, and delayed skin test reactivity, can then be used to further define and classify the degree of undernutrition and evaluate the response to nutrition support.

Metabolic response is the stereotypical response of the body to stress and is often proportional in magnitude to the severity of the injury. The temporal sequence of metabolic events following injury has two phases, namely, the ebb and flow phases of the postinjury response. The ebb phase occurs during the first 12–24 h after injury and is characterized by a decrease in cardiac output, oxygen consumption, and hypothermia associated with hemodynamic instability. In addition, elevated levels of glucagon and cathecholamines lead to hyperglycemia, increased circulating free fatty acids, and a corresponding decrease in circulating insulin. The subsequent flow phase follows after successful resuscitation of the patient. In contrast to the ebb phase, the flow phase is characterized by an increase in both cardiac output and metabolic rate as the body attempts to preserve various organ functions.

CASE STUDY: PART 1

AW is a 48-year-old man with a history of hypertension who presented to the emergency department (ED) with a 4-day history of increasing diffuse abdominal pain, associated with several episodes of vomiting, and constipation, alternating with diarrhea over the past week. He denied fever or chills. He has no known allergies and takes no medications at home. On physical examination, the abdomen was distended, diffusely tender with hypoactive bowel sounds. Radiographic findings of the abdomen revealed dilated bowel loops with multiple air fluid levels. He was admitted to the surgical service and underwent exploratory laparotomy, with lysis of adhesions and resection of 25 cm of jejunum with primary anastomosis, and upon recovery was transferred to the ICU.

This phase is further characterized by a neuroendocrine response and release of inflammatory mediators that lead to increased turnover of carbohydrates, proteins, and lipids. The increased circulating amino acids and fatty acids released during this period are utilized as alternative energy sources. The duration of the flow phase is dependent upon the nature of the injury.

The term specialized nutrition support (SNS) refers to the provision of specially formulated nutrient products to maintain or improve a patient's nutritional status via the enteral or parenteral route. Enteral nutrition (EN) is the provision of SNS by nonvolitional delivery by a tube into the gastrointestinal tract. Increasing use of this modality, also referred to as tube feeding, has followed innovations in both access and formulas. Parenteral nutrition (PN) is the provision of some or all nutrients through a central vein. Product osmolality and volume limit the effective administration of PN by peripheral vein. Still one of the most complex prescription drug products in terms of dosing and compatibility, PN has in the past been referred to as hyperalimentation and total parenteral nutrition.

Enteral nutrition (EN) is administered into the GI tract and parenteral nutrition (PN) into a vein.

PATHOPHYSIOLOGIC CONSIDERATIONS

Undernourished State

The dynamics of fuel utilization by the body can best be understood by studying energy utilization during fasting. In the normal nonfasting condition, glucose is the main energy source of the body and is supplied by the breakdown of daily ingested food. During fasting in healthy subjects, serum glucose is maintained by the breakdown of hepatic glycogen stores, a process known as glycogenolysis. However, the glycogen store of the body is limited and is rapidly depleted within a 24-h period. During a prolonged fasting state, the body's energy utilization shifts from glucose to ketones, which are generated by the oxidation of body fat stores. Body tissues with an obligate need for glucose as the sole source of energy obtain their supply via hepatic gluconeogenesis. In this process, lactate, glycerol, and amino acids from muscle proteins provide the substrates for glucose production. In addition to the change in the pattern of energy utilization, the body also decreases energy expenditure by about 20%. As is discussed later, this is in stark contrast to energy expenditure during sepsis. In critically ill patients such as those with severe burns, trauma, or sepsis, energy expenditure remains high both during periods of adequate nutrition support and during periods of temporary suspension of nutrition intake. Indeed, the body's energy balance remains negative even with aggressive nutrition support.

Hypermetabolic State

Recent understanding of the body's metabolic response to injury and the possible role of the gastrointestinal tract in the genesis of systemic inflammatory response has led to the practice of early nutrition support in critically ill patients. During periods of stress, as seen in patients with sepsis, trauma, and burns, energy consumption may increase as much as 100% above baseline depending on the severity of injury. This increase in metabolic rate and energy expenditure commonly seen following injury is known as the hypermetabolic state. The

Physiologic changes in the body following injury are high serum levels of catecholamines and glucagon, relative tissue insensitivity to insulin, increased energy consumption, and tissue catabolism.

The hypermetabolic state results from altered neuroendocrine response of the body during stress and is defined by increased tissue catabolism and energy expenditure.

hypermetabolic state is characterized by severe catabolism of muscle protein, resulting in a net negative balance of body nitrogen that may eventually lead to organ failure. As seen during fasting, the fuel utilization of the body shifts from carbohydrate to fat as the glucose stores are rapidly depleted and as the synthesis of glucose by the liver cannot keep up with the body's high energy needs. Unlike malnutrition, where nutrition support is enough to induce positive nitrogen balance, the metabolic derangement following injury can be reversed only by providing adequate nutrition support while treating the underlying disease process.

This altered fuel utilization and hypermetabolic state is largely brought about by a neuroendocrine response involving macromediators (e.g., catecholamines, cortisol, glucagon) and additional responses coordinated by micromediators such as cytokines, eicosanoids, and reactive oxygen and nitrogen species at the level of the leukocyte and endothelium. The systemic inflammatory response syndrome, identified in many critically ill patients despite varying initial clinical presentations, may be considered the clinical manifestation of dysregulation of the mediators of the injury response. Aside from being a direct consequence of the primary insult, multiple organ dysfunction may result from prolonged or uncontrolled systemic inflammation. Poor control of the underlying etiology of inflammation, ischemia and reperfusion, altered gastrointestinal permeability, and other causes have been suggested as explanations for progression to organ dysfunction. A patient's outcome may also relate to the premorbid nutritional status, which can partly determine the severity of response at the cellular–molecular level. Although the response itself may be detrimental, use of nutrition may dampen the response and optimize outcome (e.g., wound healing, immune function, musculoskeletal strength).

The hormonal milieu in these patients favors gluconeogenesis, despite hyperinsulinemia, and lipolysis, although triglyceride clearance may be reduced. Although protein synthesis per se may increase, the rate of proteolysis is greater, and amino acid efflux from skeletal muscle supports the acute-phase response and gluconeogenesis. The resulting clinical picture is one of a hyperglycemic, hypertriglyceridemic, azotemic, and often edematous patient.

The goal of managing the response in these patients is to modulate it in hopes of decreasing morbidity and mortality. Although maximizing oxygen delivery and minimizing infectious complications therapeutically may improve outcome, nutrition support is just as necessary, in organ or visceral resuscitation, by minimizing the detrimental effects on nutritional stores and providing substrate to the tissues.

Nitrogen Balance

Negative nitrogen balance occurs when the rate of protein breakdown exceeds protein synthesis.

The amount of nitrogen in the diet and the amount of nitrogen excreted in the urine plus the small amount of nitrogen lost through the gastrointestinal tract determine nitrogen balance, or the overall metabolic balance of the individual. A positive nitrogen balance means that the body's structural proteins are rebuilding and is a desired endpoint of all forms of nutrition support. In normal subjects, a negative nitrogen balance up to approximately 4 g/day can be expected. In any kind of injury or stress, the negative nitrogen balance invariably increases severalfold beyond normal depending on the severity and duration of injury. In malnourished subjects, negative nitrogen balance increases to about twice normal, reflecting a loss of body cell mass to catabolism. In essence, the body is using its available fuel reserves (i.e., muscles and adipose tissue) as energy sources. In severe injury, as exemplified by a greater than 40% burn injury, a negative nitrogen balance can approach 27 g/day. Because 6 g of protein contains approximately 1 g of nitrogen, burn patients can lose as much as 162 g protein/day. If this hypermetabolic rate goes on unabated, or is only partially attenuated by aggressive nutrition support, severe malnutrition will occur within 2 weeks.

It is possible to achieve zero nitrogen balance in normal subjects by providing enough daily calories and protein to meet energy expenditure and obligatory protein losses from ongoing metabolic processes. A zero or positive nitrogen balance can be similarly achieved in malnourished patients when enough calories and nitrogen are supplied. Unfortunately, the negative nitrogen balance that occurs during sepsis and severe injury is resistant to even the most aggressive nutritional supplementation. A zero nitrogen balance can eventually be achieved as recovery from the initial injury is achieved. Some studies suggest that enteral feeding is more effective in attenuating the metabolic response to injury compared to parenteral nutrition. Whether this is due to maintenance of gut integrity and prevention of bacterial translocation during enteral feeding or some other factor remains to be confirmed.

Protein Metabolism

Structural body protein serves as a large, readily available energy reserve that can be mobilized by the body during fasting or following injury. The amino acids released during catabolism of muscle proteins are mainly used as a substrate for gluconeogenesis and are made available for the synthesis of new proteins for tissue repair and immune response and for the synthesis of acute-phase proteins by the liver. In addition, the release of branched chain amino acids serve as nitrogen donors for the synthesis of glutamine, which is the preferred fuel source of rapidly dividing cells such as intestinal mucosa or white blood cells. However, the increase in protein catabolism during injury is not without side effects. The increase in amino acid efflux from skeletal muscle results in increased urinary nitrogen excretion and a negative nitrogen balance. Because food intake immediately following injury is often limited, and because of the hypermetabolic state following injury, an increased negative nitrogen balance invariably follows injury and, if not reversed by nutrition support and treatment of injury, the condition results in severe malnutrition.

Amino acids from protein breakdown are used for gluconeogenesis.

Glucose Metabolism

During injury, altered fuel utilization and perturbation in hormonal milieu commonly results in hyperglycemia, despite elevated levels of insulin. Specifically, increased hepatic gluconeogenesis coupled with decreased glucose uptake by insulin-sensitive tissues such as skeletal muscle and adipose tissue are the main reasons for increased blood glucose levels following injury. The decreased uptake of glucose by muscle cells and adipose tissue is caused by stress-induced insulin resistance, thought to be mediated by elevated levels of antiinsulin hormones (cortisol, catecholamines, glucagon) and cytokines released during stress by inflammatory cells.

Stress-induced hyperglycemia caused by increased circulating catecholamines and relative tissue insensitivity to insulin.

Hyperglycemia following injury is thought to be a biologically adaptive mechanism designed to provide adequate supply of glucose to poorly vascularized wounds. In addition, the brain obtains almost all its energy from glucose oxidation.

Lipid Metabolism

Adipose tissue is the major fuel reserve of the body. During mild to moderate trauma, an increase in free fatty acids and glycerol can be seen as early as 2 h following injury. Fat becomes the predominant source of energy as the supply of glucose becomes limited. The respiratory quotient, that is, the ratio of carbon dioxide production to oxygen uptake ($VCO_2/\dot{V}O_2$) is lower during stress compared to baseline, indicating preferential use of lipids as an energy source; this may be advantageous because lipid has a sparing action on protein catabolism. The increased free fatty acids serve as a fuel source for tissues, except the red blood cells and the central nervous system. The increased rate of lipolysis is thought to result from a continuous stimulation of the sympathetic nervous system during injury.

In patients with severe trauma, both free fatty acids and ketones are decreased while the level of glycol remains unchanged. This apparent discrepancy in the rate of lipolysis between mild to moderate trauma on the one hand and severe trauma on the other hand is probably caused by decreased perfusion of adipose tissue in severe injury.

Ketones derived from fatty acids serve as an alternate fuel source during stress.

NUTRITION ASSESSMENT

Malnutrition is unfortunately still prevalent in the hospitalized patient and increases the risk for morbidity and mortality. Poor premorbid nutritional status, or changes in nutritional status as a result of concurrent disease, may affect wound healing, immunocompetence, musculoskeletal strength, and cardiopulmonary function. There is no single presenting sign or symptom, biochemical marker, or physical examination finding that defines nutritional status, least of all in the critically ill patient.

Poor nutritional status influences patient outcome from critical illness.

CASE STUDY: PART 2

Initial ICU data included:

- Medications: vancomycin 1 g IV daily, ciprofloxacin 400 mg IV q12h, metronidazole 500 mg IV q12h, famotidine 20 mg IV daily, lorazepam 2 mg IV prn, morphine 2 mg IV prn, and D5W/0.45 NaCl with 20 mmol KCl/l at 80 ml/h
- Vital signs: T_m, 100. °F; BP, 135/88 mmHg; HR, 90/min; RR, 12/min
  Height, 5′9″; weight, 84 kg (usual weight, 88 kg; preop weight, 83 kg)
- Pertinent findings: sedated but arousable; intubated and mechanically ventilated; nasogastric tube to suction with over 600 ml out in the first few hours postop; abdominal distension; dressing intact; no bowel sounds or flatus/stool noted; adequate urine output; total fluid in/out 3100/2800 ml; left subclavian triple lumen catheter in place centrally as confirmed by chest X-ray
- Pertinent lab results: Na, 138 mmol/l; K, 4.1 mmol/l; Cl, 106 mmol/l; CO_2, 22 mmol/l; BUN, 18 mg/dl; Cr, 0.9 mg/dl; glucose, 128 mg/dl; triglycerides, 240 mg/dl; albumin, 2.8 gm/dl; WBC, 9 k/mm^3; Hb, 9.5 g/dl; platelets, 240 k/mm^3; INR 1.1

Use the history, physical examination, and lab markers for nutrition assessment.

A nutritional assessment includes a good history (as available), a nutritionally focused physical examination, along with careful interpretation of height and weight, and laboratory markers. The history should be able to identify chronic disease states, most of which impact nutritional status: gastrointestinal (GI) disorders, poor appetite, dental and oral health, surgeries, and recent weight changes. Serum albumin has traditionally been used as a marker of nutritional status. However, in critically ill patients with reprioritization of hepatic protein synthesis and changes in fluid compartmentalization, hypoalbuminemia is common regardless of nutritional status. Prealbumin, with a shorter half-life than albumin, can be used as a protein status marker along with C-reactive protein. The latter helps distinguish the presence of an acute-phase response from poor nutritional status as a cause for hypoprealbuminemia. All the subjective and objective data available are then evaluated to make the best clinical assessment of nutritional status. By definition, the severely ill patient with sepsis, organ dysfunction, extensive surgery, burns, or traumatic wounds has altered nutritional status by virtue of their altered metabolism.

The metabolic response to injury impacts nutrient metabolism and nutritional requirements.

INDICATIONS FOR NUTRITION SUPPORT

Specialized nutrition support (SNS) is indicated in patients with altered nutritional status who are unable to improve their status on their own.

The goal of SNS is to limit the comorbidity of malnutrition.

Many institutions have a nutrition support team or individuals (physician, nurse, dietitian, pharmacist) specializing in nutrition support available to the intensivist. As previously noted, a patient's nutritional status is evaluated on the basis of specific subjective and objective data. The potential risks versus benefit from SNS depend on nutritional status and estimated time until resumption of usual diet. Generally, SNS may be required for patients with an alteration, or potential for an alteration, in nutritional status who are otherwise unable to improve or maintain their nutritional status on their own. The critically ill patient may also be evaluated based on severity of illness and premorbid nutritional status. The patient with adequate premorbid nutritional status who is expected to improve clinically and eat within a week is not likely to require SNS. However, the patient with significant illness or injury, not expected to recover within a week, may need nutrition support. The threshold is especially low for the patient with poor nutritional status on admission to the ICU, including undernourished and obese patients as well as those with imbalances in specific nutrients. The goal of providing SNS is to minimize the comorbid effects of malnutrition and to prevent or manage specific nutrient imbalances. When an indication for SNS is established, the timing, route, and dosing become important.

TIMING OF NUTRITION SUPPORT

When indicated, SNS is best administered as soon as possible in a hemodynamically stable patient with safe access.

When indicated, SNS should be initiated as early as feasible to minimize the adverse systemic effects of the injury response. Data suggest that delay for more than 48 h significantly increases the risk of infection, length of stay, and mortality in burn and trauma patients. A patient should first be hemodynamically stable with a safe enteral or parenteral access device in place. Timing of SNS along with the degree of malnutrition may influence outcome. Postoperative PN is no better than intravenous fluids in well-nourished or mildly malnourished patients, and may actually be worse than fluids postoperatively if the patient is not severely malnourished. The best outcome (fewer postoperative complications) results from initiating PN preoperatively in severely malnourished surgical patients. Trauma patients do better, in terms of infectious morbidity and mortality, with initiation of EN within 24 h compared with waiting 5 days before initiating. Generally, early SNS (enteral or parenteral) is better than later in those with an indication. There is a trend toward fewer infections and less systemic inflammation in the critically ill burn, trauma, and gastrointestinal surgical patients with EN initiated early. There are no data to support any advantage to delaying SNS when it is indicated. Once indicated, the next decisions involve determining the route, access, and duration of SNS.

EARLY
trauma → ↓ infect.
+/- mortality
burn → ↓ SIRS
↓ infect"

ROUTE AND ACCESS OF NUTRITION SUPPORT

The enteral or the parenteral route is available to deliver SNS formulations. Decision making about the route of SNS involves evaluation of gastrointestinal (GI) tract function, anticipated duration of SNS, and the relative benefits of EN versus PN.

> The function of the GI tract and expected duration of therapy help determine the route and access for SNS.

Although assessment of premorbid status and severity of illness determines initiation of SNS, the function of and access to the gastrointestinal tract determine the route of administration. The function of both the upper and lower gastrointestinal tract should be determined. Whenever a functional gastrointestinal tract can be safely accessed in a patient with an indication for SNS, the enteral route should be used. Adequate function requires absence of anorexia, nausea, vomiting, or excessive drainage from a naso/orogastric tube. The presence of 200 ml or more of gastric output over 4–6 h (100 ml or more if gastrostomy) or documented tracheal aspiration of gastric contents would preclude using the gastric route for EN. The abdominal exam should also reveal no distension or tenderness, with the presence of flatus or passage of stools; the value of bowel sounds, present or absent, is limited. Surgery on the gastrointestinal tract does not preclude the use of EN per se, but the presence of sig-

CASE STUDY: PART 3

On postoperative day 2 (POD 2), the patient was febrile and somewhat more agitated despite adequate analgesia. The same drug regimen had been continued and the patient had required increasing amounts of saline boluses to maintain adequate circulatory pressures. A pulmonary artery catheter was placed via the right subclavian vein for hemodynamic monitoring.

- Vital signs: T_m, 101.8°F; BP, 128/68 mmHg; HR, 108/min; RR, 18/min; CVP, 6 mmHg; PAOP, 12 mmHg, CI, 3.6 l/min · m^2; SVR, 850 dynes · s/cm^5.
- Pertinent findings: nasogastric suction, ~1000 ml today; (pH 3.5); abdominal distension, without flatus or stool; decreasing urine output, fluid in/out 4200/1800 ml.
- Pertinent lab results: Na, 141 mmol/l; K, 3.8 mmol/l; Cl, 110 mmol/l; CO_2, 20 mmol/l; BUN, 22 mg/dl (UUN 7); Cr, 1.4 mg/dl; glucose, 160 mg/dl; Mg, 1.1 mg/dl; P, 2.1 mg/dl; Ca, 7.5 g/dl; albumin, 2.1 g/dl; WBC, 14 k/mm^3.
- Nutrition support assessment/plan: Given a 6% weight loss before admission, NPO status for at least 6 days with a worsening clinical condition, and no expectation of resuming oral diet in the next few days, this patient was a candidate for SNS. The GI tract could not be used because of poor gastric emptying and no access to the small bowel. The patient was a candidate for short-term PN via a lumen of the central catheter. Nutrient dosing was based on the metabolically active weight of 74 kg. His caloric goal was 2000 kcal/day (27 kcal/kg) based on an estimated basal energy expenditure of 1667 and an activity factor of 1.2. The calories provided by dextrose and lipid should not exceed 440 g/day and 75 g/day, respectively. The empiric protein goal is 110 g/day (1.5 g/kg). Maintenance fluid needs are approximately 2200 ml/day. The 1000-ml PN, initiated at 42 ml/h, contained 60 g protein, 200 g dextrose, and 40 g lipid (providing 1080 nonprotein kcal). If tolerated, the goal volume can be ordered the following day at 1800 ml at 75 ml/h containing 108 g protein (17 g nitrogen), 360 g dextrose, and 72 g lipid (providing 1944 nonprotein kcal/d), including 80 mmol NaCl, 60 mmol potassium acetate, 5 mmol calcium gluconate, 12 mmol magnesium sulfate, and 24 mmol sodium phosphate in those 1800 ml along with 10 ml 12-multivitamin product, 1 mg vitamin K (not included in the multivitamin), 3 ml 5-trace-element product, and 40 mg famotidine (discontinuing the intermittent IV famotidine).

nificant ileus, obstruction, peritonitis, hemorrhage, high-output fistula, necrotizing pancreatitis, ischemic bowel, short bowel syndrome, documented malabsorption, or intractable vomiting or diarrhea suggest the parenteral route for many patients. The small bowel is still capable of nutrient absorption despite the presence of poor gastric emptying, and consideration may be given to directly accessing the proximal small bowel for EN.

The small bowel may be considered for EN delivery even in the presence of poor gastric emptying.

Assuming safe access to the GI tract, there may be differences between gastric and intestinal feeding. Aspiration risk is greater for bolus feeding as opposed to continuous gastric feeding. Data do not consistently support the contention that the risk of tube feed aspiration is lower in patients fed post pylorus; however, the intestinal administration of an appropriate formulation reduces the time to achieve the goal dosing rate and lowers the risk of diarrhea. Duodenogastric reflux may contribute to gastric volume, but reflux is less likely when the distal end of the feeding tube is beyond the ligament of Treitz. No one finding predicts success with the enteral route, but with a functional GI tract, the best test of EN tolerance is a trial of EN before committing to the parenteral route. If the GI tract cannot be safely accessed, then PN is appropriate until the enteral route is usable. The weakest link in using EN is safe access, although there are a number of techniques to place EN access devices in critically ill patients.

Devices exist for obtaining enteral and vascular access. Placement of enteral access may be guided by endoscopy, fluoroscopy, laproscopy, or surgically as well as by blind placement. Anticipating the duration of EN helps determine the most appropriate and comfortable enteral access for the patient. Generally, for short-term use (<3 weeks), the transnasal/transoral route is sufficient. If treatment for longer than 3 weeks is anticipated, percutaneous access of a gastrostomy, transgastric jejunostomy, or jejunostomy may be considered whether placed endoscopically, fluoroscopically, or surgically. A silicone or polyurethane tube of at least 10 French with adequate internal diameter can be used for the transnasal/transoral access device.

The transnasal/transoral route is sufficient for short-term EN; percutaneous tube placement is considered for long-term EN.

An intravascular catheter placed in a central vein, ideally a triple lumen catheter placed through the subclavian vein with the distal tip in the vena cava, is required for PN administration. A peripheral venous access may be used for the short-term (<5 days) administration of PN in the absence of a central access or while titrating the rate of the EN to goal dosing. Correct placement of both enteral and parenteral access devices should be confirmed before use. Placement of long-term indwelling catheters for continued PN administration at an alternate care site may be considered if transfer from the ICU with that therapy is possible. The use of either the enteral or parenteral route for SNS does not preclude the adjunctive use of the other route to best meet an individual patient's needs.

Although the etiology is unexplained, infectious complications are usually fewer with EN than PN.

PN has a higher incidence of infectious complications than does EN, even when line-related infections are excluded. This difference may result from altered GI mucosal permeability and mucosal lymphoid tissue at the respiratory and gastrointestinal tracts. Whether this is a direct result of the route of administration or of the nutrient composition by that route (with subsequent impact on gene expression and regulation of nutrient flow by the GI tract) remains unclear. The substrate delivered in parenteral formulations may be incomplete or unbalanced for that route of delivery. The clearest evidence for an outcome advantage of EN over PN comes from trials in abdominal trauma; an advantage in favor of PN is suggested in head-injured patients, but otherwise the evidence is inconsistent in terms of clinical outcome. Interestingly, studies that reveal no significant difference in rate of infection between patients receiving EN or PN have dosed calories at the recommended levels and hypoglycemia is rare. On a more basic level, EN regimens often are less costly than PN regimens. PN is often included among the most costly drugs provided by an institution when usage is significant.

ADMINISTRATION OF NUTRITION SUPPORT

Enteral

Critically ill patients tolerate EN best when administered continuously into the stomach or proximal small bowel using a pump. The head of the bed should be elevated to 30°–45°, and the feeding can be administered at full strength starting at 10–20 ml/h. The dosing rate may

CASE STUDY: PART 4

On POD 3, infusions of morphine, lorazepam, and cisatracurium were initiated to facilitate ventilatory management. Dopamine and norepinephrine infusions were started to maintain adequate perfusion. Antimicrobials were appropriately modified. An indirect calorimetry reading, under adequate conditions, provided a resting energy expenditure of 2164 kcal/day for this patient.

- Vital signs: T_m, 101°F; BP, 180/20 mmHg; MAP, 78 mmHg; PAOP, 15 mmHg; CI, 4.4 l/min; SVR, 760 dynes · s/cm^5.
- Pertinent findings: weight, 90 kg; poor GI function continued (gastric pH 4.5); renal function stabilized; fluid in/out 3900/2000 ml.
- Pertinent lab results: Na, 142 mmol/l; K, 4.2 mmol/l; Cl, 110 mmol/l; CO_2, 21 mmol/l; BUN, 20 mg/dl; Cr, 1.4 mg/dl; glucose, 190 mg/dl; Mg, 2 1.1 mg/dl; P, 2.3 mg/dl; Ca, 7.7 g/dl; WBC, 17 K/mm^3, CRP, 24; prealbumin, 8.
- Nutrition support assessment/plan: Patient continues to require SNS via the parenteral route. Increased weight likely reflects fluid retention. The low prealbumin likely reflects both poor nutritional status and the response to inflammation. PN is well tolerated with titration to the goal rate. The empiric caloric dosing goal is similar to results of indirect calorimetry so there is no need to alter the regimen, especially given ventilatory status and hyperglycemia. Consider initiating an insulin infusion if serum glucose exceeds 200 mg/dl, with a goal of 180 mg/dl during the inflammatory response.

be titrated up by another 10–20 ml/h every 6–12 h toward the goal rate as tolerated. The goal rate would be the hourly volume of a formulation that over the course of a day would provide the patient's nutrient dosing needs. Patients who have been nil per os (npo) for a week or longer, or those with severe malnutrition on presentation, may need to be advanced toward goal rate more slowly. Unfortunately, because of slow advancement, inappropriate stoppages, and underdosing, half of critically ill patients do not meet their nutrient requirements during a course of EN therapy. Additives to the EN formulation are to be avoided to limit risk of contamination and because of limited compatibility data. A pharmacist should be consulted before administering any medication through the same access device as the EN formula. The ideal order for EN includes the product name, the volume, and accompanying rate with the patient's dosing weight. The administration bag and set should be changed every 8–12 h, and any remaining formula should be discarded. Because of its propensity to support microbial growth, a volume of EN should not remain in a bag for more than 8–12 h.

EN is initiated at 10–20 ml/h and titrated to goal as tolerated.

Slow advancement and stopping of infusion results in many critically ill patients not meeting their requirements.

Parenteral

The PN formulation is prepared on a daily basis and administered in a single container at a rate not to exceed 42 ml/h for the first day and advanced to the goal rate by the second or third day, as tolerated to limit complications involving volume, glucose, or electrolytes. The PN should be infused through a catheter port dedicated for this purpose, with no breaks in technique for blood draws or to administer another medication or blood product, to limit infectious complications and interactions. Additional nutrients and medications may be prescribed that the pharmacy can include in the PN formulation if supported by both clinical and pharmaceutical data. For reasons of PN instability or institutional policies, occasionally the lipid portion of the formulation is administered separately from the rest of the PN; in those instances, an infusion pump should be used to administer the lipid dose over at least 20 h. The ideal PN order includes the volume and accompanying rate, and the daily dose of each nutrient requested, with the patient's dosing weight. Transition from PN to EN (or oral diet) requires overlap of both routes, tapering the parenteral infusion rate as the patient tolerates EN. Once the patient tolerates at least 50% of energy and protein requirements by the enteral or oral route, PN can be discontinued.

PN can be initiated at 1 l the first day and advanced to goal by the second or third day as tolerated.

Limit infectious complications and interactions by using a dedicated catheter port for PN.

DOSING AND FORMULATION ISSUES

The dosing of macronutrients and micronutrients via SNS is based on patient requirements and may differ with the route of administration and the formulation, given issues of bioavailability, physiologic regulatory mechanisms, and physicochemical characteristics of enteral or parenteral products.

Macronutrients

Generally, critically ill patients require 25–30 nonprotein kcal/kg and 1.5–2 g protein/kg daily.

General recommendations for dosing macronutrients in critically ill adult patients include 25–30 (nonprotein) kcal/kg/day and 1.5–2 g protein/kg/day regardless of route, although it is less likely that these needs could be met via a peripheral vein. The calories are delivered as carbohydrate and lipid, with dosing limitations of no more than 5–6 g/kg/day and ≤1 g/kg/day, respectively. Fluid maintenance is estimated at 30–35 ml/kg/day, individualized to a patient's fluid balance and solute load. The dosing weight of each patient should be documented in the medical record and on the label of the nutrient formulation. The patient's actual body weight can be used if it is less than or similar to ideal body weight and does not represent recent fluid imbalance. For an obese patient, dosing should be based on a metabolically active weight estimated as [(actual weight − ideal weight)(0.25) + ideal weight]. Of course, changes in fluid status must be taken into account when evaluating recorded weights. The aforementioned dosing guidelines are empiric, based on population parameters. The specific requirements of an individual patient may vary with their clinical state and can be ascertained when clinically necessary. Basal energy requirements can be estimated using the Harris–Benedict predictive equations, which take into account weight, height, age, and gender:

An appropriate dosing weight should be used.

Empiric energy requirements may be estimated by predictive equations or measurements of energy expenditures.

$$\text{Men: } 66.5 + (13.7 \times \text{weight in kg}) + (5 \times \text{height in cm}) - (6 \times \text{age in years})$$

$$\text{Women: } 65.5 + (9.6 \times \text{weight in kg}) + (1.8 \times \text{height in cm}) - (4.7 \times \text{age in years})$$

These equations estimate energy expenditure at rest and necessitate a factor to account for the patient's level of activity and hypermetabolism, which when multiplied with the basal requirement provides an estimate of total energy expended (kcal/day). Factors may be of the order of 1 in the sedated patient to 1.6 in the agitated patient with significant burn injury. Energy requirements can also be based on a calculated expenditure using the Fick equation or measured energy expenditures as determined by indirect calorimetry.

The Fick equation requires use of a functional pulmonary artery catheter for the parameters needed to calculate oxygen consumption ($\dot{V}O_2$). Energy expenditure (kcal/day) is then estimated as $\dot{V}O_2$ (ml/day) × 7. This equation holds best for the hemodynamically stable, spontaneously breathing patient and poorest for unstable, mechanically ventilated patients. Indirect calorimetry is preferred for this patient population.

Indirect calorimetry uses a portable, open-circuit calorimeter to measure the volume and concentration of inspired and expired oxygen and carbon dioxide. The calorimeter uses the data to calculate $\dot{V}O_2$ and carbon dioxide production (VCO_2), which are proportional to substrate utilization and energy expenditure. The relationship has been simplified into the following equation: energy expenditure (kcal/day) = ($\dot{V}O_2$ in l/day) (3.9) + (VCO_2 in l/day) (1.1). The findings from indirect calorimetry should take into account any limitations inherent in the methodology or calorimeter. Limitations may be based on unmet assumptions such as that all O_2 and CO_2 exchange occurs across the lung, is associated with ATP synthesis, and no O_2 or CO_2 is stored or retained. Measuring energy expenditures using indirect calorimetry may be of most benefit in obese critically ill patients or those not responding as expected to empiric dosing of macronutrients.

Empiric protein requirements can be based on nitrogen losses.

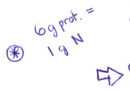

Patient-specific protein dosing can be based on the level of nitrogen elimination, which serves as a marker of the degree of hypercatabolism. The quantity of urea nitrogen eliminated in the urine of a patient with adequate renal function can be used to determine the catabolic index: urinary urea nitrogen (g/day) − [(nitrogen intake (g/day) × 0.5) + 3]. A value of 0–5 indicates mild catabolism and a value >5 indicates severe catabolism requiring higher doses of protein. As steady state is approached following several days of SNS, nitrogen balance can be determined: (nitrogen intake (g/day) − [urinary urea nitrogen (g/day) + 4]. A value of 0 to +4 is ideal, but unrealistic in a critically ill patient. Values better than −10 are considered an interim success in the ICU.

EN products vary in nutrient content, source, and cost.

A large number of commercially prepared enteral formulations exist, varying in nutrient content, nutrient source, osmolality, and cost. Guidelines for use depend on access to the

TABLE 21-1

SELECTED ENTERAL NUTRITION FORMULAS

CATEGORY	PATIENT CHARACTERISTIC	EXAMPLES
Intact:		
Isotonic	Functional gastrointestinal tract	Isocal, Isocal HN, IsoSource, IsoSource HN, Nutren 1.0, Osmolite, Osmolite HN; (fiber containing) Fibersource, FiberSource HN, Jevity, Jevity Plus, Nutren 1.0 with Fiber, ProBalance, Ultracal
Concentrated	Fluid restricted, increased metabolic requirements	Deliver 2.0, Magnacal, Nutren 1.5, Nutren 2.0, ReSource Plus, Two Cal HN
Hydrolyzed:	Maldigestion, malabsorption, or intolerance to intact formulas	AlitraQ, Criticare HN, Crucial, Peptamen, Reabilan, Reabilan HN, Subdue, Vital HN, Vivonex TEN
Disorder Specific:	Critically ill/immune	Advera, AlitraQ, Crucial, ImmunAid, Impact, Perative, Promote, Replete, TraumaCal
	Organ dysfunction	AminAid, HepaticAid II, Magnacal Renal, Nepro, NutriHep, NutriVent, RenalCal, Pulmocare, Respalor
	Diabetes	DiabetiSource, Glucerna, Glytrol

gastrointestinal tract and patient tolerance. The various products can be classified into several categories (Table 21-1). Each health care institution or system carries only a select number of products on their formulary. Intact macronutrient (polymeric) and hydrolyzed macronutrient (monomeric/oligomeric) formulas are always represented. Polymeric formulas are divided into those that are isotonic, some containing fiber, which usually provide about 1 kcal/ml, and those that are more concentrated in calories or protein and often provide 1.2–2 kcal/ml. The more concentrated a formulation is, the less free water it contains, which may be of value in fluid-restricted patients. The hydrolyzed formulas are typically reserved for patients with malabsorption. The role of formulations designed for specific disorders remains unclear on the basis of current data. These specialized products vary in caloric density and composition, including the presence of hydrolyzed macronutrients. A formula is selected that meets a patient's energy, protein, and fluid needs most closely. Additional factors include the patient's past medical history and organ function, as well as the physicochemical characteristics of available enteral formulas.

EN products are selected to most closely meet a patient's requirements.

The PN admixtures are prepared aseptically by a pharmacy from commercially available stock solutions on a daily basis for the ICU patient. Some health care institutions develop standard base formulations that contain amino acids, dextrose, lipids, and water in defined proportions to which the remaining micronutrients are added as clinically necessary and pharmaceutically appropriate. Although somewhat more expensive, parenteral formulations allow the flexibility for meeting patient-specific dosing requirements as stability and compatibility allow. PN formulations can be maximally concentrated when necessary. The choice of specific EN or PN formulations should also consider the patient's organ function.

PN formulations can be manipulated to closely meet a patient's requirements.

Micronutrients

The dosing of electrolytes, vitamins, and trace elements for critically ill adult patients follows general guidelines for use of SNS available in the literature. Tables 21-2 through 21-4 provide guidelines for dosing micronutrients. For enteral dosing, the adult recommended dietary allowance/adequate intake levels established by the Institute of Medicine are used as an initial guide, although they are intended for otherwise healthy individuals obtaining nu-

Micronutrient dosing is based on published guidelines.

TABLE 21-2

DAILY ELECTROLYTE REQUIREMENTS

ELECTROLYTE	ENTERAL	PARENTERAL
Sodium	500 mg (22 mmol)[a]	1–2 mmol/kg
Potassium	2 g (51 mmol)[a]	1–2 mmol/kg
Chloride	750 mg (21 mmol)[a]	As needed to maintain acid–base balance with acetate
Calcium	1200 mg (30 mmol)	5–7.5 mmol
Magnesium	420 mg (17 mmol)	4–10 mmol
Phosphorus	700 mg (23 mmol)	20–40 mmol

[a] Estimated minimal requirements for healthy adults

trients from a mixed oral diet and vary with age and gender. Commercially available EN formulations contain fixed micronutrient levels that often meet guidelines when administered in volumes of 1–3 l daily. Parenteral dosing guidelines are intended for patients with increased requirements. The dosing level for nearly each micronutrient in a PN formulation can be altered if clinically necessary. Individual patient requirements may vary with clinical condition and monitoring parameters.

EN products may contain a greater variety of nutrients than do PN formulations.

Overall nutrient composition differs between EN and PN, with the latter being far from complete. The EN products are much more comprehensive in included nutrients. For example, intravenous lipid products used in the United States for making PN consist of soybean oil, which contains significant amounts of $\omega 6$ fatty acids, considered to be immunosuppressive and enhancers of the stress response. In contrast, EN formulations may contain a better balance of $\omega 6$ and $\omega 3$ fatty acids, which may dampen the response to injury and limit immunosuppression. The clinically relevant ratio or dose of each class of fatty acid is not yet clear.

Pharmacology

Specific nutrients may have a role in modulating the injury response at pharmacologic doses in subgroups of the critically ill.

Use of nutrients for pharmacologic effects rather than meeting nutrient requirements has been termed nutritional pharmacology or nutrient pharmacotherapy. This term refers to tailor-made SNS targeted for a specific pharmacologic effect in a disease process or organ system dysfunction. Immunonutrition describes an aspect of nutrient pharmacotherapy for formulations designed to enhance immune cellularity and function. Although based in large part on immunologic changes in vitro or in vivo, the clinical benefits have begun to be more seriously examined in critically ill patients. As just suggested, certain substrates (lipids, amino acids, micronutrients) may modulate injury response.

TABLE 21-3

DAILY VITAMIN REQUIREMENTS

VITAMIN	ENTERAL	PARENTERAL
Thiamine	1.2 mg	3 mg
Riboflavin	1.3 mg	3.6 mg
Niacin	16 mg	40 mg
Folic acid	400 μg	400 μg
Pantothenic acid	5 mg	15 mg
Vitamin B_6	1.7 mg	4 mg
Vitamin B_{12}	2.4 μg	5 μg
Biotin	30 μg	60 μg
Choline	550 mg	Not well defined
Ascorbic acid	90 mg	100 mg
Vitamin A	700–900 μg	1000 μg
Vitamin D	15 μg	5 μg
Vitamin E	15 mg	10 mg
Vitamin K	90–120 μg	1 mg

TABLE 21-4

DAILY TRACE ELEMENT REQUIREMENTS

TRACE ELEMENT	ENTERAL	PARENTERAL
Chromium	25–35 μg	10–15 μg
Copper	0.9 mg	0.3–0.5 mg
Fluoride	3–4 mg	Not well defined
Iodine	150 μg	Not well defined
Iron	8–18 mg	Not routinely added
Manganese	1.8–2.3 mg	60–100 μg
Molybdenum	45 μg	Not routinely added
Selenium	55 μg	20–60 μg
Zinc	8–11 mg	2.5–5 mg

Some SNS formulations have been enriched with one or more specific substrates for a targeted therapeutic effect, although widespread acceptance is limited by the published data. Most work in using substrate-enriched formulations to enhance patient outcome has been with EN products. The greatest benefit appears to be a reduction in major infectious complications. Data in trauma patients suggest fewer infections, less antibiotic use, fewer days on mechanical ventilation, and shorter length of stay. The specific nutrient and dosing parameters are not yet clear, but benefit seems to require 4–6 days of treatment. Widespread use awaits results from head-to-head trials of various substrate-enriched formulations in defined critically ill subpopulations. Specific nutrients and metabolites include amino acids (e.g., arginine, cysteine, glutamine), fatty acids (e.g., γ-linolenic acid, α-linolenic acid, eicosapentanoic acid, docosahexanoic acid), and others (e.g., nutrient antioxidants, glutathione, ornithine α-ketoglutarate, nucleotides). As with any other therapeutic intervention, vigilant monitoring is necessary to assess progress whether using traditional or substrate-enriched SNS.

MONITORING NUTRITION SUPPORT

Regardless of the route or rationale for providing nutrition support, such patients must be appropriately monitored. Monitoring is an ongoing process in the critically ill patient receiving SNS to assess both efficacy and the potential complications of the regimen. Sub-

Therapeutic and adverse effects of SNS need to be monitored regularly.

CASE STUDY: PART 5

On POD 5, The patient went to the OR yesterday for open drainage of intraabdominal fluid collections (identified on CT scan). Intestinal tissue appeared healthy without anastomotic leak. A dual-lumen, nasojejunal feeding tube was placed intraoperatively above the anastomosis to replace the nasogastric tube. Clinical improvement continued postoperatively, weaning down requirements for norepinephrine; cisatracurium discontinued as ventilatory status improved. Plan to reduce sedation and analgesia as tolerated.

- Vital signs: T_m, 100°F; BP, 105/70; HR, 85/min; PAOP, 14 mmHg; CI, 3.2 l/min; SVR, 920 dyne · s/cm^5.
- Pertinent findings: nasogastric output below 600 ml, abdomen less distended, patient noted to pass flatus, urine output continues to improve, in/out 3600/3200 ml.
- Pertinent lab results: Na, 141 mmol/l; K, 4.2 mmol/l; Cl, 108 mmol/l; CO_2, 22 mmol/l; BUN, 20 mg/dl (UUN 13); Cr, 1.2 mg/dl; glucose, 180 mg/dl; Mg, 2.1 mg/dl; P, 2.4; Ca, 7.7 mg/dl; WBC, 12–14 K/mm^3.
- Nutrition support assessment/plan: The patient has improved clinically, and is less catabolic, based on a catabolic index of 1.5. Although the patient is still unable to initiate an oral diet, an attempt at initiating EN is practical at this time. The enteral access device placed allows small bowel feeding with simultaneous gastric decompression. PN will continue to meet the patient's needs until tolerance of EN can be determined. A concentrated, polymeric formula (1.2 nonprotein kcal/ml, 65 g protein/l) is initiated at 10 ml/h via the nasojejunal tube. The administration rate may be advanced to 20 ml/h after 12 h in the absence of nausea, vomiting, increased intragastric volumes, abdominal distension, cramps, or diarrhea. The patient may be advanced to the goal administration rate of 70 ml/h (providing 2016 nonprotein kcal and 109 g protein). The goal will only provide about 1350 ml of free water; the remaining 850 ml can be provided by IV fluids and/or water flushes via the tube.

jective and objective data are collected at baseline and routinely during the course of therapy as dictated by clinical status. Physical findings including vital signs, hemodynamics, and fluid status are readily available, and the status of the gastrointestinal tract, access devices, and access sites should also be obtained daily. Laboratory findings include a comprehensive metabolic panel at baseline to include serum electrolytes (consider ionized calcium and ionized magnesium if available), serum urea nitrogen, creatinine, glucose, albumin, prealbumin, C-reactive protein, triglycerides, a complete blood count, and INR. Until the patient is stable, obtain serum electrolytes, urea nitrogen, creatinine, and glucose (or fingerstick glucose) on a daily basis. Serum electrolytes should be maintained in the normal range. A weekly serum prealbumin and triglyceride along with body weight is valuable in monitoring the SNS regimen. The arterial blood gas may be used to evaluate pCO_2 as an indicator for excessive caloric dosing with an inability to eliminate the metabolic by-product. Other markers including urinary nitrogen and electrolytes can be obtained as clinically necessary.

Therapeutic Effect

The effect on clinical outcome of providing metabolic substrate, or of modulating the injury response with nutrients, in critically ill patients requires further investigation. The general goal is to maintain or improve nutritional status as determined by body weight and serum protein markers, but in the critically ill patient, supporting metabolism during the injury to limit associated morbidity and mortality is the predominant goal. Benefits that are sought in these patients include improved weaning from mechanical ventilation, wound healing, fewer infections, shorter ICU length of stay, and return to oral diet. More specific markers may include a serum prealbumin above 10–15 mg/dl and a nitrogen balance between −10 and 0 g, although renal dysfunction may falsely elevate both parameters. There appears to be a strong correlation between the C-reactive protein/prealbumin ratio within the first 5 days and severity of subsequent organ dysfunction: best at <1, worse at >4.

Adverse Effects

Address or prevent the complications of SNS, which may be mechanical, infectious, or metabolic.

Complications can occur with both EN and PN. Complications of EN may be classified as mechanical, infectious, metabolic, or gastrointestinal. Complications of PN may be classified as mechanical, infectious, and metabolic. Management of complications is specific to the varied etiologies and patient variables.

The access device used for EN may cause local irritation, be misplaced or become dislodged, alter the risk for aspiration, become clogged, or be involved in gastrointestinal obstruction. The EN formulations are excellent growth media for microorganisms and care should be taken when administering them (e.g., discard remaining formula, bag, and administration

CASE STUDY: PART 6

POD 7, the patient is resting comfortably while completing his course of antimicrobials. He has been weaned from vasopressors and continuous infusion sedation and analgesia, requiring only intermittent IV doses. A ventilator weaning trial is under way. The patient continues a similar PN formulation at 42 ml/h, while also continuing EN at 55 ml/h.

- Vital signs: T_m, 99°F; BP, 132/84; HR, 94/min; RR, 18/min.
- Pertinent findings: nasogastric output minimal today on intermittent suction; the abdomen is nontender, nondistended; two stools passed yesterday; incisional wound is healing well; urine output is adequate, fluid in/out 2900/2500 ml.
- Pertinent lab results: Na, 142 mmol/l; K, 4 mmol/l; Cl, 106 mmol/l; CO_2, 28 mmol/l; BUN, 20 mg/dl; Cr, 1 mg/dl; glucose, 172 mg/dl; Mg, 2.2 mg/dl; P, 2.5; Ca, 7.8 mg/dl; WBC, 10 K/mm^3.
- Nutrition support assessment/plan: The patient continues to require SNS to maintain nutritional status as the inflammatory response resolves. He is tolerating the enteral route, now at 80% of goal dosing. The PN may be discontinued to avoid overfeeding and associated hypercarbia, which may hinder weaning from the ventilator. Once the patient has been successfully extubated, the enteral device may be removed, and the patient may begin a trial of oral soft diet and liquids. If he has no difficulty in swallowing, he can be advanced to a normal healthy diet.

set every 8–12 h; do not add anything to the formulation or access the feeding tube unnecessarily). Metabolic complications include poor glycemic control, and dehydration often manifests with rising serum sodium and urea nitrogen/creatinine ratio. Patients with severe malnutrition are particularly at risk for the refeeding syndrome in which drastic intracellular shifts of potassium, magnesium, and phosphorus occur acutely following reinstitution of feeding (enteral or parenteral) to support tissue anabolism. Adverse gastrointestinal effects include nausea, vomiting, elevated gastric residual volumes, abdominal cramps, bloating, distension, constipation, and diarrhea.

Both the mechanical and infectious adverse effects associated with PN result from the intravenous access device and can be significant. Complications include pneumothorax, hemothorax, vascular injury, air emboli, fracture, thrombosis, malposition, and line-related infection. Metabolic complications to be prevented or managed include hypertriglyceridemia (triglycerides >400 mg/dl), hyperglycemia (glucose >150–180 mg/dl), electrolyte abnormalities, gallbladder stasis, and gut atrophy.

SUMMARY

Specialized nutrition support can play a significant role in managing selected critically ill patients. When appropriate, the nutrition support regimen should be optimized in terms of timing, route, and dosing to maximize the benefits and minimize complications. Available nutrition support expertise in the institution should be utilized, whether as a formal consulting service or an individual physician, dietitian, nurse, or pharmacist. Regardless of the route or rationale for providing SNS to critically ill patients, this pharmacotherapeutic modality must be monitored for both therapeutic and adverse effects. Placing nutrition support as a priority and being vigilant in its appropriate use may help identify individual patient and population outcomes.

REVIEW QUESTIONS

1. **Physiologic changes in the body in response to injury include:**
   - A. Increased serum glucagon
   - B. Increased serum cortisol
   - C. Increased lipolysis
   - D. Increased protein catabolism
   - E. All of the above

2. **Nutritional support is indicated in each of the following ICU patient situations except:**
   - A. Poor premorbid nutritional status and nil per os for 7 days since admission
   - B. Adequate premorbid nutritional status and expected to eat within 5 days of admission
   - C. Adequate premorbid nutritional status, now with multiple organ dysfunction following extensive small bowel resection
   - D. Poor premorbid nutritional status, now ICU day 4 following severe head injury

3. **The best time to initiate nutrition support in a burn or trauma patient who is unable to improve nutritional status on their own is:**
   - A. Before the patient is hemodynamically stable
   - B. Within 48 h of the injury
   - C. After 5 days of conventional management
   - D. Following completion of any antibiotic regimens

4. **The major determinant of the route of administration chosen for nutrition support is:**
   - A. Function of the GI tract
   - B. Cost of therapy
   - C. Anticipated duration of therapy
   - D. None of the above

5. **The appropriate amount of nonprotein calories to provide empirically in a critically ill patient who has no known glucose or lipid disorders is:**
   - A. 2000–2200 kcal/day
   - B. 100–120 kcal/kg
   - C. 25–30 kcal/kg/day
   - D. 5–6 kcal/kg/day

6. **Which of the following adverse effects may be associated with either enteral or parenteral nutrition therapy?**
   - A. Hyperglycemia
   - B. Hypokalemia
   - C. Hypertriglyceridemia
   - D. Hypomagnesemia
   - E. All of the above

ANSWERS

1. The answer is E. The typical neurohormonal response of the body during period of stress or body injury is characterized by increased blood levels of stress hormones, including glucagon and cortisol. Fat is mobilized via lipolysis as an alternative fuel source.
2. The answer is B. In patients with adequate nutritional status, withholding nutritional support for a few days has no negative clinical effect, especially if they are expected to eat within a few days. In all other patient situations, such as inpatients who have poor premorbid nutritional status before hospitalization (choice A), those in a hypermetabolic state such as patients with multiorgan dysfunction (C), and patients who are expected to have a protracted recovery, early nutritional support is recommended.
3. The answer is B. In patients with severe injury as in multiple trauma, severe burn, or sepsis, nutritional support is recommended as soon as hemodynamic stability is achieved.
4. The answer is A. Enteral nutrition is preferred if gastrointestinal function is intact to maintain gut integrity and prevent bacterial translocation. Moreover, the risks associated with central venous access (infection, thrombosis, bleeding, pain) required for total parenteral nutrition are avoided.
5. The answer is A. In patients who are critically ill, the amount of nonprotein calories is adjusted higher commensurate with the level of stress. Providing adequate nonprotein calories promotes the utilization of proteins for rebuilding the body instead of being utilized as a fuel source.
6. The answer is E. Hypokalemia, hypomagnesemia, and hypophosphatemia may occur during the refeeding syndrome or because of inadequate replacement of electrolytes. Hypertriglyceridemia may occur during lipid infusion, especially in patients with diabetes mellitus or pancreatic insufficiency. Hyperglycemia commonly occurs in ICU patients as a result of elevated stress hormones.

SUGGESTED READING

A.S.P.E.N. Board of Directors. Guidelines for the use of enteral and parenteral nutrition in adult and pediatric patients. J Parent Enter Nutr 2001;25:(in press).

Beale RJ, Bryg DJ, Bihari DJ. Immunonutrition in the critically ill: a routine review of clinical outcome. Crit Care Med 1999;27:2799–2805.

Cerra FB, Benitez MR, Blackburn GL, et al. Applied nutrition in ICU patients. A consensus statement of the American College of Chest Physicians. Chest 1997;111:769–778.

Hawker FH. How to feed patients with sepsis. Curr Opin Crit Care 2000;6:247–252.

Kinney JM. Metabolic responses of the critically ill patient. Crit Care Clin 1995;11:569–585.

Lipman TO. Grains or veins: is enteral nutrition better than parenteral nutrition? A look at the evidence. J Parent Enter Nutr 1998;22:167–182.

Rombeau JL, Rolandelli RH (eds) Clinical Nutrition: Enteral and Tube Feeding, 3rd Ed. Philadelphia: Saunders, 1997.

Rombeau JL, Rolandelli RH (eds) Clinical Nutrition: Parenteral Nutrition, 3rd Ed. Philadelphia: Saunders, 2000.

Souba WW. Nutritional support. N Engl J Med 1997;336:41–48.

CHAPTER 22

Joseph Crocetti and Samuel Krachman

Oxygen Content, Delivery, and Uptake

CHAPTER OUTLINE

LEARNING OBJECTIVES

After studying this chapter, you should be able to:

- Understand the principal determinants of oxygen content and appreciate the concepts of oxygen delivery and consumption.
- Understand the normal physiologic relationship between oxygen delivery and consumption.
- Understand oxygen supply dependency in critically ill patients.
- Understand goal-directed therapy and the controversies that surround it.

Normal cellular function in the body is critically dependent on oxygen. Therefore, it is important for the body to be able to deliver oxygen to the cells and for the cells to utilize the oxygen once it has arrived. A change in either of these variables could lead to the development of cellular hypoxia and result in end-organ failure and possibly death. In many disease states, changes in oxygen delivery (DO_2) and oxygen consumption ($\dot{V}O_2$) are noted to occur and may be responsible for the clinical presentation of these patients. Meeting the metabolic demands of the cells is thus an important component of therapy in the critically ill patient.

A change in oxygen delivery or consumption can result in cellular hypoxia.

OXYGEN UTILIZATION

At the cellular level, the most efficient means of generating ATP is through oxidative phosphorylation, which is a series of oxidation–reduction reactions in which oxygen serves as the terminal electron acceptor (Figure 22-1). In the absence of oxygen the cell must depend on glycolysis, which is a very inefficient process to generate ATP, or depend on limited high-

CASE STUDY: PART 1

G.C. is a 47-year-old alcoholic college professor who complained of 2 days of shaking chills, fever, cough productive of yellow sputum, and left-sided chest pain. Initial examination in the emergency room revealed an acutely appearing man with a respiratory rate of 36, pulse of 122, and blood pressure of 90/42. His initial chest radiograph showed a left lower lobe infiltrate; arterial blood gas analysis demonstrated a metabolic acidosis and a respiratory alkalosis. His CBC was significant for a WBC of 22.0 with 24% bands and hemoglobin of 10. The patient was treated empirically for community-acquired pneumonia with a third-generation cephalosporin and given 2 liters of normal saline intravenously.

energy stores in the body such as creatine phosphate. The critical level of oxygen required by the cells for oxidative phosphorylation is unknown, yet it has been shown that mitochondria can continue to function normally so long as the partial pressure of oxygen (PO_2) is maintained at greater than 0.5 mmHg. In intact animals and in humans, the critical level of oxygen appears to be an arterial PO_2 (P_aO_2) of 20 mmHg, as evidenced by changes in end-organ function and changes in the level of ATP. Such findings suggest that humans are able to tolerate severe hypoxia before cellular and end-organ dysfunction develop. In disease states such as sepsis or in the acute respiratory distress syndrome (ARDS), however, cellular hypoxia and end-organ dysfunction can occur at much higher levels of P_aO_2, possibly because of the changes in DO_2 and oxygen utilization at a mitochondrial level that occur with these disorders.

> The critical level of oxygen in normal humans is P_aO_2 of 20 mmHg.

> In disease states, cellular hypoxia occurs at higher values of P_aO_2.

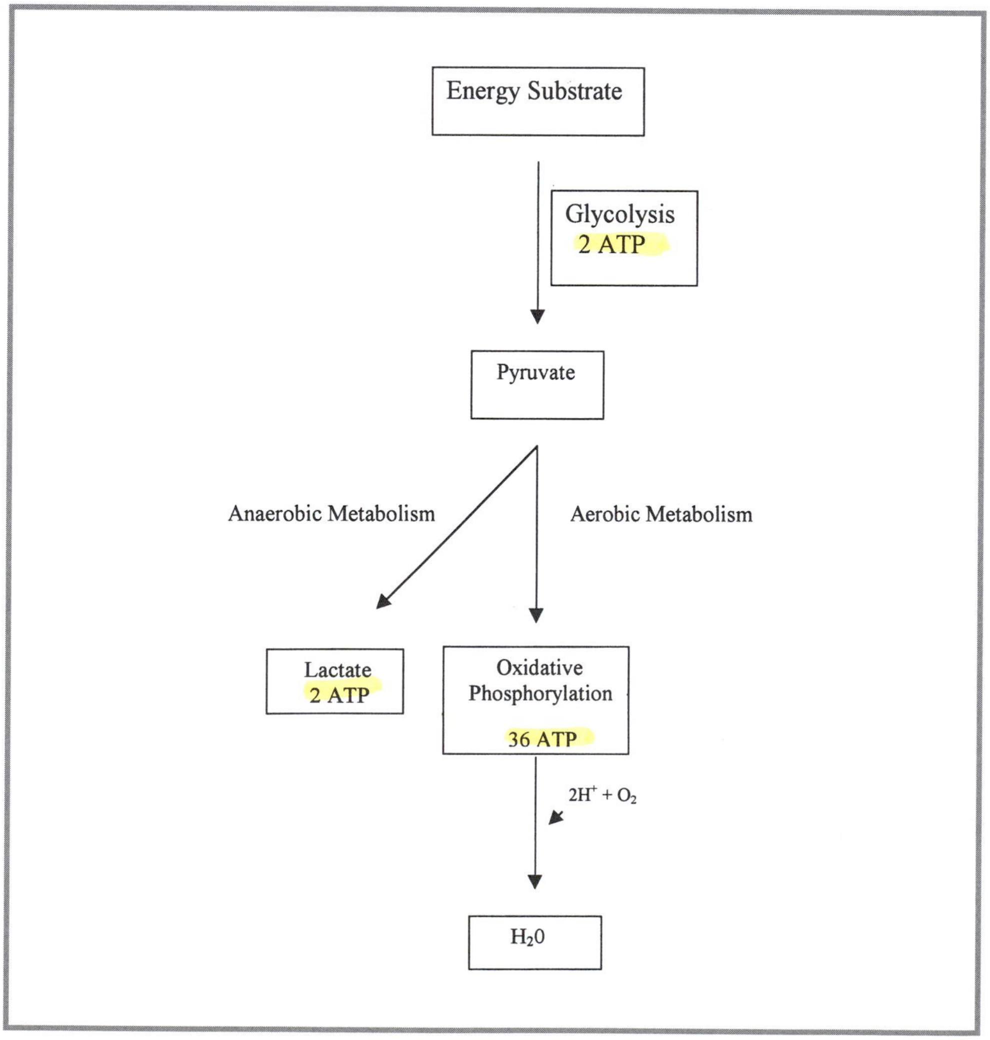

FIGURE 22-1

At the cellular level, the most efficient means of generating ATP is through oxidative phosphorylation, which is a series of oxidation–reduction reactions in which oxygen serves as the terminal electron acceptor. Under anaerobic conditions, pyruvate is converted to lactate, which is a very inefficient mechanism for ATP production.

TABLE 22-1

DISTRIBUTION OF BLOOD FLOW AND OXYGEN UTILIZATION

ORGAN	CARDIAC OUTPUT (l/min)	OXYGEN DELIVERY (ml/min)	OXYGEN UPTAKE (ml/min)	RESISTANCE (mmHg/min)
Brain	14	840	52	7
Heart	5	300	34	20
Splanchnic bed	28	1680	83	3.6
Kidney	23	1380	19	4.4
Skeletal Muscle	16	960	57	6.3
Skin	8	480	12	12.4

OXYGEN REQUIREMENTS OF THE VARIOUS TISSUES

Each organ system in the body has different oxygen requirements that must be met to function properly and maintain normal homeostasis (Table 22-1). To meet the oxygen demands of the different organ systems, changes occur in cardiac output and microcirculatory flow. The microcirculatory system consists of the arterioles, capillaries, and the venous system. Although 80% of the blood in circulation is stored in the venous system, local control of DO_2 to the organ systems occurs at two levels: (1) the small muscular arterioles, which are the major resistance vessels in the body and dilate in response to tissue hypoxia; and (2) the precapillary sphincters, which regulate the number of capillaries that are available for gas diffusion into the tissue cells. It would be ideal if we could directly measure the DO_2 to each organ system to ensure that it is adequate. Unfortunately, this is not possible, and at present we can only obtain measurements of total body DO_2 and $\dot{V}O_2$ and thereby indirectly assess overall body oxygen requirements from these less sensitive and specific values.

Local control of DO_2 occurs at the arterioles and precapillary sphincters.

OXYGEN CONTENT

The oxygen content of arterial blood (CaO_2) is the sum of two components, the oxygen bound to hemoglobin and the oxygen dissolved in blood:

$$CaO_2 = (1.3 \times Hb \times SaO_2) + (0.003 \times PaO_2)$$

where Hb is hemoglobin, SaO_2 is the arterial oxygen saturation, and PaO_2 is the arterial partial pressure of oxygen. The first part of the equation states that each 1 g of hemoglobin binds 1.3 ml of oxygen when the hemoglobin is completely saturated ($SaO_2 = 100\%$). The second part of the equation measures the amount of oxygen that is actually dissolved in the blood, which is of the order of 0.003 (ml/dl/mmHg). As can be seen, under normal physiologic conditions the oxygen that is dissolved in the blood contributes little to CaO_2. Most of the oxygen in the blood is bound to hemoglobin, and thus SaO_2 is the most important blood gas variable for assessing the CaO_2 of arterial blood. Assuming a Hb of 14 g/dl, SaO_2 of 98%, and a PaO_2 of 100 mmHg, CaO_2 (Table 22-2) can be calculated as:

Most of the oxygen in the blood is bound to hemoglobin.

$$CaO_2 = (1.3 \text{ ml/g} \times 14 \text{ g/dl} \times 0.98) + [0.003 \text{ (ml/dl)/mmHg} \times 100 \text{ mmHg}]$$

$$CaO_2 = 18.1 \text{ ml/dl}$$

OXYGEN DELIVERY

Global oxygen delivery is calculated as the product of the cardiac output (Q) and the CaO_2:

$$DO_2 = Q \times CaO_2 \quad \text{or} \quad DO_2 = Q \times (1.3 \times Hb \times SaO_2) \times 10$$

where DO_2 is oxygen delivery and Q is cardiac output. The equation is multiplied by 10 to convert volumes percent to ml/min. A DO_2 index (DO_2I) can be calculated by substituting

***

TABLE 22-2

OXYGEN DELIVERY AND CONSUMPTION VARIABLES

VARIABLES	EQUATION	NORMAL VALUE
Oxygen content (CaO_2)	$CaO_2 = (1.3xHbxSaO_2) \times (0.003xPaO_2)$	16–22 ml/dl
Mixed venous content ($C\bar{v}O_2$)	$M\bar{v}O_2 = (1.3xHbxSvO_2) \times (0.003xP\bar{v}O_2)$	12–17 ml/dl
Oxygen delivery (DO_2)	$DO_2 = QxCaO_2$	460–650 ml/min
Oxygen uptake ($\dot{V}O_2$)	$\dot{V}O_2 = Qx(CaO_2 - C\bar{v}O_2)$	96–170 ml/min
Oxygen extraction ratio (O_2ER)	$O_2ER = \dot{V}O_2/DO_2$ $O_2ER = CaO_2 - C\bar{v}O_2/CaO_2$	22%–32%
Arterial oxygen tension (PaO_2)	Measured	95 ± 5 mmHg
Arterial saturation (SaO_2)	Measured	$97\% \pm 2\%$
Mixed venous oxygen tension ($P\bar{v}O_2$)	Measured	40 ± 5 mmHg
Mixed venous saturation ($M\bar{v}O_2$)	Measured	$75\% \pm 5\%$
Systemic vascular resistance (SVR)	(Mean arterial pressure – central venous pressure)/Qx80	800–1200 dyne/s/cm^{-5}
Pulmonary vascular resistance (PVR)	(Mean pulmonary artery pressure – pulmonary wedge pressure)/Qx80	150–250 dyne/s/m^{-5}

the cardiac index (CI) for the cardiac output, which is simply the cardiac output divided by the body surface area (BSA):

$$DO_2I = Q/BSA \times (1.3 \times Hb \times SaO_2) \times 10$$

Assuming a cardiac output of 5 l/min, hemoglobin of 14 g/dl, and SaO_2 of 98%, a normal DO_2 (see Table 22-2) can be calculated as:

$$DO_2 = 5 \text{ l/min} \times (1.3 \text{ ml/g} \times 14 \text{ g/dl} \times 0.98\%) \times 10 \text{ (scaling factor)}$$

$$DO_2 = 900 \text{ ml/min}$$

Using a cardiac index of 3 l/min, a normal DO_2I (Table 22-2) can be calculated as:

$$DO_2I = 3 \text{ l/min/m}^2 \times (1.3 \text{ ml/g} \times 14 \text{ g/dl} \times 0.98\%) \times 10 \text{ (scaling factor)}$$

$$DO_2I = 540 \text{ ml/min} \cdot \text{m}^2$$

Thus, from the foregoing equation it can be seen that oxygen delivery is simply the product of three main variables: arterial oxygen saturation, hemoglobin, and cardiac output.

Oxygen delivery is the product of arterial oxygen saturation, hemoglobin, and cardiac output.

OXYGEN CONSUMPTION

Oxygen consumption is defined as the quantity of oxygen consumed per unit time. Total body $\dot{V}O_2$ can be measured by two different techniques: the reverse Fick equation or indirect calorimetry using a metabolic cart. $\dot{V}O_2$ can be affected by many variables, including fever, anxiety, pain, and shivering, and thus it is important for the patient to be relatively stable at the time the measurements are obtained.

VO_2 can be measured by the reversed Fick equation or by indirect calorimetry.

The indirect Fick equation calculates $\dot{V}O_2$ by using the equation:

$$\dot{V}O_2 = Q \text{ l/min} \times (CaO_2 \text{ ml/dl} - C\bar{v}O_2 \text{ ml/dl})$$

where Q is cardiac output and $CaO_2 - C\bar{v}O_2$ is the arteriovenous difference in oxygen content. $C\bar{v}O_2$ is the venous oxygen content $[(1.3 \text{ ml/g} \times Hg \times S\bar{v}O_2\%)]$ and $S\bar{v}O_2$ is the saturation of venous blood. The indirect Fick method is usually employed in critically ill patients through the use of a pulmonary artery catheter. The cardiac output is determined by thermodilution technique. Mixed venous oxygen saturation ($S\bar{v}O_2$) is determined by a blood sample from the distal port of the pulmonary artery catheter; and SaO_2 is obtained by co-oximetery. The equation can be rearranged as:

$$\dot{V}O_2 = Q \text{ l/min} \times (1.3 \text{ ml/g} \times Hb \text{ g/dl}) \times (SaO_2\% - S\bar{v}O_2\%)$$

Using a cardiac output of 5 l/min, hemoglobin of 14 g/dl, SaO_2 of 98%, and $S\bar{v}O_2$ of 75%, a normal $\dot{V}O_2$ (see Table 22-2) can be calculated as

$$\dot{V}O_2 = 5 \text{ l/min} \times (1.3 \text{ ml/g} \times 14 \text{ g/dl}) \times (0.98 - 0.75) \times 10 \text{ (scaling factor)}$$

$$\dot{V}O_2 = 244 \text{ ml/min}$$

The equation is again multiplied by 10 to convert volumes percent to ml/min.

Indirect calorimetry uses a metabolic cart to obtain measurements of expired gas volumes of both O_2 and CO_2 and then calculate $\dot{V}O_2$ according to the formula:

$$\dot{V}O_2 = (F_iO_2 \times V_I) - (F_EO_2 \times V_E)$$

where F_iO_2 is the fraction of inspired oxygen, V_I is the inspired minute volume, F_EO_2 is the mixed expired oxygen concentration, and V_E is the expired minute volume. As is discussed later, this method has the advantage of actually measuring rather than calculating $\dot{V}O_2$ as is done using the indirect Fick method. Although indirect calorimetry may be more accurate in obtaining the $\dot{V}O_2$, it is also more cumbersome at the bedside and thus is not frequently done in the intensive care unit setting.

OXYGEN EXTRACTION RATIO

The oxygen extraction ratio reflects the tissue's avidity for oxygen.

The oxygen extraction ratio (O_2ER) is the fractional uptake of oxygen by the tissues from the capillary bed and thus reflects the tissue's avidity for oxygen. Under normal physiologic conditions, the tissues extract about 25% of the oxygen that is bound to hemoglobin in the circulation. A normal extraction ratio of 25% results in a $S\bar{v}O_2$ of 75%. The extraction ratio can be calculated as:

$$O_2ER = CaO_2 - C\bar{v}O_2/CaO_2 \times 100$$

$$0.25 = (20 \text{ ml/dl} - 15 \text{ ml/dl})/20 \text{ ml/dl}$$

where O_2ER is oxygen extraction ratio, CaO_2 is arterial oxygen content, and $C\bar{v}O_2$ is venous oxygen content. Another equation that can be used to calculate the oxygen extraction ratio is

$$O_2ER = \dot{V}O_2/DO_2 \times 100$$

If a normal $\dot{V}O_2$ of 250 (ml/min)/m^2 and DO_2 of 1000 (ml/min)/m^2 are assumed, a normal oxygen extraction ratio (Table 22-2) can be calculated as

$$O_2ER = 250 \text{ (ml/min)/m}^2/1000 \text{ (ml/min)/m}^2 \times 100$$

$$O_2ER = 0.25 \text{ (ml/min)/m}^2$$

NORMAL PHYSIOLOGIC RELATIONSHIP BETWEEN DO_2 AND $\dot{V}O_2$

Under normal conditions, DO_2 is determined by the oxygen requirements of the tissue cells and thus their $\dot{V}O_2$. Increases in cellular metabolic demand, as seen during exercise, are met by increases in both cardiac output and local perfusion to the associated organs. At maximal exercise, DO_2 can increase to 4 to 5 times the resting level. This increase in DO_2 may not be sufficient to meet the cellular demands for oxygen, however, with increases to as high as 10 fold during maximal exercise. The cells attempt to compensate for this inadequate DO_2 by increasing their oxygen extraction from a basal level of 25% to as high as 80% during maximal exercise, but at some point the oxygen demands of the cells can no longer be met and anaerobic metabolism begins. This point is referred to as the anaerobic threshold, and

CASE STUDY: PART 2

Despite volume resuscitation, the patient developed worsening hypotension with a blood pressure of 70/40 mm/Hg. The patient's urine output decreased, and his work of breathing increased requiring mechanical ventilation. A Swan–Ganz catheter was then placed, which showed right atrial pressure, 6 mmHg; pulmonary artery pressure, 16/10 mmHg; and pulmonary capillary wedge pressure (PCWP), 12 mmHg. Cardiac output was elevated at 8 l/min, systemic vascular resistance was decreased at 510 ml/kg/min, and mixed venous saturation was 68%; oxygen content was 12.8 ml/100 ml, oxygen delivery was 1024 ml/min, oxygen uptake was 300 ml/kg/min, and oxygen extraction ratio was 30%.

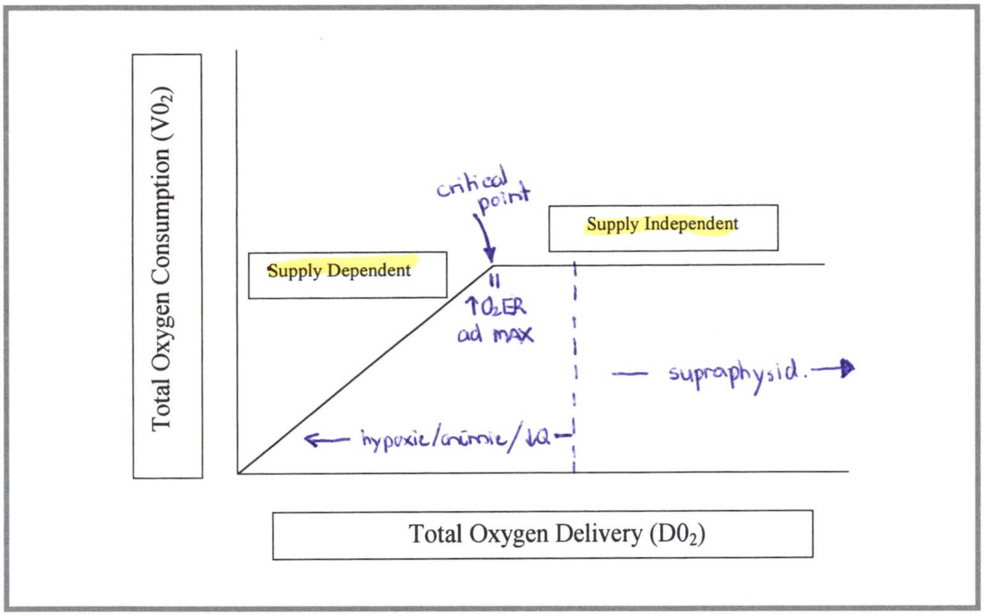

FIGURE 22-2

When DO_2 is the independent variable, $\dot{V}O_2$ remains unchanged in response to an increase in DO_2 (as with inotropic medications increasing cardiac output) for the oxygen supply to the cells is already adequate (supply independent). When DO_2 is decreased (as with anemia or a decreased cardiac output), however, a biphasic response in $\dot{V}O_2$ is observed. Initially, as DO_2 decreases the cells respond by increasing oxygen extraction to maintain $\dot{V}O_2$. A point is reached at which the cells can no longer increase their extraction of oxygen (critical DO_2), and $\dot{V}O_2$ becomes dependent on DO_2 (supply dependent).

in normal individuals it can occur when $\dot{V}O_2$ is as low as 40% of maximum. The inefficient use of anaerobic sources of ATP leads to the production of such by-products as lactate and the development of a metabolic acidosis. Thus, under normal conditions $\dot{V}O_2$ is the independent variable with changes in DO_2 occurring in response to the oxygen needs of the tissue.

> The anaerobic threshold occurs when the oxygen demands of the cells are no longer being met.

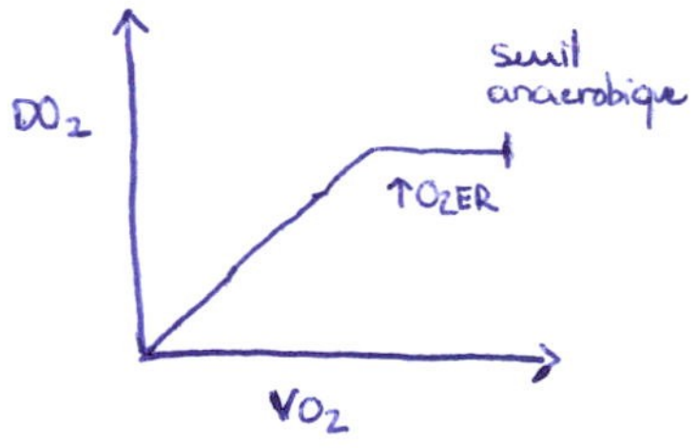

A different relationship between DO_2 and $\dot{V}O_2$ can be observed in situations where DO_2 is the independent variable; this occurs when DO_2 is either decreased, as with anemia, hypoxemia, or decreased cardiac output, or increased, as when cardiac output is increased with inotropic medications. Under these conditions, a biphasic relationship between $\dot{V}O_2$ and DO_2 is observed (Figure 22-2). In normal individuals, increases in DO_2 do not result in a significant increase in $\dot{V}O_2$ because the cells do not require any additional oxygen. When DO_2 decreases, the cells initially are able to compensate by increasing oxygen extraction to meet their metabolic demands. Yet, as DO_2 decreases further a point is reached, referred to as the "critical point" (DO_2 crit), where maximal oxygen extraction can no longer meet cell oxygen demands and $\dot{V}O_2$ begins to decrease linearly with DO_2; this is referred to as supply dependency. In healthy animal models in which DO_2 was slowly decreased, values for DO_2 crit have been found to be 6–10 ml/kg/min.

OXYGEN SUPPLY DEPENDENCY IN THE CRITICALLY ILL

> The normal biphasic relationship in DO_2 and $\dot{V}O_2$ is not observed in the critically ill.

In contrast to normal animals where supply dependency is noted only at very low values of DO_2, critically ill patients with sepsis and ARDS demonstrate supply dependency at much higher levels of DO_2. In addition, the normal biphasic relationship between DO_2 and $\dot{V}O_2$ is not observed (Figure 22-3). A number of mechanisms have been proposed to explain the linear relationship between DO_2 and $\dot{V}O_2$ observed in these patients. One such scheme suggests that the DO_2 crit is much higher than normal in these critically ill patients. Because of their disease state, these patients may not be able to increase DO_2 sufficiently to reach the supply-independent portion of the curve; a point where the increased oxygen demands of the cells can be met. Another explanation proposed for the observed supply dependency is the inability of cells to adequately increase extraction of oxygen to meet the increased demand. In other words, the extraction ratio remains unchanged whether DO_2 increases or decreases, and thus the relationship between DO_2 and $\dot{V}O_2$ remains linear (Figure 22-3). This

FIGURE 22-3

The *dotted line* represents pathologic supply dependency observed in patients with sepsis or the acute respiratory distress syndrome (ARDS). Oxygen consumption is observed to be continuously dependent on oxygen delivery with no evidence of a critical DO_2, above which a supply-independent state would exist.

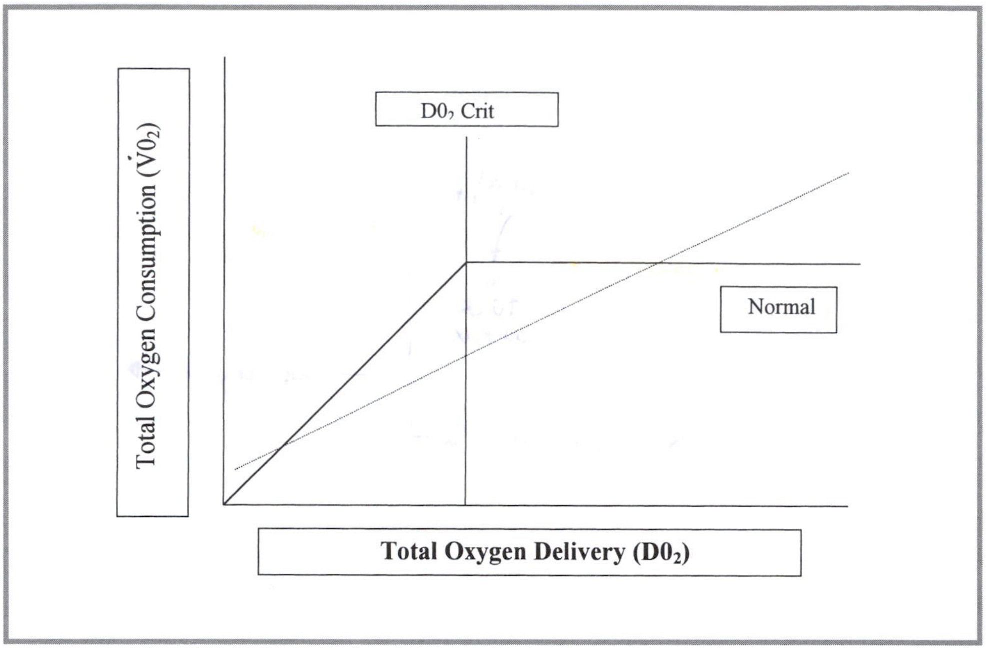

Impaired O_2 extraction may result from direct endothelial or parenchymal cell injury.

inability to increase oxygen extraction can result from two main mechanisms: (1) alteration in organ blood flow distribution and (2) direct endothelial or parenchymal tissue injury.

Alteration in Blood Flow Distribution

An altered blood flow to the capillary beds could produce changes in the DO_2–$\dot{V}O_2$ relationship similar to that observed in sepsis by means of several mechanisms, including a redistribution of cardiac output to organs with low oxygen extraction ratios. This change can occur when there is loss of the normal microvascular tone and the major muscular arterioles are no longer able to control blood flow distribution to the organs with the highest oxygen requirements (Figure 22-4). Changes can also occur in the precapillary sphincters that control local organ blood flow. Despite compelling clinical evidence, neither of the proposed mechanisms for altered organ blood flow has been observed in animal models of septic shock.

FIGURE 22-4

Alteration in blood flow distribution may lead to a decrease in blood flow to organs with increased oxygen demands, which may contribute to a state of supply dependency. (Reprinted with permission from Dorinsky PM, Gadek JE. Mechanisms of multiple nonpulmonary organ failure in ARDS. Chest 1989;96:885–892).

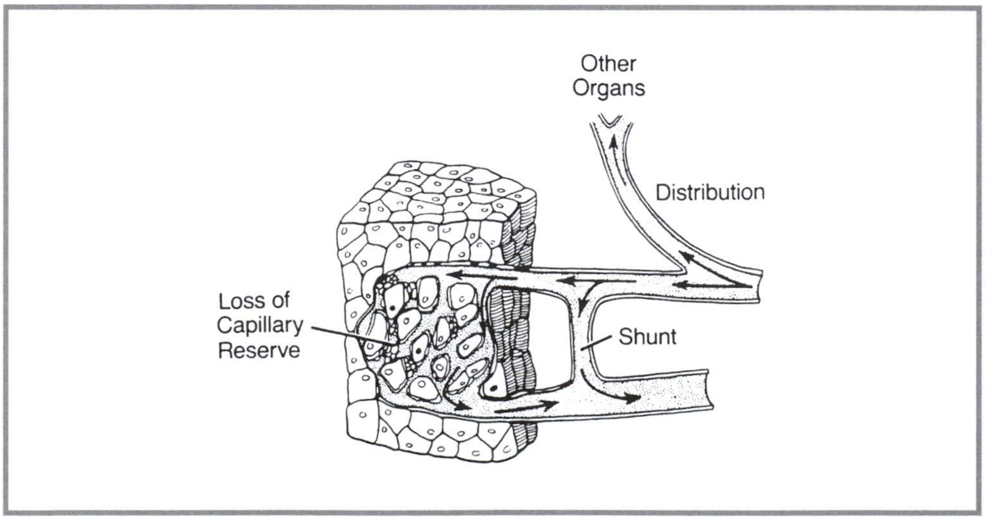

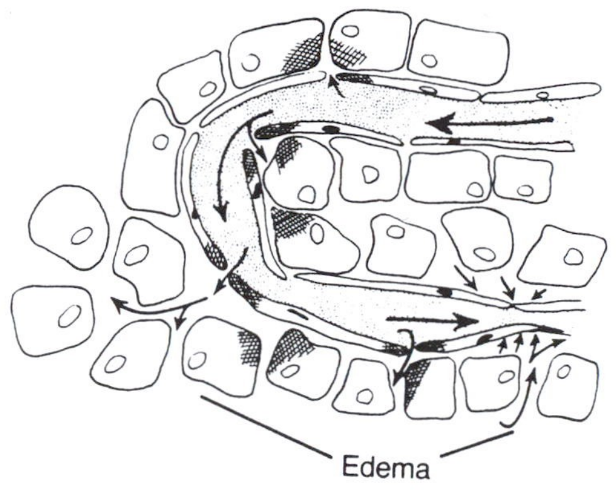

FIGURE 22-5

Oxygen extraction may be impaired secondary to endothelial or parenchymal cell injury, which may lead to a state of supply dependency. (Reprinted with permission from Dorinsky PM, Gadek JE. Mechanisms of multiple nonpulmonary organ failure in ARDS. Chest 1989;96:885–892).

Endothelial and Parenchymal Injury

Direct injury to the endothelium can impair the ability of the cells to directly extract oxygen from the blood (Figure 22-5). This impairment can occur in disease states that cause a systemic inflammatory response, such as sepsis and ARDS. The normal mixed venous oxygen levels observed in these disease states could be explained by this mechanism. Despite an apparently adequate DO_2, the injured endothelium cannot extract the amount of oxygen needed to meet cellular demand. Another proposed mechanism involves direct injury to the parenchymal cells themselves, which may impair oxygen utilization at any level of DO_2.

Studies Demonstrating Oxygen Supply Dependency

Earlier animal studies demonstrated that sepsis and not isolated lung injury was responsible for the apparent oxygen supply dependency. In dog models, it was shown that both bacteremia and endotoxemia, but not isolated lung injury, were responsible for the significantly increased DO_2 crit from 8 to 12 ml/kg/min. More important, the oxygen extraction ratio at the point where oxygen consumption became supply dependent fell from 70% to 51% in the bacteremic dogs. This result suggests a problem with end-organ tissue oxygen utilization rather than a primary respiratory process. Since these early animal experiments there have been numerous studies in patients with respiratory failure and sepsis demonstrating oxygen supply dependency.

Bahari et al. studied the effects of increasing DO_2 in 27 critically ill ARDS patients. In those patients who died, there was a significant increase in $\dot{V}O_2$ and O_2 ER in response to an increase in DO_2, whereas there was only a small increase in $\dot{V}O_2$ and an actual decrease in O_2ER in those who survived (Figure 22-6). This finding suggested an existing oxygen debt in those patients who died, with the tissue cells deprived of the required oxygen needed for optimum aerobic metabolism. In contrast, those patients who survived appeared to have adequate oxygen delivery to the cells for aerobic metabolism and thus remained on the supply-independent portion of the DO_2–$\dot{V}O_2$ curve. Other investigators have noted that additional markers suggesting an existing oxygen debt, such as the presence of a metabolic acidosis or increased serum lactate, predicted an oxygen supply-dependent state.

Thus, based on clinical studies suggesting the existence of an oxygen supply-dependent state in critically ill patients, treatment strategies were designed with the aim of increasing DO_2 to supranormal values. It was hoped that by correcting any existing oxygen debt, multisystem organ failure could be prevented and mortality decreased.

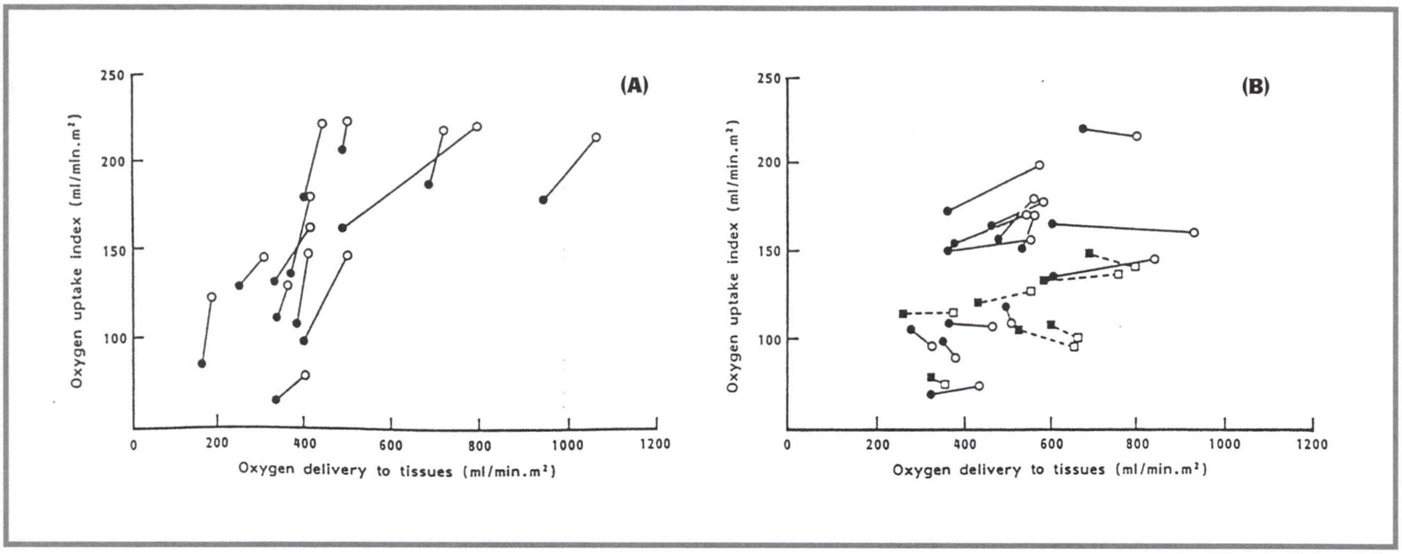

FIGURE 22-6

Effects of prostacyclin infusion on oxygen delivery and oxygen uptake in 27 patients with acute respiratory failure (*circles*) and 7 controls (*squares*). In the 13 patients who died **(A)**, there was a significant increase in oxygen uptake in response to an increase in oxygen delivery. A similar increase in oxygen uptake was not seen in those patients who survived, as well as the controls **(B)**. (Reprinted with permission from Bihari D, Smithies M, Gimson A, Tinker J. The effects of vasodilation with prostacyclin on oxygen delivery and uptake in critically ill patients. N Engl J Med 1987;317:397–405).

GOAL-DIRECTED THERAPY

In the early 1970s, Shoemaker et al. described a group of critically ill surgical patients with improved survival when supranormal values for DO_2 and $\dot{V}O_2$ were observed. Since then, studies have been designed for goal-directed therapy in which DO_2 and $\dot{V}O_2$ are increased to these previously noted supranormal values. This approach is based on three tenets: (1) that critically ill patients die of multisystem organ failure and that tissue hypoxia may be partially responsible for its development; (2) that tissue hypoxia may persist in critically ill patients despite early resuscitation to normal hemodynamic endpoints; and (3) that increasing oxygen delivery can reverse tissue hypoxia. Since this original observation by Shoemaker et al. there have been 13 randomized trials to evaluate goal-directed therapy. Six studies demonstrated favorable results, but most concerned trauma or surgical patients, and supranormal values for DO_2 and $\dot{V}O_2$ were obtained before hemodynamic compromise or the development of organ dysfunction. There is also concern in that improved outcome was based on a post hoc comparison of subgroups of patients who were able to reach supranormal values for DO_2 and $\dot{V}O_2$ regardless of whether they received goal-directed therapy to achieve these supranormal values.

There have also been seven studies in critically ill medical and surgical patients that failed to demonstrate improved survival with goal-directed therapy. In fact, in one study the control group actually had a lower mortality than the goal-directed group, in which dobutamine was used to increase DO_2 (Figure 22-7). Of note, in these studies only approximately 60% of the patients were able to reach these supranormal values for DO_2 and $\dot{V}O_2$ with therapy, while some of the control patients were able to meet these goals without intervention. In the largest study, Gattinoni et al. randomized 762 critically ill medical and surgical patients to three groups with different hemodynamic goals: (1) a normal cardiac index group (2.5–3.5 l/min/m²), (2) a supranormal cardiac index (>4.5 l/min/m²), and (3) a normal mixed ve-

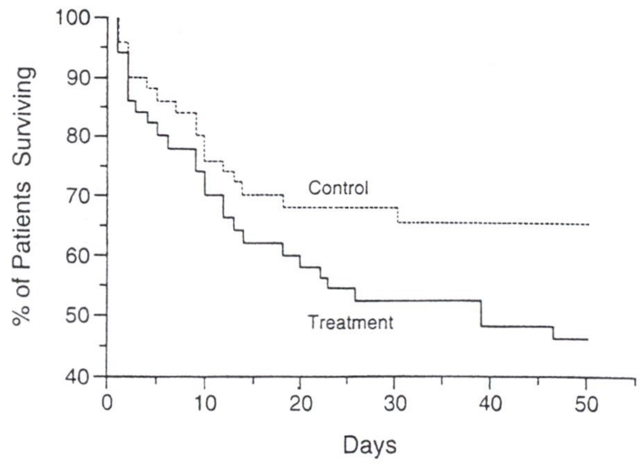

FIGURE 22-7

In-hospital survival was significantly better in the control group compared to the treatment group, which met certain hemodynamic goals in regards to oxygen delivery. (Reprinted with permission from Hayes MA, Timmins AC, Yau EHS, Palazzo M, et al. Elevation of systemic oxygen delivery in the treatment of critically ill patients. N Engl J Med 1994;330:1717–1722.

nous oxygen saturation group ($S\bar{v}O_2 \geq 70\%$); 94% of the normal cardiac index group, 45% of the supranormal cardiac index group, and 60% of the normal mixed venous saturation group were able to reach their goals. There was no difference in survival or the development of organ dysfunction among the groups, even when only those patients who were able to obtain their assigned goals were analyzed.

The relative lack of success with goal-directed therapy may be partially explained by the results of a recent study by Ronco et al. These investigators identified the DO_2 crit in nine septic and eight nonseptic patients by measuring DO_2 and $\dot{V}O_2$ as life support was being discontinued. They noted a significantly lower DO_2 crit than that previously found in animal experiments and in humans using pooled data. In addition, there was no difference in the DO_2 crit values for those patients with and without sepsis, at 3.8 and 4.5 ml/kg/min, respectively. Those studies that attempted goal-directed therapy had patients with baseline values for DO_2 that were much greater than the DO_2 crit noted in the Ronco et al. study. In addition, Ronco et al. noted no difference in the O_2ER at DO_2 crit in those with and without sepsis, at 0.61 and 0.59, respectively, which are values similar to those at maximal exercise. These findings suggest that DO_2 is most likely adequate in the majority of critically ill patients, even those with sepsis. In addition, sepsis does not appear to significantly impair the tissue's ability to extract oxygen. Therefore, attempting to increase DO_2 to supranormal levels in all or nonselected critically ill patients to increase $\dot{V}O_2$ may be without benefit.

Increasing DO_2 to supranormal values may be without benefit.

CONTROVERSIES REGARDING OXYGEN SUPPLY DEPENDENCY

The presence of oxygen supply dependency, which has been reported in a number of studies, should be interpreted with caution for the following reasons. First, concerns have been raised in regard to the methods used to determine $\dot{V}O_2$, which may produce an artifactual correlation between DO_2 and $\dot{V}O_2$. In many of these studies $\dot{V}O_2$ was calculated using the reverse Fick equation. Therefore, both DO_2 and $\dot{V}O_2$ were calculated using the shared variables of cardiac output and CaO_2. An increase or decrease in either variable could cause DO_2 and $\dot{V}O_2$ to change in the same direction, producing a linear relationship between the two variables and the appearance of a supply-dependent state. Since these initial studies, five investigations have directly compared the $\dot{V}O_2$ obtained with the reverse Fick equation to that measured using a metabolic cart. In all these studies, no correlation was found between the calculated $\dot{V}O_2$ values and those obtained using the metabolic cart. Also, although there appeared to be a supply-dependent state when $\dot{V}O_2$ was calculated using the reverse Fick equation, this was not evident when $\dot{V}O_2$ was measured using the metabolic cart.

Using the Fick equation, DO_2 and $\dot{V}O_2$ are calculated using shared variables.

CASE STUDY: PART 3

The diagnosis of pneumonia with systemic inflammatory response syndrome was made. At this point the patient was placed on maintenance IV fluids and started on dopamine. As a result, the patient's PCWP increased to 14 mm/Hg and his SVR increased to 876 dyne/s/m^5; cardiac output decreased to 5 l/min and oxygen content remained at 12 mm/Hg. These values resulted in oxygen delivery of 600 ml/kg/min and oxygen consumption of 120 ml/kg/min, with an extraction ratio of 20%.

The patient's mean arterial pressure stabilized and his urine output increased. Subsequently, his blood cultures grew *Pneumococcus* and the patient completed a 14-day course of antibiotics for bacteremia and sepsis. The patient was able to be weaned and extubated on the third ICU day and the dopamine eventually was weaned off with no significant changes in his oxygen delivery, oxygen consumption, or extraction ratio.

Another concern regarding the notion of supply dependency is that under normal conditions spontaneous changes in O_2 demand result in changes in DO_2, as seen with exercise. In a number of studies involving septic and ARDS patients, data had been collected over a period of time (hours to days) and appeared to demonstrate a supply-dependent state, but this finding may represent only appropriate changes in DO_2 occurring in response to changing O_2 demands. Finally, it should be noted that many of these studies, including those that attempted goal-directed therapy, were conducted without any knowledge of what is a normal DO_2 crit value in either healthy individuals or critically ill patients.

LACTIC ACIDOSIS

There has also been controversy regarding the significance of lactic acidosis in patients with sepsis. It has been assumed that the increased arterial lactate is the result of a decreased DO_2 and a tissue oxygen debt, resulting in anaerobic metabolism (see Figure 22-1). There is recent evidence, however, that arterial lactate increases as a result of an increase in glycolysis. Sepsis is characterized by a hypermetabolic state with increased glucose uptake by cells. This increased uptake appears to be mediated by the Glut-1 membrane transporter, which is not insulin dependent. Glut-1 production increases in sepsis, with increased mRNA production for the Glut-1 glucose transporter, a process thought to be mediated by cytokines. The increase in cellular glucose leads to an increase in the production of pyruvate. If the oxidative metabolic pathway is unable to metabolize the increased pyruvate, the cells will convert it to lactate. Thus, unlike an anaerobic state in which the lactate/pyruvate ratio is elevated, in sepsis, it remains unchanged, with lactate being produced solely because of an increase in the substrate pyruvate. A number of studies have reported this preserved lactate/pyruvate ratio in septic patients despite the presence of an elevated arterial lactate. These findings strongly suggest that arterial lactate is not an accurate marker for the presence of anaerobic metabolism in sepsis.

In sepsis, the lactate/pyruvate ratio remains unchanged.

Serum lactate is not an accurate marker for anaerobic metabolism in sepsis.

RECOMMENDATIONS

Initial management involves establishing hemodynamic stability.

The primary objective in the initial management of the critically ill patient is to establish hemodynamic stability and thus organ perfusion (Figure 22-8). Organ perfusion can be gauged by several clinical indexes such as mentation, urinary output, skin perfusion, and blood pressure. When perfusion is subnormal, treatment is targeted at the pathophysiologic cause (i.e., cardiac performance, vascular resistance, or inadequate filling pressure). The initial treatment for most patients is volume (crystalloid, colloid, or blood), and treatment is guided by the response to therapy, such as increased urine output, improved mentation, and increased mean arterial pressure. If there is no response to initial therapy, clinical assessment may be supplemented by invasive hemodynamic monitoring, which allows measurement of specific parameters that can be addressed with volume, if the pulmonary capillary artery pressure is

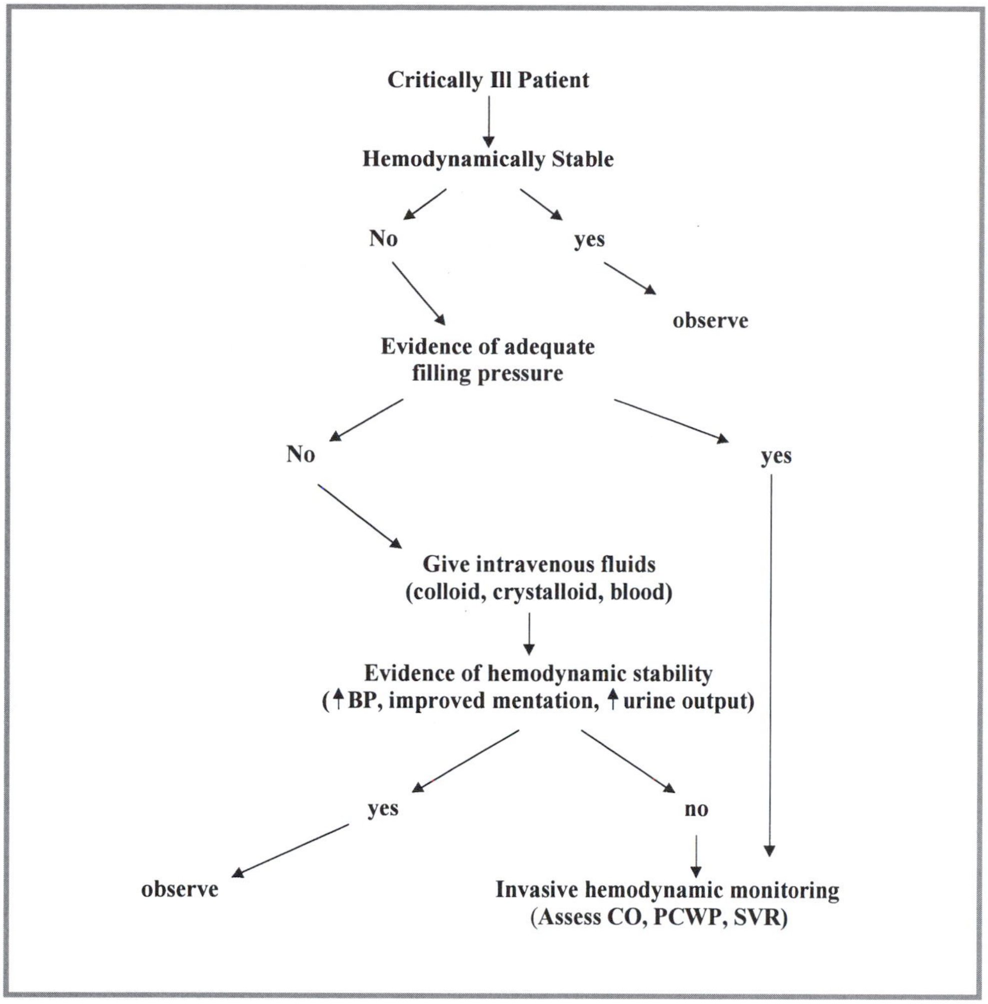

FIGURE 22-8

Algorithm for the treatment of the hemodynamically unstable critically ill patient.

low, or specific vasoactive therapy. DO_2 and $\dot{V}O_2$ are among the parameters that can be monitored in these patients during hemodynamic stabilization. Interventions aimed at optimizing DO_2 to values within the normal range should be the goal; this should result in adequate tissue oxygenation and metabolism as measured by O_2ER and $\dot{V}O_2$, respectively. The limitations of these measurements should be understood, because they are global measurements and because there are technical concerns in regard to shared variables. At the present time there are no data to support improved outcome in critically ill medical or surgical patients with the indiscriminate use of goal-directed therapy.

Interventions aimed at optimizing DO_2 to within the normal range should be the goal.

No data support the indiscriminate use of goal-directed therapy.

SUMMARY

Adequate oxygen delivery is crucial for normal cellular function. In critically ill patients, the normal relationship between DO_2 and $\dot{V}O_2$ is often disturbed and may be responsible for increased morbidity and mortality. Initial management should include efforts to normalize DO_2 to ensure that oxygen demands are met at the cellular level. Therapeutic interventions aimed at increasing DO_2 to supranormal levels in unselected patients have not been shown to improve survival. Maintaining hemodynamic stability and treatment of the underlying disease process thus remain the primary goals in the management of the critically ill patient.

REVIEW QUESTIONS

1. **What is the least important component of oxygen delivery?**
   A. Hemoglobin
   B. Oxygen saturation
   C. Oxygen dissolved in blood
   D. Cardiac output

2. **Which of the following has been associated with improved survival in septic patients?**
   A. Increasing oxygen content
   B. Increasing delivery
   C. Decreasing oxygen consumption
   D. None of the above

3. **The normal physiologic response to an increased oxygen uptake during exercise is to?**
   A. Increase oxygen delivery by increasing cardiac output
   B. Decrease oxygen extraction
   C. Increase oxygen content of the blood by hyperventilating
   D. All of the above

4. **A 47-year-old woman with toxic shock syndrome remains hypotensive despite volume resuscitation with 2 l normal saline. The house staff decides to place a Swan–Ganz catheter; the initial numbers are CVP = 5 mmHg, RAP = 12/7 mmHg, PAP = 13/8 mmHg, PCWP = 8 mmHg, MAP = 40 mmHg, CO = 5.5, and SVR = 509 dyne/s/m^5. The next intervention for hemodynamic support would be to:**
   A. Add epinephrine to increase SVR.
   B. Add dobutamine to increase cardiac output.
   C. Administer more volume to increase the PCWP.
   D. All of the above.

ANSWERS

1. The answer is C. The least effective way to increase oxygen delivery (DO_2) is by increasing PaO_2. Recalling the equation for oxygen content as [$CaO_2 = (1.3 \times Hgb \times SaO_2) + (0.003 \times PaO_2)$], note that PaO_2 contributes little to CaO_2. DO_2 is simply the cardiac output $\times$ CaO_2. Thus, SaO_2 and hemoglobin make up most of the CaO_2, and these two variables should be normalized in managing septic patients to ensure an adequate DO_2.
2. The answer is D. Large prospective randomized trials have shown no benefit of increasing DO_2 to supraphysiologic levels to improve outcome for septic patients. To the contrary, trying to achieve these levels has actually been shown to increase mortality. Optimizing DaO_2 by maintaining $SaO_2 > 90\%$ and hemoglobin at 7–10 g/dl, and decreasing oxygen consumption ($\dot{V}O_2$) by controlling hyperthermia and using sedation when indicated, is recommended. Even these measures have not been shown necessarily to affect survival.
3. The answer is A. The normal physiologic response to increasing $\dot{V}O_2$ during exercise is to increase DO_2 by increasing cardiac output up to 4–5 fold that seen at rest. Increased oxygen extraction occurs when cardiac output is unable to meet the increasing oxygen requirements, with $\dot{V}O_2$ noted to increase up to 10 fold at maximal exercise.
4. The answer is C. The following patient has toxic shock syndrome that can manifest with profound circulatory shock. Many of these patients have profound volume depletion secondary to capillary leak and vasculature dilatation and need large amounts of volume for hemodynamic support. In the following example, the initial 2 l of volume given was not sufficient to stabilize the patient. The numbers obtained from the Swan–Ganz catheter showed that the preload of the left ventricle was suboptimal and that the patient needed more volume. In this case, I recommend more volume until the PCWP is 12–14 mmHg, and a concomitant increase in the MAP and CO is desirable. If increasing the PCWP to normal values has no effect on organ perfusion (as evidenced by increases in the MAP, CO, and urine output), at this point I would add vasopressors.

   Initial treatment with epinephrine in this patient may be effective, but with the suboptimal PCWP, volume infusion would be the recommended first intervention. If there was hemodynamic instability after optimizing the PCWP, epinephrine may be added. The administration of dobutamine will increase cardiac output but may also decrease SVR, and for this reason this would not be the first intervention.

SUGGESTED READING

Bihari D, Smithies M, Gimson A, Tinker J. The effect of vasodilation with prostacyclin on oxygen delivery and uptake in critically ill patients. N Engl J Med 1987;317:397–403.

Chittock DR, Ronco JJ, Russell JA. Monitoring of oxygen transport and oxygen consumption. In: Tobin MJ (ed) Principles and Practice of Intensive Care Monitoring. New York: McGraw-Hill, 1997: 317–343.

Gattinoni L, Brazzi L, Paolo P, et al. A trial of goal-oriented hemodynamic therapy in critically ill patients. N Engl J Med 1995;333: 1025–1032.

Hotchkiss RS, Karl IE. Reevaluation of the role of cellular hypoxia and bioenergetic failure in sepsis. JAMA 1992;267:1503–1513.

Ronco JJ, Fenwick JC, Tweeddale MG, et al. Identification of the critical oxygen delivery for anaerobic metabolism in critically ill septic and nonseptic humans. JAMA 1993;270:1724–1730.

Shoemaker WC, Montgomery ES, Kaplan E, Elwyn DH. Physiologic patterns in surviving and nonsurviving shock patients. Arch Surg 1973;106:630–636.

VADIM LEYENSON

Circulatory Shock

CHAPTER OUTLINE

LEARNING OBJECTIVES

After studying this chapter, you should be able to:

- Define circulatory failure.
- Recognize the major mechanisms of circulatory failure.
- Recognize the signs and symptoms of circulatory failure.
- Recognize the different types of circulatory failure.
- Know the major algorithms of circulatory failure treatment.

Circulatory failure, or shock, is a state of inadequate perfusion relative to the tissue demands. It is always characterized by low blood pressure and dysfunction of key vital organs. The presentation of shock can vary depending on its nature and severity. It also depends on the vital organs involved. Virtually every aspect of shock, from its definition to treatment, remains controversial. In this chapter we attempt to cover the most established principles of the pathophysiology and therapy of circulatory failure. We also define circulatory failure, review the major pathophysiologic mechanisms, and provide major algorithms of treatment.

DEFINITION OF SHOCK

Shock is very difficult to define because of the range of its presentation and the complexity of its pathophysiology. One definition of shock is "a syndrome which is characterized by an acute generalized disturbance in the normal perfusion pattern resulting in hypoperfusion and profound dysfunction of critical organs." Symptoms of shock include confusion, hypotension, oliguria, and tachycardia. However, the spectrum of symptoms is not limited to these

> The key features of shock are hypotension and hypoperfusion.

CASE STUDY: PART 1

A 67-year-old woman presented with a 3-day history of tracheobronchitis. She did not have any significant past medical history. Over the past several days she had complained of intermittent fever, chills, and shortness of breath. She was treated by her family M.D. with oral antibiotics. Today, her family found the patient pale, shivering with warm extremities, and changed in mental status. She was evaluated in the emergency room and found to have a heart rate of 60 beats/min and blood pressure of 80/60 mmHg. She had no urine output.

The physical signs and manifestations of circulatory failure depend on the underlying disease and the cause of the shock.

few; a variety of other symptoms may occur (Table 23-1). The clinical presentation of circulatory failure may vary depending on the type of organ failure. Metabolic acidosis frequently occurs, especially in severe shock, but it is not essential to the definition of the syndrome.

PATHOPHYSIOLOGY OF SHOCK

Hypoperfusion leads to intracellular hypoxemia. Liposomal disruption is a point of irreversible damage.

The cascade of pathophysiologic mechanisms involved in shock is shown in Figure 23-1. Shock affects different organs by altering their functional integrity. Organ failure occurs by two major mechanisms, hypoperfusion and the inability to utilize oxygen. Hypoperfusion seems to be the initiating event. Because of decreased delivery of oxygen, adenosine triphosphate (ATP) production diminishes. Also, because of hypoperfusion, the permeability of cell membranes is increased. All these changes lead to endoplasmic reticular swelling, which is the initial presentation of intracellular hypoxemic damage. The second organelles to be affected are the mitochondria; continuous hypoperfusion and oxygen debt lead to progressive mitochondrial swelling; which further potentiates a disruption in oxidative metabolism and further worsening of oxygen debt. Eventually, with continuation of cellular hypoxemia, liposomal rupture leads to the release of multiple degradative enzymes that further perpetuate a vicious cycle of intracellular damage. Most likely, liposomal disruption is a point of irreversible damage.

Neurohumoral Responses

All responses, including neurohumoral responses, are directed toward protecting cells in organs against the effects of hypovolemia, hypoperfusion, and oxygen death. In normal individuals, any fall in blood volume causes an increase in afferent impulses from carotid and aortic baroreceptors and from mechanical receptors within the right atrium. This increase, in turn, leads to increased sympathetic activity, which causes cardiac stimulation and vasospasm. This response is also potentiated by the release of adrenocorticotropic hormone (ACTH) and antidiuretic hormone (ADH), as well as increased production of epinephrine and cortisol. The kidneys respond by increasing the secretion of renin-angiotensin. The major

TABLE 23-1

CLINICAL MANIFESTATIONS OF CIRCULATORY FAILURE

ORGAN/SYSTEM	SYMPTOMS
Central nervous system	Mental status changes, tremor, seizures
Heart	Hypotension, tachycardia, chest pain, new murmurs, arrhythmia, ↑ JVD
Respiratory	Tachypnea, hypoxemia, ↑ WOB
Renal	Oliguria, change in urine color
Gastrointestinal	Nausea, vomiting, diarrhea, ileus
Skin	Cold, clammy

JVD, jugular venous distension; WOB, work of breathing

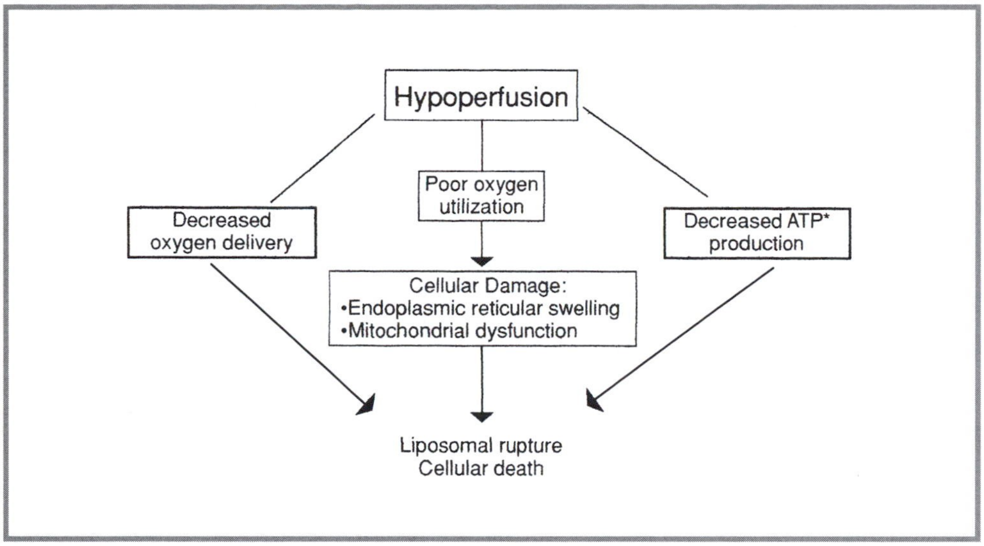

FIGURE 23-1

The key pathophysiologic mechanisms of circulatory failure. The core of pathophysiology of shock is hypoperfusion, leading to insufficient oxygen delivery and utilization and eventually to cellular death. *ATP*, adenosine triphosphate.

effect of all these alterations is directed toward maintaining blood pressure and retaining salt and water. However, in severe hypovolemia, these compensatory mechanisms may be ineffective, and eventually end-organ deterioration occurs.

The major effect of neurohumoral changes is to maintain adequate perfusion status.

Figure 23-2 demonstrates the effects of a variety of hormonal and nonhormonal substances that are released into the circulation during shock, including prostaglandins, histamine, bradykinin, serotonin, beta endorphins, and myocardial depressant factors. These substances alter blood flow distribution to the organs by increasing various organ vascular wall permeability, or by inducing changes in blood flow by affecting blood cell rheology. Hormones, such as the polypeptide hormone cachexin or tumor necrosis factor, are released from macrophages in response to endotoxemia. These hormones plus platelet-activating factors slow blood flow by promoting platelet aggregation and potentiate inflammation by promoting macrophage mobilization. These hormones appear to have a major role in the development of septic shock.

Vasoactive substances released in shock affect blood flow, vascular wall permeability, and inflammatory response.

Nonhormonal vasoactive chemicals, such as nitric oxide (NO), are capable of producing significant vasodilatation and are also probably very important in the development of shock.

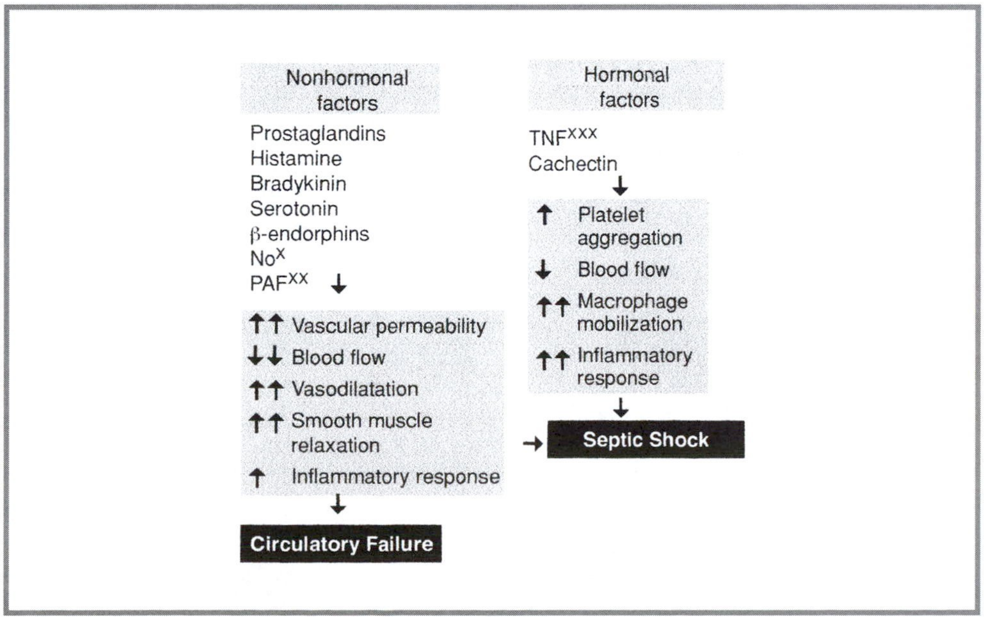

FIGURE 23-2

Hemodynamic, cellular, and inflammatory responses to a variety of hormonal and nonhormonal substances released into the circulation during shock. *NO*, nitric oxide; *PAF*, platelet-activating factor; *TNF*, tumor necrosis factor.

FIGURE 23-3

Major metabolic responses in circulatory failure. Decreased insulin availability and increased insulin resistance, secondary to enhanced production of glucocorticoids and catecholamines, lead to lactic and ketoacidosis.

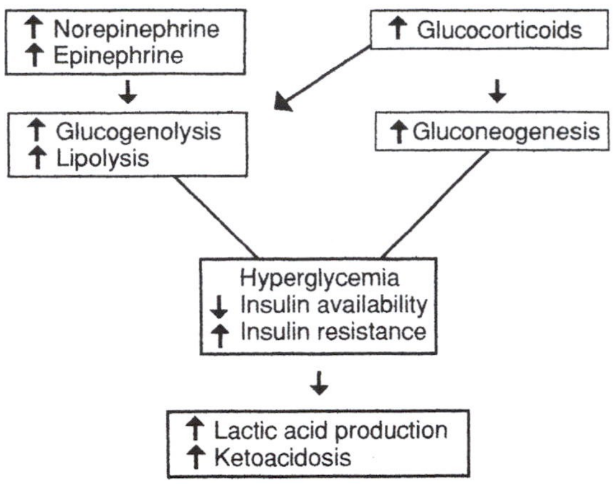

The several potential sources of NO include the vascular endothelium, neutrophils, smooth muscle cells, platelets, mast cells, and fibroblasts. Besides smooth muscle relaxation, which potentially plays a role in hypotension in patients with circulatory failure, NO participates in platelet inhibition, the inflammatory response, and neurotransmission. High concentrations of NO and its precursors have been found in patients with septic shock.

Metabolic Responses

The pathophysiology of shock is extremely complicated and consists of a cascade of neurohumoral and metabolic changes.

Neurohumoral alterations lead to immediate metabolic responses (Figure 23-3). A significant release of catecholamines decreases insulin secretion, which leads to increased glycogenolysis and lipolysis. Glucocorticoids potentiate the effect of the catecholamines and promote gluconeogenesis, which further decreases insulin availability. Both mechanisms lead to hyperglycemia. Because of limited oxygen availability, hyperglycemia contributes to lactic acid production, which eventually inhibits glyconeogenesis, further limiting the availability of energy resources for normal cellular function. At some point, ketone bodies and the branched chain amino acids can be used as alternative fuel sources. However, without adequate oxygen supplementation, these sources become inefficient.

Certain types of shock, such as septic shock, have different metabolic responses. For example, in contrast to hypovolemic shock, patients with septic shock develop an early proteolysis while lipolysis remains relatively inhibited. Specific metabolic responses are discussed later when the different types of circulatory failure are described.

CAST STUDY: PART 2

Following presentation, the patient was started on intravenous fluid resuscitation. A Swan–Ganz catheter was inserted, revealing a high cardiac output, low systemic vascular resistance, and relatively normal wedge pressure. After several hours of fluid resuscitation, the patient's blood pressure remained 70/50 mmHg and her pulse at 150 beats/min. The patient remained anuric and eventually developed respiratory failure. A chest X-ray showed pulmonary edema. The patient subsequently required intubation and mechanical ventilation.

EFFECTS OF SHOCK ON SPECIFIC ORGANS

Heart

Shock introduces an additional requirement for myocardial oxygen extraction thereby leading to increased cardiac work. Increased cardiac work may result from reflex sympathetic stimulation and peripheral vasoconstriction. However, these increased metabolic requirements must be met by increased coronary blood flow. Because of hypotension, coronary perfusion is compromised and cardiac function may suffer. Certain chemical substances released during shock states such as myocardial depressant factor, platelet-activating factor, and nitric oxide may also play roles in some forms of shock. Obviously, underlying cardiac disease further adds to cardiac dysfunction. Cardiac output also can be affected by the extent of underlying coronary artery disease, sympathetic stimulation, certain medication administration, hypoxemia, and acidosis.

The heart may fail secondary to increased metabolic requirements.

Respiratory System

Respiratory failure is commonly associated with circulatory failure. However, hypoperfusion is not the main mechanism leading to gas exchange abnormalities because the lungs have a vast blood supply. The most common cause of respiratory failure in shock is pulmonary edema; this may occur from increased hydrostatic pressures or increased lung capillary permeability. The initial therapy of shock with massive fluid resuscitation or multiple blood transfusions may also contribute to the development of pulmonary edema.

Respiratory failure occurs because of increased demands secondary to enhanced metabolic load or iatrogenic interventions.

Brain

The brain is extremely sensitive to changes in perfusion because it almost exclusively depends on perfusion to meet its oxidative metabolic demands. Therefore, compensatory mechanisms are directed toward preserving brain perfusion. Several factors play a key role in regulation of brain perfusion. These factors are regional carbon dioxide and oxygen tensions, and contraction or dilation of vascular smooth muscle in the presence of increased or decreased intravascular pressures. These factors may be affected by common metabolic changes related to circulatory failure as well as by drug administration and cellular edema. However, irreversible changes in brain cellular structure occur relatively late and, fortunately, rarely result in irreversible brain dysfunction.

The brain is relatively spared in circulatory failure.

Kidney

Oliguria is one of the major manifestations of shock. Hypoperfusion is not the only mechanism of shock-related oliguria because blood flow to the kidney rarely drops below 40%–50% of normal. Additional mechanisms play an important role in the reduction of glomerular filtration; these include sympathetic overstimulation, circulating catecholamines, angiotensin, and prostaglandins, all of which contribute to arterial vasoconstriction and redistribution of blood flow away from the renal cortex to the medulla. Additionally, there is increased salt and fluid reabsorption in the distal tubule secondary to increased aldosterone and ADH production, compensatory mechanisms that preserve intravascular volume but ultimately lead to diminished urinary output. Mechanisms causing oliguria can be further amplified by using vasoconstricting agents or by ischemic injury to the nephron. However, renal failure caused by shock is not limited to glomerular dysfunction. Significant damage may also occur at the tubular level.

Hypoperfusion is the main, but not the only, cause of renal failure.

Three major pathologic mechanisms of tubular dysfunction are the following:

1. Tubular necrosis with poor diffusion of glomerular infiltrate.
2. Tubular obstruction by casts, cellular debris, and tubular damage due to hypercalcemia

or the direct toxic effect of substances such as myoglobin. Because of tubular epithelial damage, interstitial edema and tubular collapse also occur.

3. Ischemic injury of the tubular apparatus leads to a severe impairment in its concentrating ability, eventually causing decreases in salt retention and urine osmolarity that further decrease intravascular osmotic pressure and promote a loss of intravascular volume.

Gastrointestinal Tract, Liver, and Pancreas

Ischemic injury is the major mechanism of GI tract dysfunction in shock.

Ischemic damage to the gastrointestinal (GI) tract has a significant role in the pathogenesis of shock. Substances that are released from the damaged GI tract contribute to many complications of shock.

Injury to the Gut

The earliest manifestation of ischemic gut injury is fluid sequestration, hemorrhage, or necrosis of gut mucosa. Later, ulcer formation can occur. The most prominent site of ischemic injury is the stomach. Patients with underlying atherosclerotic disease of the mesenteric artery are especially prone to developing ischemic injury. Because of hypoperfusion, breakdown of the gut mucosa leads to excessive permeability and provides a port of entry for bacteria or for bacterial toxins, both of which have a pivotal role in septic shock.

Liver

Liver injury is not usually apparent in the initial stages of shock. Later, hepatic cell death occurs. Earlier indications of hepatocyte damage include the release of characteristic enzymes such as serum glutamic oxaloacetic transaminase or, sometimes, in cases complicated by biliary obstruction, elevations in bilirubin, and alkaline phosphatase. Impaired hepatic clearance contributes to increases in serologic vasoactive substances that can perpetuate circulatory failure. The reticuloendothelial (RES) system can also be impaired as well. However, the role of RES dysfunction in shock states is not clear.

Pancreas

The role of pancreatic damage in shock is not clearly established. Some data suggest that a myocardial depressant factor is released from the pancreas. It is possible that ischemia or infections may adversely affect islet cell function and thereby contribute to diminished insulin production. It is possible that the same factors may also contribute to the increased production of vasoactive substances.

BLOOD AND COAGULATION

Disseminated intravascular coagulation (DIC) is a common feature of septic shock.

Blood viscosity increases significantly, especially during the late stages of shock, and may significantly impair the microcirculation. Higher levels of platelet-activating factor lead to platelet dysfunction, thereby further decreasing circulation by means of excessive platelet activation. Disseminated intravascular coagulation (DIC) is especially common in septic shock and contributes significantly to microcirculation hypoperfusion. Platelet damage leads to the release of many vasoactive substances, including prostaglandins and platelet-activating factor. These substances may be responsible for many of the manifestations of shock. In shock, the hemoglobin–oxygen dissociation curve shifts to the right because of a reduction in 2,3-diphosphoglycerate and metabolic acidosis. This shift leads to enhanced unloading of oxygen at the tissue level and serves as a compensatory mechanism to compensate for decreases in cardiac output and arterial oxygen.

TABLE 23-2

COMMON HEMODYNAMIC PROFILES IN SHOCK

TYPE	CO	SVR	PAOP	PAP	SAP
Hypovolemic	↓ or N	↑	↓	↓	↓
Cardiogenic	↓	↑	↑	↑	↓
Septic	↑	↓	↓ or N	↓ or N	↓

CO, cardiac output; SVR, systemic vascular resistance; PAOP, pulmonary artery occlusion pressure; PAP, pulmonary artery pressure; SAP, systemic arterial pressure; N, normal

TYPES OF SHOCK

Detailed descriptions of different types of shock are provided in other chapters. We discuss here the characteristic features that distinguish one form of shock state from another. Common hemodynamic patterns of shock are demonstrated in Table 23-2.

Cardiogenic Shock

The main types of shock are hypovolemic, cardiogenic, and septic.

Cardiogenic shock is caused by pump failure. Pathophysiology of cardiogenic shock is caused by decreased ventricular contractility.

Cardiogenic shock results from cardiac pump failure. It is defined by the presence of an inappropriately low cardiac output, despite normal or high right atrial pressures. Cardiogenic shock is usually diagnosed when the cardiac index is less than 2.0 $l/min/m^2$ and the pulmonary artery occlusion pressure is ≥18 mmHg. The pathophysiology of cardiogenic shock results from decreased left ventricular contractility. The end-diastolic pressure stroke volume relationship is shifted downward and to the right (Figure 23-4) and, therefore, despite the same level of ventricular preload, the ejection fraction is reduced. To compensate for this, the diastolic ventricle becomes more compliant, thereby allowing the stroke volume to increase at the same end-diastolic pressure. According to the Frank–Starling relationship, therefore, cardiac output increases by increasing end-diastolic volume or preload. Eventually, even with increased preload, the left ventricle is unable to maintain its function, which leads to pulmonary edema, a reduction in mixed venous oxygen saturation, and pulmonary shunt.

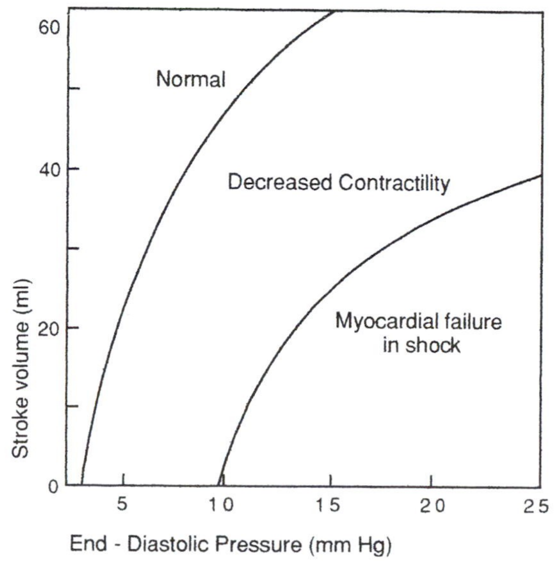

FIGURE 23-4

The Frank–Starling relationship between preload and contractility in normal state and in circulatory failure. The pathophysiology of cardiogenic shock results from decreased left ventricular contractility. The end-diastolic pressure stroke volume relationship is shifted downward to the *right*; therefore, despite the same level of ventricular preload, stroke volume, is reduced.

Arterial desaturation aggravates the lower oxygen delivery that results from the reduced cardiac output.

Myocardial infarction or ischemia is the most common cause of left ventricular failure leading to shock. From 10% to 20% of patients with transmural myocardial infarction experience circulatory failure. Infarction of more than 40% of the myocardium usually leads to cardiogenic shock. Anterior infarction is more likely than inferior or posterior myocardial infarction to be associated with shock.

Certain conditions cause cardiogenic shock by increasing diastolic stiffness, such as ischemia, pericardial tamponade, prolonged hypovolemic or septic shock, and ventricular hypertrophy or restricted cardiomyopathy. These conditions cause not only systolic but also diastolic dysfunction. When systolic contractility is decreased and cannot be compensated for by increases in left ventricular end-diastolic pressure, circulatory failure occurs.

Valvular dysfunction may also cause LV dysfunction. The most frequent cause of valvular dysfunction is acute mitral regurgitation because of rupture of the chordae tendinae or the papillary muscle; it is usually due to ischemic injury. Acute mitral regurgitation significantly raises left ventricular end-diastolic pressure and produces symptoms of acute pulmonary edema and cardiogenic shock.

Cardiac arrhythmias may aggravate hypoperfusion and either contribute to or cause a shock state. Ventricular arrhythmias are most commonly associated with cardiogenic shock. Sinus tachycardia and atrial tachycardia may be seen in hypovolemic or septic shock.

Hypovolemic Shock

Venous return to the heart may be inadequate for several reasons. Decreased intravascular volume may result from hemorrhage, dehydration, decreased vascular tone, and sepsis, and rarely may be secondary to increased resistance to venous return, such as with obstruction of the inferior vena cava. Venous return may also be reduced when the right arterial pressure is significantly increased despite normal ventricular function, such as in situations when the pressure surrounding the heart is elevated by pericardial tamponade.

Intravascular volume contraction leads to marked decrease in filling pressures. Hypovolemic shock is caused by decreased venous return.

Hypovolemia is the most common cause of shock caused by decreased venous return. Intravascular volume is decreased, leading to a marked decrease in filling pressures. Because cardiac output depends on end-diastolic ventricular pressure, cardiac output will be reduced. Sympathetic stimulation increases catecholamine production and temporarily compensates for decreased end-diastolic pressure by increasing heart rate and therefore increasing cardiac output. However, if approximately 40% of intravascular volume is lost, sympathetic stimulation can no longer maintain mean systemic pressure, resulting in decreased venous return and clinical shock. After sufficient time or severity (40% of loss of intravascular volume) irreversible change or development of the "no reflow phenomenon" occurs. This phenomenon implies that stagnant neutrophils become adherent to endothelial surfaces, even after adequate fluid resuscitation, and may block capillary beds, thereby causing tissue hypoxemia. Further damage occurs with cardiac ischemic and systemic release of inflammatory mediators. Also, cardiac dysfunction caused by diastolic stiffness during hypovolemic shock further impairs ventricular filling, leading to more severe hypoperfusion.

The most impressive example of hypovolemic shock occurs in trauma. Intravascular volume may be decreased because of a loss of blood volume and significant redistribution of intravascular fluid to the extravascular compartment, that is, third spacing of fluid. The mechanism of cardiac dysfunction in trauma includes direct cardiac injury, myocardial contusion causing diastolic stiffness, and the presence of high levels of circulating myocardial depressant factors.

Septic Shock

Septic shock, the most common example of shock, is characterized by reduced arterial muscular tone and an abnormal redistribution of blood flow. The most common organisms causing septic shock are gram-negative bacilli, which are found in approximately two-thirds of all sepsis cases, or one-third of patients presenting with septic shock. Recently, however, gram-positive bacteria as a cause of sepsis and septic shock have been reported more frequently. Characteristic features of septic shock are large pulse pressures, warm extremities, good capillary refill, and low diastolic and mean blood pressures. Septic shock also is often associated with fever, elevated heart rate, and high white blood cell counts.

Features of septic shock are large pulse pressures, warm extremities, good capillary refill, and low mean arterial pressure.

Complex pathophysiologic mechanisms contribute to inadequate organ system perfusion in septic shock and are hallmarked by mismatches in oxygen supply and demand in various organ beds. Some organs and tissues receive more blood and oxygen delivery than usual whereas other organs are unable to maintain aerobic metabolism and normal function.

Depression of systolic contractility is the key cardiovascular abnormality observed in septic shock. The depression in contractility may be partially caused by a change in oxygen or other substrate metabolism. Most likely, the heart extracts less oxygen as a result of cellular inability to extract oxygen. Therefore, in sepsis, myocardial cell oxygen consumption is decreased while the oxygen demands are elevated. At least part of the depression in systolic contractility results from the presence of myocardial depressant factors.

If the patient recovers, decreased systolic contractility is reversible over 5–10 days. The ventricles of survivors of septic shock have been noted to be able to adequately dilate as part of the normal compensatory response to a decrease in ventricular contractility. In nonsurvivors, the ventricle does not dilate and, as a result, stroke volume and cardiac output decrease because of impaired diastolic filling.

Another important feature of septic shock is decreased arterial resistance, which is almost always observed. The lowered arterial resistance in circumstances of high cardiac output is caused by impaired arterial vasoregulation. A variety of factors, such as bacterial toxin production and circulating vasoactive substances, affect arterial autoregulation. Redistribution of blood flow to a lower resistance circuit such as the skeletal muscles results in decreased resistance and decreased venous return. Because of these factors, cardiac output may be increased, although cardiac function is decreased by decreased contractility. Eventually, increased vascular permeability leads to the redistribution of fluid outside of the intravascular compartment and decreased venous return may occur; this further contributes to a decrease in ventricular contractility.

Abnormalities in the microcirculation also contribute to fluid redistribution in septic shock. The microcirculation is affected by the increased numbers of leukocytes adhering to the endothelial surface, altered red blood cell distribution, and the presence of disseminated intravascular coagulation.

Less Common Types of Shock

There are a few other types of hypovolemic shock, not so frequently observed as those already described. One of these types is anaphylactic shock, which occurs as a result of the attack of mediators such as histamine on the heart, circulation, and peripheral tissue. As in septic shock, cardiac contractility increases and vascular tone decreases. Blood flow is redistributed to lower-resistance vascular beds such as the skeletal muscles. Significant endothelium permeability may also occur, resulting in extravascular vascular compartment expansion and, consequently, intravascular compartment hypovolemia. Venous tone and consequently venous return to the heart are simultaneously reduced, contributing to decreased cardiac contractility.

Neurogenic shock is uncommon. In general, there is impaired neurogenic regulation of cardiovascular tone, which often occurs in clinical situations associated with significant blood loss.

Certain endocrinologic conditions may result in shock. States associated with inadequate catecholamine production, such as Addison's disease (i.e., adrenocortical deficiency) may result in shock or may be a contributing factor to other forms of shock. Hypothyroidism and hyperthyroidism may be contributing factors in extreme presentation of thyroid dsyfunction for the development of shock. Pheochromocytoma may result in shock by significantly increasing vascular afterload and therefore redistributing volume from the intravascular into the extravascular compartment.

Several poisons such as carbon monoxide, cyanide, and others that are also associated with circulatory failure are discussed elsewhere in this volume.

TREATMENT OF CIRCULATORY FAILURE

The major goals of resuscitation in shock are to reverse hypotension and to provide adequate perfusion of vital organs and tissues.

In this chapter we discuss only the general approach to the therapy of circulatory failure. Specific therapies are discussed in their appropriate chapters.

The goals of therapy in patients with circulatory failure can be summarized as follows: maintaining cardiac output and oxygen delivery, reversing hypotension, and correcting hypovolemia. One must realize that at times the therapy can be associated with undesirable effects. For example, extremely aggressive fluid resuscitation may lead to pulmonary edema because of excessive permeability of the vascular bed, low intravascular osmotic pressure, and increased hydrostatic pressure due to decreased left ventricular contractility. Therapy, therefore, should be directed toward maintaining adequate mean arterial pressure, which is usually between 60 and 70 mmHg, a level sufficient for perfusion of the heart and the brain, while simultaneously seeking the lowest ventricular filling pressure to achieve these goals.

FLUID THERAPY

The initial therapeutic measure for treatment of circulatory failure is fluid resuscitation.

Our approach to hemodynamic management is summarized in Figure 23-5. If a patient presents with signs of hypotension or hypoperfusion, an initial fluid challenge of 250–500 ml normal saline or colloid-containing solution can be given for about 30 min and repeated as necessary. If blood pressure does not respond to this therapy, and the patient shows signs of developing pulmonary edema, a right heart catheter (i.e., Swan–Ganz) should be inserted. If patient is still hypovolemic, and the pulmonary capillary wedge pressure is less than 12 mmHg, further fluid resuscitation with normal saline, plasma, or packed red blood cells (PRBC) should be continued.

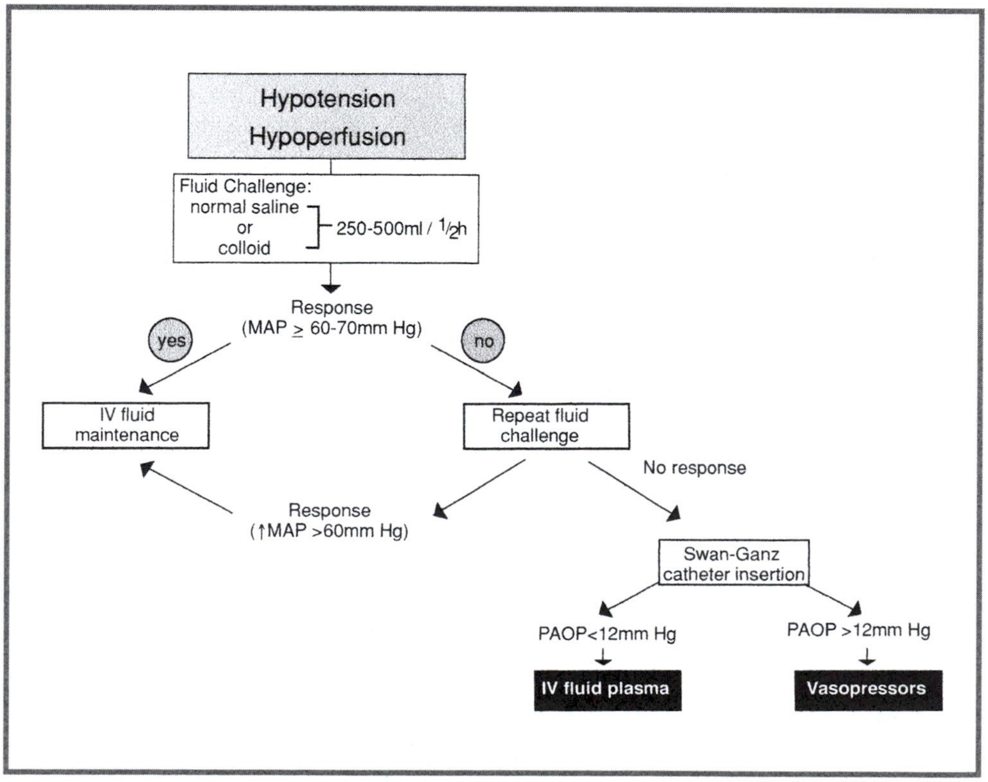

FIGURE 23-5

Hemodynamic management of shock. *MAP*, mean arterial pressure; *PAOP*, pulmonary artery occlusion pressure.

Plasma transfusion provides significant volume reexpansion. PRBC transfusions may theoretically improve the blood oxygen-carrying capacity and enhance oxygen delivery more effectively than saline resuscitation when the patient is severely anemic. One should remember that there is no proof that one type of the replacement fluid is superior to another for resuscitation purposes alone in circulatory failure. If the patient is normovolemic, with pulmonary capillary wedge pressures of 12–15 mmH_2O, and continues to be hypotensive, vasopressors should be started. We usually recommend starting dopamine at 5 mcg/kg/min and titrating to a mean arterial pressure between 60 and 70 mmHg, which should be sufficient for adequate perfusion of vital organs (i.e., brain and heart). If a high dose of dopamine ($>$10 mcg/kg/min) is reached and there are still signs of poor perfusion and hypotension, norepinephrine, a primary alpha agonist with mild beta$_1$ activity, can be added at 1–12 mcg/min and titrated to an adequate perfusion state. If a patient presents with primary cardiogenic shock (low cardiac output, high afterload), inotropic support with dobutamine or amrinone, agents that increase contractility and reduce arterial afterload, can be added.

In summary, adequate circulatory volume must be ensured before a vasopressor medication is started. The type of replacement fluid should be selected on the basis of need for blood transfusion, nature of the type of fluid lost from the vascular space, and the acuity of the problem, as well as potential risks of the product to the patient.

SUMMARY

Shock has a range of presentations and complexities that develop in critically ill patients admitted to the intensive care unit. A better understanding of the pathophysiologic mechanisms and of the metabolic and humoral disturbances associated with the shock state enables the clinician not only to choose appropriate diagnostic tests but also to apply therapeutic interventions logically to support vital organ function.

REVIEW QUESTIONS

1. **The major symptoms that define the state of shock include the following except:**
   A. Hypotension
   B. Oliguria
   C. Tachycardia
   D. Fever

2. **Which of the following substances is released from macrophages in response to endoxemia in septic shock?**
   A. Tumor necrosis factor
   B. Prostaglandins
   C. Serotonin
   D. Histamine

3. **All the following metabolic responses occur in shock except:**
   A. Glycogenolysis
   B. Gluconeogenesis
   C. Lactic acid production
   D. Increased insulin availability

4. **The initial therapy for patient in state of shock is:**
   A. IV fluid bolus
   B. IV dopamine
   C. IV norepinephrine
   D. IV dobutamine

ANSWERS

1. The answer is D. The major symptoms of shock—hypotension, oliguria and tachycardia—are caused by severe hypoperfusion, which is the core pathophysiologic component of shock. Fever can be present in septic shock but is not characteristic for other types of shock.
2. The answer is A. The major source of tumor necrosis factor is the macrophage. Sources of other vasoactive products listed in this question are platelets, smooth muscle and endothelial cells, and mast cells.
3. The answer is D. Enhanced glycogenolysis and gluconeogenesis occur due to a surge in cathecholamine and glucocorticoid release during the state of shock. Insulin production and release usually are not sufficient to meet increased metabolic demands. Increased lactic acid production reflects the inadequate oxygen delivery and utilization in shock.
4. The answer is A. Because the major pathophysiologic event in shock is hypoperfusion, efforts should be directed to restore adequate intravascular volume. Therefore, fluid infusion should be the first step in therapy.

SUGGESTED READING

Bartlett RH. Critical Care Physiology. Boston: Little, Brown, 1996.

Hall JB, Schmidt GA, Wood LDH. Principles of Critical Care, 2nd Ed. New York: McGraw-Hill, 1998.

Lodato RF. Cardiovascular derangement in septic shock and nitric oxide. J Crit Care 1996;11:151–154.

CHAPTER 24

Francis C. Cordova, Maria Roselyn Lim, and Gerard J. Criner

Neuromyopathies in the Critically Ill

CHAPTER OUTLINE

LEARNING OBJECTIVES

After studying this chapter, you should be able to:

- Be aware of the different neuromuscular disorders that may be encountered in the ICU.
- Know the effect of neuromuscular dysfunction on the respiratory system.
- Know the proper initial evaluation and management of patients with neuromuscular dysfunction and respiratory failure.
- Be familiar with neuromuscular disorders commonly encountered in the ICU.

Neuromuscular disorders are increasingly recognized as a significant contributor of morbidity and mortality in the intensive care unit (ICU). This recognition is largely brought about by the increased awareness of acquired neuromuscular dysfunction following acute life-threatening illness. Indeed, the development of acquired neuromyopathy during the course of treatment of life-threatening illness such as acute myopathy and critical illness polyneuropathy has replaced traditional causes of neuromyopathy (Guillain–Barré syndrome, myasthenia gravis) as the most common origin of muscle weakness in the ICU.

Although neuromuscular diseases are varied in etiology and pathogenesis, all can potentially lead to life-threatening respiratory failure, primarily by affecting the pump function of

TABLE 24-1

NEUROMUSCULAR DISEASES CAUSING MUSCLE WEAKNESS IN THE ICU SETTING

LEVEL OF THE MOTOR UNIT	DISORDER
Motor neuron	Amyotrophic lateral sclerosis
	Poliomyelitis
Peripheral nerve	Guillain–Barré syndrome
	Critical illness polyneuropathy
	Shellfish poisoning
	Porphyric neuropathy
Neuromuscular junction	Myasthenia gravis
	Botulism
	Hypermagnesemia
	Lambert–Eaton syndrome
Muscle	Acquired disorders
	Myoglobinuric myopathy
	Hypokalemic paralysis
	Toxic myopathy
	Acute myopathy of intensive care
	Congenital disorders
	Acid maltase deficiency
	Mitochondrial myopathy

In the ICU setting, neuromuscular dysfunction usually presents as acute respiratory failure, acute or chronic respiratory failure, or failure to wean from mechanical ventilation.

the respiratory muscle and by impairing its ability to generate effective cough. Thus, neuromuscular dysfunction typically presents in the ICU setting as either an acute respiratory failure, acute or chronic respiratory failure, or failure to wean from mechanical ventilation after the resolution of the acute illness. Acute respiratory failure can be caused by respiratory muscle weakness or, in most cases, precipitated by an infection, usually a community-acquired pneumonia. In patients who fail to wean from mechanical ventilation, the incidence of neuromuscular dysfunction has been reported as 10%–25% in various ventilator rehabilitation units across the country.

The severity of respiratory muscle dysfunction caused by neuromuscular diseases depends on the pattern and extent of respiratory muscle involvement (inspiratory or expiratory muscle involvement) and availability of effective medical therapy (plasmapheresis in Guillain–Barré syndrome; anticholinergic agents in myasthenia gravis). Moreover, the respiratory pump may be impaired at the level of the central nervous system, spinal cord, peripheral nerve, neuromuscular junction, or respiratory muscles. Neuromuscular disorders seen in the ICU setting are listed in Table 24-1.

A thorough understanding of the neuroanatomic and pathologic changes caused by the different neuromuscular disorders is important in their diagnosis and treatment. In this chapter, the etiology, pathophysiology, and treatment of selected neuromuscular diseases commonly seen in the ICU are discussed in detail.

PATHOPHYSIOLOGY OF NEUROMUSCULAR DISEASES THAT AFFECT RESPIRATORY FUNCTION

Neuromuscular disease becomes a life-threatening illness when it affects the function of the respiratory system. In certain neuromuscular diseases, such as congenital myopathies, cardiomyopathy may lead to congestive heart failure. However, the changes that occur in the respiratory system in patients with neuromuscular disorders are, by far, the most common reason for an admission into the ICU.

Different neuromuscular diseases can impair the different functional components of the respiratory system. Some diseases may affect the cortical center of breathing whereas others predominantly affect the function of the respiratory muscle and the chest wall as a mechanical pump to drive air in and out of the lungs. In addition, weakness of the upper airway muscles can lead to swallowing difficulty and frequent aspiration of oropharyngeal contents, further impairing lung function. The end result of these pathophysiologic changes imposed

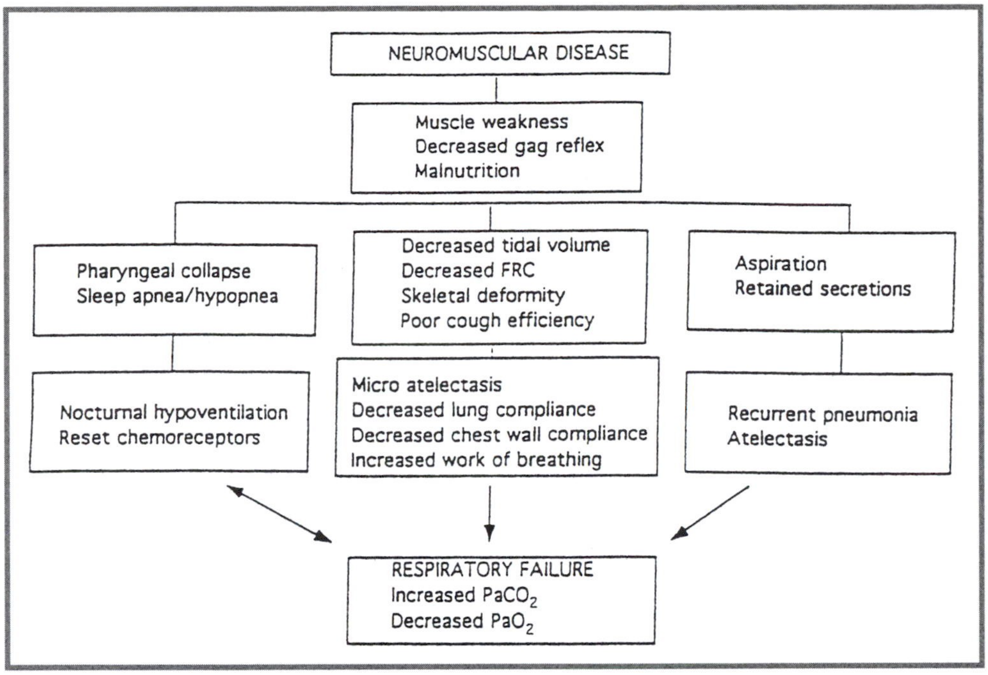

FIGURE 24-1

Schematic diagram of pathologic changes induced by neuromuscular disease on the respiratory system. The severity of these pathologic changes depends on the type and clinical stage of the neuromuscular disorder. FRC, functional residence capacity.

on the respiratory system by neuromuscular weakness is respiratory failure (Figure 24-1). The typical changes in the respiratory system that are commonly observed in patients with moderately advanced chronic neuromuscular dysfunction are listed in Table 24-2. All these pathologic changes are further magnified during sleep and exercise.

Control of Breathing

Chronic respiratory insufficiency in patients with chronic neuromuscular disorder is mainly the result of respiratory muscle weakness. However, several studies have shown that some patients afflicted with congenital myopathies exhibited hypoventilation out of proportion to the severity of the respiratory muscle weakness, suggesting the presence of impaired central respiratory drive.

Respiratory muscle weakness in the most common cause of chronic respiratory failure.

Several studies have shown the ventilatory response to hypoxia and hypercapnia is blunted in patients with congenital myopathies. In normal individuals, the relationship between oxygen desaturation and ventilation is linear; that is, a fall of oxygen saturation by 1% is approximately associated with a 1 l/min increase in minute ventilation. A much steeper linear increase in minute ventilation is seen during hypercarbic challenge. For every 1 mmHg rise in PCO_2, ventilation increases by 2.5–3 l/min. This normal predictable increase in minute ventilation in response to hypoxia and hypercapnea may be disturbed in neuromuscular disorders.

However, definite conclusions could not be drawn from these early studies because ventilatory response to metabolic stress is not a good index of central respiratory drive in the presence of respiratory muscle weakness. The blunted ventilatory response to hypoxic and

TABLE 24-2

PATHOPHYSIOLOGIC EFFECTS OF NEUROMUSCULAR DISORDERS ON THE NEURORESPIRATORY AXIS

CONTROL OF BREATHING	NORMAL/INCREASED PM_{100}
Respiratory muscle function	Decreased PI_{max} and PE_{max}
Lung and chest wall mechanics	Decrease in lung and chest wall compliance
Gas exchange abnormalities	Hypercapnia and hypoxemia
Sleep-related breathing disorder	Nocturnal hypercapnia and hypoxemia with normal daytime arterial blood gas

hypercapnic challenge seen in patients with chronic neuromuscular disease may be related to other factors such as respiratory muscle dysfunction and abnormal chest wall and lung mechanics and does not necessarily imply a decrease in central ventilatory output.

Mouth occlusion pressure, or Pm_{100}, is the maximum amount of negative pressure generated during early inspiration and is an index of central respiratory drive.

A better test of the central respiratory drive, one that is independent of respiratory mechanics, is the mouth occlusion pressure, or Pm_{100}. Pm_{100} refers to the maximum negative mouth pressure generated during the first 100 ms of inspiration with complete airway occlusion. Because the Pm_{100} is obtained during early inspiration with only a fraction of total inspiratory time, it is not influenced by conscious alteration in respiration. Similarly, because the Pm_{100} is only a fraction of the maximum inspiratory muscle strength, the result remains valid even in the presence of moderately severe respiratory muscle weakness.

Pm_{100} is normal or increased in patients with mild to moderately advanced neuromuscular disorder.

In studies using Pm_{100}, central respiratory drive has been found to be normal or increased in patients with neuromuscular disease despite substantial muscle weakness. Indeed, several studies have shown that despite significant reduction in respiratory muscle strength, the Pm_{100} in patients with Duchenne's muscular dystrophy, myotonic dystrophy, and a variety of neuromuscular diseases is one- to twofold higher than in normal controls. Similar increases in Pm_{100} were observed in normal volunteers after severe muscle weakness induced by curarization. Thus, it appears that central respiratory drive as measured by Pm_{100} is usually preserved in most patients with neuromuscular disease.

Respiratory Muscle Function

The respiratory muscles consist of the upper airway muscles, diaphragm, chest wall muscles, and abdominal muscles. The respiratory muscles can be further divided functionally into inspiratory and expiratory muscles. The inspiratory muscles produce rib cage expansion and negative intrathoracic pressure, allowing inspiratory airflow. During rest, exhalation is passive and is driven by the recoil pressure of the lung and chest wall. However, the expiratory muscles become active during periods of increased expiratory airflow as in coughing and exercise and in patients with airflow limitation. The innervation of the different respiratory muscle groups and their functions are shown in Table 24-3.

Respiratory muscle weakness may present clinically as exertional dyspnea, fatigue, poor cough, and recurrent respiratory tract infections.

Patients with moderate to severe respiratory muscle weakness due to a neuromuscular disease often complain of fatigue, poor sleep quality, and dyspnea, especially on exertion. Moreover, because of ineffective cough, recurrent respiratory infections, acute or chronic respiratory failure, and pulmonary hypertension are common. However, a significant percentage of these patients may be asymptomatic despite moderate to severe weakness of the inspiratory and expiratory muscles. In one study, 27% of patients with moderately advanced neuromuscular disease who had severe reduction in both inspiratory and expiratory muscles had no respiratory complaints. In another report, 50% of patients with severe respiratory muscle weakness due to chronic neuromuscular disease were asymptomatic. It is unclear

Many patients with significant respiratory muscle dysfunction are asymptomatic.

TABLE 24-3

INNERVATION OF THE RESPIRATORY MUSCLES

MUSCLE GROUP	NERVE
Upper airway	
Palate, pharynx	Glossopharyngeal, vagus, spinal accessory
Genioglossus	Hypoglossal
Inspiratory	
Diaphragm	Phrenic
Scalenes	Cervical C4–C8
Parasternal intercostals	Intercostal T1–T7
Sternocleidomastoid	Spinal accessory
Lateral external intercostals	Intercostal T1–T12
Expiratory	
Abdominal	Lumbar T7–L1
Internal intercostals	Intercostal T1–T12

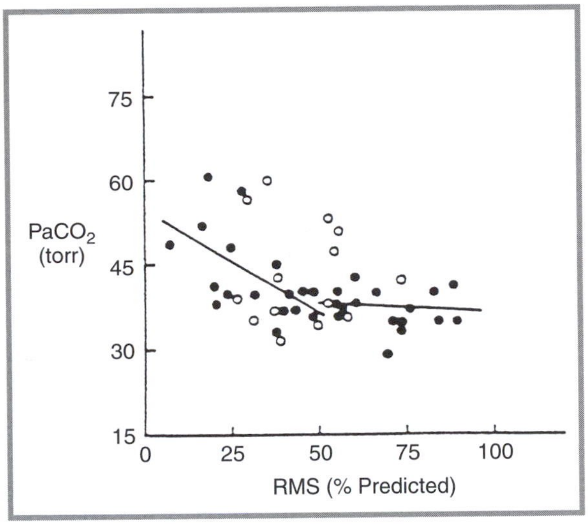

FIGURE 24-2

In patients with neuromyopathies, the relationship of respiratory muscle strength (RMS) and PCO_2 is discontinuous. Hypercapnia is likely to occur only when respiratory muscle strength is less than 30% of predicted.

why there is such a poor correlation between the extent of respiratory muscle weakness and the clinical symptoms reported by the patients. It is possible that the presence of significant respiratory muscle weakness is masked by concomitant generalized muscle weakness and a sedentary lifestyle.

The severity and the pattern of involvement of the respiratory muscles by the different neuromuscular disorders is not uniform. Some diseases cause global respiratory muscle dysfunction whereas others cause preferential weakness of the inspiratory or expiratory muscles. Moreover, a decrease in both inspiratory and expiratory muscle strength may not correlate with the general muscle strength assessment. Primary muscle diseases such as the polymyosities cause more significant impairment of the respiratory muscles in comparison to neuropathies. The relationship between inspiratory muscle strength and the onset of ventilatory insufficiency is not linear. Once maximum inspiratory mouth pressure decreases to less than 30% of predicted, hypercapnea ensues (Figure 24-2).

Neuromyopathies may lead to different degrees of inspiratory and expiratory muscle weakness.

Respiratory failure ensues when maximum inspiratory pressure is <30% of predicted.

Lung and Chest Wall Mechanics

Lung volume studies in patients with chronic respiratory muscle weakness often show a restrictive ventilatory pattern with a reduction in forced vital capacity (FVC) and preserved forced expiratory volume in 1 s/forced vital capacity ratio (FEV_1/FVC). Lung volume studies typically reveal a moderate reduction in total lung capacity and functional residual capacity with a normal or elevated residual capacity. A moderate fall in both inspiratory and expiratory reserve volume occurs. The decline in FVC is mainly caused by respiratory muscle weakness, and the decrease in FVC, in the absence of obstructive lung diseases, parallels the progression of the underlying respiratory muscle function. A significant reduction in lung compliance may also contribute to decreased FVC in these patients. The exact causes of reduced lung distensibility in these patients remains speculative and may be in part caused by (1) failed maturation of normal lung tissue in congenital neuromuscular diseases, (2) the presence of micro- or macroatelectasis, (3) an increase in alveolar surface tension caused by breathing chronically at low tidal volume, and (4) alteration in lung tissue elasticity.

Patients with neuromuscular disease have a rapid shallow breathing pattern similar to patients with interstitial lung disease. The exact mechanism of this abnormal breathing pattern is unclear but is thought to be caused by changes in lung and chest wall elastic recoil. Similar to the changes seen in the lungs, a significant reduction in chest wall compliance has also been reported in patients with chronic neuromuscular disease. The mechanisms of reduction in chest wall compliance are not clear but may be due to increased rib cage stiffness caused by fibrotic changes in the chest wall (i.e., tendons, ligaments, and costovertebral and costosternal articulations).

Lung and chest wall compliance decreases in patients with neuromyopathies.

FIGURE 24-3

In patients with neuromyopathies, hypercapnia is likely to occur when the vital capacity (VC) is less than 55% of predicted.

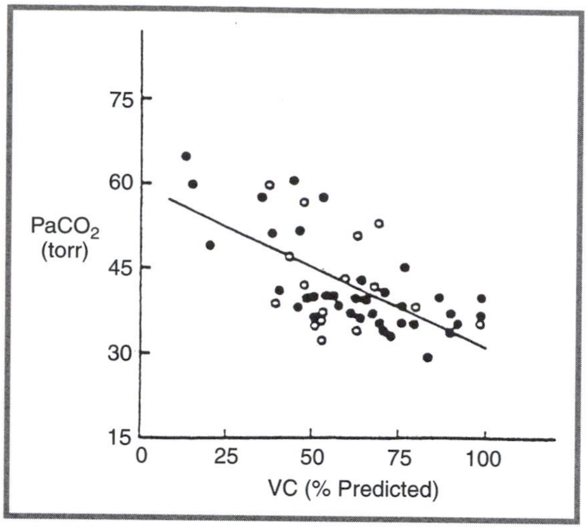

Gas Exchange Abnormalities

Hypoxemia and hypercapnia caused by ventilation/perfusion inequality are common in advanced disease.

Hypercapnia and hypoxemia are late findings in patients with stable chronic neuromuscular disease. Hypercapnia with a relatively normal FVC and static maximum respiratory pressures should suggest sleep-related breathing disorders (obstructive sleep apnea, obesity hypoventilation syndrome), the presence of parenchymal lung diseases such as chronic obstructive airway disease, problems with central respiratory drive such as the chronic hypoventilation syndrome, or hypothyroidism (as previously discussed). Even if daytime gas exchange parameters are normal, significant hypoxemia and alveolar hypoventilation may occur during sleep, especially during REM sleep when the activity of the accessory respiratory muscles is diminished. In advanced chronic neuromuscular disease, evidence of alveolar hypoventilation on blood gas examination is likely when the FVC is less than 55% of predicted and maximum inspiratory mouth pressure (PI_{max}), and maximum expiratory mouth pressure (PE_{max}) are less than -30 cmH_2O (Figure 24-3). However, the onset of hypercapnia in advanced neuromuscular disease may be abrupt. Ventilation perfusion inequality due to atelectasis is the most common cause of hypoxemia in these patients.

Effect of Neuromuscular Disease on Sleep

Hypoxemia and hypercapnia caused by nocturnal hypoventilation may occur in the absence of daytime gas exchange abnormalities.

Sleep-related breathing disorders such as impaired sleep quality and REM-related hypopnea are common in patients with respiratory muscle weakness caused by various neuromuscular diseases. Indeed, significant gas exchange abnormalities may be present and unsuspected even in the absence of daytime hypoxemia and hypercapnia.

Effects of REM sleep on respiratory physiology are alveolar hypoventilation, irregular breathing pattern, and upper airway obstruction due to decreased bulbar muscle tone.

Several physiologic changes in the respiratory system occur during sleep, particularly REM sleep, which can explain the predisposition of patients with poor pulmonary reserve in general, and respiratory muscle weakness in particular, to gas exchange abnormalities during sleep. Among the physiologic changes occurring during sleep are alveolar hypoventilation, inhibition of accessory inspiratory muscle activity, and development of a chaotic breathing pattern during REM sleep that causes significant hypoventilation in patients with diaphragm weakness. In addition, pharyngeal muscle weakness, which is present in some neuromuscular diseases, may aggravate the physiologic loss of upper airway tone during REM sleep, thereby increasing the predisposition to obstructive sleep apnea and hypopnea in these patients.

If nocturnal hypoventilation is severe and remains clinically unrecognized, daytime hypercapnia and hypoxemia might ensure even in the absence of severe respiratory muscle dysfunction. Nocturnal gas exchange abnormalities usually precede and occur much earlier than abnormalities in daytime arterial blood gas. Indeed, patients with normal nocturnal gas exchange are unlikely to have abnormal daytime values.

Daytime gas exchange abnormalities and a decrease in FVC are useful in predicting patients with neuromuscular disease who are at risk for severe oxygen desaturation during sleep. In a study involving 20 patients with a variety of moderately advanced neuromuscular diseases, the degree of arterial oxygen desaturation during REM sleep was directly related to the severity of daytime hypercapnia and hypoxemia. Both percent predicted FVC and the decrease in FVC from the sitting to supine positions were also found to correlate with the minimum oxygen saturation measured during REM sleep. Mean decrease in FVC from the seated to the supine positions in this study was 21%. Interestingly, the maximum static respiratory pressures were not predictive of nocturnal hypoventilation.

Upper Airway Dysfunction

Upper airway dysfunction, manifesting as the inability to handle oral secretions, recurrent aspiration, hoarseness, or stridor, is common in patients with neuromuscular dysfunction, especially when respiratory muscle weakness is present. Airway intubation and mechanical ventilation are often required to protect the airway and prevent aspiration once upper airway dysfunction is present.

The flow–volume loop is useful in excluding significant upper airway dysfunction. Indeed, an abnormal flow–volume loop has a high sensitivity and specificity in predicting bulbar and upper airway involvement in patients with neuromuscular dysfunction. A typical flow–volume loop in a patient with motor neuron disease with bulbar involvement is shown in Figure 24-4. A sawtooth pattern of the flow contour has been described in patients with Parkinson's disease. In addition, variable extrathoracic obstruction that reverses with drug therapy has been described in patients with myasthenia gravis.

The flow–volume loop is helpful in detecting upper airway dysfunction.

EVALUATION OF PATIENTS WITH NEUROMUSCULAR DISEASE

Clinical History

The diagnosis of neuromuscular disease should be suspected in all patients who are admitted to the ICU with unexplained acute or chronic hypercapnic respiratory failure. Unless a high index of suspicion is used in the diagnosis of neuromyopathy, the diagnosis will be missed or delayed because the presence of a neuromuscular dysfunction is often masked by

Neuromuscular disorders should be suspected in patients with respiratory failure and sensorimotor symptoms.

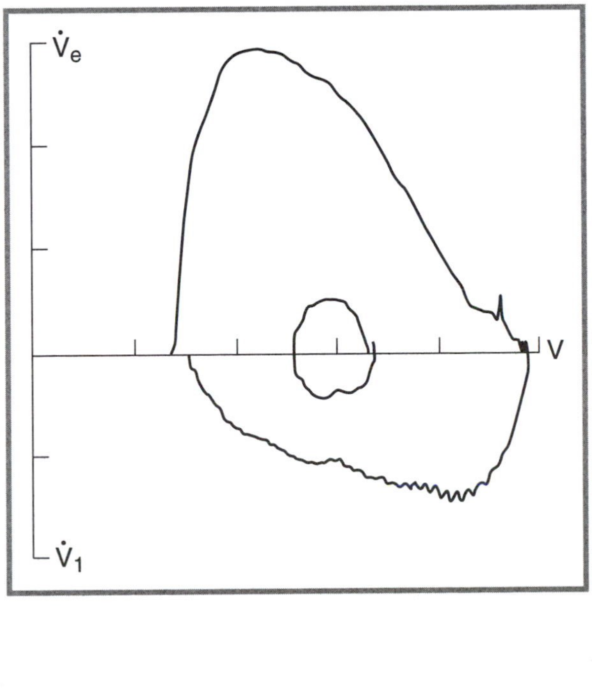

FIGURE 24-4

Upper airway obstruction caused by bulbar muscle involvement is common in patients with neuromuscular disease. The flow–volume loop may show a plateau of the inspiratory loop, suggesting extrathoracic upper airway obstruction.

CASE STUDY: PART 1

N.C., a 38-year-old self-employed businessman, sought neurology consultation for progressive limb numbness and weakness over the past week. His symptoms started 10 days before consultation when he experienced numbness and a tingling sensation in both feet. Because he had never been sick and had always lived a healthy lifestyle, he ignored the symptoms and attributed them to the tight new moccassins his wife had given him on their 10th wedding anniversary. However, 2 days later, he began to have difficulty climbing stairs and doing his usual 10K run. Three days before consultation, he experienced the same symptoms and weakness in both hands. He denied any swallowing difficulty. His past medical history was unremarkable except for a bout of diarrhea 2 months ago following a business trip to China.

the precipitating illness. Moreover, detailed neurologic history is often not available in the ICU setting because the patients are often intubated or are too breathless or confused to provide an accurate detailed history. In some cases, respiratory muscle weakness caused by a neuromuscular disease comes to light only after the patient has failed multiple weaning trials. Nevertheless, accurate historical details can often be obtained from significant others, primary caregivers, and medical records.

Inquiries about a preexisting neuromuscular disease are very important. Several neuromuscular diseases may cause sudden clinical deterioration, especially in advanced disease. Patients with congenital myopathies may develop cardiorespiratory failure or increased diaphragm weakness in the latter phases of their illness. The pattern of skeletal muscle weakness may suggest a particular diagnosis. Acute ascending paralysis of the lower extremities suggests Gullain–Barré syndrome; waxing and waning of neurologic symptoms is commonly seen in multiple sclerosis; and skeletal muscle weakness with repetitive action of a particular muscle group is highly suspicious of myasthenia gravis unless proven otherwise.

A detailed history of dietary intake over the last 48 h and drug and toxin ingestion should be obtained if possible. Acute shellfish poisoning (saxatoxin) may lead to skeletal muscle weakness. A history of consumption of home-canned goods suggests botulinum toxin poisoning. Several commonly used drugs such as cholesterol-lowering agents, colchicine, cyclosporin, chloroquin, and L-tryptophan can cause myotoxicity.

Diseases that predominantly affect the pump function of the respiratory system (i.e., phrenic nerve injury) present as dyspnea on exertion, weak cough, and recurrent respiratory tract infections whereas diseases that affect primarily the limb muscles (i.e., congenital myopathy, amyotrophic lateral sclerosis [ALS]) present as the inability to lift heavy objects, difficulty standing after sitting on a chair, or difficulty walking. However, some neuromuscular diseases such as ALS or mitochondrial myopathy can present initially as acute respiratory failure. Once the respiratory muscles are affected in advanced neuromuscular disease, respiratory failure may occur abruptly, due to an intercurrent illness, or slowly over months or years, finally culminating in hypercapnic respiratory failure. In most neuromuscular diseases, respiratory muscle weakness usually occurs insidiously and is typically associated with weakness of other skeletal muscle groups. However, as many as 50% of patients with significant respiratory muscle weakness are asymptomatic until they develop respiratory failure.

CASE STUDY: PART 2

On physical examination, the patient appeared anxious but was not in any distress. Except for mild tachycardia, his vital signs were within normal limits. Cardiopulmonary examination was within normal limits. His hands and feet were cool to the touch. On neurologic examination, he had normal mental status. His cranial nerves were normal. On sensory examination, he had decreased touch sensation on both lower extremities and loss of propioception at the toes bilaterally. His muscle strength in both upper and lower extremities was 4/5 and 3/5, respectively. His reflexes were 1+ in the upper extremities, and no knee jerks could be elicited on both lower extremities. No ankle jerks were present.

TABLE 24-4

DIFFERENTIATION BETWEEN UPPER AND LOWER MOTOR NEURON LESIONS

LEVEL	SYMPTOM
Upper motor neuron	Weakness Spasticity Hyperreflexia Babinski sign
Lower motor neuron	Weakness Atrophy Flaccidity Hyporeflexia Fasciculation

Physical Examination

A thorough physical examination and a detailed neurologic assessment may reveal a previously undiagnosed neuromuscular disorder. However, physical examination may be limited by sedation, the use of neuromuscular blocking agents, or the presence of edema. Certain neurologic findings are helpful in differentiating upper motor neuron versus lower motor neuron lesions (Table 24-4) and in differentiating neuropathy versus myopathy (Table 24-5).

In patients with early or mild neuromuscular weakness, respiratory muscle weakness may not be detected on routine physical examination. Tachypnea at rest is very common with the onset of respiratory muscle weakness. As respiratory muscle weakness progresses, the increase in respiratory rate may then followed by signs of increased respiratory distress such as nasal flaring, recruitment of the accessory muscles, and intercostal as well as subcostal retractions. Progressive weakness of the respiratory muscles eventually leads to paradoxical inward motion of the rib cage and outward displacement of the abdomen during inspiration. Abnormal paradoxical motion of the rib cage and abdomen may indicate either impending respiratory failure or diaphragm weakness. Indeed, paradoxical inward movement of the abdomen on inspiration that worsens with the recumbent position is typically seen in diaphragm weakness.

Signs of respiratory muscle weakness are tachypnea, use of accessory muscles of respiration, and paradoxical movement of the thorax and abdomen during breathing.

Ancillary Tests

Arterial Blood Gases

Abnormalities in arterial blood gases occur late in patients with severe respiratory muscle weakness and may not be present before the need to implement ventilatory support. Hypoxemia is commonly the result of microatelectasis due to ineffective cough and retained secretions, causing ventilation–perfusion mismatch or intrapulmonary shunting. More importantly, alveolar hypoventilation caused by respiratory muscle weakness or decreased central respiratory drive may also contribute significantly to hypoxemia. Hypoxemia mainly

TABLE 24-5

DIFFERENTIATION BETWEEN MYOPATHY AND POLYNEUROPATHY

	CLINICAL CHARACTERISTICS	NERVE CONDUCTION	EMG
Neuropathy	Distal weakness Flaccidity Hyporeflexia Bulbar involvement Sensory and autonomic changes	Diminished	Denervation potentials in axonal neuropathies
Myopathy	Proximal weakness Normal reflexes No sensory and autonomic changes Pain	Normal	Small motor unit potentials

caused by alveolar hypoventilation is supported by a normal alveolar-arterial oxygen gradient. Pulse oximetry, which is a measure of arterial oxyhemoglobin saturation, is useful in detecting hypoxemia but is not a sensitive indicator of hypoventilation.

Hypoxemia and hypercapnia are late findings in patients with respiratory muscle weakness.

Hypercapnia is a late finding in severe respiratory muscle weakness. In fact, hypercapnia does not occur until the respiratory muscle strength is less than 50% of predicted. Careful analysis of the pH and bicarbonate level is helpful in determining acute from chronic hypercapnic respiratory failure. Sleep-induced breathing disturbances may also lead to hypercarbia and should be carefully studied in susceptible patients.

Pulmonary Function Tests

Spirometry and lung volume studies are helpful in the initial evaluation as well as in follow-up of patients with neuromuscular disease during therapy. In general, spirometry produces a restrictive pattern characterized by a reduction in FVC and a normal FEV_1/FVC ratio. Moreover, there is a decrease in effort-dependent expiratory flow such as peak expiratory airflow measurement whereas FEV_1 and measurement of midexpiratory flow rates (FEF_{25-75} or FEF_{50}) are often greater than normal predicted values because of increased elastic recoil. The increase in elastic recoil pressure results from decreases in both lung and chest wall compliance. The lung volume study typically shows a decrease in total lung capacity (TLC) and an increase in residual volume (RV) due to expiratory muscle weakness. Diffusion capacity is usually normal.

The usual pulmonary function test results in patients with respiratory muscle weakness are decreased expiratory flow rates (FVC, FEV_1), increased RV, and decreased TLC.

Serial measurements of FVC are helpful in following the progression of respiratory muscle weakness and in evaluating the need for partial or full ventilatory support. In patients with rapidly progressive respiratory muscle weakness, as seen in Guillain–Barré syndrome, daily measurement of FVC (<10 ml/kg or <1 l) helps to determine when to consider elective airway intubation and mechanical ventilation. Alternatively, FVC can also be used as one of the criteria for the initiation of weaning trials and liberation from mechanical ventilation.

Serial FVC measurement is a useful bedside test in predicting impending respiratory failure in patients with rapidly progressive neuromyopathies.

Upper airway dysfunction is commonly seen in chronic neuromuscular diseases and may be detected easily by analyzing the flow–volume curves. For example, the inspiratory plateau of the flow waveform is indicative of extrathoracic upper airway obstruction. In patients with Parkinson's disease, instability of the upper airway muscles is reflected in "sawtoothing" of the contour of the flow–volume loop. An abnormal flow–volume loop in patients with neuromuscular disease is both highly sensitive and specific in predicting bulbar dysfunction.

Abnormal flow–volume loop indicates upper airway muscle dysfunction.

Radiographic Assessment

Radiographic findings in patients with neuromuscular disease are helpful in detecting pneumonia, atelectasis, and other parenchymal lung disease. Although small lung volumes on chest x-ray may suggest the possibility of inspiratory muscle weakness, this is a very nonspecific finding in the ICU setting because portable chest x-rays are often used and a film at maximum inspiration may not be obtained. Nevertheless, in the right clinical setting, small lung volumes on chest radiograph and the presence of bilateral basal bandlike atelectasis suggest chronic volume loss that may be the result of weak respiratory muscles as seen in bilateral hemidiaphragm paralysis. However, this radiographic picture could also be easily dismissed as a poor inspiratory effort. On the other hand, unilateral hemidiaphragm paralysis can be easily recognized on a routine chest radiograph as a unilateral elevated hemidiaphragm. The elevation of a hemidiaphragm due to weakness or paralysis can be confirmed by performing a "sniff test" under fluoroscopy, which may demonstrate paradoxical upward movement of the affected hemidiaphragm during a rapid sniff maneuver or lack of contraction during ultrasonographic imaging.

Chest radiographic findings suggestive of respiratory muscle weakness are small lung volumes, bilateral basal atelectasis, and elevated hemidiaphragm.

Maximum Mouth Pressures

Maximum static respiratory pressures, measured at the airway opening during a voluntary contraction against an occluded airway, are the most sensitive tests to assess respiratory muscle dysfunction in patients with neuromuscular disease even in the absence of symptoms and

TABLE 24-6

SELECTED NORMAL MAXIMUM STATIC AIRWAY PRESSURES VALUES IN ADULTS

STUDY	SEX	PI_{MAX} CMH_2O	PE_{MAX} CMH_2O
Black,	Male	124 ± 22	233 ± 42
Hyatt, 1969	Female	87 ± 16	152 ± 27
Rochester,	Male	127 ± 28	216 ± 41
Arora, 1983	Female	91 ± 25	138 ± 39
Leech, et al.	Male	114 ± 36	154 ± 82
1987	Female	71 ± 27	94 ± 33

SOURCE: Black LF, Hyatt RE. Maximal respiratory pressures normal values and relationship to age and sex. Am Rev Respir Dis 1969;99:969–702. Rochester DF, Arora NS. Respiratory muscle failure. Med Clin North Am 1983;67: 573–598. Leech JA, Ghezzo H, Stevens D, Becklake MR. Respiratory pressures and function in young adults. Am Rev Respir Dis 1983;128:17–23

normal ventilatory function. The extent of respiratory muscle weakness can be quantified by measuring the maximum inspiratory (PI_{max}) and expiratory pressures (PE_{max}) that can be generated by the respiratory muscles. It should be remembered that measurement of static mouth pressures are affected by lung volumes. Thus, PI_{max} is measured near RV when the inspiratory muscles are at their greatest mechanical advantage; PE_{max} is measured near TLC when the inward recoil pressure of the respiratory system and the ability of the expiratory muscles to generate force is greatest. Table 24-6 shows normal maximum static inspiratory and expiratory muscle strength in adults. Reported values vary widely in different studies and may be due to differences in techniques utilized or to learning effect in individual subjects after repeated measurements.

PI_{max} and PE_{max} are used to measure global inspiratory and expiratory muscle strength, respectively.

In chronic neuromuscular diseases, measurement of both maximum static inspiratory pressures and expiratory pressures (PI_{max} and PE_{max}) are frequently decreased. Here, PI_{max} and PE_{max} usually range from 37% to 52% of normal depending on disease severity and the type of neuromuscular disease. In a study of 16 patients with various chronic neuromuscular diseases, the mean static inspiratory pressure measured with the esophageal balloon was 43% of predicted. In patients with proximal myopathies, hypercapnic respiratory failure has been reported to occur when PI_{max} and PE_{max} were less than 30% or if the FVC was less than 55% of predicted. Even in patients with only mild generalized muscle weakness, profound reduction in maximum static respiratory pressures may occur. In another study of 30 patients with stable chronic neuromuscular weakness, 30% of patients with relatively good general muscle strength had unsuspected severe respiratory muscle weakness (less than 50% predicted). Because of the frequent involvement of the respiratory muscles in neuromuscular diseases, the measurement of maximum static respiratory pressures should be routine in the assessment of neuromuscular disease patients, regardless of the severity or stage of the disease.

Respiratory insufficiency occurs when PI_{max} and PE_{max} are $<30\%$ of predicted.

The PI_{max} and PE_{max}, in addition to FVC, are useful parameters to monitor the progression of respiratory muscle weakness in patients with acute neuromuscular disease who are admitted to the ICU. These tests are reproducible, cheap, and easy to perform serially at the bedside to predict impending respiratory failure in patients with respiratory muscle weakness and the need for ventilatory support. Ventilatory support is often required when VC is less than 10–15 ml/kg or PI_{max} is less than 20–25 cmH_2O. In certain circumstances such as pneumonia, atelectasis, or inability to clear secretions, mechanical ventilation may be required before these parameters are obtained.

Serial measurement of FVC, PI_{max}, and PE_{max} provides useful parameters to follow in the ICU to predict need for ventilatory support.

Although measurement of maximum static respiratory pressures is useful in quantifying global respiratory muscle strength, it does not distinguish selective weakness of a particular respiratory muscle group and it does not provide any information on respiratory muscle endurance.

Transdiaphragmatic Pressure Measurement

In contrast to maximum static pressures, which measure global respiratory parameters, transdiaphragmatic pressure (P_{di}) specifically measures diaphragm strength. Although transdiaphragmatic pressure measurement is more invasive and not readily available in clinical

Transdiaphragmatic pressure measures diaphragm muscle strength.

practice, it may be useful in certain clinical conditions when phrenic nerve injury is suspected, as can be seen following cardiac surgery or trauma.

Measurement of diaphragm strength is made by estimating esophageal (P_{es}) and gastric (P_{ga}) pressures via balloon-tipped catheters placed in the midesophagus and in the stomach, respectively. The P_{di} is then calculated as the algebraic sum of P_{es} from P_{ga} ($P_{di} = P_{ga} - P_{es}$). Several maneuvers with varying degree of difficulty have been used during the measurement of P_{di} to obtain maximal voluntary activation of the diaphragm. The P_{di} obtained during a maximal sniff maneuver is the easiest to perform whereas $P_{di\ max}$ obtained after a Mueller maneuver combined with an active expulsive maneuver appears to be the most reproducible and maximal transdiaphragmatic pressures. The measurement of transdiaphragmatic pressure is limited by the need for an invasive procedure and the large variation in P_{di} values even in normal individuals. The wide intrasubject variability of P_{di} may be attributed to the patient's submaximal efforts and to activation of the intercostal and accessory muscles, which causes upward displacement of the diaphragm, resulting in falsely low P_{di} values.

Direct stimulation of the phrenic nerve, by consistently obtaining maximal stimulation of the diaphragm, avoids the variability in measured P_{di} when only volitional effort is used. The phrenic nerve can be easily stimulated in the neck as it traverses the posterior border of the sternocleidomastoid muscle at the level of the cricoid cartilage. Phrenic nerve stimulation may be performed with either a transcutaneous electrode or a magnetic coil. Use care to ensure supramaximal stimulation as indicated by monitoring the maximum diaphragm muscle action potential (DMAP). This technique is currently used only in the research setting.

SPECIFIC NEUROMUSCULAR DISORDERS

Amyotrophic Lateral Sclerosis

Amyotrophic lateral sclerosis (ALS) is a progressive neurodegenerative disorder of the skeletal muscles.

Amyotrophic lateral sclerosis (ALS) is a progressive neurodegenerative disorder of both upper and lower motor neurons leading to the loss of skeletal muscle function. The incidence of ALS is 1–2 per 100,000 people. The majority of cases are sporadic (classical ALS), but 5%–10% of cases result from autosomal dominant inheritance (familial ALS). There is a male predilection with a male to female ratio of 2:1. Death is usually the result of progressive respiratory failure and respiratory infections. Mean survival from the initial onset of symptoms is 3–4 years.

The exact etiology of ALS is unknown. A gene mutation encoding copper–zinc superoxide dismutase, a free oxygen radical scavenger, has been identified in 10%–15% of familial ALS patients. This finding suggests that the disease may be triggered by the susceptibility of the neurons to oxidative stress. Recent evidence suggests that the motor neurons are susceptible to glutamate-induced neurotoxicity. Glutamate is the principal excitatory neurotransmitter in the brain. The decreased uptake of glutamate is thought to lead to overstimulation of the glutamate receptors, which increases intracellular calcium. The increase in intracellular calcium activates the proteolytic enzymes, causing cell membrane injury.

Progressive weakness of distal extremities is the most common complaint in patients with ALS.

The usual clinical presentation in two-thirds of ALS patients is progressive weakness of the distal extremities, although early involvement of the bulbar muscles occurs in 25% of cases. Clinical staging criteria of ALS are listed in Table 24-7. Early involvement of the phrenic nerve neurons in some patients with ALS can lead to acute respiratory failure or nocturnal hypoventilation even before other symptoms become clinically evident.

TABLE 24-7

CLINICAL STAGING CRITERIA OF AMYOTROPHIC LATERAL SCLEROSIS (ALS)

Stage I	Symptoms limited to one limb, bulbar or respiratory musculature
Stage II	Symptoms in an additional site
Stage III	Inability to walk, or involvement of all limbs
Stage IV	Wheelchair-bound more than 50% of time
Stage V	Bedbound
Stage VI	Death from ALS

Although respiratory muscle impairment is usually only evident in advanced disease, abnormalities in pulmonary function tests are apparent even in patients with only mild weakness of the extremities. Serial lung function studies in ALS patients invariably show progressive reduction in FVC and maximum voluntary ventilation as well as a progressive increase in residual volume (RV). The decline in FVC correlates with poor outcome. Both the maximum inspiratory pressure (PI_{max}) and maximum expiratory pressure (PE_{max}) are reduced, to about 34% and 47% of predicted, respectively. In symptomatic patients with relatively preserved pulmonary function, MIP and MEP are frequently abnormal. An MIP of less than -60 cmH_2O is 100% sensitive for predicting less than 18-month survival.

Progressive decline in FVC and maximum inspiratory pressure (MIP) has a poor prognosis.

The shape of the flow–volume curve may identify a subset of patients with greater weakness of the expiratory muscles. In patients with severe weakness of the expiratory muscles, the flow–volume loop shows concavity of the maximal expiratory curve with a sharp drop in flow at lower lung volume. This group of ALS patients have lower maximal expiratory pressures, smaller vital capacities, and higher residual volumes compared to patients with normal flow–volume loops.

A flow–volume loop with a concave-shaped maximum expiratory curve suggests expiratory muscle weakness in patients with ALS.

Adequate oxygenation is usually well maintained even with severe abnormalities in spirometry. Monitoring of arterial blood gas is not useful in early disease. Spirometry, however, is still important in the initial evaluation of patients with ALS because impairment in ventilatory function is frequently underestimated even by an experienced examiner.

The comprehensive management of ALS patients should include measures to alleviate symptoms and specific drug therapy to alter the progressive clinical course of ALS. Riluzole, an antiglutamate drug, is FDA-approved for the treatment of ALS. Riluzole is the only treatment that has been shown to prolong survival in ALS. It should be given to patients once a diagnosis of ALS is made. Other antiglutamate drugs, such as gabapentin, or neurotrophic factors, such as insulin-like growth factors and glial-derived neurotrophic factor, are under investigation.

Noninvasive positive pressure ventilation (NPPV) and an antiglutamate drug, riluzole, have been shown to prolong survival in ALS.

Despite optimal medical therapy, disease progression invariably occurs, resulting in respiratory insufficiency requiring some form of ventilatory assistance. The onset of respiratory failure often signals the rapid decline in global functional status as well. The need for mechanical ventilation should be discussed with the patient and family early on to prevent rapid decline in lung function. In a survey of ALS patients, patients with early disease are more receptive to long-term ventilatory support compared to patients with advanced disease. ALS patients who develop respiratory symptoms, or have moderate reduction in lung function or a rapid decline in lung function, should be offered noninvasive ventilation such as Biphasic (inspiratory and expiratory) positive airways pressure (BIPAP). In patients who can tolerate nasal noninvasive positive pressure ventilation (NPPV), the risk of death is decreased a factor of 3.1. Recently, 122 patients with ALS were offered BIPAP therapy once they developed dyspnea, or FVC less than 50%, or a fall of more than 15% in FVC in 3 months follow-up. Those patients who used BIPAP more than 4 h/day not only showed a slower decline in lung function but also had decreased mortality rates. Some patients with acute respiratory decompensation may have partial improvement in respiratory muscle strength after a period of ventilatory assistance. Theophylline may improve respiratory muscle strength in these patients. One study has shown that theophylline significantly increases respiratory muscle strength after resistive breathing. In that study, the negative inspiratory pressure, FVC, and peak inspiratory flow increased by 28%, 10%, and 12%, respectively.

Phrenic Nerve Injury

Unilateral or bilateral diaphragm weakness can follow phrenic nerve injury. Reported causes of phrenic nerve injury are listed in Table 24-8. In most cases of diaphragm weakness, the exact diagnosis remains elusive. In diaphragm dysfunction following cardiac surgery, phrenic nerve injury may occur secondary to cold exposure or to mechanical stretching during surgery.

Cold exposure and mechanical stretching of the phrenic nerve are the two causes of phrenic nerve injury during open heart surgery.

The diagnosis of bilateral diaphragm weakness is frequently delayed. The symptoms of diaphragm weakness are often nonspecific, and the routine physical findings are insensitive and unreliable. In the absence of parenchymal lung disease or heart failure, dyspnea that is made

Unilateral diaphragm weakness usually does not cause any symptoms. Bilateral diaphragm weakness causes dyspnea that is aggravated by lying down.

TABLE 24-8

CAUSES OF PHRENIC NERVE INJURY

Thoracic surgery	Motor neuron disease
Chest trauma	Myopathies
Mediastinal tumors	Neuropathies
Mediastinal and pleural infection	Myelopathies
Forceful neck manipulation	

worse by lying down is an important clue to the diagnosis. The cephalad displacement of the abdominal contents in the supine position further increases the workload of the already weakened diaphragm. Significant diaphragmatic weakness can often be confirmed during physical examination by the presence of thoracoabdominal paradox in the recumbent position.

Pulmonary function test (PFT) findings in bilateral diaphragm weakness are decreased FVC, RV, and TLC. FVC is reduced by more than 50% from sitting to supine position.

Unilateral diaphragm weakness, in contrast, is usually well tolerated even if the pulmonary function test (PFT) reveals a mild reduction in FVC and TLC. The diagnosis of unilateral diaphragm weakness is often suspected only on routine chest radiograph that is ordered for other clinical indications. Extensive workup is usually not warranted unless severe symptoms point to other cardiopulmonary conditions.

Elevated unilateral or bilateral diaphragms may be seen on chest x-ray. Diaphragm weakness can be confirmed by visualizing diaphragm movement on the fluoroscopy sniff test or by measuring P_{di}.

Once the diagnosis of diaphragm weakness is clinically suspected, measurement of respiratory muscle strength and fluoroscopic findings on the sniff test may help confirm the diagnosis. On routine pulmonary function testing, bilateral diaphragm paralysis reveals a restrictive ventilatory defect characterized by a decrease in FVC, RV, and TLC. The VC is typically reduced to less than 50% of predicted in the erect posture and is further reduced in the recumbent posture. In the upright posture, contraction of the abdominal muscles during expiration and relaxation during early inspiration result in outward motion of the abdomen and facilitates the passive descent of the diaphragm. In the recumbent posture, diaphragm function is further impaired by the increase in the inspiratory workload imposed by the cranial displacement of the abdominal visceral contents. As in any other neuromuscular disease, chronic hypercapnic respiratory failure may be seen in moderate to severe bilateral diaphragm weakness.

Radiographic findings in patients with diaphragm weakness typically show either unilateral or bilateral elevated hemidiaphragm depending on the location of the phrenic nerve injury. However, parenchyma and pleural diseases such as atelectasis, pulmonary fibrosis, subpulmonic fluid collection, or atelectasis may also show the same radiographic picture. A fluoroscopic technique to evaluate diaphragmatic excursion known as the sniff test is helpful in further evaluating the presence of diaphragm paralysis. As described earlier, the paralyzed diaphragm exhibits an upward paradoxical movement into the chest cavity because of the development of negative intrapleural pressures during the sniff maneuver. The sniff test is not useful in the evaluation of bilateral diaphragm paralysis and may result in an apparently false-normal study. Both hemidiaphragms may appear to descend normally during a sniff maneuver, despite profound weakness, due to sudden relaxation of the abdominal muscles. In addition, a positive sniff test should also be interpreted with caution because this can be seen in up to 6% of normal individuals. Paradoxical diaphragm movement should be at least 2 cm to increase the test's specificity.

Measurement of transdiaphragmatic pressure (P_{di}), despite its limitations discussed earlier (e.g., intersubject variability, invasive procedure, need for full patient cooperation) is useful in the diagnosis and quantitation of diaphragm weakness. Total diaphragm paralysis is diagnosed when there is no pressure difference across the two sides of the diaphragm ($P_{di} = 0$) during a forced inspiratory maneuver against an occluded airway.

Recovery of diaphragm weakness depends on the etiology. In phrenic nerve injury following cardiac surgery, 80% of patients recover nerve function in 6 months and 90% in 1 year.

Guillain–Barré Syndrome

Guillain–Barré syndrome (GBS) is an acute idiopathic polyneuritis that is usually preceded by a viral illness.

Guillain–Barré syndrome (GBS) is an acute idiopathic polyneuritis that usually presents clinically as a rapidly ascending paralysis of the lower extremities which often leads to bulbar and respiratory compromise. Although the exact etiology is unknown, several risk factors

CASE STUDY: PART 3

Initial laboratory examination showed a normal hemogram and routine blood chemistries. Cerebrospinal fluid examination revealed WBC of 4/mm^3, RBC of 0/mm^3, glucose of 55 mg/dl, and protein of 96 mg/dl. EMGs of both lower and upper extremities showed prolonged sensory and motor latencies with decreased conduction velocities. A diagnosis of Guillain–Barré syndrome was made. The patient was admitted to the neurology service and was immediately started on intravenous immunoglobulin. On admission, his FVC was 2.8 l and his PI_{max} was 110 cmH_2O. An arterial blood gas showed a pH of 7.39, $PaCO_2$ of 42 mmHg, PaO_2 of 80 mmHg, and HCO_2 of 24 mEq/dl. He appeared comfortable, and he denied any shortness of breath. On the third hospital day, he complained of shortness of breath after going to the bathroom. A repeat FVC was 2.0 l, a notable decrease compared to admission. He was transferred to the ICU for closer monitoring.

have been identified, among which are viral illnesses (cytomegalovirus, Epstein–Barr virus, HIV), *Mycoplasma pneumoniae* infection, influenza vaccination, recent surgery, trauma, and malignancy (lymphoma). A recent study has shown a strong association between antecedent *Campylobacter jejuni* infection and Guillain–Barré syndrome.

The clinical signs and symptoms of GBS are shown in Table 24-9. The symptoms typically begin with a sensory phase consisting of numbness and tingling in the fingers, toes, and trunk lasting 7–10 days. Pain over the extremities or flank is commonly reported as a "charley horse," but objective sensory impairment is minimal despite complaints of paresthesias. This stage is followed classically by an ascending pattern of limb weakness from the lower to upper extremities. The extent of motor weakness is variable, ranging from mild paresis to complete paralysis. In 50% of GBS cases, weakness of the lower extremities usually peaks within several days of diagnosis. The muscle weakness usually does not progress beyond 4 weeks. Autoimmune dysfunction is very common. Other variants of Guillain–Barré syndrome with asymmetric involvement of the extremities, presence of ataxia, or the absence of paresthesia have been described. The Miller–Fisher variant of GBS refers to the syndrome of ophthalmoplegia, ataxia, and areflexia. In these patients, 95% have a polyclonal antibody to ganglioside GQ1b. In more than half the cases, the syndrome is preceded by a history of recent upper respiratory tract infection, flu-like symptoms, or diarrheal illness 1–3 weeks before the onset of symptoms. Abnormal CSF examinations and nerve conduction studies are confirmatory for the diagnosis of Guillain–Barré syndrome. Cerebrospinal fluid (CSF) examination characteristically shows increased CFS fluid protein without an increase in cell count. This CSF finding is commonly referred to as albuminocytologic dissociation. Nerve conduction study typically shows multifocal demyelination. The proposed diagnostic criteria for typical Guillain–Barré syndrome are shown in Table 24-10.

Acute respiratory failure is one of the well-recognized complication of GBS. In 15%–30% of cases of acute GBS, acute respiratory failure is profound and requires mechanical ventilation. The incidence of acute respiratory failure increases by twofold once respiratory mus-

The symptoms caused by GBS peak at 4 weeks after onset of symptoms.

The Miller–Fisher syndrome consists of ophthalmoplegia, ataxia, and areflexia.

Cerebrospinal fluid (CSF) findings in GBS: high protein content with few cells, referred to as albuminocytologic dissociation. EMG findings in GBS: multifocal demyelination.

Acute respiratory failure occurs in 15%–30% of patients with GBS.

TABLE 24-9

USUAL CLINICAL SIGNS AND SYMPTOMS OF GUILLAIN–BARRÉ SYNDROME

SYMPTOMS	INCIDENCE
Ascending paralysis of the lower extremities	95%
Paresthesias	85%
Facial muscle weakness	60%
Oropharyngeal muscle weakness	50%
Ocular muscle weakness	15%
Autonomic dysfunction	65%
Cardiac arrhythmia	
Blood pressure lability	
Gastrointestinal dysfunction	
Pupillary dysfunction	
Sweating abnormalities	
Urinary retention	

TABLE 24-10

DIAGNOSTIC CRITERIA FOR TYPICAL GUILLAIN–BARRÉ SYNDROME AS PROPOSED BY ASBURY AND CORNBLATH

Features required for diagnosis	Progressive weakness of both upper and lower extremities Areflexia
Features strongly supporting the diagnosis	Progression of symptoms over days to 4 weeks Symmetry of symptoms Mild sensory symptoms or signs Cranial nerve involvement, especially bilateral weakness of facial muscles Recovery beginning 2–4 weeks after progression ceases Autonomic dysfunction Absence of fever at the onset Elevated protein concentration in CSF with fewer than 10 cells/ml^3 Typical electrodiagnostic features
Features making the diagnosis doubtful	Sensory level Marked, persistent asymmetry of symptoms or signs Severe and persistent bladder and bowel dysfunction More than 50 cells/ml^3 in CSF
Features excluding the diagnosis	Diagnosis of botulism, myasthenia, poliomyelitis, or toxic neuropathy Abnormal porphyrin metabolism Recent diptheria Purely sensory syndrome without weakness

cle dysfunction is detected and the patient requires ICU care. Other common complications are pneumonia, recurrent aspiration, and pulmonary thromboembolic disease.

Indications for ventilatory support: FVC $<$ 12–15 ml/kg, upper airway dysfunction, and hypoxemia and hypercapnia

All patients suspected of having GBS and showing signs of respiratory muscle dysfunction should be transferred to the ICU for closer monitoring. Other clinical indications for admission to the ICU are listed in Table 24-11. Severe weakness of diaphragm force-generating capacity is shown by a marked reduction in maximum transdiaphragmatic pressures during acute ventilatory failure and during recovery from the illness. Serial FVC is the most useful test in predicting the need for mechanical ventilation and should be performed daily, or twice daily depending on the clinical condition of the patient. Figure 24-5 shows the changes in respiratory function with the progressive decline in FVC and its suggested treatment. Several studies have shown that a FVC of 12–15 mg/kg is a sign of imminent respiratory failure. In patients who develop respiratory failure due to Guillain–Barré syndrome, FVC measured serially decreased from a mean of 2.5 l to 0.9 l within 2 weeks. Other indications for intubation and ventilatory support include respiratory distress, inability to handle oral secretions, hypoxemia ($PaO_2 < 70$ mmHg on room air or alveolar-arterial O_2 difference >300 mmHg with FiO_2 of 100%) and hypercapnia. Blood gas analysis is used to ensure adequate oxygenation and ventilation. Hypercapnia is a late sign of ventilatory failure and should not be relied upon for need for mechanical ventilation. The average $PaCO_2$ at the time of intubation when FVC is less than 12 ml/kg was 43 mmHg in two large series of GBS patients.

CASE STUDY: PART 4

In the ICU, the patient was started on subcutaneous heparin for deep venous thrombosis prophylaxis. Daily range-of-motion exercises were also performed to prevent development of limb contractures. Over the next 2 days in the ICU, his FVC decreased further, to 1.5–1.6 l (weight, 100 kg). In addition, his limb weakness continued to worsen despite repeated plasma infusion. He was now unable to get out of the bed without nursing assistance. His chest x-ray showed bibasilar atelectasis and mild pulmonary vascular congestion. Because of his continued clinical deterioration and a chest radiographic findings of fluid overload, plasma infusion was stopped and he was started on plasmapheresis. On the third hospital day, he was noted to have a nasal voice and complained of difficulty in swallowing liquids. A repeat arterial blood gas showed pH 7.35, $PaCO_2$ 45 mmHg, PaO_2 70 mmHg, and HCO_2 22 mEq/dl. He was electively intubated and placed on mechanical ventilation.

TABLE 24-11

CLINICAL INDICATIONS FOR ADMISSION TO THE ICU IN PATIENTS WITH GUILLAIN–BARRÉ SYNDROME

C	Conduction block, bradycardia, asystole
R	Rapid progression of motor weakness
I	Infection
T	Tachyarrhythmias
I	Intensive care monitoring of respiratory and autonomic dysfunction
C	Complications of critical illness: pulmonary embolism, myocardial infarction
A	Airway: ventilatory failure, bulbar weakness
L	Labile blood pressure: hypertension/hypotension

The word "critical" is used as a mnemonic for the different indications

Upper airway dysfunction due to bulbar muscle dysfunction in GBS may cause inability to swallow oral secretions and increases the risk of aspiration. Clinical signs of bulbar muscle dysfunction such as nasal voice, abnormal gag reflex, dysarthria, and poor mobility of pharyngeal muscles must be closely monitored. In addition, swallowing dysfunction can be assessed at the bedside by asking the patient to drink sips of water and observing for coughing. Early intubation may be necessary to protect the airway even if respiratory muscle strength is still adequate.

Weaning may be started once FVC exceeds 8–10 ml/kg, adequate oxygenation can be achieved with FiO_2 of 40% or less, and patients are able to double their minute ventilation. The maximum inspiratory force at the time of successful weaning is usually greater than 40 cmH_2O. The average duration of mechanical ventilation in two large series was 50–55 days. Some patients may require tracheostomy because of the need for prolonged mechanical ventilation and better pulmonary toilet. In patients who have shown favorable response to treatment, tracheostomy may be delayed up to 10 days to avoid the procedure in patients who rapidly improve.

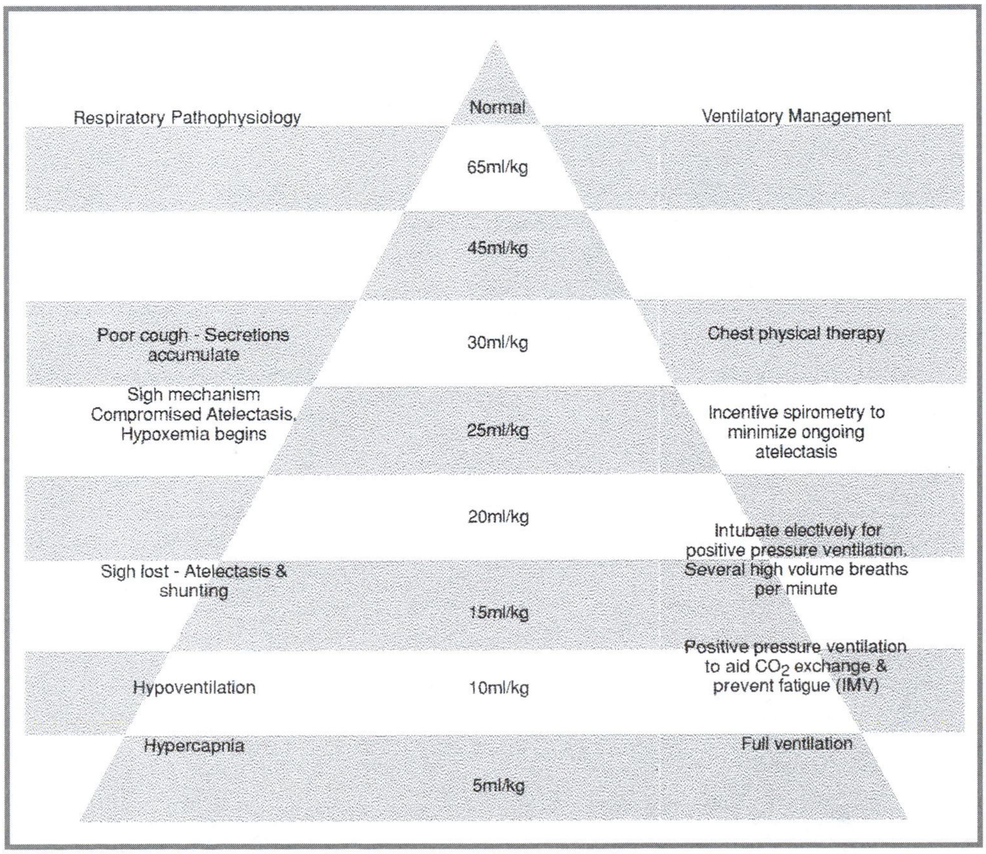

FIGURE 24-5

Progressive decline in forced vital capacity (FVC) due to respiratory muscle weakness in patients with acute or chronic progressive neuromuscular disease is reflected in a similar decline in respiratory system function. Serial FVC can be used to institute timely intervention to avert or delay the onset of respiratory failure.

CASE STUDY: PART 5

On the sixth ICU day, the patient showed signs of motor strength recovery. Both hip and knee flexion and extension were 4/5. Similar increases in muscle strength were observed in his upper extremities. Weaning parameters showed FVC of 2.2 l, maximum negative inspiratory pressure of 38 cmH_2O, and a minute ventilation of 6 l/min. He was successfully extubated after 2 h of T-piece weaning trials. He was transferred from the ICU the following day without further incident.

Aggressive pulmonary toilet is indicated to prevent as well as treat atelectasis. Atelectasis may require repeated bronchoscopy and may decrease the incidence of nosocomial pneumonia. Subcutaneous heparin is the preferred therapy for deep venous thrombosis prophylaxis compared to pneumatic boots to avoid prolonged foot drop due to compression of the peroneal nerve. Corticosteroids are not beneficial and may be harmful.

Treatment for GBS: supportive care, ventilatory support, and intravenous immunoglobulin or plasmapheresis.

In two multicenter trials, plasmapheresis (250 ml/kg every 2 days for a total of 5 treatments) using either albumin or fresh-frozen plasma as replacement fluids showed short-term benefits in early motor recovery and ambulation, reduced the number of patients who required assisted ventilation, and shortened the duration of mechanical ventilation. Immunotherapy should be started within 2 weeks of onset of symptoms or as early as possible. However, in patients with rapidly deteriorating clinical symptoms, plasmapheresis may still offer some benefits even if the duration of the disease is more than 3 weeks. Intravenous immunoglobulin (IVIG) given within 2 weeks is as effective as plasma exchange therapy.

Factors associated with poor prognosis with GBS: older age, mean compound muscle action potential amplitudes <20%, need for ventilatory support, and rapid progression of symptoms.

With the advent of modern ICU care, mortality from Guillain–Barré syndrome dropped from 15% in the 1970s to 3%–4% in the 1980s. Prognosis is good but only 15% of patients will have no neurologic residual; 50%–65% of patients will have persistent mild neurologic dysfunction such as mild distal weakness or numbness. Factors associated with poor prognosis are age greater than 60 years, mean compound muscle action potential amplitudes from distal stimulation less than 20% of normal, need for ventilatory support, and rapid progression to severe weakness (less than 1 week).

Critical Illness Polyneuropathy

Sepsis and multisystem organ failure are the two most common causes of acquired acute weakness syndrome in the ICU.

Critical illness polyneuropathy should be suspected in patients who fail weaning from mechanical support, develop areflexic limbs weakness, or have a complicated ICU course as a result of sepsis.

Acute weakness syndrome acquired in the ICU is now increasingly recognized as a common sequela of sepsis and multiorgan failure since its initial description about two decades ago. The syndrome can be divided into four categories (Table 24-12). The syndrome is often initially suspected because of failure to wean from mechanical ventilation as the patients recover from the critical illness or the development of flaccid and areflexic limbs. Patients with this syndrome have no prior history of neuropathy or myopathy. They usually have a prolonged complicated course in the ICU, often with sepsis as one of the complications, and clinical and laboratory data that suggest multisystem organ failure. Possible etiologies of critical care polyneuropathy include toxic metabolic causes such as hyperglycemia, causing nerve ischemia by endovascular shunting, or nerve toxins resulting from multiorgan system fail-

TABLE 24-12

ACUTE WEAKNESS SYNDROME IN THE ICU

Myopathy	Acute necrotizing myopathy Disuse atrophy
Neuromuscular junction abnormalities	Myasthenia-like syndrome Prolonged neuromuscular blockade
Neuropathy	Critical illness Polyneuropathy Acute motor neuropathy
Polyneuromyopathy	Combination of neuropathy and myopathy

ure (MSOF). Possible causes of myopathy include delayed clearance of 3-desacetyl metabolite of vecuronium due to renal failure, steroid-induced myopathy, and protracted use of neuromuscular blocking agents.

The diagnosis of critical care polyneuropathy is confirmed by EMG studies that show primary axonal polyneuropathy rather than a demyelinating process, as suggested by the reduction in the amplitude of the compound action potential without significant prolongation of the latency. For those patients who survive their critical illness, the clinical course of ICU-acquired polyneuropathy or myopathy is usually benign; although clinical recovery of nerve function often is prolonged, it is usually complete in 6 months to 1 year. About one-third of patients have difficulty weaning from the ventilator while 70% have evidence of peripheral neuropathy.

EMG is the ancillary test of choice to confirm the diagnosis of critical care polyneuropathy and to exclude other causes of weakness. Primary axonal polyneuropathy is the EMG finding in critical illness polyneuropathy (CIP).

Myasthenia Gravis

An autoimmune disorder characterized by impaired transmission of neural impulses across the neuromuscular junction due to the destruction of the postsynpatic acetylcholine receptors, myasthenia gravis is the most common disorder of neuromuscular transmission with a prevalence of 0.5–14.2 per 100,000. The disease typically affects younger women between 20 and 30 years and older men between 50 and 70 years of age. Thymic tumors are seen in 10% of cases, mostly in older men.

The typical presentation of the myasthenic patient is fluctuating weakness of the involved voluntary muscles and its improvement with rest and with administration of anticholinesterase agents (Tensilon test). Ocular, facial, and neck muscles are commonly involved. Asymmetric ptosis and extraocular muscle weakness occur in 70% of patients. However, only 15% of the patients have weakness limited to the ocular muscles. The majority of patients develop generalized weakness involving the oropharyngeal, diaphragm, and other respiratory muscles and limb weakness within the first 2 years of the onset of symptoms. Respiratory muscle weakness is seen in one-third of patients and may occur in the absence of peripheral muscle weakness. On physical examination, fatigability of the involved muscles can be elicited by asking the patient to do repetitive or sustained muscle activity such as looking upward for several minutes to see if there is lid or ocular muscle weakness.

Weakness due to myasthenia gravis is characterized by progressive weakness from repetitive use of a particular group of muscles and by improvement of muscle strength with rest.

Ocular, facial, and neck muscles are commonly involved in myasthenia gravis. Respiratory muscle weakness may occur as the primary symptom.

The Tensilon test is a simple test that can be done at the bedside to confirm the diagnosis of myasthenia gravis. Tensilon (edrophonium), a short-acting inhibitor of acetylcholinesterase, is given intravenously to elicit transient improvement in muscle weakness. Atropine should be available if bradycardia should occur. Vital signs should be carefully monitored during the duration of the test. A test dose of 2 mg tensilon is initially given to the patient to monitor for signs of clinical improvement in muscle strength during the next 3–5 min. The presence of adverse reaction such as bradycardia, nausea, and increased salivation should be carefully monitored. A second dose of 8 mg tensilon may be given if no effect is seen following the test dose. A positive Tensilon test is highly suggestive of myasthenia gravis, but a positive test has been reported in patients with Lambert–Eaton syndrome, botulism, and ALS. In patients with moderately generalized myasthenia gravis, performance of pulmonary function tests before the administration of Mestinon reveals mild reduction in FVC and moderate reduction in both MIPS (46% of predicted) and MEPS (48% of predicted). There is no evidence of restrictive and obstructive lung disease. As in other chronic neuromuscular diseases, the breathing pattern is rapid and shallow. After mestinon treatment, FVC, FEV_1, MIP, and MEP significantly improve, although respiratory muscle strength does not normalize. Arterial blood gas examination is frequently normal even with severe impairment of transdiaphragmatic pressures (P_{di}). Arterial blood gas is, therefore, not useful in monitoring the severity of respiratory muscle dysfunction.

Diagnosis of myasthenia gravis: abnormal tensilon test, acetylcholine receptor antibodies, and abnormal EMG.

Pulmonary function test in moderately advanced myasthenia gravis: decrease in forced expiratory flow rates and maximum static inspiratory pressure and normal arterial blood gas.

A serologic test may also be used to support the diagnosis of myasthenia gravis. Antibodies to acetylcholine receptors are seen in 80% of patients with generalized myasthenia and 60% with ocular myasthenia. The concentration of the acetylcholine receptor antibodies does not correlate with the severity of disease activity. Acetylcholine receptor antibodies have been found in Lambert–Eaton syndrome and in systemic lupus erythematosus.

Electrodiagnostic study is nonspecific for myasthenia gravis, but a decrease of 10%–15% in the amplitude of the action potential during slow repetitive nerve stimulation is seen in 77% of myasthenic patients. Single-fiber EMG is abnormal in 92% of the patients and is thought to be the most sensitive test, even in patients with negative serum antibody against acetylcholine receptor or normal repetitive nerve stimulation test.

Acute respiratory failure usually occurs in the setting of either a myasthenic, cholinergic, or brittle crisis or as the initial presentation of the disease. Myasthenic crisis refers to worsening of the basic underlying disease process that results in respiratory and oropharyngeal muscle weakness requiring ventilatory support, which is usually precipitated by discontinuation or decrease in the dosage of anticholinergic medications, surgery (thymectomy), administration of neuromuscular-blocking medications (aminoglycosides, curare-like drugs), or emotional crisis. Myasthenic crisis can be confirmed by performing a Tensilon test that results in improvement in muscle strength. Cholinergic crisis refers to the worsening of motor weakness by an excess of anticholinesterase medication that causes depolarizing blockade at the myoneural junction. This syndrome can be diagnosed and differentiated from myasthenic crisis by the presence of muscarinic symptoms such as hypersalivation, sweating, increased bronchial secretions, nausea and vomiting, and diarrhea. Moreover, symptoms will become worse with the Tensilon test. Nicotinic symptoms such as fasciculations and cramps are rare. Brittle crisis occurs when the disease is difficult to treat and the patient alternates between myasthenic and cholinergic crises.

Causes of myasthenic crisis: discontinuation of the anticholinergic drugs, surgery, neuromuscular blocking drugs, and emotional crisis.

Cholinergic crisis is the worsening of the neurologic symptoms in myasthenia gravis from excess of anticholinesterase medications.

The most common cause of respiratory failure is surgery, usually after thymectomy, followed by myasthenic and cholinergic crisis. In a series of 22 patients reported, the mean duration of mechanical ventilation was 8 days, with 6 patients (32%) requiring tracheostomy for prolonged mechanical ventilation. Postoperative monitoring is important because respiratory failure occurs within 24 h of surgery in more than 50% of patients. Serial measurements of FVC and maximum static respiratory pressures are helpful in detecting the onset of respiratory failure. The dosing schedule of anticholinesterase medications will affect the measurement of these respiratory parameters. The maximum improvement in respiratory muscle strength occurs about 2 h after the drug is given and slowly declines before the next dose is given. Consequently, FVC, PI_{max}, and PE_{max} should be measured 30 min before the next dose of anticholinesterase agents. When FVC is below 15 ml/kg and the maximum static respiratory pressures are less than ± 30 cm, assisted ventilation is probably required. Recurrent aspiration due to bulbar involvement and atelectasis are frequent respiratory complications of myasthenia gravis. Upper airway obstruction can occur in myasthenia gravis due to vocal cord paralysis. Flow–volume loop may show variable extrathoracic airway obstruction with the characteristic inspiratory plateau. The major cause of death is pulmonary infection.

Respiratory complications of myasthenia gravis: acute respiratory failure, upper airway obstruction, and sleep-related breathing disorders.

Several clinical parameters have been proposed as predictors of postoperative respiratory failure after thymectomy. Severity of disease, especially with the presence of bulbar symptoms and low VC, appear to be the most important factor in predicting postoperative respiratory failure.

Clinical predictors of postoperative respiratory failure in myasthenia gravis: bulbar muscle involvement and low vital capacity.

Sleep-related breathing disturbances might occur in patients with myasthenia gravis. Patients should be asked about sleep-related symptoms such daytime hypersomnolence, nocturnal and early morning awakening, and morning headaches. Older patients with moderate obesity, daytime alveolar hypoventilation, and restrictive lung defect should undergo a sleep study to screen for sleep apnea and nocturnal hypoventilation. Sleep studies in patients with myasthenia gravis reveal mixed central apneas and hypopneas.

Treatment of myasthenia gravis: anticholinesterase agents, corticosteroids, plasmapheresis, and thymectomy.

Treatment of myasthenia gravis includes anticholinesterase agents, high-dose corticosteroids, and plasmapheresis in patients who are refractory to steroids and immunosuppressive therapy. Anticholinesterase agents are the first line of treatment. Most patients improve significantly with this treatment but only a few patients regain normal function. Remission can be induced in up to 80% of patients with corticosteroids. However, initiation of corticosteroids therapy may cause temporary worsening of muscle weakness, usually on the 6th to 10th day of therapy. Close observation for signs of respiratory insufficiency is advisable. Other immunosuppressive agents (azathioprine, cyclosporin) are also useful in myasthenia gravis, either alone or in combination with steroids. Even in the absence of thymoma, thymectomy has also been shown to improve survival and clinical symptoms in patients with myasthenia gravis compared to patients who were treated medically. Up to 80% of patients with no thymoma improved clinically following thymectomy, but the response may be delayed. Thymectomy is indicated in young patients (<55 years old) and in patients with thymoma because of the risk of malignant transformation. Plasmapheresis may be beneficial in patients with fulminant myasthenia gravis who are not responding to conventional treatment.

Steroid Myopathy

Acute Steroid Myopathy

Acquired ICU myopathy is increasingly recognized as an important cause of weakness in the ICU, contributing to failure to wean from mechanical ventilation. In a recent retrospective study evaluating the causes of neuromuscular weakness in the ICU, 89 of 92 patients who had an EMG study had evidence of neuromuscular disorder. The most common cause of weakness was myopathy (46%), followed by peripheral neuropathy (28%). Only 4 of the patients had a preexisting myopathy that contributed to their admission to the ICU. Various neuromuscular diseases such as Guillain–Barré syndrome, myasthenia gravis, amyotrophic lateral sclerosis, and myopathy (acquired before ICU admission) accounted for only 28% of all patients. Thus, 73% of the patients studied in this series had acquired ICU weakness syndrome. Similar to previous studies, sepsis and multiple organ dysfunction are risk factors for the development of critical care myopathy and polyneuropathy. In addition, organ transplant recipients who suffered organ rejection also appeared to be risk for ICU-acquired myopathic syndrome. Intravenous corticosteroids and prolonged used of neuromuscular blockade have been implicated in ICU acquired myopathy. Biopsy of the involved muscle usually reveals muscle fiber atrophy, vacuolar muscle necrosis, and loss of myosin thick filaments.

Acute myopathy is the most common acquired neuromyopathy in the ICU.

Risk factors for the development of acute ICU myopathy: sepsis, multisystem organ failure, and prolonged use of neuromuscular drugs.

Chronic Steroid Myopathy

Unlike the acute myopathy recently described in the ICU setting, chronic steroid myopathy results from prolonged used of corticosteroids, usually manifesting as proximal limb and girdle muscle weakness. Thus, affected patients have difficulty combing their hair, reaching overhead for an object, and climbing stairs. Muscle enzymes are usually normal. EMG is either normal or reveals only slight myopathic changes. Muscle biopsy usually shows loss of type IIa muscle fibers with no evidence of inflammation or fiber necrosis. There is poor correlation between total dose of steroid and the severity of muscle weakness. However, gradual improvement in muscle strength follows with the discontinuation and reductions in corticosteroids.

Characteristics of chronic steroid myopathy: proximal muscle weakness, normal muscle enzymes, mild myopathic changes on EMG, and loss of type IIa muscle fiber on muscle biopsy.

TREATMENT OF NEUROMUSCULAR DYSFUNCTION IN THE ICU

The specific medical therapy for each of the neuromuscular disorders has been discussed previously. The proper care of these complicated patients often requires a multidisciplinary team of health care workers consisting of pulmonary specialist, neurologist, respiratory therapist, physiatrist, physical therapist, and nutritionist. Once the acute life illness has resolved, some patients who have experienced difficulty weaning from the ventilator require prolonged care in a respiratory rehabilitation unit. Frequent family interaction with the health care team is beneficial to facilitate the transition of care from the ICU to a stepdown unit.

TABLE 24-13

INDICATIONS FOR MECHANICAL VENTILATION IN PATIENTS WITH NEUROMUSCULAR DISORDERS

Acute respiratory failure	Severe dyspnea Marked accessory muscle use Inability to handle secretions Unstable hemodynamic status Hypoxemia refractory to supplemental O_2 Acute respiratory acidosis
Chronic respiratory failure	
Nocturnal hypoventilation	Morning headache Lethargy Nightmares Enuresis
Nocturnal oxygen	SaO_2 <88% despite supplemental O_2
Desaturation	Due to hypoventilation with $PaCO_2$ >45 mmHg, pH <7.32
Cor pulmonale	

Mechanical Ventilation

Common causes of respiratory failure in neuromyopathy include progressive respiratory muscle weakness, pneumonia, and inability to handle upper airway secretions and recurrent aspirations.

Ventilatory insufficiency leading to chronic respiratory failure is a common sequela of progressive neuromuscular diseases, but acute respiratory failure is common and often precipitated by recurrent aspiration, lower respiratory tract infections, or other acute illness that places an additional burden on an already limited ventilatory reserve. Pneumonia is the most common cause of increased morbidity and mortality in patients with advanced chronic neuromuscular disease. Once impending respiratory failure is recognized, mechanical ventilation should be used early to support spontaneous breathing until the acute precipitating event is identified and treated promptly. The indications for mechanical ventilation are shown in Table 24-13. In patients who present with onset of severe dyspnea, acute hypercapnea with respiratory acidosis, or moderate to severe hypoxemia, and in the presence of hemodynamic instability, translaryngeal intubation and mechanical ventilation are often necessary and are preferred over noninvasive mechanical ventilation. In certain clinical situations, noninvasive positive pressure ventilation (NPPV) may be used to augment minute ventilation in patients who present with acute hypercapnic respiratory failure who remain alert and cooperative with intact upper airway function and minimal airway secretions. All the patients described previously should be treated in intensive care units, even those patients who tolerated initial application of noninvasive positive pressure ventilation for closer monitoring. Invasive and noninvasive mechanical ventilation are compared in Table 24-14.

Noninvasive ventilation is the preferred mode of ventilatory support in patients with advanced neuromyopathies.

Noninvasive ventilation can be delivered two ways: as noninvasive positive pressure ventilation (NPPV) or as negative pressure ventilation.

Noninvasive ventilation has been shown to attenuate the decline in lung function and improve gas exchange, cognitive function, and survival in patients with neuromuscular disease. Noninvasive mechanical ventilation can be delivered as either NPPV or negative pressure ventilation (NV). The benefits and limitations of both forms of noninvasive mechanical ventilation are listed in Table 24-15.

Negative pressure ventilation, the iron lung in particular, was the first widely used method of mechanical ventilatory support in the management of respiratory failure due to neuro-

TABLE 24-14

COMPARISON OF CLINICAL FACTORS FAVORING INVASIVE VS. NONINVASIVE MECHANICAL VENTILATION IN PATIENTS WITH NEUROMUSCULAR DISEASE

Invasive ventilation (endotracheal intubation)
- Copious secretions
- Upper airway dysfunction
- Inability to tolerate or failure of noninvasive ventilation
- Impaired mental status
- Unstable vital signs

Noninvasive ventilation
- Awake, cooperative patient
- Intact upper airway function
- Minimal secretions
- Stable vital signs

TABLE 24-15

ADVANTAGES AND DISADVANTAGES OF POSITIVE AND NEGATIVE PRESSURE VENTILATION USED IN PATIENTS WITH NEUROMUSCULAR DISEASE

TYPE	ADVANTAGES	DISADVANTAGES
Negative pressure ventilators	Dependable	Cumbersome
Tank	Airway cannulation not required	Predisposes to obstructive apnea
Pulmowrap	Minimal hemodynamic effect	Limits nursing care
Cuirass	Maintenance of speech	Controlled ventilation
Positive pressure by mask or mouthpiece	Avoids upper airway obstruction	Aerophagia
	Pressure preset, compensates leak	Pressure sores
	Patient-initiated machine breaths	Leaks
		Problems with interface

muscular diseases. During the poliomyelitis epidemics in the 1930s, negative pressure was highly effective in augmenting alveolar ventilation and decreasing the mortality due to poliomyelitis. The early success of negative pressure ventilation (NV) in the treatment of acute respiratory failure due to poliomyelitis has since been repeated in patients with chronic respiratory failure from other forms of neuromuscular and chest wall diseases.

In recent years, NPPV has become the first choice of ventilatory support in patients with chronic respiratory failure due to a wide variety of neuromuscular diseases who have associated upper airway dysfunction. Because of the limitations of NV discussed earlier, it is now used only in patients unable to tolerate NPPV or is used during the daytime in combination with NPPV. In the ICU setting, we prefer NPPV over NV because of the ease of use and access to patients, its portability, and the maintenance of upper airway patency during sleep. Different types of masks may be used (nasal, oronasal, full facemask) for the application of NPPV depending on the patient's comfort and preference, as well as to provide proper fit to minimize air leak. In patients with significant air leaks from mouth, chin straps may help close the mouth. Alternatively, an oronasal or full facemask often solves the problem of mouth leak and patients who are mouth breathers. Occasionally, facial ulcers or erythema may develop due to contact pressure from a particular mask interface. In this situation, using two different mask interfaces and rotating their use may promote healing of the facial ulcers and prevent recurrence, or allowing a longer rest period between applications of NPPV may be of benefit.

Common problems with NPPV: air leaks, facial contact ulcers, and aerophagia.

Common problems with negative pressure ventilation: upper airway obstruction, limited portability, and limited nursing care access to patient.

Once a proper mask interface has been chosen, a wide variety of positive pressure ventilators may be used to deliver NPPV. In the intensive care setting, we prefer to use standard ICU ventilators because of the option of using either assist/control or pressure support mode or the combination of the two, depending on the clinical situation and patient preference. For example, synchronous intermittent mandatory ventilation (SIMV) combined with pressure support is useful in patients with nocturnal hypoventilation with decreased spontaneous respiratory rate as may occur during sleep. Some useful features available in standard ventilators that are useful in the acute care setting are the ability to monitor respiratory pattern and to supply different amounts of supplemental oxygen. In patients with acute or chronic respiratory failure who are otherwise hemodynamically stable, small pressure-limited, flow- or time-cycled portable ventilators (bilevel positive airway pressure) have been used with success. These devices are particularly useful in partial chronic ventilator support in patients with progressive neuromuscular dysfunction once their acute illness that requires ICU care has resolved.

The initial setting of the ventilator, whether tidal volume or inspiratory pressure, should start low and ramp up slowly, usually every 3–5 min as the patient can tolerate, to achieve an increase in assisted tidal volume of 30%–50% above baseline or a decrease in 5–10 mmHg in $PaCO_2$. The expiratory airway pressure on BIPAP is usually set at 4 cm to ensure continuous flow of gas during expiration, thus flushing out the expired gas. If supplemental oxygen is required, oxygen tubing is connected to the ventilator tubing using a T-connector. The expiratory airway pressure may also be titrated up to increase FRC and improve gas exchange. The initial duration of ventilatory assistance depends on the severity of respiratory failure and patient tolerance. In acute setting, ventilatory assistance of 20 h may be needed.

In a chronic setting, we allow the patient to use NPPV during the daytime for a few hours, followed by nocturnal use of 6–8 h once they are accustomed to the NPPV setting.

SUMMARY

The diagnosis of neuromuscular dysfunction should be considered in all patients with unexplained acute hypercapnic respiratory failure, acute on chronic hypercapnic respiratory failure, and in patients who fail to wean from ventilatory support after resolution of their acute illness. In patients with rapidly worsening respiratory weakness, FVC less than 12–15 ml/kg indicates impending respiratory failure and the need to initiate ventilatory support. Other indications for ventilatory support include upper airway dysfunction, abnormal gas exchange, and hemodynamic instability. Noninvasive positive pressure ventilation may be used to provide partial ventilatory support in neuromuscular patients with hypercapnic respiratory failure who are awake, cooperative, hemodynamically stable, and with preserved upper airway function. The prognosis of patients with neuromuscular dysfunction who require ICU admission depends on the clinical stage and type of neuromuscular disease, nature of the precipitating medical illness, and response of the patient to available therapy. In most cases of neuromuscular disorder, therapy is mainly supportive and is directed to avoid complications arising from chronic illness.

REVIEW QUESTIONS

1. **Neuromuscular diseases may lead to respiratory failure due to which of the following mechanisms?**
   A. Respiratory muscle weakness
   B. Upper airway dysfunction
   C. Recurrent aspiration
   D. Sleep-related breathing disorder
   E. All the above

2. **Which of the following statements about respiratory failure due to neuromyopathies is false?**
   A. Nocturnal hypoventilation may occur in the absence of perturbation in daytime gas exchange.
   B. Serial forced vital capacity (FVC) and maximum static inspiratory pressure (PI_{max}) are helpful in timing the need for ventilatory support.
   C. Ventilatory support should only be instituted when hypoxemia and hypercapnia occur.
   D. Noninvasive positive pressure mechanical ventilation is the preferred mode of ventilatory support in patients with chronic respiratory failure caused by advanced neuromuscular disease.

3. **The common causes of muscle weakness in the ICU following life-threatening illness are these, except:**
   A. Acute myopathy
   B. Critical illness polyneuropathy
   C. Protracted use of neuromuscular blocking agents
   D. Aminoglycoside-induced neuromuscular blockade

4. **Typical pulmonary function test findings in patients with moderately advanced neuromyopathies are the following, except:**
   A. Low FVC, FEV_1, and FEV_1/FVC
   B. Low TLC, high RV
   C. Low peak expiratory flow rate
   D. Normal diffusion capacity (when connected to lung volume)
   E. Low maximum voluntary ventilation

5. **Factors associated with poor outcome in Guillain–Barré syndrome are:**
   A. Older age
   B. Mean compound action potential amplitudes <20% of normal
   C. Need for ventilatory support
   D. Rapid clinical course
   E. All the above

ANSWERS

1. The answer is E. Neuromuscular disease may potentially affect the different components of the respiratory system. It primarily leads to respiratory muscle weakness, which when severe enough in turn leads to respiratory failure. In some diseases, bulbar involvement results in upper airway dysfunction and recurrent aspiration of oropharyngeal contents. Sleep-related breathing disorders, such as nocturnal hypoventilation and obstructive sleep apnea, are commonly seen in patients with moderately advanced neuromuscular disease. Severe nocturnal hypoventilation and obstructive sleep apnea, if left untreated, eventually lead to abnormalities in daytime hypercapnia and hypoxemia as well.
2. The answer is C. Abnormalities of arterial blood gas are late findings in patients with neuromuscular disease. In patients with acute demyelinating polyneuropathy such as Gullain–Barré syndrome, ventilatory support should be instituted when FVC is <12–15 ml/kg to avoid complications during the periintubation period. In chronic respiratory failure caused by chronic progressive neuromyopathy, intermittent ventilatory support with noninvasive mechanical ventilation is usually started when FVC is <50%.
3. The answer is D. Aminoglycosides may potentiate muscle weakness in susceptible patients with neuromuscular disorders. Acquired weakness in the ICU is most commonly the result of acute myopathy and critical illness polyneuropathy. Risk factors commonly associated with these conditions are sepsis, multisystem organ failure, shock, and prolonged use of neuromuscular blocking agents, especially in the presence of renal and hepatic failure.
4. The answer is A. Pulmonary function tests in patient with moderate respiratory muscle weakness due to chronic neuromyopathies typically show restrictive lung defect characterizes by low FVC and FEV_1, but with normal or high FEV_1/FVC ratio. In contrast to patients with interstitial lung disease where both TLC and RV are both reduced, the lung volume study in patients with neuromyopathy usually shows reduced total lung capacity and increased residual lung volume due to expiratory muscle weakness. Peak expiratory flow rate and maximum voluntary ventilation are similarly reduced in these patients because of respiratory muscle weakness. The diffusion capacity is usually normal when corrected to lung volume.
5. The answer is E. All these factors have been found to correlate with poor outcome in patients with Guillain–Barré syndrome.

SUGGESTED READING

Braun NMT, Arora NS, Rochester DF. Respiratory muscle and pulmonary function in polymyosities and other proximal myopathies. Thorax 1983;38:616–623.

Ellis ER, Bye PTP, Bruderer JW, Sullivan CE. Treatment of respiratory failure during sleep in patients with neuromuscular disease. Am Rev Respir Dis 1987;135:148–152.

Gibson GJ. Diaphragmatic paresis: pathophysiology, clinical features, and investigation. Thorax 1989;44:960–970.

Kelly BJ, Luce JM. The diagnosis and management of neuromuscular disease causing respiratory failure. Chest 1991;99:1485–1494.

McCool FD, Mayewski RF, Shayne DS, Gibson CJ, Griggs RC, Hyde RW. Intermittent positive pressure breathing in patients with respiratory muscle weakness. Chest 1986;90:546–551.

McKhan GM, Griffin JW, Cornblath DR, Mellits ED, Fisher RS, Quaskey SA, et al. Plasmapheresis and Guillain-Barré syndrome: analysis of prognostic factors and the effects of plasmapheresis. Ann Neurol 1988;23:347–353.

Plasma Exchange/Sandoglobulin Guillain-Barré Trial Group. Randomized trial of plasma exchange, intravenous immunoglobulin, and combined treatments in Guillain-Barré syndrome. Lancet 1997;349:225–230.

Rochester DF, Esau SA. Assessment of ventilatory function in patients with neuromuscular disease. Clin Chest Med 1994;15(4):751–763.

Ropper AH. The Guillain-Barre syndrome. N Engl J Med 1992;326(6): 1130–1136.

Unterborn JN, Hill NS. Options for mechanical ventilation in neuromuscular diseases. Clin Chest Med 1994;15(4):765–781.

van der Meche FGA, Schmitz PIM, the Dutch Guillain-Barré Study Group. A randomized trial comparing intravenous immune globulin and plasma exchange in Guillain-Barré syndrome. N Engl J Med 1992;326:1123–1129.

CHAPTER 25

FREDERIC H. KAUFFMAN

Disorders of Thermoregulation

CHAPTER OUTLINE

LEARNING OBJECTIVES

After studying this chapter, you should be able to:

- Discuss the major mechanisms of normal thermoregulation.
- Define heatstroke and list predisposing factors.
- Describe the clinical manifestations of heatstroke and its treatment modalities and goals.
- List the major factors that affect prognosis in heatstroke.
- Define malignant hyperthermia and list the ways in which it differs from heatstroke.
- Define hypothermia and differentiate the general clinical manifestations associated with declining core temperature.
- Describe various clinical procedures used to lower core temperature.
- Know the clinical significance of core afterdrop, the situations in which it occurs, and ways to avoid it.
- Interpret arterial blood gas results in a clinically useful manner.

The body's ability to maintain core temperature within a very precisely defined range is truly remarkable. Intricate physiologic mechanisms are constantly at work to prevent wide swings in body temperature despite the effects of changing environmental conditions. These mechanisms take place subconsciously and are vital to the preservation of normal subcellular, cellular, organ, and total body function. Significant alterations in these mechanisms, resulting in profound elevation or depression of core temperature, may be life threatening. Heatstroke and profound hypothermia are the two major medical emergencies of disordered thermoregulation encountered in clinical practice, with malignant hyperthermia representing a special case of elevated core temperature.

NORMAL THERMOREGULATION

Maintenance of normal core body temperature requires that mechanisms designed to promote heat loss and heat conservation respond to constantly changing environmental conditions. Such conditions also are affected by exercise and gender. Control of body temperature is dependent on hypothalamic and peripheral temperature-sensitive neurons that allow for the appropriate dissipation or conservation of heat. A basic understanding of normal thermoregulation is essential to the logical management of both heatstroke and profound hypothermia.

Hypothalamic and peripheral temperature-sensitive neurons are required for normal control of core body temperature.

Mechanisms of Heat Loss

In the presence of heat stress peripheral mechanisms respond to blood temperature perfusing the hypothalamus. Cutaneous vasodilation, coupled with sweat gland activation, promotes heat loss via convection and evaporation. Cardiovascular responses in the form of increased stroke volume and heart rate are critical to the delivery of increased blood flow to the peripheral circulation. Evaporation is the most critical mechanism by which heat is lost when environmental temperature exceeds core temperature but is limited in the setting of high environmental humidity. Radiation plays a role when skin is exposed, prompting heat loss to the environment. Conduction plays only a minor role in the dissipation of heat, except when the body is exposed to substances with high conductivity. For example, water has a conductivity 25–50 times that of air and plays a major role in the precipitous loss of heat in submersion accidents.

The evaporation mechamism of heat loss is limited in the setting of high environmental humidity.

The heat conductivity of water is far greater than that of air.

Mechanisms of Heat Conservation

Cutaneous cold-sensitive neurons initiate the normal physiologic responses to a cold environment. Afferent impulses directed to the hypothalamus initiate shivering, a heat-generating mechanism, and piloerection, a heat-conserving mechanism. Shivering increases heat production by 100%–400%. Subsequent efferent sympathetic fiber impulses from the hypothalamus promote peripheral vasoconstriction, a heat-conserving mechanism, and mobilization of glucose and fat stores. Utilization of increased fuel stores increases endogenous heat production.

Shivering is a heat-generating mechanism.

Peripheral vasoconstriction promotes heat conservation.

Effects of Exercise and Gender

Quite a number of physiologic responses occur in the setting of exercise, most of which alter core temperature in an upward direction, and as such may play a role in the development of heat illness syndromes. Respiratory rate and minute ventilation increase, resulting in respiratory alkalosis. Lactic acidosis also occurs due to conversion to anaerobic metabolism, and pH levels as low as 7.0 have been documented during strenuous exercise. In addition, there is a normal increase in core body temperature during exercise, first documented during the Boston Marathon of 1903. Transient temperatures as high as 107°F have been documented in athletes undergoing strenuous exercise in the setting of significant environmental heat stress. With normal elevations in body temperature, cellular metabolism and heat production increase, thereby predisposing the athlete to heat illness. A number of cardiovascular processes also come into play. Peripheral vascular resistance decreases. Stroke volume, heart rate, and cardiac output all increase. There is a normal loss of sodium and potassium through loss of body fluids, and athletes experience a mild to moderate degree of dehydration during exercise. Renal blood flow is decreased and transient myoglobinuria, proteinuria, hematuria, and pyuria may be noted. Transient leukocytosis and mild coagulation abnormalities also develop.

Increased core temperature is a normal response to strenuous exercise.

Dehydration occurs in the setting of exercise and predisposes to the development of heat illness.

Of great interest is the observation that gender affects the physiologic response to heat stress. It is extremely rare for females to develop exercise-induced heatstroke. Sweating is

Males are much more prone to the development of heat illness than females.

CASE STUDY 1: PART 1

A 75-year-old male boarding home occupant was found unresponsive by his son in the patient's fourth-floor room. It is not known when he last left his apartment, or when he last ate or drank. His son informed the paramedics that his father has a history of hypertension and congestive heart failure, and that in addition to a calcium channel blocker and diuretic, he takes phenothiazines for chronic schizophrenia. The son also commented that his father "drinks a bit." All windows in the apartment are shut and there is no functioning air conditioning. The local region has experienced a heat wave over the past 2 weeks, with daily environmental temperatures between 92° and 100°F. Vital signs include a pulse of 120/min, blood pressure of 90/palp., respirations of 8–10/min, and a rectal temperature of 106°F.

less profound in females, and evaporation mechanisms are postulated to be more efficient than in male counterparts. The greater surface area to mass ratio in females allows for more efficient transfer of heat to the environment. And finally, it is well known that females develop lower baseline core temperatures during the preovulatory phase of their menstrual cycles. All these mechanisms are believed to protect females against the development of heat illness syndromes, especially during strenuous exercise in a hot and humid environment.

HEATSTROKE

Diagnosis

> No specific temperature defines heatstroke, but most victims have core temperatures in excess of 104°F.

> Major central nervous system dysfunction is essential to the diagnosis of heatstroke.

Heatstroke is the only heat illness syndrome in which normal thermoregulatory mechanisms are lost, thereby resulting in significant morbidity and mortality. Three essential elements must be present for a diagnosis of heatstroke: (1) the patient must have been exposed to a major form of heat stress, (2) core body temperature must be elevated, usually greater than 104°F, and (3) the patient must display major central nervous system dysfunction. It must be emphasized that no specific temperature defines heatstroke, but in the presence of the other two features, a profoundly hyperthermic patient must be treated as if they have heatstroke. In addition, at the time of presentation to the emergency department, not all patients with heatstroke will have core temperatures greater than 104°F. Such may be the case when treatment has been initiated in the field, or when evaporation is maximized in route to the hospital, thereby resulting in a fall in core temperature. In such cases, prehospital personnel are invaluable in assisting with establishment of the diagnosis. The most common forms of central nervous system dysfunction seen in patients with heatstroke are seizures and alteration in mental status. However, any form of central nervous system dysfunction can occur, including tetanic contractures, oculogyric crisis, delirium, psychosis, stupor, coma, and focal neurologic findings. A common misconception is that patients who sweat do not have heatstroke; in reality, many heatstroke patients are noted to sweat appropriately at the time of presentation. The presence of sweating should never be used to exclude the diagnosis.

Predisposing Factors

A veritable multitude of factors predispose to the development of heat stroke. General categories include environmental factors, cardiovascular disorders, increased endogenous heat load, altered dissipation of heat, various drug families, lack of acclimatization, and a history of heatstroke. Table 25-1 delineates these factors in greater detail, and Table 25-2 details common drug families known to predispose to the development of heatstroke.

Lack of acclimatization and a history of heatstroke deserve special attention. Acclimatization is the process by which individuals who undergo strenuous exercise on a regular basis over a period of several weeks to months develop tolerance to heat stress. Such individuals display physiologic effects similar to those of well-conditioned athletes. During exercise in the setting of heat stress, the acclimatized individual has a lower temperature and physical exertion threshold for sweating, sweats more profusely, develops less rise in core tempera-

TABLE 25-1

FACTORS PREDISPOSING TO HEATSTROKE

Environmental factors	Altered heat dissipation
High temperature	Scleroderma
High humidity	Cystic fibrosis
Low wind velocity	Drugs (see Table 25-2)
Cardiovascular disorders	Lack of acclimatization
Congestive heart failure	History of heat stroke
Coronary artery disease	Extremes of age
Increased endogenous heat load	Male gender
Status epilepticus	
Febrile illnesses	
Overt psychosis	

ture, and demonstrates decreased oxygen utilization and increased oxygen consumption compared to the unacclimatized individual. As such, the unacclimatized individual who exercises strenuously during periods of high environmental temperature and humidity is at significantly greater risk for the development of heatstroke.

Whether an individual with a history of heatstroke is forever intolerant to heat stress is a matter of some debate. Based upon prior studies, heat intolerance does exist after an episode of heatstroke, but other researchers have found that over time (5–12 months) most victims of exertional heatstroke regain heat tolerance. Nonetheless, any patient with a history of heatstroke who returns to settings of significant heat stress would be prudent to be extravigilant in heatstroke prophylaxis.

Clinical Manifestations

Heatstroke effects nearly every organ system in the body. In addition to a dramatic increase in core body temperature, patients with heatstroke have major alterations in their central nervous system function. Cardiovascular manifestations may be variable; the elderly commonly demonstrate a hypodynamic response, whereas younger healthy individuals often present with tachycardia, increased cardiac output, and decreased systemic vascular resistance. The presenting circulatory state is determined by the patient's underlying volume status and cardiac function, and represents the patient's ability to respond to the hemodynamic stresses of heat stroke. Pulmonary vascular resistance in patients with heatstroke is quite variable, and central venous pressure monitoring generally reflects accurately the state of the central circulation. Electrocardiographic findings are nonspecific, and autopsy findings have yielded varying degrees of myocardial fiber degeneration, necrosis, and hemorrhage.

Gastrointestinal symptoms are quite common, frequently including nausea, vomiting, diarrhea, and gastrointestinal hemorrhage. Signs and symptoms of liver injury typically occur several days after presentation, though frank hepatic failure is uncommon. Classically, transaminitis with normal bilirubin and alkaline phosphatase is seen.

Bleeding disturbances are multifactorial in etiology and when present denote a poor prognosis. Elevated prothrombin time and thrombocytopenia may be demonstrated as early as 30 min after presentation but do not necessarily herald the development of disseminated intravascular coagulation.

Rhabdomyolysis, although not universal, is very common in heatstroke victims. Acute tubular necrosis is seen in greater than 30% of patients with heatstroke attributable to exertion, though it is less common in the elderly. Other renal findings that may not be directly

Exertional heatstroke often is associated with severe rhabdomyolysis.

TABLE 25-2

DRUG FAMILIES THAT PREDISPOSE TO HEATSTROKE

Anticholinergics: impair sweat glands/evaporation
Sympathomimetics: decrease cutaneous heat loss and increase endogenous heat production
Myocardial depressants: decrease cardiac output/cutaneous heat loss
Diuretics: decrease cardiac output
CNS stimulants/depressants: alter behavioral response to heat stress

TABLE 25-3

CLASSIC VERSUS EXERTIONAL HEATSTROKE

FEATURE	CLASSIC	EXERTIONAL
Age	Elderly	Young
Rhabdomyolysis	Moderate	Severe
ATN	<5%	>30%
DIC	Mild	Severe
Epidemic	Yes	No
Chronic illness	Yes	No

ATN, acute tubular necrosis; DIC, disseminated intravascular coagulopathy

associated with acute tubular necrosis include proteinuria and evidence of myoglobinuria and interstitial nephritis. Other common metabolic derangements include hyperglycemia, hypernatremia, hypokalemia, hypophosphatemia, hypocalcemia, hyperuricemia, lactic acidosis, and respiratory alkalosis.

Classic heatstroke tends to occur in the elderly and generally occurs during heat wave epidemics.

Heatstroke is classified into two different, although not always distinct, categories: classic heatstroke and exertional heatstroke. Table 25-3 indicates the typical differences between these two classifications of the disorder.

Treatment

Rapid cooling is the most essential aspect in preventing morbidity and mortality in the patient with heatstroke.

As with all patients, the initial priority of management is stabilization of the airway. Many, although not all, patients with heatstroke require endotracheal intubation as a first-line tool of stabilization. Oxygen is administered to all patients, and appropriate intravenous access established, with drawing of necessary laboratory values. The patient must be totally undressed to allow full medical assessment and to facilitate cooling techniques. Once the ABC's are evaluated and stabilized, immediate and aggressive cooling is imperative if morbidity and mortality are to be avoided. All patients with heatstroke should be cooled to a core temperature of no more than 101°F utilizing evaporation, or immersion techniques, or both. Although some debate still exists as to the optimum technique of cooling, the essential point is that the given institution be prepared, educated, and inserviced in advance for the cooling of such patients. Personal preference is to combine both techniques simultaneously, although many authorities espouse one or the other technique. Whichever approach is utilized, all efforts must be undertaken to achieve adequate cooling in the shortest amount of time possible. An important fact is that antipyretics do not have a role in the management of heatstroke.

Aggressive monitoring, not only of core temperature but also of all vital functions is essential to optimal treatment planning. Respiratory management is guided by the usual prin-

CASE STUDY 1: PART 2

Airway assessment revealed lack of airway tone and loss of protective reflexes; the patient was intubated and placed on 100% oxygen on a ventilator. Multiple large-bore intravenous lines were placed and 0.9% normal saline solution administered wide open. Cardiac monitor revealed sinus tachycardia, and pulse oximetery revealed an oxygen saturation of 99% on the ventilator. General inspection revealed evidence of dehydration and no evidence of trauma. Lung exam was clear, cardiac exam was remarkable only for the tachycardia, and abdominal exam revealed diminished bowel sounds without organomegaly. Rectal exam revealed normal tone and stool was negative for occult blood. Neurologic exam revealed pupils to be 3 mm, equal, and reactive to light; corneal reflexes were intact, and the patient had spontaneous respirations. There was no response to verbal stimuli, and deep painful stimuli initiated decorticate posturing. Deep tendon reflexes were normoreactive and symmetric; plantar response was downgoing bilaterally. Immediate cooling techniques were instituted; the patient's torso was packed in ice, all other exposed skin surfaces were sprinkled with water, and large fans were run at the bedside to promote evaporation. Core body temperature declined to 101.6°F within the first 20 min of resuscitation; pulse decreased to 100/min, and blood pressure rose to 128/72 mmHg.

ciples of critical care, with frequent utilization of arterial blood gas (ABG) measurement to guide oxygenation and ventilation therapy. Rarely do patients with uncomplicated heatstroke require more than 2 l of intravenous fluid for stabilization; ideal management includes placement of a CVP line to guide initial therapy, with pursuit of other causes of hypotension should it persist. Consideration should be given to the administration of $D_{50}W$ and thiamine initially, and blood should be drawn to evaluate electrolytes, renal function, liver function, coagulation parameters, and complete blood count at a minimum.

Complications of heatstroke should be anticipated, including violent shivering, seizures, renal failure, rhabdomyolysis, acid–base disturbances, and cardiac dysrhythmias. Most of these problems respond to aggressive cooling. Should shivering be problematic (it promotes increased heat production), benzodiazepines are the treatment of choice. In the past, phenothiazines were used, but their use no longer is recommended because of their slow onset of action, propensity to produce hepatotoxicity, reduction of the seizure threshold, and exacerbation of hypotension. Volume status must be optimized if renal failure is to be avoided or minimized. The use of bicarbonate or mannitol therapy to prevent or treat rhabdomyolysis-induced acute tubular necrosis is controversial.

Most complications of heatstroke respond to aggressive cooling.

Prognosis

The prognosis in patients with heatstroke is related to several factors. The level and duration of hyperthermia play the most important role, along with the duration of coma. Patients who have prolonged coma, disseminated intravascular coagulation, and acute renal failure generally die within several days from multisystem organ failure. Patients who have coma less than 10 h in duration have a reasonable chance of survival. Their hepatic and renal function tends to be less severe, but permanent central nervous system damage is common. Coma that lasts less than 3 h generally indicates a good prognosis. Recent data from the 1995 heat wave in Chicago revealed a 21% hospital mortality, with overall 1-year mortality of 36%. Significant neurologic impairment was seen in 76% of survivors. Pooled data from many studies indicate mortality rates of 30%–80%.

The most important prognostic factors in heatstroke are the level and duration of hyperthermia and the duration of coma.

MALIGNANT HYPERTHERMIA: A SPECIAL CASE

A very rare congenital disturbance of calcium regulation in striated muscle, malignant hyperthermia develops following exposure to general anesthetics, depolarizing muscle relaxants, or, rarely, extreme exertion. Uncontrolled calcium influx into the sarcoplasmic reticulum of striated muscle following exposure to one of these agents gives rise to severe muscle rigidity, increased endogenous heat production, and profound hyperthermia. Dantrolene sodium is the treatment of choice for malignant hyperthermia, although it has not been demonstrated to have any beneficial effects above and beyond standard treatment principles for patients with heatstroke.

Dantrolene sodium is the treatment of choice for malignant hyperthermia but is not effective in the management of heatstroke.

CASE STUDY 2: PART 1

A 35-year-old homeless man was found unresponsive on a sidewalk during a rainstorm. His clothing was soaked and he was not wearing a coat or hat. An empty bottle of wine was found beside him. Environmental temperature is 38°F. The patient was brought to the emergency department by concerned citizens. On examination the man appeared somewhat cachectic, wet, and not shivering. Vital signs included an irregularly irregular pulse of 46/min, blood pressure of 75/palp., respirations of 8/min, and a rectal temperature of 83°F. There was no evidence of trauma. The patient only groaned in response to verbal stimuli. Pupils were 6 mm, equal, and sluggishly reactive to light. Corneal reflexes were intact, as were gross extraocular movements. The neck was supple. Lung exam was clear. Cardiac exam revealed an irregularly irregular pulse without murmur or rub. Abdominal examination was remarkable only for absent bowel sounds, and stool exam was negative for occult blood. Deep tendon reflexes were absent throughout, and plantar response was downgoing bilaterally.

HYPOTHERMIA

Diagnosis

Hypothermia is defined as a core temperature less than 95°F.

Metabolic activity and tissue oxygen requirements decline as core temperature decreases.

Clinical criteria for brain death do not apply in the setting of hypothermia.

Perhaps the most overlooked vital sign in the acute resuscitation phase of the critically ill patient is core temperature. The foregoing case illustrates just how important is accurate measurement of the core temperature to diagnosis and management of such patients. Typically hypothermia is defined as a core temperature less than 95°F. The diagnosis of hypothermia is essential in that many patients have achieved meaningful survival despite profound drops in core temperature (as low as 48°F in controlled settings) once hypothermia is clinically recognized and the patient is rewarmed appropriately. In addition, as temperature declines, metabolic activity and tissue oxygen requirements decline, thereby rendering a protective effect to vital organs. Cerebral autoregulation is preserved, thereby providing central nervous system protection even in the setting of profound hypothermia. As such, it is imperative to understand that traditional clinical criteria for brain death are not applicable in the hypothermic patient, leading to the clinical adage that "no patient is dead until warm and dead."

Causes

Although environmental exposure is a common cause of profound hypothermia, many other causes and contributing factors must be entertained. Table 25-4 lists factors in the differential diagnosis of hypothermia, many of which play a contributing role in the cited case.

Clinical Manifestations

The clinical findings in patients with hypothermia are fairly predictable, depending on the degree of depression of core temperature. Hypothermia can be divided into three categories based upon core temperature; such categorization is useful not only for description of clinical manifestations but for therapeutic decision making as well.

TABLE 25-4

DIFFERENTIAL DIAGNOSIS OF HYPOTHERMIA

- Environmental exposure
- Massive fluid and blood administration
- Decreased heat production
  - Malnutrition
  - Hypoglycemia
  - Hypopituitarism
  - Hypothyroidism
  - Hypoadrenalism
  - Cholinergic drugs
  - Beta-blockers
- Increased heat loss
  - Erythrodermas
  - Ethanol
- Loss of central regulation
  - CNS trauma
  - Cerebrovascular accident
  - Uremia
  - Drugs: benzodiazepines, phenothiazines, barbiturates, opiates, carbon monoxide, cyclic antidepressants
- Loss of peripheral regulation
  - Spinal cord injury
  - Alpha-blockers
  - Phenothiazines
- Miscellaneous
  - Sepsis
  - Malignancy

Mild Hypothermia (90°–95°F)

Patients with mild degrees of hypothermia typically present with no immediately life-threatening complications but often feel rather uncomfortable because of the change in their body temperature. Such patients maintain their shivering mechanism and maintain stable vital signs in the absence of other complicating factors. Mental status may be normal, although typically such patients exhibit varying levels of amnesia, coupled with mild ataxia and dysarthria.

Moderate Hypothermia (80°–90°F)

Hypothermia in the moderate range characteristically begins to alter vital signs and function and must be treated carefully to avoid life-threatening complications. General depression of vital function takes place, with progressive decline as core temperature continues to fall. Now shivering, a normal heat-producing response to hypothermia, is abolished. Mental status continues to decline, with varying levels of confusion and eventual obtundation. Cardiovascular status now becomes altered significantly. As core temperature drops, an initial increase in heart rate and cardiac output will be followed by a steady decline in pulse and blood pressure. A critical threshold for the development of atrial fibrillation occurs at 86°F and for ventricular fibrillation at 83°F. Of importance is that atrial fibrillation, once it develops, typically is slower than expected for patients with new-onset atrial fibrillation, even in the absence of conduction system disease. Respiratory function also is affected, with initial increase in respiratory rate followed by progressive decline in minute ventilation and the loss of protective reflexes. Bronchorrhea also is noted as core temperature drops.

Severe Hypothermia (<80°F)

Severe hypothermia represents an immediate threat to life. Mental status is profoundly altered, with nearly universal development of stupor and coma. Cardiovascular deterioration continues with more profound degrees of bradycardia and hypotension; ventricular fibrillation is a feared complication at this stage and often extremely difficult to treat. Ultimately, asystole develops. Respiratory function and airway protection also diminish significantly.

> Progressive bradycardia and hypotension develop as core temperature declines.

> Ventricular fibrillation is a major contributor to death in the setting of hypothermia but responds poorly to traditional treatment in the absence of rewarming.

Common Laboratory and EKG Findings

There are no diagnostic or pathognomonic laboratory findings in hypothermia, but many abnormalities must be anticipated and treated within the special confines of hypothermia; this is particularly true for arterial blood gas assessment, which is discussed separately.

Insulin production and release are impaired in hypothermic patients, as is end-organ effect. The net result is the finding of hyperglycemia. Rewarming alone will reverse these effects and often returns the patient to a euglycemic state. Overly aggressive administration of insulin before rewarming is very likely to result in hypoglycemia as the patient is rewarmed and must be avoided.

> Hyperglycemia should be treated with caution in hypothermia because of altered insulin release and end-organ effect.

CASE 2: PART 2

The patient was carefully intubated and placed on a ventilator with 100% oxygen. Two large-bore intravenous catheters were placed, appropriate blood studies obtained, and a Foley catheter placed. Administration of $D_{50}W$, naloxone, and thiamine resulted in no change in the patient's clinical status. An arterial blood gas was sent to the laboratory. Cardiac monitoring revealed atrial fibrillation and what appeared to be Osborn waves; EKG confirmed these findings. Portable chest x-ray suggested early noncardiogenic pulmonary edema. Warming measures initially instituted included administration of warmed, humidified oxygen and warmed intravenous fluids. Preparation was made to institute warmed thoracostomy lavage and peritoneal lavage should initial rewarming techniques prove inadequate. In addition, the cardiothoracic service was notified of the patient's condition, and discussions entertained the use of extracorporeal rewarming should clinical deterioration ensue.

Expect the need for volume repletion in the hypothermic patient.

Sodium and water resorption are impaired in hypothermia, the latter because of a decreased renal response to antidiuretic hormone (ADH). The resultant "cold diuresis" is very common in profoundly hypothermic patients, and the need for volume repletion should be anticipated in all patients. In addition, renal failure may ultimately ensue and generally is multifactorial in etiology, being caused by volume depletion, rhabdomyolysis, or associated sepsis.

Hemoconcentration is a common finding as a result of fluid losses and plasma shifts. In addition, leukopenia and thrombocytopenia may be severe in the setting of severe hypothermia. Disseminated intravascular coagulation, although not common, may develop as well.

The acid–base changes that occur in the setting of hypothermia are complex and vary from patient to patient, but certain alterations often are quite characteristic. Respiratory rate and tidal volume initially rise, and then fall progressively as the level of hypothermia worsens, giving rise to a respiratory alkalosis. Increased lactate production and decreased hepatic and renal clearance of acid loads contribute to a metabolic acidosis. The solubility of carbon dioxide rises as core temperature falls; the subsequent decline in the partial pressure of carbon dioxide gives rise to a respiratory alkalosis. As would be predicted, many patients with hypothermia develop mixed acid–base pictures.

Osborn waves are characteristic of profound hypothermia.

As noted, the EKG findings in the setting of hypothermia are progressive and quite interesting. After an initial rise in heart rate, a progressive change from tachycardia to bradycardia occurs. Atrial fibrillation and atrial flutter typically start to occur around 86°F, and demonstrate lesser degrees of relative tachycardia than in the euthermic patient. The threshold for ventricular fibrillation is lowered starting at 83°F and asystole is nearly universal by 64°F. Before the development of ventricular fibrillation, prolongation of the PR, QRS, and QT intervals typically occurs. ST-T wave changes are variable, but may suggest myocardial ischemia due to hypothermia-induced alterations in coronary autoregulation. Below 86°F, terminal elevation and widening of the QRS complex may be seen; these J-wave abnormalities, known as Osborn waves, are quite characteristic of profound degrees of hypothermia. Cardiac dysrhythmias solely caused by hypothermia (and not related to underlying heart disease) typically resolve with rewarming.

Treatment Principles and Techniques

Careful intubation is safe in the setting of hypothermia and should be performed as indicated by the usual criteria.

Appropriate clinical management in the setting of significant hypothermia is based upon the accurate diagnosis of the disorder, coupled with the findings at the bedside. As with all critically ill patients, the primary goal of resuscitation is to stabilize airway, breathing, and circulation (the ABC's). Indeed, it is well known by clinicians experienced with managing hypothermic patients that physical manipulation of the patient may precipitate ventricular fibrillation, a dreaded complication of hypothermia that is very hard to treat. This fear has led some clinicians to be hesitant to provide aggressive airway protection, such as endotracheal intubation, in patients who otherwise would be candidates for the procedure. It has been well documented in animal studies that endotracheal intubation, performed carefully by skilled clinicians, is a safe and often life-saving procedure. As such, the assessment of airway protection and management should proceed in the usual, albeit careful, fashion; 100% oxygen should be administered to all patients, along with $D_{50}W$, naloxone, and thiamine in the appropriate settings. Intravenous access is essential, and should a central venous catheter be necessary, it should be placed without touching the myocardium and risking the precipitation of ventricular fibrillation. The use of prophylactic lidocaine or bretylium before procedural manipulation has been suggested by some but has never proven to be effective in preventing hypothermic-induced lethal dysrhythmias. Finally, during the initial resuscitation phase, volume depletion should be anticipated and treatment begun with warmed intravenous normal saline solution.

Many potential rewarming techniques are available to the treating physician. The choice of which techniques, and in what combination, should be determined not only by the patient's absolute core temperature but also by their overall clinical condition. In general, however, the more profound the degree of hypothermia, and the greater the degree of clinical deterioration, the more aggressive the rewarming techniques.

Passive rewarming is appropriate for patients who are clinically stable with mild levels of hypothermia. All patients should be dried thoroughly, to avoid heat loss due to the conductivity of water, and covered with dry blankets. Underlying causes of hypothermia should be sought and corrected. Intravenous fluids, warmed to 109°–111°F, empirically are sensible and may be given safely but should not be relied upon for aggressive rewarming of any patient. Further, the use of warmed nasogastric, bladder, and colorectal lavage tends to be ineffective.

Active external rewarming includes the use of heating blankets, hot water bottles, and total immersion of the patient in warm water. Such techniques have a tendency to produce core afterdrop (discussed later) and generally are not used.

Patients with more severe levels of hypothermia are treated more aggressively. The use of warmed humidified oxygen (temperatures up to 111°F can be administered without threat of tracheal damage) is a standard treatment modality that has withstood the test of time. This technique takes advantage of the large pulmonary surface area, but care must be taken to measure the oxygen temperature at the point of entry to the patient and not at the point of oxygen source on the wall. The use of warmed humidified oxygen is particularly effective in the intubated patient but can be delivered through less invasive devices in the nonintubated patient.

Warmed humidified oxygen administration is a useful rewarming therapy for most hypothermic patients.

Warmed peritoneal lavage also is an effective means to rewarm the hypothermic patient. Potassium-free dialysate is used, warmed to 111°F. Due to volume shifts and clod diuresis, coupled with the volume deficits associated with doing peritoneal dialysis, aggressive fluid therapy and monitoring are essential.

Warmed thoracostomy lavage is a relatively new, yet effective, technique described primarily in the case report literature. Although formal studies have not appeared in the literature, descriptive case studies consistently indicate effective rewarming. Once again, lavage fluid warmed to 111°F may be used safely. Two chest tubes are placed on the same side of the patient, the higher one for influx of warmed fluid and the lower one for fluid efflux. Careful attention to input and output volumes is essential to avoid iatrogenic hydrothorax. This technique, along with warmed peritoneal lavage, is particularly useful for hemodynamically compromised or deteriorating patient when extracorporeal rewarming is not available.

Active core rewarming is indicated in the profoundly hypothermic, unstable, or deteriorating patient.

Extracorporeal rewarming, via traditional cardiopulmonary bypass or continuous arteriovenous rewarming, is the most aggressive technique available to rewarm the severely hypothermic patient. Once instituted, rewarming takes place within minutes. Because technical expertise and a team approach are required, this technique is reserved for the most critical of patients. As would be predicted, it is not available at all institutions and is not always immediately available at institutions that posess the capability. Thus, all support staff should be alerted as soon as a potential patient candidate is identified.

Avoidance of Core Afterdrop

Core afterdrop is the paradoxical fall in core body temperature despite the institution of rewarming techniques. As already noted, cardiovascular instability is directly related to fall in core temperature, thereby giving rise to concern of potential worsening complications should core temperature continue to drop after patient presentation to the hospital. Several causative factors probably contribute to the development of core afterdrop. The classic reason given for its development, found in many textbooks to this day, is that as the peripheral circulation is vasodilated via active external rewarming techniques, cold blood and lactic acid are returned to the central circulation, thereby promoting a further fall in core temperature and a worsening of metabolic acidosis. No doubt this mechanism plays some role in the development of core afterdrop, but it is of more than just academic interest to realize that a vascular system is not necessary for this phenomenon to occur in experimental models. In addition, core afterdrop does not occur in patients who have acquired hypothermia over many hours to days; rather, it tends to occur only in patients who have experienced a rapid and precipitous drop in core temperature (e.g., submersion victims).

Development of core afterdrop does not require a vascular tree; transfer of heat along temperature gradients plays a key role in its development.

Experimental models of hypothermia have been developed using gelatin molds and legs of beef with temperature thermisters placed at progressively deeper levels relative to the central core of the model. The systems were then placed in a surrounding bath that allowed cooling and rewarming of the surrounding environment, thus simulating submersion with rapid cooling, followed by external rewarming. These systems demonstrated a fall in core temperature (i.e., core afterdrop) so long as a temperature gradient existed between the surface of the model and the central core. Once the temperature gradient was abolished, core temperature began to rise with further heating of the surrounding bath. As such, core afterdrop developed in the absence of a circulatory system and was caused solely by the temperature gradients established between the surface and core of the experimental model. In victims who have acquired hypothermia over many hours to days, enough time has elapsed for the temperature gradients to be abolished, and during rewarming core afterdrop is not observed. Clearly, when core afterdrop is a potential concern (i.e., in victims with rapid development of hypothermia), core rewarming techniques as noted here prevent dangerous core afterdrop and its potentially lethal complications.

Interpretation of Arterial Blood Gases

The interpretation of arterial blood gas values in the profoundly hypothermic patient represents one of the great dilemmas for critical care practitioners. The pH of water increases as temperature decreases because of inhibition of dissociation of water molecules. The pH change of blood exactly parallels this change in electrochemically neutral water, and as such the pH gradient between the inside of the cell and its external environment remains constant despite changes in temperature. In addition, the partial pressures of both oxygen and carbon dioxide decrease with falling temperature despite the lack of change in absolute blood content of these gases. The net result is that arterial blood gas values in a hypothermic patient, measured at patient temperature rather than at 98.6°F, yield a marked respiratory alkalosis (assuming no change in metabolic parameters).

Arterial blood gases are best interpreted without temperature correction in the hypothermic patient.

If one assumes, however, that the critical aspect of cellular survival in hypothermia is the maintenance of the intracellular to extracellular pH gradient, such "abnormal" values would be perfectly appropriate. Thus, the conventional wisdom in managing hypothermia is to maintain the aforementioned gradient, utilizing uncorrected or euthermic arterial blood gas values and treating the acid–base status of the patient as if they were euthermic. This approach also prevents the development of hypoventilation, alveolar collapse, and subsequent impairment in oxygenation. The literature suggests that this maintenance of ventilation yields lesser degrees of hypothermic-induced myocardial irritability and necrosis. One final exception, however: it is not clear that uncorrected values of partial pressure of oxygen should be used. Most authorities err on the side of accepting the lower, corrected value, thereby working more aggressively to improve the oxygenation status of the patient.

Treatment "Pearls"

Management of the hypothermic patient requires an individualized approach. Not all patients respond in identical fashion to the same level of hypothermia or to the same treatment mo-

TABLE 25-5

TREATMENT "PEARLS" IN HYPOTHERMIA

1. Always stabilize the ABC's.
2. If you need to intubate, you need to intubate.
3. Avoid jostling the patient: this may precipitate full cardiac arrest.
4. Make sure the patient is dry: the conductivity of water is very high.
5. Search for underlying causes of hypothermia.
6. Expect the need for volume expansion because of "cold diuresis."
7. Atrial fibrillation and bradycardia are best treated by rewarming alone. An organized rhythm is a good sign in hypothermia, whereas ventricular fibrillation is to be feared.
8. Avoid chest compressions with an organized rhythm, so long as the degree of bradycardia correlates with the degree of hypothermia.
9. Do not miss occult trauma.
10. Arterial blood gas values need not be corrected for temperature (except, perhaps, for pO_2).
11. Patients are not dead until warm and dead.

dality. Patient prognosis is most closely correlated with underlying disease and not with the absolute degree of hypothermia. Isolated hypothermia yields mortality rates as low as 0%–10%, whereas mortality rates may rise as high as 90% in the presence of serious underlying medical conditions. Despite these variables, certain principles of evaluation and management are important for all patients. These clinical "pearls" are listed in Table 25-5.

SUMMARY

Core temperature is one of the many vital parameters normally maintained within a narrow range by the human body. Profound alterations in core temperature, be they upward or downward, may represent life-threatening syndromes that require a firm understanding of thermoregulation, differential diagnoses and etiologies, and treatment options. Fortunately, aggressive resuscitation can be, and often is, lifesaving when coupled with full supportive care techniques. No body system is immune from damage caused by alterations in core temperature, and all systems must be monitored and treated aggressively to optimize patient outcome.

REVIEW QUESTIONS

1. **Which of the following statements is true?**
   - **A.** Conduction is the most critical mechanism of heat loss during times of high environmental temperature.
   - **B.** Heat loss due to evaporation is limited by high environmental humidity.
   - **C.** The conductivity of water is 25-40 times that of air.
   - **D.** Shivering is a heat-generating mechanism capable of increasing heat production upward of 400%.

2. **The diagnosis of heatstroke involves all the following except:**
   - **A.** Exposure to significant environmental heat stress
   - **B.** Lack of sweating
   - **C.** Elevation in core body temperature, generally greater than 104°F
   - **D.** Manifestation of major central nervous system dysfunction

3. **Which of the following statements regarding hypothermia is not true?**
   - **A.** Hypothermia is defined as a core body temperature less than 95°F.
   - **B.** Traditional clinical criteria for death do not apply in the setting of hypothermia.
   - **C.** Avoid chest compressions with an organized bradycardic rhythm if the degree of bradycardia corresponds to the degree of hypothermia.
   - **D.** Shivering is abolished, even in the setting of mild hypothermia.

4. **Severe hypothermia:**
   - **A.** Is defined as a core temperature less than 80°F only if an immediate threat to life exists.
   - **B.** Nearly always is accompanied by stupor and coma.
   - **C.** Indicates clinical death in the setting of asystole.
   - **D.** Generally is associated with cardiovascular collapse but not profound respiratory dysfunction.

5. **Treatment modalities for severe hypothermia include:**
   - **A.** Warmed humidified oxygen
   - **B.** Warmed peritoneal lavage
   - **C.** Warmed thoracostomy lavage
   - **D.** Extracorporeal rewarming
   - **E.** All the above

ANSWERS

1. The answer is B, C, and D. Conduction plays a critical role in the dissipation of heat when the body is exposed to substances of high conductivity, such as water. During times of high environmental temperature exceeding core temperature, evaporation becomes the most critical mechanism of heat loss.
2. The answer is B. It is a common misconception that patients who sweat do not have heatstroke. The presence of sweating should never be used to rule out the diagnosis of heatstroke.
3. The answer is D. Shivering is a normal heat-generating mechanism that is maintained in mild hypothermia, defined as core tem-

peratures between 90° and 95°F. Shivering is not abolished until core temperature drops below mild levels of hypothermia.

4. The answer is B. Severe hypothermia is defined as a core temperature less than 80°F and always represents an immediate threat to life. The typical indicators of clinical death cannot be relied upon in the setting of severe hypothermia; many patients have been resuscitated successfully from profound depressions in core temperature. Cardiovascular and respiratory deterioration are quite common in the setting of severe hypothermia.

5. The answer is E. Severe hypothermia must be treated aggressively because it is an immediate threat to life. The initial resuscitation goals are to stabilize airway, breathing, and circulation and to restore core temperature to at least mild levels of hypothermia. The choice of rewarming techniques depends upon the level of hypothermia, the clinical status of the patient, and the availability of techniques at a given institution. In the setting of severe hypothermia, multiple rewarming techniques often are used simultaneously.

SUGGESTED READING

Danzl DF, Pozos RS. Accidental hypothermia. N Engl J Med 1994;331: 1756–1760.

Delaney KA, Vassallo SU, Goldfrank LR. Thermoregulatory principles. In: Goldfrank LR, Flomenbaum NE, Lewin NA, et al. (eds.) Goldfrank's Toxicologic Emergencies. Norwalk, CT: Appleton and Lange, 1994.

Dematte JE, O'Mara K, Buescher J, et al. Near-fatal heat stroke during the 1995 heat wave in Chicago. Ann Intern Med 1998;129: 173–181.

Kauffman FH. Profound accidental hypothermia. Trauma Q 1989;6: 7–11.

Tek DA, Olshaker JS. Heat illness. Emerg Med Clin North Am 1992; 10:299–309.

Vicario SJ, Okabajue R, Haltom T. Rapid cooling in classic heat stroke: effect on mortality rates. Am J Emerg Med 1986;4:394.

CHAPTER 26

GREGORY J. ROSSINI AND WISSAM CHATILA

Infections in the Intensive Care Unit

CHAPTER OUTLINE

LEARNING OBJECTIVES

After studying this chapter, you should be able to:

- Understand the pathophysiology of specific infections in the ICU.
- Identify infectious complications in critically ill patients.
- Conduct appropriate diagnostic workup for infections encountered in the ICU.
- Develop a systematic approach for managing ICU-related infection.
- Execute effective measures to prevent infectious complications in the ICU.
- Understand how to effectively work up and treat patients with sepsis.
- Choose the appropriate antimicrobial regimen for either empiric or culture-focused treatment of ICU Infections.

Nosocomial infections are associated with high mortality in ICU patients.

ACUTE BACTERIAL MENINGITIS

Acute bacterial meningitis (ABM) is a life-threatening and severe infection involving the membranes of the central nervous system (CNS). ABM often presents in fulminant fashion with multiple complications and a high fatality rate despite the availability of potent antimicrobial therapy. The annual incidence of ABM is approximately 3.0 cases per 100,000 population in the United States but varies greatly according to risk factors such as geography, race, and gender. Mortality rates also vary according to the same risk factors and depend on the type of invading pathogen, ranging from 6% for *Haemophilus influenzae* meningitis to 35% for nosocomial meningitis. Currently, two issues dominate the field of ABM: first, the change in epidemiology effected by the introduction of *H. influenzae* type b vaccine, and second, the emergence of multidrug-resistant *Streptococcus pneumoniae* as a

Only 20–30% of patients with sepsis have a definitive source of infection.

new pathogen. Recognition of pathogens based on age and prompt initiation of antimicrobial therapy are the cornerstones of ABM management.

Pathogenesis and Microbiology

Recognition of pathogens based on age group is important for initiation of proper antibiotic regimen.

Entry into the central nervous system is accomplished through direct extension or hematogenous spread.

If treatment is delayed during the first 48 h, the development of pus can lead to adhesions and hydrocephalus.

The pathogenesis of ABM depends on both host factors and the nature of the invading pathogens (Figure 26-1). Direct extension from adjacent structures (middle ear, paranasal sinuses) and hematogenous spread are the two routes of bacterial entry into the CNS; however, the exact mechanism of bacterial penetration through the blood–brain barrier (BBB) remains undetermined. Once the subarachnoid space has been penetrated, bacterial cell wall components stimulate the formation of various inflammatory cytokines, thus activating the inflammatory cascade that further perpetuates disruption of the BBB. Inflammatory and cytokine responses have been reported to differ according to the invading organism, which may explain the variability in complication rates among various CNS pathogens. In meningococcal meningitis, if treatment is delayed, a thin layer of pus forms around the meninges within 48 h after onset of the infection, resulting in adhesions around the brain and cerebral hydrocephalus.

Following the widespread use of vaccines against *H. influenzae* capsular type b in the United States, there has been a steady decline in the incidence of meningitis caused by this organism. Countries that have not adopted the widespread use of this vaccine, however, continue to observe higher rates of infection with *H. influenzae*. In adults, *Neisseria meningitidis* and *Streptococcus pneumoniae* are far more common causes of meningitis than *H. influenzae* (Table 26-1). Adult *H. influenzae* infections usually are associated with one or more predisposing factors including otitis media, sinusitis, pneumonia, head trauma with cerebrospinal fluid (CSF) leak, immune deficiency, and asplenia. On the other hand, *N. meningitidis* infections are more often found in children and young adults, and at times occur in epidemics in schools and on college campuses. For both *N. meningitidis* and *H. influenzae*, nasopharyngeal carriage is thought to facilitate initiation of the meningitis. Persons with complement deficiencies (C5–C8) are also known to be at far greater risk to develop neisserial infections.

Pneumococcal infections share the same risk factors as *H. influenzae* infection. In addition, they are frequently associated with distant active infections such as pneumonia and en-

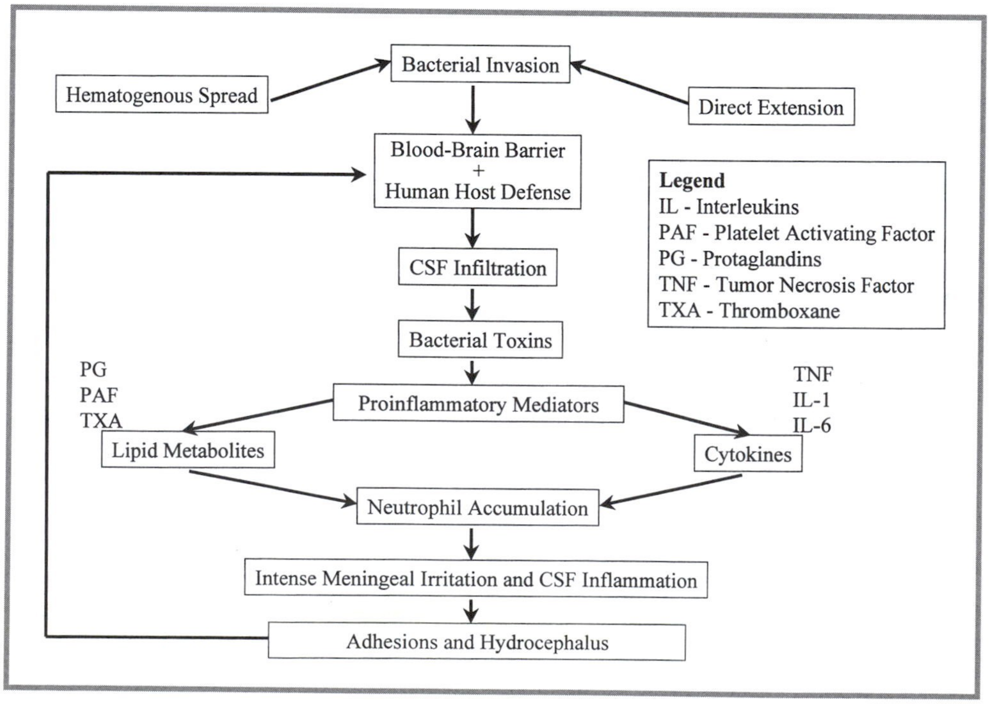

FIGURE 26-1

The pathogenesis of acute bacterial meningitis depends on host anatomic and immunologic factors as well as bacterial virulence factors.

TABLE 26-1

BACTERIAL PATHOGENS CAUSING MENINGITIS IN ALL AGE GROUPS

0–3 months	Group B streptococci
3 months–18 years	
18–50 years	
50 years	Gram-negative rods
Impaired immunity	Gram-negative rods
Trauma/neurosurgery	Staphylococci Gram-negative rods

docarditis. *Listeria monocytogenes* is encountered in the extreme age groups (neonates and elderly) and in debilitated patients including cancer patients, alcoholics, and immunosuppressed adults. Immunosuppressed adults and those who undergo neurosurgical procedures are also predisposed to develop meningitis resulting from aerobic gram-negative rods and *Staphylococcus aureus*. *Staphylococcus epidermidis* infections are mostly observed in patients with cerebrospinal shunts.

Neisseria meningitidis and *Streptococcus pneumoniae* are the most common causes of meningitis in adults.

Haemophilus influenzae meningitis has a strong association with otitis, sinusitis, pneumonia, head trauma, and asplenia. *N. meningitidis* occurs more commonly in young adults and in college campus outbreaks. Nasopharyngeal carriage is believed to cause initiation of the meningitis with either organism.

Presentation and Diagnosis

Most patients with ABM have fever, headache, meningismus (meningeal irritation), rigors, vomiting, myalgias, and occasionally signs of cerebral dysfunction. Elderly, immunocompromised, and debilitated patients may have a less fulminant presentation consisting of change in mental status (confusion, delirium, or lethargy), absence of fever, and a great variability in the degree of meningismus. Severe meningismus is accompanied by Kernig's sign (resistance to passive extension of the legs) and Brudzinski's signs (passive flexion of the neck causing flexion of the hips and knees), which can be elicited in half the patients with ABM. Less often, patients present with cranial nerve palsies, new-onset seizures, focal neurologic deficit, or signs of increased intracranial pressure such as severe hypertension, bradycardia, and coma. Meningococcal septicemia may also manifest with a hemorrhagic skin rash, acute adrenal insufficiency (Waterhouse–Friderichsen syndrome) caused by adrenal hemorrhage, and disseminated intravascular coagulation (DIC).

Listeria monocytogenes causes meningitis in elderly patients, neonates, and debilitated or immunosuppressed patients.

Fever, headache, and meninigismus are typical manifestations of acute bacterial meningitis (ABM); however, in the elderly or immunocompromised the presentation may be more subtle.

Prevention and Management

Patients should receive their first antibiotic dose immediately after clinical evaluation establishes the suspicion for ABM, ideally within 30 min of their initial presentation to the emergency room. There is no excuse for any delay in therapy; delaying antimicrobial therapy until after a CT scan of the brain is completed increases mortality and complications (Figure 26-2). Selection of an empiric antibiotic is based on the patient's age and risk factors. Large doses of bactericidal antibiotics with good CSF penetration are usually given to control this overwhelming infection (Table 26-2). Appropriate antimicrobial therapy should sterilize the CSF within 24–36 h. Once susceptibility of the organism is known, antimicrobial therapy can be directed according to the pathogen. Penicillin-susceptible strains of *S. pneumoniae* and *N. meningitidis* are treated with penicillin G 4 million units q4h. *L. monocytogenes* is sensitive to ampicillin, and usually an aminoglycoside is added for the first several days of therapy. Methicillin-sensitive staphylococcal infections should be treated with

Kernig's sign is increased resistance to passive leg extension. Brudzinski's signs are associated flexion of the hips and knees with passive neck flexion.

Lumbar puncture is diagnostic of ABM in 60%–90% of cases, and is associated with elevated CSF pressure and elevated CSF white blood cells.

nafcillin or oxacillin; vancomycin has poor CSF penetration compared to nafcillin and should be reserved for resistant infections. For infections caused by highly resistant *S. pneumoniae* [minimal inhibitory concentration (MIC) > 2 g/ml], vancomycin with rifampin and a third-generation cephalosporin (cefotaxime or ceftriaxone), together with a repeat lumbar puncture after 24–36 h of therapy, have been suggested for optimal management. Recent reports on meropenem, a new carbapenem antibiotic, show that it has an increased activity against resistant *S. pneumoniae* as well as against *L. monocytogenes*; its effectiveness remains to be determined in clinical studies.

Brain imaging with CT or MRI can exclude intracranial and parameningeal processes or complications related to meningitis.

Antibiotic therapy should be administered when clinical evaluation establishes suspicion of meningitis, and antibiotics should be given within 30 min from initial presentation.

Adjunctive therapy with steroids has been shown to be useful in neonates, but such therapy in adults has been controversial. Some studies support the use of dexamethasone (0.15 mg/kg q6h for up to 4 days) 30 min before the first dose of antibiotic for pediatric patients. Treatment with dexamethasone in pediatric patients is intended to prevent devastating neurologic complications. Despite controversy regarding the use of steroids in adults, several studies suggest adjunctive corticosteroids for certain high-risk patients who have significantly elevated intracranial pressure with cerebral edema. Additionally, seizures should be treated aggressively to prevent further neurologic damage.

Prevention is directed toward persons who were exposed to patients infected with either *H. influenzae* or *N. meningitidis*. One dose of ciprofloxacin (500 or 750 mg) or rifampin twice a day for 2 days (10 mg/kg; not exceeding 600 mg/day) is recommended and is effective in eradicating nasopharyngeal carriage of *N. meningitidis* for close contacts. Ceftriaxone (250 mg IM) has been administered as alternative meningococcal chemoprophylaxis for pregnant women and persons intolerant of ciprofloxacin. All contacts of a patient with *H. influenzae*, including health care providers, should receive daily rifampin (20 mg/kg, not exceeding 600 mg/day) as chemoprophylaxis for 4 days.

INFECTIVE ENDOCARDITIS

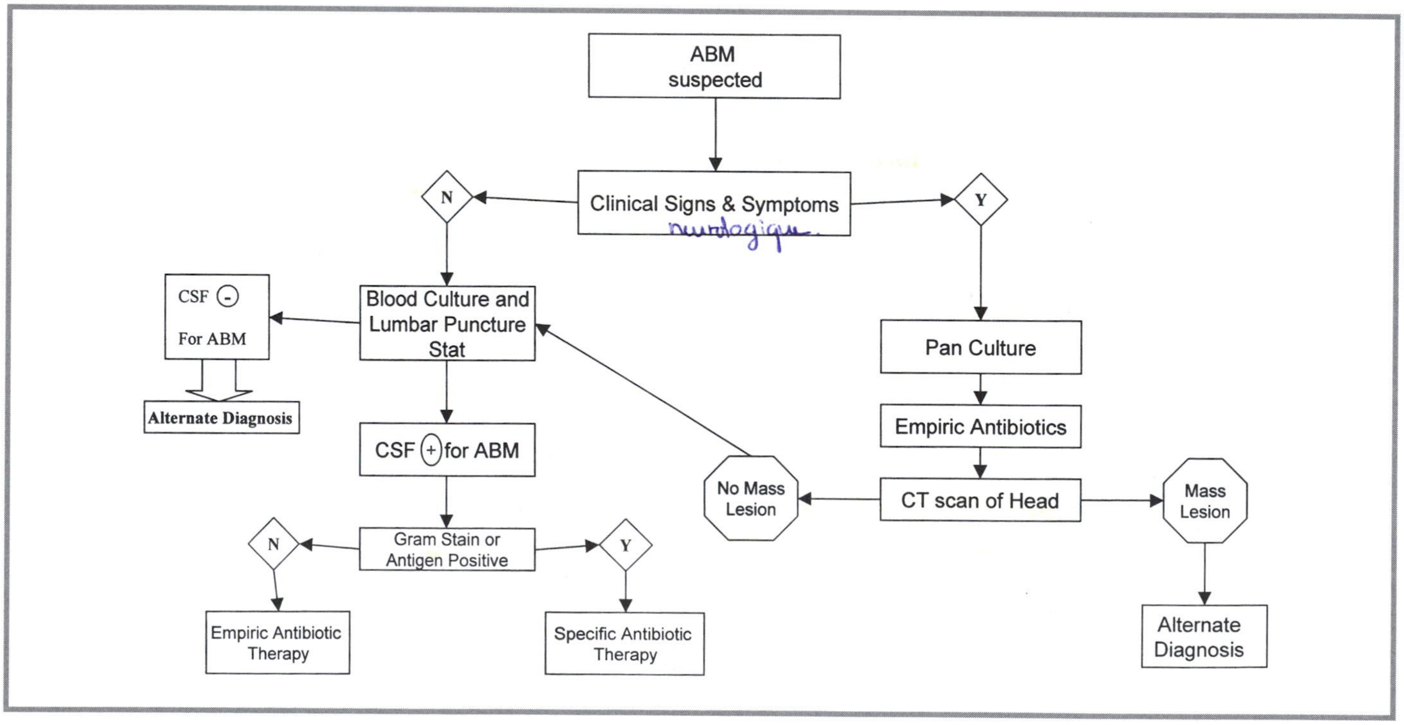

FIGURE 26-2

The patient with suspected acute bacterial meningitis (ABM) should receive careful assessment, with a low threshold for starting antibiotics early. Lumbar puncture should also be done immediately if there are no focal neurologic signs.

TABLE 26-2

CHOICES AND DOSAGES OF EMPIRIC ANTIBIOTIC THERAPY FOR BACTERIAL MENINGITIS

Adult immunocompetent	Cefotaxime or	2 g q4h
	Ceftriaxone	2 g q12h
	Vancomycin	1 g q12h
	Rifampin	300 mg BID
Over 50 years or with impaired immunity	Ampicillin	2 g q4h
	Cefotaxime or Ceftriaxone	
	Vancomycin	
	Aminoglycoside[a]	
Nosocomial or postneurosurgery	Vancomycin	1 g q12h
	Ceftazidime	4 g q8h
	Aminoglycoside[a]	

[a] Gentamicin, amikacin, or tobramycin if *Pseudomonas* is suspected; patients with gram-negative meningitis who fail systemic therapy should be considered for intrathecal or intraventricular aminoglycoside therapy

Infective endocarditis (IE) is defined as a cardiac endothelial infection that causes a systemic febrile syndrome and may lead to multiple endocardiac or endovascular complications. Classic manifestations of IE are not always seen in the ICU because of the acuity of the disease. Acute IE, particularly with right-sided heart valve endocarditis seen in intravenous drug abuse (IVDA) patients, does not have the same immunologic vascular sequelae displayed by subacute IE. In hospitalized patients, IE has been linked to intravascular nosocomial infections complicating their primary disease. Despite the lack of specific signs for IE, clinical clues and risk factors should help prompt recognition, which is essential for good outcome. Mortality from IE has been reported to be approximately 15%, increasing to 25% for patients who require surgical interventions.

Sterilization of the CSF can be obtained within 24–36 h of administration of bactericidal antibiotics with good CSF penetration.

Pathogenesis and Risk Factors

Development of IE requires transient bacteremia, allowing pathogens to adhere to the endocardial surface with subsequent nidus formation within a fibrin layer. Any condition that facilitates bacterial access to the bloodstream may lead to IE, especially in patients with predisposing heart disease (aortic and mitral valve disease, previously infected valves, prosthetic valves, ventricular septal defect, patent ductus arteriosus, coarctation of the aorta). Dental trauma, urologic manipulation, or more serious infections, such as sepsis and catheter-related infection, are well-known causes of IE. Streptococci (mostly viridans) from the oral flora, staphylococci from the skin flora, and enterococci from the intestinal flora are most commonly associated with IE because they are more adherent to the endocardium compared to other organisms (Table 26-3). Patients with prosthetic valves and IVDA using contaminated intravenous injections are susceptible to IE caused by less adherent gram-negative organisms and fungi. In non-IVDA patients, aortic and mitral valve infections are far more common compared with tricuspid valve involvement, which is more commonly found in IVDA.

Presentation and Diagnosis

Fever, constitutional symptoms, and heart murmurs are the most common signs and symptoms encountered with IE. Right-sided endocarditis is frequently associated with pulmonary emboli; left-sided valvular involvement is associated with systemic emboli causing neurologic deficit, mesenteric ischemia, splenic infarct, or renal insufficiency. Mycotic aneurysms, caused by infection of the vessel walls mostly at arterial branching points, are also encountered in IE and have variable manifestations.

Cardiac endothelial infection with a systemic febrile component may lead to endocardial and endovascular complications. The typical manifestations of subacute infective endocarditis are not always seen in the ICU setting.

Presentation of mycotic aneurysms depends on the location of vessels involved. Most aneurysms are asymptomatic unless they rupture. Focal neurologic signs suggest intracranial hemorrhage, and abdominal pain may be related to hepatic artery or abdominal aortic mycotic aneurysms, which may erode and cause aortoenteric fistulae. Occasionally there is a

Mortality from IE can be as high as 25% for patients who require surgical interventions.

direct extension from the infected vessel into adjacent vertebrae, resulting in osteomyelitis. Another dramatic presentation of IE is severe acute mitral regurgitation, causing fulminant acute pulmonary edema that may be mistakenly attributed to cardiac ischemia. The classic manifestations of subacute IE, including petechiae (seen in the conjunctiva, soft palate, and distal extremities), splinter hemorrhages (under nails), Osler's nodes (2–5 mm tender and erythematous subcutaneous lesions on the finger pads), Janeway lesions (painless and erythematous lesions on palms and soles), and Roth spots (retinal vascular hemorrhages), are seldom seen in ICU patients. In contrast, laboratory abnormalities are frequently observed in most patients. Anemia, leukocytosis, thrombocytopenia, elevated sedimentation rate, and hematuria are commonly present but are nondiagnostic for IE. Because many hospitalized patients present with nonspecific signs, symptoms, and laboratory findings, the diagnostic workup for IE should be performed in all patients with bacteremia or fungemia of unclear origin, particularly if they have endocardial abnormalities or prosthetic devices.

> Any condition that allows bacterial access to the bloodstream may lead to IE.

> Conditions associated with IE include dental trauma, urologic manipulation, and catheter-related infections.

The most important test for the diagnosis of IE is blood culture, which should always be obtained before initiating antimicrobial therapy. Three sets of blood cultures improve the yield to isolate the causative organism; the evidence of persistent bacteremia is consistent with the diagnosis of IE. Negative blood cultures despite IE may be related to administration of antimicrobials before drawing blood cultures, poor microbiologic technique, or IE caused by fastidious organisms (the HACEK group, *Legionella*, *Chlamydia*, *Brucella*, *Bartonella*, *Coxiella*, anaerobes, fungi). Delaying blood cultures until after the first dose of antibiotic reduces the yield for recovering the organism from 90%–95% to 35%–40%. A diagnostic strategy called the Duke criteria has recently proven to have better clinical applicability and sensitivity than the older criteria (the Beth Israel criteria) (Table 26-4). Duke criteria stratify patients into three categories and combine echocardiographic findings with various clinical data (Figure 26-3). Transthoracic echocardiography (TTE), performed first in patients suspected to have IE, has a 60% sensitivity in detecting valvular vegetations. Transesophageal echocardiography (TEE) has surpassed TTE in the diagnosis of IE, having a sensitivity greater than 90%, but TEE is usually reserved for patients with complicated endocardial infections and those with negative or poor quality TTE still suspected to have IE. CT scanning is usually reserved to investigate the presence of leaky mycotic aneurysms or distant abscesses, and angiography is performed to confirm the diagnosis of aneurysms.

> Fever, constitutional symptoms, and heart murmurs are the more commonly encountered symptoms and signs of IE.

> Left-sided complications of IE include systemic emboli causing renal insufficiency, mesenteric ischemia, or neurologic deficits. Right-sided complications include septic emboli to the lung.

> Mitral regurgitation often has a severe fulminant presentation with acute pulmonary edema.

Management

Hospitalized and critically ill patients suspected of having IE should be started on empiric antibiotics after obtaining all blood cultures. Acute-onset native valve infections, prosthetic valve infections, and IVDA endocarditis are treated empirically with nafcillin (or oxacillin) and gentamicin, pending culture results. Gentamicin causes a more rapid clearing of bacteremia without affecting the overall cure rate and is recommended because of its synergy with nafcillin. For patients allergic to penicillins and beta-lactams, and in hospitals where methicillin-resistant *Staphylococcus aureus* and *Staphylococcus epidermidis* (MRSA,

> Diagnostic workup for IE should be performed in all patients with bacteremia or fungemia of unknown etiology.

TABLE 26-3

COMMON PATHOGENS CAUSING BACTERIAL ENDOCARDITIS

Streptococcal species	Coagulase-negative staphylococci
Enterococcal species Gram-negative rods Culture-negative endocarditis HACEK organisms: species	Gram-negative rods Streptococcal species Enterococcal species Fungal pathogens

TABLE 26-4

MAJOR AND MINOR DUKE CRITERIA FOR CLINICAL INFECTIVE ENDOCARDITIS

Typical microorganism in two separate blood cultures (B/C)	Predisposing cardiac disease or intravenous drug abuse
Persistently positive blood cultures (3 positive blood cultures)	Fever 38.0°C (100.4°F)
Echocardiogram evidence of vegetation, abscess, or prosthetic valve dehiscence	Evidence of valvular embolic disease or mycotic aneurysm
New valvular regurgitation	Immunologic evidence of endocarditis (i.e., glomerulonephritis, Osler nodes, Roth spots, rheumatoid factor)
	Blood culture positive (3 sets)
	Echocardiographic evidence consistent with endocarditis (not meeting major criteria for echocardiographic evidence of IE)

IE, infective endocarditis
SOURCE: Modified from Durak DT, et al. Am J Med 1994;96:200

MRSE) infections are prevalent, vancomycin (30 mg/kg/day, or doses adjusted according to renal function to yield vancomycin levels 1 h post dosing of 30–45 mg/ml) substitutes for nafcillin. Once the organism has been identified, antibiotics should target the organism according to its susceptibility (Table 26-5). The majority of cases of IE require prolonged parenteral antibiotic therapy to achieve a cure. Methicillin-sensitive strains of staphylococci should be treated with nafcillin (or oxacillin) because vancomycin has a lower efficacy compared with nafcillin. Similarly, patients who are allergic to penicillin but not to beta-lactams should receive cefazolin (2 g IV q 8 h) and not vancomycin. For streptococcal prosthetic valve endocarditis, duration of therapy should be extended to 6 weeks with gentamicin given for at least the first 2 weeks. For documented methicillin-resistant staphylococcal prosthetic valve endocarditis, rifampin (300 mg PO q8h) should be added to vancomycin and gentam-

Three sets of blood cultures improve the yield to isolate organisms. Negative blood cultures in clinical IE suggest administration of antimicrobials, poor microbiologic technique, or infection with HACEK organisms.

Clinical criteria allow stratification to aid the management of IE.

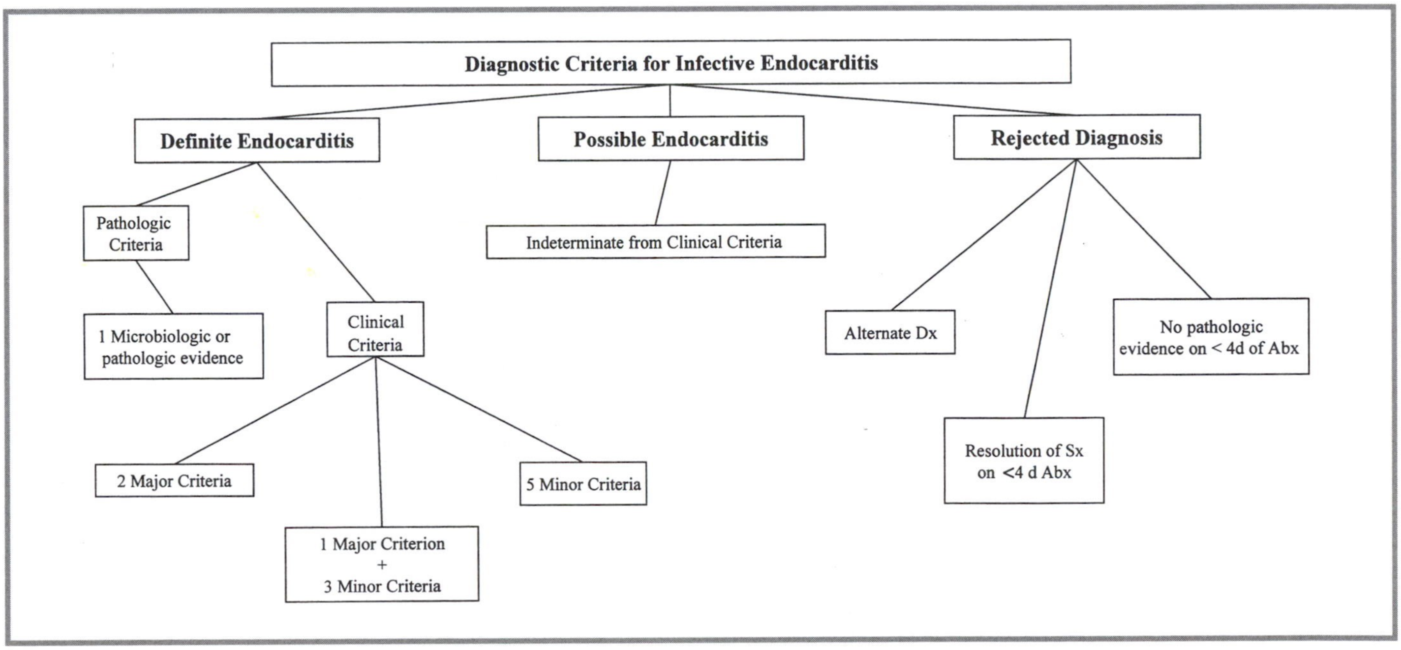

FIGURE 26-3

A risk-stratifying approach to the diagnostic evaluation of the patient with infective endocarditis.

Transesophageal echocardiography (TEE) is more sensitive than transthoracic echocardiography (TTE) to detect valvular vegetations.

For all patients suspected of having IE, empiric antimicrobials should be started after blood cultures have been obtained.

icin (keep in mind the need to increase coumadin dosing because of drug interaction with rifampin).

The only effective way to prevent the complications of IE is to prevent IE itself by using prophylactic antibiotics for certain patients with known predisposing risk factors for IE who are undergoing procedures (recommendation by American Heart Association and the Infectious Disease Society of America (IDSA); JAMA 1997;277:1794). Unfortunately, although complications decrease after starting antimicrobial therapy, once IE is established, catastrophic events cannot be fully prevented. Devastating complications may involve any part of the systemic circulation. Septic emboli to lungs, coronary arteries, spleen, bowel, and extremities are encountered in 22%–50% of case, and up to 65% of emboli involve the central nervous system. Most emboli tend to occur within 2 to 4 weeks of antimicrobial therapy, but some have been reported to occur as late as 15–30 weeks because of nonhealing vegetations. The size and number of vegetations, the involved valve, and the infecting organism may all contribute to the risk of embolization. Large vegetations (>1 cm) on the anterior leaflet of the mitral valve caused by staphylococcal or fungal infections are more likely to embolize. There is no specific therapy for septic emboli, and anticoagulation is not recommended (except for patients with prosthetic valves already receiving anticoagulation). Two major emboli, excluding cutaneous emboli, occurring after institution of appropriate antibiotics is generally accepted as an indication for valve replacement surgery to prevent further embolization. Other indications for valve replacement surgery include new-onset heart failure, fungal endocarditis, failure of therapy (persistent bacteremia, increase in size of the vegetation, perivalvular extension of IE, or formation of myocardial abscesses), and unstable prosthetic valve. Urgent surgical therapy can be lifesaving, especially for acute severe heart failure, and is usually superior to medical treatment for fungal and prosthetic valve endo-

TABLE 26-5

ANTIBIOTIC REGIMENS FOR INFECTIVE ENDOCARDITIS ACCORDING TO PATHOGEN

ORGANISM	ANTIMICROBIAL	DURATION[a]
Penicillin-sensitive streptococci (MIC 0.1 μg/ml)[b]	Pen[c] 12–18 million units/day	4 weeks
	Ceftriaxone 2 g qd	4 weeks
	Pen 12–18 million units/day gentamicin 1 mg/kg q8h[d]	2 weeks
Intermediately penicillin-sensitive streptococci (0.1 MIC 0.6 μg/ml)	Pen 18 million units/day gentamicin 1 mg/kg q8h	4 weeks
Highly penicillin-resistant streptococci (MIC 0.6 μg/ml)	Pen 18–30 million units/day gentamicin 1 mg/kg q8h	4–6 weeks
	Ampicillin 12 g/day gentamicin 1 mg/kg q8h	4–6 weeks
MSSA or MSSE[e]	Nafcillin (or oxacillin) 12 g/day	4–6 weeks
	gentamicin 1 mg/kg q8h	3–5 days
Tricuspid valve MSSA endocarditis (in IVDA)	Ciprofloxacin 750 mg po bid	4 weeks
	Rifampin 300 mg po bid	2 weeks
	nafcillin tobramaycin	
MRSA or MRSE[f]	Vancomycin 30 mg/kg (2 g/day) rifampin 300 mg po q8h[g] gentamicin 1 mg/kg q8h[g]	4–6 weeks
HACEK group	Ceftriaxone 2 g qd or Ampicillin 12 g/day Gentamicin 1 mg/kg q8h	4 weeks
Fungi[h]	Amphotericin B 0.8–1.0 mg/kg/day flucytosine 100–150 mg/kg/day	

[a] For native valve endocarditis (refer to text for prosthetic valve endocarditis)
[b] Minimal inhibitory concentration (MIC)
[c] Aqueous penicillin G
[d] Achieve a peak serum level of 3 μg/ml
[e] Methicillin-sensitive *Staphylococcus aureus* and methicillin-sensitive *Staphylococcus epidermidis*
[f] Methicillin-resistant *Staphylococcus aureus* and methicillin-resistant *Staphylococcus epidermidis*
[g] Usually added for inadequate response to vancomycin; ciprofloxacin, minocycline, and trimethoprin-sulfamethoxazole are other alternatives to gentamicin
[h] Surgery is almost always required

carditis. Management of mycotic aneurysms depends on the site of the infected vessel. For example, resection of the involved abdominal aortic aneurysm is indicated. On the other hand, intracranial mycotic aneurysms may heal with antibiotics and are either treated with antimicrobial therapy alone, or with surgical excision, which is often reserved for bleeding or enlarging accessible aneurysms.

SEPSIS

Sepsis is a syndrome whereby a serious infection induces a cascade of deranged inflammatory events causing nonspecific systemic manifestations and often leading to multiorgan dysfunction (Table 26-6). Clearly any infection can cause such a presentation, and the severity of illness may vary considerably in the presence of these nonspecific findings, hence the heterogeneity of the sepsis syndrome. The same presentation is observed in certain diseases without any evidence of infections, such as acute pancreatitis and major trauma. This noninfectious inflammatory pattern, which mimics sepsis, has been termed the systemic inflammatory response syndrome (SIRS). Despite the availability of advanced life-supportive care and the introduction of newer antimicrobial therapy, sepsis is among the leading causes of ICU admissions and continues to be the most common complication seen in critically ill ICU patients. Moreover, sepsis remains associated with a mortality rate of 30%–40% and is the most common cause of death in most ICUs in the United States and Europe. Great resources have been allocated for sepsis research, resulting in a worthy understanding of its pathogenesis, but no major specific therapeutic breakthroughs have yet been introduced.

> Septic emboli occur in a significant number of patients. The size and number of vegetations, the valve, and the infecting organisms all contribute to embolization risk.

Pathogenesis and Microbiology

> Surgical therapy can be lifesaving in acute severe heart failure.

A more detailed discussion of the pathogenesis of sepsis is covered in Chapter 18. In brief, an infectious stimulus or one of its by-products triggers the release of proinflammatory cytokine mediators (tumor necrosis factor-alpha, interleukin-1, interleukin-8), which initiates a systemic inflammatory response. Initial hypotheses regarding sepsis suggested that unimpeded proinflammatory responses contributed to the clinical features of this syndrome. Current evidence supports the hypothesis that sepsis results from derangements in the host immune response, that is, an imbalance between proinflammatory and antiinflammatory cytokines (interleukin-1 receptor antagonist, interleukin-4, interleukin-10, tumor necrosis factor receptor antagonist) (Figure 26-4). In such an uncontrolled inflammatory milieu, other mechanisms such as redistribution of regional blood flow, reduction in oxygen supply, oxidant injury, and alterations in intermediary metabolism contribute to tissue ischemia and injury, resulting in organ dysfunction. The difference between sepsis and SIRS lies only in the precipitating stimulus; in SIRS, the initial insult is thought to be noninfectious.

> Sepsis is a syndrome resulting from a cascade of deranged inflammatory events caused by serious infection. It is associated with nonspecific systemic manifestations that often lead to multiple organ system failure.

Any serious infection can lead to sepsis, and no single organism predominates. The spectrum of pathogens involved in sepsis varies according to the host and the affected organ. The most common site of infection giving rise to severe sepsis is the lung (e.g., pneumonia), followed by the abdominopelvic region (e.g., cholecystitis), then the urinary tract (e.g., pyelonephritis). Staphylococcal infections and infections with enteric gram-negative organisms are frequently associated with nosocomial sepsis. Immunocompromised patients, whether presenting from the community or already hospitalized, are at risk for developing sepsis secondary to bacterial as well as viral and fungal pathogens. The history, physical ex-

> Despite better understanding of the pathophysiology of sepsis, mortality approaches 30%–40%.

TABLE 26-6

CLINICAL FEATURES OF SEPSIS

Clinical presentation	Laboratory
Fever or hypothermia	Leukocytosis or granulocytopenia
Tachypnea	Thrombocytopenia
Tachycardia with or without hypotension	Respiratory alkalosis/hypoxemia
Oliguria	Hyperglycemia
Confusion or obtundation	Lactic acidosis

aminations, and initial workup often establish a suspected source of infection, although only 30% of patients have positive blood cultures and 20%–30% of patients have no identifiable source of infection.

Presentation and Diagnosis

An infectious stimulus triggers the release of proinflammatory cytokines such as tumor necrosis factor, interleukin-1, and interleukin-8.

Sepsis is currently thought to result from an imbalance between proinflammatory and antiinflammatory cytokines.

The most common sites of infection associated with sepsis are the lung, abdominopelvic region, and urinary tract.

Sepsis represents a continuum of clinical presentations, and the infection can arise in any body region. Sepsis is a clinical diagnosis in patients with suspected infection who present with fever or hypothermia, tachypnea, tachycardia, leukocytosis, or leukopenia. The diagnosis of sepsis is confirmed by abnormalities in central hemodynamics. An elevated cardiac output, low systemic vascular resistance, and low to normal pulmonary artery occlusion pressure (or wedge pressure) are characteristic of sepsis. During the early stages of sepsis, clinical features may be more specific and may vary according to the host and the affected organ; hypoxemia and dyspnea would suggest pneumonia as the cause of sepsis. In elderly and immunocompromised patients or with the progression of sepsis, the site of infection tends to be less evident because of poor host response or multiple organ dysfunction. For instance, hypoxemia and dyspnea may reflect diaphragmatic dysfunction or acute respiratory distress syndrome (ARDS) in a patient who has abdominal sepsis. Eventually, some patients develop septic shock and multiorgan failure despite appropriate antimicrobial therapy, regardless of the precipitating event.

A clinical picture suggesting sepsis should always prompt a diagnostic workup that is directed toward identifying a source of the infection and isolating the pathogen. A sepsis workup is incomplete if it does not include a white blood cell count with a peripheral smear, chemistry profile, blood cultures, and urine cultures. Additional testing is usually guided by the history and physical examination. A chest radiograph, sputum Gram stain, and cultures are obtained when the clinical scenario is consistent with pneumonia. CT of the abdomen or head, paracentesis, and lumbar puncture are performed if an intraabdominal or a central nervous system infection, respectively, is suspected. It is generally recommended to sample any fluid collec-

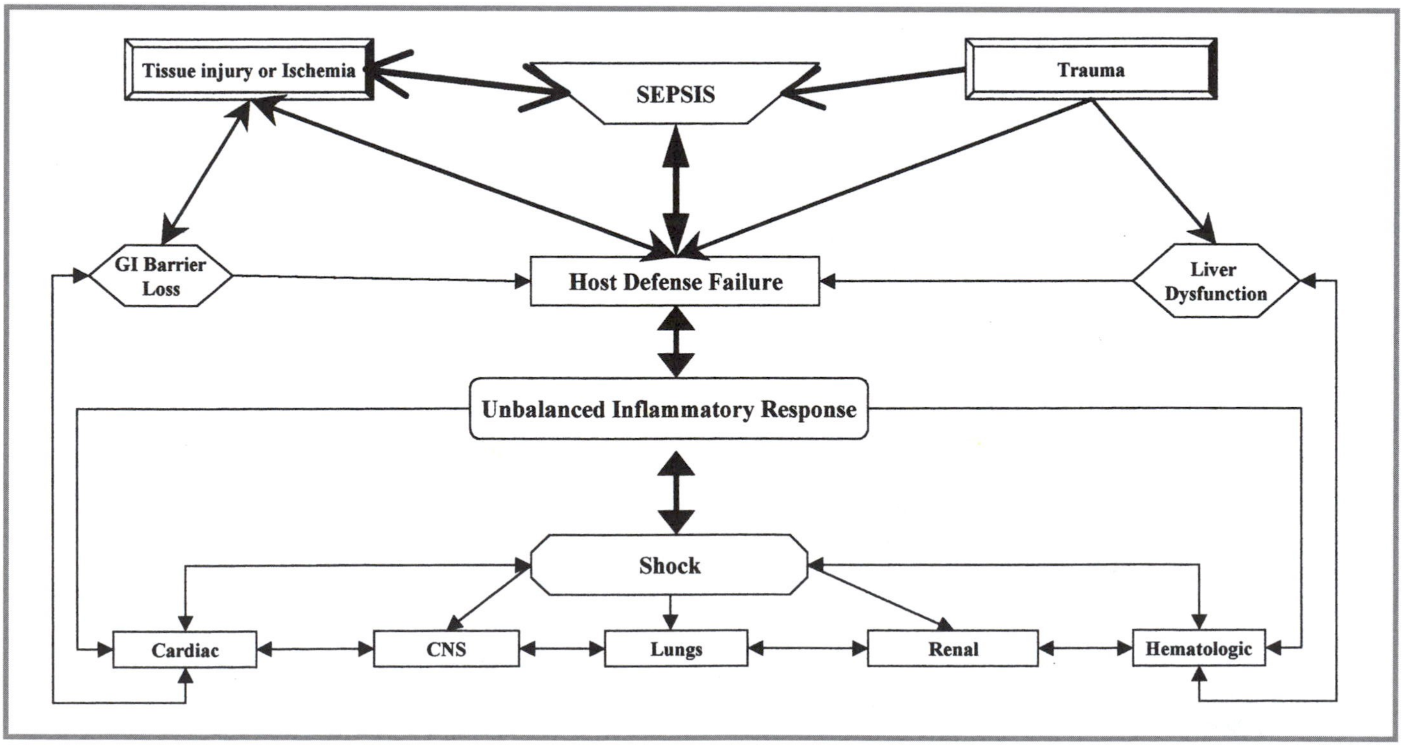

FIGURE 26-4

The complex pathophysiologic process of sepsis is initiated by tissue injury and perpetuated by an unbalanced inflammatory response.

tion that is found on diagnostic imaging because it may be the source of infection. Moreover, to optimize the microbiologic yield, all cultures should be obtained before administering antibiotics. Assessment of risk factors and comorbidities helps in the diagnostic workup and the selection of antimicrobial therapy; however, if the primary site of infection is not readily identifiable, a systematic search for infection should cover the respiratory, gastrointestinal, biliary, and genitourinary tracts, along with the central nervous and cardiovascular systems.

Positive blood cultures are seen in 30% of patients and about 20%–30% have no identifiable source of infection.

Patients already in the hospital or in the ICU are vulnerable to developing secondary sepsis from either failure of their therapy or superimposed nosocomial infections. Sepsis is frequently encountered in hospitalized patients, debilitated patients, and those at risk for the development of nosocomial infections. Specific nosocomial infections, which add significantly to the morbidity and mortality of patients, are discussed in more detail in this chapter. Often it becomes difficult to isolate the offending organism and ascertain whether the systemic inflammatory process is infectious or noninfectious in patients with prolonged hospitalization who become colonized with numerous pathogenic organisms, particularly in patients receiving multiple antibiotics or systemic glucocorticosteroids and those presenting with an intraabdominal inflammatory process. For example, a patient with a colonized indwelling catheter may be diagnosed with a line sepsis to explain his clinical deterioration, but the actual cause of sepsis is in fact mesenteric ischemia, which is often identified arduously. Nonbacterial infectious pathogens are uncommon in most ICUs but may vary depending on geographic location and host susceptibility. These pathogens, along with the noninfectious causes of sepsis-like syndrome, should be considered in patients whose illness has no clear etiology (Table 26-7).

Sepsis can be confirmed by right heart catheterization. The usual findings include elevated cardiac output, low systemic vascular resistance, and low to normal pulmonary capillary wedge pressure.

With a high clinical suspicion for sepsis, conduct a diagnostic workup directed at locating an infectious source and a specific pathogen.

Management

Antimicrobials and drainage (surgical or nonsurgical, depending on the primary site) of abscesses when present are the cornerstone of therapy for eradicating all septic foci. Findings from the history, physical examination, and initial diagnostic workup usually lead to a presumptive diagnosis and guide the initial choice of empiric antimicrobial therapy. Any uncertainty about the cause of sepsis, site of infection, or type of pathogen justifies the use of aggressive broad-spectrum antibiotics (Table 26-8). A 10%–15% increase in mortality is observed in patients who receive delayed or inappropriate antimicrobial therapy. The ideal scenario is to start antibiotics very early in sepsis, immediately after obtaining all cultures, then identifying the cause of the infection and directing the therapy according to the sensitivity of the organism. Unfortunately, not all patients present early in the course of their disease, and many progress to septic shock and die despite adequate antibiotic coverage.

Fluid collections found on imaging studies should be sampled before administration of antibiotics, if possible, to assure the highest yield.

Assessment of risk factors and comorbid conditions aid the diagnostic workup and subsequent antimicrobial choice.

Sepsis is commonly encountered in hospitalized, debilitated patients and those at risk to develop nosocomial infections.

When perpetuation of tissue injury is related to an inappropriate immune response and hypoperfusion, therapy for septic shock is directed to restore adequate oxygen tissue delivery, support failed organs, and prevent complications. Aggressive fluid resuscitation (up to 10 l of crystalloid solution over 24 h may be needed) is recommended to regain organ function because effective intravascular volume is reduced by vasodilatation and increased permeability. Usually the goal of hemodynamic resuscitation is to maintain a mean arterial pressure above 60 mmHg and a cardiac index greater than 2.8 $l/min/m^2$. Although there is current debate on the use of pulmonary artery catheters, many clinicians depend on central hemodynamic monitoring to guide therapy especially if septic shock is refractory to fluid resuscitation. For patients who continue to be hypotensive and have evidence of organ dysfunction despite fluid resuscitation, vasoactive agents (dopamine, phenylephrine, dobutamine, norepinephrine, or epinephrine) are used in an attempt to restore tissue perfusion and an acceptable mean arterial blood pressure.

There is some evidence, although inconclusive, that monitoring gastric intramucosal pH with gastric tonometry reflects gut mucosal perfusion. This measurement may be a better marker of tissue perfusion than the measurements of central hemodynamic parameters. In addition, gauging therapy to prevent gastric intramucosal acidosis may reduce mortality in septic patients. Early mechanical ventilatory support is recommended for shock-related respiratory failure. Resting the respiratory muscles and delivering adequate FiO_2 and positive end-expiratory pressure (PEEP) ensures better alveolar ventilation (to optimize CO_2 removal),

Management of sepsis should focus on early institution of antimicrobial therapy and drainage of any abscesses.

TABLE 26-7

UNUSUAL CAUSES OF SEPSIS OR SEPSIS-LIKE SYNDROME

Bacterial infections
- Mycobacterial: tuberculosis, *Mycobacterium avium* complex

Nonbacterial infections
- Viral: dengue, enteroviruses, hepatitis A or B, influenza, cytomegalovirus, herpes zoster viruses
- Rickettsial: Rocky Mountain spotted fever, ehrlichiosis
- Malarial
- Fungal

Noninfectious
- Drug-related: anaphylaxis, neuroleptic malignant syndrome
- Drug intoxication: cocaine, organophosphate
- Drug withdrawal: alcohol
- Anaphylaxis
- Systemic vasculitis: polyarteritis nodosa, systemic lupus erythematosus
- Acute pancreatitis
- Acute hepatic failure
- Heatstroke
- Rhabdomyolysis

prevents hypoxemia, and diverts cardiac output from the respiratory muscles to hypoperfused vital organs. Aggressive organ-specific support, such as hemodialysis for renal failure, replacement of blood components for coagulopathy and bleeding, and nutritional support (enteral feeding is likely more beneficial than parenteral nutrition) are often needed while awaiting the reversal of sepsis.

Septic shock and sequential organ failure portend a poor prognosis, and currently there is no adjunctive therapy that has been proven to alter the outcome of sepsis. Numerous investigations have evaluated targeted therapy along the inflammatory cascade to modulate host immune response and microcirculatory changes, and so far, only activated protein C has shown a reduction in morbidity and mortality. Accordingly, and until clinical investigations demonstrate an effective approach to monitor and to modulate the host inflammatory

TABLE 26-8

EMPIRIC ANTIBIOTIC SELECTION FOR SEPSIS

Life-threatening sepsis	■ Aminoglycoside (gentamicin, tobramycin or amikacin) plus one of the following: ■ Third-generation cephalosporin (cefotaxime or ceftriaxone) ■ Antipseudomonal penicillins (piperacillin-tazobactam or ticarcillin-clavulanic acid) ■ Carbapenams (imipenem) ■ Suspected MRSA: add vancomycin rifampin
Intraabdominal or pelvic infections	■ Metronidazole or clindamycin + aminoglycocide ■ Piperacillin–tazobactam, ticarcillin–clavulanic acid, imipenem or second-generation cephalosporin (cefoxitin or cefotetan) aminoglycoside
Billiary tract sepsis	■ Piperacillin or mezlocillin metronidazole aminoglycoside ■ Piperacillin–tazobactam or ampicillin–sulbactam aminoglycoside
Urosepsis	■ Third-generation cephalosporin (cefotaxime or ceftriaxone) aminoglycoside ■ Piperacillin–tazobactam or ticarcillin–clavulanic acid aminoglycoside ■ Imipenem aminoglycoside
Neutropenia	■ Ceftazidime aminoglycoside ■ Imipenem aminoglycoside ■ Cefepime aminoglycoside ■ Piperacillin–tazobactam amikacin (single daily dose) ■ Ceftriaxone amikacin (both as a single daily dose)

SOURCE: Adopted and modified from Med Lett 1998;40:33

response, meticulous bedside care assuring optimal hemodynamic interventions to prevent secondary organ injury and complications offer the best hope for patient survival.

NOSOCOMIAL INFECTIONS

Nosocomial infections are defined as infections acquired in the hospital after patients are exposed to the hospital microflora. Nosocomial infections are a heavy economic burden on hospitals, and, more important, they are a major cause of morbidity and mortality in patients who are already compromised. Susceptibility of hospitalized patients to such infections is not uniform and, in general, depends on severity of illness, the degree of patient immune dysfunction, and patient exposure to various high-risk interventions. For example, intubated patients on mechanical ventilation support are frequently sedated and require intravascular catheters and bladder cannulation, all of which predispose to ventilator-acquired nosocomial pneumonias, line infections, and genitourinary sepsis with resistant hospital organisms. This section is limited to the discussion of serious and frequently encountered nosocomial infections: nosocomial pneumonia, nosocomial sinusitis, line infections, and *Clostridium difficile* colitis. Many of these infections are preventable, and although general infectious precautions such as washing the hands after examining each patient should be always followed, one cannot overemphasize the specific preventative strategies for each nosocomial infection.

Initial therapy for septic shock relies on fluid resuscitation followed by vasoactive agents such as dopamine if the mean arterial blood pressure has not improved.

Close monitoring for evidence of organ dysfunction is important for optimizing perfusion and possible prevention of multiple system organ failure.

Despite development of many investigational therapies, exceptional bedside care and optimal hemodynamic support remain vital for management.

Nosocomial Pneumonia

Pneumonia is defined separately from other infections of the lower respiratory tract. Nosocomial pneumonia is a specific type of pneumonia that occurs in patients who have been hospitalized for more than 48 h. The incidence of nosocomial pneumonia is 0.5%–1% of all hospital admissions, 15%–20% of ICU admissions, and 18%–60% of mechanically ventilated patients. In addition, pneumonia is associated with the greatest mortality of any nosocomial infection: attributable mortality ranges from 27% to 33% and increases to 50%–70% in mechanically ventilated patients. Pathophysiology of nosocomial pneumonia is complex and varies between different patient populations in the hospital. Although risk factors can help identify patients with nosocomial pneumonia, management of such infections remains extremely challenging because of emerging resistant organisms, lack of a gold standard for diagnosis of pneumonia, and associated morbidities.

Pathogenesis and Risk Factors

Nosocomial infections are associated with high mortality, prolonged hospital stay, and excessive use of resources.

Risk factors for nosocomial pneumonia are either intrinsic or extrinsic. Intrinsic factors include severity of illness, associated comorbidities, malnutrition, and advanced age. Extrinsic factors are related to interventions that interfere with the integrity of the host defense mechanisms; such factors include nasogastric tubes, mechanical ventilation via endotracheal or nasotracheal intubation, and heavy sedation or neuromuscular blockade. Most extrinsic risk factors impair swallowing and leave the upper airway unprotected from aspiration. Bacteria invade the lower respiratory tract via aspiration, inhalation of contaminated aerosols, or hematogenous spread. Overt or covert aspiration (at times referred to as microaspiration) of oropharyngeal or gastric flora is thought to be the most common route of organism delivery to the lower respiratory tract. In critically ill patients, the oropharynx becomes colonized with gram-negative organisms a few days after admission to the hospital, especially if the patients have been exposed to antimicrobial therapy (Table 26-9). Once an inoculum of pathogenic organisms reaches the lower respiratory tract, advanced disease, medical disease processes that reduce host immunity, and violation of the host anatomic barriers make the ideal milieu for a pneumonia to flourish (Figure 26-5).

Nosocomial pneumonia is associated with the highest mortality of all nosocomial infections in the ICU.

Presentation and Diagnosis

The criteria for diagnosing pneumonia include clinical, radiographic, and laboratory evidence of infection. Classical signs and symptoms of pneumonia are often present and in-

Mortality for nosocomial pneumonia is as high as 70% in mechanically ventilated patients.

clude cough with new onset of purulent sputum or change in character of sputum. Fever, tachypnea or dyspnea, tachycardia, hypoxemia, leukocytosis, crackles, or dullness to percussion are often present. In addition, one may find new or progressive infiltrate on chest radiographs and organisms isolated from sputum or blood cultures. Nonetheless, clinical evaluation is frequently limited in critically ill patients, and there are many noninfectious processes that mimic lower respiratory tract infections; thus, it is common to overdiagnose nosocomial pneumonia and mistreat patients (Table 26-10). Isolation of organisms from blood or pleural fluid cultures in the right setting is highly specific for pneumonia, but the prevalence of bacteremia in patients with nosocomial pneumonia is relatively low (8%–15%). On the other hand, the microbiology of sputum and tracheal aspirate is nonspecific for the diagnosis of nosocomial pneumonia because the majority of hospitalized patients are colonized with a number of potentially pathogenic organisms.

Intrinsic risk factors are severity of illness, comorbid conditions, malnutrition, and advanced age.

Extrinsic risk factors are related to violations of host defense integrity.

Although debatable, many intensivists favor using an invasive diagnostic technique that some investigators believe to be more accurate than clinical diagnosis of nosocomial pneumonia. This technique uses fiberoptic bronchoscopy (FOB) or nonbronchoscopically placed small-caliber catheters to obtain uncontaminated samples from the lower respiratory tract. The most extensively studied sampling methods are the fiberoptic bronchoscopic performance of bronchoalveolar lavage (BAL) and protected specimen brushing (PSB) with quantitative culture techniques. The diagnostic threshold for quantitative cultures, to differentiate infections from colonization, has been established at 10^3 colony-forming units (cfu) for BAL and 10^4 cfu for PSB. Specificity of quantitative BAL and PSB for the diagnosis of nosocomial pneumonia is reported as high as 90%; however, this result has not been reproduced in all investigations. Poor FOB technique, early pneumonia, poor BAL return, and use of antibiotics may reduce sensitivity and specificity of the bronchoscopic diagnosis. The use of invasive quantitative diagnostic methods remains controversial, and their clinical utility remains to be determined. On the other hand, invasive testing is the accepted standard for the diagnosis of pneumonia in immunocompromised patients; BAL and PSB have a superior yield and a higher accuracy compared to noninvasive techniques in immunocompromised patients due to a higher prevalence of nonbacterial pathogens in these patients. Yield from the cultures is significantly reduced if the patient is already on antibiotic therapy; therefore, all cultures should be obtained before initiation of therapy regardless of the diagnostic technique used to obtain respiratory secretion samples.

Microbiologic evaluation via sputum or tracheal aspirate is nonspecific for diagnosing nosocomial pneumonia because a positive culture may reflect colonization.

Microbiology

The knowledge that critically ill patients have an altered oropharyngeal and gastrointestinal flora and that aspiration is the most common route of pathogen entry into the lower respiratory tract contributes to understanding the pathogenic differences between nosocomial pneumonia and community-acquired pneumonia. Nosocomial pneumonia has been most commonly associated with enteric gram-negative bacilli (50%–70%), but pneumonias caused by resistant gram-positive pathogens, such as *Staphylococcus aureus*, are becoming more prevalent in many ICUs. A variety of other organisms are known to cause nosocomial pneumonia (Table 26-11). *Staphylococcus epidermidis* is often isolated from endotracheal aspirates, but it is not known to have significant pulmonary pathogenic potential and can be ignored. Tuberculosis and aspergillosis are rare causes of nosocomial pneumonia and occur in epidemics among susceptible patients. Prevalence of specific pathogens causing nosocomial pneumonia varies among ICUs (because of variability in ICU microflora) and with the diagnostic technique used (e.g., BAL vs. endotracheal aspirate).

TABLE 26-9

PREEXISTING CONDITIONS ASSOCIATED WITH PHARYNGEAL COLONIZATION BY GRAM-NEGATIVE BACTERIA

Prolonged hospitalization	Coma
Antibiotic exposure	Pulmonary disease
Major surgery	Renal disease
Diabetes mellitus	Neutropenia

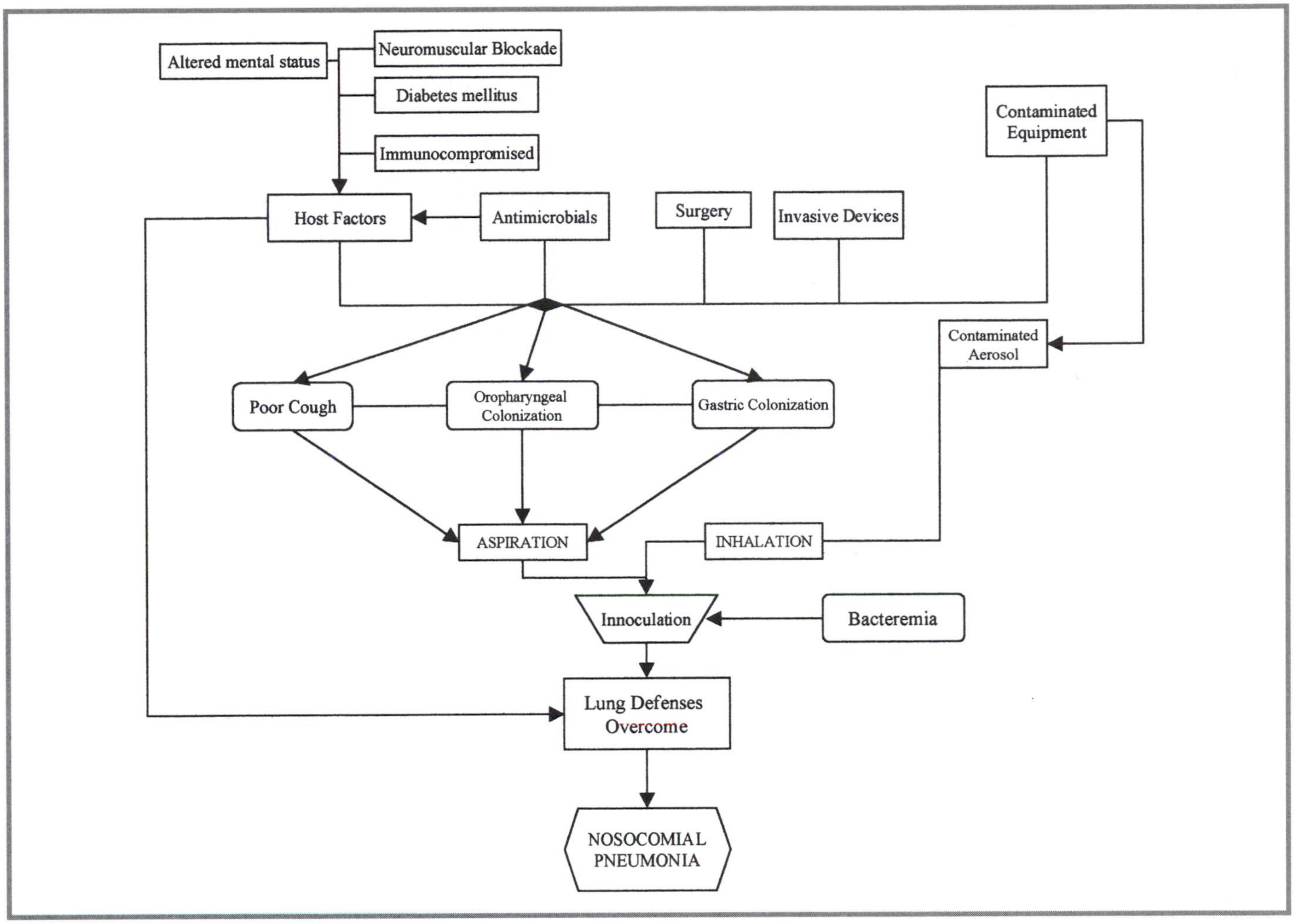

FIGURE 26-5

The pathogenesis of nosocomial pneumonia involves an interplay between multiple host-dependent and nonhost-dependent factors.

Management and Prevention

It is obvious that accurate diagnosis is critical for optimal antimicrobial therapy. Hospital microflora, timing of onset of the nosocomial pneumonia, type of risk factors, and severity of the patient's illness guide initial empiric antibiotic therapy pending the diagnostic workup. Supportive therapy, including ventilatory, hemodynamic, and nutritional support, together with the appropriate antimicrobial coverage are the cornerstones of successful treatment of nosocomial pneumonia. Inadequate antibiotic regimens, even if changed later in the course of the illness, are consistently found to be a significant risk factor for poor outcome in patients with nosocomial pneumonia. Table 26-11 summarizes guidelines for empiric treatment of nosocomial pneumonia based on recommendations of the American Thoracic Society. Un-

Lower respiratory tract secretions obtained via bronchoscopic sampling are more specific than tracheal aspirates.

Poor bronchoscopic technique, early pneumonia, and use of antibiotics may reduce the sensitivity and specificity of bronchoscopic sampling.

TABLE 26-10

RADIOGRAPHIC MIMICS OF PNEUMONIA

Atelectasis (most common)	Pulmonary infarct
Aspiration	Asymmetric pulmonary edema
Pleural effusions	Pulmonary hemorrhage
Acute respiratory distress syndrome	Bronchiolitis obliterans organizing pneumonia
Pulmonary contusion	

Critically ill patients have altered oropharyngeal and gastrointestinal flora, and aspiration is the most common portal of entry into the lower respiratory tract.

fortunately, even with correct choice of antibiotic, overall mortality from nosocomial pneumonia remains substantial (25%–50%); hence, prevention of such infection will have the greatest impact on outcome of hospitalized patients.

Maintaining a semiupright position and contact precautions for selected transmittable organisms (*Staphylococcus aureus*, group A streptococci, *Neisseria meningitidis*, penicillin-resistant *Streptococcus pneumoniae*, multiple resistant gram-negative bacilli, *Mycobacteria tuberculosis*, and viral exanthems) are the most important maneuvers shown to be effective in reducing incidence of nosocomial pneumonia. Avoiding gastric distension and high residuals from tube feeding minimizes the risk for further aspiration. It is uncertain whether the use-specific ulcer prevention strategy (sucralfate vs. H2-blockers) has an impact on the development of nosocomial pneumonia; most of the evidence shows no significant differences between the two strategies. In addition, some investigators suggest that continuous aspiration of subglottic secretions via specially designed endotracheal tubes decreases the incidence of ventilator-acquired pneumonia; however, limited data are available on such interventions. Indiscriminate use of selective decontamination of the oropharynx and the digestive tract with topical antibiotics has not been found to be effective.

Nosocomial Sinusitis

Inappropriate antibiotic choice is a significant risk factor for mortality in nosocomial pneumonia.

Sinusitis in ICU patients presents as a complicated and severe sinus infection or, more frequently, as an indolent nosocomial infection frequently seen in mechanically ventilated patients. This discussion is limited to nosocomial sinus infections. Recent investigations have highlighted a potential role for nosocomial sinusitis in the pathogenesis of ventilator-acquired

TABLE 26-11

ETIOLOGIC ORGANISMS OF NOSOCOMIAL PNEUMONIA, ASSOCIATED RISK FACTORS, AND EMPIRIC ANTIBIOTIC THERAPY

RISK FACTORS	ORGANISMS	ANTIBIOTIC THERAPY
No prior antibiotic therapy	Core organisms[a]	■ Second- and third-generation cephalosporins (ceftriaxone) ■ Fourth-generation cephalosporins (cefepime) ■ Quinolones (levofloxacin)[b]
Prior antibiotic therapy	Core organisms species	■ Same as above ■ Antipseudomonal penicillins (pipercillin) ■ Cephalosporins (ceftazidime or cefepime) ■ Carbapenem (imipenem) ■ Quinolones (ciprofloxacin) ■ Vancomycin for suspected MRSA ■ Amphoteracin B or fluconazole for suspected fungal infection
Corticosteroid therapy	Core organisms species	Same as in patients with prior antibiotics
Diabetes mellitus	Core organisms	Same as in patients with prior antibiotics
Prolonged mechanical ventilation or tracheostomy	Core organisms	Same as in patients with prior antibiotics
Aspiration	Gram-negative organisms Oral anaerobes	Core antibiotic coverage clindamycin or extended-spectrum penicillin (pipericillin)
Coma	Core organisms	Core antibiotic coverage vancomycin if MRSA is suspected
Prior influenza	Core organisms	Core antibiotic coverage vancomycin if MRSA is suspected

MRSA, methicillin-resistant *Staphylococcus aureus*
[a] Core organisms include *Enterobacter* species, *Escherichia coli*, *Haemophilus influenzae*, *Klebsiella* species, *Proteus* species, *Serratia* species, and *Staphylococcus aureus*
[b] Preferred for treatment of suspected *Legionella* or atypical pathogens

pneumonia and the development of sepsis with bacteremia. For these reasons, nosocomial sinusitis must be considered a potentially serious complication in ICU patients.

Pathogenesis and Risk Factors

The airspaces within the sinuses are normally sterile, and secretions in these spaces are drained through the ostia into the nasal cavity. In most people, the maxillary sinus has one ostium (2.5 mm in diameter and 6 mm in length) that serves as the only nondependent outflow tract for drainage. Other ostia from the frontal and ethmoid sinuses are located near the maxillary ostia in the ostiomeatal complex (Figure 26-6). Any localized process at the ostiomeatal complex leads to obstruction in several ostia, which in turn causes intracavitary negative sinus pressure and decreased oxygen tension, promoting the influx and growth of bacteria in the sinuses. The most important cause of obstructed ostia is mucosal swelling and placement of foreign objects into the nasal cavity (nasotracheal and nasogastric tubes). Even patients with endotracheal intubation, without intranasal devices, are at risk for the development of nosocomial sinusitis possibly because of pooling of nasopharyngeal secretions, increased adherence of virulent bacteria to the nasopharyngeal mucosa, and the absence of nasal airflow needed to maintain normal sinus gas exchange. Clinical studies have confirmed nasotracheal intubation, nasogastric tubes, and duration of endotracheal intubation or nasogastric cannulation as significant risk factors for development of maxillary sinusitis. Rouby and colleagues reported a 96% incidence of radiographic sinusitis in nasotracheally intubated patients and 22.5% in orally intubated patients. Other nonanatomic risk factors include facial trauma, heavy sedation, and supine position.

Semiupright position and contact precautions are the most effective maneuvers to prevent nosocomial pneumonia.

Presentation and Diagnosis

The classic signs of acute purulent sinusitis, consisting of facial tenderness, purulent nasal discharge, and headache, are often absent or difficult to elicit in the critically ill patient. Unexplained fever or sepsis should initiate the workup of nosocomial sinusitis. CT scanning of the sinuses has replaced plain radiographs because of better accuracy in evaluating all sinuses and because CT scanning provides an anatomic guide if surgery is required. In addition, CT affords the added benefit of being able to detect adjacent structural complications. The only limitation for CT scan is that patients must be transported to the radiology department, which carries certain risks for the critically ill. CT demonstration of air–fluid levels and opacification in sinuses defines radiographic sinusitis. In contrast, mucosal thickening

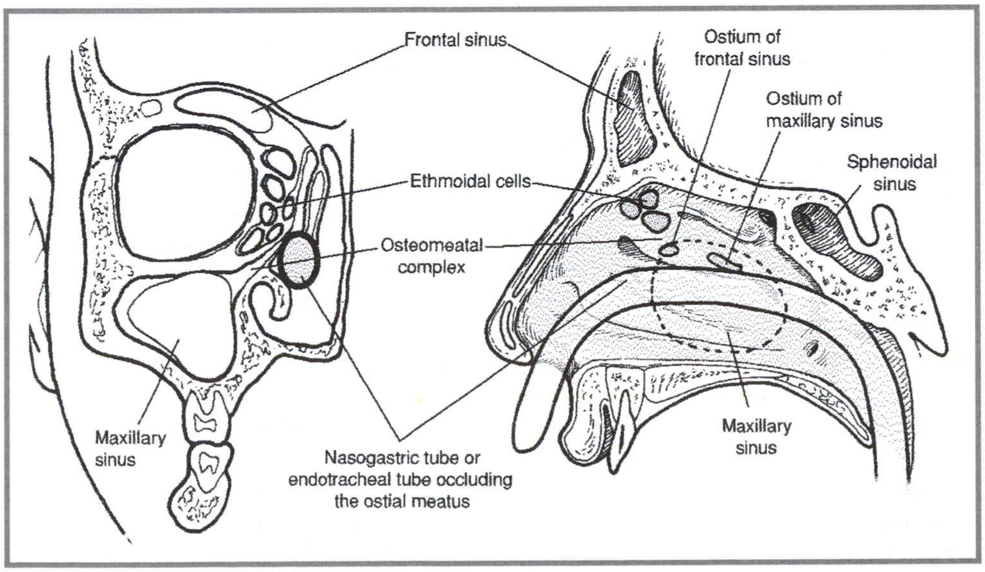

FIGURE 26-6

The cause of paranasal sinusitis is related to impaired drainage of the osteomeatal complex.

is not always suggestive of acute sinusitis as 9%–43% of the general population have this radiographic finding.

The most important predisposing risk factor for the development of nosocomial sinusitis is placement of nasal tubes.

When radiographic sinusitis is identified on CT scan, sinus aspiration should be performed because only 30%–50% of patients with these CT abnormalities have infectious sinusitis. The nasal cavity is highly contaminated; therefore, adequate nasal disinfection should be done before obtaining quantitative cultures from sinus drainage. A growth of 10^3 cfu/ml is accepted as the diagnostic threshold for infectious sinusitis, although lower counts and even negative cultures are observed in patients already on antibiotic therapy. Some investigators have suggested the presence of more than five altered neutrophils per high-power field combined with positive qualitative cultures to diagnose nosocomial sinusitis in patients receiving antibiotics.

Microbiology

Unlike sinusitis in the outpatient setting, where *Streptococcus pneumoniae* and *Haemophilus influenzae* are most commonly encountered, ventilator-dependent patients are infected with a wide spectrum of nosocomial gram-positive (*Staphylococcus aureus*, *S. epidermidis*, enterococcus species), gram-negative (*Enterobacter* species, *Klebsiella pneumoniae*, *E. coli*, *Pseudomonas aeruginosa*, and others), and fungal organisms. Moreover, nosocomial sinusitis is distinguished by frequently being polymicrobial (25%–100%) compared to other nosocomial infections (Table 26-12).

CT scanning of the sinuses is preferred to plain radiographic techniques.

Air–fluid levels and opacification on CT define radiographic sinusitis.

Prevention and Management

Prevention of nosocomial sinusitis starts by avoiding nasal cannulation with nasotracheal or nasogastric tubes. Patients identified with sinusitis should receive topical vasoconstrictors, such as oxymetazoline or phenylephrine, to relieve the mucosal swelling and to improve sinus drainage. Empiric antibiotic therapy without sinus aspiration may mean there is an inherent risk of treating radiographic rather than infectious sinusitis. In addition, this approach may inadequately address resistant organisms and may interfere later with diagnosis because antibiotics alter sensitivity of the quantitative cultures; sinus aspirate cultures should guide antimicrobial therapy, keeping in mind that sinus drainage may be needed for a complete response. Recent investigations suggest that 47% of patients with signs of sepsis respond to maxillary drainage without antibiotic therapy. This latter approach should be reserved for less critically ill patients until such findings are confirmed. Finally, some patients with pansinusitis, involving the ethmoid, sphenoid, and maxillary sinuses, may not improve with adequate antibiotic and maxillary drainage. Under these circumstances, a more radical sinus surgery for drainage may be required for complete eradication of the infection.

Intravascular Catheter-Related Infection

Intravascular catheter infection is a serious complication resulting from intravascular access. Bacteremias secondary to peripheral venous catheter infections are rare (<0.2%); in contrast, central venous catheters account for more than 90% of all catheter-related bacteremias. Before describing the pathogenesis and management of catheter-related infections, it is important to know the phraseology used in this setting. First, the site of the catheter is said to be colonized when a certain number of organisms grow from the catheter. Although colonization is frequently a prerequisite to develop a line infection, it does not present with local or systemic signs of infection and is not equivalent to an exit site infection. Second, catheter-related infection may present as an exit site infection (local cellulitis and abscess formation), without bacteremia, or as catheter-related bacteremia (or sepsis). Catheter-related bacteremia is correlated with significant colonization, even in the absence of local infection, and is defined as bacteremia originating from the catheter site; therefore, this diagnosis is based on isolation of the same organism from the catheter and the blood. Third, a blood culture is said to be contaminated because of improper sterilization technique while obtaining the blood sample and does not represent colonization or infection.

Avoid nasal cannulation, the dependent position, and indiscriminate antibiotic use.

TABLE 26–12

INFECTIOUS PATHOGENS CAUSING NOSOCOMIAL SINUSITIS

Polymicrobial (about 25%–50%)
Yeast ( )
Anaerobes

Pathogenesis and Risk Factors

There are basic mechanisms for the development of catheter-related infections (Figure 26-7). Contamination of the hub from inappropriate handling during tubing changes or blood draws and infection of the dermal tunnel from migration of organisms along the subcutaneous tunnel formed after catheter insertion are the most common cause of catheter-related infections. Heavy skin colonization at the insertion site is strongly associated with catheter-related bacteremias and is a reason why many clinicians avoid cannulation of femoral veins; the inguinal region may be difficult to sterilize. Less commonly, the catheter tip is seeded hematogenously from a distant source after a transient bacteremia. Within 24–48 h of catheter insertion, a fibrin sheath forms around the intravascular surface of the catheter. During bacteremia, this fibrin sheath serves as a nidus for attachment and growth of organisms. Fibrin sheath formation and adherence of bacteria to catheters is related to the smoothness and thrombogenicity of the catheter. Polyvinylchloride catheters are more thrombogenic than polyurethane or silicone catheters, and adherence of organisms occurs less with Teflon and silicone rubber (silastic) catheters. The fourth mechanism is infusate infection; once in the system, the infection will persist despite changing the intravenous bags. In general, laxity in following aseptic techniques during insertion and handling of catheters can eventually lead to catheter-related infections.

Central venous catheters cause 90% of catheter-related bacteremias.

Presentation and Diagnosis

Diagnosis of catheter-related bacteremia is based on the isolation of the same organism from the catheter and the blood.

Fever and leukocytosis with or without other signs of sepsis is a common scenario in ICUs. Complicated line infections often involve bacteremias with septic emboli and secondary seeding of intravascular prostheses, if present. In patients with intravascular access and this clinical presentation, catheter-related infections should always be suspected. Inspection of catheter sites should be part of the daily evaluation of hospitalized patients; paradoxically, an inflamed and erythematous site may be sterile but a normal-appearing site may be significantly colonized. It should be remembered that signs of local inflammation at the insertion site are neither sensitive nor specific to detect catheter-related bacteremias or colonization. Clinical suspicion should be always coupled with laboratory criteria to reach the final diagnosis of catheter-related infections. Traditionally, blood cultures are obtained percutaneously from a distant site and from the catheter, which is then removed and sent for culture.

The most common cause of catheter-related bacteremia is dermal tunnel infection due to migration of organisms from contaminated or endogenous skin flora.

Skin colonization at the insertion site is strongly associated with catheter-related bacteremias.

Two accepted methods for culturing catheters yield meaningful information. The first method is the semiquantitative culture method (the Maki technique) in which a segment of the catheter is rolled on a culture medium. Because approximately 80% of catheter-related infections are caused by dermal tunnel infections, care should be taken to culture the intradermal segment (0.5 cm below the skin to 3 cm distally), not only the tip of the catheter. Positive cultures by this method, that is, patients having a catheter-related infection, are defined as 15 or more colony-forming units (cfu); fewer than 15 cfu on semiquantitative cultures indicate insignificant colonization and is less likely to account for bacteremia. The second method, the quantitative culture method (the Brun–Buisson technique), counts the number of organisms grown from catheter segment cultures after sonification of the catheter. Positive quantitative cultures are defined as more than 10^3 organisms in the broth and are associated with bacteremia. Catheter-related bacteremia is diagnosed when the same organism is isolated from blood cultures and catheter cultures in the absence of another active source of infection. A positive culture from purulent exudate at the site of insertion is also accepted as a sign of catheter-related infection. Interpretation of blood cultures obtained from the same catheter suspected to be infected rather than from a distant site is always fraught with uncertainty; blood cultures may be positive because of contamination (poor technique obtaining the blood) or colonization, even in the absence of a true bacteremia. In catheter-

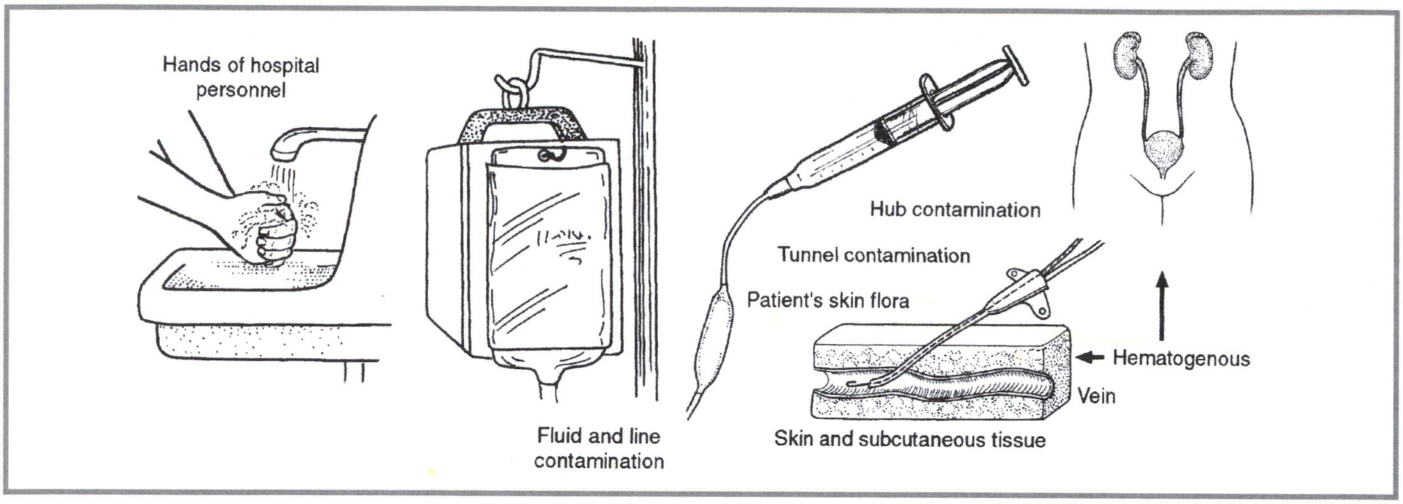

FIGURE 26-7

Anatomic factors that play a role in catheter-related bacteremias.

Inspection of the catheter site is important but local inflammation at the insertion site is not very specific for colonization of the catheter.

related bacteremia, the infusate or the hub usually is not cultured unless the results are important for characterizing a specific infectious epidemic.

In contrast to semiquantitative and quantitative techniques used to establish the diagnosis of colonization and catheter-related infections, two newer methods obviate removing the catheter; the sepsis may be related to another source, and many lines are uninfected. The first method consists of obtaining simultaneous blood samples from the catheter and from a peripheral vein for paired quantitative blood cultures. The finding of 5 to 10 times more colonies from blood drawn through the catheter compared to the peripheral site suggests catheter-related bacteremia. The second method relies on time required for blood cultures (also drawn concurrently from the catheter and a peripheral vein) to become positive. In catheter-related bacteremia, there is a positivity time differential between the two samples; blood cultures drawn through the catheter become positive at least 2 h earlier than the peripheral blood inoculum because of the higher organism count in the former.

Both catheter tip and intradermal segment should be cultured. For the semiquantitative method, positive cultures are defined as growth of more than 15 colony-forming units (cfu).

Microbiology

Coagulase-negative *Staphylococcus* species (*S. epidermidis*) and coagulase-positive staphylococcus (*S. aureus*) bind easily to the surface of catheters and the fibrin sheath; thus, they are the most common cause of line infections. The second most common organisms to cause catheter infections are enteric gram-negative organisms (*Enterobacter*, *Klebsiella*, and *Serratia* species), followed by *Candida* species (*C. albicans*). Immunocompromised patients may be more at risk to develop catheter-related infections with unusual organisms such as *Stenotrophomonas maltophilia*, *Flavobacterium* species, enterococcus species, *Corynebacterium* species, other *Enterobacter* species, and *Malassezia furfur*.

Prevention and Management

Most catheter-related infections are preventable if stringent aseptic precautions are always followed. Prevention strategies are appropriate selection of the catheter and insertion site, aseptic precautions during insertion of the catheter, and meticulous care of the catheter site and the delivery system. Cannulating the subclavian vein is associated with the lowest incidence of infection but has a higher risk for other noninfectious complications. Avoiding multilumen thrombogenic catheters and using cuffed or bonded catheters with antiseptics or antimicrobials will reduce, but not eliminate, the risk of catheter-related infections. Applying chlorhexidine (2% aqueous or 0.5% tincture) at the insertion site reduces cutaneous bacterial colonization and thus dermal tunnel infections. Dry gauze or permeable dressings are more effective than transparent dressings for site care in decreasing the cutaneous flora. Changing the dressing daily and using topical antimicrobials also reduce the rate of skin colonization and catheter-related infections. Avoiding frequent interruptions to the delivery system, especially with total parenteral nutrition (TPN), minimizes risks of contamination. Changing catheters routinely over a guidewire does not prevent line infections; in the presence of dermal tunnel colonization or infection, this practice does not sterilize the tunnel. Finally, some clinicians advocate removal of high-risk catheters following an episode of bacteremia to prevent seeding of the catheter.

Once catheter-related infection is documented, the catheter should be removed, except for uncomplicated *Staphylococcus epidermidis* line infections. In contrast, infections of surgically implanted, long-term indwelling catheters (Broviac, Hickman, or Cook catheters) are commonly left in place unless the bacteremia is caused by *Staphylococcus aureus* or if they are complicated by expanding cellulitis, septic thrombophlebitis, or resistant bacteremia despite appropriate antibiotics. Often, when a line infection is suspected in a seriously ill septic patient (those with hypotension, organ dysfunction, septic thrombosis, or persistent fever and bacteremia), the catheter is removed and is sent for semiquantitative or quantitative cultures and empiric therapy with vancomycin to cover *Staphylococcus* species is started. For critically ill patients and when gram-negative organisms are suspected, additional empiric antigram-negative coverage should be included (third- or fourth-generation cephalosporins, quinolones, aminoglycosides, beta lactam-beta lactamase inhibitors, penicillinase-resistant penicillins, or carbapenems). By the time the results from blood and catheter (or site) cultures become available, most patients with catheter-related infection are improved. If the site is not colonized or the patient does not respond to therapy, another source for the infection should be sought and treated accordingly.

Catheter-related infections are preventable with strict aseptic techniques, proper choice of insertion site, and meticulous local care.

Local colonization without bacteremia usually responds to line removal, and unless there is an expanding cellulitis or the patient is immunocompromised, antimicrobial therapy can be discontinued. Catheter-related infection with bacteremia caused by organisms other than *Staphylococcus aureus* are treated for 5–7 days after line removal; *S. aureus* catheter-related bacteremia is treated for 14 days. Unfortunately, some patients continue to have evidence of sepsis despite these measures and under such circumstances one should consider line infections with resistant organisms, complications such as septic emboli and prosthetic endovascular infections, or another source of infection. Nonneutropenic patients on antimicrobial therapy for more than 14 days, receiving TPN, and showing growth of *Candida* from two or more sites, patients with a complicated intraabdominal surgery, and neutropenic patients with persistent fever (>3 days despite empiric antibiotics) are at risk for candidemia. Such patients, if stable, should be started on fluconazole 400 mg/day and, if candidemia is confirmed, treatment should be continued for 10 days after line removal. Unstable patients and those already on fluconazole who do not improve should be treated with amphotericin B.

Treatment for catheter-related bacteremia involves removal of the central venous catheter in seriously ill patients and *Staphylococcus aureus* infection. Removal of a surgically implanted catheter is not always required.

Clostridium difficile Colitis

Clostridium difficile is an anaerobic gram-positive bacterium that commonly causes antibiotic-associated colitis in hospitalized patients. The clinical presentation of *Clostridium difficile* infections is variable, ranging from asymptomatic carriage or a simple self-limited watery diarrhea to a severe pseudomembranous colitis resulting in sepsis or toxic megacolon. Toxic megacolon is a severe complication that often results in acute peritonitis and even death. Although diarrhea is the most common manifestation of *C. difficile* colitis, it is not invariably present, especially in the most critically ill patients. It is unclear why *C. difficile* does not always cause symptomatic infection; however, old age, malnutrition, intestinal malignancies, use of antispasmodics, and bowel ischemia have been identified as risk factors for the development of severe *C. difficile* infection.

Pathogenesis and Risk Factors

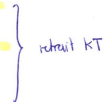

Clostridium difficile colonizes the gastrointestinal tract in 1%–3% of normal healthy adults, in 10%–20% of hospitalized adults, and in 40% of neonates. It is hypothesized that antibiotics alter the colonic flora, facilitating the uncontrolled growth of anaerobic bacteria, including *C. difficile*. Antibiotic-associated colitis may result from any antimicrobial agent but most frequently follows treatment with clindamycin and cephalosporins. In addition, cancer chemotherapeutic agents have been reported to cause *C. difficile* colitis. *C. difficile* can also be transmitted after exposure to patients or staff who are infected or colonized with *C. difficile* or who are carrying the bacteria. Pathogenic strains of *C. difficile* elaborate two protein exotoxins, toxin A and toxin B. Strains that do not produce these toxins are not pathogenic. Severe inflammatory enterocolitis is in part mediated by activation of monocytes by both toxins and by the neutrophilic chemoattractant response to toxin A.

Clostridium difficile colitis presentation ranges from self-limited diarrhea to severe toxic megacolon.

Diagnosis and Management

Clostridium difficile infections can be diagnosed in patients with an appropriate clinical history by a variety of tests. Endoscopy demonstrating pseudomembranes and mucosal injury can establish the diagnosis of *C. difficile*-induced colitis most quickly and accurately. Pseudomembranes are yellow-white plaques, composed of mucus, inflammatory cells, and fibrin exudate that loosely adheres to the inflamed mucosa. These pseudomembranes are seen in 14%–25% of patients with mild disease and 87% of patients with more fulminant disease. Radiographic findings are often nondiagnostic and nonspecific; thickening or distension of the colon can be suggestive of pseudomembranous colitis. Pneumatosis coli and intrahepatic portal venous air have been described in patients with severe *C. difficile* colitis. On the other hand, the laboratory diagnosis of *C. difficile* colitis has become more accurate and is based on the demonstration of bacterial toxins in stool samples.

Antibiotics, by altering intestinal flora, allow overgrowth of anaerobic bacteria, including *C. difficile*.

The gold standard for laboratory diagnosis is the tissue culture cytotoxicity test; however, most hospitals use rapid enzyme immune assays (enzyme-linked immunosorbent assay, or ELISA). The ELISA methods rely on the use of monoclonal or polyclonal antibodies against both toxins A and B. ELISA testing has a slightly lower sensitivity of specificity than the culture cytotoxicity test; therefore, a negative test does not exclude the diagnosis, and if the index of suspicion is high then colonoscopy should be performed. Colonoscopy is more useful than sigmoidoscopy because the disease may spare the rectum and the pseudomembranes may be found beyond the sigmoid colon.

Enterocolitis is mediated by monocyte activation by *C. difficile* toxins A and B and by neutrophilic chemoattractant response to toxin A.

Management of *C. difficile* infections depends on the severity of illness. Mild diarrheal illness often responds to discontinuation of the offending antibiotic. In contrast, critically ill patients require treatment with either vancomycin (125 mg PO q.i.d) or metronidazole (500 mg PO t.i.d.). Usually when *C. difficile* colitis is suspected, empiric therapy with metronidazole or vancomycin is administered orally, pending results of diagnostic workup. Both vancomycin and metronidazole for 10–14 days, when given via the enteral route, appear to be equally effective in the treatment of *C. difficile* colitis, but cost issues favor use of metronidazole. Clinical improvement is usually noted within 3 days. For severe complicated *C. difficile* colitis, subtotal colectomy may be required to prevent a fatal outcome if medical management fails. Although intravenous metronidazole is used to treat *C. difficile* colitis because it reaches adequate fecal concentration, its efficacy has not been established. The parenteral route is used mostly in postoperative patients or those with ileus. Intravenous vancomycin is not advocated, however, because it is not excreted in the gastrointestinal lumen. Some intensivists prefer the use of oral vancomycin for severe *C. difficile* colitis or for the treatment of relapse. Because the efficacy of intravenous metronidazole has not been proven, vancomycin enemas have been suggested, together with intravenous metronidazole in patients with severe infections and altered gastrointestinal motility.

Pseudomembranes, which are loosely adherent yellow-white exudative mucosal plaques, are found in about 25% of patients with mild disease and 87% of patients with severe disease.

The tissue culture cytotoxicity test is the gold standard for the laboratory diagnosis of *C. difficile* colitis; however, most hospitals use ELISA tests for both toxins A and B.

SUMMARY

Infections are encountered almost routinely in the ICU, and nosocomial infection is one of the most common diagnoses. Nosocomial pneumonias or ventilator-acquired pneumonias, along with intravascular catheter-related infections, are the most commonly encountered infections and account for most mortality associated with ICU infections. An understanding of the mechanisms involved in the development of infection in the patient admitted to the ICU is the cornerstone for management and the prevention of devastating complications. More important, meticulous examination of each patient, assessment of patient risk factors, and knowledge of the types of organisms specific to the clinical scenario allow early and appropriate empiric therapy. Early institution of appropriate antibiotic therapy is important for the prevention of sepsis and its fatal sequelae. On the other hand, antibiotic therapy must be tempered by judicious use based on clinical information and on the severity of the patient's condition, thus blunting the perpetuation of antibiotic resistance.

Treatment is usually oral metronidazole or vancomycin, but surgical intervention may be required to prevent mortality in more severe cases that do not respond to medical management.

REVIEW QUESTIONS

1. **Which of the following is the most appropriate management plan for a 45-year-old man with hypotension, fever of 39.5°C, headache, nuchal rigidity, and somnolence?**
   - **A.** Computed tomography (CT) scan of the head
   - **B.** Lumbar puncture with Gram stain of the cerebrospinal fluid
   - **C.** Initiation of antibiotic therapy with ceftriaxone 2 gq12, concomitant lumbar puncture, and admission to the ICU
   - **D.** Admission to the ICU followed by performing lumbar puncture and starting dopamine

2. **A 65-year-old man with steroid-dependent chronic obstructive pulmonary disease and coronary artery disease is post-coronary artery bypass graft day 4. The patient has failed multiple attempts at weaning and continues to be on mechanical ventilatory support. The patient received cefazolin prophylaxis for 2 days postoperatively and treated with cefotaxime for a urinary tract infection. Over the next 24 h he developed a fever of 39°C, progressive hypoxemia requiring increased oxygen supplementation, and progressive right lower lobe infiltrates on chest radiograph. Which management plan is best?**
   - **A.** Obtain blood and sputum cultures, continue cefotaxime, and wait for the culture and sensitivities before changing antibiotic therapy.
   - **B.** Repeat urinalysis, remove the indwelling bladder catheter, and continue current antibiotic regimen.
   - **C.** Start additional antibiotic therapy to include coverage of gram-negative organisms, including *Pseudomonas* species, and persistent gram-positive organisms, including MRSA, after obtaining sputum, blood, and urine cultures.
   - **D.** Perform fiberoptic bronchoscopy with segmental right lower

lobe lavage, obtain blood culture, continue cefotaxime, and wait for culture and sensitivity.
E. Remove all central lines, send catheters for quantitative culture, and start vancomycin.

3. **Risk factors for the development of nosocomial sinusitis in patients who are mechanically ventilated include all the following except?**
A. Presence of a nasogastric feeding tube
B. Orotracheal intubation
C. Recumbent position for prolonged periods
D. Enteral nutrition

4. **A 55-year-old man with a long history of alcoholism was admitted with hypotension, hypothermia, leukocytosis, left lower lobe consolidation, and right middle lobe consolidation on radiograph after being found stuporous in an alley behind a local cafe. The patient was admitted to the ICU for bilobar pneumonia where he was intubated because of poor gas exchange and progressive infiltrates on chest x-ray. At that point he was started on clindamycin for suspected aspiration pneumonia. On day 5 in the ICU, he started having fever up to 39°C and profuse diarrhea, and on day 6 he became lethargic, hypotensive, and was noted to have bloody diarrhea. The appropriate management for this patient includes:**
A. Treat with immodium (an antidiarrheal) and dietary fiber supplementation.
B. Obtain blood, sputum, urine cultures, and stool specimen for *Clostridium difficile* toxin assay and initiate empiric treatment with oral metronidazole and intravenous vancomycin for the remainder of the antibiotic course.
C. Stop clindamycin and start broad coverage antibiotics to treat nosocomial-acquired pneumonia.
D. Obtain CT scan of head and lumbar puncture, continue clindamycin if cerebrospinal fluid is negative for meningitis, and obtain transthoracic echocardiography to look for endocarditis.

ANSWERS

1. The answer is C. Acute bacterial meningitis is a fulminant fatal process, especially if recognition of the disease and institution of therapy are delayed. Often, there is concern about potential brain herniation if a lumbar puncture is performed in patients who have mental status changes and unsuspected brain masses; therefore, most clinicians obtain a CT scan before doing the lumbar puncture. However, CT scan of the brain is never considered a valid reason to delay antimicrobial treatment in patients suspected to have acute bacterial meningitis. Lumbar puncture with fluid analysis is necessary in this scenario, but treatment with appropriate antibiotics should be instituted as soon as the diagnosis is suspected and after obtaining blood cultures. It may be true that this patient needs ICU care, but that should not delay the workup and treatment of acute bacterial meningitis.
2. The answer is C. This patient has developed a ventilator-associated pneumonia that has led to clinical deterioration in the setting of antibiotic therapy for a urinary tract infection. Although the patient may have an inadequately treated urinary tract infection, he has worsening respiratory status and a chest radiographic finding suggesting ventilator-acquired pneumonia. The patient's new infection is likely due to a resistant organism; therefore, to continue his daily antibiotic regimen with cefotaxime while waiting for culture and sensitivity is inappropriate. Although some clinicians advocate the use of fiberoptic bronchoscopy to obtain quantitative bronchoalveolar lavage on protected specimen brush cultures, it is an accepted practice to obtain sputum and blood cultures while waiting for culture and sensitivity results and change to antimicrobial treatment to include treatment for MRSA and pseudomonas. With this practice, fiberoptic bronchoscopy is reserved for later if patients fail the current antibiotic regimen.
3. The answer is D. Known risk factors for the development of hospital-acquired sinusitis include any devices that are placed in the nasopharynx and obstruct the normal drainage of the paranasal sinuses; these include nasogastric feeding tubes, endotracheal tubes inserted orally or nasally, and the recumbent position for long periods. Enteral nutrition is not known to be a risk factor for the development of nosocomial sinusitis unless it is given via a nasogastric tube.
4. The answer is B. The patient developed signs of sepsis and deteriorated despite improvement of his pneumonia. His sepsis workup should include *C. difficile* toxin assay because of the diarrhea. Other sources of infection may be his urinary tract, central indwelling catheter, spontaneous bacterial peritonitis, or meningitis. Endocarditis should be suspected if he has a new cardiac murmur or persistent bacteremia. The change in mental status in this patient is likely related to sepsis, and although CT scan of the brain and lumbar puncture may be required, other antibiotics should be added to clindamycin to treat his new sepsis. Indiscriminate use of antidiarrheals without first ruling out infection in a patient with fevers may lead to severe complications, including toxic megacolon. Intravenous fluids with potassium supplementation would be appropriate in this patient with profuse diarrhea. Flexible sigmoidoscopy may be helpful in diagnosing pseudomembranous colitis. In this patient with aspiration pneumonia, empiric metronidazole and stool analysis for *C. difficile* toxin are most appropriate.

SUGGESTED READING

Acute Bacterial Meningitis:

Quagliarello VJ, Scheld MW. Treatment of bacterial meningitis. N Engl Med J 336:708–716.

Tunkel AR, Scheld MW. Bacterial infections of the central nervous system. In: Hall JB, Schmidt GA, Wood LD (eds.) Principles of Critical Care, 2nd Ed. New York: McGraw-Hill, 1998:1275–1292.

Infectious Endocarditis:

Cobbs GC, Carr MB. Endocarditis and other intravascular infections. In: Hall JB, Schmidt GA, Wood LD (eds.) Principles of Critical Care, 2nd Ed. New York: McGraw-Hill, 1998:1232–1248.

Sepsis:

Light B. Approach to sepsis of unknown origin. In: Hall JB, Schmidt GA, Wood LD (eds.) Principles of Critical Care, 2nd Ed. New York: McGraw-Hill, 1998, 1159–1171.

Wheeler AP, Bernard GR. Treating patients with severe sepsis. N Engl J Med 1999;340:207–214.

Nosocomial Pneumonia:

Lode HM, Schaberg T, Rouby JJ. Nosocomial infection in the critically ill: The lung as a target organ. Anesthesiol 1996;4:757–759.

Mandell LA, Campbell GD. Nosocomial pneumonia guidelines: an international perspective. Chest 1998;113:188S–193S.

Rello J, Rue M, Jubert P, et al. Survival in patients with nosocomial pneumonia: impact of the severity of illness and the etiologic agent. Crit Care Med 1997;25:1862–1867.

Clostridium difficile Colitis:

Chatila W, Manthous CA. *Clostridium difficile* causing sepsis and an acute abdomen in critically ill patients. Crit Care Med 1995;23: 1146–1150.

Catheter-Related Infections:

Maki DG, Stolz SM, Wheeler S, Mermel LA. Prevention of central venous catheter-related bloodstream infection by use of an antiseptic-impregnated catheter: a randomized controlled trial. Ann Intern Med 1997;127:257–266.

Pearson ML. Guideline for prevention of intravascular device related infections: Part 1. Intravascular device-related infections: an overview. Am J Infect Control 1996;24:262–277.

Raad I. Intravascular catheter-related infections. Lancet 1998;351:893–898.

CHAPTER 27

Clarke U. Piatt and Kathleen J. Brennan

Critical Care Endocrinology

CHAPTER OUTLINE

LEARNING OBJECTIVES

After studying this chapter, you should be able to:

- Differentiate diabetic ketoacidosis from hyperosmolar nonketotic coma and understand the management strategies for each disorder.
- Identify thyroid disorders in the intensive care unit by use of clinical findings and laboratory data and review of appropriate therapy.
- Review the clinical findings and the diagnostic evaluations of adrenocortical excess and insufficiency.
- Understand the pathogenesis and treatment of diabetes insipidus and the syndrome of inappropriate antidiuretic hormone secretion.

DISORDERS OF GLUCOSE METABOLISM

Diabetic ketoacidosis and hyperosmolar nonketotic coma are acute and life-threatening disorders of glucose metabolism. Both conditions may present with acute changes in mental status that can progress to coma; however, they vary greatly in their pathophysiology and treatment.

Diabetic Ketoacidosis

Patients with type I diabetes mellitus have an overall lack of insulin.

Diabetic ketoacidosis (DKA) generally occurs in type I diabetes mellitus and results from lack of insulin combined with excess glucagon.

Diabetes mellitus type I occurs in patients with inadequate production of insulin as the result of an autoimmune destruction of beta cells in the exocrine pancreas. Diabetic ketoacidosis (DKA), a complication of type I diabetes mellitus, is associated with a profound insulin deficit with the presence of increased concentrations of glucagon and other insulin counterregulatory hormones. Triggers for DKA and insulin insufficiency include insulin noncompliance and conditions that may increase insulin requirements (Table 27-1).

Serum glucose levels rise as insufficient insulin reduces the peripheral tissue uptake of glucose and the glucagon excess causes an increase in hepatic production of glucose through

TABLE 27-1

TRIGGERS FOR DIABETIC KETOACIDOSIS (DKA)

Infection	Alcohol or drug ingestions
Injury	Insulin noncompliance
Emotional stress	Myocardial infarction

the stimulation of gluconeogenesis and glycogenolysis (Figure 27-1). Protein breakdown in the peripheral tissues provides amino acids for further glucose production by the liver. The combination of a lack of insulin with excessive circulating catecholamines causes lipolysis of adipose tissue, which results in the liberation of free fatty acids from fat. In the liver, the free fatty acids are ultimately converted to ketone bodies, which include the strong organic ketoacids acetoacetic acid and β-hydroxybutyrate. An elevation in ketoacids causes a fall in serum pH that is initially tempered by the buffering effect of serum bicarbonate and an elevated anion gap. The anion gap ($NA^+ - CL^- + HCO_3^-$) normally represents anions that are not usually measured, such as polyanionic plasma proteins (albumin), inorganic phosphates, sulfates, and organic acids. The elevation in ketoacids observed in DKA contributes to these unmeasured ions and elevates the anion gap, truly reflecting the severity of the episode. As continued ketoacids are produced, metabolic acidosis progresses and the buffering capacity of available bicarbonate is exceeded. Compensation for metabolic acidosis occurs in the form of increased alveolar ventilation and CO_2 excretion, renal excretion of H^+, and increased renal HCO_3^- production. Ketoacid production, however, can exceed these compensatory mechanisms, and a rapid progression of metabolic acidosis may ensue.

Ketone bodies, which include acetoacetic acid and β-hydroxybutyrate, are produced in the liver.

The anion gap represents unmeasured anions and is elevated in DKA as a result of ketoacid production: anion gap = Na − (Cl − HCO_3^-).

Elevated serum glucose and ketones result in a significant osmotic diuresis that results in dehydration. Sodium, phosphate, and potassium are lost in the urine as sequelae of the osmotic diuresis.

Patients with type II diabetes mellitus continue to produce adequate amounts of insulin to prevent lipolysis. However, insulin production is insufficient to allow adequate glucose uptake by peripheral tissues or to stop hepatic overproduction of glucose; this results in hyperglycemia and subsequent osmotic diuresis with resulting hypovolemia and dehydration, without the metabolic acidosis seen in DKA. However, some patients with very poor diabetic control combined with severe insulin resistance can develop DKA.

Patients with type II diabetes mellitus have peripheral resistance to insulin.

Clinical Findings

Patients can present after several hours or days of worsening diabetic control. The examination is notable for dehydration with dry skin and mucous membranes. Altered mental sta-

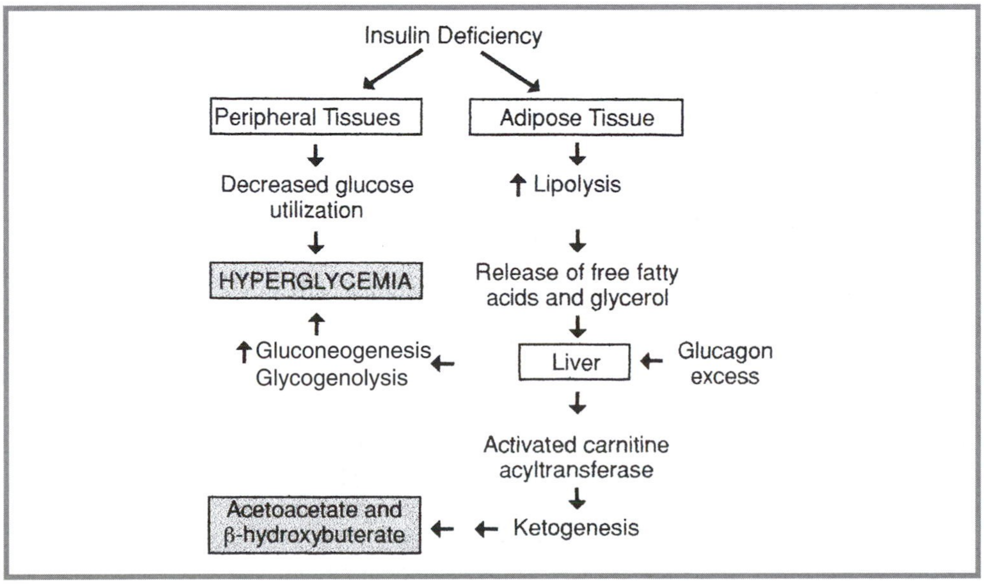

FIGURE 27-1

Pathogenesis of diabetic ketoacidosis (DKA). Insulin deficiency results in decreased uptake of glucose by peripheral tissues and subsequent hyperglycemia. The lack of insulin also leads to loss of inhibition of lipoprotein lipase in adipose tissue and increased release of free fatty acids (FFA) and glycerol. FFA and glycerol are taken up by the liver and synthesized into ketoacids (beta-hydroxybutyrate, acetoacetate, and acetone), which are released into the blood, resulting in an anion gap acidosis.

tus is also common. The initial symptoms are polyuria, nausea, vomiting, and abdominal pain. The odor of acetone, the breakdown product of ketoacids, may be detected on the patient's breath. Patients may have a pattern of rapid and deep breathing known as Kussmaul's respirations in an effort to maximize exhaled carbon dioxide.

Diagnosis

β-Hydroxybutyrate is the most common ketoacid but is not measured; only acetoacetate is measured.

Serum glucose levels are elevated, often exceeding 500 mg/dl with an elevation in serum ketones. A metabolic acidosis is present as a result of the elevation in ketoacids. Patients with renal insufficiency have higher anion gaps and serum ketoacids as a result of decreased urinary ketoacid excretion. β-hydroxybutyrate is the most common serum ketoacid; however, only acetoacetate is commonly measured. Most available laboratory tests for ketoacids utilize nitroprusside, which has significant colorimetric and quantifiable reactions to acetoacetate only. Acidosis causes an extravascular shift of potassium with initial high serum levels measured despite total body potassium deficit as a result of renal losses. Blood urea nitrogen and creatinine may be elevated as a result of severe dehydration. Urinalysis reveals concentrated urine with the presence of glucose and ketones.

Management

Insulin replacement and volume resuscitation are the principal therapy in DKA.

Precipitating factors for DKA must be excluded.

Serum potassium may be initially elevated, but total body stores are low.

The principal therapy is insulin repletion therapy to increase the utilization of glucose in the periphery, to decrease fatty acid production, and to counter the effects of glycogenolysis in the liver. An initial bolus dose of intravenous insulin is given at 10–20 units followed by 0.1 U/kg/h maintenance therapy. Fluid deficits in most patients presenting with DKA are approximately 5–10 l, and initial fluid resuscitation is necessary to restore intravascular volume and lower serum glucose levels through hemodilution. Two to three liters of isotonic saline (0.9%) is administered in the first 3 h with cautious use in patients with underlying cardiac or renal disease. Precipitating factors of DKA, such as infection, stroke, or myocardial infarction, should be considered during patient evaluation. Serum glucose is measured hourly, and dextrose-containing fluids are added when glucose levels fall below 200–300 mg/dl. Electrolytes and anion gap are measured routinely. As the acidosis is corrected, serum potassium levels often begin to fall, reflecting total body depletion; potassium chloride supplements are added to intravenous fluids when serum levels begin to normalize. Normalization of the pH and resolution of the anion gap indicates the metabolism of ketoacids. The patient may be given a subcutaneous intermediate-acting insulin preparation with discontinuation of continuous intravenous insulin as they can tolerate an oral, calorie-controlled diet.

Complications of DKA include cerebral edema, acute respiratory distress syndrome (ARDS), and arterial thrombosis.

DKA remains a life-threatening disorder with mortality as high as 50% in the elderly. Complications of DKA include cerebral edema as a result of hyperosmolarity, which can cause progressive neurologic impairment. Acute respiratory distress syndrome (ARDS) has been rarely reported in cases of refractory DKA. Arterial thrombosis is a recognized complication of DKA that may present as stroke, myocardial infarction, or other organ ischemia. Lactic acidosis may also be present with ketoacidosis that presents with shock, sepsis, or prior metformin use.

Hyperosmolar Nonketotic Coma

Hyperosmolar hyperglycemic nonketotic coma (HHNC) generally occurs in type II diabetes mellitus.

Hyperosmolar hyperglycemic nonketotic coma (HHNC) is a metabolic derangement that occurs mainly in adults with type II diabetes. It has distinct clinical and laboratory findings that distinguish it from DKA (Table 27-2). HHNC is characterized by hyperosmolarity, hyperglycemia, and minimal ketosis. Despite the name, coma is present in less than 10% of cases. Patients present with severe dehydration and focal or global neurologic deficits. Mortality has been reported at 50%. HHNC commonly presents in the sixth decade of life.

Severe dehydration caused by hyperglycemia and osmotic diuresis is the hallmark of HHNC.

HHNC results from insulin resistance and relative insulin deficiency producing hyperglycemia. Hyperglycemia and the resulting hyperosmolarity lead to osmotic diuresis and an osmotic shift of fluid into the extravascular space, resulting in volume depletion and dehydration. Unlike DKA, ketoacidosis does not commonly develop.

TABLE 27-2

COMPARISON OF PRESENTATION OF DIABETIC KETOACIDOSIS (DKA) AND HYPEROSMOLAR HYPERGLYCEMIC NONKETOTIC COMA (HHNC)

PARAMETER	DKA	HHNC
Type of diabetes mellitus (DM)	Type I	Type II
Blood glucose	usually <600 mg/dl	usually >900 mg/dl
Primary therapy	Insulin	Volume repletion
Serum ketones	Extreme elevations	Normal to mildly elevated
Anion gap	Usually >20	Normal
Osmolarity	Mild elevation	Extreme elevations
Treatment	Insulin replacement	Fluid resuscitation

Clinical Findings

Many HHNC patients have a known history of diabetes, usually of the adult-onset type. However, in at least one-third of patients, the development of HHNC heralds the onset of diabetes mellitus. There is often a preceding illness that results in several days of increasing dehydration. The preceding event may be difficult to determine but is frequently an infection, especially a pneumonia or urinary tract infection. A wide variety of other major illnesses may serve to initiate HHNC, primarily through limiting mobility and access to water; these include an acute stroke, intracranial hemorrhage, acute myocardial infarction, and gastrointestinal bleeding. The stress response to any acute illness also tends to increase serum cortisol, catecholamines, glucagon, and other hormones with effects opposite to those of insulin. A variety of drugs that raise serum glucose, inhibit insulin, or cause dehydration may also cause HHNC. Drugs and other iatrogenic causes of HHNC include alcohol, beta-blockers, phenytoin, H2 blockers, corticosteroids, diuretics, dialysis, total parenteral nutrition, and glucose- or dextrose-containing fluids. Noncompliance with oral hypoglycemic agents or insulin therapy can also result in HHNC.

On presentation, a wide variety of focal and global neurologic changes may be present that include drowsiness, delirium or coma, focal or generalized seizures, visual changes, hemiparesis, or sensory deficits.

Alterations in mental status are often the presenting symptoms of HHNC.

Diagnosis

Hyponatremia or hypernatremia may be present. The measured serum sodium should be corrected upward 1.6 mEq/L for every 100 mg/dl increase in serum glucose to determine the true sodium level (Table 27-3). Total body potassium is likely to be low regardless of its measurement; a low measured serum K^+ suggests profound total body losses as a result of osmotic diuresis. An elevated anion gap metabolic acidosis may be present as a result of dehydration but is usually less profound than that observed in DKA. Serum measurement of creatinine is elevated initially due to volume depletion; when possible it should be compared to previous values as many diabetics have renal insufficiency at baseline. Serum glucose is usually dramatically elevated, often more than 800 mg/dl.

Serum osmolarity is nearly always greater than 320 mOsm/dl. If the calculated value is significantly lower than the measured value, toxic alcohol ingestion should be considered. Serum ketones may not be found in pure HHNC but may be present in cases of HHNC where DKA or starvation ketosis concomitantly occur. Urinalysis will reveal an elevated specific gravity, glucosuria, ketonuria, and possible evidence of urinary tract infection.

TABLE 27-3

CRITICAL CALCULATIONS IN DIAGNOSIS AND MANAGEMENT OF DKA AND HHNC

$$\text{Anion gap} = [NA^+] - ([Cl^-] - [HCO_3^-])$$

$$[NA^+]_{\text{corrected}} = [NA^+ + 1.6\left(\frac{\text{serum glucose} - 100\text{ mg/dl}}{100}\right)$$

$$\text{Serum Osmolality} = 2[NA^+] + [K^+] + \frac{\text{serum glucose mg/dl}}{16} + \frac{\text{Blood urea nitrogen mg/dl}}{32}$$

$$\text{Free water deficit} = 0.6(\text{patient's weight in kg}) \times \left(\frac{\text{plasma }[NA^+]}{140} - 1\right)$$

Creatine phosphokinase (CPK) with isoenzymes should be determined as rhabdomyolysis may occur in HHNC. Acute myocardial infarction is also frequently associated with HHNC.

Management

Intravascular volume resuscitation is the principal therapy in HHNC.

Intravenous access with crystalloid fluid resuscitation is the immediate goal of therapy. Fluid deficits in HHNC are large, with fluid requirements often greater than 10 l. As in DKA, administration of 2–3 liters of normal saline in the first few hours is appropriate, with slower initial rates in patients with significant underlying cardiac or renal disease. Although many patients with HHNC respond to fluids alone, intravenous insulin in dosages similar to those used in DKA can facilitate correction of hyperglycemia.

THYROID DISORDERS

Hypothyroidism, Myxedema Coma, and Euthyroid Sick Syndrome

Hypothyroidism is a deficiency of circulating thyroid hormones that may be caused by the failure of the thyroid gland to synthesize or secrete thyroid hormones (primary hypothyroidism) or by decreased release of thyroid-stimulating hormone (TSH) from the pituitary (secondary hypothyroidism) (Figure 27-2).

Chronic thyroiditis is the most common cause of spontaneous hypothyroidism in the United States. Other etiologies include idiopathic atrophy of the thyroid, thyroid ablation following treatment for Graves' disease, disruption of the hypothalamic pituitary axis, and iodine deficiency. Symptoms of hypothyroidism may be initially nonspecific and slowly progressive (Table 27-4).

Myxedema coma may present as hypothermia, hypoglycemia, shock, and hypoventilation.

In the critically ill patient, thyroid insufficiency may present with more dramatic symptoms. Myxedema coma is a manifestation of severe hypothyroidism with initial findings that may include hypothermia, hypoglycemia, shock, hypoventilation, or ileus. Precipitating factors for myxedema coma include cold exposure, illness, infection, trauma, and drugs that suppress the central nervous system. The mortality rate in myxedema coma approaches 50%–70%.

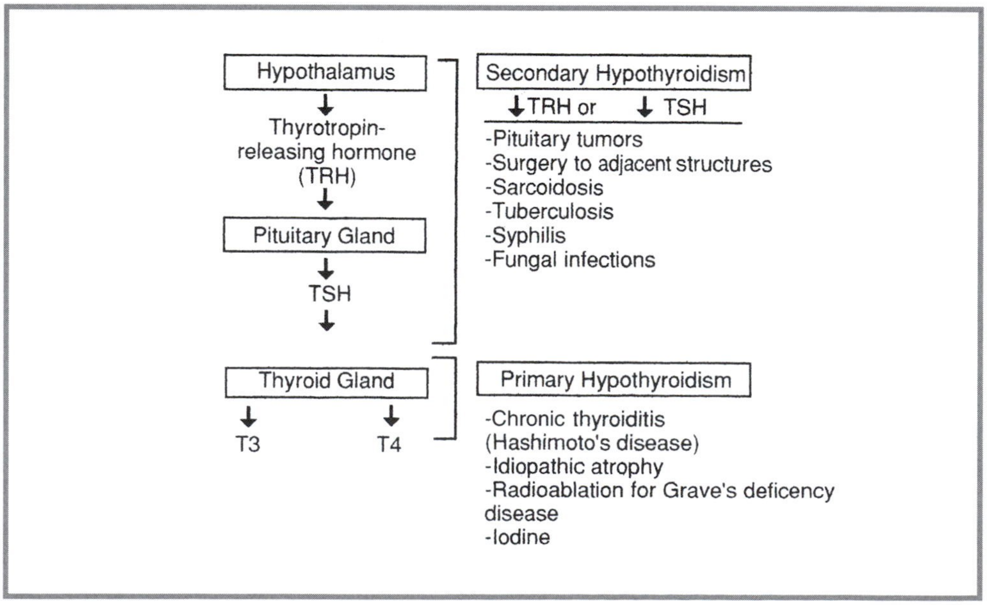

FIGURE 27-2

Etiology of hypothyroidism.

TABLE 27-4

CLINICAL FINDINGS OF HYPOTHYROIDISM

Symptoms	Physical examination
Weakness, lethargy, and fatigue	Dry, yellow skin
Dry skin and coarse hair	Hypothermia
Puffy eyelids, face, and hands; swollen legs	Bradycardia
Cold intolerance	Nonpitting edema
Constipation	Slow, deep tendon reflexes
Weight gain	Loss of lateral eyebrow
Hoarseness	Hypoventilation
Menorrhagia	
Hearing loss	

Diagnosis

The diagnosis of thyroid dysfunction is based on clinical findings and the results of thyroid function testing. Initial laboratory screening evaluation includes serum thyroid-stimulating hormone (TSH), which is low in secondary hypothyroidism and elevated in primary hypothyroidism. Abnormal TSH levels should be confirmed with measurement of serum triiodothyronine (T_3) and thyroxine (T_4) levels, which are decreased in both primary and secondary hypothyroidism (Table 27-5).

Thyroid-stimulating hormone (TSH) is the initial screening test for thyroid insufficiency.

Euthyroid sick syndrome (ESS) commonly occurs in the critically ill patient. Patients have normal thyroid function, but thyroid function studies show low values for T_3/T_4 and normal to slightly elevated TSH levels. In ESS, the abnormalities in thyroid function studies result from severe underlying systemic illness with decreased peripheral conversion of T_4 to T_3 and decreased binding of thyroid hormones to thyroid-binding globulin. Therapy is directed at treating the underlying illness.

Euthyroid sick syndrome (ESS) is characterized by low T_3/T_4 and normal to elevated TSH but normal thyroid function.

Management

Patients who initially present with mild to moderate symptoms of hypothyroidism may be started on 0.05 mg of oral synthetic L-thyroxine with slow upward titration in dose to the targeted maintenance dose over a 6- to 12-week period. Patients with moderate to severe hypothyroidism and those with underlying cardiovascular disease may be at higher risk for complications during initial therapy. Initial doses of thyroid replacement should be reduced to 0.025 mg in these patients, with appropriate monitoring for sequelae including arrhythmias and angina.

Myxedema coma requires rapid replacement with a 200–500 μg IV bolus dose of L-thyroxine, followed by 50–150 μg IV daily until the patient is able to tolerate oral replacement therapy. Hydrocortisone 100 mg every 8 h is recommended during rapid treatment because adrenal failure may be precipitated during thyroxine therapy. Supportive care may include intubation and mechanical ventilation for hypoventilation. Slow external warming is indicated for associated severe hypothermia; however, excessive peripheral vasodilitation may lead to vascular collapse. Pulmonary artery catheterization may be required in patients with hemodynamic instability whose intravascular volume status is unclear or who may have a component of cardiogenic shock.

Myxedema coma requires intravenous L-thyroxine, consideration of initial hydrocortisone replacement therapy, and supportive measures.

TABLE 27-5

INTERPRETATION OF THYROID FUNCTION STUDIES

DIAGNOSIS	T_4	T_3	TSH	T_3 UPTAKE
Primary hypothyroidism	↓	↓/N	↑	↓/N
Secondary hypothyroidism	↓	↓	N	–
Euthyroid sick syndrome	↓/N	↓	N/slightly ↑	N/↓

TSH, thyroid-stimulating hormone; ↓, decreased; ↑, increased; N, normal

TABLE 27-6

SYSTEMIC MANIFESTATIONS OF THYROTOXICOSIS

Cardiovascular
Arrhythmias
High output congestive heart failure
Hypertension
Pulmonary
Increased work of breathing
Respiratory muscle weakness
Neurologic
Seizures
Altered mental status (delirium to coma)

Thyrotoxicosis and Thyroid Storm

Levels of thyroid hormone that are greater than required for normal physiologic function may result in thyrotoxicosis. Hyperthyroidism results from excessive stimulation of thyroid follicular cells in Graves' disease, an autoimmune disorder associated with the production of immunoglobulins that bind to and stimulate TSH receptors. Excessive ingestion of synthetic thyroid hormone may also produce similar findings (see Levothyroxine Overdose, later in this chapter). Destruction of follicular cells as a result of inflammation as is observed in conditions such as nodular toxic goiter or subacute thyroiditis from viral infections can cause excessive thyroid hormone release. Less commonly, hyperthyroidism may result from excessive production of TSH from the pituitary (i.e., tumors) or from teratomas of the ovary (struma ovarii).

Elevated thyroid hormone levels cause an increase in adrenergic stimulation that results in an increase in metabolic demand, increased O_2 consumption, hyperdynamic circulation, and increased work of breathing. The manifestations of hyperthyroidism may have more pronounced implications for critically ill patients (Table 27-6).

Thyroid storm is a life-threatening complication of thyrotoxicosis with tachycardia, hypertension, and altered mental status.

Thyroid storm is a rare and life-threatening complication of severe thyrotoxicosis that is associated with marked fever, tachycardia, and agitation that can lead to cardiovascular collapse. Precipitating factors include infection, surgery, acute psychiatric illness, diabetic ketoacidosis, pulmonary embolus, bowel infarction, parturition, trauma, withdrawal of antithyroid medication, radioactive iodine therapy, and iodine-containing contrast agents.

Clinical Findings

Symptoms of mild to moderate hyperthyroidism include a history of heat intolerance, weight loss, weakness, oligomenorrhea, and anxiety (Table 27-7). The clinical findings in severe hyperthyroidism often include tachycardia, hypertension, hyperpyrexia, and altered mental status; however, all these findings may not be present during thyroid storm. The patient's symptoms can rapidly progress with risk for cardiovascular collapse as a result of high-output heart failure. Diagnosis is suspected by the presence of clinical symptoms, and established by measuring elevated serum levels of T_4 or free T_4.

Therapy

In the critical stages of thyrotoxicosis and thyroid storm, the therapeutic goals are to reduce the levels of thyroid hormone and to minimize or treat systemic effects. Propylthiouracil

TABLE 27-7

PHYSICAL FINDINGS OF HYPERTHYROIDISM

Hyperpyrexia	Exophthalmus with stare and lid lag
Tachycardia with possible ectopy/arrhythmias	Proximal muscle weakness
Tachypnea	Resting tremor
Respiratory fatigue	Warm and moist skin
Elevated pulse pressure	Fine and silky hair
Goiter	
Dermopathy	

(PTU) and methimazole are oral agents that inhibit the synthesis of thyroid hormone. PTU also inhibits the conversion of T_4 to T_3 in peripheral tissues. The onset of action of PTU is immediate, but serum thyroid hormone levels will take several weeks to normalize. PTU is initially given as a dose of 300 mg orally every 6 h. Side effects include rash, agranulocytosis, and hepatotoxicity. Patients with contraindications to antithyroid agents can receive iodine with oral cholecystographic agents (ipodate or iopanoate) that inhibit 5′-deiodination and decrease the conversion of T_4 to T_3.

Therapy for thyroid storm includes propylthiouracil (PTU), Lugol's solution, and β-adrenergic antagonists.

A further reduction in thyroid-stimulating hormone can be achieved by the addition of iodine as Lugol's solution, a saturated solution of potassium iodide. It is given 2 h after the first dose of PTU at a dosage of 1–2 drops orally every 12 h. Patients intolerant to iodine can receive lithium carbonate or perchlorate, which decrease iodine uptake by the thyroid gland.

Propranolol or other β-adrenergic antagonists are given for symptom relief or in patients with tachycardia, angina, or myocardial infarction. β-Adrenergic antagonists should be used with caution in the setting of thyroid storm because they can precipitate cardiopulmonary instability. These drugs should be avoided in the elderly, asthmatics, and patients with cardiomyopathy. If required, verapamil or short-acting beta-blockers such as esmolol may be used instead.

Thyroid storm requires supportive care, which may include fluid resuscitation and cooling measures for hyperpyrexia. Adrenal insufficiency may accompany thyroid storm, and patients with hypotension should be considered for treatment with hydrocortisone 100 mg every 8 h until a diagnosis is established.

Levothyroxine Overdose

Levothyroxine, a commonly prescribed medication, accounts for frequent accidental or intentional overdoses with as many as 5000 cases reported annually. The symptoms begin approximately 24 h after ingestion with the conversion of T_4 to T_3. Immediate treatment is gastric lavage with administration of activated charcoal and sorbitol. Propranolol is added if patients have with mild symptoms, and PTU and prednisone are given to patients with severe symptoms or large ingestions with delayed or ineffective gastric lavage.

DISORDERS OF PARATHYROID GLAND FUNCTION

Parathyroid hormone (PTH) works in conjunction with vitamin D to regulate total body calcium. PTH is secreted in response to hypocalcemia and stimulates renal tubular calcium resorption and phosphate excretion. It also stimulates the conversion of 25-hydroxyvitamin D to 1,25-dihydroxyvitamin D, the active form of vitamin D, which stimulates calcium and phosphate absorption from the gastrointestinal (GI) tract.

Parathyroid hormone (PTH) stimulates renal calcium reabsorption and phosphate excretion.

Hyperparathyroidism

Primary hyperparathyroidism, as a result of parathyroid adenomas, hyperplasia, or carcinoma, represents the majority of evaluations for hypercalcemia in the outpatient population. In hospitalized patients, malignancy is the predominant source of severe elevations in serum calcium as a result of humoral release of PTH-related peptide or by direct bony destruction by tumor. The PTH-related peptide uses the PTH receptors but is not detected by traditional PTH immunoassays.

Clinical Findings

The majority of symptoms are not present unless serum calcium is greater than 12 mg/dl, and most symptoms result from rapid elevations in serum calcium. Clinical findings of hyperparathyroidism may include nephrolithiasis, polyuria, anorexia, nausea, vomiting, and constipation. Neurologic manifestations may progress from weakness and fatigue to coma. The electrocardiogram may demonstrate a shortened QT interval.

Patients taking digoxin are at greater risk for digoxin toxicity with hypercalcemia. Polyuria with decreased oral intake and vomiting can lead to marked dehydration. A history of hypercalcemia greater than 6 months without evidence of underlying cause or the presence of nephrolithiasis suggests hyperparathyroidism. Measurement of PTH by intact molecule or by fragment of PTH (C-terminal assay) can be used to differentiate primary hypercalcemia from secondary causes.

Therapy

Until the diagnosis is established, initial management of symptomatic hypercalcemia includes volume repletion with isotonic saline (0.9%) followed by promotion of a saline diuresis with 100–150 ml/h isotonic saline to promote calcium excretion via the kidneys. For severe hypercalcemia, pamidronate at 60–90 mg may be given over 4 h in isotonic saline infusion to inhibit bone reabsorption. Response to pamidronate may be observed within results seen within 48–72 h. Calcitonin, which also inhibits bone reabsorption, may be given at 4–8 IU/kg intramuscularly or subcutaneously and may provide a more rapid response in lowering serum calcium 1–3 mg/dl over several hours. If malignant hypercalcemia is suspected, other treatments could include the administration of plicamycin, glucocorticoids, or gallium nitrate. The only effective long-term treatment of symptomatic hyperparathyroidism remains parathyroidectomy.

Hypoparathyroidism

Hypoparathyroidism is often only diagnosed during the evaluation of unexplained hypocalcemia. Hypoparathyroidism remains relatively uncommon in the general population of the United States, with an incidence of approximately 0.6%. Hypoparathyroidism may be congenital or idiopathic in origin, but infiltrative diseases, immunosuppressive agents, and a high incidence of neck surgeries may make it a more common finding in the intensive care unit patient (Table 27-8).

Clinical Findings

Symptoms of severe hypoparathyroidism include muscular tetany, altered mental status, and seizures.

Hypocalcemia produces acute symptoms when ionized calcium is less than 2.5 mg/100 ml. Neurologic symptoms predominate secondary to hyperexcitability of neuronal membranes. Mild muscular fatigue and numbness or tingling about the face, hands, and feet are common

TABLE 27-8

ETIOLOGIES OF HYPOPARATHYROIDISM

Congenital:
- Parathyroid aplasia
- DiGeorge syndrome: dysgenesis of thymus and parathyroid glands

Iatrogenic: (the most common cause of hypoparathyroidism is surgery)
- Surgical resection postparathyroid adenoma resection (usually transient, secondary to suppression of other parathyroid glands)
- Surgical resection: post-total parathyroidectomy or disruption of the vascular supply during thyroidectomy

Infiltration or destruction:
- Sarcoidosis
- Wilson's disease: inherited, copper overload
- Hemachromatosis: inherited, iron overload
- Metastatic carcinoma
- Infarction
- Radiation

Suppression of the parathyroid gland:
- Hypomagnesemia: pancreatitis, aminoglycosides, pentamidine, loop diuretics, cisplatin, and amphotericin B
- Hypermagnesemia
- Drugs: aluminum, asparagine, doxorubicin, cytosine arabinoside, cimetidine

Multiple endocrine neoplasia

Idiopathic

TABLE 27-9

CLINICAL FINDINGS OF HYPOPARATHYROIDISM AND HYPOCALCEMIA

Hyperreflexia
Tetany
Chvostek's sign: twitching of the facial muscles when the facial nerve is tapped anterior to the ear
Trousseau's sign: development of carpal spasm when a blood pressure cuff is inflated on an arm for 3 min
Seizures
Altered level of consciousness
Heart failure

with mild hypercalcemia. Severe hypocalcemia causes overt tetany with muscle twitching and cramping and occasional carpopedal spasm. Chvostek's sign may signify hypocalcemia if twitching of the facial muscles is observed when the facial nerve is tapped anterior to the ear. Trousseau's sign is another physical finding in hypocalcemia and describes the development of carpal spasm in an arm where a blood pressure cuff is inflated for more than 3 min.

Laryngeal stridor may also occur in hypocalcemia. Cardiac effects are limited, because cardiac tetany occurs at levels of hypocalcemia lower than those needed for neurologic effects and ECG changes to be observed. Neurologic effects include extremity and periorbital paresthesias, muscle cramps, altered mental status, and seizures (Table 27-9).

Evaluation

Serum calcium levels should first be corrected for serum albumin levels. Because approximately half of serum calcium is bound to albumin, decreased levels of albumin result in a lower total serum calcium level although the free calcium levels may be normal. Free calcium levels can be adjusted for the effect of reduced serum albumin by adding 0.8 mg/dl calcium for every 1 g/dl reduction in serum albumin below 4 g/dl. In addition to history and examination findings, hypocalcemia and hyperphosphatemia are consistently present in hypoparathyroidism. Several disorders may produce similar laboratory and clinical findings (Table 27-10). A decreased serum PTH level may help establish the diagnosis.

Treatment

Severe hypocalcemia is treated with intravenous calcium gluconate.

In emergent situations in which severe hypocalcemia is suspected and seizures, tetany, life-threatening hypotension, or cardiac arrhythmia are present, empiric treatment with elemental calcium is recommended. An initial 180 mg dose of calcium gluconate as a 10% solution can be given over 10 min (one ampule of 10% calcium gluconate equals 90 mg/10 ml); this raises the ionized calcium by approximately 0.5–1.5 mM. Following the initial dose, a continuous infusion of 0.3–2.0 mg elemental calcium/kg/h is administered over 6–8 h with subsequent adjustments based on serial serum calcium measurements every 2–4 h. Hypomagnesemia may also be present and must be treated to correct hypocalcemia. Chronic management consists of 1–2 mg elemental calcium daily with vitamin D supplementation.

ADRENAL GLAND DISORDERS

The adrenal cortex produces glucocorticoids and mineralocorticoids.

The adrenal cortex produces several types of hormones that are synthesized from cholesterol, including the glucocorticosteroids and mineralocorticosteroids. The glucocorticoids cortisol and corticosterone act on carbohydrate metabolism, while the mineralocorticoids al-

TABLE 27-10

DIFFERENTIAL DIAGNOSIS OF HYPOCALCEMIA

Hypoparathyroidism	Malabsorption
Pseudohypoparathryoidism	Vitamin D deficiency
Hypoalbuminemia	Acute pancreatitis
Renal failure	Hypomagnesemia

The adrenal medulla produces dopamine, epinephrine, and epinephrine.

dosterone and dehydroepiandrosterone regulate renal sodium and potassium secretion. The adrenal medulla synthesizes the catecholamines dopamine, norepinephrine, and epinephrine under the control of the sympathetic nervous system. In response to increased stress or physiologic demands, products of the adrenal medulla influence cardiac output and vascular tone.

Adrenocortical Insufficiency

Adrenal insufficiency results from adrenal gland failure or adrenocorticotropic (ACTH) insufficiency.

Adrenocortical insufficiency is characterized by the deficiency of cortisol with or without a deficiency of aldosterone. Primary adrenal insufficiency (Addison's disease) is a result of intrinsic adrenal gland failure with deficiency of both cortisol and aldosterone. In response to low serum cortisol, secretion of adrenocorticotropic hormone (ACTH) by the anterior lobe of the pituitary gland is increased with elevated serum levels. Secondary adrenal insufficiency results from inadequate or absent secretion of ACTH from the anterior lobe of the pituitary gland. In the critically ill patient, adrenocortical deficiency is a frequently encountered diagnosis, identifying a group of patients who often are at increased risk because of severe underlying disease (Table 27-11).

Clinical Findings

Adrenal deficiency includes symptoms of generalized fatigue, nausea, or vomiting. Exam findings include orthostatic hypotension, truncal obesity, and abdominal striae (Table 27-12). In primary adrenal failure, aldosterone insufficiency results in decreased potassium excretion and sodium reabsorption in the distal renal tubules. Significant renal wasting of sodium and water results in hypovolemia and azotemia; hyperkalemia is often present and may precipitate arrhythmias. ACTH excess causes skin hyperpigmentation.

Adrenal crisis may result from a significant deficiency or inadequate response to acute stressors including infection or surgery. Patients on chronic steroid therapy for adrenal insufficiency or other illnesses (chronic obstructive pulmonary disease, asthma, or connective tissue diseases) are at risk secondary to absent or diminished adrenal response to stress. Findings may include rapid clinical deterioration with marked hypotension, fever, abdominal pain, and altered mental status. In the critically ill, adrenal insufficiency should be considered in patients who manifest hypotension that is unexplained or is not responsive to therapy.

Diagnosis

Low serum cortisol suggests adrenal insufficiency, but ACTH stimulation is used for definitive diagnosis.

Laboratory findings include hyponatremia, hyperkalemia, hypoglycemia, eosinophilia, and azotemia. A reduced random serum cortisol level does not confirm a diagnosis of adrenal insufficiency, but a low serum cortisol level in patients with a consistent clinical presentation may be suggestive. ACTH stimulation testing establishes the diagnosis. For the rapid ACTH test, serum cortisol is measured before and 30 min after IV or IM injection of cosyntropin (synthetic ACTH) at 250 μg. Serum cortisol level should rise at least 7 μg/dl and

TABLE 27-11

ETIOLOGIES OF ADRENAL FAILURE

Primary adrenocortical insufficiency	Secondary adrenocortical insufficiency
Autoimmune	Vascular
Mycobacterium tuberculosis	Pituitary surgery
Hemorrhage	Irradiation
AIDS	Head trauma
Metastatic carcinoma	Infection
Drugs	Autoimmune disorders
Sarcoidosis	Sarcoidosis
Amyloidosis	Histocytosis x
Hemachromatosis	Hemochromatosis
Glucocorticoid therapy	Lipid storage disease
Tumors	Isolated ACTH deficiency
	Congenital conditions

TABLE 27-12

CLINICAL FINDINGS IN ADRENAL INSUFFICIENCY

Orthostatic hypotension
Weakness/fatigue
Gastrointestinal complaints (anorexia, nausea, vomiting)
Hyponatremia
Dehydration
Eosinophilia
Increased skin pigmentation (primary adrenal insufficiency)

should reach 18 μg/dl in normal patients. Serum ACTH levels are elevated in primary adrenal insufficiency. For patients with a nondiagnostic rapid ACTH stimulation test with consistent history, standard ACTH testing should be performed in which 25–40 μg cosyntropin is given over 8 h with the 24-h measurement of free cortisol or 17-hydroxycorticosteroid levels before and after the infusion. A three- to fivefold increase in urinary cortisol and a 15–40 μg/dl rise is serum cortisol is normal (Table 27-13).

Treatment

Suspicion of adrenal crisis requires immediate glucocorticoid repletion. If the diagnosis is not established, 10 mg dexamethasone is administered intravenously followed by ACTH stimulation testing. Following testing or if the patient with known adrenal insufficiency, 100 mg hydrocortisone is administered every 8 h. After improvement in the patient's symptoms, conversion to equivalent oral hydrocortisone doses may be achieved. A gradual taper over 1–2 weeks of the prednisone dose to maintenance requirements may begin after resolution of the stress trigger.

Addisonian crisis requires prompt hydrocortisone replacement therapy.

Glucocorticoid replacement is given as hydrocortisone in a twice-daily dose of 20 mg in the morning and 10 mg at night. Although hydrocortisone has some mineralocorticoid effect, patients with primary adrenal failure will likely require additional mineralocorticoid replacement in the form of fludrocortisone 0.05–0.2 mg daily for the clinical findings of persistent orthostatic hypotension, hypernatremia, and hyperkalemia. In all patients on chronic adrenocorticoid replacement therapy, dosages must be increased before expected stressors (surgery) or during illness.

Adrenocortical Excess

In the general population, pituitary microadenomas that secrete excessive amounts of ACTH account for 80% of endogenous adrenocortical excess (Cushing's syndrome). Hypersecretion of glucocorticoids by adrenal tumors and ectopic ACTH production are less common. The most common of adrenocortical excess in the intensive care unit is iatrogenic, occurring in patients with exogenous glucocorticosteroid requirements.

Excess glucocorticoid administration is the most common cause of adrenocorticoid excess.

Clinical Findings

Physical examination findings include truncal obesity and a rounded face in patients with chronic adrenocortical excess (Table 27-14). Mild to moderate hyperglycemia may be present.

TABLE 27-13

SERUM CORTISOL AND ADRENOCORTICOTROPIC HORMONE (ACTH) STIMULATION TESTING

Serum cortisol
>14 μg/ml in normal conditions
>22 μg/ml during stress conditions
ACTH stimulation testing
Obtain serum cortisol
Administer 250 μg synthetic ACTH IV
Obtain serum cortisol 1 h later
>7 μg increase indicates normal adrenal function
<7 μg increase indicative of adrenal failure

TABLE 27-14

CLINICAL FINDINGS OF ADRENOCORTICAL EXCESS

Truncal obesity
Rounded face
Fat deposits in the supraclavicular fossae and over the posterior neck
Hirsutism
Amenorrhea
Psychiatric disorders/depression
Thin skin
Easy bruising
Reddish striae
Proximal muscle weakness
Osteoporosis

Diagnosis

Serum cortisol is not useful in diagnosis.

Positive overnight dexamethasone suppression test is followed by the low-dose dexamethasone suppression test to establish the diagnosis.

Random serum cortisol levels are not useful for diagnosis because cortisol secretion may vary at time of collection. Urinary cortisol measured from a 24-h specimen can be used to establish cortisol excess but may be nondiagnostic with borderline values. Screening tests include overnight dexamethasone suppression test and 24-h urine cortisol test. The overnight dexamethasone suppression test utilizes 1 mg dexamethasone given at 11 P.M. with collection of plasma cortisol at 8 A.M. Normal plasma cortisol levels are less than 5 μg/dl with higher levels suggesting cortisol excess. An abnormal screening test indicates the need to perform a low-dose dexamethasone suppression test with 0.5 mg dexamethasone administered every 6 h for 48 h with urine cortisol measurement in the last 24 h. Failure to suppress urine cortisol to less than 20 μg/24 hours is diagnostic of Cushing's syndrome (Table 27-15).

TABLE 27-15

LABORATORY TESTING FOR ADRENOCORTICAL EXCESS

Plasma control:
- Normal:
  - 5–25 μg/dl in early morning
  - $<$10 μg/dl in evening
- Cushing's syndrome:
  - Episodic secretion makes
    - Interpretation difficult

Urinary cortisol:
- Normal, 20–100 μg/24 h
- Cushing's syndrome, $>$120 μg/dl

Dexamethasone suppression testing:
- a. Overnight dexamethasone suppression testing
  - 1 mg dexamethasone at 11 P.M.
  - Serum cortisol at 8 A.M.
    - Normal, $<$5 μg/dl
    - Suggestive of cortisol excess, $>$5 μg/dl
- b. Standard dexamethasone suppression testing
  - Day 1: measurement of 24-h urinary 17-hydroxycorticosteroid and evening cortisol levels
  - Day 2 and 3: dexamethasone 0.5 mg every 6 h with measurement of 24-hour urinary 17-hydroxycorticosteroid and evening cortisol levels each day
  - Day 4 and 5: dexamethasone 2 mg every 6 h with measurement of 24-h urinary 17-hydroxycorticosteroid and evening cortisol levels each day

Normal:
- Evidence of suppression:
  - Urinary 17-hydroxycorticosteroid $<$3 mg/24 h
  - Serum cortisol $<$5 μg/dl
- Cushing's disease:
  - Suppression with high dose
- Adrenal tumor or ectopic ACTH:
  - No suppression seen

Therapy

In the intensive care unit, patients on prolonged glucocorticoid therapy should be monitored for its clinical consequences and frequently reassessed for possible dose reduction. As for other etiologies, such as ACTH-secreting pituitary adenoma or hypersecreting adrenal adenomas, a primary goal of intensive care unit therapy is supportive care until patients may stabilize to undergo definitive diagnosis or treatment.

DIABETES INSIPIDUS AND SYNDROME OF INAPPROPRIATE ANTIDIURETIC HORMONE SECRETION

Arginine vasopressin or antidiuretic hormone (ADH) is produced in the supraoptic nucleus of the hypothalamus and travels down the pituitary stalk where it is stored in the pituitary gland's posterior lobe. At the level of the renal collecting ducts, ADH promotes water reabsorption. Disorders of the neurohypophysis or the kidneys can result in marked alteration of the body's ability to control urine concentration.

Antidiuretic hormone (ADH) is produced by the supraoptic nucleus of the hypothalamus.

ADH promotes water reabsorption in the renal collecting ducts.

Diabetes Insipidus

Diabetes insipidus (DI) is a disorder that is characterized by excretion of large quantities of dilute urine and results from an absolute deficiency of ADH (central DI) or renal resistance to the effects of ADH (nephrogenic DI). Primary central DI results from an inherited or idiopathic reduction in the number of hypothalamic nuclei; secondary DI results from a variety of pathologic lesions to the neurohypophysis. DI may be a temporary or permanent condition depending on its etiology. The resistance to ADH at the kidney in nephrogenic DI can result from an X-linked inherited disorder or may be acquired by damage to the renal medulla or distal nephrons.

Diabetes insipidus (DI) is characterized by large quantities of dilute urine.

Central DI results from damage to the neurohypophyseal system and decreased ADH.

Nephrogenic DI results from renal resistance to ADH.

Clinical Findings

Patients present with polyuria and have 3–30 l of urine volumes daily as a result of the inability to reabsorb water or concentrate urine. Patients complain of nocturia and thirst as a reaction to urinary losses. Dehydration and hypovolemia can develop rapidly in these patients and may be the presenting event in the intensive care unit.

Diagnosis

Serum osmolarity (>280 mOsm/kg) is elevated, reflecting free water losses, with urine osmolarity less than 200 mOsm/l. The water deprivation test is the principal test for establishing the diagnosis of DI. Measurements of serum and urine osmolarity and weight are taken at baseline. Water intake is withheld and urine output and osmolarity are measured hourly. During the test, the urine of a patient with DI remains dilute despite water deprivation. The diagnosis of DI is established when the patient has manifestations of hypotension, tachycardia, and a body weight less than 5% of baseline, or the urine osmolarity does not change over 3 h. To distinguish central from nephrogenic DI, 5 U aqueous vasopressin or 1 μg desmopressin are given subcutaneously with measurements of urine osmolarity taken at 30 min and 1 h later. In central DI, the response is an increase in urine osmolarity greater than 50% or greater than 700 mOsm/l. Patients with partial DI (diminished ADH production) show a slow rise in urine osmolarity greater than 9%. There is no change in urine osmolarity in patients with nephrogenic DI.

Serum osmolarity is elevated with urine osmolarity <200 mOsm/l.

The water deprivation test can establish diagnosis of DI.

Injected synthetic ADH is used to distinguish central from nephrogenic ADH after water deprivation.

Management

Vasopressin may be used to treat both acute and chronic DI.

Partial DI may be treated with thiazide diuretics or sodium restriction alone.

ADH-releasing drugs may be used as an additional agent in partial DI.

Patients with nephrogenic DI do not have improvement with vasopressin replacement therapy or ADH-releasing drugs, treatment with thiazides, and sodium restriction.

For central DI, treatment focuses on reversible causes and hormonal replacement therapy. Hormonal replacement therapy with aqueous vasopressin at 5–10 U every 4–6 h SC or IM is used for acute presentations of central DI in the intensive care unit. Synthetic vasopressin (DDAVP or desmopressin) has prolonged antidiuretic activity and can be given as a nasal spray, 10–40 μg twice daily, for long-term replacement therapy.

Patients with partial DI may benefit from alternative therapies that include thiazide diuretics and ADH-releasing drugs. Thiazide diuretics paradoxically reduce urine volume by decreasing extracellular volume while increasing proximal tubule water reabsorption, with urine volumes falling 25%–50%. Limiting salt intake in these patients reduces their solute load and urine output. ADH-releasing drugs, chlorpropamide (3–5 mg/kg po daily), clofibrate (500–1000 mg bid) or carbamazepime (100–400 mg po bid), may be also used in patients with partial DI and in combination with thiazide diuretics.

Patients with nephrogenic DI may be treated with thiazide diuretics and by limiting salt intake. Indomethacin or other prostaglandin inhibitors may also be effective in reducing urine output by decreasing renal blood flow and glomerular filtration rate.

Syndrome of Inappropriate ADH Secretion

Syndrome of inappropriate antidiuretic hormone secretion (SIADH) is characterized by water retention and concentrated urine.

ADH may be elevated secondary to increased plasma osmolarity and in response to volume depletion.

SIADH is caused by excess release by ADH by the neurohypophysis or ectopic production.

In contrast to DI, certain conditions cause an elevation in circulating ADH that precipitates increased renal water retention and results in concentrated urine. ADH may be elevated as a physiologic response to rising plasma osmolarity in the setting of sodium retention in congestive heart failure, cirrhosis, nephrosis, or myxedema and in response to sodium-retaining drugs (e.g., nonsteroidal antiinflammatory agents, fludrocortisone). Patients with the syndrome of inappropriate ADH secretion (SIADH) have a pathologic excess of ADH that is not a physiologic response to excess serum sodium or hypovolemia. In these patients, ADH is overproduced by the neurohypophysis in response to local injury, inflammation, or drugs. Ectopic production from neoplasms or inflammatory lung disease is another source of elevated ACTH.

Symptoms

The retention of water by the kidney with resulting hyponatremia and hypoosmolarity is responsible for the type of symptoms exhibited by the patient. In mild SAIDH, serum sodium levels are 130–135 mmol/l, usually with the absence of symptoms. As serum sodium levels fall with ongoing water retention, cerebral edema may develop and precipitate alterations in mental status that range from confusion to coma.

Diagnosis

Water load testing can be used to establish the diagnosis.

The diagnosis is suspected in patients who demonstrate progressive hyponatremia, a concentrated urine with osmolarity greater than 300 mOsmol/kg, and have an altered mental status. Other etiologies for the hyponatremia must be excluded, such as conditions that would cause volume overload (heart failure with sodium retention and compensatory water retention to correct for rising plasma osmolarity) or volume depletion (adrenocortical deficiency with renal salt wasting and compensatory water retention). When other etiologies have been excluded, the diagnosis can be established with a water load test. The test is performed on those with a serum sodium greater than 125 mmol/l to prevent cerebral edema (patients may be water restricted before the test to elevate serum sodium to a safe level). Water is given to the patient as an initial load of 20 ml/kg up to 1500 ml, and urine osmolarity is measured hourly for 5 h. In normal patients, 65% of free water should be excreted in 4 h and 80% in 5 h, with a urine osmolarity less than 100 mOsm/kg by the second hour. In the intensive care unit, however, the presence of many stimuli for ADH release makes a definitive diagnosis difficult. Conditions of stress, hypovolemia, hypotension, and pain elevate ADH levels that may invalidate the water load test.

Treatment

Restriction of free water intake to a total of 800–1000 ml per day remains the primary initial treatment. In patients with severe hyponatremia with serum sodium less than 115 mEq/l, serum osmolarity less than 230 mOsm/kg, and symptoms of hyponatremia, hypertonic saline (3%) is cautiously administered because rapid serum sodium correction can result in central pontine myelinolysis (CPM). CPM results in quadriplegia and weakness of the lower face and tongue with permanent damage. The lesion may spread dorsally, compromising the sensory tracts and resulting in a "locked-in" syndrome. To avoid this complication of therapy, plasma sodium should not be increased more than 1 mEq/l in 1 h and no greater than 10 mEq over 24 h. A loop diuretic may also be given during hypertonic fluid administration if volume overload develops.

Water restriction is the primary therapy for SIADH.

Hypertonic saline can be given in severe hyponatremia but can induce central pontine myelinolysis (CPM) if corrected too rapidly.

For patients with chronic SAIDH, ADH inhibition with demeclocycline may be useful in addition to water restriction. Demeclocyline is given at 600–900 mg/day and is a potent inhibitor of ADH at the renal tubule. However, patients are at risk for renal failure, bacterial superinfections, and drug-induced water loss with hypernatremia and hypovolemia.

SUMMARY

Endocrine disorders remain a common finding in the intensive care unit patient. Clinical and laboratory findings help distinguish patients with diabetic ketoacidosis from those with hyperosmolar nonketotic coma. Both disorders require specific and aggressive treatment. Thyroid, parathyroid, and adrenal gland disorders may have profound systemic effects, ranging from alteration in mental status to hemodynamic instability. Alterations in ADH secretion or renal response to ADH may result in DI or SIADH.

REVIEW QUESTIONS

Questions 1 and 2.

A 37-year-old woman with a history of insulin-dependent diabetes mellitus (type I) presented to an emergency room with complaints of fatigue and progressive right flank pain. On physical examination, she had a temperature of 102.2°F with a heart rate of 120 beats/min, respiratory rate of 18/min, and blood pressure of 110/70 mmHg. Her skin and mucous membranes were dry. The lung exam was clear, and the cardiac exam showed regular tachycardia without murmurs or rubs. Her right flank was tender to percussion. Extremities were dry.

Laboratory tests showed a white count of 14.5 × $10^3/\mu l$ with hemoglobin of 11.5 g/dl, hematocrit of 38%, and platelets of 336 × $10^3/\mu l$. Chemistry total panel showed sodium of 150 mmol/l, potassium 3.4 mmol/l, chloride 110 mmol/l, bicarbonate 12 mmol/l, blood urea nitrogen (BUN) 60 mg/dl, creatinine 1.9 mg/dl, and glucose 1100 mg/dl. Urinalysis showed 40 plus white blood cells per high-power field with white cell casts, glucose ++++, protein +, positive leukocyte esterase, and positive nitrates. Her arterial blood gas was pH 7.01; $Pa{CO_2}$ 32 mmHg, and $Pa{O_2}$ 78 mmHg.

1. **What would be the most appropriate primary therapies?**
   A. Aggressive fluid resuscitation with normal saline and antibiotics
   B. Correction of acidosis with one ampule of sodium bicarbonate given in 250 ml of normal saline
   C. Subcutaneous insulin at the patient's usual outpatient dose
   D. Potassium repletion with 40 mEq in 250 ml normal saline
   E. Insulin bolus followed by continuous insulin infusion

2. **After initial therapy, the patient exhibited a persistent elevated anion gap acidosis but her blood sugar had decreased to 100 mg/dl. The most appropriate response is to:**
   A. Decrease the insulin infusion
   B. Increase the insulin infusion and change IV fluids to 5 or 10% dextrose
   C. Start enteral feeding
   D. Administer one ampule of dextrose intravenously

3. **A 79-year-old man with type II diabetes mellitus and chronic renal insufficiency presented to the emergency room reporting frequent falls and increased confusion. He awakens to voice but is somnolent and does not follow commands. His family reported that he had eaten little by mouth during the past 3 days. His temperature was 101°F with a heart rate of 110 beats/min and blood pressure of 100/70 mmHg. His skin and mucous membranes are dry. Laboratory values are notable for sodium 155 mmol/l, chloride 16 mmol/l, bicarbonate 21 mmol/l, and glucose 750 mg/dl. A urine dipstick indicated glucose, ketones, and concentrated urine. The most appropriate initial therapy would be:**

A. Insulin administration by continuous infusion
B. Aggressive fluid resuscitation with 0.9% saline
C. Aggressive fluid resuscitation with 5% dextrose with 0.45 saline
D. Repletion of potassium

4. **A 55-year-old woman with type II diabetes mellitus presented to the emergency room with dyspnea and cough productive of yellow sputum. Her temperature was 102°F with heart rate 100 beats/min and blood pressure 70/40 mmHg. Intravascular volume resuscitation and dopamine were initiated. Her chest x-ray demonstrated left lower lobe consolidation. She was started on antibiotics for presumed community-acquired pneumonia. The laboratory reported white cell count 15 with 15% band forms and 12% eosinophils, hemoglobin 11 g/dl, sodium 130 mmol/l, potassium 5.2 mmol/l, and glucose 60 mg/dl. A pulmonary artery catheter was placed, revealing pulmonary capillary wedge pressure of 16 mmHg with a cardiac output of 5 l/min. The diagnosis of adrenal insufficiency was considered. What is the next most appropriate step?**
A. Obtain a random serum cortisol level.
B. Obtain a serum ACTH level.
C. Perform a rapid ACTH stimulation test.
D. Inject hydrocortisone 100 mg IV.

ANSWERS

1. The answer is A and E. In DKA, the initial serum potassium levels are elevated but total body stores of potassium are decreased. Initially potassium repletion is not indicated, but with correction of acidosis and intracellular shifts potassium may be required. Subcutaneous insulin is not indicated in the acute management of DKA. Bicarbonate administration has been used in cases of acidosis with pH <7.00 but with the risks of inducing alkalosis and hypokalemia. Parenteral insulin and volume resuscitation are the most important therapies in the initial management of DKA. Since the patient has evidence of a urinary tract infection, starting empiric antibiotics along with urine cultures would also be appropriate.
2. The answer is B. Diet or enteral feeding should resume when acidosis and anion gap have resolved. The patient had a continued insulin requirement; decreasing the insulin infusion would worsen DKA. The insulin dose should be increased. Parenteral glucose should be given as 5%–10% dextrose continuous infusion to maintain blood sugars.
3. The answer is B. Unlike DKA, patients with HHNC do not have a marked requirement for insulin. Total serum potassium may be reduced secondary to renal losses, but repletion is not usually part of initial therapy. HHNC is associated with marked volume depletion and primary therapy is volume resuscitation.
4. The answer is D. ACTH levels are used to distinguish primary from secondary adrenal insufficiency and would not be relevant for the acute presentation. Random cortisol levels can be used to screen patients with suspicion for adrenal insufficiency. The diagnosis is unlikely if a random cortisol is greater than 20 μg/dl. The rapid ACTH test can be used to establish the diagnosis in acute presentations, but in this unstable patient immediate treatment with replacement hydrocortisone was indicated.

SUGGESTED READING

Bardin C. Current Therapy in Endocrinology and Metabolism, 6th Ed. Chicago: Mosby-Year Book, 1997.

Braverman L. Diseases of the Thyroid, 1st Ed, Vol 2. Totowa, NJ: Humana Press, 1997.

Davidson M. Diabetes Mellitus: Diagnosis and Treatment, 4th Ed. Philadelphia: Saunders, 1998.

Grossman A. Clinical Endocrinology, 2nd Ed. London: Blackwell, 1998.

Patrick K. Endocrinology of Critical Disease, 1st Ed, Vol 5. Totowa, NJ: Humana Press, 1997.

Philip F. Endocrinology and Metabolism, 4th Ed. New York: McGraw-Hill, 2001.

Wilson J. Williams Textbook of Endocrinology, 9th Ed. Philadelphia: Saunders, 1998.

CHAPTER 28

FREDERIC H. KAUFFMAN AND THOMAS NUGENT

Evaluation and Management of Toxicologic Emergencies

CHAPTER OUTLINE

LEARNING OBJECTIVES

After studying this chapter, you should be able to:

- List the methods available for decreasing toxin absorption in the gastrointestinal tract, with the indications, contraindications, and potential complications of each method.
- Describe toxin exposures for which enhancing toxin elimination is possible, with the specific means to do so.
- Describe the limitations of toxicologic drug screening, with indications for its use in specific clinical scenarios.
- Know those toxin exposures for which specific antidotes exist, with the indications and potential complications of their use.
- Identify the principles by which an exposure can be determined to be nontoxic and have a working knowledge of the many household items that are nontoxic.
- Describe mechanisms by which unknown compounds can be identified.

Despite the temptation to manage and treat the toxin-exposed patient from the perspective of the toxin ingested, the astute clinician understands that it is imperative to have a patient-centered approach to patient management. The old adage, "treat the patient and not the disease," is nowhere more relevant than in the field of toxicology. Knowing with the specific toxin(s) ingested is, indeed, important to patient management, but most patients will not benefit from administration of a specific antidote. In fact, the majority of patients benefit

Treat the patient and not the disease.

CASE STUDY: PART 1

An 18-year-old male was noted to be quieter than usual at breakfast. Later that morning, after playing basketball, his sister noted that he was sweating profusely and complaining of abdominal pain. That same evening his mother found him lethargic and lying on the floor. He was rushed to the emergency room. Family members stated that before this episode the patient was healthy, had no significant past medical or surgical history, and did not take illicit drugs. They denied the presence of prescription drugs in the household.

Physical examination revealed a lethargic, diaphoretic, disoriented male appearing his stated age. Temperature was 98°F, pulse 116/min and regular, BP 160/90 mmHg, and respirations 60/min, and room air pulse oximetry 100%. There was no evidence of trauma. Pupils were 4 mm, equal, and reactive to light. Optic disks were sharp bilaterally. Neck was supple. Breath sounds were clear bilaterally. Cardiac exam was normal except for tachycardia. Decreased bowel sounds were noted, along with right lower quadrant tenderness without rebound. Rectal exam was normal except for heme-positive stool. Extremities were normal. Neurologic exam was significant for disorientation to person, place, and time but was otherwise nonfocal.

The patient was placed on a cardiac monitor (sinus tachycardia) and large-bore intravenous access was obtained. Intravenous naloxone resulted in no clinical change. Bedside glucose measurement was 40 mg/dl. Administration of one ampule of $D_{50}W$ resulted in the patient becoming intermittently agitated. Blood was sent for electrolytes, blood urea nitrogen, creatinine, complete blood count, and comprehensive drug screen; arterial blood gas on room air revealed PaO_2 121 mmHg, $PaCO_2$ 22 mmHg, and pH 7.39. A Foley catheter was placed and a urine sample sent to the laboratory.

most from an organized management approach based upon sound toxicologic principles guided by working knowledge of the ABC's, gastric decontamination, enhancement of drug elimination, and the recognition of nontoxic levels of exposure.

Develop an organized approach when treating overdose patients.

Rarely will a patient with a toxic exposure be managed initially by a physician trained and board certified in toxicology. More often, the treating physician and health care team are emergency or critical care specialists. It is essential that such individuals have sound knowledge regarding generic toxicologic principles, plus an understanding of what types of exposures require consultative input from a toxicologist, generally found via the regional poison control center. Knowing what you do not know is just as important as knowing what you do. By selectively utilizing the expertise provided by regional poison control centers, the emergency or critical care specialist can provide optimal patient care based upon the latest scientific advances and at the same time facilitate ongoing toxicologic research.

ABC represents the evaluation of a patient's airway, breathing, and circulation.

Toxicology has become a highly specialized field with rigorous training and credentialing guidelines. It is impossible to duplicate a text of toxicology in this chapter. Rather, generic principles of poison management are emphasized, with some detailed information on some of the more commonly required specific antidotes. It is hoped that the information found in this chapter provides a solid foundation for future study with the clinical basis by which to treat most poisoned patients.

INITIAL TREATMENT OF THE PATIENT WITH ALTERED MENTAL STATUS AND SUSPECTED TOXIN EXPOSURE

Repeat the ABC's frequently during the evaluation.

Review vital signs including pulse oximetry.

The management of all seriously ill patients, regardless of etiology, begins with addressing the ABC's. Evaluation for airway compromise, breathing difficulties, and circulatory problems should be done quickly, with attention to the possibility of head or cervical trauma in the patient in whom trauma cannot be excluded initially. Adequacy of the frequency and depth of respirations must be assessed quickly, with early decision regarding the need for intubation. Once the airway is stabilized and oxygenation established, all vital signs should be obtained, including the often-neglected core temperature. Any life-threatening conditions identified by vital sign assessment (including pulse oximetry) should be treated immediately, including hypotension, hypertension, significant bradycardia or tachycardia, dysrhythmias, hypoxemia, and profound hyperthermia or hypothermia. Establishment of large-bore intra-

TABLE 28-1

INITIAL TREATMENTS FOR THE PATIENT WITH ALTERED MENTAL STATUS AND SUSPECTED DRUG OVERDOSE

100% oxygen
Hypertonic dextrose, 0.5–1.0 g/kg as $D_{50}W$ in the adult or $D_{10}W$ in the child
Thiamine 100 mg by slow IV administration
Naloxone 2 mg IV

venous access and cardiac monitoring is essential to clinical management. Blood samples should be sent for electrolytes, blood urea nitrogen, creatinine, glucose, and complete blood count. Extra red-top tubes of blood should be collected and held pending subsequent need for specialized laboratory studies. The role of drug screens in this setting is discussed later in this chapter, and their use should be guided by individual clinical assessment with the knowledge that the results often do not affect patient management. History and physical assessment should guide the need for specific drug levels, such as acetaminophen, salicylates, lithium, digoxin, and theophylline. Arterial blood gas analysis is indicated early to assess adequacy of oxygenation and ventilation, along with the possibility of certain toxic–metabolic etiologies for altered mental status (e.g., elevated anion gap metabolic acidosis secondary to volatile alcohol ingestion). A Foley catheter should be inserted, if clinically indicated, and urinalysis performed for potential clues as to the substance ingested (e.g., calcium oxalate crystals in ethylene glycol poisoning). Indications for naso-orogastric tube placement and gastric lavage are discussed next.

> Acquire intravenous access with the largest bore needle obtainable.

> Blood samples should be taken after the ABC's are evaluated.

In the initial management of patients with altered mental status, readily correctable causes must be entertained, including hypoxemia, hypoglycemia, thiamine deficiency, and opiate overdose. Administration of 100% oxygen is indicated initially, along with intravenous hypertonic dextrose solution, thiamine, and naloxone (Table 28-1). The presence of focal neurologic findings does not rule out hypoglycemia as a potential etiology. If bedside glucose monitoring is utilized to assess serum glucose values, it is imperative that such instruments be quality controlled on a regular basis to ensure accuracy of readings in the clinical setting. Case reports of anaphylaxis associated with large, rapid intravenous boluses of thiamine do exist, but the likelihood of this complication is exceedingly rare and can be avoided by careful, slow administration with simultaneous vital sign monitoring. Some authorities recommend naloxone be reserved for patients with clinical or historical evidence of opiate toxicity, such as miosis, respiratory/neurologic depression, or fresh cutaneous track marks. The presence of any of these findings does, in fact, identify the overwhelming majority of opiate-intoxicated patients, but the margin of safety and potential clinical benefit of the drug mandate its very liberal use in patients with altered mental status.

The remainder of the physical examination should be completed after the foregoing antidotes have been administered, ABC's and vital signs have been reassessed, and life-threatening conditions have been treated. Specific attention should be paid to evidence for head, neck, trunk, or extremity trauma; focal neurologic findings; abnormal pupillary responses; unusual breath or skin odors; cardiorespiratory abnormalities; and specific toxicologic syndromes (Table 28-2). In addition, historical details that might provide clues as to specific toxins ingested should be aggressively sought. Family members, friends, and witnesses should be questioned concerning past medical history, social history, prescribed medications, toxic substances accessible to the patient, empty pill bottles, suicide notes, and past toxic ingestions.

> Inquire about coingestions such as acetaminophen and salicylates.

> Initial evaluation of a patient with an altered mental status should include scanning for needle marks, spot glucose testing, and examination of the pupils for miosis.

> Interview family and friends for additional information.

DECREASING GASTROINTESTINAL ABSORPTION

Despite the long-term utilization of various techniques designed, in theory, to decrease the absorption of orally ingested toxins, no other "dogma" of medical toxicology has been more controversial or more extensively challenged. For example, the once-routine use of syrup of ipecac to induce emesis and thereby decrease toxin absorption has been relegated to a minimally used decontamination modality. Clinical trials of various decontamination strategies, looking at clinical outcome parameters, have served to rigorously evaluate just what thera-

TABLE 28-2

TOXIC SYNDROMES AND THEIR PHYSICAL FINDINGS

TOXIN	BP	P	RR	T	PUPIL SIZE	BOWEL SOUNDS	DIAPHORESIS
Mental status							
Adrenergic agonists	Inc Abnl	Inc	Inc	Inc	Inc	Inc	Inc
Anticholinergics	± Abnl	Inc	±	Inc	Inc	Dec	Dec
Cholinergics	± Abnl	±	NC	NC	±	Inc	Inc
Ethanol/sedative hypnotics	Dec Abnl	Dec	Dec	Dec	±	Dec	Dec
Opioids	Dec Abnl	Dec	Dec	Dec	Dec	Dec	Dec
Withdrawal							
Ethanol/sedative hypnotics	Inc Abnl	Inc	Inc	Inc	Inc	Nl or Inc	Inc
Opioids	Inc Nl	Inc	NC	NC	Inc	Inc	Inc

BP, blood pressure; P, pulse; RR, respiratory rate; T, temperature; Inc, increased; Abnl, abnormal; Dec, decreased; NC, no charge; NL, normal

peutic modalities truly do make a significant difference in the overdose patient. This scientific effort has led to a more rational basis for the management of such patients. No longer are simplistic guidelines that apply one strategy to all situations appropriate. Each patient must be considered individually, and therapy must be tailored to the individual circumstances (e.g., patient age, weight, specific ingestion, time of ingestion, and clinical signs and symptoms) for clinical outcome to be maximized.

Gastric Emptying

Gastric emptying is indicated when coingestions cannot be ruled out or when an ingestion of highly toxic substances has occurred.

The decision to proceed with gastric emptying must be guided by several principles and questions (Table 28-3). First, the clinician must evaluate the risk of the ingestion to the patient. What compound was ingested? Is the compound potentially lethal? When was the compound ingested? How much was ingested? Gastric emptying is not indicated for the ingestion of nontoxic compounds or nontoxic amounts of some potentially toxic compounds. The all-too-common practice of gastric emptying just to "teach the patient a lesson" has absolutely no place in clinical management. Gastric emptying is indicated when potentially toxic coingestions cannot be ruled out or when compounds with extreme clinical risk (e.g., cyanide) have been ingested. Obviously, such clinical decision making requires a careful clinical history and physical examination.

Second, the clinician must decide if gastric emptying will remove enough compound to produce clinically favorable results. Most drugs, other than those that delay gastric emptying (e.g., anticholinergics and sedative-hypnotics) or form pyloric concretions (e.g., iron and enteric-coated aspirin), are unlikely to be recoverable after 2–4 h post-ingestion.

TABLE 28-3

FACTORS THAT INCREASE THE LIKELIHOOD THAT GASTRIC EMPTYING WILL IMPROVE OUTCOME

Ingested compound has high risk of toxicity (e.g., salicylates, theophylline, cyclic antidepressants)
Clinical evidence of toxicity
Lack of effective antidote
Recent ingestion (less than 1–2 h)
Ingested compound not adsorbed by activated charcoal (e.g., heavy metals)
Ingestion of sustained release compound
Ingested compound delays gastric emptying (e.g., anticholinergics)

Third, has gastric emptying been studied for the given ingestion, and have clinical benefits to gastric emptying been demonstrated? Clinical benefit to gastric emptying is maximized when the ingested compound is potentially very toxic and emptying takes place within 1 h of ingestion.

Fourth, will gastric emptying itself pose a significant clinical risk to the patient? Although gastric emptying techniques are, overall, safe and carry little risk of complication when performed appropriately, some patients may not be suitable candidates for the procedure. Potential risks of gastric emptying include esophageal tears, pharyngeal injury, tracheal placement of lavage tubes, pneumothorax, and pulmonary aspiration.

Most ingestions are not recoverable by gastric lavage after 2 h.

Fifth, are there alternatives to gastric emptying that carry less risk and greater potential clinical benefit to the patient? For example, many authorities have stated that in the setting of minimal benefit from gastric emptying and great potential benefit from a specific antidote (e.g., the patient presents to the emergency department 6 h post ingestion of a toxic dose of acetaminophen), gastric emptying simply delays the administration of effective therapy.

Potential complications of gastric lavage include esophageal tears, pharyngeal injury, tracheal placement of lavage tubes, pneumothorax, and pulmonary aspiration.

Orogastric Lavage Versus Emesis

During the past two decades, considerable research has compared the use of orogastric lavage to syrup of ipecac in overdose patients. Questions asked included: Which technique removes more toxin? Does the time of ingestion effect toxin removal? Which technique is more effective in preventing toxin absorption? Does effectiveness of either technique differ depending on whether the toxin is a solid or a liquid? How large an orogastric tube is necessary to be effective? Does the anticipated use of an antidote affect the decision making process? Simplistic answers to these and other questions have, generally, not been forthcoming. However, such analysis has refined the clinical principles that guide the treatment of patients.

Consider inducing emesis when the pill size is larger than the lavage tube.

In general, orogastric lavage and emesis appear to be comparable in terms of decreasing toxin absorption, but it must be emphasized that great individual variation in absorption occurs when studying these techniques. The range of toxin absorption measured can be tremendous, even under similar design situations, making clinical assumptions in a given patient quite difficult.

Lavage tube size is another variable to consider, along with the size of the pill or compound ingested. In children, lavage tube size may be limited, and emesis may be more effective in removing certain compounds. When emesis is contraindicated, however, even a small-diameter lavage tube may be considered in trying to remove at least some ingested particles.

Probably the most frequent risk affecting the choice of gastric emptying technique is the risk of pulmonary aspiration. Any patient unable to protect their airway during the process of gastric emptying must be intubated before gastric lavage, and emesis is contraindicated; included is ingestion of compounds such as cyclic antidepressants, isoniazid, propoxyphene, camphor, and beta-blockers. In addition, ingestion of materials likely to obstruct the airway in the setting of emesis is another contraindication to emesis.

Emesis carries a risk of aspiration and loss of airway control.

The role and clinical importance of oral activated charcoal in the setting of drug ingestion has greatly expanded in recent years. Ipecac-induced emesis takes time to be effective and is often followed by a protracted course of nausea and vomiting, thereby delaying the effective administration of activated charcoal. Orogastric lavage generally is a safe and rapid technique of emptying the stomach that can be followed immediately by the administration of activated charcoal via the lavage tube.

Ipecac-induced emesis plays little role in the management of the poisoned patient in the hospital setting. However, syrup of ipecac may play a clinically useful role as a gastric decontaminate in the home setting under physician or poison control center guidance and in children in whom large-bore orogastric tubes cannot be placed.

Syrup of ipecac is best used in the home setting under the guidance of poison control or a physician.

Activated Charcoal

Probably the greatest advance in recent years in the management of the poisoned patient has been the greater understanding of the positive role played by the use of activated charcoal.

Activated charcoal works best when used in a 10:1 ratio (activated charcoal to drug).

Multiple-dose activated charcoal (every 2–6 h) can be used with large-quantity ingestions or extended-release medications.

Multiple doses of activated charcoal can be given with drugs using the enterohepatic circulation (i.e., aminophylline).

When ingestion amount is unknown, activated charcoal can be given at 1–2 g/kg of body weight.

Activated charcoal has long been recognized as an effective adsorbent of many compounds. Carbonaceous material is first pyrolyzed and then oxidized at high temperature, thereby increasing its adsorptive capacity via a maze of internal pores, resulting in a large adsorptive surface area. Efficacy depends in large part on the timing of administration and the rate of drug absorption. Therefore, for drugs with rapid absorption via the gastrointestinal tract, early administration of activated charcoal is essential. Adsorptive capacity of activated charcoal is limited by the ratio of activated charcoal to drug, and in vitro and in vivo studies suggest that a ratio of 10 to 1 (activated charcoal to drug) maximizes effect.

Multiple-dose activated charcoal, typically given every 2–6 h, enhances the total body clearance of many drugs in experimental animal and human studies. Not only does the charcoal adsorb drug on first pass through the gastrointestinal tract, but it also may enhance adsorption beyond that of single-dose charcoal when very large quantities of drug are ingested, drug absorption is delayed or release is prolonged (e.g., enteric-coated or sustained-release products), drug reabsorption via enterohepatic circulation can be prevented, or enteroenteric circulation can be enhanced. This latter benefit explains the utility of multiple-dose charcoal in enhancing the elimination of intravenously administered drugs such as aminophylline.

Initial oral dosing of activated charcoal should take into account both patient size and amount of drug ingested (if known). An activated charcoal to drug ratio of 10 to 1 is ideal. If the amount of drug ingested is not known, 1–2 g/kg body weight is recommended. There is no universal standard for subsequent oral doses of activated charcoal; recommendations vary from 0.25 to 0.5 g/kg every 1–6 h. In settings where activated charcoal is poorly tolerated, slow continuous infusion via nasogastric tube may prove helpful.

Cathartics

Whole bowel irrigation should be used instead of cathartics for sustained-release or insoluble toxins.

Over the years, cathartics have been recommended in the management of poisoned patients. In theory, cathartics have been thought to hasten the elimination of orally ingested compounds, thereby limiting systemic toxin absorption. In adding cathartics to the use of activated charcoal, it also has been theorized that charcoal-induced constipation is minimized and elimination of charcoal-bound drug is enhanced. Unfortunately, despite the widespread use of cathartics, little evidence substantiates their clinical efficacy. In fact, significant adverse effects can occur with aggressive use of cathartics, including dehydration, hypokalemia, metabolic alkalosis, hypermagnesemia, hypocalcemia, and hyperphosphatemia. As such, cathartics should not be used routinely in the management of the poisoned patient. Evacuation of sustained-release or insoluble toxins not adsorbed to activated charcoal is better and more safely accomplished through the use of whole bowel irrigation.

Whole Bowel Irrigation

Do not use whole bowel irrigation instead of charcoal.

Polyethylene glycol or equivalent should be given at 0.5–2.0 l/h depending on patient body size.

Contraindications for whole bowel irrigation include an ileus, gastrointestinal perforation, or gastrointestinal obstruction.

Rapid bowel evacuation, a minimum of fluid and electrolyte shifts, and reduction in bioavailability of ingested toxin are the goals of whole bowel irrigation. Initial trials involved solutions that unfortunately caused dramatic fluid and electrolyte shifts, making the technique unacceptable in the management of most overdose patients. With the development of polyethylene glycol and electrolytes solution (PEG-ELS), a nonabsorbable solution that causes minimal fluid and electrolyte shifts, renewed interest arose in the toxicologic concept of whole bowel irrigation. The current clinical role for whole bowel irrigation in the poisoned patient remains to be rigorously tested, although its use has become more widespread in patients who may benefit from its use, such as those who have ingested sustained-release drugs (e.g., theophylline and verapamil), drugs that are not adsorbed to activated charcoal (e.g., heavy metals and sustained-release lithium), and drug packets (e.g., cocaine body packers). It should be emphasized that whole bowel irrigation should not preclude administration of activated charcoal in patients who have coingested substances that are well adsorbed by activated charcoal. The oral or nasogastric dose of PEG-ELS is 0.5 l/h in small children and 2 l/h in adults, for 4–6 h or until the rectal effluent is clear. Contraindications to the use of whole bowel irrigation include the presence of an ileus, gastrointestinal perforation, or gastrointestinal obstruction.

CASE STUDY: PART 2

Pending laboratory results, the patient became intermittently lethargic and agitated, at one point punching a nurse in the face. Attempts at orogastric tube placement and administration of activated charcoal were unsuccessful. Due to increasing lethargy the patient was intubated and gastric lavage performed, followed by administration of activated charcoal.

Laboratory results were significant for sodium 149 mmol/L, potassium 4.6 mmol/L, chloride 108 mmol/L, bicarbonate 18 mmol/L, blood urea nitrogen 14 mg/dl, creatinine 1.4 mg/dl, glucose 43 mg/dl (pre-D_{50}), hemoglobin 18 gm/dl, white blood cell count 25,500 K/μL with left shift, and no coagulopathy. Follow-up arterial blood gas on 100% oxygen revealed PaO_2 468 mmHg, $PaCO_2$ 60 mmHg, and pH 7.13.

Shortly thereafter the patient became febrile to 106°F. Initial supraventricular tachycardia rapidly deteriorated into bradyasystole unresponsive to advanced cardiac life support protocol and cardiopulmonary resusitation. An autopsy was obtained.

ENHANCING TOXIN ELIMINATION

In theory, once clinical strategies have been initiated to inhibit systemic toxin absorption, strategies to enhance toxin elimination from the body are sensible. However, such techniques are indicated only in a minority of patients. Enhanced elimination techniques should be considered when patients fail to respond to appropriate and full supportive care; when renal or hepatic function are compromised and normally would represent the major route of toxin elimination; when serum toxin levels indicate the potential for serious morbidity or mortality; or when scientific research suggests that significant toxin elimination can be achieved. Table 28-4 lists the more commonly utilized methods of toxin elimination. The first four methods listed (forced diuresis, alteration of urinary pH, multiple-dose activated charcoal, and whole bowel irrigation) are techniques that can be instituted quite readily in the Emergency Department when clinically appropriate. The remaining methods fall under the purview of intensivists and consultants, in which case the emergency physician provides initial supportive care, coupled with prompt identification of toxin exposure potentially amenable to these methods of elimination.

THE ROLE OF TOXICOLOGIC DRUG SCREENING

A question infrequently asked before ordering a toxicologic drug screen is, "How will this information help in the clinical management of the patient once it is received?" In reality, most clinical decisions are made before drug screen results are available. Toxicologic drug screens rarely determine the additional need for specific therapeutic modalities. Appropriate decontamination procedures and supportive care are the cornerstone of successful clinical management in most poisoned patients. Finally, toxicologic drug screens are costly, especially when plotted against clinical utility when ordered routinely. As such, toxicologic drug testing should be undertaken only when diagnostic uncertainty persists or knowledge from the testing will affect clinical management (Table 28-5). In general, urine is the preferred specimen for qualitative, comprehensive assessment; serum is preferred when quantitative drug assessment correlates with clinical effect and management decisions or when serial levels will assist clinical monitoring. Although not universally accepted, some authorities argue that routine serum testing for acetaminophen and salicylate should be undertaken

Toxic drug screens should be completed if the results will change management.

N-Acetylcysteine is used in acetaminophen overdose.

TABLE 28-4

METHODS USED TO ENHANCE TOXIN ELIMINATION

Forced diuresis	Hemofiltration
Alteration of urinary pH	Exchange transfusion
Multiple-dose activated charcoal	Plasmapheresis
Whole bowel irrigation	Toxin-specific antibody fragments
Peritoneal/hemodialysis	Chelation therapy
Charcoal hemoperfusion	

TABLE 28-5

CLASSES OF COMPOUNDS INCLUDED IN MOST COMPREHENSIVE DRUG SCREENS[a]

Alcohols	Antidepressants	Opioids
Barbiturates	Antihistamines	Nonopioid analgesics
Benzodiazepines	CNS stimulants	Antiarrhythmics
Anticonvulsants	Neuroleptics	

[a] Specific compounds tested for vary from laboratory to laboratory; when requesting a comprehensive or drug-specific screen, it is essential to know exactly which drugs your laboratory is capable of testing

in all patients suspected of intoxication. This strategy incorporates the facts that such testing is inexpensive and readily available, these compounds are found frequently in combination with other over-the-counter preparations, and that missed identification of these intoxications carries a risk of significant morbidity and mortality.

SPECIFIC ANTIDOTES FOR SPECIFIC TOXINS

The acetaminophen toxicity nomogram is only used in acute ingestion.

Most poisoned patients benefit not from a specific antidote but rather from sound clinical management based upon general principles of poison management. However, in very specific settings where the toxin ingested is amenable to antidote therapy, the timely and knowledgeable use of a specific antidote may be lifesaving. Thus, a working knowledge of a select group of antidotes is an important part of the medical armamentarium for the emergency and critical care practitioner.

History of ingestion of more than 150 mg/kg of acetaminophen should prompt administration of *N*-acetylcysteine.

A list of commonly utilized antidotes follows. For each antidote, we discuss the toxin that it counteracts, its mechanism of action, clinical indications, dosing information, contraindications to use, and potential complications of treatment. This approach may provide a useful reference for the treatment of patients encountered in the clinical setting.

N-Acetylcysteine

Toxin

Acetaminophen.

Mechanism of Action

Patients with liver disease require less acetaminophen to become toxic.

In acetaminophen ingestion, approximately 60% of the drug is metabolized to acetaminophen glucuronide and 30% to acetaminophen sulfate, both of which are nontoxic metabolites eliminated in the urine. Less than 5% of the drug is eliminated unchanged in the urine and is thought to be nontoxic. Between 5% and 15% of the drug is oxidized by the P-450 system to *N*-acetyl-*p*-benzoquinoneimine (NAPQI). In the presence of adequate stores of glutathione, NAPQI is complexed with glutathione and converted to nontoxic cysteine and mercaptate conjugates. In acetaminophen overdose, glutathione stores are depleted and free NAPQI binds to hepatic cellular proteins, with resultant cell death and hepatic necrosis. *N*-Acetylcysteine (NAC) serves primarily as a glutathione precursor, thereby maintaining or replenishing stores of glutathione and allowing continued detoxification of NAPQI. NAC

CASE STUDY: PART 3

The autopsy revealed no evidence of trauma or chronic medical conditions. Initial drug screen subsequently returned positive for salicylates; no other drugs were found. Quantitative analysis revealed a salicylate level of 125 mg% (therapeutic, 15–30 mg%.) Cause of death was determined to be acute salicylate intoxication.

can serve as a substitute for glutathione, can increase sulfation of acetaminophen to nontoxic metabolites, and may directly limit the extent of hepatotoxicity.

Clinical Indications

History of acute acetaminophen ingestion greater than 150 mg/kg suggests a potentially toxic exposure, as does an acetaminophen level that falls on or above the toxicity line of the acetaminophen toxicity nomogram. NAC is most effective if given within 8 h of ingestion. Chronic ingestion is more problematic, and the nomogram cannot be used in this setting. Hepatotoxicity is a concern in adults ingesting more than 4 g/day or children ingesting more than 75 mg/kg/day. In such circumstances, signs or symptoms of hepatotoxicity, elevated hepatic enzymes, or acetaminophen levels greater than 10 μg/ml 4 h after the last dose should prompt NAC therapy.

Loading dose of *N*-acetylcysteine is 140 mg/kg followed by 70 mg/kg given every 4 h for 17 doses.

Dosing Information

Currently, only oral NAC is FDA approved. A loading dose of 140 mg/kg is administered by mouth or nasogastric tube, followed by a maintenance regimen of 70 mg/kg to be given every 4 h thereafter for an additional 17 doses.

Contraindications

No specific contraindications exist to the use of NAC in acetaminophen toxicity. Teratogenic data for NAC are not available, but the risk of not treating a potentially fatal overdose far exceeds fetal risk of treatment.

Potential Complications

Oral NAC is quite foul tasting and may induce vomiting. NAC is rapidly absorbed but should be readministered if vomited within 1 h of ingestion. Oral NAC has not been reported to cause anaphylactoid reactions, although intravenous NAC, still considered experimental in the United States, has caused such reactions.

Antivenin: Snakes

Toxin

Venom from rattlesnakes, water moccasins, copperheads, coral snakes, and some South American pit vipers and Asian snakes.

Rattlesnake bites almost always require administration of crotalid antivenin.

Mechanism of Action

The two commercially available antivenins in the United States are crotalid and elapid. These antivenins are refined and concentrated preparations of equine serum globulin. Crotalid is a polyvalent IgG antibody created after equine exposure to a group of pit vipers found in the Western Hemisphere. Similarly, elapid is an IgG antibody created after equine exposure to the Eastern and Texan coral snake. Crotalid and elapid antivenins act by coating the offending antigen with IgG antibody. The systemic effects of the venom are thereby neutralized or blunted by this immunologic therapy. The lifesaving effectiveness of these antivenins has been proven in animal models, but the specific effect on human morbidity and mortality is not known.

Clinical Indications

The horse-derived serum is an impure solution containing not only venom-specific IgG but also other serum proteins that could induce allergic responses. These responses include ana-

Serum sickness occurs in up to 50% of patients receiving antivenin.

phylactoid reactions, serum sickness, and immediate or delayed hypersensitivity responses. The use of antivenin is based upon symptomatology and snake type. Prophylactic administration is usually discouraged. In general, rattlesnake bites almost always require antivenin (crotalid), whereas water moccasin bites occasionally need the elapid antivenin and the relatively benign bite of a copperhead requires only supportive care. Most snakebites cause pain and swelling over an area to 6 in. in diameter. Symptoms warranting consideration of antivenin usage include tissue necrosis, anaphylaxis or shock, bleeding or any kind of coagulopathy, weakness, paralysis or paresthesias, dizziness, sweating, nausea, vomiting, hypothermia, or tachypnea. The need for skin testing before administration of antivenin is debatable because the test is inaccurate and potentially dangerous.

Dosing Information

Mix snake antivenin vials with normal saline in a 1:10 to 1:100 ratio.

Patients with mild symptomatology should not be given antivenin, except in the case of rattlesnake bites. Bites from a rattlesnake can create dangerous systemic effects without causing significant local reactions. Reconstituted antivenin should be diluted to 1:10 to 1:100 in 0.9% sodium chloride solution and given intravenously. The initial infusion of the antivenin solution should be 25–50 ml/h. The infusion rate can be increased if no allergic reactions are noted. Ultimately, 2–10 vials per hour can be infused if needed. Usually the infusion is completed within 24 h, but there is yet no standard protocol; therefore the rate and duration of infusion is symptom guided.

Contraindications

Antivenin skin testing and prophylactic antivenin usage should be discouraged, except in the case of a documented Mojave rattlesnake bite because the systemic effects may not be preceded by local symptoms. Patients with previous anaphylactic responses to horse serum or horse serum-derived products should be discouraged from receiving antivenin.

Potential Complications

Anaphylaxis with subsequent death can result. There is also an approximate 50% chance of developing serum sickness within 3–20 days of receiving antivenin.

Antivenin: Scorpion and Spider

Toxin

Bites from the *Centruroides* scorpion species and the black widow spider warrant consideration of antivenin if systemic symptoms are present.

Venom from scorpion stings and spider bites. The only clinically important indigenous species of scorpion located in the United States are the *Centruroides* species of the southwestern desert. The most troublesome arachnoid venom comes from the black widow spider.

Mechanism of Action

As with snake antivenin, the antivenins for scorpion stings and arachnoid bites are derived by immunizing animals to the toxin and creating an IgG serum that can be intravenously instituted into victims. The serum decreases symptomatology and aids in the treatment of patients who cannot be quickly transported to a facility that can provide maximal supportive care. This scenario usually applies to small children who are not located near an institution appropriately equipped for pediatric critical care. Antivenin to the *Centruroides* scorpion species is available through the Antivenin Production Laboratory at Arizona State University, Tempe (APL-ASU) and is distributed throughout Arizona despite lack of FDA approval. Its use is restricted to the state of Arizona, and its transport across state lines is prohibited. The use of antivenin to black widow spider bites is usually not necessary and is again limited to patients who have the potential for systemic complications or symptoms.

Clinical Indications

These antivenins should only be used in patients who develop serious systemic symptoms. Proper usage of the antivenins requires a working knowledge of the venoms and their clinical expressions. The venom from *Centruroides* scorpion species is predominantly a neurotoxin, but other proteins in the inoculum can cause hemolysis, local tissue destruction, or hemorrhage. The sting causes local pain, numbness, and swelling, as well as possibly increasing sensitivity to tactile stimuli. It should be noted that the local symptoms seen after a scorpion sting do not correlate well with systemic toxicity. Systemic symptoms may include anxiety, restlessness, muscle spasms, nausea, vomiting, excessive salivation, sweating, pruritis, hyperthermia, blurred vision, pseudoseizures, hypertension, hemiplegia, syncope, cardiac dysrhythmias, or respiratory arrest. As with most intoxications, children and the elderly are at a greater risk of severe reactions.

Increasing infusion rate and cumulative dose of antivenin positively correlate with the likelihood of developing serum sickness.

The black widow spider has a venom composed of both protein and nonprotein compounds that paralyze prey and liquefy tissues for subsequent ingestion by the arachnid. The paralyzing protein in the spider's venom produces its toxic effect by destabilizing neuronal membranes and causing depletion of acetylcholine from presynapic nerve terminals. Usually the patient initially notes a pinprick sensation followed by local swelling and erythema. The clinician may notice two small fang marks in the area of redness. A dull crampy pain that is usually felt at the initial bite site spreads to a generalized cramping which predominates in the abdomen. Other symptoms may include dizziness, restlessness, ptosis, nausea, vomiting, headache, pruritis, dyspnea, conjunctivitis, profuse sweating, weakness, dysarthria, anxiety, and cramping pain in all muscle groups. The patient is usually hypertensive, and cerebrospinal fluid pressure may be elevated. There may be electrocardiographic changes similar to those produced by digitalis. The symptoms are usually more severe in children or small adults because the inoculum to volume of distribution is higher.

Dosing Information

Scorpion antivenin is shipped from APL-ASU to the hospital as fresh immune serum. The 5-ml vials are usually instilled over 15 to 30 min. Black widow antivenin is dispensed in 2.5-ml vials and should be diluted in 50 ml of saline for intravenous use. The infusion rate and the cumulative dose administered positively correlate with the likelihood of developing toxic side effects. In other words, an increase in dose amount and a faster infusion rate are associated with more adverse side effects.

Contraindications

There are no absolute contraindications to usage of antivenin to scorpions or black widow spiders. Any administration of these products should be preceded by serious consideration of the benefit-to-risk ratio, and toxicologic consultation is advisable to those unfamiliar with their administration.

Potential Complications

See potential complications associated with snake antivenin.

Calcium

Toxin

Calcium channel blockers, fluoride, ethylene glycol, magnesium, and potassium.

Mechanism of Action

Normal calcium balance is needed for proper muscle and nerve function. The aforementioned toxins create an absolute or relative imbalance of calcium in different ways. Calcium

After a calcium channel blocker overdose, calcium infusion should be started for bradycardia, atrioventricular blockade, altered mental status, or idioventricular rhythm.

Follow serum calcium levels in ethylene glycol or fluoride ingestions.

Consider calcium infusion in patients with hypermagnesemia or hyperkalemia and any cardiac conduction disturbance.

channel blockers create a relative intracellular hypocalcemia. Infusing calcium can attenuate overblockade of calcium channels in a calcium channel overdose. Calcium infusion increases its extracellular concentration, thereby augmenting its transcellular gradient and facilitating its movement intracellularly. In fluoride and ethylene glycol overdoses, calcium complexes with the toxin to create a salt. Eventually, an absolute hypocalcemia ensues, and a calcium infusion is needed to maintain and restore homeostatic levels. High serum levels of potassium or magnesium can destabilize cardiac membrane potentials with resultant arrhythmias. The added positively charged ions outside the cell membranes create a less negative and more excitable membrane potential. Calcium infusion counteracts this destabilization of membrane potentials by providing extra intracellular cations that drive the membrane potential in a negative direction toward a more secure resting potential.

Clinical Indications

Calcium infusion during calcium channel overdose is indicated for bradycardia, any atrioventricular blockade, altered mental status, or idioventricular rhythm. Calcium infusion can also be given if hypotension ensues, but its clinical efficacy in this situation has never been proven. In the presence of hypocalcemia, calcium infusion can aid in the effectiveness of atropine administration. Intravenous calcium salts should also be administered with symptomatic hypocalcemia as a result of ethylene glycol or fluoride intoxication. The clinical manifestations of hypocalcemia include perioral paresthesias, tingling of the fingers and toes, seizures, laryngeal spasm, and spontaneous or latent tetany. Other manifestations of hypocalcemia include Chvostek's sign, Trousseau's sign, prolongation of the Q-T interval, and changes in the QRS complex and ST segments that may mimic alterations seen in an acute myocardial infarction. Hypermagnesemia and hyperkalemia should be treated with calcium infusion if any signs of cardiac arrthymias are noted.

Dosing Information

In calcium channel overdose, 1 g of calcium chloride or 3 g of calcium gluconate can be administered every 10–20 min as needed to reverse symptoms. Monitoring patients for iatrogenic hypercalcemia is prudent in those without life-threatening complications. The acutely administered cumulative dose should not exceed 45 mEq because of the dangerous possibility of hypercalcemia. Skin exposure to hydrogen fluoride in concentrations greater than 20% usually requires an intradermal injection of 10% calcium gluconate. Exposures to hydrofluoride with a concentration less than 20% respond to coverage with calcium carbonate tablets mixed with a water-soluble jelly. In fluoride burns of the digits, an intraarterial calcium infusion can be attempted. Intravenous calcium, in the form of calcium chloride or calcium gluconate, should be given in doses sufficient to reverse EKG abnormalities (QT or QRS prolongation) associated with ethylene glycol overdose, hypermagnesemia, or hyperkalemia. Intravenous calcium should not exceed a rate of 1.8 mEq/min unless the patient is in a life-threatening situation.

Contraindications

The development of hypercalcemic toxicity. If digitalis toxicity exists, or the patient is currently taking digoxin, extreme caution should be taken. In cases of concomitant hyperphosphatemia, the serum calcium times the phosphate product should not exceed 66 mg/dl.

Potential Complications

Hypercalcemia. Symptoms include nausea, vomiting, constipation, hypertension, shortening of the QT interval, polyuria, altered mental status, hyporeflexia, and coma.

Cyanide Antidotes

Toxin

Cyanide.

Mechanism of Action

Cyanide has a high affinity for the ferric ion. The binding of cyanide to the ferric ion disrupts intracellular aerobic metabolism by removing it from the cytochrome oxidase complex; this results in hypoxemia. The only commercially available FDA-approved antidote in the United States, the Lilly Cyanide Kit, contains amyl nitrate pearls, 3% sodium nitrite, and 25% sodium thiosulfate. The exact mechanism by which nitrites work is not known, but the use of cyanide induces methemoglobinemia. Methemoglobin converts to cyanomethemoglobin under normal physiologic conditions. Cyanomethemoglobin then reacts with thiosulfate and the enzyme rhodenase to form thiocyanate, which is then excreted in the urine.

A cyanide kit contains all the antidotes needed in a cyanide overdose.

Ideally, a methemoglobin level of 30% should be attained before giving thiosulfate.

Clinical Indications

In cases of moderate to severe overdoses associated with clinical deterioration not amenable to supportive care.

Dosing Information

Amyl nitrite pearls should be broken into a gauze sponge and placed so the patient can inhale the fumes for at least 30 s of each minute if the sodium nitrite solution is not immediately available. Three percent sodium nitrite solution can be diluted in approximately 100 ml solute and infused intravenously over 2–4 min. The goal is to produce a methemoglobin level close to 30%. Subsequently, 50 ml of 25% thiosulfate solution can be given intravenously. Follow methemoglobin levels and redose if symptoms reappear within 1 h of initial dosing. If symptoms reappear, the aforementioned procedure should be reinstituted with pharmacologic doses at 50% of the original amount.

Methemoglobin levels are available on arterial blood gases.

Contraindications

Caution should be used in patients with cardiovascular disease.

Potential Complications

Nitrites may worsen hypoxemia in patients with concomitant elevated carboxyhemoglobin levels. Thiocyanate can cause nausea, vomiting, arthralgias, muscle cramps, and psychosis. Nitrites can produce hypotension and methemoglobinemia. Worsening hypoxemia can result from the administration of nitrites. Methemoglobin levels greater than 30% can produce symptomatic cyanosis, whereas levels greater than 70% can be lethal.

Deferoxamine

Toxin

Iron, aluminum.

Mechanism of Action

Deferoxamine has a high binding affinity for iron and aluminum and therefore it complexes with the metals. The deferoxamine complex is then excreted from the body.

Deferoxamine binds aluminum and iron.

Clinical Indication

All symptomatic patients with a serum iron level greater than 300 μg/dl should receive deferoxamine. Other indications include lethargy, significant abdominal pain, hypovolemia, acidosis, or patients having more than one episode of emesis or multiple soft stools. Intravenous deferoxamine therapy should be given to all these aforementioned presentations. Patients with mild toxicity can receive intramuscular injections. Deferoxamine can also be used to treat aluminum-associated dialysis encephalopathy and osteomalacia.

Dosing Information

Intravenous infusion rates have been recommended not to exceed 15 mg/kg/h, and duration of therapy should not exceed 24 h; 2 g deferoxamine can be given during the last half hour of dialysis to aid in aluminum detoxification.

Contraindications

Deferoxamine should not be given to patients with anuria or end-stage renal disease.

Severe renal disease, or anuria in patients not receiving dialysis, because most of the chelate is excreted in the urine.

Potential Complications

Hypotension, pulmonary toxicity (ARDS), ocular and ototoxicity, and infection.

Digoxin-Specific Antibody Fragments

Toxin

Digoxin, digitoxin, oleander, squill toad venom.

Mechanism of Action

Digibind half-life is 15–20 h in patients with normal renal function.

Redosing of digibind should be considered if signs of digoxin toxicity have not reversed within 30 min.

Digoxin-immune antigen-binding fragment (Fab) (digibind) is derived from specific antidigoxin antibodies produced from sheep after digoxin exposure. Digibind is administered intravenously and binds free digoxin intravascularly and in the interstitial space. The Fab–digoxin complex is predominantly removed from the body via the kidneys. Digibind's half-life appears to be about 15 h, and clinical improvement is seen within 30 min of administration. It is unclear what effect renal impairment has on Fab–digoxin removal.

Clinical Indications

Serum levels of digoxin are probably inaccurate after the initial dosing of digibind.

The indications for using digoxin-specific antibody fragments depend on the signs of digoxin toxicity. Digoxin serum levels may not correlate well with impending life-threatening toxicity because the drug concentrates in tissues before equilibrating in the serum. The time of distribution of digoxin is approximately 6–8 h. Serum concentrations of digoxin greater than 15 ng/ml usually require digoxin-specific antibody fragments regardless of clinical signs of toxicity. Signs of digoxin toxicity include first-, second-, or third-degree heart block as well as ventricular tachycardia and fibrillation. Other indications for digibind usage include patients with known digoxin ingestions greater than 10 mg or an elevated potassium level greater than 5.0.

(3)

Dosing Information

Each vial of digibind contains 38 mg of digoxin-specific Fab fragments, which bind approximately 0.5 mg of digoxin or digitoxin. The dose of digibind given to neutralize digoxin can be based on either the ingestion amount, if a reliable history is given, or the serum amount, if the serum level was drawn at least 4 h after the ingestion. Basing the digibind dosing on history enables the clinician to multiply the total dosage of digoxin ingested by

0.80, which is the bioavailability of the drug. Doubling this product generates the number of vials of digibind needed. When basing digibind dosing on serum levels of digoxin, the clinician can multiply the serum concentration of digoxin by the patient's weight in kilograms and divide that product by 100 to calculate a dosing amount. The antibody fragment should begin to show signs of reversing the digoxin-induced toxicity within 30 min. If signs of toxicity persist, an additional dose of digibind should be given. Digibind is primarily excreted in the urine, and its half-life appears to be 15–20 h in patients with normal renal function. The half-life of digoxin is 1.5–2 days; therefore, a rebound in serum digoxin levels can occur 12 h after digibind administration. Readministration of digibind should again be based on signs of digoxin toxicity. It should be noted that the measurement of digoxin levels after dosing of digibind may not be clinically useful. Most laboratories are not equipped to measure free digoxin levels and therefore report the total digoxin amount, which includes both the free and digibind-bound amounts.

*

Hyperkalemia can herald impending digoxin toxicity.

Contraindications

There are no contraindications for digoxin-specific antibody fragments.

Potential Complications

Serum potassium levels must be closely monitored when digibind is administered. Digoxin acts on the Na-K-ATPase pump, which increases intracellular levels of Ca^{2+} and Na^{+} as well as extracellular levels of K^{+}. High serum potassium levels can herald digoxin toxicity; however, a high potassium level may not accurately assess the total body amount of potassium because a higher proportion of potassium may be extracellular. The high serum potassium amounts eventually leads to added excretion because there is an increase in renal handling and clearance, which could result in lowering of total potassium body stores. The administration of digibind could therefore cause reshifting of potassium intracellularly. This intracellular potassium shift could result in the development of hypokalemia and its associated complications.

Hypokalemia can occur after digibind dosing.

Ethanol

Toxin

Methanol, ethylene glycol.

Mechanism of Action

Ethanol competitively inhibits both methanol and ethylene glycol conversion to toxic metabolites by antagonism of the enzyme alcohol dehydrogenase. Inhibiting conversion of ethylene glycol and methanol allows passage of the unchanged substrate into the urine.

Clinical Indications

Ethanol should be administered immediately if the patient history suggests ingestion of either methanol or ethylene glycol. Ethylene glycol is most commonly found in antifreeze, whereas methanol can be found in de-icing solutions, windshield washing fluid, carburetor cleaners, shellac, and paint removers or paint thinners. An inebriated patient with a normal ethanol level should also raise suspicion of methanol or ethylene glycol intoxication and should result in ethanol treatment. Other situations suggesting methanol or ethylene glycol overdose include an unexplained metabolic acidosis or a high anion gap. Note that a normal anion gap does not rule out ethylene glycol or methanol overdose because it is the metabolites of these substances that induces the acidosis. In other words, the time between the exposure and measurement of arterial pH and serum electrolytes may be insufficient to produce a high anion gap acidosis. Ethylene glycol or methanol overdose will cause an elevated osmolar gap. Serum levels of the toxins may also be used to help guide therapy. Any serum

Ethylene glycol is found in antifreeze.

Methanol can be found in de-icing solutions, shellac, and paint thinners.

level of methanol or ethylene glycol above a trivial amount should result in ethanol administration. Serum levels of methanol or ethylene glycol greater than 25 mg/dl should result in the use of ethanol along with immediate dialysis.

Dosing Information

Ethanol can be given in oral or intravenous form. Oral ethanol delivery is preferred, but patient noncompliance or incapacity to safely ingest the alcohol often results in the need to administer the treatment intravenously. Obtaining a blood ethanol level of 100–150 mg/dl provides sufficient competitive blockade of alcohol dehydrogenase to allow methanol and ethylene glycol to pass in the urine relatively unchanged. Achieving an ethanol to methanol or ethanol to ethylene glycol ratio of 1:4 also provides sufficient protection from conversion of the primary alcohol to its toxic metabolites. A loading dose of 0.8 g/kg IV given in 10% ethanol solution usually results in a rapid attainment of appropriate serum ethanol levels. An IV maintenance dose of 130 mg/kg/h of ethanol should keep serum levels at an acceptable range. Interpatient differences in the metabolism of ethanol necessitate periodic monitoring of serum levels. Because of increased ethanol clearance, patients undergoing hemodialysis require a maintenance dose of 250–350 mg/kg/h to maintain appropriate serum ethanol levels. In patients with a significant metabolic acidosis, renal clearance of toxins is improved by adding bicarbonate. In addition, thiamine and pyridoxine should be given to patients with ethylene glycol ingestion and folic acid should be given to those with methanol ingestion.

A normal anion gap does not rule out ethylene glycol or methanol overdose.

Contraindications

There are no absolute contraindications to ethanol usage in severe ethylene glycol or methanol overdose.

Potential Complications

The administration of ethanol could cause worsening CNS depression, hypoglycemia, pancreatitis, and dehydration. Patients receiving ethanol orally have the added risk of aspiration and therefore require close monitoring in an ICU setting. Intravenous infusion of ethanol can cause venous irritation at the infusion site; consequently, it should be diluted with solute to at least a 10% solution. A 10% ethanol solution is hyperosmolar and can cause undesirable fluid shifts in a patient.

Serum levels of ethylene glycol or methanol >25 mg/dl require dialysis.

Flumazenil

Toxin

Benzodiazepine.

Mechanism of Action

Flumazenil competitively inhibits the benzodiazepines at the benzodiazepine receptor.

Clinical Indication

There are no absolute indications in the use of flumazenil. It can be used to reverse oversedation created by benzodiazepines.

Dosing Information

Flumazenil doses >2–3 mg are rarely needed.

Flumazenil can usually be given safely at a rate of 0.1 mg/min and the total dose rarely needs to exceed 2–3 mg. The onset of action occurs within a few minutes and the duration of action is approximately 1 h. The patient should be followed over time to see if redosing of flumazenil is needed because the half-life of flumazenil is considerably shorter than that of some long-acting benzodiazepines.

Contraindications

Flumazenil can induce seizures in patients who have a history of seizures or who are currently being treated for seizures with benzodiazepines. Some studies have noted an increase incidence of adverse events with patients receiving flumazenil concomitantly with tricyclic antidepressants; therefore, patients receiving tricyclics either chronically or as an overdose should not receive flumazenil. Caution should also be used in giving flumazenil to patients with any long-term usage or dependency on benzodiazepines.

Potential Complications

Flumazenil can potentially cause seizures in patients with a known seizure disorder. The possibility of cardiac arrhythmias also exists. Reversal of the benzodiazepine effect can also result in confusion, restlessness, and agitation.

Naloxone

Toxin

Opiod intoxication.

Mechanism of Action

Naloxone is a narcotic antagonist. The exact mechanism of action of naloxone is not known, but it is thought to competitively antagonize opiates at receptor sites.

Naloxone can be given IV, IM, or SC.

Clinical Indications

Opiate overdose resulting in clinically significant respiratory depression, hypotension, or potential loss of airway control by the patient.

Dosing Information

Initial dosing of naloxone is 0.4–2.0 mg.

The usual starting dose of naloxone is 0.4 mg in a nonopioid-dependent patient. This initial dose can be as high as 2.0 mg if the opioid overdose amount is known to be substantial. The starting dose for opioid-dependent patients should probably be 0.1 mg because higher doses can potentially induce withdrawal. Naloxone can be given intravenously, intramuscularly, or subcutaneously. Oral administration is not effective because of the substantial first-pass metabolism of the liver. The onset of action occurs within 2 min of administration when given intravenously. The onset of action via intramuscular or subcutaneous injection is only slightly longer in a patient with a normal integument and muscle mass. The half-life after parenteral administration is 30–81 min. Repeated dosing or continuous infusion may be needed if the half-life of the narcotic is substantially longer than that of naloxone. The maintenance dose of naloxone can be determined by infusing two-thirds of the initial effective bolus dose on an hourly basis, which can be accomplished by giving hourly scheduled injections of naloxone or by diluting naloxone in saline and delivering the solution over the course of an hour or hours.

Contraindications

Known hypersensitivity to naloxone.

Potential Complications

Caution should be used when giving naloxone to long-term users of narcotics because of the possibility of withdrawal. Patients may also awaken confused, disoriented, or angry. Naloxone has also been associated with hypertension, cardiac arrhythmias, pulmonary edema, and seizures.

Physostigmine

Toxin

Initial dosing of physostigmine is 1–2 mg.

Anticholinergics, including atropine, and phenothiazines.

Mechanism of Action

Physostigmine reversibly inhibits central and peripheral cholinesterases, resulting in higher acetylcholine concentrations at the postsynaptic nerve terminal.

Clinical Indications

The half-life of physostigmine is approximately 18 min.

Physostigmine is used to reverse the life-threatening clinical effects of an anticholinergic overdose. Symptoms of anticholinergic toxicity include lack of salivation and perspiration, mydriasis, confusion, hallucinations, restlessness, and tachycardia. Other sequelae of anticholinergic overdoses include coma, severe hypertension, or seizures.

Dosing Information

Physostigmine can be administered intravenously or intramuscularly. The dose to reverse a cholinergic intoxication is 1–2 mg. Physostigmine should be given over several minutes under close monitoring. The onset of action is within minutes and half-life is approximately 18 min, but interpatient pharmacokinetics vary widely. Repeat dosing of physostigmine may be necessary because the half-life of physostigmine might be shorter than that of the anticholinergic.

Contraindications

Physostigmine should be given with extreme caution.

Physostigmine is contraindicated in patients with asthma, diabetes, cardiovascular disease, obstruction of urinary or gastrointestinal tract, and those receiving a depolarizing neuromuscular blocking agent. Overdose or fast administration of physostigmine can cause hypotension, bradycardia, hypersalivation, seizures, nausea, vomiting, defecation, and urination. Asystole has been reported in patients with tricyclic overdose.

Potential Complications

Physostigmine augments acetylcholine levels and therefore can increase vagal tone, cause hypersalivation, diarrhea, bradycardia, and seizure. The possibility of physostigmine overdose and its potential for lethal effects make the cost-to-benefit profile high and should caution its use.

Sodium Bicarbonate

Toxin

Tricyclic antidepressant, salicylates, rhabdomyolysis, ethylene, and methanol intoxication.

Method of Action

Bicarbonate should be considered in cyclic antidepressant overdose with a QRS complex >0.10 s in duration.

Sodium bicarbonate may decrease the affinity of tricyclic binding to the cardiac myocyte sodium ion channels, ultimately resulting in less lethal cardiac arrhythmias. Salicylate toxicity is altered by alkalinization with sodium bicarbonate by shifting a larger proportion of the salicylate into the ionized form and thereby lessening its ability to cross the blood–brain barrier and cause neurotoxicity. Alkalinization also helps increase renal excretion of salicylates. Myoglobin dissociates into globin and ferrihemate, which is toxic to renal tubules, at urine pH below 5.6. Preventing a urinary pH below 5.6 permits the safe passage of myogloblin into the urine without significant release of the toxic ferrihemate. Sodium bicarbonate administration in methanol intoxication may decrease ocular toxicity by changing the distribution of the offending metabolite, formic acid. Animals poisoned with ethylene glycol showed a fourfold increase in the lethal dose by using sodium bicarbonate alone.

Clinical Indications

Some authors advocate starting bicarbonate in tricyclic overdoses when the QRS complex duration is greater than 0.10 s. Sodium bicarbonate should be given as soon as patients show signs of systemic toxicity during salicylate overdoses and when the urinary pH falls below 6.0 in a patient with rhabdomyolysis. Sodium bicarbonate should be administered to an ethylene glycol or methanol overdose patient whose acidosis results in a serum pH below 7.30.

Dosing Information

In tricyclic overdose, the goal is to narrow the QRS complex while keeping the blood pH between 7.50 and 7.55; this can be accomplished by rapidly infusing 1–2 mEq/kg sodium bicarbonate as a bolus and then setting up a maintenance infusion by instilling several 50-ml ampules of sodium bicarbonate in D_5W solution. In a salicylate overdose the bicarbonate is titrated until the urinary pH approaches 7.5, whereas in rhabdomyolysis the goal should be urinary pH of 6.5. During toxic alcohol poisonings, the blood pH should be titrated upward to a pH greater than 7.30.

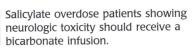

Salicylate overdose patients showing neurologic toxicity should receive a bicarbonate infusion.

Contraindications

Sodium bicarbonate loading and maintenance dosing requires the institution of large amounts of volume into the vascular space. Patients who have heart failure, renal failure, or currently have pulmonary edema with respiratory compromise should be given bicarbonate with caution. Bicarbonate can also increase the carbon dioxide load on the respiratory system; therefore, caution and close monitoring are warranted for patients with an inability to increase their minute ventilation.

Potential Complications

As previously stated, the patient could have respiratory failure from a large volume load or the increased demand on minute ventilation. A blood pH alkalinized to greater than 7.55 could cause seizures or arrhythmias. Hypocalcemia can occur with sodium bicarbonate administration in ethylene glycol intoxication; therefore, calcium should be monitored. Hypokalemia can occur by shifting of potassium ions from the extracellular to the intracellular compartment with changes in serum pH.

Urinary pH should be maintained above 6.0 in rhabdomyolysis.

Vitamin K

Toxin

Coumarins and indandiones. The coumarins include warfarin and the superwarfarins present in some rodenticides.

Mechanism of Action

Coumarin depletes the reduced form of vitamin K, which is essential in the activation of coagulation factors 2, 7, 9, and 10. Infusing vitamin K overwhelms this coumarin-induced depletion of coagulation factors.

IV administration of vitamin K should be avoided.

Clinical Indications

Bleeding resulting from or complicated by a prolonged prothrombin time. Vitamin K can also be used in patients with substantially elevated prothrombin times who are currently not bleeding but who are at high risk of bleeding. Characteristics associated with an increased risk of bleeding during warfarin therapy include age above 65; a history of cerebrovascular disease, stroke, or gastrointestinal bleeding; heart disease; concurrent aspirin therapy; and hypertension.

Maximum pharmacologic activity of vitamin K is obtained with q6h dosing.

Efficacy of oral vitamin K is dependent on an intact hepatobiliary circulation.

Dosing Information

The amount of vitamin K needed to reverse the effects of a coumarin or an indandione overdose is dependent on the cumulative dose of poison ingested and the half-life of the toxin preparation. The initial prothrombin time and the degree of normalization of the prothrombin time should also influence the dosing and route of administration. Vitamin K can be administered intravenously, intramuscularly, orally, or subcutaneously. Oral administration is preferred. Its absorption time from the gastrointestinal tract is 2–3 h and its peak onset of action is approximately 12 h. The absorption of orally received vitamin K depends on the availability and competence of the hepatobiliary circulation; therefore, patients with biliary obstruction, pancreatitis, steatorrhea, or cholestasis may have decreased absorption and efficacy. Starting doses can range from 1 to 50 mg, and the greatest pharmacokinetical activity is obtained with administration of the vitamin every 6 h. The number of doses needed to reverse the toxin depends on the half-life of the poison and the efficacy of previous doses. The duration of action of warfarin can be as long as 2–5 days, whereas some superwarfarins present in rodenticides can have a period of action lasting several months. Therefore, ingestion of a superwarfarin may require several months of vitamin K dosing. Subcutaneous administration of vitamin K has similar pharmacokinetics as the oral preparation except there is a slightly faster onset of action. Aqueous solutions are dispensed in 2 mg/ml and 10 mg/ml preparations. Subcutaneous injections of vitamin K are limited to 5 ml per injection site (or 50 mg). Injections greater than 5 ml have variable absorption. Intramuscular injections of vitamin K should be avoided because of the potential for intramuscular bleeding. Intravenous injections of vitamin K have resulted in the death of several patients. Therefore, the use of intravenous vitamin K should always be questioned. Although the onset of action of intravenous administration is slightly better than the subcutaneous route, its risk-to-benefit ratio should preclude its use in almost every situation. In the case of severe life-threatening hemorrhage, intravenous vitamin K has been shown to increase the activity of coagulation factors 2, 7, 9, and 10 to only 50% of normal levels after 4 h. This slow improvement in coagulation factors provides reason for treating hemorrhage in the acute setting with blood products such as fresh-frozen plasma. If a situation arises that demands the administration of vitamin K intravenously, steps should be taken to minimize potential complications. The solution should be diluted in normal saline or a preservative-free dextrose solution and administered slowly at a rate that should not exceed 1 mg/min in adults.

Contraindications

Vitamin K_1 has no contraindications.

Potential Complications

Overcorrection of the prothrombin time can present a problem for patients at high risk of developing thrombi. Vitamin K administered intravenously has resulted in several reported deaths; therefore, its use should always be questioned. Rapid intravenous administration may be associated with facial flushing, diaphoresis, chest pain, hypotension, or dyspnea with or without an anaphylactoid reaction. Subcutaneous injections of vitamin K can result in a local skin reaction. Intramuscular injections in patients with a propensity to bleed can cause development of a hematoma.

Protamine

Toxin

Heparin.

Method of Action

Heparin is an acidic compound that complexes with the basic compounds antithrombin III and protamine. Heparin induces its anticoagulation effect by binding and complexing with antithrombin III. Protamine, a stronger base compound than antithrombin III, has a greater electrochemical affinity to complex with heparin than antithrombin III. As such, protamine removes heparin from the heparin–antithrombin III complex and creates a neutralized protamine–heparin complex.

Protamine complexes with heparin, creating a neutralized compound.

Clinical Indications

Protamine is most often used after cardiopulmonary bypass surgery to reverse the effects of heparin after the patient is removed from the bypass pump. Its use in the intensive care unit setting should be limited to life-threatening bleeding complications resulting from heparin overdosing.

Dosing Information

Heparin diffuses quickly from the circulation; therefore, the protamine dose needed to reverse heparin-induced anticoagulation relates to the time dosing of the heparin. One milligram of protamine neutralizes approximately 100 units of heparin given within the previous 15 min. Approximately 0.5 mg and 0.25 mg of protamine can be given per 100 units of heparin administered within the previous 1 and 2 h, respectively. The total dose of protamine should not exceed 50 mg during 10 min. Repeat dosing can be based on the partial thrombin times drawn approximately 15 min after the completion of the protamine infusion. Overshooting the protamine needed to neutralize heparin should be avoided because protamine has been shown to have weak anticoagulant effects when given in the absence of heparin.

Contraindications

Any patient with a known allergy to protamine should be given protamine with extreme caution. Because protamine should only be given in life-threatening heparin-induced bleeding, the use of protamine in an allergic patient should be based on clinical judgment. Because protamine is derived from salmon sperm, there is a theoretically increased risk of adverse reactions in patients with fish allergies and previous vasectomies. Patients previously exposed to protamine also have an increased risk of developing anaphylactoid reactions. Patients who could have been exposed to protamine include those who underwent cardiopulmonary bypass surgery and diabetics using protamine-containing insulin preparations, which include NPH Iletin I-II, Lispro, and Umuline Protamine Isophane.

Potential Complications

Documented adverse reactions include bradycardia, hypotension, hypertension, thrombocytopenia, leukopenia, anticoagulant effects, and anaphylactoid and anaphylactic reactions. The hypotensive and bradycardic events are believed to be infusion rate-related complications. Therefore, protamine should not be given at a rate greater than 50 mg over 10 min. Supportive care for a possible anaphylactic or anaphylactoid reaction should be readily available before administering the protamine dose.

TABLE 28-6

COMMONLY ENCOUNTERED NONTOXIC ITEMS

Bath oils	Ballpoint pen ink	Most antibiotics
Body conditioners/shampoos	Crayons	Corticosteroids
Cosmetics	White glue/paste	Candles
Shaving cream	Play-doh	Cigarettes
Toothpaste	Silly Putty	Latex paint
Laundry detergent	Clay	Motor oil
Chalk	Antacids	

NONTOXIC EXPOSURES

A surprisingly large and varied number of products commonly encountered in everyday life are either nontoxic in any amount or route of exposure or are nontoxic in limited amounts. Patient and parental anxiety, along with overall health care cost, can be limited when identification of a nontoxic exposure can be made. When absolute product identification of a single, nontoxic ingestant can be made, a reliable estimate of amount and route of exposure is available, the patient is symptom free, and reliable patient observation and follow-up are assured, the exposure can be classified as nontoxic. If any of these factors is deemed unreliable, the patient should be instructed to seek immediate medical evaluation. Table 28-6 provides a partial list of commonly encountered items that are nontoxic.

SUMMARY

Sound principles of supportive care are the foundation for the clinical management of the poisoned patient. Establishment of an adequate airway, ensuring breathing and oxygenation, and maintaining adequate circulation are the first and foremost therapeutic priorities in these patients. A thoughtful approach to gastric decontamination and toxin elimination will supplement care and improve clinical outcome. A working knowledge of some of the more commonly used antidotes is helpful (and mandatory in the case of oxygen, naloxone, glucose, and thiamine), and can always be supplemented by contact with the nearest poison control center (Table 28-7). A careful history may identify nontoxic exposures, thereby eliminating the need for potentially noxious treatment.

REVIEW QUESTIONS

1. **Which overdose may not benefit from a bicarbonate infusion?**
   A. Cyclic antidepressant overdose
   B. Salicylate overdose
   C. Methanol ingestion
   D. Ethylene glycol ingestion
   E. Digoxin overdose

2. **Which of the following choices is not an indication for giving digibind?**
   A. Serum potassium level >5.0
   B. Serum calcium <7.0
   C. A known ingestion >10 mg
   D. Any degree of heart block
   E. Digoxin serum concentration >15 ng/dl

3. **Redosing of digibind should be based on which of the following criteria?**
   A. A digoxin level of 20 ng/dl after initial dosing of digibind
   B. A digoxin level of 30 ng/dl after initial dosing of digibind
   C. Second-degree heart block
   D. Atrial fibrillation
   E. Fifteen hours after the initial dose (the half-life of digibind) of digibind and a normal sinus rhythm

4. **Which of the following choices is not a contraindication for flumazenil usage?**
   A. Diazepam dependency
   B. A patient receiving gabapentin for neuralgia
   C. Concomitant tricyclic antidepressant overdose
   D. A patient currently taking doxepin for depression
   E. A patient receiving diazepam for a seizure disorder

TABLE 28-7

SUMMARY OF TOXINS AND ANTIDOTES

TOXIN	ANTIDOTE	DOSAGE	CLINICAL INDICATION	CONTRAINDICATIONS
Aluminum	Deferoxamine	2 g 0.5 h during dialysis	Encephalopathy, osteomalacia	None
Atropine	Physostigmine	1–2 mg/5 mm	Overdose not responsive to supportive care	Asthma, GI/GU obstruction, diabetes, cardiovascular disease
Benzodiazepines	Flumazenil	0.1 mg/min starting dose	No absolute indications	hx/o seizures, cyclic antidepressants, benzodiazepine dependency
Calcium channel blocker	Calcium	1 g CaCl or 3 g Ca gluconate	Hypotension, conduction abnormalities	Hyperphosphatemia, hypercalcemia
Coral snake venom	Elapid	See crotalid	Tissue necrosis, systemic symptoms	Horse serum sensitivity
Coumarins	Vitamin K	Based on INR	Bleeding	None
Cyanide	Lilly cyanide kit	Amyl nitrite pearls and/or 3% sodium nitrite, then 25% sodium thiosulfate	Moderate to severe overdose not amenable to supportive care	See text
Digitoxin	Digibind	1 vial/0.5 mg digoxin	See digoxin	None
Digoxin	Digibind	1 vial/0.5 mg digoxin	Digoxin level >15 ng/mL, AV blockade, K^+ >5.0, digoxin ingestion >10 mg	None
Ethylene glycol (+ thiam pyridoxin)	Calcium	CaCl or Ca gluconate	Hypocalcemia	Hyperphoshatemia, hypercalcemia
	Ethanol	0.8 g/kg bolus, then 130 μg/kg/h		
	Sodium bicarbonate	1–2 mEq/kg bolus then 1 amp in D_5W	Blood pH <7.30	Volume overload
Fluoride	Calcium	10% Ca gluconate injection or $CaCO_3$ mixed with jelly	Tissue necrosis, systemic hypocalcemia	Hyperphosphatemia, hypercalcemia
Heparin	Protamine	0.5 mg within 1 h of heparin 0.25 mg within 2 h of heparin	Bleeding	Protamine sensitivity
Hyperkalemia	Calcium	CaCl/Ca gluconate	Hypocalcemia	Hypercalcemia
Hypermagnesemia	Calcium	CaCl/Ca gluconate	Hypocalcemia	Hypercalcemia
Indandiones	Vitamin K	Based on INR	Bleeding	None
Iron	Deferoxamine	<15 mg/kg/h not to exceed 24 h	Serum Fe >300 μg/dl	Anuria, renal insufficiency
Methanol (+ ac. folique)	Ethanol	See ethylene glycol	See text	None
	Sodium bicarbonate	1–2 mEq/kg bolus then 1 amp in D_5W	Serum pH < 7.30	Renal or heart failure
Myoglobin	Sodium bicarbonate	1–2 mEq/kg bolus then 1 amp in D_5W until urinary pH>6.5	Urinary pH < 6.0	Volume overload
Oleander	Digibind	1 vial/0.5 mg digoxin	See digoxin	None
Opioids	Naloxone	0.4–2.0 mg starting dose	Hypotension, respiratory depression	
Phenothiazines	Physostigmine	1–2 mg/5 min		See above
Pit viper venom	Crotalid	25–50 N ml/h 1:10 dilution	Rattlesnake bites, tissue necrosis, systemic symptoms	Horse serum sensitivity
Salicylates	Sodium bicarbonate	1–2 mEq/kg bolus then 1 amp in D_5W	CNS symptoms	Volume overload
Scorpion venom	APL-ASU antivenin	5-ml vials over 15–30 min	Systemic symptoms	Serum sensitivity
Spider venom	IGG spider antivenin			Serum sensitivity
Squill toad venom	Digibind	1 vial/0.5 mg digoxin	See digoxin	None
Cyclic anti-depressants	Sodium bicarbonate	1–2 mEq/kg bolus then 1 amp in D_5W	QRS complex >0.10	Volume overload

INR, international normalization ratio

5. **In which patient scenario is an ethanol infusion not absolutely necessary?**
   A. A patient receiving dialysis for a methanol overdose
   B. A patient who admits to taking only a small amount of paint thinner
   C. An unconscious patient with an unexplained osmolar gap and a blood pH without any metabolic derangements
   D. An inebriated patient who is found unconscious at home
   E. A child found unconscious near an empty container of antifreeze

ANSWERS

1. The answer is E. It is generally recommended that a person being treated for a cyclic antidepressant overdose be given a bicarbonate infusion when their QRS complex exceeds 0.10 s. The bicarbonate infusion should be continued until the QRS complex narrows or the blood pH attains a level between 7.50 and 7.55. Salicylate intoxication with systemic toxicity (i.e., confusion, etc.) should prompt a bicarbonate infusion. The goal is a urinary pH approaching 7.50. Alkalinization to a blood pH greater than 7.30 may also help patient outcome in a methanol or ethylene glycol poisoning. An overdose with digoxin would not benefit from a bicarbonate infusion and therefore would be considered the correct answer.
2. The answer is B. Indications for digibind dosing in a digoxin overdose include a potassium level greater than 5.0, a known ingestion of greater than 10 mg, any first-, second-, or third-degree heart block, ventricular tachycardia and fibrillation, or a digoxin concentration greater than 15 ng/dl. There is no clear benefit in supplementing calcium in a patient with a digoxin overdose.
3. The answer is C. Redosing of digibind should be based on signs of toxicity such as cardiac conduction delays, ventricular tachycardias, or fibrillations. Therefore, the reemergence of a second-degree heart block should prompt redosing of digibind. The serum concentration level of digoxin is usually not useful after the initiation of digibind because most serum assays are unable to discriminate between digibind and digoxin. Consequently, digibind redosing based on digoxin concentration levels received after the initial antidote dose is incorrect. Although the half-life of digibind is considerably shorter than digoxin, redosing of digibind should be based on clinical signs and symptoms.
4. The answer is B. Patients who have a seizure disorder who receive benzodiazepines for control of their disorder, as well as those patients who are on benzodiazepines long term, should only be given flumazenil with extreme caution, and some authors would argue that the benefits might not outweigh the potential harm. Patients who are receiving tricyclic antidepressants chronically or concomitantly in an overdose should not receive flumazenil. Gabapentin is occasionally used to treat seizures, but the drug itself does not preclude the usage of flumazenil.
5. The answer is D. Ethanol should be used in any patient with suspected methanol or ethylene glycol ingestion. Ethylene glycol is found in antifreeze, whereas methanol can be found in de-icing solutions, shellac, paint removers and thinners, windshield washer fluid, and carburetor cleaners. Serum methanol or ethylene glycol levels greater than 25 mg/dl should result in immediate dialysis along with the administration of ethanol. Patients with methanol or ethylene glycol ingestion may not have a metabolic acidosis, but they will have an osmolar gap. The anion gap and metabolic acidosis created by an ethylene glycol or methanol overdose may not be evident at presentation because it is the active metabolites that create these metabolic derangements. Therefore, a patient with an unexplained osmolar gap and a history or physical exam compatible with an ethylene glycol or methanol overdose should probably receive an ethanol infusion until the serum levels of these toxins return and confirm or refute the preliminary diagnosis of an ethylene glycol or methanol overdose. Any child with a suspected ingestion of antifreeze should receive an ethanol infusion until the potential threat of an overdose can be ruled out. A patient without suggestion of a methanol or ethylene glycol ingestion should not receive an ethanol infusion prophylactically.

SUGGESTED READING

Ellenhorn's Medical Textbook of Toxicology, 2nd Ed. Baltimore: Williams & Wilkins, 1997.

Goldfrank's Toxicologic Emergencies, 6th Ed. East Norwalk, CT: Appleton & Lange, 1998.

CHAPTER 29

NOAH BRAD SCHREIBMAN AND GERALD M. O'BRIEN

Metabolic Disturbances of Acid–Base and Electrolytes

CHAPTER OUTLINE

LEARNING OBJECTIVES

After studying this chapter, you should be able to:

- Use a systematic approach to identify the nature and chronicity of acid–base disorders.
- Be proficient in calculating the anion gap as well as the delta:delta equations.
- Differentiate between common causes of the anion gap and nonanion gap acidosis.
- Identify common causes of metabolic alkalosis.
- List the common causes, clinical symptoms, and physical examination signs of:
  - Hyponatremia
  - Hypernatremia
  - Hypokalemia
  - Hyperkalemia
  - Hypocalcemia
  - Hypercalcemia
  - Hypomagnesemia
  - Hypermagnesemia
  - Hypophosphatemia
  - Hyperphosphatemia
- Determine the treatment options for the foregoing electrolyte disorders.

A wide range of acid–base and electrolyte disorders are encountered daily by the clinician caring for critically ill patients. The goal of this chapter is to supply the reader with a systematic strategy that can be used when confronted with abnormal serum chemistry and blood gases so that one can successfully arrive at a precise assessment, diagnosis, and therapeutic plan. Several case studies illustrate and help guide this discussion. This chapter does not dwell on the basic pathophysiology of each disorder, but we encourage the reader to refer to the Suggested Reading list at the end of the chapter to learn more about specific areas.

METABOLIC DISORDERS OF ACID–BASE METABOLISM

Terminology

Clinical disorders of acid–base balance are classified according to which of two variables, $PaCO_2$ or serum bicarbonate, HCO_3^-, is altered by underlying pathologic process. A primary change in the $PaCO_2$ is referred to as either a respiratory acidosis or alkalosis. Metabolic disorders are the result of primary changes in the serum concentration of bicarbonate. A decrease in the serum bicarbonate is referred to as metabolic acidosis; an increase in the serum concentration of bicarbonate is referred to as metabolic alkalosis.

A mixed acid–base disorder occurs when two independent pathophysiologic processes result in an alteration of serum bicarbonate or $PaCO_2$ or both.

Primary alterations of the serum bicarbonate result in a series of metabolic events that attempt to maintain the acid–base equilibrium and normal pH. A simple acid–base disturbance is present when one pathologic process results in an alteration of the HCO_3^- (or $PaCO_2$) along with the compensatory alteration of the reciprocal variable. A mixed acid–base disorder is said to occur when two independent pathophysiologic processes result in an alteration of the serum bicarbonate or $PaCO_2$ or both.

Systematic Approach

A step-by-step approach to the analysis of acid–base chemistries is required because two or more disorders may exist simultaneously and one may be dangerously overlooked. This approach should be used every time one is confronted with an abnormal set of electrolytes and blood gases.

Step 1: Identify the Most Obvious Disorder and Check for Internal Consistency

Vérifier si pH / BIC/ pCO2 ont du bon sens...

The mathematical relationship between the $[H^+]$, serum bicarbonate, and $PaCO_2$ can be used to eliminate conflicting findings between the $PaCO_2$ on the blood gas and the measured bicarbonate on the serum electrolyte panel. A few moments of checking for internal consistency can save valuable time and effort.

$$[H^+] = 24 \times PaCO_2/\text{measured } [HCO_3^-]$$

The pH is the negative log of the serum hydrogen ion concentration.

The pH is the negative log of the serum hydrogen ion concentration ($[H^+]$). A normal pH of 7.4 corresponds to a blood hydrogen ion concentration ($[H^+]$) of 40 nanoequivalents per liter. It is important to remember that as $[H^+]$ increases, pH value decreases and vice versa. This relationship is nonlinear (Figure 29-1), but it is nearly linear over the narrow range of pH values normally clinically encountered (7.1–7.5). Within these limits, the pH can be calculated by assuming the pH will change by 0.01 units (up or down) for every 1 nEq/l change in $[H^+]$ (above or below 40 nEq/l). A more accurate estimate of $[H^+]$ is required over the wider range of pH because the slope of the relationship of pH and $[H^+]$ is steeper below

CASE STUDY 1: PART 1

A 19-year-old girl was brought to the emergency room by her mother with complaints of severe nausea and vomiting for several days. She had a history of insulin-dependent diabetes mellitus and chronic depression with a prior attempted suicide and alcoholism. Physical examination showed her to be lethargic, with a temperature of 98.0°F. Respirations were 34/min; heart rate and blood pressure were BP 120/80 mmHg and HR 120/min, supine, and BP 100/70 mmHg and HR 160/min, upright. Laboratory values were Na^+, 136 mEq/l; Cl^-, 70 mEq/l; K^+, 3.6 mEq/l; HCO_3^-, 19 mEq/l; BUN (blood urea nitrogen), 21 mEq/l; serum blood glucose, 580 mg/dl; serum osmolarity, 315 Osm; and ABG (arterial blood gas): pH, 7.58; PaO_2, 104 mmHg; $PaCO_2$, 21 mmHg.

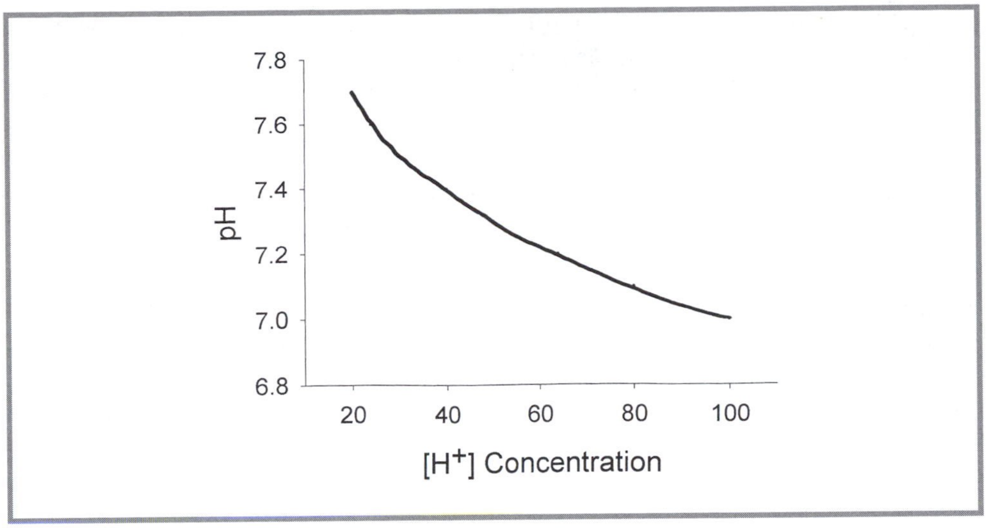

FIGURE 29-1

Relationship of pH to [H^+]. The relationship is nearly linear from pH 7.1 to 7.5, values normally clinically encountered. At pH extremes, the relationship becomes more curvilinear.

7.4. The pH can then be calculated by assuming that the pH will change by 0.008 units for every 1 nEq/l change in the [H^+] above 40 nEq/l and that the pH will change by 0.0125 units for every 1 nEq/l change in the [H^+] below 40 nEq/l. If the calculated pH does not closely agree with the measured pH, then an accurate assessment of the patient's acid–base status cannot be determined. The reasons for this may be laboratory error or that the two tests were drawn at different times and reflect temporal changes in body chemistry.

Step 2: Assess the Compensatory Response

The body's homeostatic mechanisms serve to return the ratio of serum bicarbonate and $PaCO_2$ toward normal and thus normalize the pH. However, there are certain rules that one can apply to help determine the acid–base disturbance. First, the compensatory response always creates a second laboratory abnormality. Second, the compensatory mechanisms fail to fully return the pH to normal. (The only exception to this rule is chronic respiratory alkalosis.) The primary disturbance can then be determined by simply looking at the pH. The absence of compensation can result from (1) a secondary pathophysiologic process, (2) insufficient time for compensatory mechanisms to act, or (3) dysfunction in the renal or respiratory systems.

Compensatory mechanisms never fully return pH to normal.

The expected respiratory compensation for either a metabolic acidosis or alkalosis can be predicted by the following formulas: a $PaCO_2$ that lies outside the predicted limits defines a coexisting respiratory disorder.

$$\text{Metabolic acidosis: } PaCO_2 = 1.5([HCO_3^-]) + 8 \pm 2$$

$$\text{Metabolic alkalosis: } PaCO_2 = 40 + 0.6(\Delta[HCO_3^-])$$

CASE STUDY 1: PART 2

The pH from the arterial blood gas tells us that this patient is alkalemic. The respiratory rate and low $PaCO_2$ suggest a simple respiratory alkalosis. Calculation of the [H^+] using the modified Henderson–Hasselbach equation ([H^+] = 24 × ($PaCO_2/HCO_3^-$), or 24 × 21/19 = 26 mEq. The pH can be calculated by assuming that the pH will change by 0.0125 units for every 1 nEq/l change in the [H^+] below 40 nEq/l. In this case, 0.0125 × 14 = 0.18, giving a calculated pH of 7.40 + 0.18 = 7.58. Therefore, the calculated and the measured pH correlate, which in fact shows internal constancy, as the gases and serum electrolytes were drawn simultaneously.

Thus far, in the case described, the patient has been demonstrated to have a respiratory alkalosis. Despite the fact that the patient's serum bicarbonate is low, as one might expect in compensation for a respiratory alkalosis, it is subsequently demonstrated that a different phenomenon occurred.

Step 3: Determine the Serum Bicarbonate Concentration and the Anion Gap Metabolic Acidosis (Low Serum Bicarbonate)

Calculating the anion gap is the most important step in assessing a metabolic acidosis.

Metabolic acidosis is defined by low serum bicarbonate, which results from either the accumulation of nonvolatile acids or the loss of bicarbonate through the gastrointestinal tract or kidney. The most important step in assessing a metabolic acidosis is to calculate the anion gap (AG). This maneuver should become routine when assessing serum electrolytes as it quickly identifies the presence of an acid–base disturbance, which may occur even in the presence of normal serum bicarbonate concentrations. The equation used to calculate the AG is:

$$AG = [Na^+] - ([Cl^-] + [HCO_3^-])$$

The total body concentration of anions equals the total concentration of cations in the body. However, this equation does not account for all ionic charges in the serum. The unmeasured anions exceed the unmeasured cations, and the difference is called the anion gap (AG). In the normal healthy state, the normal anion gap is 12(±2). Low anion gap rarely occurs in the critically ill patient, but, when present, the most frequent etiology is a change in the serum albumin. It therefore is important to take into account changes in the serum albumin level when calculating the AG. As a rule of thumb, the normal AG is corrected downward for every 1 g/dl reduction in the normal serum albumin concentration. The presence or absence of an elevated AG is used to categorize metabolic acidosis.

Metabolic Acidosis

Elevated AG Acidosis

An anion gap acidosis can be caused by either exogenous or endogenous compounds.

In a high AG acidosis, the rise in serum $[H^+]$ is accompanied by a rise in an unmeasured anion, which is often an organic acid (Table 29-1). This rise may be the result of either endogenous acid production (ketoacids and lactate) or of certain exogenous compounds (ethylene glycol, salicylates, and methanol). The identification of an "osmolar gap" is necessary to identify the presence of an unmeasured toxic substance. The osmolar gap is calculated by determining the difference between the calculated and measured serum osmolarity, which should normally be less than 10 mOsmol. The calculation for serum osmolality is:

$$\text{Serum osmolality} = 2(Na^+) + \text{glucose}/18 + \text{BUN}/2.8$$

Normal AG Acidosis

The two most common causes of normal anion gap acidosis are gastrointestinal and renal losses.

In normal AG acidosis, the fall in bicarbonate is matched by a proportional rise in the serum chloride, often referred to as a hyperchloremic metabolic acidosis. The causes of this form

TABLE 29-1

ELEVATED ANION GAP ACIDOSIS

* GAINS ANIONS *

1. Endogenous sources	II. Exogenous sources
A. Ketoacidosis	A. Salicylate poisoning
1. Diabetic ketoacidosis (DKA)	B. Ethylene glycol (glycolic and oxide acid)
2. Starvation ketoacidosis	C. Methanol
B. Lactic acidosis	D. Ethanol
	E. Paraldehyde

TABLE 29-2

NONANION GAP ACIDOSIS

I. GI losses
   A. Diarrhea
   B. Small bowel function
   C. Ileostomy
II. Urinary losses
   A. Proximal renal tubular acidosis (RTA)
   B. Distal RTA
   C. Acetazolamide obstruction
   D. Urinary obstruction
III. Rapid dilution of plasma bicarbonate by saline
IV. Hydrochloric acid addition

of metabolic acidosis are listed in Table 29-2. This form of acidosis most often results from the loss of [HCO_3^-] from gastrointestinal or renal sources. More rarely, a normal anion gap acidosis results from rapid dilution of the plasma HCO_3^- by saline or addition of hydrochloric acid (or equivalent) to the body fluids, with rapid renal excretion of the accompanying anion and replacement of [HCO_3^-] by [Cl^-].

The approach to the patient with non-AG metabolic acidosis (Figure 29-2) starts with the history and physical examination and the serum potassium concentration ([K^+]). The most common cause of normal AG acidosis is diarrheal illness, which depletes both [HCO_3^-] and [K^+]. Extracellular fluid depletion from voluminous stools results in the elaboration of renin and aldosterone, which enhances renal [K^+] secretion and further worsens the hypokalemia. Hypokalemia is also seen in nonanion gap acidosis caused by both proximal (type II) and distal (type I) renal tubular acidosis (RTA). Nevertheless, metabolic acidosis caused by gastrointestinal losses can be differentiated from RTA by the urinary ammonium ([NH_4^+]) excretion, which is typically low in RTA and high in patients with diarrhea. Urinary ammonium cannot be directly measured, but it is estimated by calculating the urine anion gap (UAG), as follows:

$$\text{Urine } [K^+] + \text{urine } [Na^+] - \text{urine } [Cl^-] = \text{urine anion gap (UAG)}$$

If the sum of the major urinary cations ([Na^+] + [K^+]) is less than the sum of major anions ([Cl^-]), then [$NH^+{}_4$] can be assumed to be present in urine (i.e., a negative urine anion gap). A positive UAG suggests the presence of a proximal RTA (type II) with a distal acidifica-

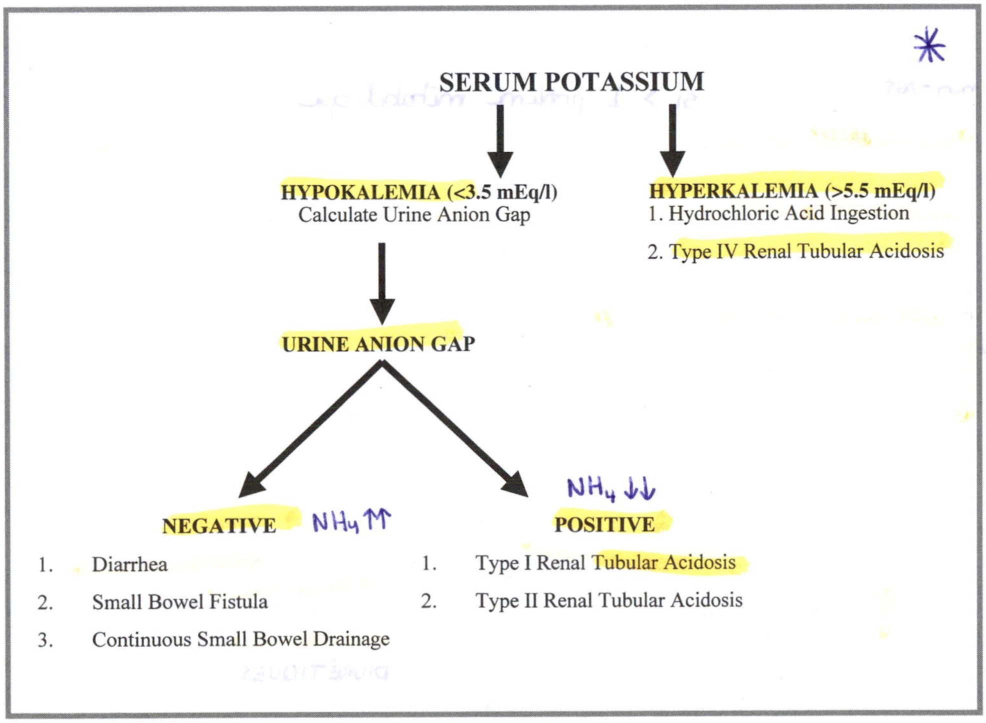

FIGURE 29-2

Algorithm for normal anion gap acidosis. Most causes of normal anion gap acidosis are associated with hypokalemia, but two conditions that occur in the setting of hyperkalemia are hydrochloric acid ingestion and type IV renal tubular acidosis. Calculating the urine anion gap estimates the urinary ammonium (NH_4^+) excretion and is used to differentiate type I and II renal tubular acidosis (positive urine anion gap) from the remaining causes of normal anion gap acidosis with hypokalemia (negative urine anion gap).

CASE STUDY 1: PART 3

The measured serum bicarbonate in this patient was low, which in contrast to the pH suggested the patient was acidotic. In a simple acid–base disorder, we would expect the $[HCO_3^-]$ and $PaCO_2$ to move in opposite directions. Here, both the $[HCO_3^-]$ and $PaCO_2$ were low, which can occur only if the patient has a mixed acid–base disturbance. Calculation of the anion gap revealed a significant gap acidosis of 47 ($[Na^+] - ([Cl^-] + [HCO_3^-])$, or $136 - (70 + 19)$). Clues to the etiology of the anion gap acidosis can be found in the history and physical exam. The history of diabetes mellitus, elevated blood sugar, and noncompliance suggested diabeteic ketoacidosis. Another possibility is alcoholic ketoacidosis. Both diagnoses can be confirmed by measuring the urine and serum ketones and a serum ethanol level. A toxic ingestion is always possible. However, there was no evidence of an osmolar gap. The calculated serum osmolality is $2(Na^+) + glucose/18 + BUN/2.8$, or $2(136) + 580/18 + 21/2.8 = 312$ Osm, the same as the measured serum osmolality. Finally, an elevated serum lactate would result from dehydration and volume depletion. Thus far, two acid–base disorders have been identified: respiratory alkalosis and an anion gap metabolic acidosis.

tion defect and inadequate $[NH_4^+]$ excretion, whereas a negative UAG suggests an extrarenal cause of the hyperchloremic acidosis (see Figure 29-2). The urine pH can also be measured to distinguish between proximal and distal (type I) RTA in which the kidney is unable to lower the urine pH below 5.3. In contrast, the metabolic acidosis caused by hydrochloric acid ingestion and RTA type IV is accompanied by an elevated $[K^+]$. RTA type IV results from generalized distal nephron dysfunction or renin-aldosterone deficiency and is most commonly seen in diabetics.

Metabolic Alkalosis (High Serum Bicarbonate)

The most common cause of metabolic alkalosis is extracellular volume depletion.

Metabolic alkalosis is the process that results in an elevated serum bicarbonate ($[HCO_3^-]$). This disorder occurs as a result of either the loss of $[H^+]$ or the gain of $[HCO_3^-]$. The kidney is extremely efficient in controlling $[HCO_3^-]$ excess, so there must also be an increase in its net reabsorptive capacity to maintain the alkalotic state. The causes of metabolic alkalosis can be divided into those associated with a high urine chloride ($[Cl^-]$) and those associated with a low urine $[Cl^-]$ (Table 29-3). The most common cause of metabolic alkalosis is extracellular volume depletion, wherein urine $[Cl^-]$ is low, and the alkalosis resolves after volume replacement. If the urine $[Cl^-]$ is high (>40 mEq/l), then mineralocorticoid excess, diuretics, or sodium bicarbonate loading are common culprits.

Step 4: Determine the Delta Anion Gap and the Delta:Delta

Using the delta:delta equations will help identify additional metabolic disorders.

This step is useful to identify additional or hidden metabolic disorders by comparing the change in the AG with the change in serum $[HCO_3^-]$. In a simple metabolic acidosis, the decrease in the serum bicarbonate (normal $[HCO_3^-]$ − measured $[HCO_3^-]$) and the increase in the AG (measured AG − 12) should be proportional. This relationship has become known as the delta:delta ($\Delta AG: \Delta[HCO_3^-]$). Another approach is to add the ΔAG to the measured serum $[HCO_3^-]$ value; a resultant value less than the normal serum $[HCO_3^-]$ is a clue that a hidden nonanion gap acidosis is present. Similarly, a resultant value that is higher than the normal serum $[HCO_3^-]$ suggests that a hidden metabolic alkalosis is present.

TABLE 29-3

CAUSES OF METABOLIC ALKALOSIS

I. Associated with low urinary chloride	II. Associated with high urinary chloride
A. Vomiting	A. Mineralocorticoid excess
B. Volume contraction	B. Exogenous $NaHCO_3^-$ therapy
C. Nasogastric suction	C. Corticosteroid abuse

CASE STUDY 1: PART 4

The calculations for determining the delta:delta in our case yielded the following information:

Determination of the Delta AG:

$AG = [(Na^+) - (Cl^- + HCO_3^-)]$

$AG = [(136) - (70 + 19)] = 47$

Normal anion Gap = 12

Delta anion Gap = 47 − 12 = 35

Determination of the Delta $[HCO_3^-]$:

Normal HCO_3^- = 24 mEq/l

Measured HCO_3^- in this patient = 19 mEq/l

Delta HCO_3^- = 24 − 19 = 5 mEq/l

The normal value for serum bicarbonate is 24 mEq/l. Adding the measured serum bicarbonate (19) to the delta anion gap (35) gives a value of 54. This value, obviously, is higher than the normal serum bicarbonate, indicating that this patient also has a severe metabolic alkalosis. Therefore, this patient was found to have a triple acid–base disorder: (1) respiratory alkalosis from hyperventilation, (2) anion gap metabolic acidosis from diabetic ketoacidosis, and (3) a metabolic alkalosis from vomiting and dehydration. She was treated with IV fluids and insulin. Her serum electrolytes and blood gases were normal by the end of 1 week.

ELECTROLYTE DISORDERS

Disorders of Water and Sodium Metabolism

Of all electrolyte disorders, by far the most common is hyponatremia. The number of etiologies and specific disorders that cause hyponatremia is vast and ever growing. However, despite the apparent complexity of the problem, the etiology of most cases of hyponatremia can be determined with a few readily accessible tests, including plasma osmolality, volume status, urine osmolality, and urine sodium.

Hyponatremia is initially classified by osmolality into hypotonic, isotonic, or hypertonic types. Some texts refer to isotonic and hypertonic hyponatremia as pseudohyponatremia. However, this chapter addresses all three osmolality states.

Hyponatremia can be hypotonic, isotonic, or hypertonic.

Hypotonic hyponatremia represents the largest group and usually the most critically ill. Hypotonicity can cause many adverse effects as a result of inevitable intracellular swelling. Among the adverse effects are seizures, neuromuscular excitability, and coma. Usually these effects are not seen early in disease. Some of the common causes of hypotonic hyponatremia, as shown in Table 29-4, can be subdivided into disorders in which renal water excretion is impaired and those in which it is normal. Once it is determined that the patient is hypotonic, the next step is determining the patient's volume status.

Hypotonic Hyponatremia

Low-volume hypotonic hyponatremia, by definition, is a loss of both sodium and water but obviously more sodium. Common causes are diuretics, GI losses, and adrenal insufficiency. A clue for adrenal insufficiency would be high potassium in conjunction with low sodium, a result of decreased aldosterone secretion. High-volume states include congestive heart fail-

CASE STUDY 2: PART 1

A 50-year-old man presented to his primary medical doctor with the complaint of weakness. He stated that for the last 6 months he had felt extremely fatigued at his job as a construction worker. On review of systems, patient also noted that he had lost 15 lb in the past year, had a slight amount of lightheadedness, and had had three episodes of hemoptysis in the last month. The physical exam showed normal vital signs and no abnormalities. Basic metabolic panel reveals a sodium of 120 mEq/l, BUN of 3 mEq/l, and osmolality of 250 mOsmol/kg.

TABLE 29-4

CAUSES OF HYPONATREMIA AND HYPOOSMOLALITY

I. Disorders of impaired renal water excretion
  A. Depleted intravascular volume
    1. Gastrointestinal losses
    2. Renal losses
    3. Skin losses: burns, cystic fibrosis
    4. Edematous states
      a. CHF (congestive heart failure)
      b. Cirrhosis
      c. Nephrotic syndrome
      d. Hypoalbuminemia
  B. Diuretics
  C. States of antidiuretic hormone (ADH) excess
    1. Syndrome of inappropriate ADH secretion (SIADH)
    2. cortisol deficiency
  D. Decreased solute intake
II. Normal renal water excretion
  A. Primary polydipsia
  B. Pregnancy
  C. Malnutrition

ure (CHF), cirrhosis, and other hypoalbuminemic states. Normal volume states are usually divided into the syndrome of inappropriate antidiuretic hormone secretion (SIADH) or psychogenic polydipsia.

Antidiuretic hormone (ADH) and the thirst mechanism are the main by-products of stimulation of osmoreceptors, which are located in the hypothalamus. ADH has its greatest effect on the collecting duct to increase water permeability back into the bloodstream. Therefore, ADH secretion should increase water reabsorption and lead to an increased urine concentration.

In patients with hyponatremia, urine osmolality indicates whether water excretion is normal or impaired.

Checking urine osmolality (UOsm) is useful to determine whether water excretion is normal or impaired. A UOsm less than or equal to 100 MOsmol/kg indicates ADH suppression. Primary polydipsia is an example of hyponatremia with a urine osmolality of less than 100 mOsmol/kg. Conversely, values greater than 100 mOsmol/kg indicate water excretion is impaired (Table 29-4), and include effective circulating volume depletion, the syndrome of inappropriate antidiuretic hormone secretion (SIADH), adrenal insufficiency, and hypothyroidism.

Various simple blood tests and a reliable history will lead the physician to the correct diagnosis from this point. One last confirmatory test is the Una, where a low (less than 25 mEq/l) value clinches the diagnosis of a depleted effective circulating volume.

Hyponatremia with a Normal or High Plasma Osmolality

Hyponatremia in these two categories is often referred to as pseudohyponatremia. Clinically, the distinction between hypoosmotic and nonhypoosmotic hyponatremia is critical because therapy in nonhypoosmotic hyponatremia is not directed toward correcting the sodium. Isotonic hyponatremia is often seen when a preponderance of either lipids or proteins displace

CASE STUDY 2: PART 2

An extensive workup of this patient's hyponatremia was begun. The patient denied any recent nausea, vomiting, or surreptitious use of diuretics. The patient had no history of heart or liver disease and no contradictory evidence on physical examination. Serum transaminases, albumin, bilirubin, and alkaline phosphatase were normal. A chest x-ray, ordered because of the patient's symptom of hemoptysis, revealed a 3 × 3 cm masslike lesion in the right middle lobe. Urine tests were also done; osmolality was 680 mOsmol/kg and urine sodium was 50 mEq/l.

CASE STUDY 2: PART 3

The patient was sent for a CT-guided needle biopsy of the lung mass. Pathology returned as small cell lung cancer. Urine chemistry tests were consistent for SIADH secondary to lung cancer causing hyponatremia. The patient began chemotherapy and water restriction to treat his lung cancer and SIADH, respectively.

sodium in the serum. Common examples are multiple myeloma and uncontrolled diabetes mellitus. Hypertonic hyponatremia is caused by infusions of glucose or mannitol. Again, the measured sodium in these cases does not represent the true sodium. For example, for each 100 mg/dl glucose increase, the serum sodium decreases by 1.6 mEq/l.

↑ 10 glucose → ↓ 3 Na⁺

Treatment of Hyponatremia

Treatment of hyponatremia is directed at two pathways: raising the low sodium itself while at the same time treating the underlying cause. Normal saline is usually sufficient in cases of hypovolemic hypotonic hyponatremia, and water restriction works well in normovolemic or edematous cases. However, in symptoms of seizure, coma, or extreme hyponatremia (<110 mEq/l), the use of hypertonic saline (3%) is indicated.

Central pontine myelinolysis is a rare but often fatal complication of too rapid sodium repletion. If sodium is replenished too quickly, the cells will shrink (from free water shifts), causing central pontine myelinolysis. There is no established rate of sodium correction, but most authors suggest the sodium correction should not exceed 1–2 mmol/h.

Central pontine myelinolysis is a fatal complication of too aggressive correction of hyponatremia.

Hypernatremia

The major difference in the diagnostic considerations between hyponatremia and hypernatremia is that all patients with hypernatremia are, by definition, hyperosmolar. Therefore, the first step in the evaluation of these patients is the determination of volume status. Regardless of the volume status of these patients, they are always free water depleted. Total body water is roughly estimated to be 60% of total weight in kilograms. The equation for free water deficit is as follows:

$$\text{Free water deficit} = (\text{total body water})(\text{measured serum Na}^+ - 145)/145, \text{ or}$$

$$\text{Free water deficit} = (0.6)(\text{body weight in kg})(\text{measured serum Na}^+ - 145)/145$$

Table 29-5 shows the main etiologies of hypernatremia. One of three circumstances must occur for hypernatremia: decreased water ingestion, water loss, or overingestion of sodium. The major categories of water loss include insensible losses (sweating, burns, fever, etc.), renal losses (including central and nephrogenic diabetes insipidus), gastrointestinal losses, hypothalamic disorders, and water loss into cells. The major cause of increased sodium in-

Hypernatremia requires either water loss, decreased water ingestion, or sodium overingestion.

CASE STUDY 3: PART 1

A 65-year-old man with a history of hypertension, diabetes, and ischemic heart disease was brought to the ER complaining of a sudden onset of crushing chest pain. His EKG was consistent with an acute anterior wall myocardial infarction (MI). Enroute to the catheterization lab, the patient went into cardiac arrest. Resuscitation efforts were successful, but only after 15 min. Despite the restoration of sinus rhythm and adequate BP, the patient remained comatose. Basic chemistries on the second ICU day showed Na 164 mEq/l, K 3.9 mEq/l, BUN 36 mEq/l, Cr 0.8 mEq/l, glucose 140 mg/dl, and POsm 332 mOsmol/kg.

TABLE 29-5

CAUSES OF HYPERNATREMIA

- I. Water loss
  - A. Insensible loss
    1. Sweating
    2. Burns
    3. Infection, fevers
  - B. Renal loss
    1. Central diabetes insipidus
    2. Nephrogenic diabetes insipidus
    3. Osmotic diuresis
  - C. GI losses
  - D. Primary hypodypsia
  - E. Water loss into cells
- II. Sodium retention
  - A. Iatrogenic NaCl or $NaHCO_3^-$ administration
  - B. Sodium ingestion

gestion is usually iatrogenic, as occurs during the often indiscriminate use of $NaHCO_3^-$ during cardiopulmonary resuscitation. This problem commonly occurs also in the administration of high-Na^+ feeding to infants.

The body has two basic defense mechanisms to combat the development of hypernatremia: ADH and thirst sensation, which is sensed by hypothalamic osmoreceptors. An interesting dynamic between the two is that, although it is generally accepted that ADH release is the first response of the body, occurring when POsm exceeds 275–285 mOsmol/kg, thirst is the more important regulator. Severe hypernatremia will not occur unless for some reason the patient is unable to ingest water or has a nonfunctional thirst reflex. Hypernatremia is very rarely observed in young alert people, and neurologic compromise is often present in patients with severe hypernatremia. Patients at risk include the physically and mentally handicapped, the elderly, or any condition wherein normal ingestion of water does not occur.

Central and Nephrogenic Diabetes Insipidus

Central and nephrogenic diabetes insipidus are two of the commonest etiologies of hypernatremia in hospitalized patients in general and in ICU patients in particular. The two conditions, however, differ greatly with respect to their causes and treatments. A basic appreciation of ADH function and origin is imperative to understanding these disorders.

ADH is produced in the hypothalamus by the supraoptic and paraventricular nuclei (Figure 29-3). It is then stored in the posterior lobe of the pituitary gland. Intravascular volume depletion is the strongest stimulus for ADH release. ADH action occurs at the collecting duct of the nephron, where it increases water permeability; this increases urine concentration.

> Central diabetes insipidus (CDI) is caused by complete or partial impairment of antidiuretic hormone (ADH) secretion, whereas nephrogenic diabetes insipidus (NDI) is caused by renal unresponsiveness to ADH.

Central diabetes insipidus (CDI) is defined as those conditions where the production and secretion of ADH is either completely or partially impaired. Table 29-6 lists the most common etiologies of CDI, which include head trauma, neurosurgery, hypoxic/ischemic insult, neoplasm, or other miscellaneous insults. All these disorders are characterized by a lack of endogenous ADH, not kidney responsiveness to it. Exogenous ADH will correct the problem in these circumstances.

Nephrogenic diabetes indipidus (NDI), on the other hand, is a disorder in which the production and secretion of ADH are normal but renal unresponsiveness to ADH causes water loss and therefore an unconcentrated urine. There are multiple causes of NDI, ranging from congenital to acquired (Table 29-7). The most common causes of NDI in adults are lithium toxicity, osmotic diuresis (seen in uncontrolled diabetes mellitus or hyperosmolar hyperglycemic nonketotic coma, HHNK), and hypercalcemia.

CASE STUDY 3: PART 2

Throughout the second and third ICU days, the patient's POsm remained 285–290 mOsmol/kg and urine output exceeded 300 ml/h. Urine studies revealed a UOsm of 130 mOsmol/kg and a urine sodium <10 mEq/l. Additionally, the patient's fractional excretion of sodium was <1%. A water restriction test was begun.

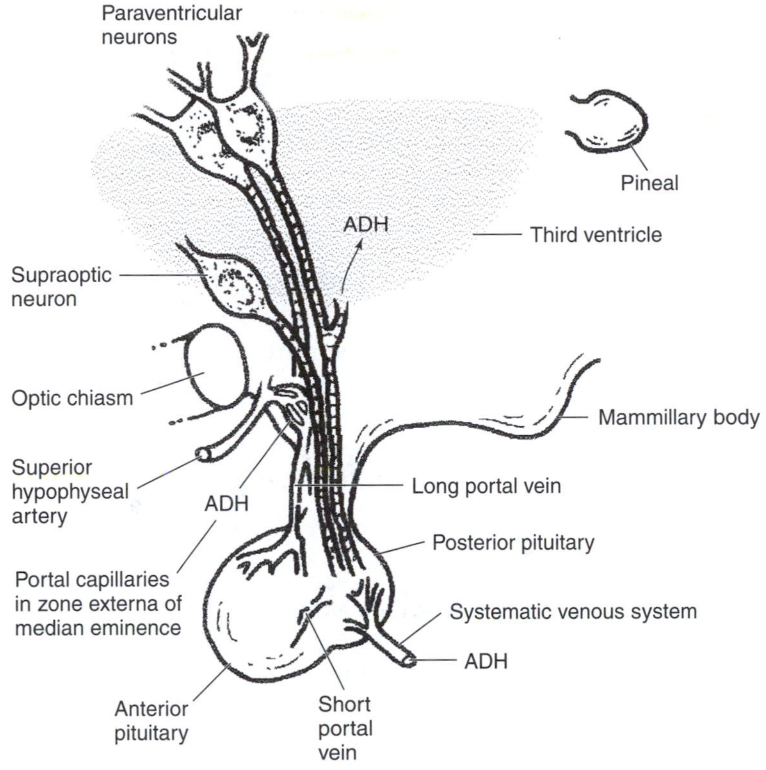

FIGURE 29-3

Production and secretion of antidiuretic hormone (ADH). ADH is produced by the paraventricular and supraoptic nuclei in the hypothalamus, transported down their axons, and secreted at three sites: the posterior pituitary gland, the portal capillaries of the median eminence, and the third ventricular CSF. (Adapted from Rose BD. Clinical Physiology of Acid–Base and Electrolyte Disorders, 4th Ed. New York: McGraw-Hill, 1994, with permission.)

NDI-associated hypercalcemia is often seen in two subsets of patients, those with primary or secondary hyperparathyroidism and those whose hypercalcemia is due to cancer. Usually calcium levels greater than 11 mg/dl are needed before NDI is apparent. The mechanism is not understood, although some investigators believe that calcium deposition in the medulla with resultant tubulointerstitial injury is the cause. The resolution of NDI follows the restoration of normal calcium, although sometimes it takes as long as 12 weeks after normal calcium is restored. Osmotic diuresis as a result of uncontrolled diabetes mellitus is another common cause of NDI. Glucosuria must be present to establish this diagnosis. Other causes of osmotic diuresis observed in the ICU include long-term high-protein enteral tube feedings and mannitol infusions (e.g., as used in cases of increased intracranial pressure).

Lithium is the medication most often implicated in causing nephrogenic diabetes insipidus. Toxic levels usually must be present for NDI, but this is not universally the case. Lithium causes NDI by directly accumulating within the collecting tubule cells, therefore decreasing the generation of cyclic AMP, which is needed for water reabsorption. This condition should be suspected in all patients with diminished mental status in whom hypernatremia is seen, particularly in young patients or those who have a psychiatric history.

> Lithium is the drug most often implicated in NDI.

The distinction between central and nephrogenic DI is not often successfully made at the time of presentation. Few hospitals have the laboratory means to measure endogenous ADH, and complicated clinical scenarios can blur the picture. The easiest and most readily available test to differentiate between CDI and NDI is the water restriction test. Reduced water

> The water restriction test is used to differentiate between CDI and NDI.

TABLE 29-6

CAUSES OF CENTRAL DIABETES INSIPIDUS

I. Idiopathic	IV. Hypoxia or ischemic encephalopathy
II. Status post-neurosurgery	V. Brain neoplasm
III. Head trauma	

TABLE 29-7

CAUSES OF NEPHROGENIC DIABETES INSIPIDUS

- I. Drugs
  - A. Lithium
  - B. Demeclocycline
  - C. Loop diuretic
- II. Osmotic diuresis
  - A. Glucose
  - B. Mannitol
  - C. Urea
- III. Electrolyte disorders
  - A. Hypercalcemia
  - B. Hypokalemia
- IV. Pregnancy (increased peripheral degradation of ADH)

intake will cause an increased plasma osmolality, which should increase ADH secretion and hence increase urine concentration. In CDI, regardless of the increase in plasma osmolality caused by water restriction, the ADH level will never increase and the urine will remain very dilute (Figure 29-4). In NDI, as the POsm rises the urine will remain dilute, but unlike CDI, the level of ADH will appropriately rise. The distinction between CDI and NDI is confirmed by a trial of ADH (vasopressin, or 1-deamino-D-Arg-8 vasopressin, DDAVP). Giving exogenous ADH will increase UOsm for CDI only, as illustrated with the patient in our case.

Symptoms of Hypernatremia

Regardless of the etiology of hypernatremia, the symptoms are quite similar and predominately neurologic in nature. It is thought that these symptoms result from the constant shifting of water in and out of brain cells because of the osmotic gradient. Headache, weakness, dizziness, irritability, and, in severe cases, even seizures and coma can be observed. Other symptoms of hypernatremia include those related to a patient's particular volume status, whether volume depleted (e.g., jugular venous distension (JVD) <5 cmH_2O, poor skin turgor, orthostatic hypotension) or volume overloaded (e.g., pulmonary or peripheral edema). Patients with diabetes insipidus with an intact mental status rarely have signs or symptoms or volume loss. Common symptoms in patients with either CDI or NDI include polyuria, nocturia, and polydypsia; this allows another use of the water restriction test, differentiating primary polydipsia for CDI or NDI. Last, patients with CDI or NDI are prone to develop hydroureter, or hydronephrosis, as a result of conscious efforts to minimize repeated urination.

Diagnosis and Treatment

Diagnosing hypernatremia depends on an increased serum Na^+ level and the appropriate clinical setting. There are some key diagnostic points to remember. First, thirst provides the main protection from hypernatremia, and so long as one has an intact thirst mechanism and access to water, hypernatremia will not develop. The second diagnostic point is the importance of checking a patient's volume status. Very few disorders cause either hypervolemic (primary hyperaldosteronism, iatrogenic $NaHCO_3^-$), or euvolemic (CDI, NDI) hypernatremia. The third and fourth diagnostic points are the utility of UOsm and the water restriction test in differentiating among various disorders.

Treatment of hypernatremia is directed toward treating both the high sodium and the underlying disorder.

Treatment of hypernatremia is directed toward treating both the high sodium and the underlying disease. Specific treatments for specific etiologies are not discussed here; most are

CASE STUDY 3: PART 3

A water restriction test was begun for this patient. After 12 h, his urine output was still 300–400 ml/h. A trial of 5 units of vasopressin was begun. After 3 h, his urine output was 35 ml/h and his measured UOsm was 450 mOsmol/kg. A diagnosis of central diabetes insipidus was made, secondary to anoxic encephalopathy suffered during cardiac arrest. A standing dose of 2 units vasopressin subcutaneously was started, with correction of his serum sodium to 142 mEq/l by the fifth hospital day. However, the patient's mental status never improved; he was placed on comfort care 1 week later, and later expired.

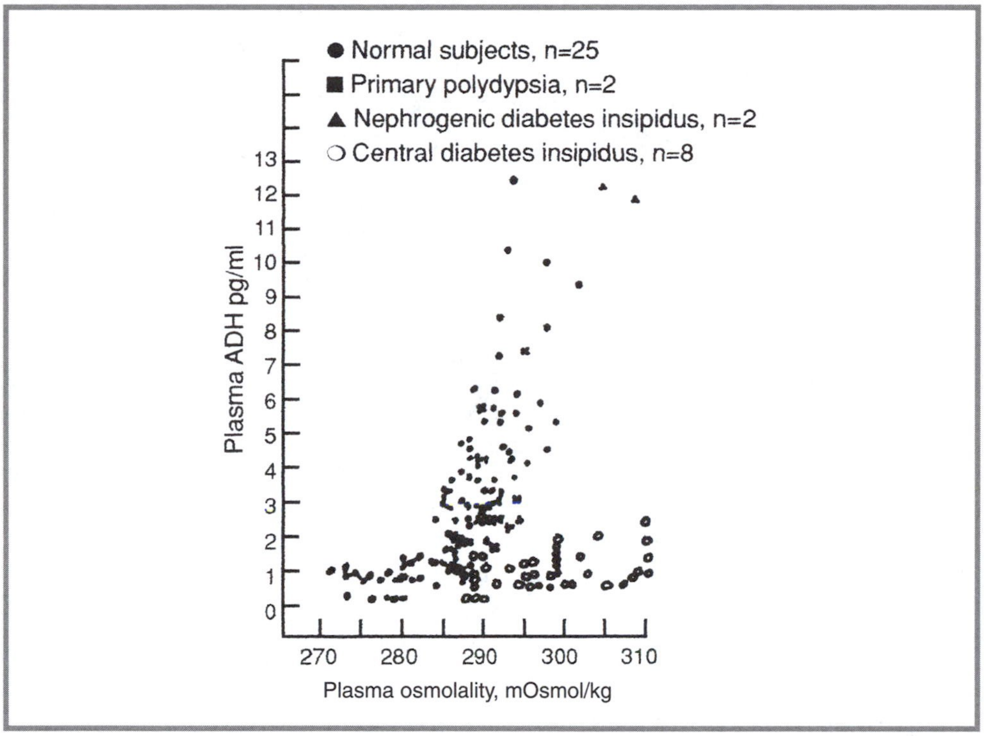

FIGURE 29-4

Response of plasma ADH to plasma osmolality. The water restriction raises plasma osmolality. In normal subjects and those with primary polydipsia and nephrogenic diabetes insipidus, plasma ADH rises in an attempt to reabsorb water. Central diabetes insipidus is defined as partial or complete impairment of ADH secretion, despite increasing plasma osmolality. (Adapted from Rose BD. Clinical Physiology of Acid–Base and Electrolyte Disorders, 4th Ed. New York: McGraw-Hill, 1994, with permission.)

obvious (e.g., DDAVP for CDI, discontinuation of lithium for NDI, fluid repletion for insensible losses). Rather, the general principles of free water repletion are discussed.

When hypernatremia is corrected too rapidly, severe fluid shifts can result in cerebral cells, causing cerebral edema, brain damage, and even death. Therefore, it is advised to correct Na^+ slowly unless the patient has significant symptoms. Lowering sodium by 0.5 mEq/h, or 12 mEq/day, has been suggested. Additionally, after calculating the free water deficit, the rate of free water repletion should be half the total projected deficit in the first 12–24 h, with slow correction thereafter. Finally, in cases of hypovolemic hypernatremia, normal saline should be used first to correct volume status before more hypotonic fluids are used to further correct the sodium concentration.

Serum Potassium Disorders

Hypokalemia

Potassium differs widely from sodium in terms of body distribution. About 98% of body potassium is intracellular. The balance between sodium and potassium is maintained by the sodium-potassium ATPase pump in the cell membrane.

About 98% of total body potassium is intracellular.

CASE STUDY 4

A 21-year-old collegiate athlete on a gymnastics scholarship complained of dizziness and leg weakness. She had had increased fatigue in both lower extremities (proximal and distal) since the athletic season started 1 month ago. She has had no recent trauma or previous episodes of lightheadedness or syncope. Physical examination revealed frequent ectopy on heart exam. Neurologic exam was unremarkable, including negative Chvostek's sign. EKG revealed frequent premature ventricular beats. Sodium, 138 mEq/l; potassium, 2.0 mEq/l.

TABLE 29-8

MAJOR CAUSES OF HYPOKALEMIA

I. Increased GI losses
II. Increased urinary losses
  A. Diuretics (loop and thiazide)
  B. Mineralocorticoid excess
  C. Sodium reabsorption with a nonreabsorbable anion
    1. Vomiting
    2. Penicillin
  D. Amphotericin B
  E. Hypomagnesemia
  F. L-Dopa
III. Intracellular shift
  A. Alkalemia
  B. Insulin excess
  C. Increased beta-agonist activity
IV. Dialysis
V. Increased sweat loss

Hypokalemia has significance in the critical care arena and a multitude of etiologies (Table 29-8). Hypokalemia can be seen with decreased net intake, increased entry into cells, increased gastrointestinal losses, increased urinary losses, increased sweat losses, and dialysis.

Diuretic use is the most common cause of hypokalemia.

Diuretic use, loop or thiazide is the most common cause of hypokalemia. High levels of both urinary chloride and potassium verify this diagnosis. Other causes of urinary potassium loss include type 1 RTA (hypokalemic, hyperchloremic acidosis), amphotericin B administration, and hypomagnesemia. Diarrhea, intestinal fistulas, tube drainage, and chronic laxative abuse are examples of gastrointestinal losses. Many conditions cause increased entry of potassium into cells, such as alkalosis, insulin, beta-agonists, and aldosterone.

Symptoms and Treatment

Hypokalemia is associated with a wide range of complications, the most serious of which are cardiovascular.

Muscle weakness and paralysis, rhabdomyolysis, hyperglycemia, renal dysfunction, and cardiac arrhythmias are signs of hypokalemia (Table 29-9). Cardiac complications include a number of reported arrhythmias, such as premature atrial and ventricular beats, sinus bradycardia, atrioventricular block, and v-tach/v-fib. Various clinical scenarios increase the risk of arrhythmias from hypokalemia, including cardiac ischemia, left ventricular hypertrophy (LVH), and digitalis use. Potassium is essential for ventricular repolarization, and with hypokalemia, many EKG changes are seen. Some are ST segment depression, appearance of "u" waves, PR interval prolongation, and widening of the QRS complex.

If left untreated, low serum potassium can have multiple deleterious effects on kidney function. Rhabdomyolysis is usually not seen unless the serum potassium level is below 2.5 mEq/l.

The main principle in the treatment of hypokalemia is that rapid administration of potassium is potentially harmful and should be used only in life-threatening situations. Intravenous potassium should be given at no more than 10–20 mEq/l/h. Oral potassium supplements are usually adequate to replete deficits in most patients. Patients with DKA who actually have a low rather than high serum potassium represent a marked deviation from this principle.

Hyperkalemia

Diabetic ketoacidosis (DKA) and digitalis overdose are two very frequent causes of hyperkalemia in the critical care arena.

The three major categories of hyperkalemia are increased intake, movement from cells into extracellular fluid, and decreased urinary excretion (Table 29-10). Examples of intraextracellular shifts are diabetic ketoacidosis (DKA), acidosis, beta-adrenergic blockade, digitalis overdose, and succinylcholine administration.

TABLE 29-9

CONSEQUENCES OF HYPOKALEMIA

I. Muscle weakness
II. Cardiac arrhythmias, exacerbated by:
  A. Digitalis
  B. Ischemia
  C. Left ventricular hypertrophy
III. Rhabdomyolysis
IV. Renal dysfunction

CASE STUDY 5: PART 1

A 25-year-old Caucasian man with no known medical history came into the emergency room complaining of nausea and vomiting for 2 days. The patient also complained of fever and rusty-colored sputum. Physical exam revealed bronchial breath sounds over the right middle lung field. Chest x-ray revealed a right middle lung infiltrate. Laboratory values were WBC, 16,000/mm^3 (84 segs, 8 bands); sodium, 130 mEq/l; potassium, 6.7 mEq/l; chloride, 103 mEq/l; HCO_3^-, 5 mEq/l; glucose, 700 mg/dl. EKG showed global peaked T waves. The patient was immediately volume resuscitated with 2 l normal saline, and an insulin drip at 10 units/h was started.

Case studies illustrates that, although the patient's acidosis and hyperglycemia led to a high level of extracellular potassium, in reality his total body potassium was depleted at the time of presentation. The insulin, by reversing his acidosis and the potassium shift out of cells, made his extracellular potassium dangerously low, precipitating the fatal arrhythmia. A critical mistake was made in not following through on the serum chemistries to guard against potassium depletion.

Symptoms, Diagnosis, and Treatment

Besides muscle weakness and cardiac arrhythmias, no other symptoms are directly related to hyperkalemia. However, these patients present with many other complaints, related to the underlying disease that caused hyperkalemia in the first place. Cardiac changes are common and usually directly related to the level of extracellular measured potassium (Figure 29-5). Peaked T wave and a shortened QT interval are among the first changes and are thought to represent rapid repolarization; these changes are seen when the serum concentration is below 7 mEq/l. Above 7 mEq/l, changes are seen that reflect delayed depolarization, including widening of the QRS complex, and, finally, the sine wave pattern, as the QRS complex merges with the T wave. Ventricular fibrillation can soon follow. These changes are not uniformly seen at these levels in all patients, mostly because of other factors (calcium, sodium, acid–base status) that influence electrical cardiac activity. Frequent EKG monitoring is a must.

A large variety of electrocardiographic changes are observed with hyperkalemia; the most serious occur when serum potassium is >7 mEq/l.

The evaluation and diagnosis of hyperkalemia begins with the history, especially information concerning kidney disease, medications (i.e., potassium-sparing diuretics, angiotensin-converting enzyme inhibitors), and muscle weakness. After physical exam, EKG, serum chemistries, and arterial blood gas are done.

The main principle of treatment of hyperkalemia is determining the severity of hyperkalemia according to the clinical scenario (Table 29-11). Life-threatening situations call for the use of IV calcium, which has been shown in various studies to have cardioprotective effects within 5 min. Other therapies, such as beta-agonists, insulin, and glucose, can be used next (although their effect is, of course, temporary). Binding resins are used for final excretion from the body. Antagonism of membrane actions, increased potassium entry into cells, and removal of excess potassium are the three major mechanisms of the therapies. In a patient with merely a high potassium but not signs of muscle weakness or EKG abnormalities, a binding resin can be used as first-line therapy, with frequent EKG monitoring.

Intravenous calcium is the first step in the treatment of life-threatening hyperkalemia.

An appreciation of total body potassium in addition to extracellular potassium is crucial to understanding and treating both hypokalemia and hyperkalemia. Cardiac arrhythmias are

TABLE 29-10

MAJOR CAUSES OF HYPERKALEMIA

I. Shift into extracellular fluid
   A. Acidosis
   B. Insulin deficiency
   C. Beta blockade
   D. Digitalis overdose
   E. General anesthesia (succinylcholine)

II. Decreased excretion
   A. Renal failure
   B. Hypoaldosteronism
   C. Type I RTA

III. Increased intake, either oral or intravenous

CASE STUDY 5: PART 2

The patient was given IV Azithromycin in addition to the volume resuscitation and continuous intravenous insulin. The patient had no further nausea or vomiting. A recent finger stick revealed a blood sugar of 250 mg/dl, so the patient's fluids were changed to $D_5{}^1/_2$ normal saline at 150 ml/h, and the insulin drip was changed to 5 units/h. At the time, the resident in charge asked the third-year medical student to obtain more serum chemistries. The patient refused blood testing, and no further changes were made in his management for the next 4 h. While in the elevator being transported to his hospital room, the patient developed ventricular fibrillation and expired.

the major complications. Treatment principles for both hypokalemia and hyperkalemia are determined by the severity of clinical signs and symptoms. Frequent cardiac monitoring is implemented because a clear correlation between measured potassium and cardiac abnormalities is not always demonstrated.

Serum Calcium, Magnesium, and Phosphate Disorders

Calcium

Parathyroid hormone, calcitonin, and vitamin D are the three main regulatory hormones in calcium homeostasis.

No electrolyte is under such complicated and multifactorial regulation as is calcium. Often found incidentally on routine blood screens in the outpatient setting, calcium abnormalities can have disastrous consequences. The three main regulatory hormones in calcium homeostasis are parathyroid hormone (PTH), calcitonin, and vitamin D (Table 29-12). These three hormones have as their major sites of action, bone, intestine, and the kidneys, respectively. One of the sterol hormones, vitamin D is synthesized in the skin by means of ultraviolet radiation. It then undergoes 25-hydroxylation in the liver and 1-alpha hydroxylation in the kidneys. The final product ($1,25(OH)_2D_3$) increases absorption of calcium and phosphate in the intestine and kidney and increases calcium resorption from bone. PTH increases resorption of both calcium and phosphate from bone, while increasing calcium resorption and decreasing phosphate resorption in the kidney. PTH also stimulates conversion of $25\text{-}D_3$ to its final product. Calcitonin has antagonistic effects toward PTH in both bone and kidney.

Hypercalcemia Etiologies of hypercalcemia include parathyroid related, malignancy related, vitamin D related, endocrine disorders, and renal failure (Table 29-13).

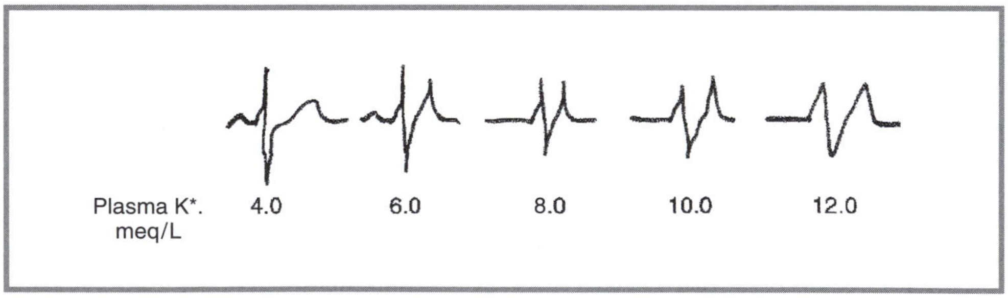

FIGURE 29-5

Electrocardiographic changes in hyperkalemia. The initial changes observed are peaking and narrowing of the T wave with a short QT interval. As hyperkalemia worsens, QRS widening, decreased amplitude, loss of the P wave, and the sine wave pattern (QRS-T wave merging) appear. These changes are observed at the approximate potassium levels illustrated, but there is substantial individual variability. (Adapted from Rose BD. Clinical Physiology of Acid–Base and Electrolyte Disorders, 4th Ed. New York: McGraw-Hill, 1994, with permission.)

TABLE 29-11

TREATMENT OF HYPERKALEMIA

I. Acute/life-threatening scenarios	II. Nonlife-threatening
A. Intravenous calcium	A. Beta agonists
B. Intravenous insulin and glucose	B. Insulin/glucose
C. Dialysis	C. Binding resins

Primary parahyperthyroidism is the most common cause of hypercalcemia. The diagnosis is made by both a high calcium and a high PTH level. About 80% of cases of primary parahyperthyroidism are caused by solitary adenomas; the remainder are caused by four-gland parathyroid hyperplasia. Hypercalcemia secondary to parahyperthyroidism is often found on routine laboratory checks in asymptomatic patients. Hypercalcemia secondary to malignancy often presents as a medical emergency. Organ systems involved include CNS (confusion, loss of memory, depression, somnolence, coma), neuromuscular (weakness), rheumatologic (joint pain, calcium pyrophosphate crystals, chondrocalcinosis), dermatologic (rash and pruritus), GI (nausea, vomiting, dyspepsia, constipation), renal (nephrolithiasis, polyuria, renal colic), and cardiovascular (hypertension, potentiation of cardiac effects of digoxin, and various EKG changes such as PR prolongation, QRS widening, QT segment shortening, and T-wave flattening).

Primary hyperparathyroidism and malignancy are the two most common causes of hypercalcemia.

Malignancies causing hypercalcemia include both solid tumors (lung, breast, kidney) and hematologic malignancies (multiple myeloma). These tumors secrete a PTH-like hormone, with a negative feedback effect on PTH secretion. These patients have high calcium in the presence of a low PTH. Other causes of hypercalcemia include granulomatous diseases such as sarcoidosis (increased vitamin D_3 production in macrophages), renal failure (e.g., diabetic nephropathy), and lithium toxicity (increased PTH threshold for negative feedback).

The standard of care for hypercalcemia starts with intravenous fluid repletion.

Treatment for hypercalcemia begins with aggressive IV repletion, usually normal saline (Table 29-14). A loop diuretic is employed once the patient is determined to be in a euvolemic state. More long-term maintenance therapies, especially in the case of malignancy-related hypercalcemia, include bisphosphonates such as pamidronate. These agents reduce bone turnover of calcium. The dose of pamidronate is 60–90 mg IV infused over 1–3 h. Other principles in the treatment of hypercalcemia include a low calcium diet and, if the patient is taking digitalis, an awareness that hypercalcemia lowers the threshold for the adverse effects of digitalis.

Hypocalcemia Hypocalcemia is defined by ionized calcium less than 1 mmol/l or total serum calcium less than 8.5 mg/dl in the presence of a normal serum albumin level. The major etiologies of hypocalcemia include parathyroid hormone related (insufficiency or suppression), vitamin D shortage, hyperphosphotemia (chelates calcium), hypoalbuminemia, hypomagnesemia, and pancreatitis.

Clinical findings predominately involve the neuromuscular system (muscle weakness, fatigue, and neuromuscular irritability in the form of spasms or seizures), cardiac manifestations (prolongation of the QT interval, resistance to digitalis, hypotension, congestive heart failure), and laryngospasm and respiratory arrest from neuromuscular weakness.

Two common clinical signs used to diagnose hypocalcemia and differentiate it from other forms of neuromuscular weakness are Chvostek's sign and Troussea's sign. Chvostek's sign

Chvostek's and Troussea's signs are two common clinical maneuvers that can identify hypocalcemia.

CASE STUDY 6

A 63-year-old man with a history of non-small cell lung cancer stage IIIa presented to the ER with a change in mental status during the preceding 2 days. His wife reported poor oral intake and weight loss over the past 2 weeks. The patient was afebrile, with evidence of volume depletion indicated by significant orthostatic changes in both heart rate and blood pressure. The measured calcium was 13 mEq/l and the measured albumin was 1.8 mEq/l.

TABLE 29-12

ACTIONS OF MAJOR CALCIUM-REGULATING HORMONES

	BONE	KIDNEY	INTESTINE
Parathyroid hormone (PTH)	Increases resorption of calcium and phosphate	Increases reabsorption of calcium; decreases reabsorption of phosphate; increases conversion of 25-OHD_3 to 1,25-$(OH)_2D_3$; decreases reabsorption of bicarbonate	No direct effects
Calcitonin (CT)	Decreases resorption of calcium and phosphate	Decreases reabsorption of calcium and phosphate; questionable effect on vitamin D metabolism	No direct effects
Vitamin D	Maintains Ca^{2+} transport system	Decreases reabsorption of calcium	Increases absorption of calcium and phosphate

SOURCE: Adapted from Greenspan FS. Basic and Clinical Endocrinology, 3rd ed. East Norwalk, CT: 1991, with permission

is elicited by tapping the facial nerve anterior to the ear lobe, slightly below the zygomatic arch. A positive response is defined by twitching of the facial muscles innervated by the facial nerve on the stimulated side. Troussea's sign involves inflating an upper extremity sphygmomanometer cuff above systolic blood pressure for a period of no less than 2 min; a positive response is defined by development of a carpal spasm.

Treatment of hypocalcemia is stratified into management for severe symptomatic versus asymptomatic patients (Table 29-15). The largest worry in patients with hypocalcemia and clinical signs of tetany (positive Chvostek's or Troussea's sign) is the development of laryngeal spasm, stridor, and loss of airway protection. Treatment options always include IV calcium in the form of calcium gluconate, corection of magnesium and phosphate abnormalities, frequent EKG monitoring, and establishment of a safe airway. Anticonvulsants may be needed in severe cases before calcium repletion is complete. Patients who are hypocalcemic secondary to excision of hyperfunctioning parathyroid glands may be vitamin D resistant and have hypocalcemia refractory to a standard level of repletion. This condition is often termed the hungry bones syndrome. These patients require increased levels of IV calcium repletion and more frequent monitoring of levels.

Laryngospasm with subsequent loss of airway protection is the gravest consequence of hypocalcemia.

Complications are sometimes observed with too aggressive repletion of calcium, such as hypercalcemia and hypercalciuria. Stone formation is a frequent problem. Thiazide diuretics are used in these cases.

Magnesium

Magnesium is an important cofactor for multiple enzymatic reactions involving energy utilization. Primarily an intracellular cation, with less than 1% found in the serum, magnesium is important for multiple processes, including Na–K ATPase channels, stability of mem-

TABLE 29-13

MAJOR CAUSES OF HYPERCALCEMIA

I. Parathyroid gland
   A. Adenoma
   B. Four-gland hyperplasia
   C. Carcinoma
II. Malignancy
   A. Lung
   B. Breast
   C. Kidney
   D. Lymphoma
   E. Multiple myeloma
III. Endocrine
   A. Hyperthyroidism
   B. Pheochromocytoma
   C. Paget's disease
IV. Vitamin D intoxication
V. Renal failure

TABLE 29-14

TREATMENT OF HYPERCALCEMIA

I. Emergent treatment	II. Nonemergent treatment
A. Normal saline (2–3 l over 3–6 h)	A. Adequate fluid intake
B. Lasix (40–100 mg every 2–4 h)	B. Bisphosphonates
C. Calcitonin	C. Oral calcium restriction
D. Bisphosphonates (60–90 mg infused over 1–3 h)	D. Knowledge of outpatient medication regimen (especially digitalis)
E. Dialysis	

branes, mitosis/meiosis, and muscle contraction. Various states in which higher levels of magnesium are needed include critical illness, pregnancy, diarrhea, or diuresis. Magnesium is absorbed in the small intestine and excreted via the kidney. In times of extreme magnesium depletion, the kidney is able to severely restrict excretion (<1 mmol/day). Hence, urinary magnesium levels are very useful in determining etiologies of hypomagnesemia.

Hypomagnesemia Hypomagnesemia is quite common in the ICU, with various studies reporting prevalence at 10%–65%. The three most common main categories of hypomagnesemia are (1) intracellular serum shifts, (2) GI losses, and (3) renal losses. Common causes of intracellular shifts include chelation by tissues during pancreatitis and rhabdomyolysis or shifts from insulin therapy. Excess GI wasting can result from malabsorption, diarrhea, nasogastric suction, or fistulas. High urinary magnesium levels in the face of hypomagnesemia suggest a primary renal cause. The most common cause of renal wasting of magnesium is drug toxicity. Cyclosporine, amphotericin B, digitalis, aminoglycosides, and diuretics (loop and thiazide) are frequent culprits.

Hypomagnesemia is very common in the critical care setting.

Hypomagnesemia affects multiple organ systems, including the cardiovascular (arrhythmias, vasospasm, angina), neuromuscular (weakness, spasms, seizures, tetany), and gastrointestinal systems (anorexia, dysphagia, nausea).

Treatment of hypomagnesemia depends on the acuteness or chronicity of the disorder. Acute hypomagnesemia requires IV repletion, in the form of magnesium sulfate. Often low potassium is present, and this should be treated. One dangerous aspect of magnesium deficiency is that cardiac arrhythmias are seen with deficient stores of magnesium not reflected in the serum levels. In life-threatening situations, 8–16 mmol should be given over 5 min; this rate is changed to over 3 h in severe depletion without cardiac arrhythmias. Chronic magnesium depletion is most commonly treated with oral magnesium.

Cardiac arrhythmias are seen with deficient stores of magnesium, even with normal magnesium serum levels.

Hypermagnesemia Hypermagnesemia is extremely uncommon in patients with normal renal function. Hypermagnesemia is often seen after ingestion of antacids or laxatives containing magnesium in patients with renal failure. Lithium intoxication, hypothyroidism, and adrenal insufficiency are other causes.

Clinical effects are not closely related to serum measurements of magnesium. CNS (change in mental status, confusion, coma), cardiovascular (prolonged PR, QRS, ST, heart block), and neuromuscular (depressed deep tendon reflexes, paralysis, respiratory muscle paralysis) changes are a few of the major consequences. Treatment modality chosen depends on the severity of organ system damage. In life-threatening cases, IV calcium is given to stabilize

Treatment of life-threatening hypermagnesemia involves intravenous calcium (for stabilization of cardiac membranes) and dialysis.

TABLE 29-15

TREATMENT OF HYPOCALCEMIA

I. Severe life-threatening
   A. Calcium gluconate (10 ml 10% solution over 10 min) or calcium chloride (10 ml 10% solution in 50 ml D_5W over 30 min
   B. 1–2 mg/kg/h of elemental calcium if symptoms persist
   C. Correct magnesium, potassium, and phosphorus abnormalities
II. Asymptomatic
   A. Calcium gluconate 2–4 g/day, divided into doses q6h
   B. Vitamin D preparation

neuromuscular and cardiac membrane instability while magnesium is removed via dialysis. In less acute cases, IV fluids (saline) and loop diuretics are given to increase elimination.

Phosphorus

Serum phosphate is under the control of both the parathyroid gland and the kidney. Clinically significant hypophosphatemia is usually less than 2 mg/dl. The kidney is quite adept at phosphate retention in states of phosphate depletion. A 24-h urine phosphate greater than 100 mg when the serum phosphate is less than 2 mg/dl suggests renal disease. Etiologies of hypophosphatemia include intracellular shifts, sepsis, alkalosis, alcoholism, DKA, and salicylate poisoning.

Hypophosphatemia often has disastrous neuromuscular complications.

Similar to magnesium and calcium, low levels of phosphorus can have disastrous neuromuscular complications, including respiratory muscle paralysis, CNS changes, and skeletal myopathy. Less commonly seen are hematologic manifestations (hemolysis and impaired platelet function.

Treatment includes IV potassium phosphate (2.5–5.0 mg/kg/q6h) for acute circumstances. Serum phosphorus, potassium, calcium, and magnesium levels should be checked every 12 h. When phosphorus levels are above 2 mg/dl, an oral sodium phosphate is used. The most important principle in treating hypophosphatemia is monitoring calcium and magnesium levels as well. In a patient with hypercalcemia, correcting the phosphate first will lead to the formation of calcium phosphate crystals, which can deposit anywhere with disastrous consequences, including irreversible joint dysfunction.

Sepsis, rhabdomyolysis, hypothermia, and tumor lysis syndrome are the most common etiologies of hyperphosphatemia encountered in the ICU.

Hyperphosphatemia (serum phosphate level >4.5 mg/dl) can be caused by increased intestinal absorption, parenteral administration, renal dysfunction, frank renal failure, hyperthyroidism, or massive extracellular shifts, such as seen in sepsis, hypothermia or hyperthermia, rhabdomyolysis, or tumor lysis syndromes, such as after chemotherapy for various lymphomas. The most common causes of hyperphosphatemia seen in the ICU are sepsis, rhabdomyolysis, hypothermia, and tumor lysis syndrome. Clinical manifestations are few. Rather, symptoms of the underlying cause (i.e., tumor lysis syndrome) predominate. First-line therapy includes calcium-containing antacids, which bind phosphorus in the gut. High rates of IV fluids and acetozolamide are effective at increasing urine phosphate excretion. Attempts are also made to restrict the patient's phosphorus intake to less than 200 mg/day. Dialysis (either hemodialysis or peritoneal dialysis) is used in cases of renal failure.

SUMMARY

Disturbances of acid–base balance and electrolytes are common in critical care. Acid–base disorders can be simple or complex, acute or chronic, incidental or life-threatening. As demonstrated by the clinical cases presented, a systematic approach is used to identify the nature of acid–base disorders, with particular emphasis given to anion gap metabolic acidosis, nonanion gap metabolic acidosis, and metabolic alkalosis.

Electrolyte abnormalities have the potential for severe clinical sequelae, and treatment for all abnormalities is based on the severity of clinical findings. Through reading this chapter, you should gain a broad appreciation of the diversity and clinical relevance of acid–base and electrolyte disorders in the critically ill patient.

REVIEW QUESTIONS

1. **Identify the acid–base disturbance in the following patients:**
   - **A.** A 25-year-old asthmatic presents acutely short of breath comes to the ER with pH 7.56, $paCO_2$ 20, HCO_3^- 24, and O_2 saturation 96%.
   - **B.** A 30-year-old woman with a history of eating disorder comes into the ER with a change in mental status and vomiting. An empty bottle of aspirin is found in the patient's bedroom. Chemistries are Na^+ 134 mEq/l, K^+ 4.3 mEq/l, Cl^- 90 mEq/l, HCO_3^- 10 mEq/l, BUN 20 mEq/l, creatinine 0.7 mEq/l, glucose 110 mg/dl; ABG: pH 7.52, $PaCO_2$ 28 mmHg, PaO_2 73 mmHg, O_2 saturation 96%.

2. **All the following are causes of anion gap metabolic acidoses except:**
   - **A.** Salicylate poisoning
   - **B.** Diabetic ketoacidosis
   - **C.** Ethylene glycol
   - **D.** Vomiting
   - **E.** Lactic acidosis

3. **All the following cause hypotonic hyponatremia except:**
   - **A.** Vomiting
   - **B.** Syndrome of inappropriate antidiuretic hormone secretion
   - **C.** Mannitol ingestion
   - **D.** Primary polydipsia
   - **E.** Congestive heart failure

4. **By accumulating in the renal collecting tubule cells, this is the drug most commonly implicated in causing nephrogenic diabetes insipidus:**
   - **A.** Lasix
   - **B.** Lithium
   - **C.** Beta-blockers
   - **D.** Thiazide diuretics
   - **E.** Haldol

5. **Diabetic ketoacidosis is a clinical scenario in which, despite initial laboratory results, the patient is actually**
   - **A.** Total body hypokalemic
   - **B.** Total body hyperkalemic
   - **C.** Total body normokalemic

6. **Why do patients with hypercalcemia secondary to malignancy have low PTH levels?**

7. **Describe the following maneuvers:**
   - **A.** Chvostek's sign
   - **B.** Trousseu's sign

8. **The first step that should be taken in the management of life-threatening hypermagnesemia is:**
   - **A.** Normal saline
   - **B.** Loop diuretic
   - **C.** IV calcium
   - **D.** Dialysis

ANSWERS

1. The answer is A. Acute respiratory alkalosis. The patient is hyperventilating, as can be observed by the fall in $PaCO_2$ and rise in pH. The serum bicarbonate level has not changed from its normal value; therefore, there is no metabolic compensation.
   The answer is B. Triple acid–base disorder. The high pH combined with a low $PaCO_2$ reveals respiratory alkalosis. However, the patient had a low serum HCO_3^-, consistent with an acidosis. The anion gap ($[Na^+] - (Cl^- + HCO_3^-]$) is elevated at 34, so the patient also has an anion gap metabolic acidosis, probably from salicylate ingestion. The patient has a delta anion gap ($34 - 12$) of 22, and if this value is added to the patient's measured HCO_3^- of 10, we get a value of 32, which is a higher than normal serum bicarbonate level of 24. Therefore, the patient also has a metabolic alkalosis, probably from vomiting after ingestion.
2. The answer is D. Salicylate poisoning, DKA, ethylene glycol, and lactic acidosis are common causes of anion gap metabolic acidosis. Excessive vomiting almost always results in a metabolic alkalosis secondary to volume contraction.
3. The answer is C. All the choices listed cause hyponatremia. However, mannitol ingestion causes hypertonic hyponatremia. This condition is a common iatrogenic cause of hyponatremia seen, for example, in cases in which mannitol is employed to treat instances of increased intracerebral hemorrhage.
4. The answer is B. Lithium is the only medication that causes nephrogenic diabetes insipidus by accumulating in renal collecting tubule cells and is the drug most commonly implicated.
5. The answer is A. Patients with diabetic ketoacidosis are total body potassium depleted, despite the high serum potassium levels. A failure to replete potassium while correcting the ketoacidosis can result in serum hypokalemia (from intracellular shift of potassium) and fatal cardiac arrhythmias.
6. Production of PTH-like hormone from the malignancy, which exerts negative feedback on PTH.
7. The answer is A. Tapping the facial nerve anterior to the ear lobe, slightly below the zygomatic arch. A positive response is defined by twitching of the facial muscles innervated by the facial nerve on the innervated side.
   The answer is B. Inflating an upper extremity sphygmomanometer cuff above systolic blood pressure for a period of no less than 2 min. A positive response is defined by development of carpal spasm.
8. The answer is C. In cases of life-threatening hypermagnesemia, IV calcium is given immediately to stabilize cardiac membranes and prevent fatal arrhythmias.

SUGGESTED READING

Blum D, Brasseur D, Kahn A, Brachet E. Safe oral rehydration of hypertonic dehydration. J Pediatr Gastroenterol Nutr 1986;5:232–235.

Greenspan FS (ed). Basic and Clinical Endocrinology, 3rd Ed. East Norwalk, CT: Appleton & Lange, 1991.

Rose BD. Clinical Physiology of Acid–Base and Electrolyte Disorders, 4th Ed. New York: McGraw-Hill, 1994.

Shapiro BA, Harrison RH, Walton JR. Clinical Application of Blood Gases, 3rd Ed. Chicago: Year Book, 1982.

Surawicz B. Relationship between electrocardiogram and electrolytes. Am Heart J 1967;73:814–834.

Zeffren JL, et al. Reversible defect in renal concentrating mechanism in patients with hypercalcemia. Am J Med 1962;33:54–63.

CHAPTER 30

MICHAEL BADELLINO AND GILBERT E. D'ALONZO

Special Problems in the Critically Ill Trauma Patient

CHAPTER OUTLINE

LEARNING OBJECTIVES

After studying this chapter, you should be able to:

- Describe the measures for determining the adequacy of resuscitation during traumatic shock.
- Appreciate the significance of the early recognition of limb compartment syndrome.
- Describe the clinical relevance of myocardial contusion.
- Discuss the importance of recognizing and treating inhalation thermal burns and toxic inhalation injuries.
- Recognize carbon monoxide toxicity and institute proper treatment.
- Recognize the importance of deep venous thrombosis as a complication in the trauma patient.
- Discuss various complications associated with massive transfusion of blood products in the trauma patient.
- Discuss abdominal compartment syndrome and its pathophysiology.

THE CONTINUUM OF SHOCK RESUSCITATION

Resuscitation consists of many interrelated and often protracted activities that are directed toward reversal of the shock state. Shock is a physiologic state, not just an abnormal hemodynamic state. It is best defined as a condition in which systemic oxygen delivery is inadequate for normal aerobic metabolic needs. Shock can be classified as hypovolemic, cardiogenic, neurogenic, or vasogenic. Traumatized patients can present in any of these states

Shock is a physiologic state, not only an abnormal hemodynamic state.

Types of shock: hypovolemic, cardiogenic, neurogenic, and vasogenic.

but most often present with hypovolemic shock secondary to acute blood loss due to bleeding, that is, hemorrhagic shock. Although resuscitation of the injured patient is usually accomplished in the Emergency Department (ED), or during emergent operative procedures, it is not uncommon for a traumatized patient to arrive in the intensive care unit (ICU) in an underresuscitated condition. Most often this is a result of inadequate volume replacement during the initial resuscitation; however, the presence of continued blood loss from occult undiagnostic injuries must always be considered.

The physiologic status of the trauma patient must be carefully determined on arrival to the ICU. For severely injured patients, or those who undergo prolonged diagnostic or therapeutic operative procedures, it is advisable to check on the condition of the patient prior to actual ICU arrival. Evidence of underresuscitation must be meticulously pursued. The initial patient evaluation should include, at a minimum, a thorough physical examination and a complete assessment of all available hemodynamic parameters, hemoglobin and arterial blood gas analysis, and a chest radiograph. Additionally, a careful summary of all resuscitative efforts must be compiled, including a tabulation of all injuries and blood loss and an accounting of infused crystalloid and blood products. This summary should include a review of the actual emergency room and anesthesia records for documentation of hypotensive episodes, acidosis, oliguria, or intraoperative use of vasoactive medications, clues that indicate that a shock state persists despite the appearance of normal hemodynamics.

Reliance on heart rate and blood pressure alone often prevents the early detection and eventual of reversal of shock.

Tachycardia is neither a sensitive nor a specific indicator of shock.

A central venous hemodynamic catheter is helpful for monitoring hemodynamic and volume status during shock that requires vasoactive therapies.

Unfortunately, reliance on gross measures of resuscitation, such as heart rate and blood pressure, often prevent early detection and eventual reversal of occult shock. Tachycardia has historically been shown to be neither a sensitive nor a specific indicator of shock. Supine arterial hypotension often is not seen until more than 30% of the circulating blood volume has been lost. Oliguria, acidosis, and lactemia are subtle but more reliable clues that tissue hypoperfusion persists. Severely injured patients or those who exhibit overt signs of underresuscitation should undergo placement of a central hemodynamic monitoring catheter (i.e., central venous pressure [CVP] line or pulmonary artery catheter) to guide further diagnosis and therapy. Although controversial, the use of an oximetric pulmonary artery catheter will facilitate serial measurements of venous filling pressures, cardiac performance, and mixed venous oxygen saturation to allow determination of tissue oxygen delivery and consumption. Once shock is correctly identified, some easily measured endpoints of resuscitation must be followed to assess the adequacy of resuscitation.

MEASURES OF THE ADEQUACY OF RESUSCITATION

Hemodynamic Monitoring

Because measures of heart rate and systemic arterial blood pressure are often unreliable in guiding resuscitation, the ICU physician may use a pulmonary artery catheter to measure a variety of hemodynamic parameters to determine vascular and cardiac status. Central venous and pulmonary artery pressures, as well as measured or calculated indices of cardiac performance, such as cardiac output and index and left ventricular stroke volume, can provide important information. Normal hemodynamics must be known; many variables affecting the trauma patient will affect these values independent of volume status (Appendix B). Temperature, acute respiratory failure, sepsis, and direct cardiac injury, to name just a few, can make these data difficult to interpret. Nonetheless, every effort should be made to normalize venous filling pressures and maintain normal cardiac output.

Often the young trauma patient will resuscitate rapidly with volume restoration, but the elderly patient and those who have experienced prolonged periods of profound hypotension or cardiac arrest may require vasoactive therapy to support and maintain an acceptable hemodynamic profile. It is axiomatic, however, that the first-line therapy for a trauma patient in shock should never be administration of vasopressor therapy unless all other causes of underperfusion, most importantly, volume depletion, have been excluded.

Urine Output

Despite its simplicity, hourly urine output remains a valuable indicator of a patient's volume status in response to fluid resuscitation. Assuming the absence of compounding factors, such as hyperglycemia, diabetes insipidus, and renal failure, a urine output greater than 1 ml/kg/h suggests euvolemia, whereas oliguria (urine output <0.05 ml/kg/h) is generally an early sign of underresuscitation. An oliguric trauma patient should have determination of serum and urine electrolytes to allow calculation of the blood urea nitrogen/creatinine ratio, urine specific gravity, and fractional excretion of sodium, to confirm a prerenal state. While awaiting these laboratory results, it is often reasonable to treat the patient without central hemodynamic monitoring with a bolus of isotonic crystalloid solution, such as lactated Ringers at 25 ml/kg, and then to assess the response. Failure to reverse oliguria with a crystalloid bolus is generally considered an indication for more invasive central monitoring such as central venous pressure or pulmonary capillary wedge pressure measurements to guide further therapy.

Hourly urine output is a valuable indicator of intravascular volume status and response to resuscitation.

Base Deficit/Acidosis

Inadequate tissue perfusion and oxygen delivery cause a shift from aerobic to anaerobic metabolism with the resultant production of pyruvate and hydrogen ions, leading to metabolic acidosis. The degree of metabolic acidosis, estimated by the base deficit, has been shown experimentally to correlate with the degree of body oxygen debt. The actual measured base deficit can predict mortality; patients having a base deficit greater than 15 mmol experience 25%–50% mortality. Patients with a progressive base deficit despite seemingly adequate resuscitation should be suspected of having continuing blood loss.

Metabolic acidosis develops during inadequate tissue perfusion during shock and correlates with survival.

The primary treatment of metabolic acidosis should be restoration of oxygen delivery by continued fluid administration or inotropic support, not pharmacologic reversal alone of serious acidosis. Only at pH levels less than 7.2 should consideration be given to the use of intravenous sodium bicarbonate, because experimental evidence suggests that, below this degree of acidosis, myocardial contractility is reduced. Thus, making serial determinations of the base deficit and pH, based on arterial blood gas sampling, a simple and reliable guide to the adequacy of resuscitation.

Acidosis that occurs during shock should be treated by fluid administration and the proper use of inotropic support, not by the pharmacologic reversal of acidosis.

Serum Lactate

Pyruvate, the end product of anaerobic glycolysis, combines with $NADH^+$ to produce lactate. Thus, in conditions favoring anaerobic metabolism (tissue hypoperfusion), serum lactate levels rise. As in the case with base deficit, serum lactate levels have been shown in some studies to correlate with oxygen debt, acidosis, and survival. Additionally, it has been suggested that the correlation of lactate levels with survival is time dependent, that is, early (less than 24 h) normalization of lactate levels (less than 2 mEq/l) enhances the chance of survival, whereas persistent (greater than 48 h) elevations in serum lactate are associated with prohibitively high (greater than 75%) mortality. Thus, serum lactate may be a useful marker for judging the adequacy of resuscitation following trauma.

In shock, serum lactate levels correlate with oxygen debt, acidosis, and survival.

Oxygen Delivery and Consumption

Considerable controversy exists concerning the utility of measuring oxygen delivery and consumption in the care of the critically ill trauma patient. Specifically, debate persists as to whether attempts at achieving either normal or supranormal oxygen delivery affect outcome. Although initial studies demonstrated an improvement in survival among patients in whom oxygen delivery was driven above normal (>600 ml/min/m^2), subsequent studies have failed to demonstrate this benefit. Theoretically, at least, the concept of matching a patient's oxygen needs to oxygen delivery remains appealing. Because shock is defined as a state in which oxygen delivery to the tissues is inadequate for normal aerobic metabolism, achieving oxygen delivery adequate for consumption should be the ultimate goal of shock resuscitation.

Although body O_2 delivery may seem to be adequate for the measured oxygen consumption, certain regional tissue beds may still be underperfused and remain a source of acidosis.

Gastric Tonometry

The technique of gastric tonometry is an evolving technology that may have promise as a real-time guide to resuscitation. The abdominal mesentery and bowel are very sensitive to changes in blood flow and are the first organ system to manifest signs of ischemia during low flow states, because the intestinal mucosa is metabolically active and is not privileged. In low flow states, flow of oxygenated blood to the mesenteric circulation may be reflexively shunted to more immediately critical organs such as the brain and heart. Because CO_2 is readily diffusible across the intestinal mucosa, intraluminal P_{CO_2} approximates intramucosal P_{CO_2}. Knowledge of the intramucosal P_{CO_2} facilitates an estimate of intramucosal pH using the the Henderson–Hasselbach equation. Several studies have demonstrated that aggressive resuscitation to restore an intramucosal gastric pH ≥ 7.35 can improve patient outcome, especially when this correction occurs within the first 12 h after injury. Although further studies are necessary, gastric tonometry may become a tool for use in the resuscitation of injured patients.

COMPARTMENT SYNDROME

A high level of clinical suspicion is needed to diagnose extremity compartment syndrome early.

Compartment syndrome is a potentially catastrophic complication that can follow crush or vascular injury of an extremity. Because this complication usually occurs several hours after injury or revascularization surgery of an extremity, it is often diagnosed in the ICU. Diagnosis and treatment must be accomplished rapidly to avoid limb loss. Therefore, careful monitoring of patients at risk and a clear understanding of the clinical presentation of this syndrome are necessary.

Pathogenesis

Following crush injury of an extremity or revascularization surgery following vascular trauma, edema caused by direct or reperfusion injury with revascularization can produce extensive accumulation of third-space tissue fluid. Although any extremity can be at risk, this syndrome is most common in the leg. The muscles of the extremities, which are encased in tough, nonelastic fascial compartments, are the areas where the process actually occurs. These noncompliant compartments will not stretch when edema develops acutely in and around the muscles. Thus, progressive edema elevates hydrostatic pressures within the muscle compartment. This pressure can ultimately rise to exceed not only venous and capillary perfusion pressures but also arterial pressure. The end result is compromise of capillary blood flow within the muscle compartment, with resultant ischemia and eventual necrosis of not only the muscle but of the nerve tissue as well.

Presentation

Classic signs of compartment syndrome are pain, paresthesias, pulselessness, pallor, poikilothermia, and paralysis.

In an awake patient, several classic signs of compartment syndrome have been recognized. These signs are often referred to as the six P's: pain, paresthesia, pulselessness, pallor, poikilothermia, and paralysis. Progression to the last four P's carries significant morbidity and suggests failure to diagnose the syndrome at its earliest and most treatable stages. Any patient at risk who complains of pain out of proportion to their injury or the beginning of paresthesias should be carefully examined for this syndrome. On examination, compartments should be palpated. Generally, they are tense, firm, and very tender as a result of the extremity swelling. Stretching of the affected muscle compartment will exacerbate pain. The foot and great toe should be flexed and extended passively to elicit pain in the involved compartment. Exacerbation of pain should prompt the immediate measurement of actual pressures in each of the compartments of the extremity. The leg, for example, has a total of four compartments. In an unconscious patient, the early signs of compartment syndrome, which are very subjective, cannot be easily determined. Thus, the diagnosis is often made late when marked tenseness in the extremity or a change in the quality of the pulse is appreciated. If the arterial pulse is missing, this is generally a very bad prognostic sign.

Compartment Pressure Measurement

Compartment pressures can be obtained with handheld monitoring devices or needles attached to pressure transducers. Some debate exists as to the exact pressure reading that establishes the diagnosis. In a normotensive patient, a compartment pressure greater than 30 mmHg is considered by most to be pathologic (some have suggested mean arterial pressure − compartment pressure > 40 mmHg). Measurements must be made in each compartment of the extremity, keeping in mind that the leg has four separate fascial compartments: anterior, lateral, deep, and superficial posterior.

Treatment and Sequelae

Immediate surgical fasciotomy is the treatment of choice for compartment syndrome.

Once established, the compartment syndrome must be treated by immediate surgical fasciotomy of all compartments in the affected extremity. In the leg, this entails decompression of all four fascial compartments. Obviously, necrotic muscle should be debrided.

Should muscle ischemia result from the compartment syndrome, systemic complications of hyperkalemia and myoglobinuria can occur. Following myocyte death, intracellular potassium and the oxygen transport protein myoglobin are released. Hyperkalemia can be initially treated with conventional measures. Myoglobinuria is toxic to the renal tubular epithelial cells and can cause tubular necrosis of the kidney with the potential for progression to acute renal failure. Once confirmed, the treatment of myoglobinuria is aimed at preventing further myocyte death in the affected limb and prevention of renal failure. All dead muscle tissue in the affected extremity must be removed; at times, this may require limb amputation. Muscles of questionable viability can be followed by serial clinical examination, including intraoperative inspection and serial serum creatinine kinase measurements. Volume loading and vigorous diuresis, preferably with an osmotic diuretic, are required to keep urine output brisk so that precipitation of myoglobin in the renal tubules can be prevented. Although commonly performed, alkalinization of the urine to further prevent precipitation of soluble myoglobin is of questionable clinical value.

MYOCARDIAL CONTUSION

Any patient who has sustained a severe blow to the chest may experience myocardial contusion.

The past 20 years have seen a radical reinterpretation of the diagnosis and management of the syndrome known as myocardial contusion. Theoretically, anyone receiving a severe blow to the anterior chest may experience significant force transmission to the heart. The rare, but very real, occurrence of blunt heart rupture testifies to the potential significance of this mechanism of injury. In reality, asymptomatic patients, despite the amount of potential force transmission to the chest, are unlikely to have suffered significant cardiac injury and, therefore are not at risk for clinically significant sequelae.

Recognition and Clinical Significance

In the past, it was recommended that patients who had suffered significant blunt trauma to the anterior chest were admitted to the ICU for up to 48 h for cardiac monitoring because life-threatening arrhythmias were sporadically observed. In addition, serial creatinine kinase measurements, echocardiography, and nucleotide heart scanning were investigated as screening tests to identify patients at risk. None of these tests proved sensitive or specific for the diagnosis of any traumatic cardiac sequela. Furthermore, perspective studies showed that any patient with a normal or near normal admission electrocardiogram was at almost negligible risk for the development of arrhythmias and even those with some abnormality on screening EKG could be observed by telemetry alone. Indeed, it is now considered that the absence of a documented abnormality on an admission EKG, or evidence of overt heart failure, makes the likelihood of myocardial contusion precipitating clinical problems unlikely. A patient with an abnormal admission EKG is monitored on telemetry. If an unexpected arrhythmia or hemodynamic instability ensues, echocardiography should be performed. Pharmacologic treatment of acute chest arrhythmias, usually tachyarrhythmias, can be treated following standard Advanced Cardiac Life Support (ACLS) guidelines. In the rare patient with myocardial contusion causing cardiac dysfunction, pulmonary artery catheterization and the use of inotropes may be necessary. Overall, myocardial contusion does not appear to increase the risk of perioperative complications in trauma patients.

CARE OF THE BURN PATIENT

Although modern care of the burn patient is routinely accomplished in a regional burn center, it may occasionally be necessary to manage an acute burn patient in an ICU before transfer. Control of the airway and evaluation for the possibility of inhalation burn airway injury are most often accomplished in the emergency room where the resuscitation usually begins. Following airway management, the major consideration in the next 24 h is continuation of fluid resuscitation.

Inhalation Injury

Inhalational injury may involve direct thermal injury to the airways and lung tissue and additional risk of toxic gas exposure.

Inhalation injury can be separated into the two distinct pathophysiologic components that differ as to the nature of the injury, timing of manifestations, and treatment. Direct thermal injury or the inhalation of toxic gases can injure the airway. Patients at special risk for inhalation injuries are those burned in a closed-space fire or exposed to petroleum-based fires.

Transfer of heat from hot gases to the airway mucosa produces direct thermal injury. Because the upper airway is a very efficient heat exchanger, direct thermal injury to the airway below the level of the larynx is uncommon. Because this injury occurs at the time of fire exposure, these patients usually exhibit signs of inhalation injury early, often in the emergency room. Signs of possible inhalation injury include carbonaceous sputum and carbonaceous deposits about the nose and mouth, singeing of facial hairs and nasal hairs, and hoarseness or stridor. For such patients, fiberoptic laryngotracheoscopy should be performed to evaluate the airway. The presence of edema, blisters, ulcerations or hemorrhage indicates the need for intubation because these lesions may progress over time and produce airway obstruction. When these findings are absent, the patient should be administered high-humidity oxygen and admitted to the ICU for monitoring oxygen saturation and periodic blood gases to evaluate for progressive hypercapnia. The use of systemic steroids in these patients remains controversial.

Signs of inhalation injury are carbonaceous sputum, singed facial hairs, hoarseness, stridor.

Airway edema, blisters, ulcers, and hemorrhage indicate a need for intubation.

Inhalation of nonheated toxic gases can also produce a delayed injury to the lower airway and lung. These patients may have stigmata of inhalation injury. Treatment is the same as just outlined; however, these patients must be followed closely in the ICU for up to 72 h as a worsening chest x-ray or PaO_2/FiO_2 ratio may signal the subsequent development of lung injury or a superimposed pneumonia.

Carbon Monoxide Poisoning

Carbon monoxide intoxication occurs in closed-space fires.

Patients exposed to a closed-space fire are at risk for the development of carbon monoxide (CO) poisoning. Because CO binds more avidly to hemoglobin than oxygen, once exposed the patients require treatment with 100% oxygen. CO toxicity may manifest as subtle to severe neurologic or cardiovascular changes; thus, a high index of suspicion for poisoning must be maintained when initially treating burn patients.

All patients at risk should have measurement of serum CO saturation levels (normally less than 3%). Smokers may have baseline CO levels of 3%–5% and firefighters on duty may have levels as high as 8%. Treatment is dependent on symptomatology. Patients with mild elevations of CO should be treated with 100% humidified oxygen and serially monitoring of CO saturation. Patients with mild neurologic symptoms are likewise treated with high-concentration oxygen and serially monitored. Patients presenting with high CO levels and severe neurologic symptoms, such as obtundation, coma, or hemodynamic instability, are best treated with hyperbaric oxygen therapy. The treatment of patients with mild neuropsychologic dysfunction is controversial. Obviously, when in doubt, high concentrations of inspired oxygen should be utilized initially in all patients at risk.

CO toxicity is treated with high-concentration oxygen and occasionally with hyperbaric oxygen.

TABLE 30-1

RECOMMENDED CALCULATIONS FOR BURN FLUID THERAPY

First 24 hours
- Lactated Ringers, 2–4 ml/kg body weight/% burn
- Half given during the first 8 h, half during the following 16 h

Second 24 hours
- Colloid as:
  - 30%–50% burn, 0.3 ml/kg body weight/% burn
  - 50%–70% burn, 0.4 ml/kg body weight/% burn
  - $>$70% burn, 0.5 ml/kg body weight/% burn
- D5W to maintain urine output $>$ 1 ml/kg/h

Fluid Resuscitation

Calculations of fluid requirements for a burn patient are made with reference to several standard formulas and take into account percentage of body surface burned and patient ideal weight. During the first 24 h, fluid resuscitation is accomplished with a crystalloid preparation, generally lactated Ringer's solution. During the next 24 h, both crystalloid and colloid infusions are utilized (Table 30-1).

The amount of initial fluid resuscitation is determined by the extent of total body surface burns.

Estimation of the percent of total body surface (TBS) area burned can be estimated by reference to the so-called rule-of-nines diagram (Figure 30-1). The anterior thorax and abdomen, the back, and each lower extremity contribute 18% each to the TBS; the head and the upper extremities, 9%; and the genitalia, 1%. A more rapid estimate can also be made with the realization that the surface area of a patient's palm is equal to approximately 1% of TBS.

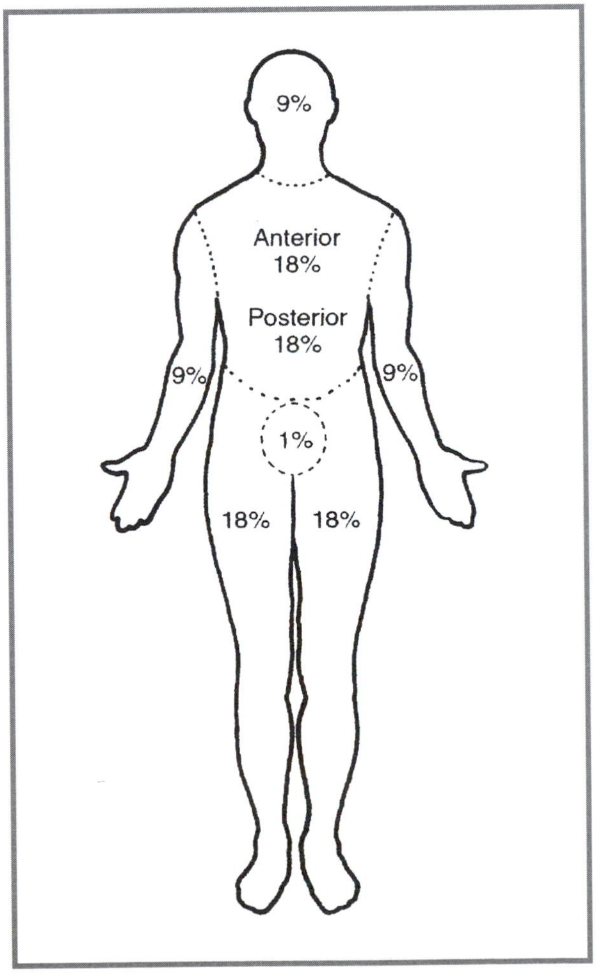

FIGURE 30-1

The rule of nines is used to calculate burned area to characterize magnitude of burn involvement.

Urine output is a reliable guide to the volume status of the burn patient; however, invasive central monitoring is desirable in patients with extensive burns (greater than 70%) and in the elderly with confounding underlying diseases. Additionally, hematocrit levels should be maintained at 30%–35%.

A unique complication observed in patients with circumferential burns of the extremities is vascular compromise secondary to compartment syndrome. Burn eschar is fibrotic, or nonelastic, in character. When edema develops in the affected extremity, a physiologic situation comparable to compartment syndrome can develop. The most useful tool to monitor the status of blood flow to an extremity with circumferential burns is a doppler flow probe and, if needed, compartment pressure measurements. Serial examinations are warranted, and loss of pulsatile blood flow is an absolute indication for urgent surgical escharotomy.

PULMONARY THROMBOEMBOLISM

Most trauma patients are at least at moderate risk for deep venous thrombosis (DVT) and pulmonary emboli (PE).

Trauma patients are at increased risk for the development of deep venous thrombosis (DVT) and pulmonary emboli (PE). The incidence of DVT and PE has been reported to be as high as 20% and 6%, respectively, following trauma. Trauma patients not only share the usual risks of the hospitalized patient for DVT, such as advanced age, recent major surgery, immobilization, and obesity, but the nature of their traumatic injuries places them at an even higher risk (Table 30-2). Indeed, regardless of the scoring system used, most trauma patients are at least at a moderate risk for DVT. Many, especially those with multiple trauma and lower extremity long-bone fractures requiring major surgery, score in the highest risk category.

Prophylaxis

Pneumatic compression devices used in conjunction with low molecular weight heparin are first-line prophylaxis for DVT in many trauma patients.

Low-dose heparin (5000 units subcutaneously every 12 h) is usually an effective prophylaxis modality in the general surgery population, but this approach does not reduce the incidence of DVT in patients with orthopedic injuries when used as a single agent, and it is often associated with bleeding complications. Furthermore, the use of unfractionated heparin is contraindicated in many trauma patients because of the nature of their injuries. For example, in patients with neurologic trauma or solid viscous injury, any degree of anticoagulation may propagate a bleeding complication that could be life-threatening. Pneumatic compression devices are very effective in reducing the risk of DVT in the general surgery population and offer the distinctive advantage of not being associated with bleeding complications; they have become the standard prophylaxis method for low to moderate risk trauma patients. Low molecular weight heparin (LMWH) appears to reduce the risk of DVT in select patients without increasing the risk of bleeding, as compared to unfractionated heparin. Thus, LMWH is being increasingly used in conjunction with pneumatic compression devices in moderate- to high-risk trauma patients.

TABLE 30-2

RISK FACTORS FOR DEEP VENOUS THROMBOSIS (DVT) IN THE TRAUMA PATIENT

Age $>$ 40 years
Obesity
Major surgery
Venous injury
Immobilization
Pelvic fractures
Glasgow score $<$ 8
Massive transfusion
Spinal cord injury
Lower extremity fracture
Femoral central venous pressure (CVP) $>$ 16

For those patients who are at highest risk for DVT, in whom neither lower extremity is available for application of a pneumatic device and who have a contraindication for heparin (e.g., combined severe head and long bone injury, head and spinal cord injury, severe pelvic and long bone fractures), placement of a prophylactic vena cava filter has been advocated. Although probably efficacious, the long-term safety and efficacy of these devices are not well established, making placement in a young trauma patient a concern although often necessary.

COMPLICATIONS OF MASSIVE TRANSFUSION

Trauma patients often require transfusion of large quantities of blood or blood products during resuscitation and operation. It is generally agreed that when more than an entire blood volume (approximately 10 units of blood or blood products) is replaced within a 24-h period, a massive transfusion has occurred. Mortality in this population approaches 50%. Complications of massive transfusion commonly observed in the ICU that contribute to mortality are hypothermia, hypocalcemia, hyperkalemia, hypokalemia, coagulopathy, and respiratory failure.

The mortality rate is very high for trauma patients who require massive transfusion.

Hypocalcemia

Anticoagulation of banked blood is accomplished with citrate, which chelates ionized calcium. Transfusions of large quantities of blood produce a large citrate load that reduces calcium in the transfusion recipient's serum. The resultant hypocalcemia is exacerbated by hypothermia and acidosis, common conditions in patients requiring massive transfusions. Hypocalcemia can lead to disturbances in coagulation and cardiac function. Therefore, both careful attention to serum calcium levels and correction of hypocalcemia are imperative.

Hyperkalemia and Hypokalemia

Both hyperkalemia and hypokalemia can occur following massive blood product transfusion. Because banked red cells release potassium during storage, as much as 8 mEq/l potassium can be infused with each unit of transfused cells. Therefore, hyperkalemia is only observed following massive transfusion. Frequent serial measurements of serum potassium are required to avoid episodes of potentially life-threatening arrhythmias.

Hypothermia

As a consequence of rapid infusion of blood and crystalloid, trauma patients are at risk for the development of hypothermia. Platelet function is directly impaired by hypothermia, probably via alterations at the level of the cell membrane. Secondary to hypothermia, platelet dysfunction can become clinically significant despite a normal platelet count. The presence of dilutional thrombocytopenia in massively transfused patients can further limit platelet function. Depletion of clotting factors is often underestimated in the cold trauma patient because routine clotting tests are performed on plasma samples warmed to 37°F.

Hypothermia is a consequence of rapid massive volume resuscitation.

Treatment is aimed at correction of any hypothermia present on emergency room arrival and prevention of further temperature loss during resuscitation, operation, and recovery. Blood- and fluid-warming devices should be used during trauma resuscitation. High ambient temperatures should be maintained in the emergency and operating rooms. Every effort should be made to utilize active rewarming devices such as warming blankets, convective air rewarmers, and radiant heat lamps. Although simple, active core rewarming by gastric and urinary bladder irrigation is somewhat inefficient. The use of extracorporal and continuous arteriovenous rewarming may be needed in the severely hypothermic patient.

Coagulopathy

Massive transfusion can lead to severe coagulopathy.

The major hemostatic defects in the massively transfused patient appear to be related to thrombocytopenia and platelet dysfunction secondary to hypothermia. Although considerable controversy exists, platelet transfusions do not appear to be justified simply because a patient has required a single blood volume replacement. In patients who have received more than 10–15 units of blood, however, and who continue to have nonmechanical bleeding, or to experience a significant drop in platelet count, platelet transfusion should be considered. Likewise, clotting factor deficiency should not arise following a single blood volume replacement. However, patients who are transfused with more than 15 units of blood and who have significant nonmechanical blood loss and a measurable coagulopathy should have blood coagulation factor replacement with the administration of fresh-frozen plasma.

ABDOMINAL COMPARTMENT SYNDROME

Intraabdominal hypertension and compartment syndrome can occur following severe visceral damage with subsequent repair.

Trauma patients often experience repeated episodes of blood loss or hypotension requiring large-volume resuscitation and may require prolonged abdominal operations. The resultant periods of ischemia and eventual reperfusion can result in massive capillary leak and diffuse abdominal visceral interstitial edema. This process in the mesentery circulation can cause significant and even massive bowel edema. Tight closure of laparotomy incisions can produce, or place a patient at risk for, the development of increased intraabdominal pressure. Additionally, the use of intraabdominal packs for hemorrhage control and postoperative intraabdominal bleeding can also increase intraabdominal pressure. Significant intraabdominal hypertension (IAH) can lead to a condition known as abdominal compartment syndrome. Recognition of this syndrome and its complications is only recently being addressed in a systematic way.

Pathophysiology

In several animal models, IAH above 20 mmHg has been shown to have a negative effect on both cardiovascular and pulmonary performance. Clinical studies have demonstrated significant improvement in cardiovascular indices once IAH has been reduced by decompressive laparotomy. Specifically, surgical decompression has been shown to increase cardiac index, oxygen delivery, and gastric mucosal pH and urine output, while reducing central venous pressure. Often, a variety of measures of pulmonary gas exchange improve and the patient requires less supplemental oxygen or positive end-expiratory pressure (PEEP) while on mechanical ventilation.

Recognition and Treatment

In patients at risk for the development of IAH, the presence of significant abdominal distension and tenseness, along with the progressive oliguria and pulmonary and cardiovascular deterioration, should trigger measurements of intraabdominal pressure to rule out abdominal compartment syndrome. Intraabdominal pressure can be reasonably and conveniently measured by monitoring urinary bladder pressure. Following the installation of 100 ml of fluid into the bladder, the Foley catheter is clamped, and, using a needle through the catheter, a transducer and manometer is affixed. Once IAH has been established (a pressure greater than 20 mmHg), surgical decompression should be immediately considered.

Decompressive laparotomy can be performed at the bedside in the ICU or in the operating room. Before decompression is carried out, optimization of volume and oxygen delivery status should be achieved along with correction of any coagulopathy. Several techniques are popular, but all include release of fascial closure, irrigation of the abdomen to remove blood clots, removal of any abdominal packs, and, if practical, reclosure of the abdomen with some type of synthetic material that will allow replacement of the bowel into the abdomen without undue tightness. A clinical measure of how much closure can be accomplished is provided by careful attention to respiratory parameters of tidal volume and peak airway pressure during closure. This procedure may need to be repeated on several occasions. Alternatively, once bowel edema subsides and IAH reverses, formal closure of the abdomen may be accomplished.

SUMMARY

Several unique situations are associated with the patient who has experienced trauma. It is paramount in critical care to pay careful attention to the resuscitation process and to be observant for the numerous complications associated with either the trauma itself or its resuscitation. Medical and surgical physicians can work carefully together to minimize these complications and ultimately improve patient survival.

REVIEW QUESTIONS

1. **Appropriate shock resuscitation includes all the following, except:**
   - **A.** Intravenous infusion of crystalloids
   - **B.** Blood transfusion
   - **C.** Vasopressor therapy
   - **D.** Intravenous infusion of sodium bicarbonate
   - **E.** All the above
2. **All the following statements are correct concerning limb compartment syndrome, except:**
   - **A.** Crush injury or limb revascularization surgery are often the causal event.
   - **B.** Limb edema is due to reperfusion.
   - **C.** The limb is always pulseless.
   - **D.** Pain and paresthesias of the limb are common.
   - **E.** Common complications include hyperkalemia and renal failure.
3. **Concerning carbon monoxide (CO) intoxication, which statement is false?**
   - **A.** It is a common complication of inhalation injury.
   - **B.** CO binds more avidly than O_2 to the hemoglobin molecule.
   - **C.** Neurologic sequelae are common.
   - **D.** O_2 therapy should be used.
   - **E.** All patients should be placed in a hyperbaric chamber.
4. **All the following are considered a complication of massive blood transfusion therapy, except:**
   - **A.** Hyperkalemia
   - **B.** Hypocalcemia
   - **C.** Hypokalemia
   - **D.** Hypothermia
   - **E.** Hypercoagulability

ANSWERS

1. The answer is C. Primary therapy does not include sodium bicarbonate solution. Sodium bicarbonate should only be used during extreme metabolic acidosis.
2. The answer is C. Compartment syndrome can be present in a limb with arterial pulses. Muscle necrosis can occur due to small vessel ischemia secondary to fascial compartment tense edema.
3. The answer is E. Hyperbaric O_2 should only be used for patients with severe neurologic symptoms or cardiovascular instability.
4. The answer is E. Patients are likely to be hypercoagulable secondary to depleted or diluted clotting factors and low or dysfunctional platelets.

SUGGESTED READING

Ivatury RR, Simon RJ. Intraabdominal hypertension: the abdominal compartment syndrome. In: Ivatury G (ed) The Textbook of Penetrating Trauma. Baltimore: Williams & Wilkins, 1996.

Knudsen MM. Coagulation disorders. In: Ivatury G (ed) The Textbook of Penetrating Trauma. Baltimore: Williams & Wilkins, 1996.

Mattox KL, Flint LM, Carrico CJ, et al. Blunt cardiac injury. J Trauma 1992;33:649–650.

McManus WF, Pruitt BA. Thermal injuries. In: Feliciano DV, More EE, Mattox KE (eds) Trauma, 3rd Ed. Stamford, CT: Appleton & Lange, 1996.

Rehm CG, Ross SE. Extremities: soft tissue. In: Ivatury G (ed) The Textbook of Penetrating Trauma. Baltimore: Williams & Wilkins, 1996.

Rutledge R, Sheldon GF. Bleeding and coagulation problems. In: Feliciano DV, Moore EE, Maddox KE (eds). Trauma, 3rd Ed. Stamford, CT: Appleton & Lange, 1996.

CHAPTER 31

John M. Travaline and Friedrich Kueppers

Ethics in Critical Care

CHAPTER OUTLINE

LEARNING OBJECTIVES

After studying this chapter, you should:

- Know the four fundamental principles of medical ethics.
- Understand the importance of obtaining informed consent.
- Know when an order for no resuscitation is appropriate.
- Understand the issues regarding withholding and withdrawing life-sustaining therapy and the concept of medical futility.
- Understand the role of ethics consultation in the critical care setting.

GENERAL PRINCIPLES

Ethical issues are common in critical care. The high degree of urgency present in managing extremely ill patients, the often sudden onset of their illness, the frequent lack of decision-making capacity of patients who are critically ill, and, for many critically ill patients, the status of being near death all contribute to ethical questions about appropriateness of therapy.

An approach to ethics in critical care can begin with consideration and understanding of four fundamental principles of biomedical ethics: (1) to do good (beneficence), (2) to do no harm (nonmaleficience), (3) to respect the patient's wishes (autonomy), and (4) to be fair (justice). Nearly all issues that arise in patient care in the critical care setting can be approached initially with one or more of these principles in mind. It is important to recognize, however, that although these principles are useful in forming arguments for debate, they remain abstract. Nonetheless, they are a foundation for ethical debate and serve as important guideposts for clinical decision making.

The four fundamental principles of biomedical ethics are beneficence, nonmaleficience, autonomy, and justice.

In this chapter, we discuss four areas of medical ethics in the context of critical care. These areas—informed consent and the use of advance directives, the do not resuscitate order (DNR), medical futility, and the withholding and withdrawing of life-sustaining medical therapy—are commonly encountered subjects of ethical discourse in this setting. In the last section of this chapter we discuss some practical matters concerning the role of ethics consultation in critical care units.

CASE STUDY

J.M. was a 79-year-old man with long-standing hypertension and chronic renal failure receiving outpatient dialysis. He had been doing well, able to live independently and to drive himself regularly to the dialysis center three times per week. During one dialysis treatment, however, he was noted to have a fever and, during dialysis, his blood pressure dropped lower than expected and could not be maintained without the use of vasopressor medication. He was transferred to the medical intensive care unit where the diagnosis of sepsis with shock was established. Appropriate and aggressive medical therapy was continued, but despite this, the patient deteriorated and needed to be intubated and placed on mechanical ventilation.

After 3 days, there was still no response to medical therapy. Moreover, routine physical examination revealed that J.M. was no longer moving any part of his left side in response to stimulation although he had been able to do so when he was admitted. Computerized tomography of the brain confirmed the suspicion that J.M. had suffered an extensive right-sided stroke. Neurologic consultation revealed that it was extremely unlikely that J.M. would survive this event. His attending physician was also concerned that, from the sepsis alone, despite continued therapy J.M. was not going to survive. Other consultant physicians involved with the case concurred.

By the fifth day of hospitalization, the attending physician was beginning to consider the withdrawal of therapy. It became more clear to her that all the medical efforts were now serving to prolong an inevitable dying process. It was obvious to her that J.M. was unable to make any decisions regarding his ongoing medical care, but she knew that he had completed an advance directive shortly after his wife died a few years earlier. This advance directive was obtained from his son; it clearly expressed J.M.'s wishes not to undergo continued life-sustaining therapy such as hemodialysis, mechanical ventilation, and vasopressor medication when his physician and other consultant physicians agreed that there was no reasonable chance for regaining mental capacity and functioning. In accordance with this directive, J.M. was withdrawn from the vasopressor supporting him and within several minutes was allowed to die as he wished. His son and other family were present as J.M. would have liked.

INFORMED CONSENT AND ADVANCE DIRECTIVES IN THE INTENSIVE CARE UNIT

One of the most important aspects of the physician–patient relationship concerns a patient's autonomy and a physician's duty to preserve it. Obtaining informed consent and acknowledgment and complying with a patient's advance directive are two major ways by which autonomy is respected.

An advance directive, in the context of health care, refers to the patient's expression of wishes regarding what they would want regarding medical care if they have lost the capacity to make decisions about such matters. Such expressions, which are generally written documents, may be very specific. For example, a patient may state that, in the event of irreversible coma and the development of cardiac arrest, "I do not want cardiopulmonary resuscitation to be performed." Other directives may simply authorize a surrogate individual to make decisions for the patient regarding medical care in the event of decisional incapacity. The appendix to this chapter shows an example of a standard advance directive that can be completed by a patient. Although this example includes commonly encountered situations and prompts an individual to select specific options, there is no absolute standard that must be followed. A patient may simply compose a letter expressing their wishes. Such a document can carry the same degree of empowerment as a more lengthy standardized document. The key element, from an ethics perspective, is to uphold the patient's autonomy by adhering to previously expressed wishes when they are known.

Another important component of interactions between physician and patient is the matter of informed consent. Informed consent is intended to uphold the principle of respect for a person's private space and self-determination. Certain procedures or interventions must be discussed with the patient, particularly when some risk is involved. The patient's consent must be documented with a form signed by the patient and the physician. Examples of some of the more common invasive procedures in the critical care setting include insertion of central venous and intraarterial catheters, thoracentesis, various types of endoscopies, and surgical procedures. Noninvasive medical therapies and procedures generally do not require a specific written consent.

> Informed consent is generally needed before performing any invasive procedure.

The informed consent document should contain certain elements: a description of the procedure and the reason(s) for doing it and a discussion of the risks, benefits, and possible alternatives. A valid consent must ensure that the patient or surrogate providing consent is competent (legally and operationally, i.e., de jure and de facto), does so voluntarily, and is informed, comprehending the relevant items for which consent is being requested. In the critical care setting, because of critical illness, a patient often lacks decision-making capacity. In such cases, physicians turn to a surrogate decision maker for the patient. The President's Commission for the Study of Ethical Problems in Medicine and Biomedical Research states that decision-making capacity requires (1) the possession of a set of values and goals, (2) the ability to understand and communicate relevant information, and (3) the ability to reason and deliberate about one's choices. It is the responsibility of the physician to determine whether these conditions are met. If the patient lacks capacity to give informed consent, the next of kin, usually the spouse, may do so. If there is no spouse, or the spouse also lacks capacity, then the following relatives in order of precedence may give informed consent: adult children, adult grandchildren, parents, brothers/sisters, nephews/nieces. Individual states, however, may have different requirements.

DO NOT RESUSCITATE ORDERS

In the 1960s, closed-chest cardiac massage was introduced to restore circulation in patients who suffered from cardiac arrest. This technique in combination with assisted ventilation was formalized as a method of cardiopulmonary resuscitation (CPR) for salvable victims of cardiopulmonary arrest. With the near contemporaneous emergence of coronary care and postsurgical units, the prototypes of intensive care units as we recognize them today, the use of CPR to restore spontaneous cardiac function became standard practice in the care of critically ill patients. As technology advanced and other resuscitative therapies became available, CPR, along with other resuscitative efforts, was routinely applied.

Over time, however, there came increasing awareness that despite these advances in technology to prolong life and the apparent success of such resuscitative maneuvers, there were circumstances in which disease processes, regardless of interventions, led to inexorable decline in a patient's condition and eventually death. With this realization, the application of CPR became more limited in such circumstances. Physician orders for "do not resuscitate" (DNR) began to appear, followed by a flurry of investigations. These studies analyzed when DNRs were written, how they were used, their implications, and whether patients desired their application. Table 31-1 lists selected studies of the DNR order in critical care.

Sometimes referred to as a "no code" order, DNR specifically requires health care providers to refrain from resuscitation of a patient in the event of cardiopulmonary arrest. It is generally not considered a limitation of other therapies, even if they are also potentially life-sustaining. Generally, DNR is established when a patient's condition is such that performing resuscitation would not likely benefit the patient, an example being terminal illness in which resuscitation will not favorably affect the course of the disease. Another circumstance is a patient who is permanently unconscious and has no meaningful interaction with others or their environment; resuscitation to restore the patient to that state is unacceptable. In critical care, DNR may be appropriate when death is inevitable even when all other life-sustaining therapies are continued; interventions aimed at restoring cardiopulmonary function in this circumstance may be considered mere prolongation of a dying process.

> Do not resuscitate (DNR) may be appropriate when death is inevitable despite continuance of all other life-sustaining therapy.

Ambiguity continues to exist in some settings with respect to "code status." To avoid confusion, it is necessary to specify clearly the goals of care for a patient and to designate the treatment level that explicitly states therapies that are to be employed or withheld. Table 31-2 lists some of the various terms regarding orders for no resuscitation.

DNR is commonly viewed as the initial step in limitation of medical therapies. Once the order is established, physicians may use this specific limitation of not performing cardiopulmonary resuscitation as a step toward limiting other therapies. A patient and their surrogate may also view this limitation as the first step in defining limits of other therapies deemed

TABLE 31-1

STUDIES CONCERNING THE DNR (DO NOT RESUSCITATE) ORDER IN CRITICAL CARE

FOCUS	DESIGN	CONCLUSION	REFERENCE
Impediments to writing DNR orders	Chart selection and panel review	Limited physician–patient relationship is major impediment	1
Overview characteristics of DNR patients the ICU	Prospective inception cohort	DNRs occur earlier and more frequently than in past in patients with poor outcomes	2
Nursing care requirements of DNR patients in the ICU	Prospective chart review	DNR patients required more nursing care	3
ICU deaths with respect to the frequency of CPR and variability in withdrawal of life support	Prospective survey; multicenter	Wide variability in end-of-life care	4
Variation in frequency of DNR orders and relationship between guidelines and qualitative observations regarding terminal care	Prospective inception cohort	DNR orders associated with patient's severity of physiologic abnormalities, age, admission diagnosis, and prior health status	5
Incidence and implications of DNR orders in medical ICU	Retrospective chart review	DNR orders occurred in older, more severely ill patients with worse prior health and poorer prognosis on ICU admission; DNR not influenced by race or socioeconomic status	6
General description of DNR orders in ICU	Multiple hospitals; retrospective chart review	DNR ordered earlier in some patients with worse prognosis; short time interval between DNR order and death or ICU discharge	7
Compared physicians' and nurses' opinions regarding DNR	Prospective opinion survey in a single hospital	Physicians and nurses agree regarding timing of DNR orders; when they disagree, physicians more likely to recommend DNR	8
Relationship between age and DNR in ICU	Large multicenter database sets	Older patients more likely to have DNR orders written independent of severity of illness	9
Patient preferences for resuscitation and the frequency and timing of DNR orders	Prospective cohort; multicentered	Frequency and timing of DNR orders is associated with patient preferences and short-term prognoses; DNR underutilization suggested	10

SOURCES:
[1] Eliasson AH, Parker JM, Shorr AF, Babb KA, Harris R, Aaronson BA, Diemer M. Impediments to writing do-not-resuscitate orders. Arch Intern Med 1999;159:2213–2218.
[2] Jayes RL, Zimmerman JE, Wagner DP, Draper EA, Knaus WA. Do-not-resuscitate orders in intensive care units. JAMA 1993;270:2213–2217.
[3] Tittle MB, Moody L, Becker MP. Nursing care requirements of patients with DNR orders in intensive care units. Heart Lung 1992;21:235–242.
[4] Prendergast TJ, Claessens MT, Luce JM. A national survey of end-of-life care for critically ill patients. Am J Respir Crit Care Med 1998;158:1163–1167.
[5] Jayes RI, Zimmerman JE, Wagner DP, Knaus WA. Variations in the use of do-not-resuscitate orders in ICUs. Chest 1996;110:1332–1339.
[6] Youngner SJ, Lewandowski W, McClish DK, Juknialis BW, Coulton C, Bartlett ET. "Do not resuscitate" orders, incidence and implications in a medical intensive care unit. JAMA 1985;253:54–57.
[7] Zimmerman JE, Knaus WA, Sharpe SM, Anderson AS, Draper EA, Wagner DP. The use and implications of do not resuscitate orders in intensive care units. JAMA 1986;255:351–356.
[8] Eliasson AH, Howard RS, Torrington KG, Dillard TA, Phillips YY. Do-not-resuscitate decisions in the medical ICU. Chest 1997;111:1106–1111.
[9] Boyd K, Teres D, Rapoport J, Lemeshow S. The relationship between age and the use of DNR orders in critical care patients. Arch Intern Med 1996;156:1821–1826.
[10] Hakim RB, Teno JM, Harrell FE, Knaus WA, Wenger N, Phillips RS, Layde P, Califf R, Connors AF, Lynn J. Factors associated with do-not-resuscitate orders: patients' preferences, prognoses, and physicians' judgements. Ann Intern Med 1996;125:284–293.

TABLE 31-2

CODE STATUS DESIGNATIONS

Code: Refers to the initation of an emergency response team to attend the patient with cardiopulmonary arrest.
No code: Refers to a patient's status when, even in the event of cardiopulmonary arrest, there is no call for an emergency response team to initiate resuscitation.
Slow code: Refers commonly to a status where it is predetermined that a patient in cardiopulmonary arrest be provided with less than maximal effort during a resuscitative attempt. This status is quite controversial and continues to be debated.
Chemical code: Refers to a resuscitative effort performed by using only drugs in the resuscitation and not initiating mechanical devices such as mechanical ventilation, pacemakers, electrocardioversion, or defibrillation.

inappropriate. It is important to recognize that such a limitation to therapy may be reversed by the patient or the surrogate.

If a patient is considered to be a candidate for DNR status, the physician should discuss with the patient, or their surrogate in cases of decisional incapacity, what DNR status means and why it may be appropriate. First, sufficient time should be provided that interruptions are minimized. It is important that both patient and surrogate have enough time to comprehend DNR status and to ask questions. Also, it is important to have enough time to explore the patient's wishes and thoughts regarding their condition, their expectations about their care and treatment, and the relevant values that influence the decision to forgo resuscitation. Second, the physician or health care provider must be sensitive in listening to and eliciting the patient's concerns, fears, and anxieties concerning their illness and the implications for the future. The patient also needs an accurate description of their medical condition, in understandable terms, so that any decision can be based upon the best information possible. The physician must also take care that his or her own values do not present a strong bias that could affect the patient's ability to come to a personal decision. Further, the patient must be reassured that DNR does not mean that either other therapies or their care will be lessened. Because patients might view the limitation of no resuscitation as involving some degree of abandonment (which may cause a patient to resist DNR), the physician must ensure that the explicit as well as implicit meaning of DNR is clearly articulated and understood by the patient. Last, in discussions concerning DNR, the patient's decision must be respected. Health care providers in critical care especially need to respect a patient's autonomy and not appear disrespectful if a patient's decision differs from that which they themselves would have made.

DNR does not mean do not treat.

DNR is compatible with aggressive, intensive care.

DNR orders should be clearly documented.

In sum, the proper establishment of DNR should ensure a sound decision by the patient or surrogate, clear understanding of DNR status by the patient, and a complete discussion of all the patient's/surrogate's questions. Written documentation of the DNR status in the medical record and communication to the physician and other health care staff must be clear to avoid miscommunication and confusion.

WITHHOLDING AND WITHDRAWING LIFE-SUSTAINING THERAPY

Withholding or withdrawing medical therapies when implementation or continuance of such therapies is determined to be of no benefit to the patient may be seen as extending a DNR order. Sometimes, despite the addition of therapy or the continuation of some therapy, a patient will continue to progress in a disease process until death. Under these circumstances, it may be appropriate to limit interventions or perhaps even withdraw previously initiated therapy that is no longer of any benefit to the patient.

Frequently, the issues surrounding withholding or withdrawing medical therapy are complex and involve ethical concerns. A patient may, by the way of an advance directive, wish no further therapy if it is of no benefit. Here the principle of autonomy is relevant. Sometimes the principle of nonmaleficience is evident in not continuing therapy that produces undue burden for a patient with no anticipated benefit. Occasionally, there are issues of justice in withholding or withdrawing therapy, particularly with scarce resources. All these factors should be carefully considered when deciding to limit life-sustaining therapy in a critically ill patient. As with the decision for do not resuscitate orders, withholding or withdrawing life-sustaining therapy requires a discussion that informs the patient or surrogate of the patient's condition and the medical appropriateness of limiting some therapy while providing assurance that the patient's best interests are the goal. These discussions frequently occur over a period of time. It is important at each time that the patient and their surrogate understand any plans for withholding or withdrawing therapy.

Discussion is of paramount importance in issues of withholding and withdrawing life-sustaining therapy.

There is no moral difference between withholding and withdrawing medical therapy.

To facilitate these decisions in critical care, professional societies have published guidelines for appropriate withdrawing and withholding of medical therapy. These guidelines underscore some important points. First, they acknowledge both a legal and ethical consensus that there is no moral difference between withholding and withdrawing medical therapy. Second, they underscore the primacy of patient autonomy in deciding to withdraw or forgo particular therapy after consultation with the patient's physician. They also emphasize the importance of a physician acting on the patient's behalf to do good and to avoid harm in making appropriate treatment recommendations based upon these principles. Communication is also stressed as a very important component of the care of patients and their families in the context of withholding or withdrawing life-sustaining therapy. It is also important to recognize that, with respect to medical therapies, physicians are not bound to provide therapy that they deem is futile.

In clinical practice, mechanisms exist to facilitate the implementation of orders to withhold or withdraw life-sustaining therapy. Although generally not as uniform as orders for no resuscitation, they share many similarities. Many institutions have a standard form listing a number of therapies often withheld. After establishing with the patient or surrogate the appropriateness of limiting therapy, the physician can check off therapies to withhold. Such therapies include transfusion of blood products and initiation of mechanical ventilation or vasopressors. At our institution, a paperless computer order entry system allows the physician to enter a pathway for the level of therapy, leading to successive screens on which a selection of specific therapies, grouped by category, can be made (Figure 31-1). Once selected, these limits of therapy appear on a daily patient summary sheet that is placed in the patient's medical record so that all caregivers may see and acknowledge the particular limits. This system procedure has facilitated patient care, promoted patient autonomy, and minimized the number of ethics consultations for clarification of clinical care issues regarding appropriate therapy. Moreover, it has eliminated most of the ambiguity formerly associated with a patient who wished to be resuscitated in the evident of cardiopulmonary arrest but did not wish intubation and mechanical ventilation. In these situations, the ability to more precisely define limits of therapy and hold the necessary discussions with the patient have provided important advances in the management of critically ill patients.

MEDICAL FUTILITY

Medical futility is frequently an elusive concept.

The concept of medical futility is quite controversial. Although it may appear to be a rather simple and straightforward concept that can be easily applied in medical practice, it is surrounded by considerable ambiguity. This ambiguity begins with its definition. Because there is no generally accepted definition of futility that answers important clinical questions which occur every day in critical care practice, many discussions concerning medical futility are frustrating and disappointing. Nonetheless, much has been written concerning the area of medical futility and many have attempted to achieve consensus on this matter. For example, a consensus statement from the Society of Critical Care Medicine's ethics committee elucidates the concept of medical futility by defining four categories for various treatments that may be considered futile: (1) treatments that have no beneficial physiologic effect, (2) treatments that are extremely unlikely to be beneficial, (3) treatments that are beneficial but are

LEVEL OF TREATMENT

YOU ARE ABOUT TO ENTER A LEVEL OF TREATMENT ORDER ON THIS PATIENT

PATIENT NAME:	DUCK, DONALD
UNIT:	MRICU
MEDICAL RECORD#:	00000000000

LEVEL 1:	DO NOT RESUSCITATE (DNR)
LEVEL 2A:	DO NOT RESUSCITATE (DNR) AND LIMITED MEDICAL THERAPY
LEVEL 2B:	LIMITED MEDICAL THERAPY
LEVEL 3:	DO NOT RESUSCITATE (DNR) AND PROVIDE COMFORT MEASURES

NO ORDER-RETURN

FIGURE 31-1

Computer screen that appears when a physician selects "level of treatment" pathway. An appropriate level of treatment can then be selected by the attending physician.

extremely costly, and (4) treatments that are of uncertain or controversial benefit. In the strictest sense of the definition, only those treatments in the first category should be considered futile; those in the other three categories are considered inappropriate and therefore inadvisable.

Discussion about futile therapy almost always involves issues of values, and the conflicts that arise as to when therapy is "futile" involve differences in values. The often-discussed example of performing CPR in a patient with metastatic lung cancer illustrates a few of the problems. Generally, a physician would recommend not performing resuscitative maneuvers in such a patient because such intervention would only prolong the inevitable process of dying. In contrast, the patient may value the prolongation of life even if for only 1 more day. In this case, resuscitation in the event of cardiopulmonary arrest may indeed be successful in restoring cardiopulmonary function; however, it may incur extreme cost and in fact be of uncertain benefit or may even lead to greater harm. These are the types of scenarios that are encountered in critical care medicine and create the need for frank discussion and counseling for patients and often their families so that appropriate therapy is provided. At many times, communication with a patient or surrogate allows the exploration of values in the context of risks and benefits for any proposed treatment so that an informed decision can be reached and the goals of therapy achieved accordingly.

In the context of debate surrounding medical futility, the physician must always first ascertain the goal of any particular circumstance and ask whether the implementation of such therapy will help achieve that goal. Communication that promotes accurate understanding of the medical facts and facilitates an affirmation of particular values will help minimize potential conflicts that arise in cases of medical futility.

Futility often engenders much emotion among health care staff. Some of these reactions are anger, frustration, sadness, and helplessness. Typically, futility cases involve a patient or family/surrogate who wishes everything to be done and a physician or health care team who deems it appropriate to not continue or provide additional therapy considered to have no benefit. The feelings of the patient or surrogate may include a sense of false optimism, distrust of health care providers to act in the best interest of the patient, religious beliefs, poor understanding, sense of entitlement, or psychologic factors such as guilt or denial. Management of such cases requires the health care team to demonstrate empathy with patients and their families, initiate and maintain effective communication, and establish clear goals of therapy, explaining these goals clearly to the patient and surrogate.

THE ROLE OF ETHICS CONSULTATION IN CRITICAL CARE

Ethics consultation may facilitate resolution of difficult ethical problems in the ICU.

Most hospitals have an ethics committee that can respond to a request for consultation when a conflict arises in the clinical realm. Consultations may be sought concerning an institution's policy. The mechanism by which an ethics committee is available for consultation varies, but in each case, the consultation should assist persons requesting their service. This assistance includes clarification of issues, retrieval of additional information, mediation of conflict, safeguarding a patient's interest, particularly in cases of decisional incapacity and the absence of a surrogate, and assurance for the appropriateness of a particular action.

SUMMARY

Conduct in the critical care setting must follow generally accepted principles of medical ethics. These principles protect the dignity of the human person and allow the application of medical science in a manner aimed at preserving life and, inasmuch as possible, ensuring a reasonable quality of living for the patient. The apparent conflicts that arise concerning the ethics of patient care in the critical care setting frequently can be minimized by explicit statement of the goals of therapy, open and honest communication among patients, families, and health care staff, and commitment to care. At times ethics consultation, may be necessary to facilitate patient management in the critical care setting and to ensure appropriate patient care.

REVIEW QUESTIONS

1. **Which of the following is not a fundamental principle in bioethics?**
   - **A.** Justice
   - **B.** Rationing
   - **C.** Beneficence
   - **D.** Autonomy

2. **Concerning an order for no resuscitation, which of the following is true?**
   - **A.** A DNR order implies no treatment.
   - **B.** DNR is incompatible with aggressive, intensive care.
   - **C.** Orders for DNR must be documented in the medical record.
   - **D.** An order for no resuscitation cannot be changed once established.

3. **Of the following, which is important to consider in approaching an ethical problem in the critical care setting?**
   - **A.** The patient's medical insurance plan
   - **B.** Duration of critical illness
   - **C.** Presence of an advance directive
   - **D.** Whether a particular therapy is futile

4. **Elements of informed consent should include at least all the following except:**
   - **A.** Assurance of a successful outcome from the proposed procedure
   - **B.** Detailed risks and benefits of proposed procedure
   - **C.** Indication for doing the proposed procedure
   - **D.** Explanation of alternative options

ANSWERS

1. The answer is B. The four fundamental principles of biomedical ethics are beneficence, nonmaleficience, autonomy, and justice.
2. The answer is C. Documentation of an order for no resuscitation must be present in the medical record of the patient. Further, the discussion(s) concerning issues of resuscitation and leading to a decision for DNR should also be clearly documented in the medical record of the patient.
3. The answer is C. An approach to an ethical problem in any setting involves many aspects. A patient's insurance plan or duration of illness are seldom important matters to consider. Similarly, determining whether a particular therapy is futile is usually not relevant. Although many cases in critical care appear to involve a question of futility, at most times this question is superficial and deeper issues, usually having to do with effective communication with patients and their families, are key. There is no consensus about medical futility and, when it can be recognized, it is thought to occur rather infrequently. A crucial aspect of many ethical problems in critical care is the existence of an advance directive.
4. The answer is A. A physician proposing to perform a procedure for a patient must obtain informed consent. At minimum, this consent must include a discussion of the risks and benefits of the proposed procedure in detail, the reason for performing the procedure, and an explanation of the potential alternatives. A physician may convey an opinion regarding the likelihood of success for a proposed procedure, but there cannot be any assurance of a successful outcome. Risks and potential complications almost always prevent giving such assurance.

SUGGESTED READING

American Thoracic Society. Withholding and withdrawing life-sustaining therapy. Am Rev Respir Dis 1991;144:726–731.

Bone RC, Rackow EC, Weg JG, and the ACCP/SCCM Consensus Panel. Ethical and moral guidelines for the initiation, continuation, and withdrawal of intensive care. Chest 1990;97:949–958.

Council on Ethical and Judicial Affairs, American Medical Association. Guidelines for the appropriate use of do-not-resuscitate orders. JAMA 1991;265:1868–1871.

Orlowski JP. Ethics in Critical Care Medicine. Hagerstown, MD: University Publishing Group, 1999.

Task Force on Ethics of the Society of Critical Care Medicine. Consensus report on the ethics of foregoing life-sustaining treatments in the critically ill. Crit Care Med 1990;18:1435–1439.

The Ethics Committee of the Society of Critical Care Medicine. Consensus statement of the Society of Critical Care Medicine's Ethics Committee regarding futile and other possibly inadvisable treatments. Crit Care Med 1997;25:887–891.

The President's Commission for the Study of Ethical Problems in Medicine and Biomedical Research. No. 040-000-00459-9. Washington, DC: U.S. Government Printing Office, 1982.

Appendix: The Medical Directive

Introduction. As part of a person's right to self-determination, every adult may accept or refuse any recommended medical treatment. This is relatively easy when people are well and can speak. Unfortunately, during serious illness they are often unconscious or otherwise unable to communicate their wishes—at the very time when many critical decisions need to be made.

The Medical Directive allows you to record your wishes regarding various types of medical treatments in several representative situations so that your desires can be respected. It also lets you appoint a proxy, someone to make medical decisions in your place if you should become unable to make them on your own.

The Medical Directive comes into effect only if you become incompetent (unable to make decisions and too sick to have wishes). You can change it at any time until then. As long as you are competent, you should discuss your care directly with your physician.

Completing the form. You should, if possible complete the form in the context of a discussion with your physician. Ideally, this should occur in the presence of your proxy. This lets your physician and your proxy know how you think about these decisions, and it provides you and your physician with the opportunity to give or clarify relevant personal or medical information. You may also wish to discuss the issues with your family, friends, or religious mentor.

The Medical Directive contains six illness situations that include incompetence. For each one, you consider possible interventions and goals of medical care. Situation A is permanent coma; B is near death; C is with weeks to live in and out of consciousness; D is extreme dementia; E is a situation you describe; and F is temporary inability to make decisions.

For each scenario you identify your general goals for care and specific intervention choices. The interventions are divided into six groups: 1) cardiopulmonary resuscitation or major surgery: 2) mechanical breathing or dialysis; 3) blood transfusions or blood products; 4) artificial nutrition and hydration; 5) simple diagnostic tests or antibiotics; and 6) pain medications, even if they dull consciousness and indirectly shorten life. Most of these treatments are described briefly. If you have further questions, consult your physician.

Your wishes for treatment options (I want this treatment; I want this treatment tried, but stopped if there is no clear improvement; I am undecided; I do not want this treatment) should be indicated. If you choose a trial of treatment, you should understand that this indicates you want the treatment *withdrawn* if your physician and proxy believe that it has become futile.

The Personal Statement section allows you to explain your choices, and say anything you wish to those who may make decisions for you concerning the limits of your life and the goals of intervention. For example, in situation B, if you wish to define "uncertain chance" with numerical probability, you may do so here.

An earlier version of this form was originally published as part of an article by Linda L. Emanuel and Ezekiel J. Emanuel, "The Medical Directive: A New Comprehensive Advance Care Document," *Journal of the American Medical Association* 261:3288–3293, June 9, 1989. It does not reflect the official policy of the American Medical Association.

Next you may express your preferences concerning organ donation. Do you wish to donate your body or some or all of your organs after your death? If so, for what purpose(s) and to which physician or institution? If not, this should also be indicated in the appropriate box.

In the final section you may designate one or more proxies, who would be asked to make choices under circumstances in which your wishes are unclear. You can indicate whether or not the decisions of the proxy should override your wishes if there are differences. And, should you name more than one proxy, you can state who is to have the final say if there is disagreement. Your proxy must understand that this role usually involves making judgments that you would have made for yourself, had you been able—and making them by the criteria you have outlined. Proxy decisions should ideally be made in discussion with your family, friends, and physician.

What to do with the form. Once you have completed the form, you and two adult witnesses (other than your proxy) who have no interest in your estate need to sign and date it.

Many states have legislation covering documents of this sort. To determine the laws in your state, you should call the state attorney general's office or consult a lawyer. If your state has a statutory document, you may wish to use the Medical Directive and append it to this form.

You should give a copy of the completed document to your physician. His or her signature is desirable but not mandatory. The Directive should be placed in your medical records and flagged so that anyone who might be involved in your care can be aware of its presence. Your proxy, a family member, and/or a friend should also have a copy. In addition, you may want to carry a wallet card noting that you have such a document and where it can be found.

FIGURE 31-1

The form on page 530 to 534 is an example of an advance directive. This particular directive is quite detailed and specific. It also prompts a person to provide a personal statement that can be helpful for guiding appropriate care for a person in the event of decisional incapacity.

MY MEDICAL DIRECTIVE

This Medical Directive shall stand as a guide to my wishes regarding medical treatments in the event that illness should make me unable to communicate them directly. I make this Directive, being 18 years or more of age, of sound mind, and appreciating the consequences of my decisions.

SITUATION A

If I am in a coma or a persistent vegetative state and, in the opinion of my physician and two consultants, have no known hope of regaining awareness and higher mental functions no matter what is done, then my goals and specific wishes—if medically reasonable—for this and any additional illness would be:

☐ prolong life; treat everything
☐ attempt to cure, but reevaluate often
☐ limit to less invasive and less burdensome interventions
☐ provide comfort care only
☐ other *(please specify)*: ______________________________

____

Please check appropriate boxes:

	I want	I want treatment tried. If no clear improvement, stop	I am undecided	I do not want
1. **Cardiopulmonary resuscitation** (chest compressions, drugs, electric shocks, and artificial breathing aimed at reviving a person who is on the point of dying).		*Not applicable*		
2. **Major surgery** (for example, removing the gallbladder or part of the colon).		*Not applicable*		
3. **Mechanical breathing** (respiration by machine, through a tube in the throat).				
4. **Dialysis** (cleaning the blood by machine or by fluid passed through the belly).				
5. **Blood transfusions or blood products.**		*Not applicable*		
6. **Artificial nutrition and hydration** (given through a tube in a vein or in the stomach).				
7. **Simple diagnostic tests** (for example, blood tests or x-rays).		*Not applicable*		
8. **Antibiotics** (drugs used to fight infection).		*Not applicable*		
9. **Pain medications, even if they dull consciousness and indirectly shorten my life.**		*Not applicable*		

SITUATION B

If I am near death and in a coma and, in the opinion of my physician and two consultants, have a small but uncertain chance of regaining higher mental functions, a somewhat greater chance of surviving with permanent mental and physical disability, and a much greater chance of not recovering at all, then my goals and specific wishes—if medically reasonable—for this and any additional illness would be:

- ☐ prolong life; treat everything
- ☐ attempt to cure, but reevaluate often
- ☐ limit to less invasive and less burdensome interventions
- ☐ provide comfort care only
- ☐ other *(please specify)*: ______________________________

____

I want	I want treatment tried. If no clear improvement, stop	I am undecided	I do not want
	Not applicable		
	Not applicable		
	Not applicable		
	Not applicable		
	Not applicable		
	Not applicable		

SITUATION C

If I have a terminal illness with weeks to live, and my mind is not working well enough to make decisions for myself, but I am sometimes awake and seem to have feelings, then my goals and specific wishes—if medically reasonable—for this and any additional illness would be:

* In this state, prior wishes need to be balanced with a best guess about your current feelings. The proxy and physician have to make this judgment for you.

- ☐ prolong life; treat everything
- ☐ attempt to cure, but reevaluate often
- ☐ limit to less invasive and less burdensome interventions
- ☐ provide comfort care only
- ☐ other *(please specify)*: ______________________________

____

____

I want	I want treatment tried. If no clear improvement, stop	I am undecided	I do not want
	Not applicable		
	Not applicable		
	Not applicable		
	Not applicable		
	Not applicable		
	Not applicable		

SITUATION D

If I have brain damage or some brain disease that in the opinion of my physician and two consultants cannot be reversed and that makes me unable to think or have feelings, *but I have no terminal illness*, then my goals and specific wishes—if medically reasonable—for this and any additional illness would be:

☐ prolong life; treat everything
☐ attempt to cure, but reevaluate often
☐ limit to less invasive and less burdensome interventions
☐ provide comfort care only
☐ other *(please specify):* ______________________
____
____

I want	I want treatment tried. If no clear improvement, stop	I am undecided	I do not want
	Not applicable		
	Not applicable		
	Not applicable		
	Not applicable		
	Not applicable		
	Not applicable		

SITUATION E

If I . . .
(describe a situation that is important to you and/or your doctor believes you should consider in view of your current medical situation):

☐ prolong life; treat everything
☐ attempt to cure, but reevaluate often
☐ limit to less invasive and less burdensome interventions
☐ provide comfort care only
☐ other *(please specify):* ______________________
____
____

I want	I want treatment tried. If no clear improvement, stop	I am undecided	I do not want
	Not applicable		
	Not applicable		
	Not applicable		
	Not applicable		
	Not applicable		
	Not applicable		

SITUATION F

If I am in my current state of health (describe briefly): ________

and then have an illness that, in the opinion of my physician and two consultants, is life threatening but reversible, and I am temporarily unable to make decisions, then my goals and specific wishes—if medically reasonable—would be:

- ☐ prolong life; treat everything
- ☐ attempt to cure, but reevaluate often
- ☐ limit to less invasive and less burdensome interventions
- ☐ provide comfort care only
- ☐ other *(please specify)*: ________

Please check appropriate boxes:

I want	**I want treatment tried. If no clear improvement, stop**	**I am undecided**	**I do not want**	
	Not applicable			1. **Cardiopulmonary resuscitation** (chest compressions, drugs, electric shocks, and artificial breathing aimed at reviving a person who is on the point of dying).
	Not applicable			2. **Major surgery** (for example, removing the gallbladder or part of the colon).
				3. **Mechanical breathing** (respiration by machine, through a tube in the throat).
				4. **Dialysis** (cleaning the blood by machine or by fluid passed through the belly).
	Not applicable			5. **Blood transfusions or blood products.**
				6. **Artificial nutrition and hydration** (given through a tube in a vein or in the stomach).
	Not applicable			7. **Simple diagnostic tests** (for example, blood tests or x-rays).
	Not applicable			8. **Antibiotics** (drugs used to fight infection).
	Not applicable			9. **Pain medications, even if they dull consciousness and indirectly shorten my life.**

MY PERSONAL STATEMENT

(Use back page if necessary)

Please mention anything that would be important for your physician and your proxy to know. In particular, try to answer the following questions: 1) What medical conditions, if any, would make living so unpleasant that you would want life-sustaining treatment *withheld*? (Intractable pain? Irreversible mental damage? Inability to share love? Dependence on others? Another condition you would regard as intolerable?) 2) Under what medical circumstances would you want to stop interventions that might already have been started? 3) Why do you choose what you choose?

If there is any difference between my preferences detailed in the illness situations and those understood from my goals or from my personal statement, I wish my treatment selections / my goals / my personal statement *(please delete as appropriate)* to be given greater weight.

When I am dying, I would like—if my proxy and my health-care team think it is reasonable—to be cared for:

- ☐ at home or in a hospice
- ☐ in a nursing home
- ☐ in a hospital
- ☐ other *(please specify)*:______________________________

CHAPTER 32

YAROSLAV LANDO AND GERARD J. CRINER

Psychologic Dysfunction in the Intensive Care Unit Patient

CHAPTER OUTLINE

LEARNING OBJECTIVES

After studying this chapter, you should be able to:

- Define the types of psychologic dysfunction found in ICU patients.
- Know the medical and psychologic problems that contribute to psychologic dysfunction in the ICU patient.
- Be aware of environmental factors contributing to psychologic impairment in the ICU patient.
- Define delirium and its treatment.

An ICU patient can develop various psychiatric disorders that can manifest either during the ICU stay or after discharge. Several factors play a role in the development of these disorders (Table 32-1). The first is the effect of the severe medical illness or its treatment on cognitive function. The second is the patient's psychologic response to their severe illness (e.g., feeling that any worthwhile life is over). A patient's worry and preoccupation about their symptoms frequently results in failure to eat or to participate in rehabilitative efforts (i.e., weaning from mechanical ventilation) and may further worsen their clinical condition. Finally, the patient's interaction with the surrounding ICU environment can result in behavior, thought, or mood disturbances. The necessary constraints imposed by an ICU environment care for critically ill patients (lights continually on, medical personnel talking, multiple beeping alarms, around-the-clock interventions) can cause sleep and sensory deprivation.

Several factors contribute to the development of psychiatric disorders in ICU patients: the severity and nature of the underlying medical illness, the patient's psychologic response to the illness, and the patient's interaction with the surrounding ICU environment.

The ICU has physical effects that may promote psychologic harm to its patients: noise, sleep deprivation, lack of orienting clues, and frequent medical interventions.

In most cases, the physical complications of the patient's medical or surgical illness are the most important factors contributing to the patient's psychiatric disorder, notably delirium. Some cases result from the emotional impact of the illness; others may have already been present, especially in those patients admitted after accidents or self-inflicted injuries. In another subset of patients, environmental factors play a more significant role.

Initial studies on this complicated topic suggested that the physical environment of the ICU played a large role in causing psychologic harm to its patients. The unique ICU environment, including constant noise, sleep deprivation, monitoring equipment, monotonous sensory input, and lack of orienting clues, was thought to precipitate psychiatric disorders in some patients. Although the independent influence of environmental factors has not been totally clarified, these early observations affected the design of modern intensive care units and the medical and nursing practice that now takes place within them. The newer-generation

TABLE 32-1

GENERAL CAUSES OF PSYCHIATRIC DISORDERS IN CRITICALLY ILL PATIENTS

1. CNS dysfunction
   - CNS hypoperfusion states
   - Hypoxemia
   - Metabolic derangements
   - Medication side effects
   - Alcohol or drug withdrawal
   - Infections
2. Subjective interpretation of the meaning of the illness
   - Feeling that life is over
   - Loss of libido
   - Sense of personal failure
3. Personal worry and preoccupation
   - Catatonia
   - Major depression
   - Withdrawal
   - Hypochondrial preoccupation with symptoms
   - Exaggerated or denied pain experience
4. Family and environmental interactions
   - Feeling that one is a burden to the family
   - Response to loss of control over activities of daily living
   - Clingy, needy response to caregivers or family
   - Response resulting in threats to leave the hospital against medical advice

> Newer-generation ICUs have been redesigned with careful attention to help maintain normal patient circadian cycles.

ICUs have been redesigned with careful attention to help maintain normal patient psyche, including efforts to reduce noise, encourage more human contact, and provide visible clocks and calendars and external windows to maintain normal circadian rhythm and ensure adequate sleep.

Recent literature now provides some insight into the long-term outcome of psychologic problems developed in the intensive care unit. Studies of patients recovering from catastrophic or exceptionally life-threatening situations have shown that such patients are prone to prolonged psychologic reactions, particularly posttraumatic stress disorder and other phobic anxiety syndromes.

> The most common psychiatric disorders that arise in an ICU patient include delirium, depression, anxiety, and behavioral problems.

The most common psychiatric disorders that arise during a patient's ICU stay include delirium, depression, anxiety, and behavioral problems (Table 32-2). The purpose of this chapter is to describe the definitions, clinical signs and symptoms, etiologic factors, interrelationships, and management of the various intensive care unit syndromes described in the literature.

CASE STUDY

J.C. is a 45-year-old man who underwent a successful kidney-pancreas transplantation 6 months ago. Following the transplant, he was started on an appropriate immunosuppressive medical regimen. He is now readmitted with a fungal infection of his left orbit. After multiple debridements were unsuccessful in eradicating the disease, J.C. underwent an anterior skull base resection in efforts to contain the infection, was placed in the ICU, and aggressive antifungal therapy was initiated. The rest of his medical regimen included broad-spectrum antibiotics, systemic steroids, prophylactic peptic ulcer and gastric motility agents, strong pain relievers, and several antihypertensive drugs. He developed mild renal insufficiency, various electrolyte disturbances, and was recovering from cytomegalovirus hepatitis. Neurologically, he was appropriate, alert, and oriented to person, place, date, and time.

Approximately 48 h after his surgery, J.C. became fidgety. He started tugging on his bladder catheter and attempted to remove his intravenous lines. He was unable to sleep for any significant length of time. His behavior varied from being asleep at one moment to climbing out of bed the next. He was unable to separate dreams from reality. J.C. would make inappropriate statements (e.g., "Since someone stole my car battery, I think I can take this IV out."). Afterward, he would usually realize he had said something inappropriate. He frequently described how his room changed colors at night and how he felt he was in a cage surrounded by stuffed animals. During neurologic assessments, however, he remained oriented and occasionally became angry at the stupidity of the staff's assessment questions regarding the date, time, and place.

TABLE 32-2

PSYCHIATRIC DISORDERS OBSERVED IN THE INTENSIVE CARE UNIT

Anxiety
Depression
Behavioral problems
Hostility
Delirium/psychosis

DELIRIUM

Delirium is by far the most common psychiatric disorder in the intensive care unit. It is defined as "transient organic mental syndrome of acute onset, characterized by global impairment of cognitive function, a reduced level of consciousness, attention abnormalities, increased or decreased psychomotor activities, and a disordered sleep–wake cycle." A classification of mental disorders uses the term delirium as the only official designation for this syndrome (Table 32-3).

Delirium is a transient organic mental syndrome of acute onset characterized by global impairment of cognitive function.

Many patients experience delirium during their hospitalization, and its presentation can be extremely variable. Although the exact incidence is unknown, it is believed that 10%–15% of hospitalized medical-surgical patients and 30%–40% of intensive care unit patients suffer from delirium. The incidence may be as high as 50% in the elderly population. Patients with delirium tend to have significantly longer hospital stays and have been shown to have higher mortality rates (up to 20%) compared with similar patients without delirium. Besides the underlying disease process contributing to the development of delirium, this tendency may be related to potentially dangerous behavior that leads to complications such as self-extubation, removal of lines and catheters, and cardiovascular stress.

Delirium may affect 30%–40% of ICU patients. Delirium may present clinically in different forms.

Recognizing delirium and patients at risk can be a challenge for clinicians. An important fact to remember is that the onset of delirium is acute, is generally transient, and rarely lasts longer than 1 month. It is manifested by a disorder of consciousness or alertness, indicating the inability to be fully aware of one's environment. Because various symptoms can represent delirium, it presents clinically in different ways. The most common variant is described as hyperactive-hyperalert. These patients tend to be restless, agitated, and even combative. Acute withdrawal from alcohol (delirium tremens) is a class example of this variant. Less

TABLE 32-3

DSM-III DIAGNOSTIC CRITERIA FOR DELIRIUM

A. Reduced ability to maintain attention to external stimuli (e.g., questions must be repeated because attention wanders) and to appropriate shift attention to new external stimuli (e.g., perseverates answer to previous question).
B. Disorganized thinking, as indicated by rambling, irrelevant, or incoherent speech.
C. At least two of the following:
   1. Reduced level of consciousness, e.g., difficulty keeping awake during examination.
   2. Perceptual disturbances: misinterpretations, illusions, or hallucinations.
   3. Disturbance of sleep–wake cycle with insomnia or daytime sleepiness.
   4. Increased or decreased psychomotor activity.
   5. Disorientation to person, place, or time.
   6. Memory impairment, e.g., inability to learn new material, such as the names of several unrelated objects after 5 min, or to remember past events, such as history of current episode of illness.
D. Clinical features develop over a short period of time (usually hours to days) and tend to fluctuate over the course of a day.
E. Either (1) or (2):
   1. Evidence from the history, physical examination, or laboratory tests of a specific organic factor (or factors) judged to be etiologically related to the disturbance.
   2. In the absence of such evidence, an etiologic organic factor can be presumed if the disturbance cannot be accounted for by any nonorganic mental disorder, e.g., manic episode accounting for agitation and sleep disturbance.

TABLE 32-4

ORGANIC CAUSES OF DELIRIUM

Drug or poison intoxication	Hypervitaminosis
Prescribed drugs	Endocrinopathies
Alcohol	Fluid and electrolyte disturbances
Illicit drugs	Errors of metabolism
Industrial poisons	Infections
Poisons of animal, plant, and mushroom origin	Intracranial
Withdrawal syndromes	Systemic
Alcohol	Head trauma
Sedatives and hypnotics	Epilepsy
Amphetamines	Neoplasm
Metabolic encephalopathies	Vascular disorders
Hypoxemia	Cerebrovascular
Hypoglycemia	Cardiovascular
Hepatic, pancreatic, pulmonary, or renal insufficiency	CNS space-occupying lesions
Avitaminosis	Hematopoietic system disorders
	Hypersensitivity disorders
	Injury by physical agents

common and often overlooked is a hypoactive-hypoalert variant of delirium. These patients are sleepy, quiet, slow to respond, and describe decreased psychomotor activity. Because they have vivid hallucinations and are absorbed in a dreamlike state, they sometimes mumble to themselves or make inappropriate gestures. Patients may also have mixed delirium demonstrating features of both these variants. Irregularly and unpredictably, they alternate between the two forms, sometimes during a single day. J.C., from our case presentation, was an example of this form of delirium. He alternated among different states; awake and agitated, asleep and having bizarre dreams, awake and hallucinating, and awake and appropriate.

Multiple etiologies of intensive care unit delirium have been identified (Tables 32-4 and 32-5). It is not difficult to understand why J.C. became delirious. He had a severe fungal infection, acidosis, renal insufficiency, electrolyte disturbance, and hepatitis. He was treated with many of the medications listed in Table 32-5. In his case, as in most others, determining the exact cause of delirium is impossible and withdrawing potential causative agents means risking improper management of the underlying medical conditions.

Although any patient in the intensive care unit (ICU) can become delirious, certain underlying factors tend to predispose patients to this condition: age 60 years or older, presence of brain damage, and presence of chronic brain disease (e.g., Alzheimer's). Of these predisposing factors, age is the most predictive. Elderly patients tend to develop significant signs of delirium with only minor physiologic derangements. Patients who are elderly and demented appear to be the most prone to the development of delirium.

> Delirium has multiple etiologies: age, psychosocial stress, sensory overload or underload, immobilization, and sleep deprivation all contribute to the development of delirium.

Other factors that can contribute to formation of delirium are psychosocial stress, sensory overload or underload, immobilization, and sleep deprivation. One study of postoperative intensive care unit delirium found more than twice as many episodes of organic delirium

TABLE 32-5

DRUGS COMMONLY USED IN THE ICU THAT ARE REPORTED TO CAUSE PSYCHOSIS AND DELIRIUM

Acyclovir	Clonidine	Nifedipine
Aminocaproic acid	Corticosteroids	Nitroprusside
Amphotericin B	Digitalis	NSAIDs
Anticonvulsants	Imipenem	Penicillin
Anticholinergic agents	Ketamine	Procainamide
Antihistamines	Ketoconazole	Propranolol
Benzodiazepines	Lidocaine	Quinidine
Captopril	Methyldopa	Ranitidine
Cephalosporins	Metoclopramide	Theophylline
Cimetidine	Metronidazole	Trimethoprim-sulfamethoxazole
Ciprofloxacin	Narcotics	

occurred in patients located in rooms without windows. Also, experimental sleep deprivation in normal subjects can reproduce the same mental status changes as observed in ICU delirium. All these factors facilitate the onset of delirium and may worsen and prolong its course. Unfortunately, most ICU patients are exposed to all these factors.

Management of the delirious patient requires recognizing the syndrome and the patients at risk, accurately observing and assessing mental function, identifying and treating the underlying causes, and treating the symptoms. This task can be difficult and requires active participation of physicians, nurses, and ancillary staff. Nursing staff have the most contact with the critically ill patient and are ultimately responsible for their safety and for providing emotional support to patient and family.

> Management of delirious patients includes recognizing the syndrome in patients at risk, observing and assessing mental function, and identifying and treating the underlying cause when treating patient symptoms.

When a patient shows hyperactive and agitated behavior, the nursing staff can usually recognize this as signs of delirium. However, if the patient lies in bed, rarely talks, has decreased motor activity, and responds slowly, delirium can easily go unrecognized, because the patient does not present management problems for the nursing staff. This patient may be experiencing confusion or hallucinations. Once delirium is recognized, simple nonpharmacologic interventions should be implemented. Timing medical and nursing interventions to allow for periods of sleep can be extremely beneficial to the patient. Other nocturnal comfort measures are avoidance of loud noise and bright light while a patient is trying to sleep. Keeping a patient awake all day so he or she can sleep all night is not recommended; this practice may worsen the problem and can contribute to more sleep deprivation.

Sensory overload is very common in the intensive care unit. Noise should be limited as much as possible, by adjusting alarm limits on monitoring devices, keeping intercom levels down, avoiding loud staff conversations around patients, and shielding patients from viewing emergent events in the intensive care unit. During patient interactions, the patient should be addressed by name and every procedure should be explained as it is performed, even if the patient is well sedated and paralyzed. This practice lessens the chance of startling the patient and perhaps causing them to become more confused. ICU lighting can contribute to a patient's delirium. Natural and artificial lighting should simulate day–night cycles, and bright overhead fluorescent lights should not be flickered on-and-off without warning the patient or protecting them from the light. Continuous bright lighting promotes further anxiety and circadian rhythm asynchrony. Last, delirium can be further exacerbated by sensory deprivation. Keeping the patient informed regarding his surroundings and providing clocks and calendars can be very helpful. Allowing liberal visits by family and significant others can further decrease this sensory underload.

> Sensory overload is a very common phenomenon in intensive care unit patients.

After nonpharmacologic interventions, the patient should be carefully reassessed for persistent signs of delirium. The agitated and hyperactive patient requires sedation to minimize risk of personal injury and allow appropriate care. Of the many choices of medications to treat delirium, some have been proven more effective. Psychotropic drugs (neuroleptics) used to control signs and symptoms of certain neurotic and personality disorders have received a great deal of attention in the treatment of agitation. Although several neuroleptic agents can be utilized, haloperidol is considered by many to be the drug of choice for the treatment of delirium in the critically ill patient. It is safe, efficacious, nonaddicting, and has few cardiovascular and pulmonary side effects. Haloperidol can be administered in various doses every 20–30 min until agitation subsides. The return of agitation indicates the need for more haloperidol.

> After nonpharmacologic interventions are implemented for the treatment of delirium, the patient should be reassessed for persistent signs of delirium.

> Psychotropic drugs may be used to control the signs and symptoms of agitation.

> Haloperidol is considered by many to be a drug of choice for the treatment of delirium in critically ill patients.

Another class of medications frequently used for sedation in the critical care setting are the benzodiazepines, which must be used with caution because they may cause respiratory and cardiac depression (especially in the elderly or severely ill patients). An efficacious "pharmacologic cocktail" to treat agitation in the critically ill patient contains haloperidol and a short-acting benzodiazepine. The combination of these two classes of agents creates synergism and allows for smaller doses of each to be used with greater efficacy and fewer side effects. Benzodiazepines are also considered agents of choice to treat alcohol and illicit drug withdrawal.

> Another class of medications used for sedation in critically ill patients are the benzodiazepines.

If the patient's agitation is secondary to pain, narcotics can be successfully used to treat those symptoms as well as delirium. Unfortunately, this class of agents can actually cause or exacerbate delirium and has profound cardiac and respiratory effects. Barbiturates have

> If the patient's agitation is secondary to pain, narcotics can be successfully used to treat these symptoms as well as delirium.

been utilized in the past for treatment of delirium, but their role has been significantly reduced because of their high incidence of side effects and long half-life. Finally, in cases of severe agitation/delirium with concerns for personal injury, neuromuscular blockers have a therapeutic role. Use of these drugs should be judicious, and should be accompanied by appropriate sedation and analgesia, because neuromuscular blockers have no ability to alter consciousness, cognition, or pain.

ANXIETY

When patients suffer life-threatening medical illnesses requiring an ICU admission, they may develop acute anxiety and fear. The initial fear is always regarding their own death. Once this fear subsides, patients tend to become preoccupied with their illness and its treatment(s). The complexity of human personality frequently is revealed in the ICU setting by the numerous manifestations that fear and anxiety can take. Some examples include paranoia, frequent calls for the nurse, silent withdrawal, outbursts of anger and impatience, and threats to leave the hospital against medical advice.

The best treatment for anxiety in the ICU patient is a combination of medication and quiet reassurance.

The best treatment for anxiety in the ICU patient is a combination of medication and quiet reassurance. If anxiety is apparent when evaluating the patient, anxiolytic treatment should be considered, and the desired endpoint should be negotiated with a cooperative patient. Benzodiazopines are the best drugs for treating the initial stages of anxiety and fear. Which agent to use depends on the desired clinical effect. For example, physicians must choose between preparations that are oral or intravenous, have shorter or longer onsets of action or half-life, and between those agents that have or do not have active metabolites. Geriatric patients are particularly vulnerable to the accumulation of the longer-acting metabolites of benzodiazopines.

A recent study from University of Iowa tested the effects of music therapy on relaxation and anxiety reduction for critically ill patients receiving ventilatory assistance. Compared to a control group, these investigators demonstrated that a single music therapy session was effective in decreasing anxiety and promoting relaxation.

BEHAVIORAL PROBLEMS

For almost 30 years, it has been known that patients demonstrate a specific chain of emotional and behavioral reactions during their ICU stay (Figure 32-1). Initially, anxiety is prominent. It is followed by increasing denial of the significance and prognosis of the illness and the stay in the ICU, as part of a reaction against the development of anxiety. Several days into the ICU admission, denial subsides and depression appears, as the impact of the patient's clinical status becomes clearer. Premorbid character traits emerge, as patients adjust to the initial shock of the crisis that resulted in their ICU admission. During this time (about 3–5 days after ICU admission), patients tend to become more passive-aggressive, irritable, and demanding. If their normal personality has a hostile edge, it will certainly manifest as their ICU stay continues. This type of behavior often leads to disruptions in their care. Members of the medical and nursing staff may begin to avoid the patient or misperceive their medical needs.

Management of the delirium patient may be complicated and require consultation with a psychiatrist.

Managing these behavioral problems can be complicated, and a consultation with a psychiatrist may be necessary to help develop therapeutic strategies. Ideally, these strategies enable the caregivers to work with the patient and provide the best ICU care possible. Treatment strategies should be individualized to each patient's psychologic makeup (e.g., firm limit setting). Physicians must clearly communicate with the nursing and ancillary staff about specific helpful interventions that will best serve the goal of rapid recovery and successful discharge of the patient from the ICU.

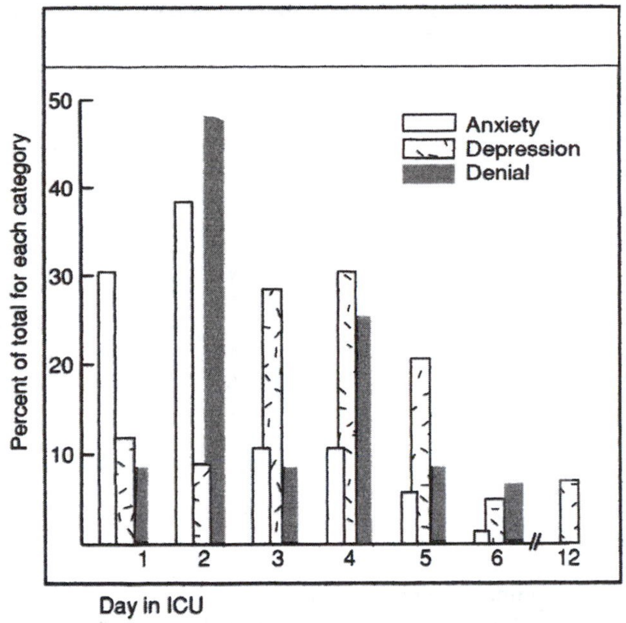

FIGURE 32-1

Typical onset of emotional and behavioral reactions of an intensive care unit patient.

TREATMENT WITH SPECIFIC PHARMACOLOGIC AGENTS

The use of specific medications to decrease patient recall of unpleasant events during the critical phases of their illness is extremely important. The medications more commonly used to treat psychiatric disorders arising in the ICU include benzodiazepines, sedative-hypnotics, antipsychotics, narcotics, anticholinergics, and antihistamines. We briefly review here the more commonly used agents in each class.

Commonly used medications used to treat psychiatric disorders in the ICU include the benzodiazepines, sedative-hypnotics, antipsychotics, narcotics, anticholinergics, and antihistamines.

Benzodiazepines

Benzodiazepines are the prototype drugs for amnesia. They also have anxiolytic, sedative-hypnotic, anticonvulsant, and muscle relaxant effects. The main effect of benzodiazepines is to produce anterograde amnesia (impairing the acquisition and storage of new information) but not to impair recall of information previously stored. This effect is ideal for ICU patients because the goal is to prevent awareness and recall of unpleasant events while leaving the patient's prior memories unaffected.

The main effect of the benzodiazepines is to produce antegrade amnesia without impairing the recall of previously stored information.

The benzodiazepines more commonly utilized in the intensive care unit are listed in Table 32-6. Diazepam, considered a long-acting benzodiazepine because of its metabolites, is used because of its rapid absorption and onset of effect in the central nervous system. Its half-life is approximately 30 h. Midazolam has a very short onset of action (5 min) and is considered a short-acting agent (half-life, 2.4 h), although it may have prolonged effects, especially in critically ill patients. Unlike diazepam, it seems to cause greater anterograde amnesia. Lorazepam is a long-acting benzodiazepine with excellent sedative and anxiolytic effects. Its peak effect is about 40 min and its amnestic effect lasts at least 4 h. Due to its lower cost and favorable pharmacokinetic properties, lorazepam has become the benzodiazepine of choice for long-term sedation in ICU patients.

TABLE 32-6

BENZODIAZEPINES USED IN THE INTENSIVE CARE UNIT

	ONSET OF ACTION	ACTIVE METABOLITE	HALF-LIFE (HOURS)	DEGREE OF SEDATION
Midazolam (Versed)	Fast	Yes	2–5	+++
Diazepam (Valium)	Fast	Yes	20–70	+++
Chlorezapate (Tranxene)	Fast	Yes	30–200	++
Fluazepam (Dalmane)	Fast	Yes	30–200	+++
Triazolam (Halcion)	Intermediate	No	1.5–5	++
Lorazepam (Ativan)	Intermediate	No	10–20	+++
Alprazolam (Xanax)	Intermediate	Yes	12–15	+
Halazepam (Paxipam)	Intermediate	Yes	12–15	++
Chlordiazepoxide (Librium)	Intermediate	Yes	5–30	++
Oxazepam (Serax)	Slow	No	5–15	+
Temazepam (Restoril)	Slow	No	9–12	++
Clonazepam (Klonopin)	Slow	No	18–50	++
Prazepam (Centrax)	Slow	No	30–200	+

Antipsychotics

Haloperidol, a potent dopamine antagonist, is the preferred antipsychotic agent in the ICU. It has little effect on the patient's cardiovascular status and respiratory drive. Acute dystonic reactions are rare in this setting. Although it is an excellent medication for agitation and delirium, it has not been shown to affect memory or recall.

Narcotics (Opioids)

Narcotic infusions (e.g., morphine, fentanyl) are often used in the ICU to provide analgesia and augment sedation. These agents are generally not amnestic and should be used with amnestic sedatives. Narcotics can, however, affect memory by modulating the learning process. Another problem with using narcotics in the critically ill patients is the significant effect of end-organ disease on metabolism of these agents.

Sedative-Hypnotics

Propofol is an ultrashort-acting general anesthetic. Although predominantly used as an induction anesthetic, it has been used as a sedative in the ICU. It seems to have significant anterograde amnestic effects when used in the operating room, but a similar conclusion has not been reached in the critical care studies.

Ketamine is another anesthetic induction agent that is generally reserved for use in patients with severe hypotension and depressed respiration. It exhibits dose-dependent analgesic, sedative, and amnestic properties. Unfortunately, ketamine can increase intracranial pressure and commonly leads to unpleasant dreams and the emergence of delirium.

Barbiturate use in the ICU is primarily reserved for anesthetic induction, to provide cerebral protection, and in the treatment of seizures. These agents have long half-lives and are not suited for routine sedation of critically ill patients. Little information exists on the amnestic properties of the barbiturates.

SUMMARY

Psychologic disorders such as delirium and anxiety are frequently seen in critically ill patients. Their etiology is not clearly understood, and these disorders can go unrecognized for days, which can lead to misdiagnosis, improper management, and often increased frustration for staff. Further research with long-term follow-up of ICU patients is required to determine the prevalence of psychologic disorders and their natural course. Etiologic factors also need to be understood. The nature of the trauma or initial illness seems to be of primary importance; however, the patient's personality plays a role, and the ICU environment may predispose to long-term psychologic problems. Detection of psychologic disorders in ICU patients is certainly worthwhile. Clinical experience suggests that early intervention improves prognosis, and that the long-term sequelae can be treated with a variety of medications, psychotherapy, desensitization, and changes in the ICU environment to improve cognitive functioning.

REVIEW QUESTIONS

1. **The most important factor contributing to psychologic dysfunction in the ICU patient is:**
   - A. Isolation
   - B. Beeping monitors
   - C. Sleep deprivation
   - D. Type and severity of underlying illness
   - E. Patient psychologic response to illness

2. **The most common psychiatric disorder observed in the ICU is:**
   - A. Depression
   - B. Anxiety
   - C. Delirium
   - D. Schizophrenia
   - E. Passive–aggressive behavior

3. **Delirium is twice as common in ICU patients who are:**
   - A. Receiving benzodiazepines
   - B. On mechanical ventilation
   - C. Housed in rooms without visible windows
   - D. With sleep deprivation
   - E. With pain

4. **The incidence of delirium in critically ill ICU patients is approximately:**
   - A. 50%
   - B. 80%
   - C. 30%–40%
   - D. 15%
   - E. 5%

5. **The psychologic disturbance associated with high mortality in the ICU patient is:**
   - A. Depression
   - B. Anxiety
   - C. Delirium
   - D. Behavioral disorder

ANSWERS

1. The answer is D. Type and severity of underlying illness. Patient isolation and beeping monitors (e.g., a form of monotonous sensory input) are important environmental factors that contribute to psychologic dysfunction in the critically ill patient. However, the type and severity of the underlying disease is the most important factor contributing to the development of delirium. Sleep deprivation and the patient's psychologic response to illness are also important factors that modify psychologic response but are not as important as the type and severity of the underlying disease in necessitating ICU care.
2. The answer is C. Delirium. Depression, anxiety, and abnormal behavior patterns are other types of psychologic disturbances observed in critically ill ICU patients, but delirium is the most common and the most important disorder. Patients with delirium tend to have longer ICU and hospital stays, higher mortality rates, and delirium can provoke dangerous behavioral patterns that lead to self-extubation and removal of needed lines and catheters, unduly contributing to cardiovascular stress.
3. The answer is C. Housed in rooms without visible windows. Benzodiazepines are a form of pharmacologic treatment for delirium, not a precipitating cause. Although the process of mechanical ventilation, which negates the patient's ability to communicate, along with sleep deprivation and pain can all contribute to patient discomfort, patients housed in ICU rooms without visible windows have twice the incidence of delirium compared to ICU patients housed in rooms with visible windows. The value of a visible window is that it allows the patient to orient themselves to time of year, and time of day, which helps to restore normal sleep–wake patterns, and reinforces patient self-monitoring of environmental cues to modify their behavioral response.
4. The answer is C. 30%–40%. Although the exact incidence of delirium is not carefully delineated, it is believed that 10%–15% of patients hospitalized on a general medical or surgical ward suffer from delirium. This incidence doubles in critically ill patients admitted to the ICU. Age may be another important factor, further increasing the incidence of delirium to approximately 50% in elderly, critically ill patients.
5. The answer is C. Delirium. Although depression, anxiety, and behavioral disorders are important issues that afflict the critically ill patient, delirium is the most important psychologic disturbance that carries with it a clear-cut increased mortality. In some respects, the 20% mortality associated with delirium reflects the severity of the underlying medical or surgical disease or signifies an acute or chronic disorder with limited physiologic patient reserve. Delirium represents lack of success in improving end-organ function due to the severity of the underlying illness or its re-

fractoriness to therapy. The development of delirium is an important factor that requires proper attention to identify the underlying disease process, maximizing optimal therapy or searching for concomitant disorders that may have been initially overlooked by attending to the primary disorder. In addition, environmental factors such as monotonous sensory input, absence of a visible window, and sleep deprivation should be sought and corrected.

SUGGESTED READING

Chlan L. Effectiveness of a music therapy intervention on relaxation and anxiety for patients receiving ventilatory assistance. Heart Lung 1998;27(3):169–176.

Geary SM. Intensive care unit psychosis revisited: understanding and managing delirium in the critical care setting. Crit Care Nurs Q 1994;17(1):51–63.

Granberg A, Engberg IB, Lundberg D. Intensive care syndrome: a literature review. Intens Crit Care Nurs 1996;XX:173–182.

Lloyd GG. Psychological problems and the intensive care unit. Br Med J 1993;307:458–459.

Sanders KM, Cassem EH. Psychiatric complications in the critically ill cardiac patient. Texas Heart Inst J 1993;20:180–187.

Schwab RJ. Disturbances of sleep in the intensive care unit. Crit Care Clin 1994;10(4):681–694.

Wagner BKJ, O'Hara AO, Hammond JS. Drugs for amnesia in the ICU. Am J Crit Care 1997;6(3):192–201.

Wilson LM. Intensive care delirium. Arch Intern Med 1972;130:225–226.

CHAPTER 33

Friedrich Kueppers

Host Defenses

CHAPTER OUTLINE

LEARNING OBJECTIVES

After studying this chapter, you should be able to:

- Understand the complexity of defense mechanisms.
- Distinguish among mechanical, biochemical, cellular, and immunologic defenses.
- Understand that defensive responses can overwhelm their controlling counterregulatory mechanisms and thereby can become harmful to the organism as a whole.

The body as a whole is built to defend itself against a potentially hostile environment. The specific features in the environment that are potential threats to the body's integrity may be mechanical, chemical, or biologic in nature. This chapter describes the most important defense mechanisms that protect against various insults including those which originate from the body itself. Situations that occur frequently in intensive care units when these mechanisms fail or are compromised are also described.

Invasion of the body by bacteria, fungi, or viruses is an ever present threat to the body's integrity. The intact skin cannot be penetrated by these organisms. However, patients who are on prolonged bedrest, particularly when they are unable to shift their body position because of paraplegia or weakness, frequently develop decubitus ulcers at pressure points, commonly the sacrum, heels, and shoulder blades. These ulcers can serve as portals of entry for organisms. The skin is also penetrated by the frequent injections that are medically necessary. Intravenous catheters that often remain in place for prolonged periods of time are other potential sites of entrance for infectious organisms.

The intact skin is essentially impenetrable for microbial pathogens.

Indwelling catheters themselves can also be sites for bacterial colonization; the bacteria, most often staphylococci, either are introduced with the catheter or may settle at the catheter site following bacteremia. The bacteria can form colonies on the catheters and give rise to bacteremia by continuously shedding bacteria into the circulation.

Mucosal surfaces are vulnerable to bacterial attacks when they are compromised by tubes or catheters. The tube can interfere with the protective mucus layer that covers the mucosa; it can also damage the mucosal cells directly by mechanical injury or indirectly by producing ischemia. These situations are common in the urinary tract with urethral catheters and in the lung with tracheal tubes when patients require mechanical ventilation. In the lung, an additional problem exists in that the endotracheal tube will interfere with mucociliary transport, an issue discussed later in more detail.

THE LUNG

The large (70–75 m^2) surface of the lung is exposed to ambient air and its contents.

The lung is particularly vulnerable to the environment because it is continuously exposed to the ambient air and its various contents. The total air-exposed alveolar surface of the lung of an adult is approximately 70–75 m^2. The amount of air that moves in and out of the lung in an adult at rest is approximately 10,000 l/24 h. With exercise, this amount increases considerably. The alveolar surface is covered by only a thin layer of lining fluid and surfactant. Dust particles, including bacteria suspended in the ambient air as well as gases and vapors, can settle directly on the alveolar surface. However, only the smallest particles, 0.3–2.0 μm, are actually carried to the alveoli. Larger particles (2–10 μm) settle on the tracheal, bronchial, and bronchiolar mucosa while particles larger than 10 μm are almost entirely filtered out in the nose and the throat.

The mucosal surface is covered with protective mucus.

Ciliated cells of the mucosa move the mucus toward the trachea and up the trachea to the larynx.

The trachea and the bronchi are covered with a layer of mucus. Any particle therefore settles on the mucus layer and not directly on the cell surface. Mucus consists of a liquid sol phase and a mucoid gel phase. The gel phase floats on the sol layer. Both components are produced by the submucosal mucous glands and, to a lesser extent, by the goblet cells that are located in the mucosal epithelium. Other cell types of the mucosal epithelium are ciliated cells and brush cells. Ciliated cells are present throughout the trachea and the bronchi, except for the smallest bronchioli, the respiratory bronchioli. Cilia are hairlike protrusions with a complex internal structure (Figure 33-1) that beat rhythmically, approximately 10–20 times per second. They beat in the liquid sol phase of mucus and, by their motion, drive the sheet of gel that is floating on the liquid phase in one direction, distally to the mouth, and therefore up the bronchial tree and the trachea. When the mucus, including bacteria and particles that have settled on it, arrives at the level of the larynx, it can either be swallowed or expectorated.

MUCOCILIARY CLEARANCE

This clearing mechanism of the lung is often referred to as the mucociliary elevator. Its efficiency is quite remarkable. It can move the mucus layer and its contents at a speed of 1–2 cm/min, and its activity is continuous because the cilia beat continuously day and night. The importance of this continuous clearing mechanism can best be appreciated when it is malfunctioning or when it experiences interference. In the immotile cilia syndrome, or ciliary dyskinesia, the cilia are defective on a genetic basis and are either completely nonfunctional or function insufficiently. The clinical consequences are frequent respiratory

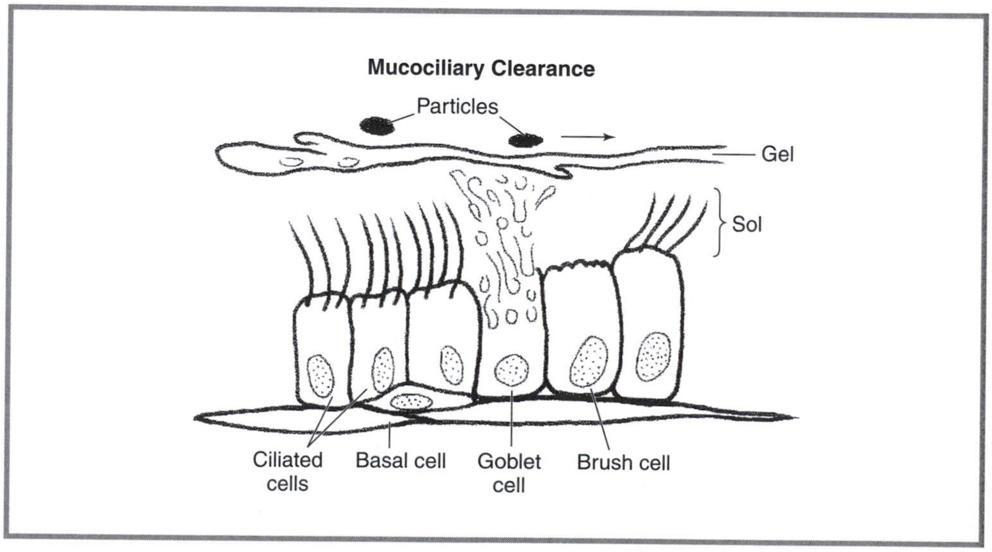

FIGURE 33-1

Schematic representation of the tracheal mucosa shows the major cell types. Note that the cilia beat within the sol phase of the respiratory secretions. The sheet of mucus (gel phase) that is being moved by the beating cilia is floating on the sol phase.

infections, chronic bronchitis, and sinusitis, to mention only the most severe symptoms. The obvious reason for these respiratory infections is insufficient clearing of respiratory secretions and bacteria that then can establish infectious colonies within the bronchi and the lung.

Some bacteria secrete substances that damage cilia and stop their activity. *Pseudomonas aeruginosa*, for example, has the ability to damage the ciliary membrane so that ATP leaks out. As a consequent, the cilia stop beating because ATP is their only source of energy. Ciliated cells can also be damaged or destroyed by chronic bronchitis, virus infections, cigarette smoke, and noxious gases, again resulting in defective mucociliary transport.

The consistency of respiratory secretions is critical for optimal functioning of mucociliary clearance. Loss of water leads to lowering of the liquid sol layer, which does not allow the cilia to function at their optimal efficiency. Too much water in respiratory secretions increases the sol layer; as a consequence, the cilia beat freely but the transfer of mechanical energy to the gel layer is insufficient, and the gel layer moves slowly or not at all. Introduction of mechanical barriers into the trachea in the form of endotracheal tubes or stents also interferes with mucus clearance and is therefore a predisposing factor for bronchitis and pneumonia. The ventilator-associated pneumonia discussed elsewhere in this textbook is a consequence of insufficient clearing of mucus, which fosters bacterial colonization.

The consistency of respiratory mucus is important for clearing efficiency.

COUGH REFLEX

The second mechanism available to clear secretions from the bronchi and trachea is cough. Cough is a complex maneuver. The first part consists of a forced expiratory motion against a closed glottis, producing high intrathoracic and intrapulmonary pressures. The glottis then opens rapidly, releasing the air from the lung. At the same time, the intrathoracic airways are compressed, forcing the noncartilagenous flaccid portion of the trachea and bronchi into the lumen, thereby decreasing the total cross-sectional area of the large airways and trachea to one-sixth of normal size at rest during tidal breathing. The velocity of air rushing through the narrowed trachea may be as high as 280 m/s as compared to 6.7 m/s with normal breathing at rest. With such a high air speed, accumulated mucus and particles on the mucosal surface can be expectorated (Figure 33-2).

Cough is the second major clearing mechanism for bronchi and trachea.

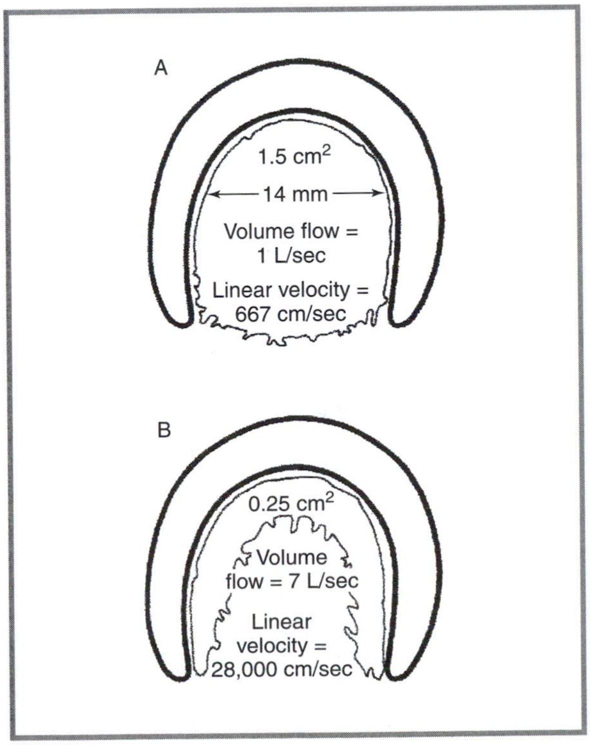

FIGURE 33-2

Changes in cross-sectional area of trachea. **(A)** Contours and dimensions of trachea during normal breathing. **(B)** During cough, the positive intrathoracic pressure inverts the noncartilaginous part of the intrathoracic trachea and decreases its cross-sectional area to 1/6 of normal; added to a 7-fold increase in flow rate, this increases the linear velocity 42 fold.

Particles 2 μm in diameter or less may settle on the alveolar surface. There are several ways such a particle may be handled.

Particles or bacteria in the alveoli are phagocytized and processed by alveolar macrophages.

1. An alveolar macrophage may phagocytize the particle. If the particle consists of organic material, it can be digested. If it is mineral dust, the macrophage can migrate out of the alveolus beyond the respiratory bronchioles and find access to the mucociliary elevator, where the phagocytized particle will be transported up the bronchi into the trachea from which it will eventually be swallowed or expectorated. The macrophage can also find access to a lymphatic vessel that will drain into a lymph node or toward the pleura. The macrophage usually dies at either of these sites, leaving the dust particle behind. The remaining dust particles can be demonstrated in hilar lymph nodes or at the pleural surface, where they form an easily visible network of dark material. Asbestos particles that are deposited close to the pleura can give rise to mesotheliomas.
2. If the offending particle happens to be a bacterium, the macrophage will also phagocytize it and process it internally. Internal processing of bacteria is initiated by the production of free oxygen radicals that oxidize the bacterial cell membrane and make it leaky and susceptible to further enzymatic attack. This initial step is essential to the killing of bacteria by phagocytic cells. Several defects are known that lead to decreased or total absence of oxygen free radical production. The result is chronic granulomatous disease that is characterized by chronic infections with *Staphylococcus aureus*, *Serratia marcescens*, *Escherichia coli*, and *Pseudomonas aeruginosa*, and formation of multiple granulomas. It is a rare disorder, but it is mentioned here to highlight the importance of this reaction in the defense against bacteria. If the macrophages are not successful in killing the invading bacteria, or if they are overwhelmed by too many organisms, the reaction may not be limited locally; instead, an inflammatory response can ensue.

THE INFLAMMATORY RESPONSE

The activated alveolar macrophage initiates the inflammatory response.

The factor that is best understood as a stimulant of macrophage activation is the lipopolysaccharide (LPS) component of the bacterial cell wall of gram-negative bacteria. LPS is released when gram-negative bacteria are lysed by macrophages or by antibiotics. LPS binds to a specific receptor (CD 14), located mainly on macrophages. A somewhat complex signaling sequence results in increased production and release of tumor necrosis factor-α (TNF-α), interleukin-1β (IL-1β), and interleukin-6 (IL-6). These factors in turn induce the production and release of other cytokines (Figure 33-3). As the number of cytokines has grown to more than 20, we discuss here only the major cytokines that have well-established functions.

TNF-α has several systemic effects: it lowers blood pressure and leads to an initial leukopenia and subsequent leukocytosis and temperature elevation. On the cellular level, TNF-α stimulates the immune response and bacteriocidal activity (see Figure 33-3). Studies in animal models have shown that complete blockade of TNF-α renders the animals unable to clear bacteria from the bloodstream and leads to death due to overwhelming bacteremia. However, prolonged elevated blood levels of TNF-α produce a sepsis-like picture. Experiments have shown that TNF-α appears within 90 min in the peripheral circulation after an injection of LPS and that it afterward disappears or is present in only very low concentrations. It is apparently no longer needed to maintain an adequate acute-phase response and an immune response.

The initial response of the alveolar macrophage is the excretion of TNF, IL-1, and IL-6.

Interleukin-1 (IL-1) has several functional similarities to TNF. Three distinct proteins are known: IL-1α, IL-1β, and IL-1ra. IL-1β is produced as a precursor peptide and only after processing by a cysteine protease (interleukin-converting enzyme) can it leave the cytoplasm. It has proinflammatory effects similar to those of TNF. The effects are mediated through binding to a receptor that is present on several cell types. A unique feature is the production of a truncated and modified form of IL-1β, known as IL-1ra, that is a separate gene product. It can bind to the IL-1β receptor and can block the action of IL-1β on the target cell. IL-1α is directly secreted by mononuclear phagocytes; it is functionally similar if not identical to IL-1β. Both interleukins are powerful inducers of the inflammatory response by directly af-

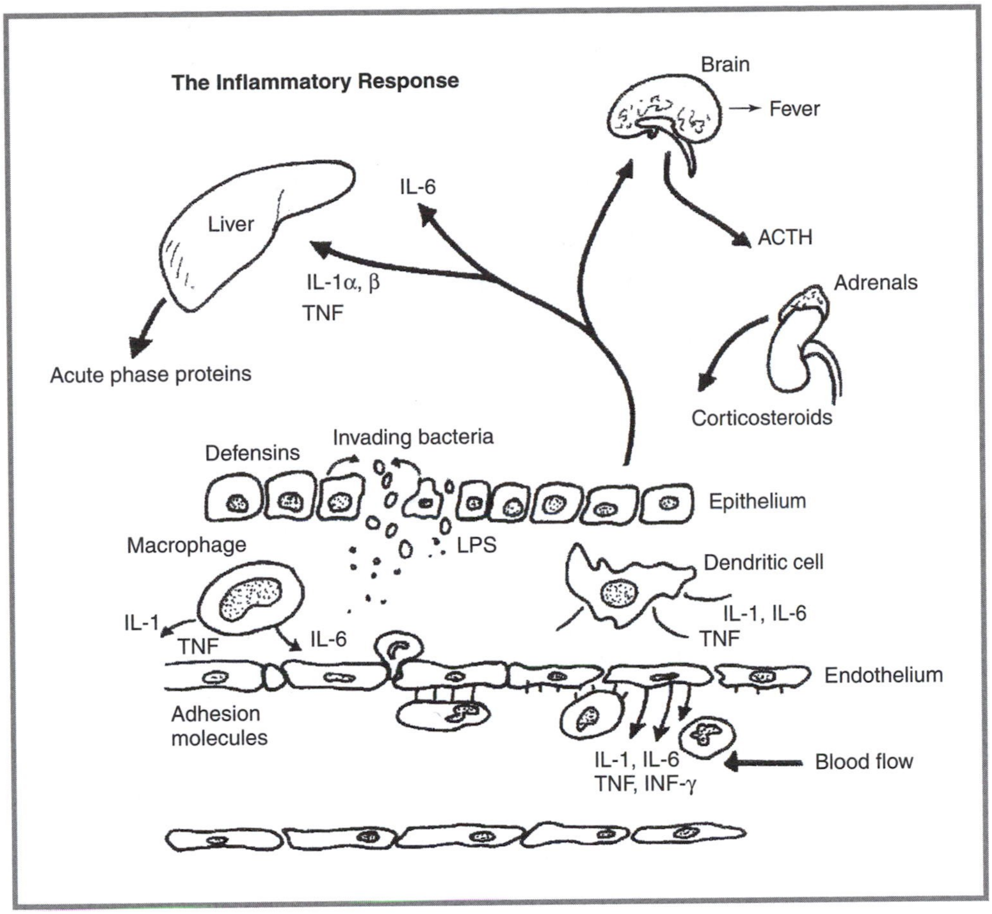

FIGURE 33-3

Bacteria have invaded the subepithelial space and release lipopolysaccharide (LPS). Inflammatory cytokines [interleukin-1 (IL-1), tumor necrosis factor (TNF), IL-6, and others] and defensins are released by the damaged epithelium, endothelial cells, dendritic cells, and macrophages. Under the influence of the inflammatory cytokines, the endothelial cells express adhesion molecules of the selectin family, which leads to initial slowing and then rolling of the polymorphonuclear neutrophils (PMNs) along the endothelial surface. Further chemokine release stimulates endothelial expression of binding proteins (I-CAM). The activated PMNs express integrins that interact with I-CAM and establish firm binding of the PMN to the endothelial wall. The PMN flattens out and penetrates the endothelial layer (diapedesis), and, following a chemokine gradient, migrates toward the site of the bacterial damage, where it will engage in phagocytosis and lysis of bacteria. The cytokines that are released into the general circulation reach the brain and the liver. The hypothalamus responds with temperature elevation; other areas of the brain may be responsible for the feeling of fatigue and malaise. The pituitary gland is stimulated to release ACTH, which in turn leads to increased release of corticosteroids from the adrenals. The liver responds to the cytokines, principally IL-6, with increased synthesis and release of acute-phase proteins: C-reactive protein, complement C3, fibrinogen, alpha-1-acid glycoprotein, alpha-1-antitrypsin, alpha-1-antichymotrypsin, haptoglobin, and alpha-2-macroglobulin.

fecting other cells to produce mediators such as other cytokines, arachidonic acid metabolites, nitric oxide, adhesion molecules, and chemotactic factors, to name just a few. These interleukins also have a direct central effect by inducing fever and fatigue (Figure 33-3).

IL-6 stimulates production of acute-phase reactant proteins by the liver.

Interleukin-6 (IL-6) is of particular importance among the various cytokines because it occupies a central role in the acute-phase response. It is a 26-kDa protein that is produced by activated macrophages but to a lesser extent is also made by lymphocytes and fibroblasts. IL-6 has a major activity on hepatocytes by stimulating the production and secretion of acute-phase reactant proteins including fribrinogen, C-reactive protein, alpha-1 acid glycoprotein, alpha-1 antitrypsin, alpha-1 antichymotryphin, alpha-2 macroglobulin, and haptoglobulin. It also stimulates immunoglobulin production by B lymphocytes and induces proliferation of T lymphocytes. Following LPS stimulation, its production and release by macrophages occurs after 4–6 h, in contrast to TNF and IL-1, which are produced within 60–90 minutes. IL-6 is elevated in septic shock as are other cytokines. A contributory etiologic role in sepsis is likely but it is not easy to separate its impact from that of other cytokines.

Similar statements can be made about other cytokines. Interleukin-8 is a chemotactic factor that is produced by several cell types including macrophages, lymphocytes, endothelial cells, and fibroblasts stimulated by LPS or IL-1 and TNF. Its principal function, is chemotactic activity for polymorphonuclear granulocytes, attracting them to the site of inflammation. High concentrations in the general circulation, however, are detrimental, as they have been associated with defective neutrophil recruitment and high mortality.

Interferons have antiviral activity.

There are three types of interferons. IFN-α and IFN-β are products of multiple cell types, whereas IFN-γ is only produced by activated T lymphocytes. The interferons have in common the ability to interfere with viral RNA or protein synthesis. However, they also promote CD8 T-cell activation and the activation of natural killer (NK) cells. High doses of IFN-α have increased mortality in mice infected with gram-negative bacteria. Blocking the IFN-α receptor with a specific antibody has been reported to protect mice from the effects of high doses of LPS. A protective effect in sepsis from gram-negative organisms has been seen in IL-10. IL-10 apparently exerts its protective effect by inhibiting the action of TNF-α, IL-1, -6, -8, IFN-α, and nitric oxide. The precise mechanism by which this is achieved has not been fully elucidated.

The inflammatory response is deregulated in sepsis.

The human body responds to invading infectious organisms with a powerful inflammatory response that is mediated by multiple cytokines such as TNF, IL-1, IL-6, and many others. These mediators act in a cascade-like fashion in that one mediator induces the production of others. Other cytokines such as IL-8 and IL-1ra and IL-10 can downregulate proinflammatory cytokines. A summary of some activities of cytokines is given in Table 33-1. In healthy individuals these mechanisms are capable of limiting a bacterial insult to a local site or, in case of a bacteremia, to eliminate the bacteria quickly by phagocytosis and lysis. However, these defense mechanisms may break down. The result is overwhelming bacteremia or a sepsis syndrome. The sepsis syndrome is apparently initially triggered by an inflammatory response that becomes so overwhelming that all natural counterregulations fail. Details of this catastrophic event are the subject of current research.

THE IMMUNE RESPONSE

The immune response is a powerful protective mechanism against invading organisms. In contrast to the inflammatory response (discussed in the previous section), which is immediate and directed against all invading organisms and agents, the immune response is adaptive in nature and can target specific organisms and offending antigens. Because its complexity is enormous, a somewhat simplified description is presented here. However, this discussion is detailed enough for understanding some of the situations important in critical care medicine.

The role of T cells in the cellular immune response is to recognize foreign antigens on cell surfaces and lyse those cells; T-cells also attract other T cells.

Two cell types are involved in the immune response: T and B lymphocytes. T lymphocytes, or simply T cells, consist of two major subgroups: cytotoxic T cells (CD8+) and helper T cells (CD4+, Th1 and Th2). Cytotoxic T cells recognize foreign antigens on cells that are infected by viruses or bacteria (Figure 33-4). They can also recognize mutated proteins on the surface of cancer cells and thus provide a continuous immune surveillance system. The offending cells are lysed directly by perforins, which are secreted by the T cells. Perforins are proteins that insert themselves into cell membranes, thereby lysing the cell. The T cells are limited in their response because they can only recognize relatively small (8–15 amino acids long) peptide antigens. Stimulated CD4+ T-helper cells secrete multiple cytokines that in turn stimulate B cells but also other T cells that have several other activities to initiate an inflammatory response (see Figure 33-3).

TABLE 33-1

ACTIVITIES OF SOME CYTOKINES

CYTOKINE	CELLULAR SOURCES	MAJOR ACTIVITIES
Interleukin-1	Macrophages	Activation of T cells and macrophages; promotion of inflammation
Interleukin-2	Type 1 (Th1) helper T cells	Activation of lymphocytes, natural killer cells, and macrophages
Interleukin-4	Type 2 (Th2) helper T cells, mast cells, basophils, and eosinophils	Activation of lymphocytes, monocytes, and IgE class switching
Interleukin-5	Type 2 (Th2) helper T cells, mast cells, and eosinophils	Differentiation of eosinophils
Interleukin-6	Type 2 (Th2) helper T cells	Activation of lymphocytes; differentiation of B cells; stimulation of the production of acute-phase proteins
Interleukin-8	T cells and macrophages	Chemotaxis of neutrophils, basophils, and T cells
Interleukin-10	Type 2 (Th2) helper T cells	Suppression of some macrophage functions, including secretion of cytokines; enhanced B-cell proliferation and Ig secretion
Interleukin-11	Bone marrow stromal cells	Stimulation of the production of acute-phase proteins
Interleukin-12	Macrophages and B cells	Stimulation of the production of interferon-γ by type 1 helper T cells (Th1) and by natural killer cells; induction of type 1 helper T cells (Th1)
Tumor necrosis factor-α	Macrophages, natural killer cell, T cells, B cells, and mast cells	Promotion of inflammation
Tumor necrosis factor-β	Type 1 (Th1) helper T cells and B cells	Promotion of inflammation
Granulocyte macrophage-stimulating factor	T cells, macrophages, natural killer cells, and B cells	Promotion of the growth of granulocytes and monocytes
Interferon-α	Virus-infected cells	Induction of resistance of cells to viral infection
Interferon-β	Virus-infected cells	Induction of resistance of cells to viral infection
Interferon-γ	Type 1 (Th1) helper T cells and natural killer cells	Activation of macrophages; inhibition of type 2 helper T cells (Th2)

SOURCE: Modified from von Andrian, HH, Mackay, CR. T-cell function and migration. N Engl J Med 2000;43:1020–1034

Macrophages and dendritic cells present antigens complexed with class II surface proteins (MHC class II) to the CD4+ helper T cells. B cells carry a large variety of immunoglobulin (Ig) molecules on their surface that recognize and bind the presented antigens. Under the influence of the stimulus by the CD4+ cells, they start to divide and to produce more Ig antibody specific for the antigen that was presented to them, leading to a full humoral immune response. The high specificity of the antibody is achieved by complex reshuffling of several components of the immunoglobin genes. Different immunoglobulins are expressed at different anatomic sites: IgG with its four subclasses (IgG-1–IgG-4) is the predominant immunoglobulin type in circulating blood and in inflammatory exudates, whereas IgA is the major immunoglobulin in the respiratory and intestinal tracts. Of all immunoglobins, IgE is present in the lowest concentration in plasma (approximately 0.05 and 0.5 μg/ml). It is also found in respiratory and intestinal secretions. Its importances lies in the fact that it has a high affinity to specific receptors on mast cells and basophilic granulocytes. In response, these cells release histamine, serotonin, and other vasoactive substances that can initiate an anaphylactic shock which can be life-threatening. The role of IgE in immune defense is probably its direct activity against some intestinal parasites.

B cells produce the humoral immune response.

It is intuitively apparent that a system of such complexity as the immune response can fail. Genetic defects are known for many steps that are necessary for a full immune response. These defects are only discussed here with respect to the pathologic outcome that may be encountered in critically ill adult patients.

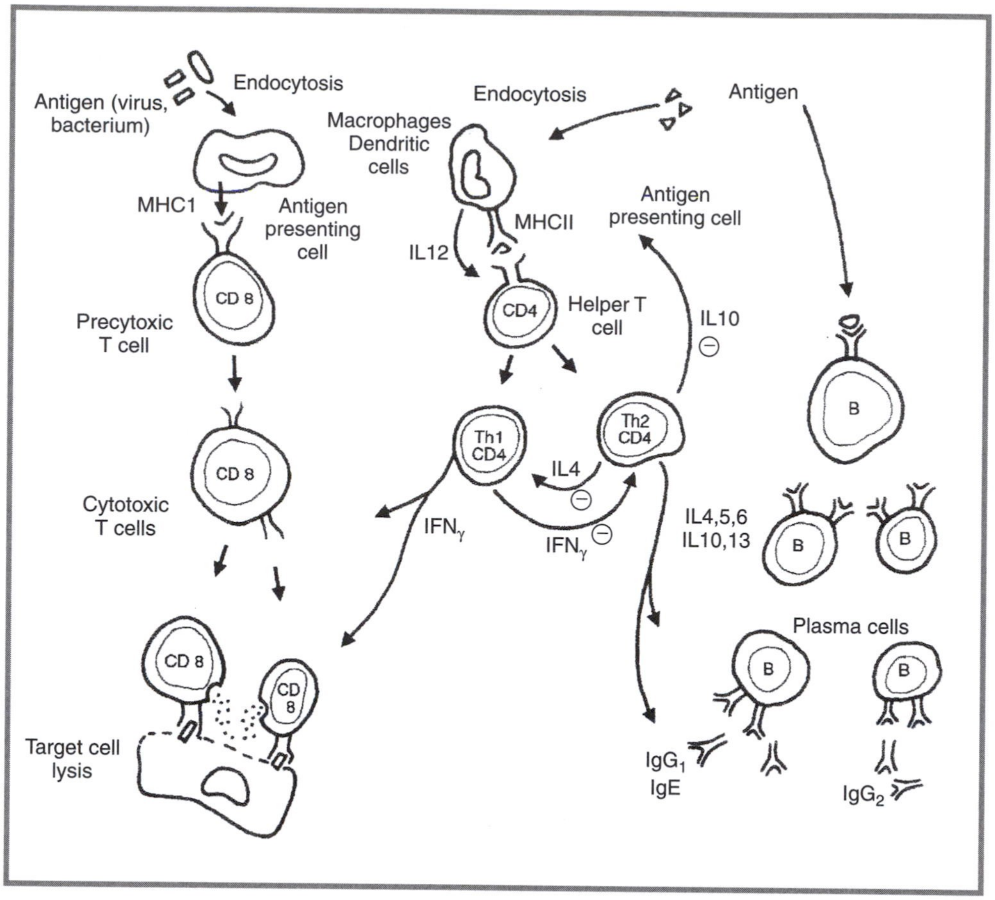

FIGURE 33-4

A macrophage or a dendritic cell encounters an antigen (a soluble protein or a virus or a bacterium). If the antigen is small (in most cases, a soluble protein), it is internalized and broken up into smaller peptides by proteases. These peptides, complexed with the major histocompatibility complex class II (MHC II), are presented to helper T lymphocyte CD4T cells. These cells become activated and are further differentiated into type 1 and 2 helper cells (Th1 and Th2). Activated Th1 lymphocytes produce predominately IFN-γ, TNF, and IL-2, which activate cytotoxic T cells (CD8T) and B cells; these B cells produce predominantly IgG-2. Th2 cells produce IL-4, -5, -6, -10, and -13, which stimulate antigen-specific B cells to produce antibody IgG-1 and IgE. If the original antigen is a virus or a bacterium, these organisms are phagocytized by macrophages or dendritic cells and internally lysed and processed. Antigens combined with the major histocompatibility complex class I (MHC I) are presented to CD8 cells. Under the influence of CD4+ helper cells, specific cytotoxic cells will recognize and lyse cells that express the original antigen combined with MHC I at their surface.

The cellular immune response or the humoral immune response can be affected. Major deficiencies of these responses usually become evident in childhood. However, there are some specific genetically determined immunodeficiencies that manifest themselves later in life.

Common humoral immunodeficiencies that are manifested in adults may be encountered in an intensive care unit.

1. In common variable hypogammaglobulinemia, the nature of the defect is not known, but its presence leads to suppression of B-cell maturation. The clinical manifestations are frequent bacterial infections, hemolytic anemia, frequent malignancies, and autoimmune diseases. The onset of symptoms occurs in the age range 20–40 years.
2. Less well understood immune defects are IgG subclass deficiencies in which one of the IgG subclasses is missing. These deficiencies can cause chronic respiratory and other in-

fections, presumably because one or several specific antibodies are simply missing from the total arsenal of antibodies.

3. Selective IgA deficiency is probably the most common inherited immunoglobulin deficiency in the U.S. white population, with a prevalence of approximately 1 in 600. A wide clinical spectrum is associated with IgA deficiency, ranging from the absence of any clinical symptoms to chronic and recurrent respiratory infections.

The cellular immune response can also be impaired by specific genetic defects. These defects manifest themselves in early childhood and are not likely to be seen in adult critically ill patients. The most prominent acquired cellular immune defect is the acquired immunodeficiency syndrome (AIDS). Although many different cells are infected by the human immunodeficiency virus (HIV-1 and HIV-2), the CD4+ T lymphocyte is the major target of the virus, leading to decrease and eventually a virtual disappearance of these cells. The patient loses the ability to eliminate infectious organisms that are normally targets of activated T cells such as *Candida albians*, *Cryptococcus neoformans*, *Pneumocystis carinii*, tubercle bacilli, and a host of viruses.

Cellular immunodeficiency in AIDS leaves the patient defenseless against many organisms that are normal T-cell targets, including *Pneumocystis*, *Candida*, and *Cryptococcus*.

The humoral immune response is also impaired, but to a lesser extent, as B cells retain the ability to produce antibodies that they made before the HIV infection, but their ability to mount an immune response to newly encountered antigens is severely weakened. AIDS is probably the most drastic example of an immunodeficiency that develops during adult life. There are, however other conditions that weaken the cellular as well as the humoral immune responses: malnutrition, chronic disease, malignancies, alcoholism, and iatrogenic regimens such as chemotherapy and, of course, immunosuppressive treatments that may be given to counteract the immunologic rejection of a transplanted allograft.

The humoral immune response is also impaired when T cells are suppressed.

A special situation is immune tolerance, which can develop when either very high doses of an antigen are infused, or low levels of an antigen are present, for prolonged periods of time. Low-dose tolerance is important because it can explain chronic carrier states for some viruses such as hepatitis B or C.

THE COMPLEMENT SYSTEM

The complement system closely interacts with the humoral immune response and thus is part of the body's defense against invading organisms. This system consists of several plasma proteins that interact in a cascade-like fashion. The complement proteins make up approximately 10% of the total plasma proteins. The usual activation process starts when an antigen–antibody complex is formed with most types of IgG molecules, or IgM. However, complexes with IgG-4, IgA, IgD, and IgE do not activate complement. The first complement component binds to a specific region of the IgG or IgM molecule in the antigen–antibody complex. This step leads to further activation of complement components C4 and C2 and, most important, C3. C3 splits into three components that are important because of their activity as anaphylatoxins. Anaphylatoxins induce degranulation and liberation of vasoactive substances and histamine from mast cells and basophilic granulocytes, thereby promoting vascular permeability and anaphylactic shock in extreme situations.

Complement binds to immune complexes.

Complement activation leads to liberation of vasoactive peptides.

The esterase of the C1–C4–C2 complex that activates C3 is regulated by a specific inhibitor (C1 INH). Genetic or acquired low concentration of this inhibitor leads to angioneurotic edema, which consists of localized extreme vascular permeability resulting in localized edema often following a trivial insult or trauma. Angioneurotic edema may occur in many soft tissues. It can be life-threatening if the larynx and vocal cords are involved.

C3b, one of the C3 products, is also important as an opsonin; that is, it favors uptake of C3b-containing immune complexes, or C3b-coated bacteria by phagocytic cells. C3 can also be activated directly, bypassing the "classical" activation cascade. The final result of complement activation is the formation of the so-called attack complex, which is a circular protein complex that inserts itself into the bacterial cell wall or the cell that was the initial target of an immune response, leading to lysis and destruction of the offending cell (Figure 33-5).

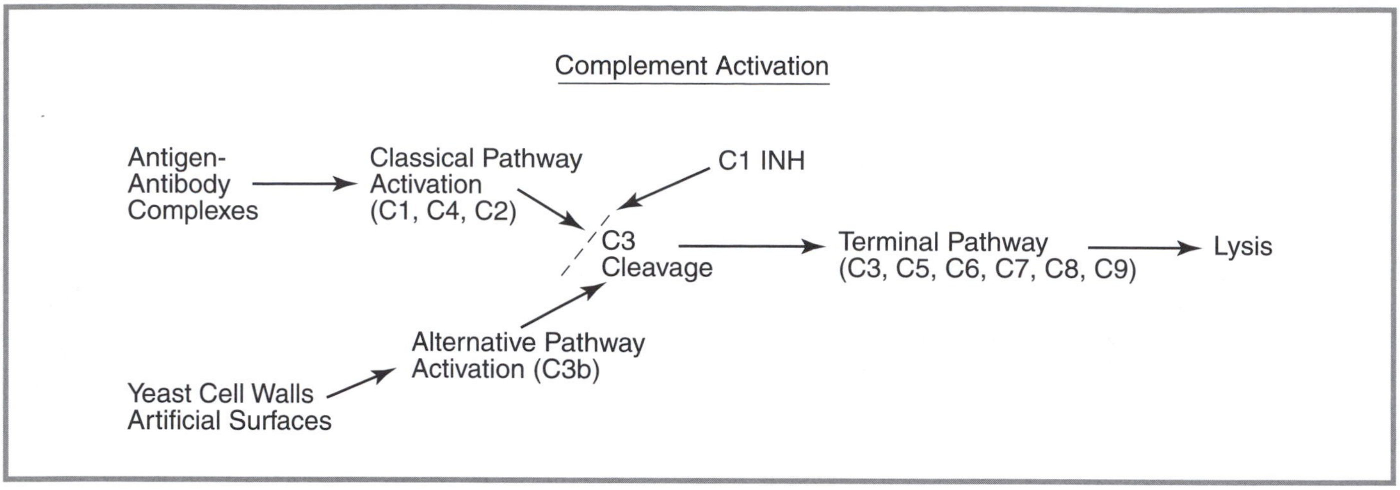

FIGURE 33-5

The complement components are labeled C with sequential numbers (C1, C2, etc.). Activation of the first three components C1, C4, and C2 by an antigen–antibody complex leads to cleavage of C3 by the activated C1 esterase in the C1–C4–C2 complex. The C1 esterase activity is regulated by a specific inhibitor (INH). By a sequence of intermediate steps, the C3 components catalyze the final attack complex, a cylindrical macromolecule that lyses a targeted cell or bacterium. C3 can also be activated directly by the alternative pathway (artificial surfaces, yeast, and other substances). Activated C3 will also lead to the formation of an attack complex.

SUMMARY

Multiple mechanisms defend the body against external and internal agents—mechanical, biochemical, and immunologic. The most important feature to understand about defense mechanisms is their redundancy; if the defense fails on one level there are several backup mechanisms that can limit the damage to the host which would otherwise occur. For example, if a bacterium settles on the alveolar surface, an alveolar macrophage engulfs the bacterium and lyses it. If this fails, polymorphonuclear granulocytes that have been attracted by cytokine signals attempt to phagocytize the offending agent. The next level is a more generalized inflammatory response involving a massive mobilization of granulocytes and production of acute-phase proteins that have antibacterial activity. The immune response that would then be activated has again multiple layers of cellular as well as humoral components.

Adding to the complexity are counterregulatory mechanisms that control almost every step in inflammation and immune response. Last, the defense mechanisms can fail or can simply be insufficient to control an overwhelming insult or they can overshoot and can become detrimental to the host, as probably happens in the sepsis syndrome and the adult respiratory distress syndrome, where massive cytokine production leads to capillary leak, hypotension, complement activation, and coagulation anomalies that characterize these catastrophic events.

REVIEW QUESTIONS

1. **Ciliated cells in the respiratory mucosa are important in pulmonary clearance because they:**
   - **A.** Adjust the hydration of respiratory secretions
   - **B.** Move mucus
   - **C.** Produce glycoproteins (components of normal mucus)
   - **D.** Absorb electrolytes

2. **Ventilator-associated pneumonia is usually caused by:**
   - **A.** Bacterial growth in the ventilator tubes
   - **B.** High humidity of the gas mixture from the vent
   - **C.** The unphysiologic O_2 concentration in the inhaled gas mixture
   - **D.** Interference with the pulmonary clearance of the vent tube
   - **E.** Aspiration of gastric content

3. **The most common genetically determined immune deficiency in the US population is:**
   - **A.** AIDS
   - **B.** Severe combined immunodeficiency
   - **C.** IgE deficiency
   - **D.** IgA deficiency
   - **E.** IgM deficiency

4. **The predominant immunogloblin in the intestinal tract is:**
   - **A.** IgG
   - **B.** IgA
   - **C.** IgM
   - **D.** IgE

5. **Dust particles that settle on the alveolar surface are readily taken up by:**
   - **A.** Mast cells
   - **B.** Type I pneumocytes
   - **C.** Type II pneumocytes
   - **D.** Alveolar macrophages
   - **E.** Polymorphonuclear granulocytes

6. **Factors that impair pulmonary clearance of airborne particles include all but one of the following:**
   - **A.** Tracheotomy
   - **B.** IgE deficiency
   - **C.** Increased water content of respiratory secretions
   - **D.** Decreased water content of respiratory secretions
   - **E.** Bronchiectasis

ANSWERS

1. The answer is B. The major function of the ciliated cells is the transport of respiratory mucus toward the trachea. In the trachea, the transport is cephalad toward the larynx.

   Brush cells are involved in fluid and electrolyte transport.

   Mucus production is by submucosal glands and goblet cells.
2. The answer is D. The endotracheal tube is a barrier to normal mucous transport. Mucus accumulates distally of the tube, and inhaled bacteria are not transported toward the larynx; they are thus able to form infectious colonies. In addition, the endotracheal tube acts as an irritant of the tracheal mucosa that responds with increased mucus production.
3. The answer is D. IgA deficiency has been found in approximately 1 of 600 persons in a white population sample. The prevalence in other populations is not known; it may be very different.
4. The answer is B. In the resting intestinal tract and in bronchial secretions at baseline, i.e., in the absence of inflammation, IgA is the predominant immunoglobulin. With inflammation, however, the basement membrane and mucosa become permeable to plasma, and IgG overtakes IgA in concentration.
5. The answer is D. Alveolar macrophages are the initial phagocytic cells. With inflammation, polymorphonuclear granulocytes move into the alveolar space and also engage in phagocytosis.
6. The answer is B. IgE deficiency alone is not associated with impairment of pulmonary clearance. Tracheotomy interferes with mucociliary transport. Increased and decreased water content of respiratory secretion lowers the efficiency of the mucociliary transport. With too much water, the sol phase is increased and the transfer of mechanical energy of the beating cilia to the gel phase decreases. Secretions that are too dry have a diminished sol phase; the cilia are compressed and cannot beat at their full efficiency.

   In bronchiectasis there is usually overproduction of secretions and loss of ciliated cells, resulting in a net transport defect.

SUGGESTED READING

Delves PJ, Roitt IM. The immune system. N Engl J Med 2000;343:37, 108, 1132.

Green GM, Akab GJ, Low RB, Davis GS. Defense mechanisms of the respiratory membrane Am Rev Respir Dis 1977;115:479–514.

Samet JM, Dominici F, Curriero FC, et al. Fine particulate air pollution and mortality in 20 US cities, 1987–1994. N Engl J Med 2000;343:1742–1749.

PART III

Specific Treatments in the Critically Ill Patient

CHAPTER 34

Clark U. Piatt, Ubaldo J. Martin, and
Gerard J. Criner

Mechanical Ventilation

CHAPTER OUTLINE

LEARNING OBJECTIVES

After studying this chapter, you should be able to:

- Understand the indications for mechanical ventilation, distinguishing hypercapnic versus hypoxemic respiratory failure.
- Recognize the various modes of mechanical ventilation and their specific indications.
- Review basic concepts of respiratory mechanics and their implications for monitoring patients receiving mechanical ventilation.
- Recognize alternate modes of mechanical ventilation and adjunctive therapies.
- Review ventilator strategies for specific diseases.
- Understand and identify complications associated with mechanical ventilation and the use of endotracheal and tracheostomy tubes.

The origins of mechanical ventilation can be traced back to Galen who initially described ventilating animals for vivisection purposes. During the eighteenth century, delivery of air to the lungs with a bellows was used to resuscitate near-drowning victims. This early technique of applying positive pressure to the victim's lungs fell in disfavor by 1827 after several experiments by Leroy identified the method with the development of pneumothorax. For the next 100 years, external devices that provided cyclical periods of negative pressure to the thorax to achieve lung inflation were developed. These initial devices led to the development of the "iron lung" by Phillip Drinker in the 1920s. The iron lung remained the mainstay of therapy for respiratory failure outside of the operating room until the 1950s, with its primary application in treating patients with poliomyelitis-induced respiratory failure.

During the 1952 polio epidemic in Denmark, the number of patients with polio and respiratory failure far outnumbered the supply of negative pressure ventilators. Ibsen, an anesthesiologist from Copenhagen, provided an alternate mode of respiratory support. He ventilated a 12-year-old girl through a tracheostomy tube by delivering positive pressure generated by manual compression of a rubber bag. As a result, positive pressure ventilation was applied to other polio patients, with teams of medical students manually providing ventilation throughout the epidemic. Mechanical ventilators were soon designed to provide positive pressure to the lungs, with the earliest machines designed by Engstrom to deliver a preset volume of gas from a piston-driven cylinder at a preset rate.

During the past 50 years, mechanical ventilation has become an instrumental therapy in medicine and is widely used to treat a diverse array of diseases causing respiratory failure. A significant evolution in mechanical ventilators has occurred during this time that has contributed to improved patient comfort and enhanced survival. This review provides the reader with basic knowledge of the mechanics and physiology of mechanical ventilation, as well as insight into the more complex modes of mechanical ventilation and their application in specific diseases.

INDICATIONS FOR MECHANICAL VENTILATION

The indications and settings of mechanical ventilation are best understood after characterizing the causes of respiratory failure into hypoxemic and hypercapnic components (Table 34-1). Hypoxemia of mild to moderate severity can often be managed by the administration

TABLE 34-1

INDICATIONS FOR MECHANICAL VENTILATION

- Hypercapnic respiratory failure
  - Increased respiratory workload
    - Increased resistive workload (i.e., asthma, airway obstruction)
    - Increased elastic workload (i.e., pulmonary fibrosis, pneumonia, or congestive heart failure)
    - Metabolic acidosis
    - Increased CO_2 production
    - Secretions
  - Impaired respiratory central drive
    - Sedation
    - Idiopathic central alveolar hypoventilation
    - Brainstem injury
  - Impaired respiratory muscle function
    - Mechanical disadvantage
      - Chest wall deformity
      - Dynamic hyperinflation (i.e., chronic obstructive pulmonary disease [COPD])
    - Muscle weakness
      - Electrolyte abnormalities
      - Myopathies
      - Neuropathies
      - Deconditioning
- Hypoxemic Respiratory Failure
  - Ventilation–perfusion imbalance
  - Right-to-left shunt
  - Alveolar hypoventilation
  - Diffusion deficit
  - Inadequate inspired oxygen

of oxygen through delivery systems ranging from a nasal cannula to facemask. With more severe hypoxemia caused by shunt or ventilation–perfusion mismatching, it may become increasingly difficult to maintain adequate oxygenation (PaO_2) and oxygen delivery (DO_2). Securing a stable airway via endotracheal intubation may be sufficient to improve oxygenation and avoid the need for ventilation in the setting of hypoxemic respiratory failure, ensuring adequate delivery of inspired oxygen and removal of airway secretions. However, in many cases of acute hypoxemic respiratory failure, institution of positive pressure ventilation is required in addition to intubation to improve oxygenation. Positive pressure ventilation, delivered either by a manual method (see Chapter 2), noninvasive ventilation (see Chapter 35), or intubation with mechanical ventilation, may recruit collapsed lung units, thereby improving ventilation and perfusion matching and decreasing the work of breathing while simultaneously decreasing oxygen utilization by unloading the respiratory muscles.

Mild to moderate hypoxemia can be managed by delivery systems such as nasal cannula or facial mask.

Endotracheal intubation provides a stable airway and may avoid the need for mechanical ventilation during hypoxemic respiratory failure.

Mechanical ventilation recruits collapsed lung units, improves ventilation and perfusion mismatching, decreases work of breathing, and unloads the respiratory muscles.

Another group of patients who are candidates for mechanical ventilation are those that are described as "tiring out" or developing respiratory muscle fatigue. These patients may have clinical findings that include nasal flaring, recruitment of the accessory muscles of respiration (sternocleidomastoid and intercostal muscles), paradoxical or asynchronous movements of the rib cage and abdomen, and an increased pulsus paradoxus. Patients develop an increased respiratory workload as a result of increased airway resistance in the setting of upper airway obstruction, copious secretions, acute asthma, or an exacerbation of chronic obstructive pulmonary disease (COPD). In COPD and asthma patients, hyperinflation may further contribute to increased work of breathing by placing the respiratory muscles at mechanical disadvantage. Decreased lung compliance as found in congestive heart failure, the acute respiratory distress syndrome, or decreased chest wall compliance as found in kyphoscoliosis or circumferential skin burns over the chest are other conditions contributing to an increased respiratory workload.

Patients developing respiratory muscle fatigue may exhibit nasal flaring, accessory muscle use, paradoxical movements of the rib cage and abdomen, and increased pulsus paradoxus.

Decreased lung and chest wall compliance contribute to an increased respiratory workload.

If the mechanical workload progressively increases, then breathing demand at some point exceeds the respiratory pump capabilities. As a result, patients are unable to sustain adequate levels of ventilation to effectively eliminate CO_2, and progressive hypercapnic respiratory failure ensues if the respiratory workload is not reduced. Under conditions of high respiratory workload, the oxygen cost of breathing may increase to more than 50% of total oxygen consumption. In this scenario, the respiratory muscles disproportionally consume oxygen at the expense of the aerobic metabolism of other organs, such as the brain, heart, and kidneys. Under these circumstances, mechanical ventilation decreases the work of breathing, decreases the oxygen cost of breathing, and redistributes oxygen delivery to the respiratory system, thereby improving oxygen delivery to other bodily organs.

At high respiratory workloads, the oxygen cost of breathing may increase to more than 50% of total oxygen consumption.

Mechanical ventilation decreases the oxygen cost of breathing.

In the setting of acute hypoxemic or hypercapnic respiratory failure, the primary goals are to maintain an adequate oxygen delivery by providing sufficient levels of oxygenation, while decreasing the work of breathing, and simultaneously providing cardiac and metabolic stability. If the underlying respiratory pathology is only transient or readily reversible, ventilation may be achieved through noninvasive modes of ventilation (see Chapter 35). Patients who exhibit altered mental status or cardiac or airway instability, or have copious secretions, are poor candidates for noninvasive ventilation and require endotracheal intubation and positive pressure ventilation.

Noninvasive ventilation is an option in patients with transient or readily reversible causes of respiratory failure.

PRINCIPLES OF MECHANICAL VENTILATION

The Ventilator

The mechanical ventilator comprises a pneumatic system that delivers breaths to the patient via flexible tubing connecting to an endotracheal or tracheostomy tube (Figure 34-1). The earliest ventilators delivered a set volume of air to the patient by means of a bellows or pneumatic piston. The pneumatic system of modern ventilators is powered by a pressurized gas source providing oxygen and medical air. To avoid harm to the patient and to minimize wear on the ventilator components, the initial pressure is regulated within an acceptable range of working pressures. A proportioning valve achieves the specific blend of oxygen and medical air chosen by the operator. Control valves then regulate the volume, pressure, and flow

Mechanical ventilator breaths are humidified, warmed, and filtered before delivery to the patient.

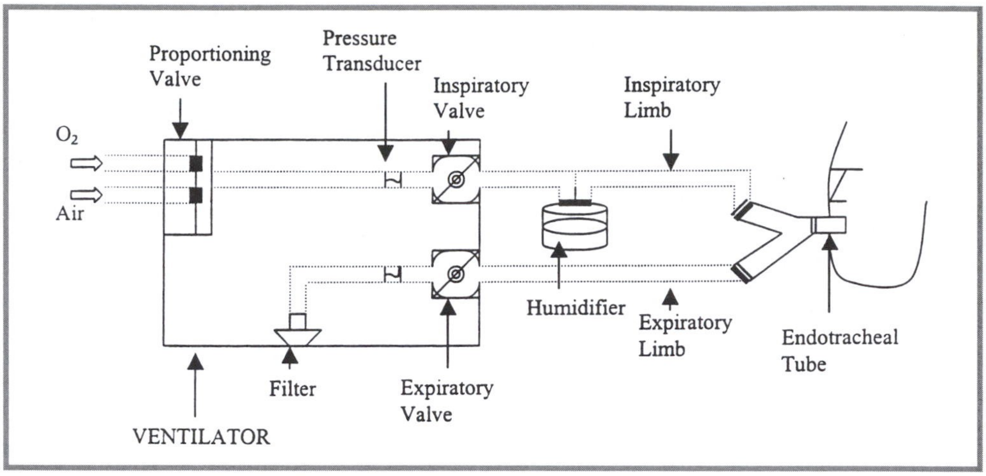

FIGURE 34-1

Schematic of a mechanical ventilator. Pressurized air and oxygen are delivered into the ventilator. A proportioning valve achieves the blend of oxygen and air specified by the operator. The amount of flow of pressure and flow delivered to the patient is controlled by one of several mechanisms (piston, compressor bellows, or proportional solenoid), in this case a flow-control valve. The mixture of air is warmed, humidified, and then delivered to the patient by an inspiratory circuit. The exhaled air is expelled through the expiratory circuit and filtered before being released to the ambient air.

from the gas source to achieve the desired mode of ventilator support. Before delivering a breath to the patient, the gas is humidified, warmed, and filtered.

The inspiratory and expiratory circuits contribute overall airway resistance. Because of the elastic nature of the inspiratory limb, a portion of energy of the ventilator breath is displaced within the tubing. The expiratory circuit remains closed during inspiration. When the inspiratory cycle is completed, a valve in the expiratory circuit opens to atmospheric pressure with the exhaled gases passing through a filter and venting outside the ventilator. The exhalation valve, which is closed during inspiration, is responsible for regulating the level of extrinsic positive end-expiratory pressure (PEEP).

Modern ventilators usually incorporate a microprocessor that controls the inspiratory and expiratory valves; the microprocessor also controls information that is monitored, displayed, and used in the alarm settings. In the event of pneumatic failure, a valve opens in the inspiratory limb, allowing the patient to breathe room air. In the event of electrical or pneumatic failure, some ventilators open both the inspiratory and expiratory valves so that gas flows throughout the circuit's inspiratory and expiratory limbs, thereby preventing CO_2 rebreathing, dynamic hyperinflation, or intrinsic PEEP.

Classification of Ventilators

To understand mechanical ventilation, it is necessary to understand some of the terms commonly used in regard to ventilators and their functions. Before discussing the available modes of mechanical ventilation, it is important to review basic concepts that allow us to classify and differentiate mechanical ventilators.

Control Variables

Control variables refer to those variables that the ventilator manipulates to deliver a breath. These variables are intimately related, and this relationship is expressed in the simplified equation of motion:

The variable that the ventilator manipulates to deliver a breath is called the control variable.

$$P_{mus} + P_{vent} = \frac{\Delta \text{ Volume}}{\text{Compliance}} + \text{Flow} \times \text{Resistance} \tag{34-1}$$

where P_{mus} is the pressure exerted by the respiratory muscles and P_{vent} is the pressure exerted by the ventilator. The right side of the equation simply states that the pressure generated by the combination of respiratory muscles and ventilator results in a volume displacement, which is opposed by the respiratory system's compliance, and flow, which is opposed by the respiratory system's resistance. The equation of motion further illustrates that ventilators can only control one variable at a time, either pressure, volume, flow, or

At a particular point in time, ventilators can only control a single variable, either pressure, flow, volume, or time.

time. The controlled variable becomes the independent variable and the others will be dependent variables. For example, if a ventilator delivers pressure, the pressure applied to the respiratory system and its opposing forces, namely resistance and compliance, will determine flow and volume. Thus, ventilators are classified as flow, pressure, or volume controllers.

Phase Variables

The period between the beginning of one breath and the beginning of the next one is called a cycle. The events within a cycle, that is, the beginning, duration, and end of a breath, are determined by so-called phase variables.

Trigger To initiate a breath, the ventilator must recognize that a preset value has been reached. The trigger or initiating variable can be time, so that after a certain amount of time has elapsed, the ventilator will deliver a breath. Ventilators can also be triggered by the patient's effort (Figure 34-2). Traditionally, ventilators have been triggered by pressure; in this case the patient must exert a predetermined amount of negative pressure to elicit a ventilator-assisted breath (-1 to -5 cmH_2O). More recently, alternatives such as flow and volume triggering have become available. In flow triggering, the patient's effort decreases the bias flow in the ventilator circuit by a determined value (1–3 l/min), which then initiates a breath. This form of triggering results in less work for the patient and a faster response time from the ventilator.

Ventilator breaths are triggered by exerting a determined pressure or by achieving a specific volume or flow.

Limit and Cycle The terms limit and cycle are frequently confused. For our purposes, if a variable such as pressure reaches a preset value and causes inspiration to end, it is called a cycle variable. If the preset value is reached without causing inspiration to end, it is called a limit variable (Figure 34-3).

Breath Types Breath types can be classified in several different ways. A breath is said to be spontaneous if the patient determines its beginning, duration, and end. If the ventilator controls any of these aspects, the breath is termed mandatory or controlled.

When a patient determines beginning, duration, and end of a breath, it is called spontaneous.

Modes of Mechanical Ventilation The mode of mechanical ventilation describes a particular set of characteristics or control and phase variables (cycle, trigger, limit) that define how ventilation is provided. It allows clinicians to communicate how ventilatory support is being delivered by a short and concise description.

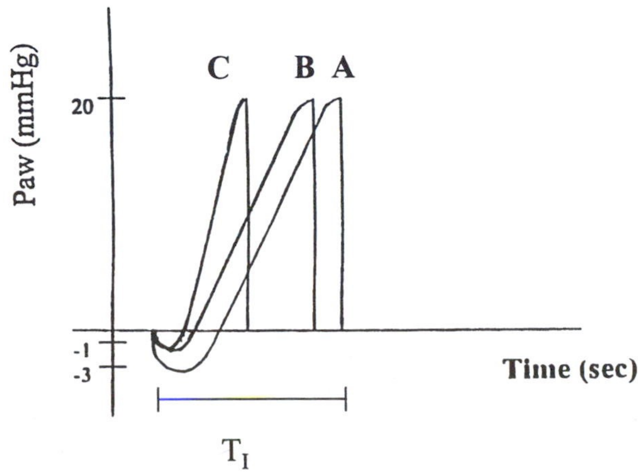

FIGURE 34-2

The effect of sensitivity and inspiratory flow rate on inspiratory time (T_I). In pressure curve *A*, the ventilator was triggered at a sensitivity of -3 cmH_2O. Curves *A* and *B* have the same inspiratory flow rate (notice the slope of the curve is the same, but the ventilator was triggered at -1.5 cmH_2O, which resulted in a shorter T_I. The sensitivity in *A* and *B* is the same, but the inspiratory flow rate is greater in *C*, resulting in a further decrease in T_I.

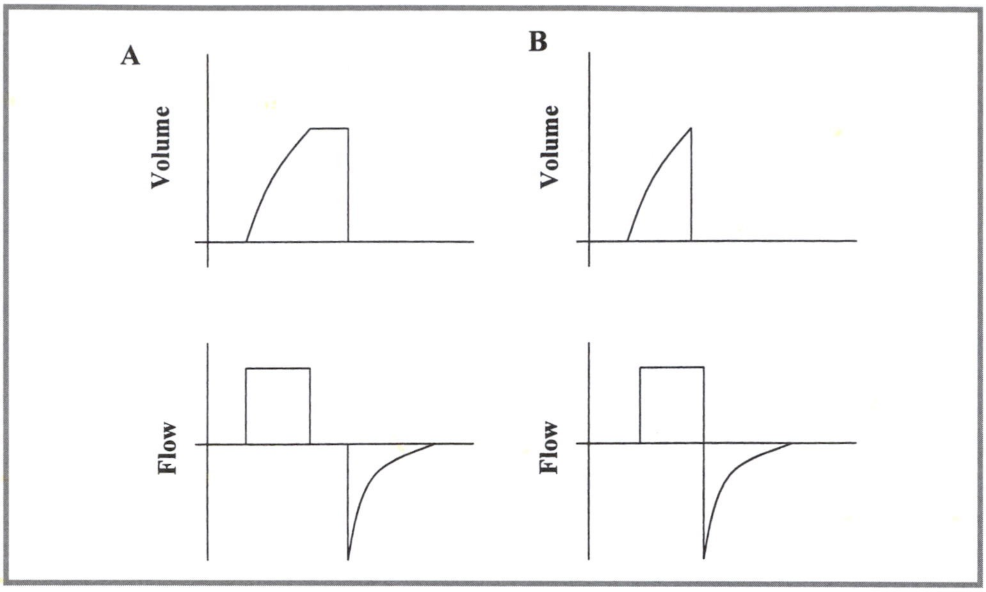

FIGURE 34-3

The difference between limit and cycle. **(A)** Both flow and volume are limited (they reach preset values before end-inspiration) and the inspiration is time cycled (after an inspiratory pause ends). **(B)** Flow is limited because it reaches its maximal value without ending the cycle, and the inspiration is volume cycled. Note expiration starts once volume has reached a preset maximum.

Setting the Ventilator

Fractional Inspired Oxygen Concentration (FiO_2)

To raise the level of PaO_2, the physician can increase the ventilator-delivered volume or increase the FiO_2.

FiO_2 should be rapidly titrated to minimize possible O_2 toxicity.

The principal means by which the physician increases PaO_2 is to raise the FiO_2 or to increase the lung volume at which the lungs are being ventilated. If a patient shows appropriate oxygen saturation with a particular level of FiO_2 before intubation, a similar FiO_2 can be used as an initial setting; otherwise, it is generally acceptable to initiate ventilatory support with an FiO_2 of 1.0. FiO_2 should be rapidly titrated to minimize the potential for possible O_2 toxicity, particularly in patients who are receiving concomitant treatment with drugs such as amiodarone or bleomycin that can enhance the toxic effects of oxygen.

Tidal Volume (V_T)

To decrease alveolar overdistension, delivered tidal volumes should be set between 6 and 10 ml/kg.

Tidal volumes of 10–15 ml/kg were traditionally used to ventilate patients. In the past decade, data have demonstrated that these volumes may cause alveolar overdistension, alveolar fracture, and ventilator-induced lung injury (VILI). Some investigators currently suggest using tidal volumes between 6 and 10 ml/kg. This caution is particularly important when ventilating patients with the acute respiratory distress syndrome (ARDS) and patients with severe bronchospasm. It is important to recognize that these new "protective ventilator strategies" may not be applicable in patients with conditions resulting in decreased chest wall compliance, such as kyphoscoliosis and obesity.

Inspiratory Flow Rate

The inspiratory flow rate, measured in liters per minute (l/min), determines how fast a V_T is delivered. The inspiratory time (T_I) is a function of V_T and flow rate:

$$T_I = V_T \text{ (l) /flow rate (l/min)} \quad (34\text{-}2)$$

The expiratory time is determined by the inspiratory time and ventilator frequency.

The inspiratory flow rate affects the inspiration–expiration ratio.

The expiratory time (TE) is determined by the inspiratory flow rate and the ventilator's frequency. For a set rate of 10 breaths/mm, the total respiratory cycle time (T_{tot}) is 6 s. The expiratory time can be determined by subtracting T_I from T_{tot}. The flow rate may also be altered during the inspiratory cycle by the use of a specific inspiratory flow pattern. Types of inspiratory patterns include rectangular, ascending ramp, descending ramp, and sinusoidal waveforms.

The relationship between inspiration and expiration is known as the inspiration–expiration (I:E) time ratio. It is clear from this that the inspiratory flow rate affects T_I and the I:E ratio.

Respiratory Rate

Once the tidal volume and FiO_2 have been set, a respiratory rate must be chosen that takes into account the patient's spontaneous rate, the patient's anticipated ventilatory requirements, and the impact of the set respiratory rate on patient–ventilator interaction (Figure 34-4).

In general, and unless the patient is sedated or paralyzed, respiratory rates below 15–20 breaths/min are poorly tolerated. Neurohumoral feedback from lung edema and inflamma-

Ventilator respiratory rates below 15–20 breaths per minute are poorly tolerated unless the patient is sedated or paralyzed.

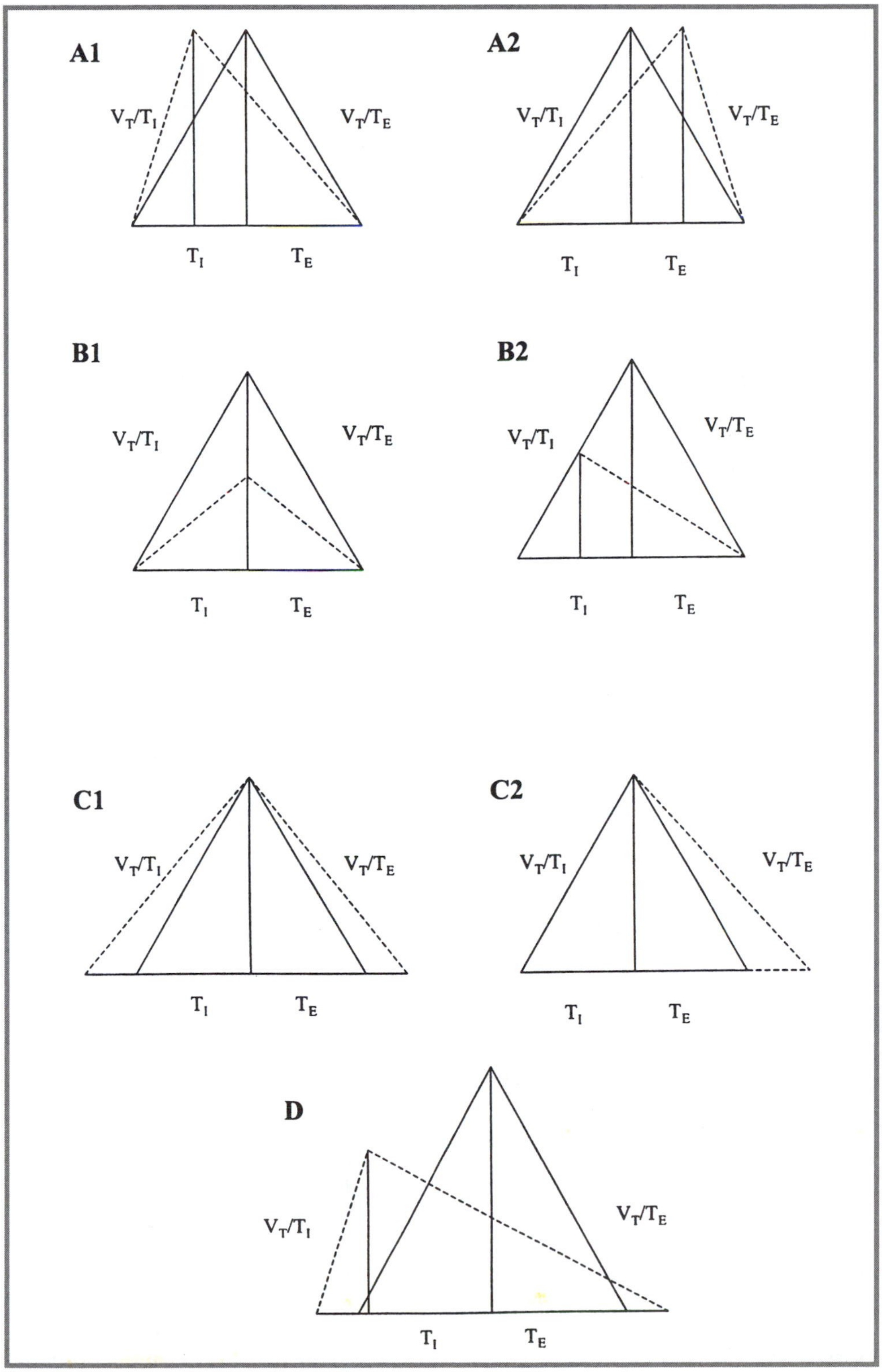

FIGURE 34-4

Relationship between tidal volume V_T), inspiratory time (T_I), expiratory time (T_E), and inspiratory flow rate (V_T/T_I). (See text)

The machine rate should be set close to the patient's own respiratory rate.

tion generally results in a rapid, shallow breathing pattern that is independent of chemoreceptive and mechanoreceptive effects on respiratory pattern. Additionally, discrepancies between actual and machine-set respiratory rates may lead to breathing patterns with inverted inspiratory to expiratory time (I:E) ratios, which are poorly tolerated. The machine rate should therefore be set close to the patient's own rate. If the actual rate is so high that effective ventilation cannot be accomplished, sedation or paralysis may be required after a careful search for rapidly reversible causes of tachypnea (pain, discomfort, fever, etc.).

I:E Ratio

Patients with asthma and chronic obstructive pulmonary disease (COPD) require a prolonged time to empty the inspired lung volume.

Increasing inspiratory flow rate with a constant respiratory rate and tidal volume results in a shorter inspiratory time and a longer expiratory time.

The relationship between the time spent in inspiration and the time spent in expiration is called the I:E ratio. The I:E ratio is not set by the operator; it results from altering the different parameters that have been previously discussed. In normal, spontaneously breathing subjects, there is abundant time to exhale the inspired tidal volume. In certain pathologic states, such as asthma and COPD, the decrement in expiratory flow may require a prolonged time to empty the inspired lung volume. How do tidal volume (V_T), respiratory rate (f), and inspiratory flow rate affect the I:E ratio? Figure 34-4 depicts how changes in these variables affect the I:E ratio. If inspiratory flow is increased and V_T and f remain constant, the inspiratory time will be shortened and the I:E ratio will be decreased (1:2 to 1:4, for example) (Figure 34-4A1). Decreasing inspiratory flow under the same conditions results in the opposite effect (Figure 34-4A2).

Decreasing V_T will have different effects, depending on the type of ventilator or ventilator mode being used. In ventilators or ventilatory modes that maintain a fixed I:E ratio and f (Siemens Servo or pressure-control ventilation), decreasing V_T will result in a decreased inspiratory flow while T_{tot} is held constant (Figure 34-4B1). If the ventilator maintains a constant inspiratory flow (Puritan Bennet 7200) and f, decreasing V_T will shorten the inspiratory time and decrease the I:E ratio (Figure 34-34B2). A decrement in respiratory rate, coupled with a fixed I:E ratio and V_T, results in an increment in T_{tot} and decreases in inspiratory and expiratory flow (Figure 34-4C1). Decreasing the respiratory rate while maintaining V_T and a constant inspiratory flow results in an increase in the duration of the cycle (T_{tot}); inspiratory time remains the same, expiratory time increases, and expiratory flow rate decreases (Figure 34-4C2).

In patients with emphysema, decreasing tidal volume, increasing inspiratory flow rate, and decreasing set respiratory rate allows more time to empty the inhaled lung volume.

Knowing the effects of altering these parameters is extremely useful. In patients with emphysema who have an expiratory flow limitation, decreasing tidal volumes, increasing the inspiratory flow rate, and decreasing the set respiratory rate will all decrease the inspiratory time and increase expiratory time. The additional expiratory time allows ventilator-delivered tidal volumes to be more completely exhaled and decreases the risk of developing intrinsic PEEP and its consequences (see Figure 34-4D).

BASIC MODES OF MECHANICAL VENTILATION

The mode of mechanical ventilation describes a particular set of characteristics or variables (cycle, trigger, limit) that define how ventilation is provided.

Assist-Control Ventilation

With assist-control (AC) ventilation, a set volume (or pressure) is given every time the ventilator is triggered.

Assist-control ventilation (ACV) is the most common mode of mechanical ventilation initially applied to patients who present with hypercapnic or hypoxemic respiratory failure. With AC ventilation, the physician sets a minimal rate and tidal volume (or pressure). The patient may trigger the mechanical ventilator at a faster rate, but the set volume (or pressure) will be delivered with each breath. Figure 34-5 is a representative tracing of AC ventilation with targeted volume. In the AC mode, the ventilator can be triggered by flow or by pressure. When the ventilator is set to be triggered by pressure, the patient must generate a certain amount of pressure (usually 1–3 cmH_2O) to open the solenoid valve and receive a ventilator-assisted breath (see Figure 34-2). If the ventilator is set to be triggered by flow, follow-

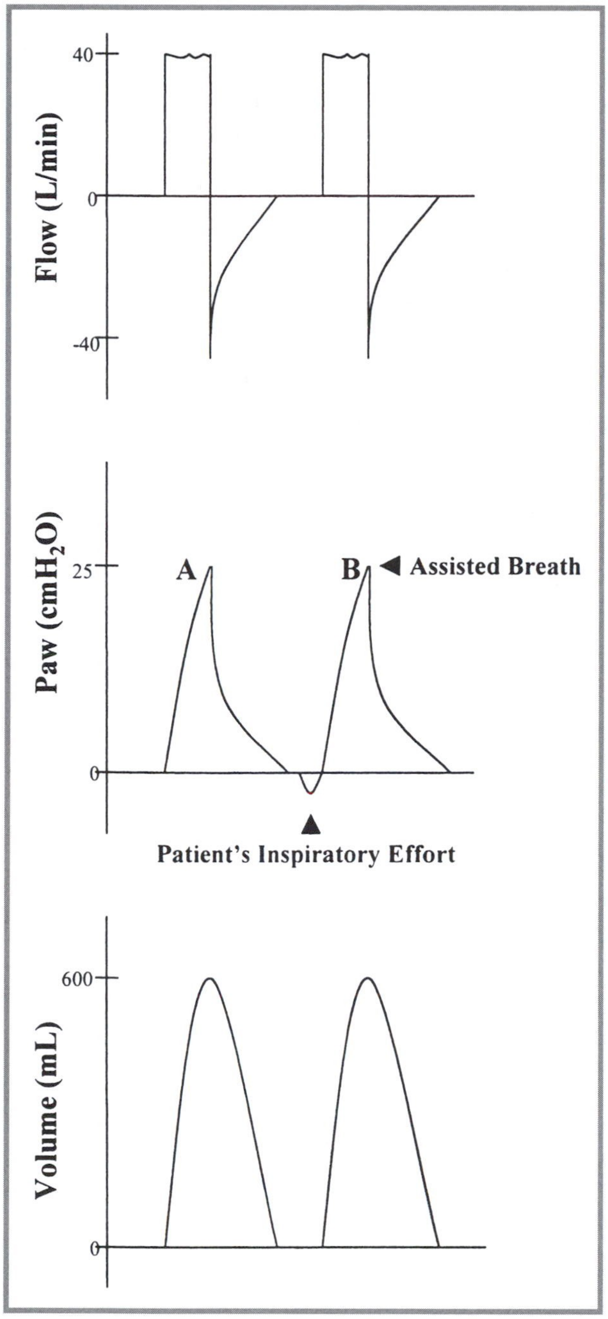

FIGURE 34-5

Pressure, flow, and volume waveforms during volume-targeted, assist-control ventilation. Breath *A* is not patient triggered. In contrast, a negative deflection is seen before breath *B*, representing the patient's inspiratory effort that triggers a ventilator breath.

ing a patient's inspiratory effort, the ventilator will sense a decrement in the circuit's baseline flow and only then deliver a breath. If the patient has no spontaneous inspiratory efforts, the ventilator will be time-triggered based on the set respiratory rate.

If the patient does not trigger the ventilator during AC ventilation, tidal volumes will be delivered at the preset respiratory rate.

Tidal volume (V_T) are generally set at 6–8 ml/kg; larger inflation volumes are avoided, as they contribute to increased intrathoracic pressures and may adversely affect cardiac output. In addition, larger tidal volumes may complicate the ventilator management of patients with heterogeneous lung pathology or regional differences in compliance. In patients with emphysema, large volumes are preferentially delivered to the most diseased and compliant areas. As a result, a larger proportion of the delivered volume will not participate in gas exchange but may possibly contribute to dynamic hyperinflation, intrinsic PEEP, decreased cardiac output, and worsening ventilation–perfusion mismatch. In patients with ARDS, who characteristically present with large regional variations in compliance, large tidal volumes will result in overdistension of the more compliant regions and may possibly contribute to

In acute respiratory distress syndrome (ARDS), large ventilator volumes may result in overdistension of the more compliant lung regions and contribute to ventilator-induced lung injury.

ventilator-induced lung injury. During ACV, changes in flow or pressure within the respiratory circuit generated by the patient's inspiratory effort trigger the beginning of the inspiratory cycle.

Controlled mechanical ventilation (CMV), the predecessor of ACV, delivers mandatory tidal volumes at a set rate delivered independent of the patient's own respiratory cycle. The major disadvantage of CMV is patient discomfort, which results from an increase in the work of breathing when mandatory breaths are asynchronous with the patient's own respiratory efforts. Patients are unable to alter their minute ventilation (V_E) if their clinical situation changes (e.g., increased $PaCO_2$, decreased PaO_2, decreased pH); therefore, maintenance of the acid–base balance is solely the responsibility of the practitioner.

Synchronized Intermittent Mandatory Ventilation

During synchronized intermittent mandatory ventilation (SIMV), between mandatory breaths the patient is allowed to breathe spontaneously from a demand valve.

Synchronized intermittent mandatory ventilation (SIMV) is a ventilator mode in which the ventilator mandatory breaths are delivered in synchrony with the patient's own inspiratory effort. Breaths are delivered at a set rate and volume. Between mandatory breaths, the patient is allowed to breathe spontaneously from a demand valve or a continuous flow of gas (Figure 34-6). Spontaneous breaths may also be supported with titrable levels of pressure support (PS) or continuous positive airway pressure (CPAP). During SIMV, each time cycle

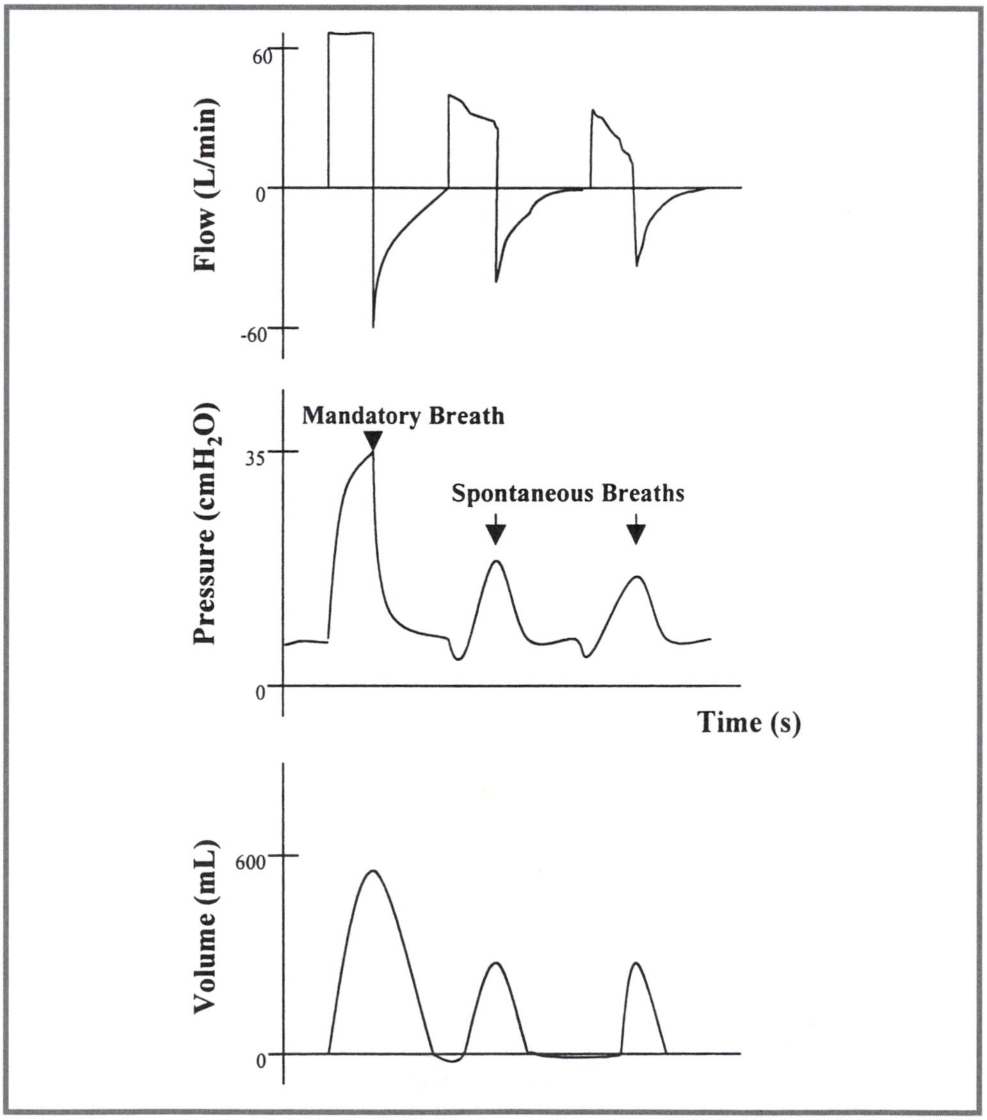

FIGURE 34-6

Pressure, flow, and volume tracings during volume-targeted, intermittent mandatory ventilation (IMV). The first breath is mandatory. The second and third breaths are spontaneous, evidencing a smaller volume displacement.

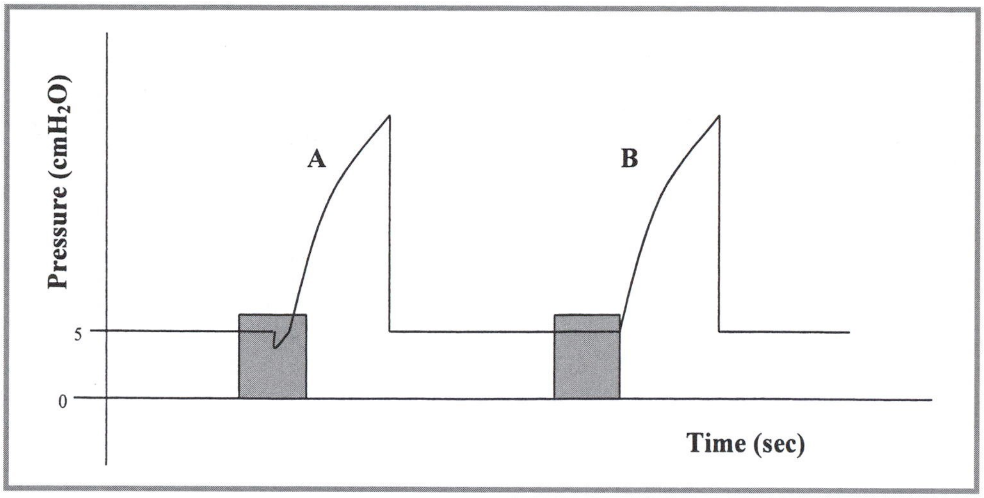

FIGURE 34-7

Pressure tracing during spontaneous intermittent mandatory ventilation (SIMV). The *shaded* areas represent the periods when the ventilator senses the patient's inspiratory effort and delivers a synchronized mandatory breath. After a preset time, if the ventilator does not sense a patient inspiratory effort it automatically delivers a preset-volume breath.

is divided into a mandatory and a spontaneous time period. If a patient is ordered an SIMV rate of 6 breaths/min, each cycle is 10 s. During the initial phase of each cycle, the ventilator, in synchrony with the patient's effort, will provide a preset tidal volume. If the patient makes no effort during this initial phase, a machine-delivered breath will be given at the beginning of the spontaneous phase to guarantee a backup rate. During the spontaneous phase, the patient's inspiratory effort will not trigger a mechanical ventilator breath, and tidal volumes are determined by the patient's spontaneous effort (Figure 34-7).

SIMV was originally postulated to improve cardiac output and stabilize blood pressure, both in contrast to ACV, because it fosters negative changes in intrathoracic pressure during spontaneous breathing. Although these effects have been demonstrated in patients with normal left ventricular function, similar effects have not been demonstrated in patients with decreased left ventricular ejection fraction. SIMV was also originally believed to facilitate weaning by avoiding alkalemia and respiratory muscle disuse atrophy, by gradually reducing the number of ventilator-assisted breaths over time. However, in contrast to these original hypotheses, two randomized-controlled trials have shown that SIMV prolongs the weaning process over T-piece or PS weans (see Chapter 36).

SIMV prolongs the weaning process over T-piece or pressure support (PS) weans.

Pressure-Support Ventilation

In contrast to ACV, pressure-support ventilation (PSV) is a pressure-preset, flow-cycled ventilator mode intended to support spontaneous respiratory efforts. With each inspiratory effort, the patient triggers the ventilator, which maintains the preset pressure level in the inspiratory circuit throughout inspiration (Figure 34-8).

During pressure-support ventilation (PSV), the patient triggers all breaths.

Pressurization of the inspiratory circuit ends when flow rate decreases at the end of the patient's inspiratory effort. Depending on the ventilator model, the inspiratory cycle ends when flow rate is less than 5 l/min or when flow rate decreases to less than 25% of the peak inspiratory flow rate. The inspiratory cycle may also be terminated by an increase in pressure above the preset value, indicating that expiration has begun. There are no set values for the amount of pressure support to be applied, but pressure is generally titrated toward achieving expired tidal volumes greater than 5–7 ml/kg, a decrease in respiratory rate (i.e., ≤35 breaths/min), and a decrement in the patient's work of breathing (i.e., decreased use of accessory inspiratory muscles). The patient retains control of the length and depth of the inspiratory cycle and may influence the percentage of the total support provided by the ventilator and the flow profile on a breath-to-breath basis. Tidal volumes are determined by a combination of PSV settings, the patient's effort, and the patient's underlying pulmonary mechanics.

The inspiratory cycle ends when flow rate decreases to less than 25% of the peak inspiratory flow rate.

During PS ventilation, the tidal volume is the result of the applied pressure, the patient's effort, and the underlying pulmonary mechanics.

Flow settings are not adjustable in the PSV mode but the speed of initial pressurization may be set in newer ventilators. PSV has been successfully used as part of a weaning strat-

FIGURE 34-8

Pressure, flow, and volume tracings for pressure-support ventilation (PSV). All breaths are being triggered by the patient. Notice that the delivered volumes vary from breath to breath.

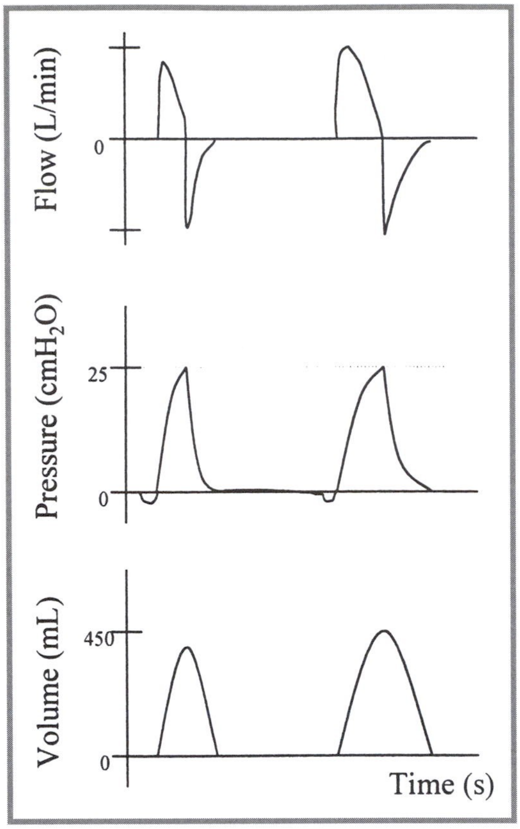

egy in patients who have adequate respiratory parameters (see Chapter 36). PSV may decrease inspiratory workload, but muscle unloading may be variable and is dependent on underlying respiratory pathophysiology. In patients with COPD, PSV may contribute to an increased work of breathing because ventilator inflation persists into the patient's neural expiratory phase. Patient–ventilator asynchrony may also result.

Pressure-Control Ventilation

> Pressure-control ventilation (PCV) is a form of pressure-limited ventilation; airway pressure is held constant and tidal volumes vary according to the respiratory system mechanics.

> In contrast to PS ventilation, breaths are initiated at a preset rate during PCV.

> PCV usually results in higher mean airway pressure and lower peak airway pressure than volume-limited ventilation.

The majority of patients receiving mechanical ventilation within current intensive care units are ventilated using various forms of volume-control ventilation; a preset tidal volume is delivered with each breath. In volume-control ventilation, the volume is held constant while airway pressure varies with changes in airway, lung, or chest wall mechanics. Pressure-control ventilation (PCV) is a form of pressure-limited ventilation in which airway pressure is held constant while tidal volume varies with changes in airway resistance or lung and chest wall mechanics. As a result, patients may receive variable tidal volumes with each respiratory effort depending on the dynamic changes in the resistive and elastic components of the respiratory system. During PCV, the rate, pressure limit, and inspiratory time are set on the ventilator. Breaths are initiated at a preset rate (time cycled), and gas flows into the patient breathing circuit until the preset pressure is reached. At this point, gas flow is reduced to the minimum flow required to maintain the airway pressure at the preset level until inspiratory time elapses (Figure 34-9). PCV has been used in clinical settings where increased peak airway pressures (implying increased alveolar pressures) are encountered and feared to predispose the patient to ventilator-induced lung injury (VILI). It also has been used in cases of ARDS where fine control of the mean airway pressure is desired and other modes have failed to adequately ventilate or oxygenate the patient. PCV usually results in a higher mean airway pressure than volume-limited ventilation but allows for lower peak airway pressures. Patients treated with PCV must often be sedated or paralyzed to achieve adequate comfort and effective ventilation.

Recently, a randomized-controlled trial compared PCV against volume-controlled ventilation. Both ventilator modes were adjusted to maintain plateau pressures below 35 cmH_2O.

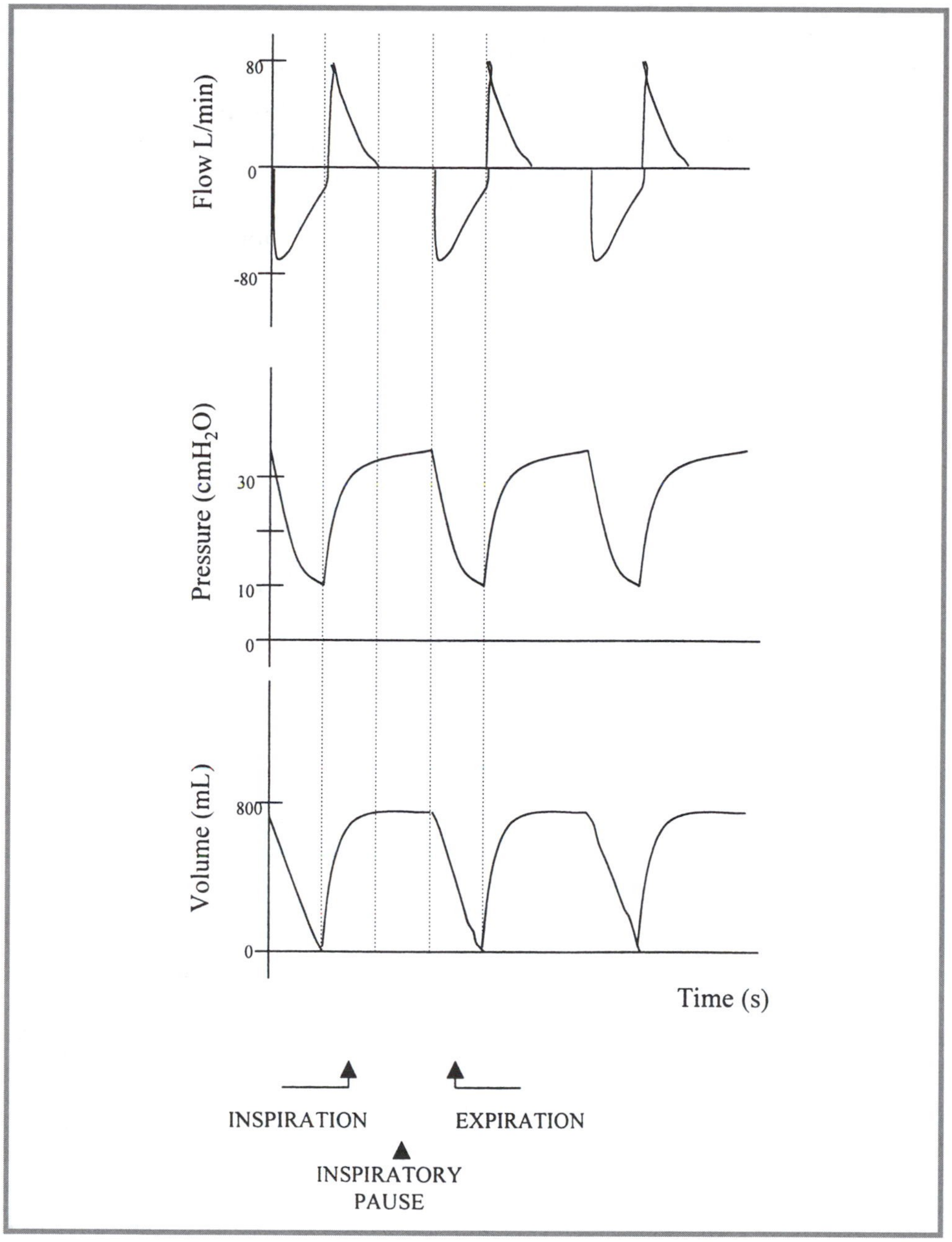

FIGURE 34-9

Pressure, flow, and volume tracings for pressure-control ventilation (PCV). In this case, an inspiratory pause has been placed, resulting in a prolonged inspiratory time and a shortened expiratory time.

The study evidenced an increment in mortality and multiorgan system failure in the volume control group, but by multivariate analysis, the ventilatory modality was not shown to be a predictor for mortality. Two prior studies also had failed to show differences in morbidity or mortality between these ventilatory modalities. Although there are theoretical advantages to PCV, the requirements for prolonged sedation and paralysis are worrisome, and the routine adoption of this mode of ventilation is not warranted at this time.

PCV generally requires sedation and paralysis and has not been shown to be superior to volume-limited ventilation in the setting of ARDS.

Continuous Positive Airway Pressure and Positive End-Expiratory Pressure

Continuous positive airway pressure (CPAP) is a mode of ventilatory support that is applied to spontaneously breathing patients. During the respiratory cycle, a constant pressure is applied to the airway throughout inspiration and expiration (Figure 34-10). The level of CPAP is the only variable that is adjusted by the physician. CPAP is commonly combined with PSV. CPAP may be used with PSV to decrease the amount of respiratory effort required to

During continuous positive airway pressure (CPAP), a constant pressure is applied to the airway throughout inspiration and expiration.

FIGURE 34-10

Pressure and volume waveforms for continuous positive airway pressure (CPAP). All breaths are spontaneously generated by the patient.

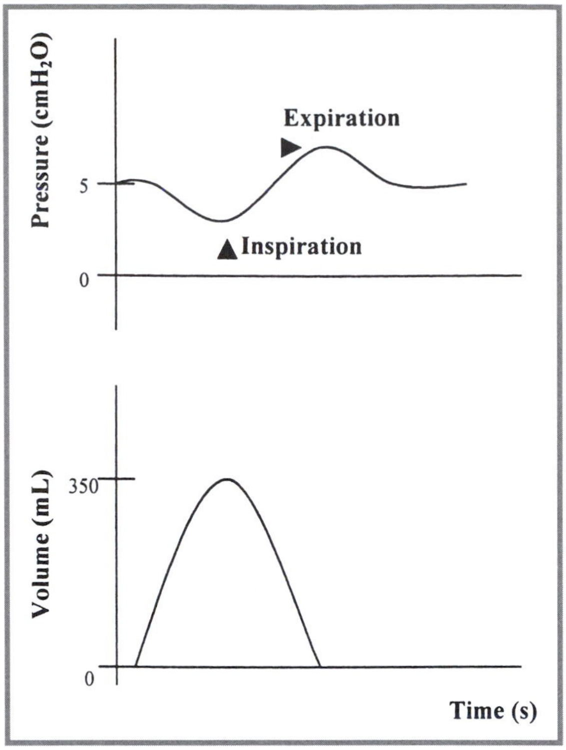

trigger a ventilator breath. CPAP has been used with PSV or alone in patients weaning from mechanical ventilation to prevent small airway collapse and atelectasis. Noninvasive CPAP delivery is commonly used to treat obstructive sleep apnea and, more recently, in the management of acute respiratory failure. For a full description of CPAP and its physiological consequences and uses, see Chapter 35.

Extrinsic positive end-expiratory pressure (PEEP) prevents alveolar collapse, recruits alveoli, and improves oxygenation by increasing end-expiratory lung volume and decreasing intrapulmonary shunt.

In the setting of respiratory failure from ARDS or congestive heart failure, decreases in lung compliance may lead to significant alveolar collapse, with an increased alveolar shunt fraction and refractory hypoxemia. Extrinsic PEEP has been used as an adjunctive technique during mechanical ventilation in these patients to prevent alveolar collapse, recruit alveoli, and improve oxygenation by increasing end-expiratory lung volume (EELV) and decreasing intrapulmonary shunt. In patients with ARDS, selection of extrinsic PEEP can be accomplished in one of two ways: (1) by titrating extrinsic PEEP upward in 2–3 cmH_2O increments while carefully following oxygenation and pulmonary mechanics; or (2) by setting extrinsic PEEP above the lower inflection point obtained by constructing a pressure–volume curve (see following). The method chosen to titrate extrinsic PEEP does not appear to have a significant impact on clinical outcome. There is a good correlation between clinically guided extrinsic PEEP and that obtained by pressure–volume curve analysis. The addition of extrinsic PEEP is also helpful in decreasing a patient's respiratory workload while on assisted or supported modes of mechanical ventilation.

Patients with intrinsic PEEP must overcome a significant amount of pressure before they can elicit flow from the ventilator, resulting in difficult ventilator triggering, delayed breath delivery, increased work of breathing, and patient–ventilator asynchrony. Some authors advocate applying extrinsic PEEP in these circumstances to facilitate triggering. Although the addition of extrinsic PEEP may decrease the workload required to initiate a ventilator breath, it is important to remember that, in many instances, hyperinflation and intrinsic PEEP are dynamic conditions which are subject to change with therapy directed at alleviating airway obstruction and decreasing the level of applied ventilation. Emphasis should be placed on therapeutic strategies aimed at relieving bronchospasm and decreasing the I:E ratio.

The application of extrinsic PEEP, however, also has distinct disadvantages. It increases intrathoracic pressure, which may decrease venous return and compromise cardiac output and O_2 delivery. Extrinsic PEEP has the most effect on the compliant regions of the lungs, and overdistension of normal lung units may occur, contributing to an increased alveolar deadspace fraction. Moreover, concern exists that extrinsic PEEP, especially at higher levels, may contribute to VILI.

Extrinsic PEEP increases intrathoracic pressure and may decrease venous return and cardiac output.

VENTILATOR STRATEGIES

Permissive Hypercapnia

Permissive hypercapnia is a ventilator strategy that allows the $PaCO_2$ to rise above normal physiologic levels by decreasing minute ventilation in selected cases of respiratory failure. It has been employed in ARDS and asthma to minimize peak and mean airway pressures and, consequently, the potential for VILI.

Permissive hypercapnia is used in ARDS and asthma to decrease peak and mean airway pressures.

The reduction in minute ventilation results in a reduction in alveolar ventilation; this, in turn, results in an increase in $PaCO_2$, a decrease in P_AO_2, and a consequent decrease in PaO_2 (see Chapter 13). Thus, higher extrinsic PEEP or a prolonged inspiratory time are frequently required to maintain oxygenation.

The acceptable degree of hypercapnia is controversial. Frequently, a minute ventilation resulting in $PaCO_2$ levels between 75 and 80 mmHg is sufficient to decrease mean airway and plateau pressures to commonly acceptable levels. Most authors recommend maintaining pH above 7.20 to minimize the adverse effects of hypercapnic acidosis. This concept may not be entirely accurate for several reasons. The deleterious effects of hypercapnic acidosis are a consequence of intracellular pH alterations. Correction of intracellular pH occurs more rapidly than correction of extracellular pH; therefore, blood pH is likely a poor surrogate for intracellular pH, and lower levels may be acceptable.

Most authors recommend maintaining pH above 7.20 to minimize adverse effects.

The potential benefits of permissive hypercapnia include a reduction in lung injury due to decreased shear forces at the alveolar level, or decreased blood flow to the injured lung, and a decreased incidence of barotrauma. Permissive hypercapnia has many downsides, however. Patients will mount a physiologic response to hypercapnia with increments in minute ventilation; therefore, sedation and paralysis are frequently required to prevent respiratory compensation and to improve patient tolerance. Acute hypercapnia may cause cerebral vasodilation and elevated intracranial pressure, and may worsen cerebral edema. Acute hypercapnic acidosis has a direct depressant effect on myocardial contraction, increases sympathetic activity, and directly causes peripheral vasodilatation. Cardiac irritation may lead to the generation of arrhythmias. Finally, hypercapnic acidosis increases pulmonary vascular resistance.

Acute hypercapnia may cause cerebral vasodilation, elevated intracranial pressure, and worsening cerebral edema.

Acute hypercapnia has a depressant effect on myocardial contractility.

Permissive hypercapnia is contraindicated in patients with cerebral edema and elevated intracranial pressures, patients with a prior history of seizures or an active seizure disorder, depressed cardiac function, and arrhythmias, and patients with increased pulmonary vascular resistance. There is currently little evidence supporting the routine use of permissive hypercapnia in ARDS or status asthmaticus. Ideally, it should be used for a short period of time to reduce mean and plateau pressures in patients at risk for VILI, particularly in those who may have a rapidly reversible cause for elevated airway pressures, while paying careful attention to its possible neurologic, cardiac, and pulmonary consequences.

Permissive hypercapnia is contraindicated in patients with cerebral edema, seizure disorder, or depressed cardiac function.

Inverse Ratio Ventilation

The inspiratory to expiratory ratio during the respiratory cycle of average adults is approximately 1:2. During inverse ratio ventilation (IRV), inspiratory time is prolonged to exceed expiratory duration to recruit additional alveolar units in situations where extrinsic PEEP is insufficient to accomplish this goal. Because the inspiratory cycle may overlap with the patient's neural expiratory phase, IRV ratios greater than 2:1 often require sedation or paralysis to maintain patient comfort. Mean alveolar pressure rises as a result of the longer inspiratory time, and rapid increases in respiratory rate can dramatically increase both peak and mean airway pressures. Patients with underlying airflow obstruction at baseline are at risk of developing severe degrees of auto-PEEP as a result of a decreased expiratory phase of respiration. Ratios greater than 2:1 have not produced improvements in oxygenation, and patients are at a greater risk for hemodynamic intolerance and VILI. IRV is commonly employed with PCV; given the dramatic nonphysiologic alterations in inspiratory and expiratory times that are required, sedation and paralysis of the patient are necessary to achieve patient comfort and effective ventilation. IRV has been used in the setting of ARDS and hypoxemic respiratory failure in an attempt to improve oxygenation, but there is insufficient evidence regarding its efficacy in reducing morbidity or mortality.

Independent Lung Ventilation

In patients with severe unilateral lung disease, independent lung ventilation allows applying different ventilation strategies to each lung.

Patients with large bronchopleural fistulas (BPF) may benefit from selective ventilation to the contralateral lung to promote closure.

Patient with severe unilateral lung pathology may require different ventilation strategies applied to each lung. In certain cases, this can only be achieved through independent lung ventilation. Patients with whole lung pneumonia, unilateral pulmonary contusion, or following single lung transplant may require extrinsic PEEP selectively delivered to the involved lung to maintain gas exchange, while simultaneously avoiding PEEP delivery to the normal or overly compliant contralateral lung. The patient with a bronchopleural fistula (BPF) and significant air leak may benefit from selective ventilation of the contralateral lung to promote closure of the BPF. In the presence of important tidal volume losses resulting from a large air leak, selective ventilation of the unaffected lung may allow for more effective ventilation.

Independent lung ventilation may be achieved through specialized endotracheal tubes. Double lumen tubes consist of two tubes; one is inserted into a main bronchus, and the other ends in the trachea. Both tubes have cuffs that ensure independent ventilation. Whenever

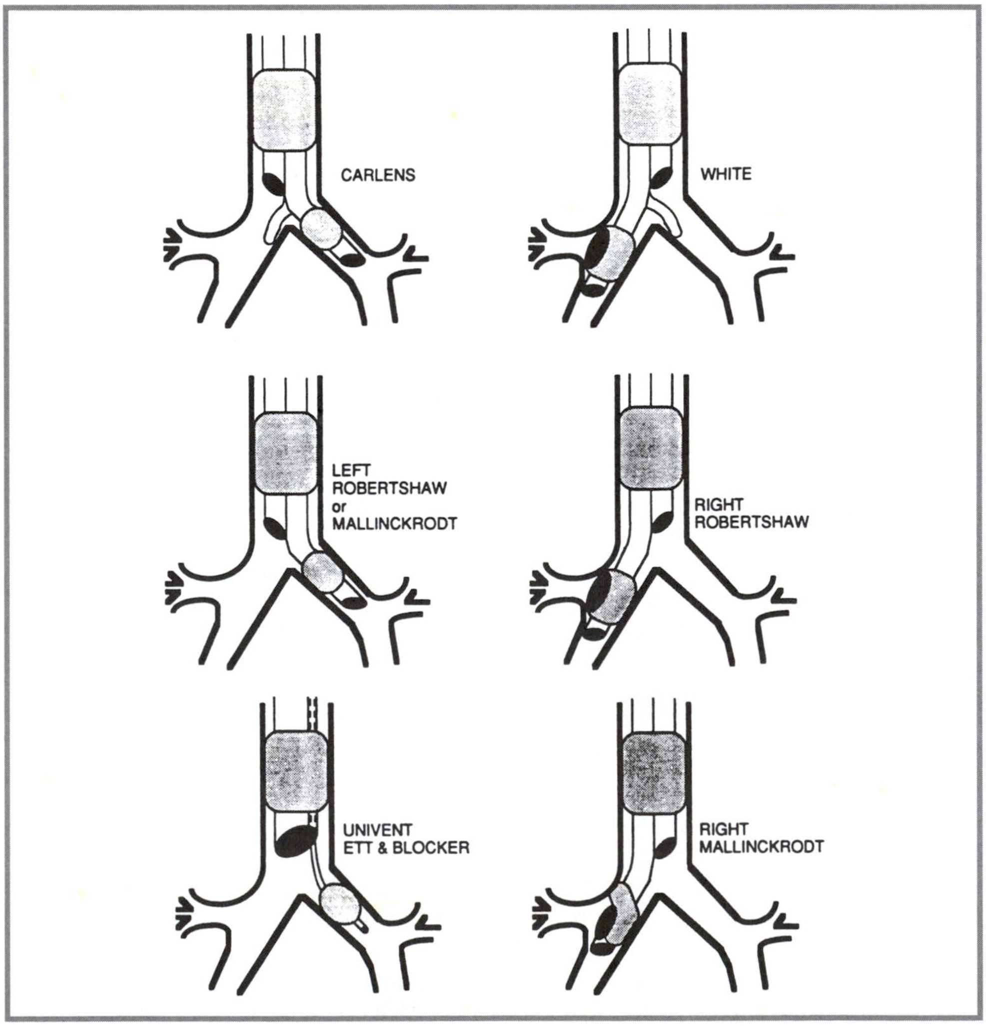

FIGURE 34-11

Common double lumen tubes.

possible, a left double tube should be placed because right double lumen tubes have a higher incidence of right upper lobe collapse. These tubes allow different ventilator strategies to be applied to each lung, such as different extrinsic PEEP levels or tidal volumes (Figure 34-11). The correct position of these tubes is paramount, and they are usually placed under bronchoscopic guidance. Minimal patient movement may cause tube misplacement; sedation and paralysis should be judiciously used in their placement and maintenance. The narrow lumens of the tube may increase the resistive workload, and the inability to effectively suction airway secretions may limit its use for prolonged periods of time. Bronchial blocking techniques are an alternative to double lumen tube placement. A balloon-tipped catheter (Magill blocker or Fogarty) is passed outside or within a conventional endotracheal tube and then inflated within the targeted main bronchus.

Independent lung ventilation can be achieved through double lumen tubes.

Prone Position Ventilation

Prone positioning of patients on mechanical ventilation has been recently described as an adjunct to improve oxygenation in selected patients with hypoxemic respiratory failure who have a poor response to conventional mechanical ventilation. The rotation of patients from a supine to prone position may have profound effects on respiratory physiology.

Prone position placement appears to decrease V/Q mismatch and improve oxygenation by recruiting functional alveoli.

In patients with severe hypoxemia who are not responsive to increases in FiO_2 or extrinsic PEEP, prone position placement may have a transient effect in decreasing ventilation/perfusion mismatch and improving oxygenation by recruiting functional alveoli. After placement in the prone position, an improvement in gas exchange is seen in 50%–70% of ARDS patients after minutes to hours. This beneficial effect appears to be transient and, because of the loss of dependent alveolar units, is lost after several hours. The patient is then returned to the supine position. The procedure is repeated as necessary to maintain an adequate PaO_2. Prone positioning should be reserved for those patients with marked hypoxia, who are not responsive to other maneuvers, as movement to the prone position itself may place the patient at considerable risks including inadvertent extubation, hypotension, desaturation, arrhythmias, and severe limitations in nursing care. Prospective randomized controlled trials examining the role of prone positioning in critically ill, hypoxemic, mechanically ventilated patients are lacking at the current time. However, one recent study reported an improvement in oxygenation with the prone position in ARDS patients, but no effect on survival.

The effect of prone position ventilation is transient and is generally lost after a few hours.

Prone position ventilation carries certain risks, such as inadvertent extubation, hypotension, and desaturation.

ALTERNATE MODES OF VENTILATION

High-Frequency Ventilation

Broadly speaking, high-frequency ventilation (HFV) is defined as mechanical ventilatory support using higher than normal breathing frequencies. This section considers techniques that use respiratory frequencies that are severalfold higher than normal (>100 breaths/min in adults and >300 breaths/min in neonate/pediatric patients). When using these frequencies tidal volumes are much smaller than in conventional mechanical ventilation, but the tidal volume–respiratory rate product is generally greater than in conventional mechanical ventilation. Two main reasons have been postulated for using HFV. First, the combination of PEEP and the small tidal volumes associated with HFV provide a conceptually ideal lung protection strategy. Second, in addition to better alveolar recruitment, the rapid flow pattern may enhance gas mixing and improve ventilation–perfusion mismatch.

High-frequency ventilatory support uses ventilator frequencies greater than 100 in adults.

High-frequency ventilation (HFV) uses small tidal volumes, frequently in conjunction with high PEEP.

High-frequency jet ventilation (HFJV) utilizes humidified gas that is delivered at a high velocity and rapid frequency (100–600 cycles per minute) within the endotracheal tube by a narrow injector. At low frequencies, jet ventilation is effective at washing out deadspace; elimination of $PaCO_2$ occurs through the principle of conductive ventilation. As the frequency of ventilation increases during jet ventilation, alveolar airway pressures approach those seen in conventional ventilation techniques. However, as the frequency of ventilation increases, conductive gas flow during jet ventilation decreases, and $PaCO_2$ may rise. High-frequency oscillators operate with a "to-and-fro" application of pressure on the airway using pistons or microprocessor gas controllers. Fresh gas is supplied with the ventilator circuit as a bias flow. HFJV has been used in patients with ARDS with the goal of reducing airway pressures and VILI, but it has not always been successful at maintaining adequate oxygen levels in this group of patients.

Potential uses for high-frequency ventilation include patients with large bronchopleural fistulas and those with cardiac dysfunction.

High-frequency ventilation can be used during bronchoscopy to provide adequate ventilatory support and lower airway pressures.

HFV has been used in neonates with the neonatal respiratory distress syndrome. Although this technique demonstrated to provide effective ventilation, no improvement in mortality was shown over conventional techniques. In the largest randomized controlled trial (NIH-HIFI), HFV was actually associated with an increased incidence of intraventricular hemorrhage. Potential uses for HFV include ventilation of patients with very large bronchopleural fistulas and of patients with cardiac dysfunction, especially by synchronizing HFV with systole to benefit stroke volume by decreasing afterload. HFV allows selected airway surgical procedures (e.g., bronchoscopy, laryngoscopy) to be performed with adequate ventilatory support and lower airway pressures.

Airway Pressure Release Ventilation and Biphasic Airway Pressure Ventilation

Airway pressure release ventilation (APRV) allows patients to breath spontaneously with the application of a high level of CPAP to the airway. The high level of CPAP allows recruiting additional alveolar units, increasing functional residual capacity, decreasing shunt fraction, and improving ventilation–perfusion matching. The elevated airway pressure is periodically reduced through a release valve, thereby allowing expiration from the higher functional residual capacity to occur before its replacement with fresh gas. The airway pressure release is set for a fixed amount of time. Thus, each mechanical breath is created by the brief interruption and restoration of airway pressure. Because each breath is provided by the release of pressure, peak airway pressures cannot exceed CPAP. Biphasic airway pressure ventilation (not to be confused with BiPAP®/noninvasive ventilation, discussed in Chapter 35) is a ventilator mode that also employs high levels of CPAP, set to decrease periodically after a preset number of respiratory cycles over specified time duration. APRV may achieve adequate oxygenation for patients with hypoxemic respiratory failure while allowing for spontaneous respiration, decreased need for sedation, and lower peak and mean alveolar pressures with a decreased risk of VILI and increased venous return. However, in patients with emphysema, the increased end-expiratory pressures may contribute to intrinsic PEEP.

Proportional-Assist Ventilation

Proportional-assist ventilation (PAV) was designed to augment the patient's respiratory efforts with varying levels of pressure support throughout the inspiratory cycle. The patient controls the inspired volume and the flow rate; the level of pressure assistance is achieved by measuring the flow and inspired volume. Pressure increases proportionately to overcome the elastic workload or the resistive workload. Unlike PSV, the degree of pressure assistance varies during the inspiratory portion of the respiratory cycle. PAV was intended to improve patient comfort and to tailor the degree of ventilator assistance based on the patient's moment-to-moment respiratory workload. However, at the current time, PAV has not been shown to improve weaning success and, like pressure-support ventilation, does not eliminate the possible development of auto-PEEP.

Partial Liquid Ventilation

Perfluorocarbon is a gas-exchanging liquid used in partial liquid ventilation.

Partial liquid ventilation is an experimental adjunct to ventilation that utilizes a gas exchanging liquid, perfluorocarbon (PFC), to fill collapsed alveolar units. Perfluro-octyl bromide is the most commonly used PFC; it is nontoxic, radiopaque, not readily absorbed into the blood, and evaporates hours to days after instillation into the respiratory tract. Technical limitations have prevented the use of complete liquid ventilation in human trials, but partial liquid ventilation in combination with gas ventilation has been employed with some degree of success. While using traditional gas ventilation techniques, PFC is instilled into the lung where it settles into the dependent portions in an amount that equals the volume of the patient's functional residual capacity. The PFC fills the alveoli during inspiration and can mimic the action of adding extrinsic PEEP by recruiting additional alveoli. Its effect on reducing alveolar surface tension serves to improve lung compliance. It is also speculated that secretion clearance is also improved as particulates float to the top of the PFC. This technique remains investigational. It most likely will not have widespread application because it is labor intensive and evidence that it improves survival in patients with hypoxemic respiratory failure secondary to ARDS is lacking.

Perfluorocarbon, used in conjunction with conventional ventilator techniques, is instilled into the lung, where it settles in the dependent portions.

ADJUNCTIVE THERAPIES

Extracorporeal Membrane Oxygenation and Extracorporeal CO_2 Removal

Extracorporeal membrane oxygenation (ECMO) is commonly performed during cardiothoracic surgery that requires cardiac arrest and blood flow and ventilation cessation. ECMO is achieved via venous cannulation. Blood is removed and drawn into an external motor driven device that provides circulatory function. Gas exchange is attained by the passage of blood across a thin, semipermeable membrane that enables oxygenation and CO_2 removal. Blood returns to the patient via an arterial cannula. Attempts made in the past to apply ECMO to patients in the ICU with hypoxemic respiratory failure secondary to ARDS have resulted in high morbidity and mortality. The high mortality observed in these patients was largely the result of an increased incidence of sepsis and bleeding events.

The use of extracorporeal membrane oxygenation (ECMO) in ARDS has not been shown to alter mortality.

Extracorporeal CO_2 removal has been attempted, often used in conjunction with permissive hypercapnia. This technique involves a venovenous circuit that diverts less cardiac output from the lung vascular bed than ECMO but it still requires heparinization, which contributes to an increased complication rate. Studies have demonstrated a reduction in $PaCO_2$ but have not shown improvement in overall survival when compared with conventional therapy; the routine use of this technique in the intensive care unit cannot be supported by medical evidence at this time. ECMO has been used successfully as an adjunct in newborns with respiratory distress syndrome, aspiration syndromes, pneumonia, and sepsis.

ECMO has been used with success as an adjunct in newborns with respiratory distress syndrome, aspiration syndromes, and sepsis.

Inhaled Nitric Oxide

Nitric oxide is a potent vasodilator and bronchodilator. In humans, it is synthesized from arginine by the enzyme nitric oxide synthase. It has a very short half-life. Clinically, nitric oxide is delivered as a gas via the ventilator circuit, resulting in selective vasodilation of the ventilated portions of the lung; this theoretically results in a decrease of V/Q mismatch by preferentially directing and increasing pulmonary circulation to the ventilated portions of the lung. These qualities led to its use in patients with ARDS. In clinical trials, the use of inhaled nitric oxide (INO) resulted in a temporary improvement in PaO_2 and a reduction in pulmonary artery pressures and pulmonary vascular resistance. A large, multicenter, randomized-controlled trial failed to show a significant reduction of mortality at 28 days in patients who received INO at different doses versus matched controls who received conventional ventilation. Problems associated with INO include the rapid inactivation of nitric oxide in a reaction with oxyhemoglobin to form methemoglobin and NO_3; therefore, methemoglobin should be routinely measured in patients receiving INO. Concern exists regarding the potential of by-products (NO_2) to be directly toxic to the lungs and cause central nervous system toxicity.

In vivo, nitric oxide is synthesized from arginine by nitric oxide synthase. It is a potent vasodilator and bronchodilator.

Patients receiving nitric oxide, especially at high concentrations, are at risk of development methemoglobinemia.

Despite the evidence that INO improves oxygenation in many patients with ARDS, clear improvement in patient survival has not been shown. The cost of INO and the need for INO delivery systems to precisely deliver the drug and monitor the development of a toxic byproduct have restricted the widespread use of this adjunctive therapy.

Inhaled nitric oxide (INO) improves oxygenation in ARDS, but improvement in patient survival has not been demonstrated.

INO has been used in the treatment of hypoxic respiratory failure of the newborn caused by persistent pulmonary hypertension, respiratory distress syndrome, aspiration syndromes, and sepsis. Persistent pulmonary hypertension of the newborn is a syndrome characterized by increased pulmonary vascular resistance, significant extrapulmonary shunting through a patent ductus arteriosus, foramen ovale, or both, and severe hypoxemia. It is the result of several different entities, including meconium aspiration, surfactant deficiency, and primary pulmonary hypertension. In several randomized trials, INO has been shown to improve oxygenation, stabilize the newborn before ECMO, and reduce the need for ECMO therapy in persistent pulmonary hypertension of the newborn. Recently, in light of the results of randomized-controlled trials, the U.S. Food and Drug Administration approved the use of INO for the treatment of hypoxic respiratory failure of the term and near-term newborn due to persistent pulmonary hypertension.

INO has been shown to improve oxygenation and reduce the need for ECMO in persistent pulmonary hypertension of the newborn.

Inhaled Heliox

Heliox is a gas mixture composed of 20%–30% oxygen and 70%–80% helium. Because of its lower density, helium allows laminar flow and decreased turbulence in the airway, resulting in lower intraluminal pressure generation. Heliox has been used in the treatment of upper airway obstruction caused by laryngospasm, tumor, edema, fibrosis, and obesity. In patients with asthma, the use of heliox has been associated with improved oxygenation and a faster improvement in forced expiratory volume (FEV_1) and peak expiratory flow rate, when compared against controls. Heliox may be useful as a bridge until the effect of systemic glucocorticoids and bronchodilators becomes apparent. One of the major disadvantages of heliox is the limitation in providing high concentrations of oxygen. If the proportion of helium is decreased below 70% of the mixture, the gas density increases and it loses its laminar flow properties; therefore, patients with high FiO_2 requirements are not suitable candidates for heliox.

Helium is less dense than air; its use thus promotes laminar flow and decreased turbulence in the airway.

Heliox has been used in the treatment of upper airway obstruction caused by tumor, edema, fibrosis, and laryngospasm.

Tracheal Gas Insufflation

Tracheal gas insufflation (TGI) is a technique whereby a low flow of fresh gas is delivered to the distal end of the endotracheal tube through a small-diameter catheter. The flow can be continuous or delivered only during exhalation. Gas can be delivered by a stand-alone catheter or by a catheter embedded in the endotracheal tube, positioned approximately 1 cm above the carina. $PaCO_2$ and endotracheal pressures must be carefully monitored while using TGI. The desired level of $PaCO_2$ determines the TGI flow that is given in addition to the ventilator's minute ventilation. TGI will result in a tracheal PEEP that is higher than the circuit PEEP; careful monitoring of tracheal pressures is necessary to avoid pressure related complications.

In one study in mechanically ventilated patients, TGI reduced $PaCO_2$ and increased pH; it also increased tracheal PEEP and mean airway pressure, thereby reducing cardiac filling. In a study in trauma patients who developed ARDS, TGI was shown to be effective in reducing $PaCO_2$ and increasing pH, although the reduction was small and its clinical relevance is debatable. It was also shown to decrease intracranial pressure resulting from permissive hypercapnia.

Although studies have not clearly shown a survival benefit from TGI in mechanically ventilated patients in whom permissive hypercapnia is employed, it may have a role in selected patients with a relatively high deadspace.

MONITORING OF RESPIRATORY MECHANICS

Pressure, airflow, and volume measurements quantify basic physiologic properties of the respiratory system, such as resistance, compliance, and work of breathing; interpreting the relationship of these variables is essential for appropriate ventilator management. These variables also provide important information regarding the patient's underlying disease.

Basic Concepts of Respiratory Mechanics

To fully understand ventilator–patient interactions, knowledge of basic respiratory mechanics is imperative. The act of breathing requires that work be performed to overcome several different impediments, the most important of which are these:

In breathing, work must be performed to overcome the elastic and resistive forces of the respiratory system.

- The elastic forces developed by the lung and chest wall when intrapulmonary volume is increased.
- Resistive forces resulting from the flow of gas through the ventilator circuit, endotracheal tube, and conducting airways.

Simple elastance/resistance models cannot fully explain the mechanical characteristics of the airway; it is clear that other forces play a lesser, yet important role. In addition to elastic and resistive forces, other factors have to be overcome, but their contribution is less important.

- Viscoelastic forces, a characteristic of certain materials that elongate when subjected to stress, followed by further elongation if stress is maintained constant. In this case adaptation to mechanical distension will occur within the lung and chest wall tissue.
- Plastoelastic forces, a characteristic of plastoelastic materials (i.e., stretchable materials), which does not follow Newtonian physics. These materials exhibit different mechanical properties at different levels of stress. Plastoelastic forces explain the difference between the inspiratory and expiratory portions of the pressure–volume (PV) curves. The lung and chest wall show a decrement in stiffness during expiration, following full lung inflation.
- The additional effect of gravitational forces and thoracic gas compressibility. These effects, however, are practically negligible.

Elementary Laws of Mechanics

A simple model of the respiratory system depicts the airway as a simple resistive element that is connected to an elastic element representing both lungs and the chest wall (Figure 34-12). In such a model the interaction between pressure, volume, and flow follow Newtonian physics. This model is particularly useful during assisted breathing on a mechanical ventilator because the applied force (or pressure) can be easily measured. In contrast, during unassisted breathing, the pressure generated by the respiratory muscles cannot be measured directly and can be calculated only if the elastic and resistive characteristics of the respiratory system are known.

In a simple analogue of the respiratory system, the pressure that is applied (P_{appl}) at any instant (t) is the sum of the elastic pressure (P_{el}) and the resistive component (P_{res}):

$$P_{appl}(t) = P_{el}(t) + P_{res}(t) \quad (34\text{-}3)$$

This equation is a simplified version of Newton's equation of motion, an application of Newton's third law of motion, which states, "For each force applied *to* a body, there is an equal opposing force *by* the body."

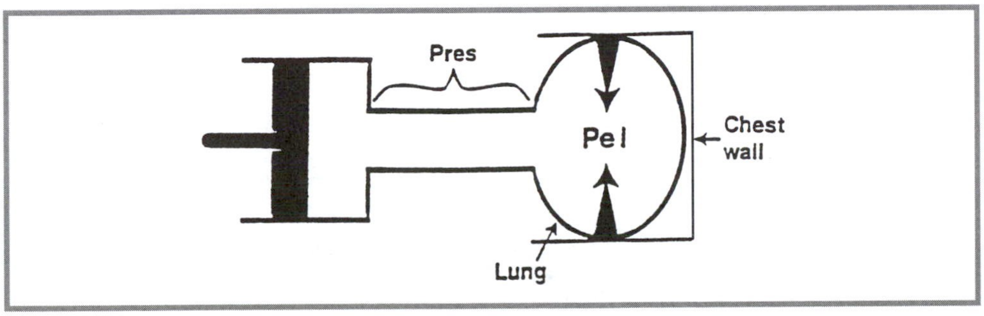

FIGURE 34-12

Simplified respiratory system model in which the airway is represented by a resistive element (Pres) and the lungs and chest are represented as an elastic element (Pel).

A change in volume is opposed by the elastance of the respiratory system, and the resistance of the respiratory system opposes flow.

How does this apply to the respiratory system? In the respiratory system, a change in volume (ΔV) is opposed by the elastance (E) of the lungs and chest wall, and flow ($\dot{V}$) is opposed by the resistance (R) of the system. Equation 34-3 can be rearranged as:

$$P_{appl} = \Delta V \times E + \dot{V} \times R \tag{34-4}$$

Notice that inertial forces are not taken into consideration by the equation of motion in the respiratory system because friction plays a negligible role in gas motion. It follows from this equation that in the absence of flow ($\dot{V}$), applied pressure (P_{appl}) to respiratory system equals elastic pressure (P_{el}), which in the relaxed mechanically ventilated patient represents alveolar pressure (P_{alv}).

$$P_{appl} = P_{el} = \Delta V \times E = P_{alv} \tag{34-5}$$

Although physiologists favor the concept of elastance (E), in practice its inverse, compliance (C) is more frequently used ($C = 1/E$).

Peak Airway Pressure

Peak airway pressure is the maximal airway pressure recorded at the end of inspiration in a relaxed patient.

Peak airway pressure or peak inspiratory pressure is the maximal airway pressure recorded at the end of inspiration during positive pressure ventilation in a relaxed patient. It represents the total pressure needed to overcome resistance related to the ventilator circuit, endotracheal tube, and airway, in addition to the elastic recoil of the lungs and chest wall (Figure 34-13).

In the completely relaxed patient without airway obstruction or significant resistance from ventilator circuit, endotracheal tube, or secretions, peak pressure may reflect alveolar pressure. Peak pressure may not always be helpful in discerning between problems affecting the resistive (asthma/COPD) or the elastic component (ARDS/pneumonia) of the respiratory system. Because peak pressure also includes the resistive properties of the circuit, endotracheal tube, and airway, it does not always reflect alveolar pressure. A large amount of energy is dissipated in the airway, especially in the presence of small-bore endotracheal tubes, significant airway obstruction, and secretions. In these cases, high peak pressures do not represent alveolar pressure and are not necessarily associated with the development of barotrauma. Additionally, increased peak inspiratory pressures are also observed when ventilating patients with increased thoracoabdominal elastic loads, such as those who are morbidly obese, extremely edematous, or having massive ascites; once again, these pressures may not pre-

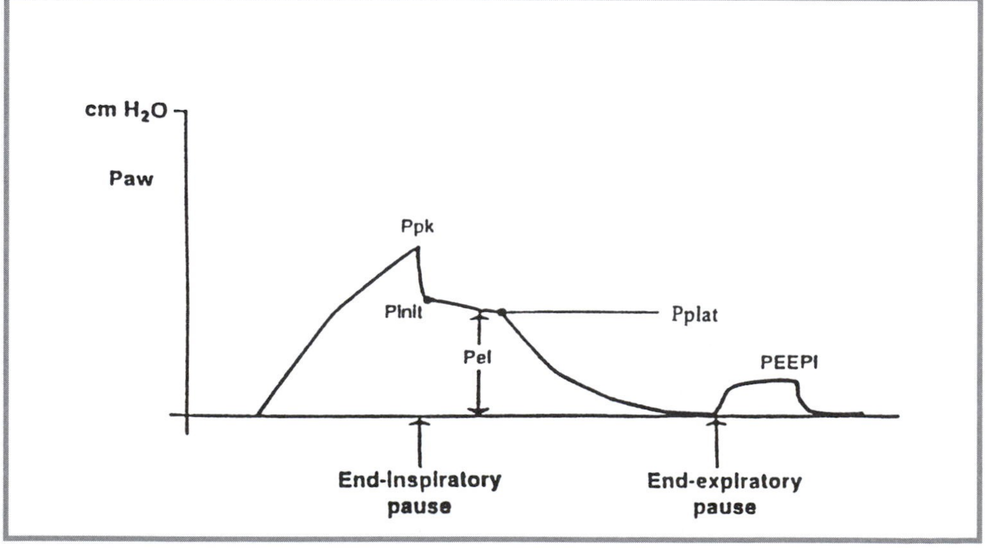

FIGURE 34-13

A typical waveform. *Ppk* represents peak pressure. If an inspiratory pause is set, a rapid drop in pressure can be observed. The initial drop in pressure at flow cessation (*Pinit*) is followed by a more gradual drop in pressure; a plateau (*Pplat*) occurs after 3–5 s. The pressure difference between Ppk and Pinit represents the pressure needed to overcome airway resistance. The difference between Pinit and Pplat reflects the viscoelastic properties of the system. Notice that at end-expiration a pause has been set, revealing the presence of intrinsic PEEP.

dispose these patients to alveolar rupture. A sudden rise in peak airway pressures should raise the suspicion of pneumothorax, significant bronchospasm, large airway atelectasis, pulmonary edema, or mucous plug formation.

A sudden increment in peak airway pressure should raise the suspicion of pneumothorax, significant bronchospasm, or a mucus plug in the airway.

Plateau Pressure

In a relaxed patient receiving assist-control ventilation, applying an inspiratory pause at the end of passive inflation (inspiration) will result in an immediate drop in airway opening pressure (P_{aw}) to a lower initial value (P_{init}). This rapid fall in pressure is followed by a more graduate decrement, until a plateau pressure (P_{plat}) is reached after 3–5 s (see Figure 34-13). The difference between peak airway pressure and the initial pressure drop (P_{init}) is thought to reflect a purely resistive component. The difference between P_{init} and P_{plat} is likely to be due to volume redistribution in areas with different time constants and viscoelastic adaptation. Hence, plateau pressure reflects lung and chest wall elastance, whereas peak airway pressure also reflects the resistive properties of the airways during inspiratory flow. High plateau pressures can be seen in patients with diffuse lung diseases, such as ARDS or multilobar pneumonia. Patients with morbid obesity or chest wall deformities (e.g., kyphoscoliosis) represent disorders with decreased chest wall compliance.

Plateau pressure reflects lung and chest wall elastance.

High plateau pressures can be seen in patients with diffuse lung diseases such as ARDS or multilobar pneumonia.

Increasing emphasis has been given to monitoring plateau pressures in mechanically ventilated patients so as to prevent ventilator-induced lung injury (VILI). In healthy lungs, a transpulmonary pressure of 35 cmH_2O would inflate the lungs to near-total lung capacity. In patients with acute lung injury or pulmonary edema, total lung capacity may be effectively reduced by alveolar loss or collapse. Therefore, the tidal volumes delivered with each ventilator-assisted breath may overdistend the more compliant regions of the lungs. The resultant higher plateau pressures may lead to alveolar overdistension of the more compliant alveolar units. Alveolar overdistension is suspected of causing "volutrauma" or VILI as a result of the shear mechanical forces applied to the alveoli as they are repeatedly opened and closed.

Alveolar overdistension is suspected to be one of the causes of ventilator-induced lung injury (VILI).

Several randomized, controlled trials have evaluated maintaining plateau pressures below 35 cmH_2O in patients with ARDS, with some studies demonstrating improved survival. Maintaining plateau pressures below 35 cmH_2O has also been shown to reduce inflammatory markers and to reduce the incidence of multiple organ failure in patients with ARDS. For ARDS patients with significant elevation of plateau pressures, pressure-control ventilation with or without permissive hypercapnia has been employed to avoid VILI. In other clinical conditions, the plateau pressure may reflect forces generated by the chest wall, abdomen, and pulmonary parenchyma. For example, patients with marked chest wall edema, abdominal distension, and pleural effusions may have abnormally elevated plateau pressures. In this clinical scenario, limiting plateau pressure to less than 35 cmH_2O may be insufficient to maintain the alveoli open, resulting in an underventilated patient. In this setting, higher plateau pressures may be necessary to achieve effective ventilation.

Maintaining plateau pressure below 35 cmH_2O has been associated with a decrease in mortality and the incidence of multiple organ failure in patients with ARDS.

Intrinsic PEEP

At the end of expiration, alveolar and airway pressures equal atmospheric pressure. Intrinsic positive end-expiratory pressure (PEEPi) or auto-PEEP occurs when alveolar pressure exceeds atmospheric pressure at the end of expiration. PEEPi results in an increased intrathoracic pressure and elevated end-expiratory lung volume. In patients with underlying airflow obstruction secondary to asthma or emphysema, the patient may not be able to completely exhale. In these circumstances, if sufficient expiratory time is not permitted to allow full exhalation, progressive hyperinflation and PEEPi occur.

Auto-PEEP occurs when alveolar pressure exceeds atmospheric pressure at the end of expiration.

In patients with underlying airflow obstruction, insufficient expiratory time will prevent full exhalation and result in progressive hyperinflation and auto-PEEP.

The increase in intrathoracic pressure may lead to profound hemodynamic consequences, such as decreased cardiac venous return and cardiac output. Moreover, dynamic hyperinflation foreshortens the respiratory muscles and places them at mechanical disadvantage, thereby contributing to an increased work of breathing.

PEEPi may occur in patients with significant airflow obstruction, in patients ventilated at high levels with a small-bore endotracheal tube in place, or when the chosen ventilator set-

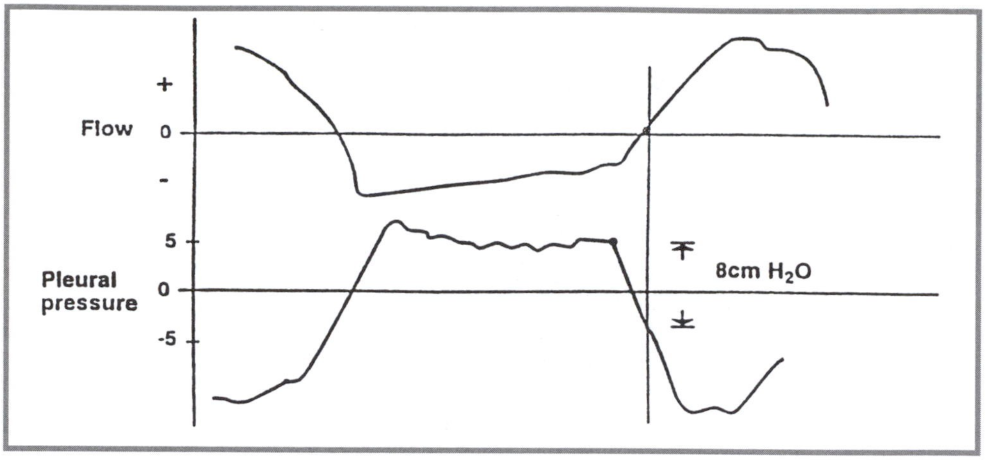

FIGURE 34-14

Dynamic intrinsic PEEP is measured by determining the difference in intrathoracic pressure (with an intraesophageal balloon) between the onset of inspiratory effort and the onset of respiratory flow. (From Haluszka et al., with permission.)

tings result in an insufficient expiratory time to allow exhalation to the resting end-expiratory lung volume. Under these conditions, patients are not able to completely exhale before the next inspiratory cycle begins, leading to progressive air trapping.

Static PEEP may be determined by occluding the ventilator's exhalation valve at end-expiration and reading the positive deflection in the pressure–time waveform.

The drop in intrathoracic pressure that is required for inspiratory flow to begin is termed dynamic PEEP.

Two methods of determining PEEPi have been described. One method is to occlude the ventilator expiratory port at the end of exhalation, which will cause the pressure in the lungs and the mechanical ventilator to equilibrate, then the level of PEEPi can be read from the ventilator's manometer or estimated from the positive deflection in the pressure–time waveform (Figure 34-13); this has been termed static PEEPi. The second method is to determine the drop in intrathoracic pressure that is required for inspiratory flow to begin (Figure 34-14). The latter measurement is called dynamic PEEPi and has been reported to be lower than static PEEPi; this is particularly true in patients with COPD and severe obstruction.

The dynamic to static PEEPi ratio appears to correlate with the difference between the initial drop (P_{init}) and final plateau pressure (P_{plat}), when a pause is set during inspiration. Because the difference between P_{init} and P_{plat} represents losses due to time constant inequalities and viscoelastic adaptation, the difference in dynamic and static PEEPi appears to be related to time–constant inequalities. It is believed that dynamic PEEPi represents the lowest regional end-expiratory pressure that must be overcome to initiate a breath, whereas static PEEPi represents the average value of PEEP present in a nonhomogenous lung tissue. Although the first method appears to be simpler, it requires precise timing with the patient's end expiration, and PEEPi may also be underestimated because of ventilator circuit compliance and abnormally elevated lung compliance resulting in pressure dissipation. Newer ventilators have software that allows automatic occlusion at the end of expiration. The second method requires the insertion of an esophageal balloon, a relatively invasive procedure, but it appears to yield more consistent results and allows for continuous measuring of PEEPi.

Dynamic PEEP determination requires the insertion of an esophageal balloon but allows more consistent results and continuous monitoring of PEEPi.

Compliance

Compliance is defined as volume change per unit of pressure change.

Compliance is defined as volume change per unit of pressure change. If airway pressure is plotted against delivered volume, the slope of the resulting curve (P–V curve) represents compliance (Figure 34-15). The curve is not linear at its extremes; the points at which a plateau is detected are called inflection points. In the curve depicted in Figure 34-15, two inflection points, a lower inflection point (LIP) and an upper inflection point (UIP), can be identified.

Compliance can be calculated as:

$$C_{tot} = V_t/(P_{plat} - \text{total PEEP}) \qquad (34\text{-}6)$$

where V_t is tidal volume and total PEEP is the sum of extrinsic PEEP and intrinsic PEEP.

Two common mistakes can lead to erroneous calculations of compliance. Because volume is dissipated by the distension of the ventilator circuit during the process of ventilation, tidal

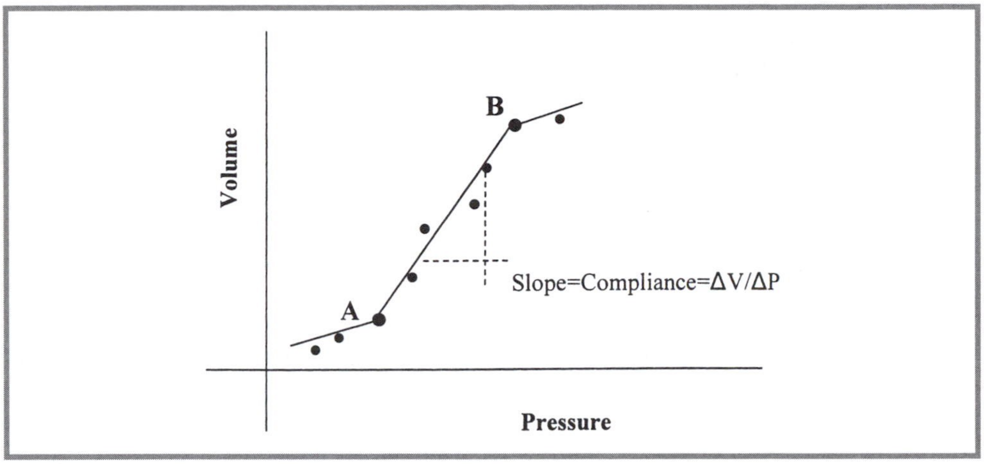

FIGURE 34-15

Schematic of a pressure–volume curve. Points *A* and *B* are the lower and upper inflection points, respectively. The slope of the curve between these two points represents compliance.

volume has to be adjusted. Each manufacturer provides compliance data for their ventilator tubing; generally 2–3 ml/cmH_2O of applied pressure is lost. Failing to include intrinsic PEEP in the equation introduces a large margin of error in the calculation of compliance, as much as 100% in patients with COPD. In a normal person, compliance is about 50–80 ml/cmH_2O.

Compliance can be partitioned into chest wall and lung components by measuring esophageal pressure (P_{es}), which reflects pleural pressure (P_{pl}). Lung compliance is calculated as:

$$C_l = V_t/(P_{plat} - P_{pl}) \qquad (34\text{-}7)$$

and chest wall compliance can be calculated as:

$$C_{cw} = V_t/P_{pl} \qquad (34\text{-}8)$$

Decreased compliance can be seen in patients with ARDS or lung fibrosis. In these cases, lung compliance is the component primarily affected (Table 34-2). Decreased compliance can also be seen in patients with morbid obesity and chest wall deformities, conditions in which the chest wall component is decreased. On the other hand, increased compliance is observed in patients with emphysema because of the decrease in lung elastic recoil.

Decreased chest wall compliance can be seen in disorders such as morbid obesity and chest wall deformities.

Increased compliance can be seen in patients with emphysema.

Resistance

Resistance is calculated as pressure in the respiratory system divided by the flow rate. Resistance of breathing comes from three sources: the airway, and lung tissue and system inertia. Airway resistance is the most important of the three. Airway resistance is caused by factors such as bronchospasm or retained secretions (Table 34-3). Airway resistance varies between inspiration and expiration; this difference is particularly important in patients with diseases such as COPD and asthma. Resistance also varies with changes in lung volume;

Resistance is calculated as pressure in the respiratory system divided by flow.

TABLE 34-2

DISORDERS ASSOCIATED WITH ABNORMAL COMPLIANCE

Decreased compliance
Acute respiratory distress syndrome (ARDS)
Congestive heart failure
Pneumonia
Pneumothorax
Chest wall deformity
Mainstem intubation
Increased compliance
Flail chest
Emphysema

TABLE 34-3

CONDITIONS ASSOCIATED WITH INCREASED AIRWAY RESISTANCE

Bronchospasm	Narrow-lumen endotracheal tube
Mucosal edema	Tracheal stenosis
Increased secretions	

expiratory resistance increases as lung volumes decrease. Airway resistance can be measured separately during inspiration and expiration.

Inspiratory resistance can be measured in relaxed patients receiving mechanical ventilation during constant flow. The driving pressure is the difference between the peak and plateau pressures. Inspiratory resistance can be calculated as:

$$R_{ins} = (P_{pk} - P_{plat})/\text{inspiratory flow} \quad (34\text{-}9)$$

It is believed that the initial drop to P_{init} (see Figure 34-13) represents a purely resistive component whereas the drop to P_{plat} also includes the lung's viscoelastic properties. It has been suggested that measurement of resistance based on the initial drop is more reflective of airway resistance whereas resistance using plateau pressures includes tissue and inertial resistance as well.

Expiratory resistance increases at lower lung volumes due to decreased airway diameter.

Expiratory resistance increases at lower lung volumes due to decreased airway diameter. Expiratory resistance can be measured using the multiple occlusion technique. The airway is intermittently occluded in stepwise fashion repeatedly during a single expiration. During each occlusion, alveolar pressure is measured and, on release, the initial flow is determined. After several data points are recorded, a pressure–flow curve is plotted, and the best-fit regression line is drawn. The slope of the regression line represents average expiratory resistance over the entire tidal volume.

Work of Breathing

To achieve normal ventilation, work has to be performed to overcome the elastic and frictional resistances of the lung and chest wall. Work is performed by patients while contracting their inspiratory muscles, by the mechanical ventilator, or by both to a variable degree. Mechanical work (W) implies that the applied pressure (P_{appl}) produces some displacement of the system, volume (V) in this case, according to the formula:

$$W = P_{appl} \times V \quad (34\text{-}10)$$

Work can be calculated from the area subtended by the applied pressure and the inflation volume.

that represents the area under the volume–pressure curve. During CMV, in relaxed patients, the work of breathing can be computed from the area subtended by the inflation volume and applied pressure (airway pressure) and calculated from Eq. 34-10. In patients who are actively breathing and share a portion of work with the mechanical ventilator, such as patients on pressure support, measurement of the patient's work of breathing requires an esophageal balloon to estimate pleural pressure (Figure 34-16). The esophageal pressure–volume loops also allow work to be separated into resistive and elastic components. Work can be expressed as work per breath, work per minute (work per breath × frequency), or work per liter (work per minute/minute ventilation). Work per liter appears to more closely reflect abnormalities in pulmonary mechanics, whereas work per minute is dependent on minute ventilation and may be lower in patients with severe airway obstruction.

Pressure–Volume Curves

A pressure–volume (P-V) curve can be constructed or plotted in paralyzed patients by measuring the airway pressure while the lungs are progressively inflated with a supersyringe (1.5–3 l). By plotting the pressure for sequential volume points, a curve such as the one de-

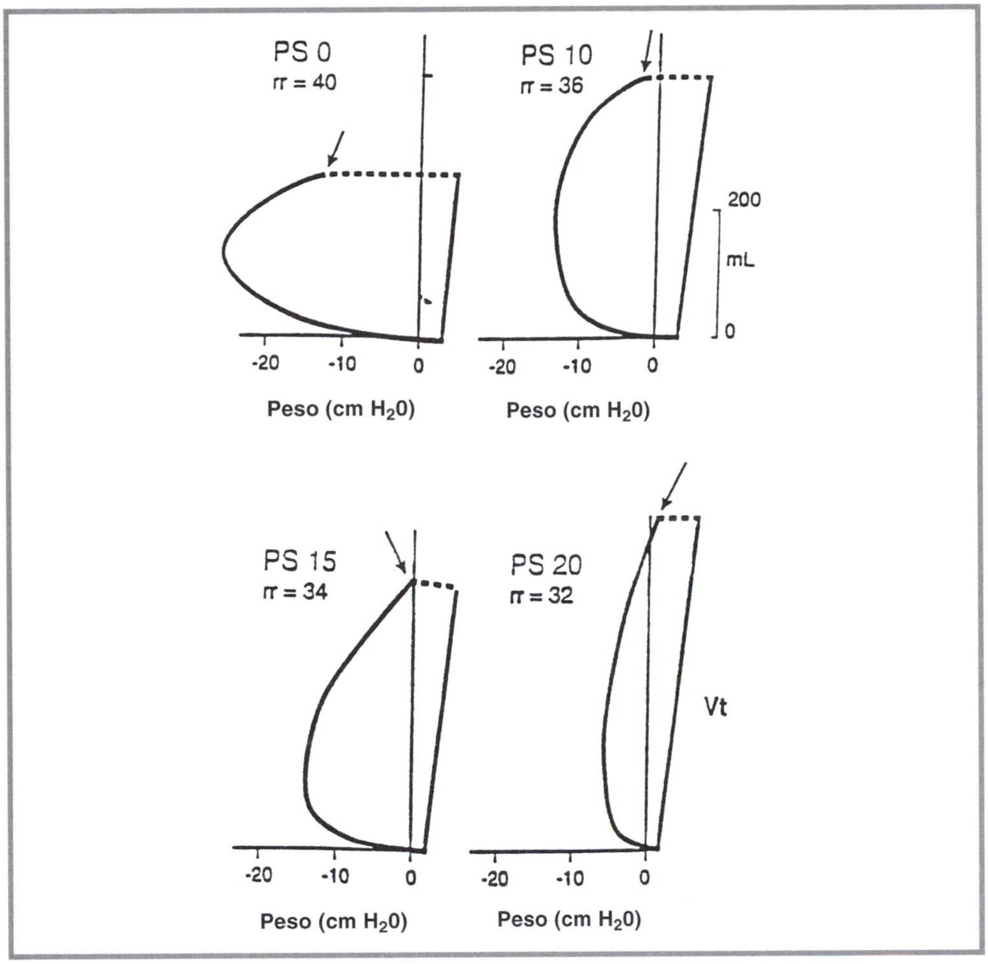

FIGURE 34-16

Loops of esophageal pressure against volume, used for the determination of work in a patient ventilated with pressure support ventilation. A progressive decrement in work per breath can be observed as pressure is increased; this also correlates with a decrement in spontaneous respiratory rate. (From Brochard et al., with permission.)

picted in Figure 34-15 is created. Compliance can be calculated from the slope of a regression line drawn over the curve.

A lower inflection point (LIP) and an upper inflection point (UIP) may be seen in a P-V curve; the LIP is thought to represent the point at which smaller airways and alveoli reopen, corresponding to closing volume. Several investigators have recommended that patients with acute lung injury and ARDS should be ventilated with PEEP set slightly above the lower inflection point. One investigator used tidal volumes of 6–8 ml/kg and individually titrated the level of PEEP in each patient, showing a decrease in mortality in patients treated in this manner. Other investigators have not reproduced these results, raising the question whether individual titration is an important factor in ARDS management. The upper inflection point (UIP) possibly reflects encroachment on total lung capacity, and inflation beyond this point may result in lung injury.

One group of investigators was able to demonstrate an upper inflection point in a group of 25 patients with ARDS ventilated with a tidal volume of 10 ml/kg and PEEP of 10 cmH_2O. The mean UIP was 26 cmH_2O for these patients, and most of the patients had higher plateau pressures. It is currently recommended that patients with ARDS be ventilated trying to maintain plateau pressures below 35 cmH_2O, which is above the upper inflection point observed by these authors. Whether this may result in VILI is unclear.

Compliance can be calculated from the slope of the pressure–volume curve.

Many investigators have recommended that patients with ARDS be ventilated with PEEP set slightly above the lower inflection point.

The upper inflection point possibly reflects encroachment on total lung capacity; inflation beyond this point may result in lung injury.

Flow–Volume Curves

Flow–volume (F-V) curves may provide useful information in ventilator-supported patients. It is important to notice that the expiratory flow contour is going to be affected by patients breathing through a fixed-diameter (endotracheal tube). Normal subjects and patients with

FIGURE 34-17

The sawtooth pattern of the flow–volume curve in a mechanically ventilated patient correlates with the presence of airway secretions. (From Jubran et al., with permission.)

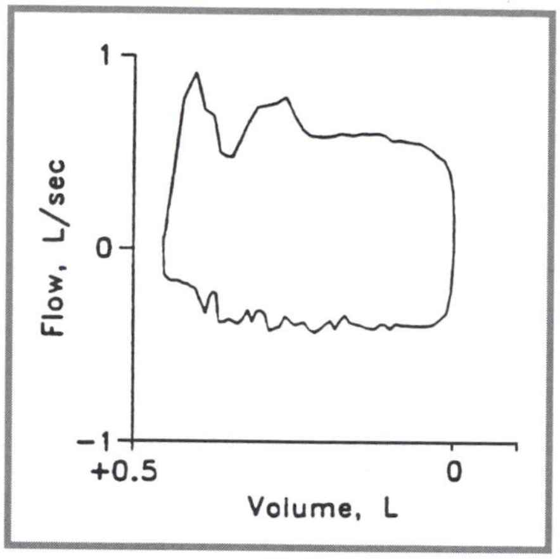

The sawtooth appearance of the flow–volume curve in mechanically ventilated patients correlates with the presence of airway secretions and the need for suctioning.

decreased compliance display a smooth decrease in flow during expiration, whereas patients with obstruction show a convex, curvilinear pattern. In patients with intrinsic PEEP, expiratory flow stops abruptly before the next mechanical breath, creating a characteristic truncated appearance on the F-V curve. In ventilator-dependent patients the appearance of sawtoothing in the flow volume curve has been associated with the presence of airway secretions and the need for endotracheal suctioning (Figure 34-17).

MECHANICAL VENTILATION FOR SPECIFIC CONDITIONS

Acute Respiratory Distress Syndrome

Recently, significant attention has been devoted to protective strategies of mechanical ventilation in patients with ARDS. The rationale behind this comes from animal studies and clinical experience suggesting that mechanical stretch and alveolar overdistension may be responsible for lesions at the alveolar-capillary level that may lead to alterations in permeability and edema. In a study examining the impact of lower end-inspiratory plateau pressures (<25 cmH_2O) in the management of patients with ARDS, 116 patients were randomized to two different groups. Tidal volume in the experimental group was about 7 m l/kg; the control group tidal volume was about 10 ml/kg. Both groups were ventilated with similar extrinsic PEEP. The low tidal volume group had a higher incidence of CO_2 retention and lower pH. Mortality did not significantly differ between groups (47% vs. 38% in the control group).

In another study, patients with limited-ventilation strategy had mortality similar to those ventilated with a conventional strategy. Interestingly, in both of these studies patients in both control and experimental groups had plateau pressures lower than 35 cmH_2O, the level that is thought to be associated with a higher incidence of alveolar overdistension and barotrauma. In contrast to these studies, a different investigative group reported a significant difference in mortality at 28 days between a group assigned to receive protective-strategy ventilation and a group receiving conventional ventilation, 38% and 71%, respectively. Protective ventilation in this group involved high extrinsic PEEP (above the LIP), tidal volumes less than 6 cmH_2O, and driving pressures less than 20 cmH_2O above the extrinsic PEEP value. The protective ventilation group also showed a higher weaning rate and a lower incidence of barotrauma. The results of this trial should be interpreted with caution because a large number of patients had parasitic disease-induced ARDS, resulting in a unique population.

ARDS patients who were ventilated with low tidal volumes (6 ml/kg) had less mortality when compared to similar patients ventilated with large tidal volumes (12 ml/kg) in a large, randomized controlled trial.

Recently, the ARDS Network, a multicenter National Institutes of Health-sponsored collaborative ARDS study group, published the results of a multicenter, randomized trial comparing ARDS patients ventilated with a tidal volume of 12 ml/kg versus patients ventilated with 6 ml/kg. The trial enrolled 861 patients and was stopped early due to an evident reduction in mortality in the low tidal volume group. This group had a 21% reduction in mortality and a significant reduction in inflammatory markers such as IL-6. The low tidal volume group had smaller plateau pressures than the traditional ventilation group. The incidence of barotrauma was similar for both groups. The results of this study have led to a new approach to mechanical ventilation in ARDS, which involves titrating extrinsic PEEP to the highest level that improves oxygenation without affecting hemodynamics, using low tidal volumes to maintain plateau pressures below 35 cmH_2O, and allowing permissive hypercapnia to occur.

Chronic Obstructive Pulmonary Disease and Asthma

Patients that present with severe bronchospasm are often difficult to ventilate and portend a significant challenge. Although asthma and COPD differ in terms of their pathophysiology, the management of these patients is similar. When treating patients with severe obstructive disease, several points must be considered. Management should focus in maintaining patient–ventilator synchrony, aggressively treating bronchospasm, and avoiding intrinsic PEEP and dynamic hyperinflation. Patients often present in acute distress and agitated, which frequently results in patient–ventilator asynchrony. Significant intrinsic PEEP, pneumothorax, and the inability to trigger are frequent causes of agitation. If these causes are not present, judicious use of sedation and, if indicated, pharmacologic paralysis is helpful in managing these patients. The use of neuromuscular blocking agents in these patients has to be carefully weighed, because most of these patients require high doses of systemic glucocorticoids and the concomitant use of these agents has been associated with the development of severe myopathy and critical care illness polyneuropathy.

> In mechanically ventilated patients with severe COPD or asthma, significant auto-PEEP, pneumothorax, and inability to trigger are frequent causes of agitation.

Aggressive treatment with bronchodilator agents and systemic steroids is the standard of care for these patients. Patients with severe airflow limitation frequently have high respiratory rates and are unable to empty their tidal volumes completely, which may lead to air trapping and development of dynamic hyperinflation and intrinsic PEEP. Initial settings should be aimed at providing the patient with enough expiratory time (decreased I:E ratio). Increasing peak inspiratory flow rate and decreasing minute ventilation by reducing either respiratory rate or tidal volume will decrease I:E ratio. These patients should initially be ventilated with a low respiratory rate and high inspiratory flow, aiming at an I:E ratio of at least 1:4 to 1:6. Peak airway pressures are generally high, but most of this pressure is dissipated in the tube and upper airway. Frequent blood gases are needed, and special attention must be paid to the development of intrinsic PEEP (see previous section). Hypercapnia can be allowed to occur so long as pH is kept above 7.20. Because of the presence of intrinsic PEEP, these patients may have difficulty triggering the ventilator. Switching from pressure triggering to flow triggering may reduce work of breathing in this particular group, resulting in improved patient comfort and patient–ventilator synchrony.

> Aggressive use of bronchodilators and systemic steroids is paramount in treating patients with severe bronchospasm.

> In patients with severe airflow obstruction, the initial ventilator settings should provide a long expiration time.

COMPLICATIONS OF MECHANICAL VENTILATION

Mechanical ventilation is a dynamic process that requires close monitoring and alteration of ventilatory parameters to prevent complications. Daily assessment for weaning should be performed because most of the complications that arise are related to the duration of mechanical ventilation.

> Most of the complications associated with mechanical ventilation are related to its duration; therefore, daily assessment of weaning should be done.

Ventilator-Induced Lung Injury

Traditional ventilation support for patients with acute respiratory failure included the use of higher tidal volumes (10–15 ml/kg). In 1974, Webb and Tierney were the first investigators to recognize that rats ventilated with high-pressure mechanical ventilation (>45 cmH_2O) developed ventilator-induced parenchymal injury, manifested by alveolar edema, hypoxemia, and decreased lung compliance. Death occurred in less than 1 h. Dreyfuss and colleagues saw histologic changes similar to those seen in humans with ARDS when they subjected rats to high-pressure mechanical ventilation. To discern whether high alveolar pressures or alveolar overdistension caused VILI, the same group conducted a study using five different ventilator strategies in rats. The control group received low-volume/low-pressure ventilation, the second group received high-pressure/high-volume ventilation, the third group received high-pressure ventilation with limited volume by means of thoracoabdominal strapping, the fourth group had high-volume/low-pressure ventilation with an iron lung, and the last group received high-pressure/high-volume and extrinsic PEEP. There were no differences between controls and the group that received high-pressure ventilation with thoracoabdominal strapping. The remaining groups developed high-permeability edema regardless of the way of administering high-volume ventilation.

The findings were substantiated by other investigators, who found a decrement in the incidence of high-permeability edema in rats ventilated with chest wall restriction. Although the mechanical ventilator-delivered volume seems to play an important role in the development of VILI, other factors, such as inflammation, may also have an important role, as is supported by studies that failed to show a progression to ARDS in neutropenic animals that were ventilated with large tidal volumes. In humans, protective lung ventilation has been associated with decreased levels of IL-6, a marker for inflammation.

Ventilator-delivered volume and concomitant inflammation are believed to be closely related to the development of ventilator-induced lung injury.

Barotrauma

Pneumothorax, subcutaneous emphysema, pneumomediastinum, and other forms of extraalveolar air are generally referred to as barotrauma. This name may be a misnomer because volume appears to be the most important cause of extraalveolar air formation in patients receiving mechanical ventilation.

Although extraalveolar air formation is usually the result of disruption of the pulmonary parenchyma, other causes are possible. Pneumomediastinum and pneumothorax can result from traumatic tracheal intubation, retropharyngeal abscess, or blunt or penetrating chest trauma, or as a complication from bronchoscopy or perforation from a foreign body in the airway. Pneumomediastinum can be seen in patients with traumatic or iatrogenic perforation of the esophagus, or in patients with spontaneous rupture of the esophagus due to vigorous retching (Boerhave's syndrome). Most commonly, in patients on mechanical ventilation, the source of the extraalveolar air lies in the pulmonary parenchyma. Although traditionally associated with elevated pressures, extraalveolar air in mechanically ventilated pressures is more likely to result from ventilation with large tidal volumes. Additional factors such as lung and chest wall compliance, underlying lung disorder, inflammation, and ventilatory mode also appear to influence the development of pneumothorax and pneumomediastinum.

In mechanically ventilated patients, the most common source for extraalveolar air is the lung parenchyma.

Because of the lack of physical signs and symptoms in ICU patients, daily chest radiographs are important. The new onset of high peak pressures in a mechanically ventilated patient should raise the suspicion of pneumothorax, especially if associated with hemodynamic instability (tension pneumothorax). The treatment of pneumothorax and bronchopleural fistula in these patients entails chest tube placement. The routine application of suction is customary in the United States, but not in other countries where suction is employed if the lung does not fully expand. The incidence of barotrauma ranges from 6% to 20% in ventilated patients. Interestingly enough, according to a recent trial, the presence of barotrauma in patients with ARDS does not appear to be an independent predictor of mortality.

The incidence of barotrauma in mechanically ventilated patients ranges from 6% to 20%.

Oxygen Toxicity

The effects of normobaric hyperoxia have been known since the eighteenth century when Lavoisier recognized that "when there is an excess of vital air (oxygen) animals undergo a severe illness." The effects of normobaric hyperoxia on the respiratory system have been extensively studied. Normobaric hyperoxia has been associated with depression of the respi-

Hyperoxia has been associated with the development of diffuse alveolar damage, hypercapnia, tracheobronchitis, absorption atelectasis, and respiratory drive depression.

ratory drive, pulmonary vasodilatation, ventilation–perfusion mismatch, hypercapnia, absorption atelectasis, acute tracheobronchitis, diffuse alveolar damage, ARDS, and bronchopulmonary dysplasia. The depression of the respiratory drive is primarily due to decreased stimulation of the hypoxia-sensitive chemoreceptors at the carotid and aortic bodies. Absorption atelectasis occurs in alveolar units with a low ventilation–perfusion ratio. In these units, the absorption of oxygen exceeds its replenishment. Oxygen may also stimulate the formation of atelectasis by interfering with the normal production of surfactant.

Oxygen may promote atelectasis formation by interfering with the production of surfactant.

The syndrome of acute tracheobronchitis and mucociliary dysfunction was described initially in normal volunteers breathing 100% O_2 for more than 24 h who developed retrosternal discomfort, cough, sore throat, nasal congestion, eye irritation, and fatigue. Bronchopulmonary dysplasia is a syndrome that develops in very low birth weight neonates; it is likely to be the result of hyperoxia, pulmonary edema, and mechanical ventilation-induced trauma. Pathologically, it is characterized by fibrosis and destruction of acinar structures, resulting in scarring and emphysematous changes.

It is still unclear at what level oxygen becomes toxic, particularly in critical care patients. The arbitrary threshold of 60% FiO_2 comes from studies in normal volunteers in the 1950s. The histologic pathology of hyperoxia-induced lung injury can be characterized by the term diffuse alveolar damage. There is abundant evidence supporting the toxic role of hyperoxia in the intensive care unit. Nevertheless, it is extremely difficult to isolate the effects of oxygen amid multiple variables such as mechanical ventilator alveolar overdistension, pneumonia, and sepsis. The combination of oxygen and volutrauma may be responsible of some for the damage reported.

In general, attempts are made to reduce F_iO_2 below 60% as soon as patients tolerate it. Achieving this goal requires a careful approach to diagnosis and treatment of conditions that interfere with adequate oxygenation, such as pneumonia, pulmonary embolism, bronchospasm, excess secretions, pleural effusions, and cardiopulmonary shunts. Decreasing oxygen consumption due to fever, infection, or patient–ventilator asynchrony is also an important step toward decreasing oxygen requirements. Finally, adequate selection of PEEP and protective ventilator strategies may also decrease oxygen requirements and result in less VILI and inflammation. Overall, when controversy arises, it is important to remember that the immediate effect of hypoxemia is far more devastating than the perspective of future oxygen lung injury.

Attempts are made to reduce FiO_2 below 60% as soon as patients tolerate it.

In specific cases, adequate selection of PEEP may aid in decreasing oxygen requirements.

Endotracheal Tube-Related Complications

Complications resulting from endotracheal tubes (ETT) can be divided according to the time in which they occur, that is, complications during ETT placement, complications occurring while the ETT tube is in place, and complications occurring after removal of the ETT.

Complications Occurring During ETT Placement

Complications during ETT placement include nasal trauma, tooth avulsion, and oral and pharyngeal laceration. Laryngeal injuries, such as glottic contusion and vocal cord laceration and hematoma, can occur during ETT placement. Tracheal laceration, perforation, or rupture are extremely uncommon. Right mainstem bronchus intubation has been reported in 3%–9% of all adult intubations. The incidence of aspiration during intubation ranges from 8% to 19% in adult nonanesthetic intubations.

Right mainstem intubation has been reported in 3%–9% of all adult intubations.

The incidence of aspiration in adult intubations ranges from 8% to 19%.

Complications Occurring While the ETT Is in Place

Sinus effusions have been reported to occur in 25%–100% of all intubated patients. Prolonged intubation predisposes to the development of sinusitis. It occurs more commonly with nasal intubation. Sinusitis is frequently missed as a cause for fever in the ICU. Up to 25% of all intubated patients will develop sinusitis; these patients frequently present with fever and rarely have purulent drainage. Computed tomography of the sinus is the preferred diagnostic method because physical findings are generally unreliable.

Up to 25% of all intubated patients develop sinusitis.

The presence of an endotracheal tube strongly predisposes patients to ventilator-acquired pneumonia (VAP).

The presence of an ETT predisposes patients to tracheobronchitis and ventilator-associated pneumonia (VAP). Endotracheal intubation may also result in laryngeal ulceration, glottic edema, tracheal ulceration, and tracheal necrosis, particularly with an overinflated cuff.

Complications Occurring After Extubation

Hoarseness is observed in more than 50% of patients early after extubation; it generally resolves in less than 7 days. Hoarseness that is present beyond 14 days suggests laryngeal injury, such as granuloma formation or vocal cord paralysis. Edema of the vocal cords and stridor can occur early after extubation. Some degree of stridor occurs in about 5% of all extubated patients. Tracheal stenosis, tracheomalacia, and tracheal dilatation are late complications of ETT placement.

Ventilator-Associated Pneumonia

Pneumonia develops in about 30% of all mechanically ventilated patients.

Late-onset VAP is defined as that occurring 72 h after tracheal intubation.

Late-onset VAP is generally associated with antibiotic-resistant bacteria such as *Pseudomonas aeruginosa* and *Acinetobacter*.

Pneumonia develops in about 30% of patients receiving mechanical ventilation. VAP refers specifically to bacterial pneumonia that develops in patients on mechanical ventilation. VAP is termed early onset if it occurs within 48–72 h after tracheal intubation; it is often related to aspiration and the intubation process. VAP that occurs after 72 h is referred to as late onset. Early-onset VAP is associated with antibiotic-sensitive bacteria, methicillin-sensitive *Staphylococcus aureus*, *Haemophilus*, and *Streptococcus pneumoniae*. Late-onset VAP is generally caused by antibiotic-resistant pathogens such as methicillin-resistant *Staphylococcus aureus*, *Pseudomonas aeruginosa*, and *Acinetobacter*.

Several strategies help prevent VAP. Handwashing, elevation of the patient's head more than 30°, oral intubation, avoidance of large gastric volumes, and continuous subglottic suctioning are some of the nonpharmacological measures that may be useful in preventing VAP. Judicious use of antibiotics is important to avoid the emergence of multiresistant pathogens. Ongoing trials are studying rotating scheduled antibiotics in the intensive care unit as a plausible measure to reduce the incidence of VAP and the appearance of multiresistant strains of bacteria. These strategies warrant further investigation.

Upper Gastrointestinal Bleeding

Patients on mechanical ventilation and patients with a history of bleeding diathesis or a history of gastrointestinal bleeding are at higher risk to develop upper gastrointestinal bleeding (GIB).

Patients on mechanical ventilation are at higher risk to develop upper gastrointestinal bleeding (GIB). Patients are also at risk if they have a previous history of upper GI bleeding, or bleeding diathesis. Significant debate exists regarding which agents to use in mechanically ventilated patients to prevent upper GI bleed. One of the theoretical concerns is that altering stomach acid production leads to bacterial overgrowth, which in turn increases the incidence of VAP. A recent study involving 1200 patients in the ICU compared ranitidine versus sucralfate. The group that received ranitidine had a significantly lower incidence of GIB. There was no difference within groups in terms of VAP, length of stay in the unit, and mortality. Ongoing trials are considering the usefulness of the new proton pump inhibitors as prophylactic agents.

Hemodynamic Alterations

Because the lungs and heart share a common space in the thorax, multiple interactions between organs are evident. Mechanical ventilation will affect the autonomic tone, pulmonary vascular pressure, heart rate, preload, afterload, and contraction. High tidal volumes have been shown to induce bradycardia. Extrinsic and intrinsic PEEP can cause a decrement in pulmonary venous return, therefore decreasing ventricular preload and cardiac output. Furthermore, because the heart is situated in the cardiac fossa, increments in pulmonary volumes and/or pressures (PEEP or hyperinflation) may lead to significant mechanical interactions resembling pericardial tamponade. Lung inflation can also release humoral factors such as prostaglandins that may have a cardiodepressive effect.

SUMMARY

Major changes in mechanical ventilation have occurred during the past several decades. These changes have been closely associated with technologic advances. The advent of computers and microprocessors has allowed more complex ventilation algorithms and new ventilatory modalities. However, a large proportion of the advances in mechanical ventilation is the direct result of better understanding of the underlying pathophysiology of the disorders causing respiratory failure. It is clear that invasive and noninvasive monitoring play an important role in managing these patients and preventing complications.

Some of the most important accomplishments in mechanical ventilation are the result of applying new ventilatory strategies while using conventional ventilatory modes, such as low tidal volumes and aggressive PEEP titration in ARDS. The use of adjunctive therapies in mechanical ventilation appears to be promising, as evidenced by the use of inhaled nitric oxide in persistent pulmonary hypertension of the neonate, but further research is needed. Finally, we have come to recognize that there is a direct relationship between the rate of complications and the duration of mechanical ventilation, which makes daily weaning assessment of utmost importance.

REVIEW QUESTIONS

1. **A 62-year-old patient with a long-standing history of COPD presents to the emergency department complaining of severe shortness of breath and wheezing that did not respond to several albuterol nebulizer treatments. He is a thin (65-kg) male, using accessory muscles, and is visibly agitated. His vital signs include respiratory rate of 28, heart rate of 112, blood pressure of 138/85, temperature of 37.1°F, and oxygen saturation of 92% on room air. He is rapidly intubated for respiratory distress. The initial settings on AC ventilation include a respiratory rate of 15, FiO_2 of 1.0, an inspiratory flow rate of 50 l/min, and a V_T of 700 ml. The patient received 4 mg lorazepam for sedation. Measured peak and plateau pressures are 35 and 25 cmH_2O, respectively. Twenty minutes later, the patient develops hypotension. His peak and plateau pressures remain unchanged. The more likely cause for hypotension in this patient is:**
   A. Overt sepsis secondary to pneumonia
   B. Hypotension secondary to sedating agents
   C. Tension pneumothorax
   D. Increased intrinsic PEEP

2. **In the patient in question 1, all the following maneuvers are likely to decrease intrinsic PEEP, except:**
   A. Decrease inspiratory flow rate
   B. Decrease tidal volume
   C. Decrease respiratory rate
   D. Decrease inspiratory time

3. **All the following statements regarding complications of mechanical ventilation are incorrect except:**
   A. Late-onset ventilator-associated pneumonia is defined as pneumonia occurring 48–72 h after endotracheal intubation and is generally caused by infection with *Streptococcus pneumoniae*.
   B. Sinusitis may be a cause of fever in the ICU, but its incidence is low.
   C. Prophylaxis for upper gastrointestinal bleed can be accomplished with H2-blockers or sucralfate.
   D. In patients with ARDS, the development of pneumothorax carries a very high mortality.

4. **A 32-year-old woman with a past medical history significant for seizure disorder is admitted to the emergency department after having a witnessed tonic-clonic seizure. Her weight is 60 kg and her height is 158 cm. In the emergency department, she suffers a second seizure and has to be intubated for airway protection. Upon intubation, gastric content is evidenced in the posterior pharynx and trachea. She is treated with lorazepam and phenytoin intravenously. A chest radiograph taken 6 h later shows right lower lobe pneumonia. She remains intubated, and appropriate antibiotic coverage is initiated. The next day she develops increasing FiO_2 requirements, her compliance is significantly decreased, and a chest radiograph reveals bilateral alveolar infiltrates. Her current ventilator settings include FiO_2 of 90%, tidal volume of 700 ml, and respiratory rate of 12 with no extrinsic PEEP. Her vital signs are stable. An arterial blood gas reveals pH of 7.37, PaO_2 of 69, $PaCO_2$ of 38, and bicarbonate of 22. Which of the following ventilator strategies is more likely to improve the patient's outcome?**
   A. Add PEEP of 5 cmH_2O, increase tidal volume to 10 ml/kg, and increase FiO_2 to 100%
   B. Tidal volume 6–8 ml/kg, titrate PEEP up to improve oxygenation while maintaining cardiovascular stability, maintain plateau pressure <35 cmH_2O
   C. Add PEEP of 5 cmH_2O, increase tidal volume to 15 ml/kg, and increase FiO_2 to 100%
   D. Pressure-control ventilation with high PEEP and inverse ratio (2:1) ventilation
   E. High-frequency jet ventilation

5. All the following statements regarding inhaled nitric oxide (INO) are correct, except:
- **A.** It reduces mean pulmonary artery pressure and pulmonary vascular resistance.
- **B.** It is indicated for persistent pulmonary hypertension of the neonate.
- **C.** It is associated with the development of methemoglobinemia in a small percent of patients.
- **D.** It significantly decreases systemic vascular resistance.

6. All the following statements regarding intrinsic PEEP (PEEPi) are correct, except:
- **A.** PEEPi may occur in patients with severe airway obstruction.
- **B.** Static PEEPi is measured by occluding the expiratory port at end-inspiration.
- **C.** It can decrease venous return and cardiac output.
- **D.** Dynamic PEEPi is determined by measuring the drop in intrathoracic pressure that is required for inspiratory flow to begin.

7. A 72-year-old patient with a history of idiopathic pulmonary fibrosis develops pneumonia and has to be intubated and placed on mechanical ventilation. Taking into consideration his underlying lung pathology, you expect to find the following lung mechanics:
- **A.** Increased peak pressure, decreased plateau pressure, increased compliance
- **B.** Increased peak pressure, increased plateau pressure, increased compliance
- **C.** Increased peak pressure, increased plateau pressure, decreased compliance
- **D.** Decreased peak pressure, decreased plateau pressure, decreased compliance

8. All the following statements regarding pressure-support ventilation (PSV) are correct, except:
- **A.** It is a pressure-preset, flow-cycled ventilatory mode.
- **B.** The patient triggers every breath.
- **C.** Tidal volumes show little or no variation from breath to breath.
- **D.** Inspiration ceases once flow decreases below 25% of peak inspiratory flow or when flow rate is <5 l/min.

9. "Permissive hypercapnia" is a ventilatory strategy that is thought to decrease mean airway pressures and consequently the incidence of ventilator-induced lung injury. Hypercapnic acidosis can be seen in this instance and is associated with which of the following conditions:
- **A.** Improved myocardial contraction
- **B.** Decreased sympathetic activity
- **C.** Cerebral vasodilation and cerebral edema
- **D.** Peripheral vasoconstriction

10. A large difference between peak and plateau pressure can be seen in all the following conditions, except:
- **A.** Tension pneumothorax
- **B.** Right mainstem bronchus intubation
- **C.** Excessive secretions and mucus plugging
- **D.** Use of small-diameter endotracheal tube

ANSWERS

1. The answer is D. The patient in Question 1 is intubated for COPD exacerbation. His initial settings include a high tidal volume, a low inspiratory flow, and a relatively rapid respiratory rate. All these parameters result in a decreased inspiratory time, which does not allow him to completely empty each tidal volume, in addition to the expiratory flow limitation imposed by his underlying disease. The end result is positive pressure at the end of expiration or intrinsic PEEP, which has the same hemodynamic consequences as extrinsic PEEP. Tension pneumothorax is unlikely in this patient because his peak and plateau pressures remained unchanged. The patient has been afebrile and hemodynamically stable until that point, which makes overt sepsis unlikely.
2. The answer is A. A decrease in flow rate, that is, the amount of volume that is delivered per unit of time, is likely to increase inspiratory time and decrease expiratory time, predisposing a patient like this to develop intrinsic PEEP.
3. The answer is C. H2-blocking agents (ranitidine, famotidine) have been shown to be as effective as sucralfate in prophylaxis for upper gastrointestinal bleeding in mechanically ventilated patients. Furthermore, recent studies failed to reveal an increased incidence of ventilator-associated pneumonia in patients treated with H2-blockers. Although late-onset ventilator-associated pneumonia is defined as occurring 48–72 h after endotracheal intubation, it is generally associated with gram-negative organisms. Sinusitis is frequently seen in intubated patients. Finally, in a large randomized trial, the occurrence of pneumothorax in patients in mechanically ventilated ARDS patients did not significantly increase their mortality.
4. The answer is B. Protective mechanical ventilation strategies using low tidal volumes, high PEEP, and maintaining plateau pressures <35 cmH2O have been shown to significantly decrease mortality in ARDS patients. Pressure-control ventilation with inverse I:E ratio has not been shown to be superior in these cases and generally requires sedation and paralysis. High-frequency jet ventilation works with very small tidal volumes and may, theoretically, reduce the incidence of VILI; up until now there has not been enough evidence to support its use in ARDS.
5. The answer is D. Inhaled nitric oxide (INO) has been shown to decrease mean pulmonary artery pressure and pulmonary vascular resistance. It has a very short half-life, and its effects on systemic vascular resistance are very small or absent. The development of methemoglobinemia is one of its complications; therefore, serial arterial blood gas determinations are made. Methemoglobinemia is infrequently seen <20 ppm. The use of INO was recently approved by the U.S. Food and Drug Administration in term and near-term neonates with persistent pulmonary hypertension, where randomized, controlled trials showed an improvement in oxygenation and a decrease in the need for ECMO.
6. The answer is B. Intrinsic PEEP (PEEPi) can be seen in patients with severe airflow obstruction, such as asthma and COPD. Its he-

modynamic consequences are similar to those caused by extrinsic PEEP. Dynamic PEEPi measurement requires placement of an intraesophageal balloon and determining the drop of intrathoracic pressure required before inspiratory flow begins. Plateau pressure is measured at the end of inspiration; static PEEPi is measured at the end of expiration.

7. The answer is C. The patient in Question 7 has an underlying disorder that is associated with decreased compliance, namely, pulmonary fibrosis. The presence of purulent secretions, debris, and inflammation caused by pneumonia will worsen compliance. The expected findings include elevated peak and plateau pressures, reflecting the altered compliance of the respiratory system.
8. The answer is C. During pressure-support ventilation, the patient triggers every breath. Pressure is preset by the operator, and the respiratory cycle is terminated once flow falls to a predetermined level, generally 25% of the initial peak inspiratory flow or <5 l/min. The delivered tidal volume is dependent on the preset pressure, the patient's effort, and the respiratory system mechanics. Variation in tidal volumes from breath to breath is expected.
9. The answer is C. Permissive hypercapnia is frequently used in the setting of ARDS and asthma exacerbation to decrease mean airway pressure. It can result in hypercapnic acidosis, which has been associated with direct myocardial depression, increased sympathetic activation, and peripheral and cerebral vasodilatation. These effects are less likely to occur if pH is maintained >7.20.
10. The answer is A. Tension pneumothorax is associated with a decreased compliance; a large difference between peak and plateau pressure is not an expected finding in this condition.

SUGGESTED READING

Amato MBP, Barbas CSV, Medeiros DM, et al. Improved survival in ARDS: beneficial effects of a lung protective strategy. Am J Respir Crit Care Med 1996;153:A531.

Appendini L, Patessio A, Zanaboni S, et al. Physiologic effects of positive end-expiratory pressure and mask pressure support during exacerbations of chronic obstructive pulmonary disease. Am J Respir Crit Care Med 1994;149:1069–1076.

Appendini L, Purro A, Patessio A, et al. Partitioning of inspiratory pressure workload and pressure assistance in ventilator-dependent COPD patients. Am J Respir Crit Care Med 1996;154:1301–1309.

Benito S, Lemaire F. Pulmonary pressure-volume relationship in acute respiratory distress syndrome in adults: role of positive end-expiratory pressure. J Crit Care 1990;5:27–34.

Brochard L, Roudot-Thoraval F, and the Collaborative Group on VT Reduction. Tidal volume (VT) reduction in acute respiratory distress syndrome (ARDS): a multicenter randomized study. Am J Respir Crit Care Med 1997;155:A505.

Feihl F. Permissive hypercapnia: how permissive should we be? Am J Respir Crit Care Med 1994;150:1722–1737.

Fleury B, Murciano D, Talamo C, Aubier M, Pariente R, Milic-Emili J. Work of breathing in patients with chronic obstructive pulmonary disease in acute respiratory failure. Am Rev Respir Dis 1985;131:822–827.

Gattnioni L, Pesenti A, Avalli L, Rossi F, Bombino M. Pressure-volume curve of total respiratory system in acute respiratory failure. Computed tomographic scan study. Am Rev Respir Dis 1987;136:730–736.

Haluszka J. Intrinsic PEEP and arterial PCO_2 in stable patients with chronic obstructive pulmonary disease. Am Rev Respir Dis 1990;141:1194–1197.

Hirschl RB. Initial experience with partial liquid ventilation in adult patients with the acute respiratory distress syndrome. JAMA 1996;275:383–389.

Jubran A. Monitoring mechanics during mechanical ventilation. Semin Respir Crit Care Med 1999;20:65–79.

Jubran A, Tobin MJ. Use of flow-volume curves in detecting secretions in ventilator-dependent patients. Am J Respir Crit Care Med 1994;150:766–769.

Jubran A, Tobin MJ. Passive mechanics for lung and chest wall in patients who failed or succeeded in trials of weaning. Am J Respir Crit Care Med 1997;155:916–921.

Marini JJ. Inverse ratio ventilation: simply an alternative, or something more? Crit Care Med 1995;23:224–228.

Nakos G. Effect of the prone position on patients with hydrostatic pulmonary edema compared with patients with acute respiratory distress syndrome and pulmonary fibrosis. Am J Respir Crit Care Med 2000;161:360–413.

Pepe PE, Marini JJ. Occult positive end-expiratory pressure in mechanically ventilated patients with airflow obstruction. Am Rev Respir Dis 1982;126:166–170.

Petty TL. An historical perspective of mechanical ventilation. Crit Care Clin 1990;6:489–504.

Ranieri VM, Guiliani R, Cinnella G, et al. Physiologic effects of positive end-expiratory pressure in patients with chronic obstructive pulmonary disease during acute ventilatory failure and controlled mechanical ventilation. Am Rev Respir Dis 1993;147:5–13.

Ravenscraft SA. Tracheal gas insufflation augments CO_2 clearance during mechanical ventilation. Am Rev Respir Dis 1993;148:345–351.

Roupie E, Dambrosio M, Servillo G, et al. Titration of tidal volume and induced hypercapnia in acute respiratory distress syndrome. Am J Respir Crit Care Med 1995;52:121–128.

Stewart TEM, Meade O, Granton J, et al. Pressure and volume limited ventilation strategy (PLVS) in patients at high risk for ARDS. Results of a multicenter trial. Am J Respir Crit Care Med 1997;155:A505.

The Acute Respiratory Distress Syndrome Network. Ventilation with lower tidal volumes as compared with traditional tidal volumes for acute lung injury and the acute respiratory distress syndrome. N Engl J Med 2000;342:1301–1308.

CHAPTER 35

Ubaldo J. Martin and Gerard J. Criner

Noninvasive Ventilation

CHAPTER OUTLINE

LEARNING OBJECTIVES

After studying this chapter, you should be able to:

- Understand the physiologic effects of noninvasive ventilation.
- Know how to apply different techniques of noninvasive ventilation, that is, negative pressure versus positive pressure ventilation.
- Understand the relative advantages and disadvantages of different types of patient–ventilator interfaces during noninvasive ventilation.
- Select the patient population that is more likely to benefit from noninvasive ventilation.
- Review the application of noninvasive ventilation in specific disease groups.
- Review and learn to manage complications associated with noninvasive ventilation.

The use of noninvasive ventilation in acute respiratory failure has received much attention in recent years because of the recognition of the important complications that result from translaryngeal intubation and also the recent development of new and different devices to perform noninvasive ventilation. Although noninvasive ventilation techniques in the form of negative pressure ventilation (e.g., tank ventilators, cuirass, rocking beds) have been used since the 1930s for the treatment of acute respiratory failure, the development of more responsive devices providing negative pressure ventilation, coupled with the recent development of noninvasive positive pressure ventilation (NPPV), have facilitated the increased use of noninvasive ventilation. Moreover, recent awareness that avoidance of translaryngeal intubation preserves upper airway function (e.g., speech, swallowing), enhances patient comfort, decreases the incidence of nosocomial respiratory infections, and appears to improve morbidity and mortality in some individuals (Table 35-1) has led to greater emphasis on noninvasive ventilation.

In this chapter, we discuss the different techniques of noninvasive ventilation, selection of appropriate candidates, the role of noninvasive ventilation in specific diseases, and pos-

TABLE 35-1

ADVANTAGES AND DISADVANTAGES OF NONINVASIVE POSITIVE PRESSURE VENTILATION (NPPV) COMPARED TO INVASIVE MECHANICAL VENTILATION

	ADVANTAGES	DISADVANTAGES
NPPV	■ Comfort ■ Preservation of upper airway functions (speech, swallowing) ■ Decreased risk of nosocomial pneumonia and sinusitis ■ Portable	■ Requires cooperative patient ■ Air leaks ■ Variable tidal volumes ■ Facial skin breakdown ■ Nasal bridge skin necrosis
Conventional mechanical ventilation	■ Patient cooperation not required ■ Control over volumes and pressures being delivered ■ Fewer air leaks	■ Complications of endotracheal tube ■ Increased risk of nosocomial pneumonia and sinusitis ■ Ventilator-induced lung injury

sible complications associated with its use. We focus on the use of noninvasive ventilation in the ICU, specifically, in the management of acute, or acute on chronic respiratory failure.

PHYSIOLOGIC EFFECTS OF NONINVASIVE VENTILATION

Noninvasive ventilation has been shown to improve gas exchange, normalize $PaCO_2$, increase PaO_2, increase pH, increase tidal volume, and decrease respiratory muscle work in acute and chronic respiratory failure. Additionally, noninvasive ventilation has been reported to stabilize metabolic parameters such as heart rate, respiratory rate, and blood pressure.

The goals of noninvasive ventilation are to improve gas exchange, decrease work of breathing, and alleviate patient dyspnea.

Negative pressure ventilation and NPPV have both been shown to assist each spontaneous breath, thereby reducing respiratory muscle work as measured by swings in transdiaphragmatic pressure, inspiratory muscle pressure–time index, or diaphragmatic electromyographic activity. The reduction in respiratory muscle work and patient effort is associated with a change in breathing pattern, towards a deeper, slower pattern, and an overall increment in minute ventilation. Both of these changes, deeper slower breathing and overall increase in total ventilation result in an increase alveolar ventilation and oxygenation while simultaneously lowering carbon dioxide tension.

Negative pressure ventilation closely mimics spontaneous respiration, and its hemodynamic effect is generally viewed as favorable when compared to positive pressure ventilation (Table 35-2). Negative pressure ventilation applied to the chest wall decreases mean intrathoracic pressure, which results in increased venous return and consequently increased cardiac output. However, negative pressure ventilation may also have a detrimental cardiovascular effect; lower intrathoracic pressures can also increase left ventricular afterload by increasing transmyocardial pressure. In some patients, the increase in venous return may lead to right ventricular dilatation and a reduction in left ventricle dimension due to shift of the interventricular septum, ultimately resulting in left ventricular diastolic dysfunction. It is clear that the cardiovascular effects of negative pressure ventilation depend on the type of negative pressure apparatus (and degree of body surface exposed to negative pressure), the patient's intravascular volume, and underlying left ventricular compliance and ejection fraction. In contrast to the hemodynamic effects of negative pressure ventilation, NPPV increases

Negative pressure ventilation causes a decrease in mean intrathoracic pressure, which results in increased venous return and consequently increased cardiac output.

Negative pressure ventilation lowers intrathoracic pressure, which may result in increased afterload due to increased transmyocardial pressure.

TABLE 35-2

HEMODYNAMIC EFFECTS OF NONINVASIVE POSITIVE PRESSURE VENTILATION (NPPV) COMPARED WITH NEGATIVE PRESSURE VENTILATION

	NPPV	NEGATIVE PRESSURE VENTILATION
Left ventricular afterload	Decreased	Increased
Right ventricular preload	Decreased	Increased
Venous return	Decreased	Increased

intrathoracic pressure, thereby decreasing venous return, preload, and cardiac output. Because NPPV exerts an effect on transmyocardial pressure opposite to that of negative pressure ventilation, a reduction in left ventricular afterload can be seen.

In patients in whom breathing against high resistive or high elastic loads has precipitated respiratory muscle fatigue, effective use of noninvasive ventilation provides respiratory muscle resting and eventual recovery. In other scenarios, noninvasive ventilation stabilizes gas exchange (increases PaO_2, decreases $PaCO_2$, increases pH) and ensures stabilization of the patient's medical status until the event precipitating respiratory failure can be treated. Noninvasive ventilation does not cure the disorder precipitating respiratory failure but rather is an adjunctive aid to provide patient stability until the precipitating disorder causing respiratory failure can be appropriately treated.

IMPLEMENTING NONINVASIVE VENTILATION

> Successful application of noninvasive ventilation is based on appropriate patient selection.

The goals of noninvasive ventilation, regardless of the device being used, are to improve gas exchange, decrease work of breathing, and alleviate the patient's dyspnea. Success in achieving these goals may obviate the need for endotracheal intubation. Successful application of noninvasive ventilation is based on appropriate patient selection, adequate sizing of the apparatus and fitting to ensure patient comfort, and proper selection of ventilatory mode (Table 35-3).

> Noninvasive ventilation for acute respiratory failure should be conducted in a monitored area such as the intensive care unit.

To maximize patient safety, it is recommended that initial treatment of patients with acute or severe forms of acute on chronic respiratory failure should begin in the intensive care unit (ICU) to ensure adequate vigilance by medical, nursing, and respiratory personnel. The choice of negative pressure ventilation rather than NPPV as the mode of delivering noninvasive ventilation depends on the expertise of the prescribing physician with the different ventilatory

TABLE 35-3

IMPORTANT FACTORS TO CONSIDER DURING APPLICATION OF NONINVASIVE VENTILATION

- Patient selection criteria
  - Awake and cooperative
  - Able to sustain short period of spontaneous ventilation
  - Intact upper airway function
  - Stable cardiovascular function
  - Absence of facial trauma
  - No excessive secretions
- Interface
  - Negative pressure ventilation
    - Tank ventilator
    - Cuirass
    - Airtight body suit
  - Noninvasive positive pressure ventilation
    - Types of facial mask
      - Nasal: advantages include less risk of aspiration and claustrophobia; disadvantages include leakage from the mouth and poor fit in edentulous patients
      - Oronasal: advantages include absence of leak from the mouth; disadvantages include increased risk of aspiration, claustrophobia, and aerophagia
    - Proper fit of mask is important in avoiding air leak
    - Chinstrap may be used to decrease mouth leaks (nasal mask)
- Modes of ventilation
  - Negative pressure ventilation
  - CPAP: initial indication for patients with cardiogenic pulmonary edema
  - BiPAP
  - Pressure support: may enhance patient's comfort
  - Assist/control mode
    - Volume preset
    - Pressure preset

CPAP, continuous positive airway pressure; BiPAP, bilevel positive airway pressure

TABLE 35-4

NONINVASIVE POSITIVE PRESSURE VENTILATION COMPARED WITH NEGATIVE PRESSURE VENTILATION: ADVANTAGES AND DISADVANTAGES

	ADVANTAGES	DISADVANTAGES
Negative pressure ventilation	No airway cannulation Significantly augments ventilation Rare hemodynamic concerns Simple devices	Cumbersome Induces upper airway obstruction Limits nursing care Controlled ventilation
Noninvasive positive pressure ventilation	Averts upper airway obstruction Patient-initiated breaths Portable	Bothersome interface Leaks Aerophagia Skin breakdown

techniques, the available equipment, the goals of ventilation, patient comfort, and unique patient factors. Expertise in providing noninvasive ventilation depends not only on the physician but also on the support staff (nurses, respiratory therapists), who continuously interact with patients while they are being evaluated for, or are being maintained on noninvasive ventilation. Both negative pressure ventilation and NPPV have distinct advantages and disadvantages (Table 35-4). Selection of a device and settings depends on minimizing side effects while simultaneously augmenting ventilation in the most efficient manner.

The first step is to decide whether a patient with respiratory failure is a candidate for noninvasive ventilation. Patients who are hemodynamically unstable, have mental obtundation (not related to hypercapnic encephalopathy), or have excessive secretions are not candidates for negative pressure ventilation or noninvasive positive pressure ventilation. If respiratory failure is associated with profound metabolic or cognitive disorders, control of the medical condition should be achieved by intubation and invasive positive pressure ventilation.

Negative Pressure Ventilation

Negative pressure ventilation is a form of noninvasive ventilation that mimics spontaneous ventilation by applying subatmospheric pressure around the thorax during inspiration, creating a pressure gradient between the atmosphere and the patient's alveoli that results in airflow and lung inflation.

Lung inflation in negative pressure ventilation occurs as a result of a pressure gradient between the alveoli and the atmosphere.

Types of negative pressure devices that have been used in the treatment of respiratory failure, especially respiratory failure caused by neuromuscular disorders, include the iron lung, cuirass, and airtight body suit ventilators (Figure 35-1). Settings for negative pressure ventilation are usually established by matching the patient's spontaneous respiratory rate and then progressively increasing the amount of delivered negative pressure until the targeted tidal volume is achieved. With the tank ventilator or iron lung, negative pressure is applied to the whole body except for the head and neck, whereas with the cuirass or the airtight body suit (poncho-wrap, pulmo-wrap, Zip suit) ventilators, negative pressure is applied to the thorax and upper abdomen. The larger the area covered by the negative pressure device, the greater the tidal volume generated. Accordingly, tank ventilators produce greater tidal volumes than body suits, which produce greater tidal volumes than a cuirass. Recently developed devices incorporate the capability for the patient to trigger the ventilator's application of negative pressure, thereby improving patient–ventilator synchrony.

The tank ventilator applies negative pressure to the whole body. The cuirass and the airtight body suits apply negative pressure to the thorax and upper abdomen.

The larger the area covered by the negative pressure device, the greater the tidal volume generated.

Negative pressure ventilation has been used in several disease categories: the neonatal respiratory distress syndrome, chronic respiratory insufficiency due to neuromuscular and chest wall diseases, and acute and chronic respiratory failure due to chronic obstructive pulmonary disease (COPD). Negative pressure ventilation can therefore be used as full ventilatory support in acute respiratory failure or as intermittent support during sleep in patients with chronic respiratory failure resulting from progressive neuromuscular or chest wall diseases.

Negative pressure ventilation can provide adequate ventilatory support in patients with chronic respiratory failure due to neuromuscular diseases and acute and chronic respiratory failure due to chronic obstructive pulmonary disease (COPD).

In the 1950s, negative pressure ventilation was reported to be effective when used in patients with acute exacerbations of chronic respiratory disease. Recent reports appear to confirm those earlier results. In a study of 20 patients presenting with acute COPD exacerbation,

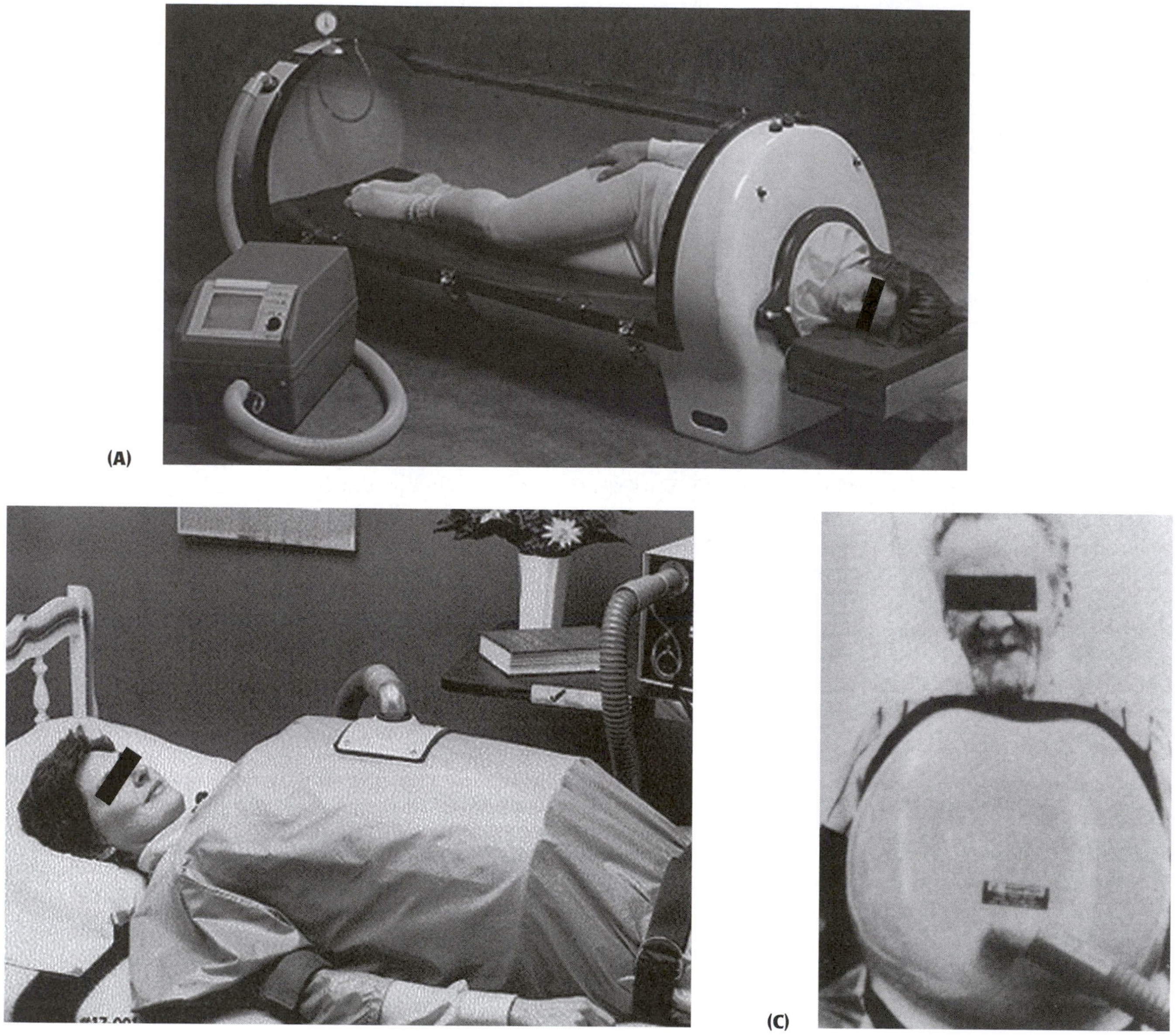

FIGURE 35-1

Negative pressure devices. The Porta-Lung® is an example of a modern noninvasive ventilating chamber. It is made in three different sizes and weighs from 33 to 53 kg. It can be interfaced with the NEV-100® (Lifecare) ventilator or the Emerson 33-CR® to provide negative pressure ventilation **(A)**. The poncho-wrap consists of an airtight body suit that surrounds a rigid frame **(B)**. The cuirass shell applies negative pressure to the chest and upper abdomen **(C)**.

the application of negative pressure ventilation for 6 h resulted in increased maximal inspiratory pressures (MIP) and decreased $PaCO_2$. In contrast, no changes in these parameters were observed during a 6-h period of sham therapy. Another study reported the clinical outcome of 105 COPD patients who also presented with acute respiratory failure. All patients were treated with standard therapy in addition to negative pressure ventilation. The mean PaO_2 and $PaCO_2$ values on admission were 34.6 $\pm$ 9.6 mmHg and 85.1 $\pm$ 16.3 mmHg, respectively. Continuous negative pressure ventilation was provided until patients had a $PaCO_2$ less than 65 mmHg or a pH greater than 7.30. Negative pressure ventilation was provided for a maximum of 2 h four times daily, or a minimum of 1 h four times per day, to achieve

$PaCO_2$ targets between 50 and 55 mmHg and a normal pH. The most common causes of acute respiratory failure in this cohort of patients were acute COPD exacerbation and pneumonia. Of 105 patients, 62 were comatose on admission, and 42 patients evidenced some degree of mental status deterioration. A total of 93 patients recovered and were discharged home; 87 patients were followed for up to 5 years. The 1-year and 5-year mortalities were 18% and 63%, respectively.

Using a case-control study design, the same authors reported the clinical outcome of 26 additional COPD patients suffering from acute respiratory failure who received negative pressure ventilation and compared their outcome to 26 matched control COPD patients who were treated with intubation and positive pressure ventilation. Mortality was similar for both groups, 23% for the negative pressure ventilation group and 27% for the control arm; however, the duration of ventilatory support was significantly shorter for the negative pressure ventilation group (16 h versus 96 h). Furthermore, there were no respiratory infections in the negative pressure group, whereas 3 patients in the control group developed respiratory infections. The results of these studies suggest that negative pressure ventilation is as effective as positive pressure ventilation in providing adequate ventilatory support in COPD patients with acute respiratory failure; however, because these studies lacked adequate controls and enrolled relatively small numbers of patients, further randomized controlled trials comparing negative pressure ventilation and invasive or noninvasive positive pressure ventilation are needed. Complications of negative pressure ventilation such as back pain and upper airway obstruction, in addition to the limitations imposed by negative pressure ventilation on providing nursing or medical care (such as placing central lines and invasive monitoring), may limit its widespread application.

Back pain and obstructive sleep apnea are complications of negative pressure ventilation.

Noninvasive Positive Pressure Ventilation

Noninvasive positive pressure ventilation can be delivered with either volume- or pressure-preset ventilatory modes. In the volume-preset mode, a tidal volume is set that increases alveolar ventilation until ventilation targets are met. In a pressure-preset mode, an inspiratory pressure boost above the end-expiratory level is chosen to augment ventilation to the chosen target.

Several preliminary steps must be implemented before noninvasive positive pressure ventilation can be instituted in the acute setting (Table 35-5). The patient should be placed in a monitored location. Monitoring should include ECG, respiratory impedance, pulse oximetry, and frequent measurement of vital signs. The patient should be sitting in bed or a chair at an angle greater than 30°. A mask should be selected and properly fit with the appropriate headgear. Ideally, several mask sizes and types should be readily available to minimize air leaks and increase patient comfort.

Noninvasive Positive Pressure Ventilation Using a Volume-Preset Mode

Volume-preset or volume-limited mode has several advantages. Almost all critical care ventilators or portable home ventilators are able to provide volume-preset ventilation, and it is

TABLE 35-5

PRELIMINARY STEPS BEFORE INSTITUTING NONINVASIVE POSITIVE PRESSURE VENTILATION IN THE ACUTE SETTING

- Select an appropriately monitored location (Intensive Care Unit, Step Down Unit, Ventilatory Rehabilitation Unit)
- Baseline vital signs and arterial blood gas
- Continuous EKG, blood pressure monitoring, continuous pulse oximetry, respiratory impedance
- Patient in bed or chair sitting at ≥30° angle
- Select and fit interface
- Apply headgear
- Select ventilation
- Connect interface to ventilator tubing and turn on ventilator

SOURCE: Modified from Mehta S, Hill N. Noninvasive ventilation. Am J Respir Crit Care 2001;163:540–577, with permission therefore readily available. Volume-preset ventilators have the capability to deliver large tidal volumes over a wide range of inspiratory flows. In this case, the volume delivered to the patient is "guaranteed" on a breath-to-breath basis. The built-in blender permits the delivery of high concentrations of oxygen. On the other hand, volume-preset ventilation can be associated with significant air leaks and cannot compensate for them by increasing the delivered volume. The presence of air leaks may also result in prolonged inspiratory times, and patient–ventilator dysynchrony may develop, thereby limiting patient tolerance.

Ventilator Settings

During noninvasive volume-preset ventilation, delivered tidal volumes are set higher (8–10 ml/kg) than during invasive mechanical ventilation to compensate for air leaks.

Setting the ventilator in the volume-limited mode to deliver noninvasive ventilation is similar to setting the ventilator for invasive ventilation (see Chapter 34). Respiratory rate is generally set at the patient's spontaneous respiratory rate. Delivered tidal volumes should be set higher than in invasive mechanical ventilation, from 8 to 10 ml/kg. Minimal trigger sensitivity should be used to allow triggering through the interface. Volume-limited noninvasive ventilation delivered through a critical care ventilator has several advantages, including the presence of alarms, the ability to use higher inspiratory fractions of O_2, and monitoring of ventilatory variables (airway pressure, inspired and expired flows, and tidal volumes).

Noninvasive Positive Pressure Ventilation Using a Pressure-Preset Mode

Pressure-preset ventilation has been shown to decrease the work of breathing, increase tidal volume, and decrease respiratory rate in patients with respiratory failure.

Pressure-preset ventilation can compensate for air leaks by maintaining a constant inspiratory pressure.

With pressure-support ventilation, the patient must trigger every breath.

A pressure-support breath is terminated after a predetermined flow has been reached, usually 25% of the initial flow.

Pressure-preset ventilation has been widely used to deliver noninvasive ventilation. This mode has been shown to decrease the work of breathing, increase expired tidal volume, and decrease spontaneous respiratory rate. Pressure-preset ventilation can compensate for air leaks by increasing ventilator flow to achieve the targeted inspiratory pressure. Two forms of pressure-preset ventilation are generally used: pressure-support ventilation (PSV) and pressure-control ventilation (PCV). With PSV, the patient must trigger every breath, and the delivered tidal volume is a result of the set pressure, patient effort, and individual pulmonary mechanics. A PSV breath is terminated after a predetermined flow has been reached, usually 25% of the initial flow. With the occurrence of air leaks during noninvasive ventilation, the ventilator's inability to appropriately sense flow decay may result in an abnormally prolonged inspiration.

During pressure-control ventilation, the physician determines delivered pressure, inspiratory time, and respiratory rate.

During PCV, the physician determines not only the pressure to be delivered but also the inspiratory time and respiratory rate. In contrast to PSV, the patient does not need to trigger each breath during PCV; moreover, if the ventilator is unable to sense a decrement in flow during pressure support, resulting in a prolonged delivery of the ventilator breath (i.e., prolonged inspiratory time), PCV can be used to set a specific inspiratory time and therefore improve patient–ventilator synchrony.

Bilevel positive airway pressure (BiPAP®) is a patient-triggered, pressure-limited, and flow- or time-cycled mode of delivering noninvasive ventilation. BiPAP® is a small, simple, portable device specifically designed for NPPV (Figure 35-2). Similar to conventional ventilators used in the ICU, BiPAP® can be set in a spontaneous mode (equivalent to the assist mode in conventional ventilators), spontaneous/time mode (equivalent to assist/control mode), or time mode (equivalent to control). The latter two modes are used to provide a backup rate and ensure a minimum mandatory minute ventilation. The spontaneous/time mode is used in patients who tend to hypoventilate during sleep, such as patients with obesity hypoventilation or severe neuromuscular disease. Both the inspiratory positive airway pressure (IPAP) and the expiratory positive airway pressure (EPAP) can be preset to specific physiologic targets. It is important to realize that the preset level of IPAP with the BiPAP® apparatus is absolute and includes the expiratory pressure. In contrast, when conventional ventilators are used to provide bilevel pressure ventilation, the IPAP is set above the EPAP, so that the total end-inspiratory pressure is the sum of the IPAP and EPAP values.

The preset level of inspiratory positive airway pressure (IPAP) in the BiPAP® ventilator is absolute and includes the expiratory pressure.

In most clinical series, noninvasive ventilatory support was administered intermittently throughout the day, but in acute respiratory failure caused by parenchymal disease, ventilatory assistance is usually required for more than 20 h/day during the first day. The duration

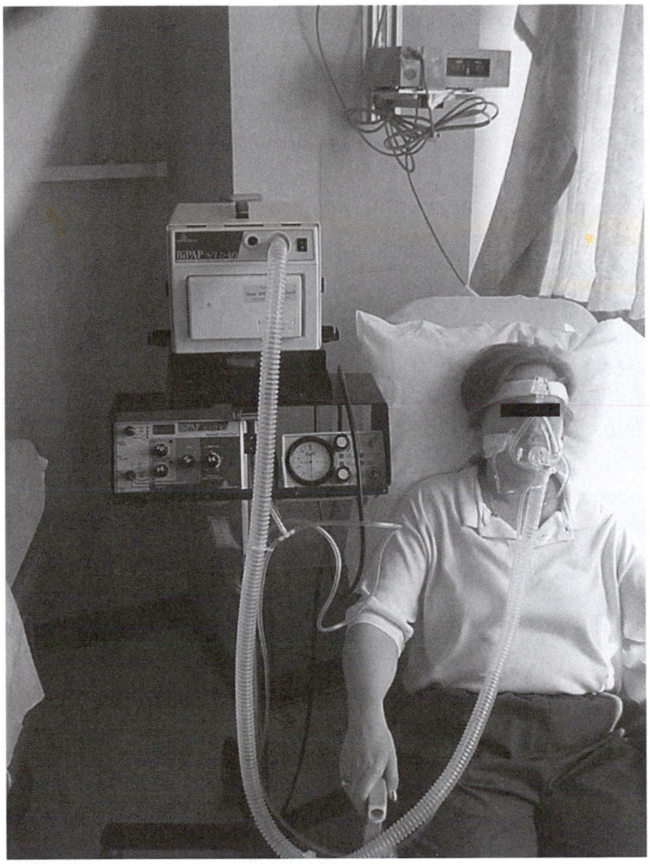

FIGURE 35-2

BiPAP® ventilator.

of NPPV is gradually reduced over subsequent days, depending on the patient's clinical status. In most studies, the overall duration of ventilatory support when treating acute respiratory failure has been relatively short, a mean of 3 ± 1 days in one study and 4 ± 0.6 days in another.

Ventilator Settings

Several options are available for pressure-preset ventilation. Pressure can be delivered by critical care ventilators or by portable positive pressure devices. If pressure support delivered by a critical care ventilator is selected, initial ventilator settings should be started low, 8–12 cmH_2O of IPAP; EPAP is generally initiated at 3–5 cmH_2O. IPAP should be titrated by 2–3 cmH_2O every 3–5 min and adjusted following parameters such as respiratory rate, exhaled tidal volume, and use of accessory muscles (see following). Critical care ventilators are able to deliver high pressures and precise oxygen mixtures.

If BiPAP® is used, it is important to remember that it consists of a single circuit for both inspiration and exhalation, which may result in rebreathing of carbon dioxide. A one-way exhalation valve is placed as close as possible to the patient, and the application of EPAP at a level of at least 3–5 cmH_2O allows a continuous flow of gas to flush CO_2 from the line and prevent significant CO_2 rebreathing. EPAP can be slowly titrated upward to increase end-expiratory lung volume and recruit collapsed alveolar units, thereby improving oxygenation. If supplemental oxygen is required, oxygen tubing can be connected to the ventilator circuit using a T-tube or bled in at a mask port.

When BiPAP® is used, 3–5 cmH_2O expiratory positive airway pressure (EPAP) provides a constant gas flow that prevents CO_2 rebreathing.

Continuous Positive Airway Pressure

Continuous positive airway pressure (CPAP) is the application of a preset positive pressure throughout the entire respiratory cycle. It does not provide a pressure boost during inspira-

Continuous positive airway pressure (CPAP) does not provide a pressure boost during inspiration to augment ventilation.

CPAP increases end-expiratory lung volume and decreases intrapulmonary shunting.

CPAP improves respiratory system compliance and decreases the work of breathing.

tion to augment ventilation (see Chapter 34). Nevertheless, CPAP has been shown to improve oxygenation by increasing end-expiratory lung volume, therefore decreasing intrapulmonary shunting. CPAP has been shown to improve respiratory system compliance, which results in a decrease in the work of breathing and improved patient comfort. This technique is useful in maintaining upper airway patency in patients with obstructive sleep apnea (OSA), in whom it is widely used.

CPAP may also be useful in decreasing the work of breathing in some patients with severe COPD caused by emphysema. With severe emphysema, a loss of lung elastic recoil leads to premature airway collapse because of loss of external traction on the conducting airways. In these patients, CPAP acts as a pneumatic stent by maintaining patency in the conducting airways and diminishes the effort required to generate intrathoracic pressure and to initiate airflow. As a result, in selected patients, CPAP reduces the work of breathing.

CPAP improves cardiac output by decreasing left ventricular afterload.

CPAP has been shown to be useful in the management of patients with acute respiratory failure resulting from cardiogenic pulmonary edema.

CPAP has also been successfully used in patients with left ventricular failure. CPAP is believed to improve cardiac output by decreasing left ventricular afterload via its effect on intrathoracic pressure. In one randomized, controlled trial, CPAP improved several cardiac and pulmonary physiologic parameters in patients with acute hypercapnic-cardiogenic pulmonary edema and decreased the rate of endotracheal intubation. Recently, however, a large randomized, controlled trial failed to demonstrate a reduction in the need for intubation or an improvement in clinical outcome in a group of patients with acute hypoxemic, nonhypercapnic respiratory failure treated with CPAP (including patients with cardiogenic pulmonary edema) compared with a group treated with conventional therapy. This study, however, did not have enough power to determine the efficacy of CPAP in the subgroup of patients with cardiogenic pulmonary edema. Based on the evidence from prior randomized controlled trials, CPAP is still considered the initial noninvasive ventilatory modality to be used in patients presenting in cardiogenic pulmonary edema.

Acutely, CPAP should be started at 3–5 cmH_2O, within range of the normal transpulmonary pressure.

In the acute setting, CPAP should be initiated at 3–5 cmH_2O, within range of the normal transpulmonary pressure. The pressure may then be titrated upward in 2-cmH_2O increments every 3–5 min while assessing patient comfort, respiratory rate, accessory muscle use, and the level of oxygenation. The optimal CPAP level reported in pulmonary edema is about 10 cmH_2O. In the setting of severe emphysema, the goal is to set the CPAP level approximately 1–2 cmH_2O below the measurable "auto-PEEP" or intrinsic PEEP (positive end-expiratory pressure). In these cases, the usual level of CPAP required is usually 5–8 cmH_2O.

APPLICATION OF NONINVASIVE POSITIVE PRESSURE VENTILATION

Patient Selection

Noninvasive ventilation provides patient stability until the precipitating disorder causing respiratory failure can be appropriately treated.

In selecting which patients will most likely benefit from noninvasive ventilation, it is important to remember that this ventilatory modality is most effective when intermittent or partial ventilatory support is required. It is also important to remember that noninvasive ventilation should be viewed as a device to prevent intubation, not to replace it.

Negative pressure ventilation may be especially suited for patients who have no need for invasive monitoring or invasive procedures.

Negative pressure ventilation may be an alternative for patients with facial deformities such that a mask cannot be properly fitted.

The first decision that the clinician must make is whether to use negative pressure ventilation or noninvasive positive pressure ventilation (NPPV). Each mode has specific advantages and disadvantages (see Table 35-4). Negative pressure ventilation has been successfully used in patients with chronic respiratory failure caused by severe neuromuscular disease and in acute exacerbations of COPD. Negative pressure may be especially suited for patients with chronic respiratory failure or acute on chronic respiratory failure that have no need for invasive monitoring or invasive procedures, such as central venous pressure measurement, pulmonary artery catheter placement, or chest tube insertion (Figure 35-3). In addition, negative pressure ventilation may be an alternative in those patients with facial deformities and a patent upper airway in whom a face mask cannot be properly fitted.

Current criteria to select patients for NPPV are based on outcome indicators and previously published entry criteria from several clinical studies. A two-step approach has been recommended (Table 35-6). The first step is to identify those patients who are at risk of re-

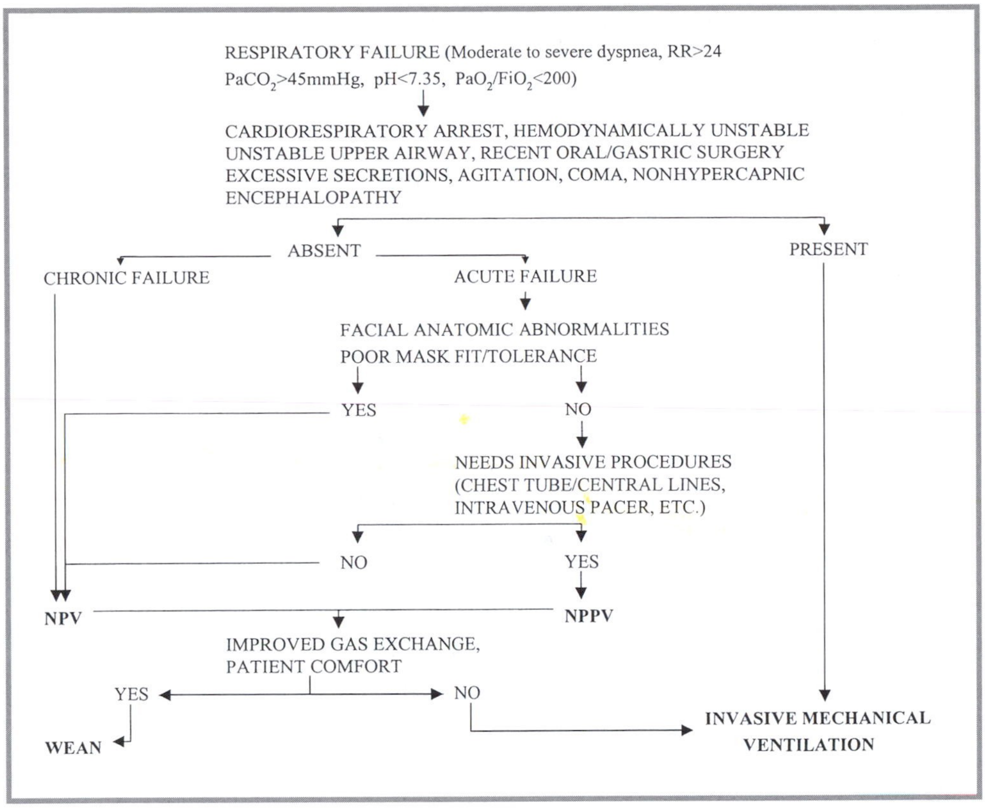

FIGURE 35-3

Selection of noninvasive ventilation in acute respiratory failure. NPV, negative pressure ventilation; NPPV (not NIPPV), noninvasive positive pressure ventilation.

quiring intubation and who are likely to benefit from ventilatory assistance. The criteria include clinical as well as gas exchange parameters. Clinical criteria include moderate to severe dyspnea, tachypnea, use of accessory muscles, and paradoxical abdominal breathing. A respiratory rate greater than 24 breaths/min is generally considered a relative indication for NPPV in patients with COPD, although higher respiratory rates have been used in hypox-

> The first step in selecting patients for NPPV is to establish which patients are at risk of requiring mechanical ventilation and who may benefit from ventilatory assistance.

TABLE 35-6

SELECTION GUIDELINES: NONINVASIVE MECHANICAL VENTILATION FOR PATIENTS WITH ACUTE RESPIRATORY FAILURE

Step 1. Identify patients in need of ventilatory assistance
- A. Symptoms and signs of acute respiratory distress
  - a. Moderate to severe dyspnea
  - b. RR $>$ 24
- B. Gas exchange abnormalities
  - a. $PaCO_2 > 45$ mmHg, pH < 7.35
  - b. $PaO_2/FiO_2 < 200$

Step 2. Exclude those at increased risk with noninvasive ventilation
- A. Respiratory/cardiac arrest
- B. Unstable clinical condition (shock, severe myocardial ischemia, life-threatening arrhythmias, status asthmaticus)
- C. Compromised upper airway (impaired cough or swallowing function, tracheal stenosis, upper airway tumors)
- D. Recent oral, esophageal, or gastric surgery
- E. Excessive secretions
- F. Agitated or uncooperative
- G. Facial trauma, burns, surgery, or anatomic abnormalities interfering with mask fit
- H. Tracheostomy in place
- I. Central nervous disorders unrelated to hypercapnic encephalopathy or hypoxemia (stroke, meningitis)

$PaCO_2$, partial pressure of arterial carbon dioxide; RR, respiratory rate; PaO_2/FiO_2, partial pressure of arterial oxygen to inspired oxygen fraction ratio

SOURCE: Modified from Mehta S, Hill N. Noninvasive ventilation. Am J Respir Crit Care 2001;163:540–577, with permission emic respiratory failure and acute pulmonary edema. The gas exchange criteria include an elevated $PaCO_2$ and worsening pH, and hypoxemia marked by a $PaO_2/FiO_2 < 200$.

Patients with imminent or actual cardiorespiratory arrest are not candidates for NPPV.

Shock, life-threatening arrhythmias, myocardial ischemia, and hemodynamic instability are contraindications to the use of NPPV.

After identifying patients who are likely to require ventilatory support, the second step consists of excluding patients in whom the use of NPPV would be considered unsafe. NPPV is not recommended in patients likely to experience imminent respiratory or cardiac arrest, and these patients should be promptly intubated. Patients with unstable conditions, such as shock, gastrointestinal bleeding, myocardial ischemia, or life-threatening arrhythmias should not be managed with NPPV. Facial trauma or facial deformities may prevent adequate fitting of a mask and are relative contraindications to the use of NPPV. The upper airway should be intact; patients with upper airway stenosis or tumors are unlikely to benefit from NPPV. Ideally, patients being considered for NPPV should be able to manage their secretions. Although it has been recommended that patients should be awake and cooperative, patients with CO_2 narcosis may benefit from NPPV. Although several studies have enrolled patients with various degrees of altered consciousness, most of these patients presented with hypercapnic encephalopathy. Patients with an altered mental status caused by conditions other than hypercapnic encephalopathy or hypoxemia (such as meningitis, subarachnoid hemorrhage, or stroke) should not receive NPPV.

Outcome Predictors

Patients with hypercapnic respiratory failure who undergo NPPV have a better prognosis than patients with hypoxemic respiratory failure.

An increase in pH and a decrease in $PaCO_2$ in the first 2 h are associated with a better outcome in NPPV.

NPPV should be promptly instituted, ideally before acidemia and hypercarbia ensue or worsen.

Several retrospective studies have found similar determinants of success, defined as avoidance of intubation, in patients receiving NPPV. Overall, hypercapnic patients appear to have better outcomes than hypercapnic patients with concomitant hypoxemia. COPD patients have a worse prognosis if they have an associated illness, especially pneumonia. Lower age, the presence of teeth (improving mask seal), and ability to coordinate breathing with the ventilator correlate with successful outcomes. Baseline levels of $PaCO_2$ and pH, as well as a decrease in $PaCO_2$, an increase in pH, and an improvement in mental status during the first 2 h of treatment with NPPV strongly correlate with success. This finding should prompt physicians to institute NPPV expeditiously before worsening acidemia and elevated levels of $PaCO_2$ occur.

Patient–Ventilator Interface

The term interface refers to the device that makes the connection between the ventilator and the patient possible. During invasive ventilation an endotracheal tube is used; in NPPV, different mask types are available; and during negative pressure ventilation, the device itself (tank, cuirass, or body suit) serves as the interface.

Negative Pressure Ventilation

Several different devices have specific advantages and disadvantages (Table 35-7). The prototypical negative pressure ventilator is the tank ventilator, also referred to as the "iron lung," a large cylindrical tank-like device with side portholes to provide nursing care and limited procedures. The patient's body is encased in the tank, but the head and neck protrude through an opening at one end. A neck collar provides an airtight seal (see Figure 35-1A).

The cuirass is a rigid shell made of fiberglass that is fitted to cover the chest wall and upper abdomen (see Figure 35-1C). A negative pressure pump generator is attached to the

TABLE 35-7

ADVANTAGES AND DISADVANTAGES OF DIFFERENT TYPES OF NEGATIVE PRESSURE VENTILATORS

TYPES	ADVANTAGES	DISADVANTAGES
Tank ventilator	Reliable, efficient	Bulky, heavy
Cuirass shell	Portable	Difficult fitting in patients with chest wall disease
Body suits	Portable, easy fitting	Back and chest wall discomfort

anterior portion of the cuirass. This device is more portable than the tank ventilator, but fitting is difficult in patients with chest wall deformities, unless it is customized. The generation of negative pressure and resulting minute ventilation are limited because of the smaller body surface that is directly in contact with this device.

Airtight body suits (e.g., "poncho wrap") use a rigid metal framework that surrounds the torso and is covered with an airtight nylon parka. The "poncho wrap" provides negative pressure over a larger body surface than the cuirass and is more portable than the tank ventilator. Backache is frequently a complication associated with the use of this device.

Noninvasive Positive Pressure Ventilation

Several different interfaces are currently available (Figure 35-4). Although designs vary greatly from manufacturer to manufacturer, four main types of masks are used to deliver NPPV: nasal prongs, and nasal, oral-nasal, or fullface masks. To optimize fit and comfort, the type of mask used should be based on the patient's facial features. The masks are secured by an elastic headgear system.

A recent study suggested that nasal masks improve patient comfort and decrease the incidence of claustrophobia, whereas nasal prongs and nasal-oral masks improve gas exchange parameters more quickly. Previous studies failed to detect significant differences in physiologic parameters between different devices. Each type of mask has advantages and disadvantages, but proper fit is crucial in minimizing air leaks and maximizing NPPV efficacy. It is recommended that several mask types and sizes should be evaluated when initiating NPPV to choose the optimal interface to the individual patient.

A proper mask fit is essential in maximizing the efficacy of NPPV.

If a nasal mask is chosen, a chinstrap may help in decreasing mouth air leaks. Air leak around the mouth is not only uncomfortable for the patients but may result in inefficient triggering and/or a prolonged inspiratory time, ultimately leading to patient–ventilator asynchrony or ineffective ventilation. Masks that fail to fit properly are also more likely to cause facial skin breakdown and nasal bridge skin ulcers. A new mask that covers the entire face (see Figure 35-4C) has recently been shown to increase comfort and significantly increase expired tidal volume, decrease $PaCO_2$, and decrease air leaks when compared with nasal and nasal-oral masks.

A chinstrap is useful in reducing mouth air leaks in patients ventilated through a nasal mask.

Monitoring Efficacy

Patients with acute respiratory failure or an acute exacerbation superimposed on chronic respiratory failure who undergo NPPV should be carefully monitored, ideally in the ICU or a similarly equipped unit. Monitoring is essential to optimize the patient's comfort and tolerance of NPPV, as well as facilitate improvements in subjective, physiologic and gas exchange parameters.

Monitoring is essential to optimize patient comfort and tolerance of NPPV.

Subjective Parameters

NPPV relieves symptoms of respiratory distress. It is therefore important to establish that the patient is comfortable by periodical clinical examination and direct questioning. Because the success of NPPV is directly related to the patient's ability to tolerate it, an effort must be made to make the patient comfortable by adjusting the mask and positioning the patient.

Physiologic Parameters

Reduction in respiratory rate and use of accessory muscles of respiration, coupled with an improvement in thoracoabdominal synchronous excursions, signal a favorable response to NPPV. An improvement in these parameters in the first 2 h portends a good prognosis. Exhaled tidal volumes are difficult to interpret because of the presence of air leaks. Most of the bilevel portable ventilators measure tidal volume by integrating the flow signal. These ventilators report the inspiratory volume accurately, but only estimate exhaled tidal volume. Blood pressure monitoring is important, especially in volume-depleted patients who may

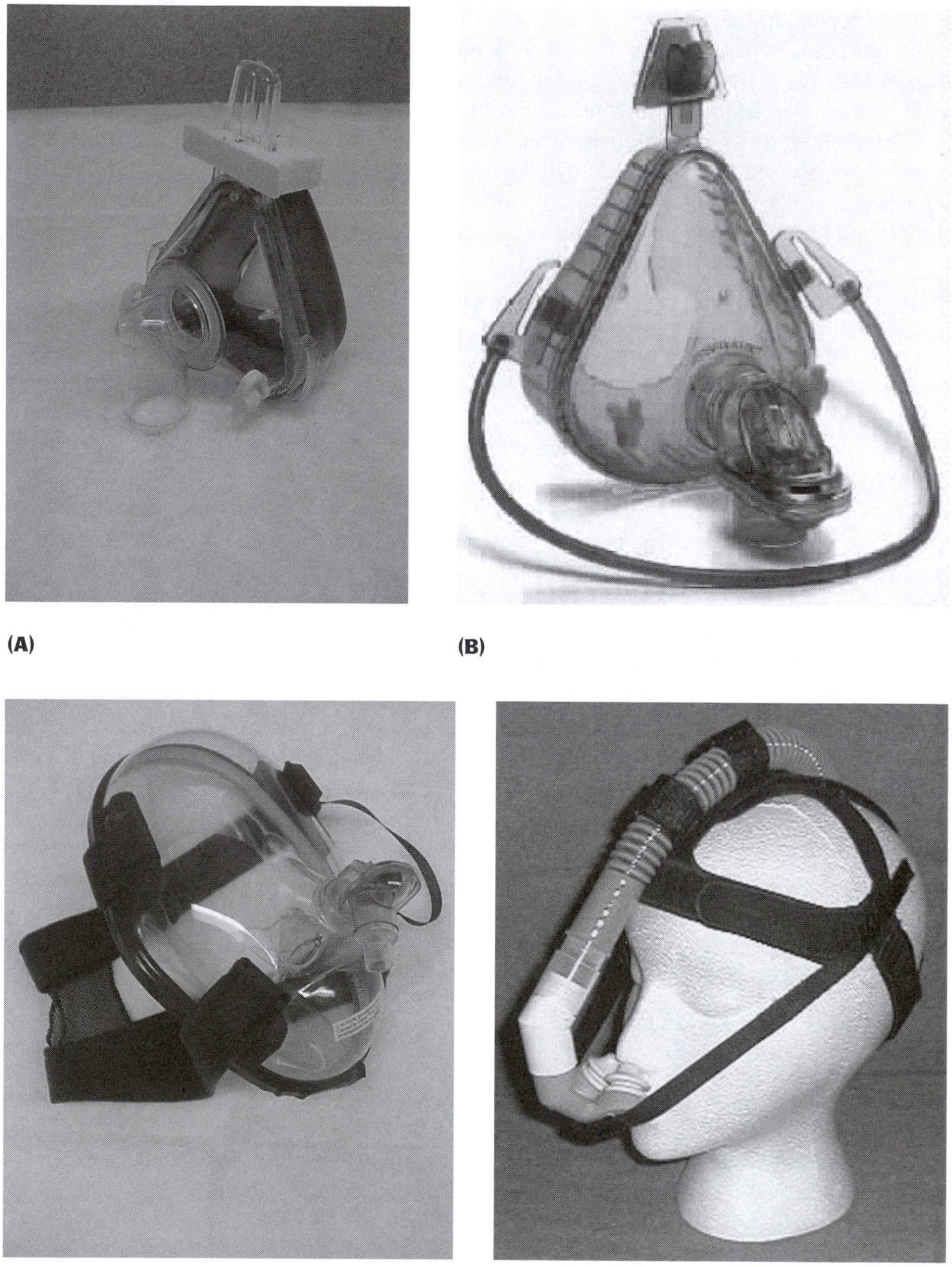

(A) (B) (C) (D)

FIGURE 35-4

Noninvasive positive pressure masks. **(A)** A nasal mask. **(B)** A nasal-oral mask. **(C)** This fencing mask may increase patient's comfort. **(D)** Nasal prongs, also known as an Adams circuit.

have a further decrease in cardiac output if NPPV reduces preload. Continuous ECG monitoring should be available. Additional parameters (i.e., FEV_1, PEFR) may need to be monitored in specific entities.

Gas Exchange Parameters

Gas exchange is monitored using continuous pulse oximetry and arterial blood gas determinations.

In the acute setting, gas exchange is monitored using continuous pulse oximetry and arterial blood gas determinations. Arterial blood gas determinations should be performed at baseline and once patients are stabilized. An initial determination should be performed 2–4 h after initiating noninvasive ventilation; thereafter, arterial blood gas sampling should be based on clinical need. Arterial blood gas determinations are useful in assessing the efficacy of a

TABLE 35-8

CLINICAL SCENARIOS WHERE NONINVASIVE POSITIVE PRESSURE VENTILATION MAY BE USEFUL

Acute respiratory failure	Postoperative respiratory failure
Cardiogenic pulmonary edema	Obesity hypoventilation syndrome
Community-acquired pneumonia	Facilitate weaning
Acute respiratory distress syndrome	COPD
Acute on chronic respiratory failure	Neuromuscular diseases
COPD	Bridge to lung transplantation
Asthma	Cystic fibrosis
Neuromuscular diseases	COPD
Chest wall diseases	

COPD, chronic obstructive pulmonary disease

particular ventilatory mode. A decrease in $PaCO_2$, an increase in PaO_2, and an increase in pH are considered markers of successful outcome. These parameters can also be used to titrate ventilator settings in specific conditions.

Arterial blood gas determinations are useful in assessing the efficacy of a particular ventilatory mode.

APPLICATION IN SPECIFIC DISEASE GROUPS

Noninvasive ventilation has been successfully applied in a wide variety of clinical scenarios (Table 35-8). The level of supportive evidence varies among different disease entities (Table 35-9). Although noninvasive ventilation is currently used in the management of both chronic and acute respiratory disorders, we would like to focus on those indications that pertain to the acute setting.

Chronic Respiratory Failure

Negative pressure ventilation and NPPV have been successfully used in patients with chronic respiratory failure; applications include thoracic cage abnormalities (e.g., chest wall deformities, kyphoscoliosis, postpolio syndrome) in addition to both rapidly and slowly progressive neuromuscular conditions (e.g., amyotrophic lateral sclerosis and a variety of myopathic/neuropathic diseases).

NPPV has become one of the cornerstones in the treatment of obstructive sleep apnea. The occurrence of upper airway obstruction during negative pressure ventilation precludes its use in patients with obstructive sleep apnea.

TABLE 35-9

USE OF NONINVASIVE POSITIVE PRESSURE VENTILATION (NPPV) IN SPECIFIC DISEASES AND THE TYPE OF SUPPORTIVE EVIDENCE

DISEASES	EFFECTIVENESS OF NPPV DURING ARF	LEVEL OF EVIDENCE
Neuromuscular and chest wall diseases	Effective	Nonrandomized, concurrent-cohort comparisons
COPD	Effective to avoid endotracheal intubation; may decrease mortality and hospital length of stay	Randomized, controlled trials
Asthma	May prevent endotracheal intubation	Nonrandomized, concurrent-cohort comparisons
Acute hypoxemic respiratory failure	Possibly effective	Randomized, controlled trials
Cardiogenic pulmonary edema	Effective	Randomized, controlled trials

COPD, chronic obstructive pulmonary disease; ARF, acute respiratory failure

Acute Respiratory Failure

Chronic Obstructive Pulmonary Disease

Negative pressure ventilation and NPPV have been used in the management of acute COPD exacerbations. In several European trials, negative pressure ventilation has been shown to decrease the duration of ventilation and the incidence of infectious complications in patients with acute COPD exacerbation. Negative pressure ventilation for acute COPD exacerbations is infrequently used in the United States where NPPV is the preferred ventilatory mode for this condition.

The largest body of evidence regarding the efficacy of NPPV in the acute setting comes from clinical studies evaluating its application in acute exacerbations of COPD. In uncontrolled trials, the success rate in avoiding intubation in acute COPD exacerbation ranges from 60% to 90%. Five randomized, controlled trials showed improvements in gas exchange and in dyspnea scores and a significant reduction in the need for intubation. Moreover, two studies showed a decrement in mortality and ICU length of stay when patients received NPPV in addition to conventional therapy for COPD in comparison to those treated with conventional therapy alone.

In 1995, a multicenter European trial randomized 85 COPD patients to receive NPPV via facial mask versus conventional therapy. The authors noted a significant decrement in the need for intubation (74% in control patients versus 26% in the NPPV group), decreased mortality (29% versus 9%), and a reduction in complications (48% versus 16%), and hospital length of stay. A recent meta-analysis concluded that the evidence from randomized controlled trial supports the use of NPPV in acute exacerbations of COPD. Although patients with severe COPD exacerbations have been shown to benefit from NPPV, this does not appear to be applicable to patients with mild to moderate exacerbations. It is important to establish that these studies used NPPV to prevent, not to substitute for, endotracheal intubation.

Patients with severe COPD exacerbation are more likely to benefit from NPPV than those with mild or moderate exacerbations.

Acute Hypoxemic Respiratory Failure

There is currently no evidence to support the use of negative pressure ventilation in patients with acute hypoxemic respiratory failure. Clinical studies evaluating the efficacy of NPPV in acute hypoxemic respiratory failure have yielded conflicting results. In an uncontrolled study, 41 patients with hypoxemic respiratory failure from a variety of causes (acute pulmonary edema, pneumonia, acute respiratory distress syndrome [ARDS]), and average initial PaO_2/FiO_2 ratios of 110 mmHg received NPPV. Despite the severity of their initial hypoxemia, only 34% of patients required intubation. In a recent randomized controlled trial, 64 patients with acute hypoxemic respiratory failure were randomized to receive NPPV or intubation. In this study, only 31% of the patients randomized to receive NPPV required intubation. In addition, this group had a lower incidence of pneumonia and sinusitis. The NPPV group had a nonsignificant trend toward decreased mortality and ICU length of stay. Other investigators have shown similar results when using NPPV in patients with hypoxemic respiratory failure resulting from postoperative solid organ transplant and ARDS.

In contrast to these favorable results, a recent report of a controlled trial of NPPV initiated in the emergency department for the treatment of a variety of disorders presenting with acute respiratory failure found no difference in the rate of intubation between patients randomized to receive NPPV or standard therapy. There was also a trend toward increased mortality in the NPPV group. This study, however, had several important limitations. It enrolled a total of 26 patients, 16 of which were randomized to receive NPPV. The distribution of patients was unequal, favoring the control group that had lower severity of illness scores. The time between admission to the emergency department and intubation was significantly increased in the NPPV group, suggesting the possibility that outcomes were related to delayed intubation and not necessarily to the ventilatory modality employed. Although there appears to be enough evidence to support the use of NPPV in hypoxemic respiratory failure, results may depend on its implementation by personnel with greater expertise. More studies are needed to further define which subgroups are more likely to benefit from this treatment modality.

Cardiogenic Pulmonary Edema

As described earlier, NPPV is best applied in conditions in which the underlying cause of respiratory failure can be reversed in 24–48 h. In acute cardiogenic pulmonary edema, NPPV provides partial ventilatory support, thereby improving gas exchange and relieving dyspnea. Additionally, NPPV unloads the respiratory muscles and prevents or delays the onset of respiratory muscle fatigue. Both CPAP and NPPV have been shown to decrease the work of breathing and intubation rates in patients suffering from cardiogenic pulmonary edema.

CPAP and NPPV have been shown to decrease the work of breathing and intubation rates in patients with acute cardiogenic pulmonary edema.

In a large controlled study by Lin and colleagues, 100 patients with acute pulmonary edema were randomized to receive CPAP and oxygen versus oxygen alone. Patients were monitored with an indwelling pulmonary artery catheter. CPAP was started at 2.5 cmH_2O and titrated up to 12.5 cmH_2O to achieve a PaO_2 greater than 80 mmHg. The CPAP group demonstrated an improvement in PaO_2 with a concomitant reduction in intrapulmonary shunt fraction and the alveolar–arterial tension gradient. The CPAP group also showed a higher cardiac stroke volume. The incidence of tracheal intubation was lower in the CPAP (8 of 50 patients) compared to the control group (18 of 50 patients). The improvement in cardiovascular function during CPAP was speculated to be caused by a reduction in left ventricular afterload.

NPPV has also been used in the treatment of cardiogenic pulmonary edema. A single randomized controlled trial in cardiogenic pulmonary edema patients compared NPPV to CPAP and showed NPPV produced a significant decrement in respiratory rate, $PaCO_2$, and dyspnea score when compared to CPAP at 30 min. Both modalities showed a similar incidence of endotracheal intubation, but the NPPV group had a higher incidence of myocardial infarction (71% versus 31%). This disparity in the incidence of myocardial infarction could be partially explained by a trend toward enrolling more patients with chest pain in the NPPV group. The difference in myocardial infarction incidence may therefore reflect baseline characteristics and not the ventilatory modality. At the present time, CPAP is recommended as the initial ventilatory mode to be used in patients with acute cardiogenic pulmonary edema unless patients present with significant hypercapnia.

CPAP is recommended as the initial ventilatory mode to be used in patients with acute respiratory failure due to cardiogenic pulmonary edema.

Immunocompromised Patients

Immunocompromised patients, regardless of the etiology of their immune disorder, are at a high risk of developing complications such as ventilator-associated pneumonia and alveolar hemorrhage during invasive mechanical ventilation. Thus, significant interest has been generated in treating these patients with NPPV to avoid endotracheal intubation. In an initial study, Meduri and colleagues reported 70% success in avoiding intubation in 11 patients with AIDS and *Pneumocystis carinii* pneumonia. In a controlled trial by Antonelli and colleagues, 40 patients with acute respiratory failure of various etiologies after solid organ lung transplant were randomized to receive NPPV or standard therapy. The NPPV group showed a significant decrease in the need for intubation and ICU mortality.

Immunosuppressed patients, regardless of the etiology of immunosuppression, are at high risk of developing complications during invasive mechanical ventilation.

More recently, Hilbert and colleagues (2001) conducted a controlled trial and randomized patients with fever, pulmonary infiltrates, and respiratory failure to receive NPPV or conventional therapy. Patients had different etiologies for immunosuppression (bone marrow transplant, solid organ transplant, AIDS). The group of patients randomized to receive NPPV had a decreased rate of endotracheal intubation and serious complications and had an increased likelihood of survival to hospital discharge. Thus, it appears that NPPV can be used as first-line therapy in selected immunocompromised patients, so long as patients are carefully monitored and promptly intubated if needed.

Postoperative Patients

Several studies have considered the use of NPPV in the perioperative setting. In a study by Pennock and colleagues, NPPV avoided intubation in more than 70% of patients that developed respiratory deterioration within 36 h of surgery. Other authors have found similar results after cardiac surgery, coronary artery bypass, and pneumonectomy. NPPV appears to improve gas exchange and decrease the need for reintubation in postsurgical patients, but most of these studies have involved few patients.

EXPANDED INDICATIONS FOR NONINVASIVE VENTILATION

Weaning from Mechanical Ventilation

Because weaning has been successfully used in providing ventilatory assistance to several groups of patients with acute and acute on chronic respiratory failure, its use has been expanded to provide ventilatory assistance to patients who fail extubation. Udwadia and colleagues were the first to report the usefulness of NPPV in facilitating the weaning process. The causes for respiratory failure included neuromuscular disease, primary lung disease (i.e., COPD), or postoperative respiratory failure following cardiac surgery. Patients were placed on NPPV once they met the following criteria: intact upper airway function, minimal airway secretions, low oxygen requirement, hemodynamic stability, ability to sustain spontaneous ventilation for 10–15 min, and functional gastrointestinal tract. NPPV was initially used for 16–20 h/day and was gradually decreased. In this study, 18 of 22 patients were successfully converted to NPPV and discharged home in a mean of 11 days. The results of this study have to be carefully interpreted, because the majority of these patients had acute on chronic respiratory failure, a significant percentage were discharged with nocturnal noninvasive ventilation, and all the patients had a tracheostomy in place, which made resuming invasive ventilatory support relatively easy.

In a study by Nava and colleagues, 40 patients with severe COPD who required mechanical ventilation and failed a T-piece trial 48 h post intubation were randomized to extubation and application of NPPV or weaning by pressure support via endotracheal tube. At 60 days follow-up, 22 of 25 patients were successfully weaned in the NPPV group compared to 17 of 25 patients in the invasive ventilation group. Patients in the NPPV group had shorter duration of mechanical ventilation, shorter ICU stay, and improved mortality at the time of discharge. None of the patients receiving NPPV developed pneumonia, compared to 7 of 25 patients in the invasive mechanical ventilation arm of the study. Girault and colleagues randomized 33 patients with acute on chronic respiratory failure to conventional pressure support weans or extubation and NPPV after they failed a 2-h T-piece trial. The NPPV group had a shorter course of mechanical ventilation and a trend toward fewer complications, but mortality, hospital length of stay, and ICU length of stay were similar among groups.

NPPV may reduce the incidence of reintubation, mechanical ventilation, and its associated complications in patients who fail a T-piece weaning trial.

NPPV appears to facilitate the weaning process in patients with acute on chronic respiratory failure, particularly in those with COPD.

The results of these trials indicate that there may be a role for NPPV in patients who fail a T-piece wean in reducing mechanical ventilation duration and its associated complications. It is important to notice that these trials enrolled patients with chronic or acute on chronic respiratory failure (Table 35-10), and that, in some cases, noninvasive ventilation was continued beyond the hospital admission. The results are therefore more likely to be applicable in patients with acute exacerbations of chronic respiratory failure, especially in those with COPD. Whether these results can be extrapolated to other patient populations is unclear at this time, and further studies are needed.

Noninvasive Ventilation in Supporting the Terminally Ill

The use of NPPV has been reported in several studies in patients who are not to be intubated but are found to have a reversible cause of respiratory failure. Benhamou and colleagues studied 30 elderly COPD patients (mean age, 76 years) for whom intubation was contraindicated or had been refused by the patients in accordance with their advance directives. Despite the severity of respiratory failure (mean $PaO_2 < 45$ mmHg), successful avoidance of intubation was reported in 60% of patients. Another study reported similar results in 26 patients with acute hypoxemic and/or hypercapnic respiratory failure who refused in-

TABLE 35-10

COMPARISON AMONG STUDIES USING NONINVASIVE POSITIVE PRESSURE VENTILATION (NPPV) FOR WEANING FROM INVASIVE MECHANICAL VENTILATION

AUTHOR	*n*	DISEASES	IPPV (DAYS)	NPPV (DAYS)	OUTCOME
Udwadia	22	CWD (9) NMD (6) Cardiac (7)	2–219	8–13	82% weaned 63% used chronic NPPV
Restrick	14	COPD (8) CWD (4)	1–229	2–60	93% weaned 21% used chronic NPPV 1 patient died
Hilbert	30	COPD	12 ± 4	5 ± 2	Compared with historical controls: ↓ Reintubation by 47% ↓ ICU LOS by 42% ↓ Duration mechanical ventilation by 54%

IPPV, invasive positive pressure ventilation; NPPV, noninvasive positive pressure ventilation; CWD, chest wall disorders; NMD, neuromuscular disorders; COPD, chronic obstructive pulmonary disease; ICU, intensive care unit; LOS, length of stay

tubation. In a retrospective analysis of mechanical ventilation in elderly patients, Benhemou concluded that NPPV offered several advantages over endotracheal intubation, such as better short-term prognosis, decreased incidence of complications, and improved gas exchange and patient comfort. These studies enrolled small numbers of patients, were based on retrospective analysis, and generally lacked adequate controls; the conclusions that can be drawn from them are therefore limited.

Regardless of the ventilatory mode used, long term-prognosis remains poor for these patients. Moreover, the use of NPPV in patients with advanced-stage diseases who refuse intubation remains controversial. Although these patients may benefit from the treatment of potentially reversible causes of respiratory failure, while retaining the ability to communicate and maintain oral intake, most authors believe that NPPV should not be used to prolong an inevitable course towards death.

COMPLICATIONS

Upper airway obstruction is a well-recognized complication of negative pressure ventilation, particularly in patients with neuromuscular disease. Although obstructive sleep apnea is not a common occurrence, the presence of nocturnal desaturation due to obstructive episodes should prompt the physician to consider the addition of CPAP or switching the patient to NPPV. Back pain, neck pain, and claustrophobia have also been reported to occur in patients receiving negative pressure ventilation. Negative pressure ventilation has also been reported to decrease lower esophageal sphincter tone in both normal and COPD patients. This problem may lead to regurgitation of gastric contents and an increased risk of aspiration; however, this condition generally responds well to agents that enhance gastric motility, such as metoclopramide. Patients with a history of gastroesophageal reflux disease and those with a prior history of gastric aspiration should be placed on promotility agents before implementing negative pressure ventilation.

The most frequently encountered complications of CPAP/NPPV are minor in magnitude and are generally related to intolerance of the mask or the degree of applied pressure. Major complications are infrequently seen (Table 35-11). A large proportion of the reported complications are related to mask pressure and include nasal pain (mucosa and over the bridge of the nose), and nasal bridge erythema and/or ulceration; these can be managed by minimizing strap tension, alternating different types of masks, applying artificial skin to the bridge of the nose, or selecting an alternate device. Common adverse effects related to airflow or applied pressures include conjunctival irritation and ear and sinus pain. Refitting the mask and decreasing pressure can treat these problems. Nasal dryness is a common complaint, but

Complications associated with mask pressure include nasal pain and nasal bridge skin ulceration.

TABLE 35-11

COMPLICATIONS OF NONINVASIVE VENTILATION

Negative pressure ventilation	Nasal bridge skin ulceration
Neck pain	Conjunctival irritation
Back pain	Ear pain
Claustrophobia	Sinus pain
Upper airway obstruction	Nasal passage dryness
Gastrointestinal reflux	Nasal congestion
Gastric content aspiration	Gastric distension
Noninvasive positive pressure ventilation	Major complications
Minor complications	Hypotension
Nasal pain	Aspiration
Nasal bridge skin erythema	Pneumothorax

so are increased nasal discharge and congestion. The former may improve by decreasing leak around the mouth and using emollients; the latter may benefit from intranasal decongestants or inhaled steroids. Gastric distension may also occur, but it is rarely reported with peak pressures less than 20 cmH_2O. Distension may respond to simethicone or providing NPPV with the patient lying on the left side, which decreases gastric compliance and thereby limits the development of gastric distension.

> Major complications of NPPV, such as pneumothorax and hypotension, are infrequent.

Major complications, which seldom occur, include aspiration, hypotension, and pneumothorax. Carefully selecting which patients should receive NPPV and maintaining at least a 30° head elevation further minimize aspiration risks. The reported incidence of pneumothorax and hypotension is less than 5%.

SUMMARY

Several options are currently available to deliver noninvasive ventilation. The choice between negative pressure ventilation and NPPV should be made based on physician and supporting staff expertise, equipment availability, patient comfort, and individual patient conditions. Negative pressure ventilation is an alternative mode of noninvasive ventilation in patients with chronic neuromuscular and chest wall diseases. It also appears to be useful in patients with acute exacerbations of chronic respiratory conditions, including COPD. In patients who require partial ventilator assistance, NPPV has been shown to improve patient comfort and decrease intubation rate and hospital length of stay. Careful attention must be paid to patient selection, proper fitting of interface devices, and adequate monitoring to increase success and the patient's tolerance of NPPV.

REVIEW QUESTIONS

1. **A 78-year-old woman presents to the emergency in respiratory distress; her respiratory rate is 36, and she is using accessory muscles. She has a long-standing history of COPD and emphysema. Her daughter, who lives with her, states that her mother's mental status has worsened over the past 2 h, and that she is less alert than usual. On her arrival to the emergency department, she develops ventricular tachycardia, and her blood pressure is measured at 60/- mmHg. The most important reason to avoid noninvasive ventilation in this patient is:**
   - **A.** Age greater than 65
   - **B.** Use of accessory muscles
   - **C.** Respiratory rate greater than 35 breaths/min
   - **D.** Change in mental status
   - **E.** Lethal arrhythmia and hemodynamic instability

2. **CPAP is thought to be useful in cardiogenic pulmonary edema because:**
   - **A.** It increases preload.
   - **B.** It increases afterload.
   - **C.** It decreases end-expiratory lung volume.
   - **D.** It decreases afterload.

3. **Complications of negative pressure ventilation include all the following, except:**
   - **A.** Upper airway obstruction
   - **B.** Claustrophobia
   - **C.** Gastric distention
   - **D.** Back pain
   - **E.** Neck pain and discomfort

4. **All the following statements regarding patient–ventilator interfaces are correct, except:**
   - **A.** Nasal masks are more likely to be associated with air leaks.
   - **B.** The use of a chinstrap may decrease air leaks in patients ventilated with nasal masks.
   - **C.** Nasal-oral masks are less effective than nasal masks in improving gas exchange.
   - **D.** Appropriate mask fitting is one of the most important steps determining successful noninvasive positive pressure ventilation.

5. **The greatest amount of evidence for NPPV's efficacy in preventing intubation has been shown in which group with acute respiratory failure?**
   - **A.** Hypercapnic patients with COPD
   - **B.** Hypoxemic patients with ARDS
   - **C.** Status asthmaticus
   - **D.** Cardiogenic pulmonary edema

ANSWERS

1. The answer is E. When considering the use of NPPV, a two-step approach has been suggested. The first step consists of determining which patients are likely to require future intubation based on respiratory signs, symptoms, and gas exchange parameters. In this case the respiratory rate and the increased use of accessory muscles are signs consistent with respiratory distress, which would make this patient a candidate for noninvasive ventilation. The second step involves determining in which patients it would be unsafe to use NPPV. In this case, the patient develops a potentially serious arrhythmia and hemodynamic instability (low blood pressure); this, along with other reasons to intubate emergently, are contraindications to the use of NPPV. The change in mental status is likely to be secondary to hypercapnic encephalopathy and is not a contraindication to NPPV. Age should not preclude the use of noninvasive ventilation.
2. The answer is D. CPAP has been shown to decrease afterload and increase stroke volume. In animal models, it has been also shown to cause increased sympathoadrenal stimulation.
3. The answer is C. Gastric distension is a relatively frequent complication in patients undergoing noninvasive positive pressure ventilation via facial mask. Back pain, neck pain, and claustrophobia have been reported in patients on negative pressure ventilation. Upper airway obstruction is a consequence of the effect of negative pressure on the pharyngeal tissue and may sometimes result in nocturnal hypoxemia in patients undergoing negative ventilation.
4. The answer is C. Most studies have shown that nasal and nasal-oral masks are equivalent in improving gas exchange. Factors such as patient comfort and proper fit are more important in determining successful NPPV. A chinstrap may be helpful in patients ventilated with a nasal mask who have persistent air leak through the mouth.
5. The answer is A. The greatest body of evidence for NPPV's efficacy in preventing intubation has been shown in patients with hypercapnic respiratory failure and COPD. The evidence is less compelling for patients with acute hypoxemic respiratory failure from other causes. There are no randomized, controlled studies suggesting that patients with status asthmaticus benefit from NPPV. Although NPPV has been used in cardiogenic pulmonary edema, the largest trial available showed an increased incidence of myocardial infarction in patients undergoing NPPV when compared to similar patients treated with CPAP. Although this trial may have introduced an imbalanced sample of patients, CPAP remains first-line treatment for cardiogenic pulmonary edema, unless patients present with hypercarbia.

SUGGESTED READING

Cordova F, Criner GJ. Using NPPV to manage respiratory failure. J Respir Dis 2000;21:342–348.

Cordova F, Criner GJ. Negative pressure ventilation, who, when, how? Clini Pulm Med 2001;8:33–41.

Evans WE, Albert RK, Angus CA, et al. International Conferences in Intensive Care Medicine: Noninvasive positive pressure ventilation in acute respiratory failure. Am J Respir Crit Care Med 2001;163:283–291.

Girault C, Daudenthun I, Chevron V, et al. Noninvasive ventilation as a systematic extubation and weaning technique in acute-on chronic respiratory failure, A prospective, randomized, controlled trial. Am J Respir Crit Care Med 1999;160:86–92.

Hilbert G, Gruson D, Portel L, et al. Noninvasive pressure support ventilation in COPD patients with postextubation hypercapnic respiratory insufficiency. Eur Respir J 1998;11:1349–1353.

Nava S, Ambrosino N, Clini E, et al. Noninvasive mechanical ventilation in the weaning of patients with respiratory failure due to chronic obstructive pulmonary disease, A randomized, controlled trial. Ann Intern Med 1998;128:721–728.

Mehta S, Hill N. Noninvasive ventilation. Am J Respir Crit Care Med 2001;163:540–577.

Lin M, Yang Y, Chiany H, et al. Reappraisal of continuous positive airway pressure therapy in acute cardiogenic pulmonary edema: short-term results and long-term follow-up. Chest 107:1379–1386.

Meduri GU, Turner RE, Abou-Shala N, et al. Noninvasive positive pressure ventilation via face mask. Chest 1996;109:179–193.

Hilbert G, Gruson D, Vargas F, et al. Noninvasive ventilation in immunosuppressed patients with pulmonary infiltrates, fever, and acute respiratory failure. N Eng J Med 2001;344:481–487.

Pennock BE, Kaplan PD, Carlin BW, et al. Pressure support ventilation with a simplified ventilatory support system administered with a nasal mask in patients with respiratory failure. Chest 1991; 100:1371–1376.

Udwadia ZF, Santis GK, Stevan MH, et al. Nasal ventilation to facilitate weaning in patients with chronic respiratory insufficiency. Thorax 1992;47:715–718.

Benhamou D, Girault C, Faure C, et al. Nasal mask ventilation in acute respiratory failure: experience in elderly patients. Chest 1992;102: 912–917.

Restrick LJ, Scott AD, Ward EM, et al. Nasal intermittent positive pressure ventilation in weaning intubated patients with chronic respiratory disease from assisted intermittent positive pressure ventilation. Respir Med 1993;87:199–204.

CHAPTER 36

UBALDO J. MARTIN AND GERARD J. CRINER

Weaning from Mechanical Ventilation

CHAPTER OUTLINE

LEARNING OBJECTIVES

After studying this chapter, you should be able to:

- Determine when a patient is ready to begin the weaning process, based on clinical history, physical examination, and routine laboratory data.
- Use bedside weaning parameters to predict weaning outcome.
- Postulate a differential diagnosis of common and uncommon causes of weaning failure.
- Understand the advantages and disadvantages of the various weaning techniques.

During the past 25 years, there has been a significant increase in the number of patients that receive mechanical ventilation as a means of life support during surgery or life-threatening medical illness. Although mechanical ventilation has clear-cut benefits, it is also associated with a significant number of complications, such as decreased cardiac output, increased intracranial pressure, ventilator-associated pneumonia (VAP), and ventilator-induced lung injury (VILI). In addition, mechanical ventilation is expensive and hinders efficient patient movement through the intensive care unit.

Weaning patients from mechanical ventilation remains one of the most challenging aspects of intensive care. Despite the advent of new and promising weaning indexes, the skills to determine which patients should be weaned and when patients are ready for weaning remain a mix of art and science. These skills appear to be greatly enhanced by experience. About 20%–25% of ventilated patients fail an initial attempt at discontinuing mechanical ventilation and will require more concentrated and prolonged attempts for discontinuance (i.e., weaning). For patients requiring prolonged mechanical ventilation, about 40% of the time spent on the ventilator is devoted to the weaning process. This percentage is even higher in patients with specific diseases such as chronic obstructive pulmonary disease (COPD), who may be undergoing active weaning attempts during as much as 60% of their time on mechanical ventilation.

In this chapter, we review clinical parameters for determining which patients are ready to begin the weaning process, the interpretation of bedside parameters in predicting weaning outcome, and the merits and disadvantages of specific weaning techniques in successfully discontinuing mechanical ventilation.

DETERMINING THE CAUSE OF RESPIRATORY FAILURE

Before withdrawing mechanical ventilation, the cause of respiratory failure must be identified.

Before mechanical ventilation can be safely withdrawn, the abnormality causing respiratory failure must be identified and show favorable signs of response to treatment. To identify the physiologic causes of respiratory failure, it is useful to separate the causes into three major categories: (1) hypoxemic respiratory failure, (2) ventilatory pump failure, and (3) psychologic factors (Table 36-1).

Hypoxemic respiratory failure can result from hypoventilation, impaired pulmonary gas exchange, or decreased mixed venous blood oxygen content. The chest radiograph, physical examination, and alveolar-arterial oxygen gradient are useful in distinguishing among intrapulmonary shunting, increased physiologic deadspace, and alveolar hypoventilation as possible causes of hypoxemic respiratory failure (see Chapter 13).

Respiratory pump dysfunction is considered the most common cause of failure to wean.

Respiratory pump dysfunction is considered by some authors to be the most common cause of failure to wean from mechanical ventilation. Failure of the respiratory system as a pump may occur whenever respiratory demand exceeds ventilatory pump capacity. Respiratory pump failure may occur because of an increased ventilatory load (even in patients with normal respiratory pump), resulting from increased deadspace, hypermetabolism due to sepsis and/or fever, increased CO_2 production due to increased carbohydrate load, or inappropriately elevated central respiratory drive. In contrast, normal or only slightly elevated ventilatory loads may not be sustained by subjects with decreased respiratory pump capacity due to impaired central respiratory drive, phrenic nerve dysfunction, or severe derangements of respiratory muscle function (i.e., underlying neuromuscular disease, electrolyte disturbances).

Abnormalities of central respiratory drive can be seen in patients with structural injury to the central nervous system, overuse of sedative agents, and metabolic alkalosis. Diaphragm dysfunction can be seen in patients with cold-induced phrenic nerve injury or direct diaphragm injury that may occur during cardiothoracic surgery. Diaphragm dysfunction has also been reported in patients following upper abdominal surgery. Impaired respiratory muscle function can also result from various underlying medical conditions.

TABLE 36-1

CAUSES OF RESPIRATORY FAILURE

- Hypoxemic respiratory failure
  - Hypoventilation
  - Impaired pulmonary gas exchange (shunt, V/Q mismatch)
  - Decreased mixed venous oxygen content
- Inadequate respiratory center output
  - Drug overdose
  - Central nervous lesions or damage (brainstem infarction, encephalopathy)
  - Severe metabolic alkalosis
- Increased respiratory workload
  - Increased minute ventilation
  - Hyperventilation
  - Increased metabolic rate (sepsis, fever, hyperthermia)
  - Increased deadspace
  - Increased elastic workload (decreased lung and/or chest wall compliance, dynamic hyperinflation)
  - Increased resistive workload (airway obstruction, secretions, endotracheal tube, ventilator circuit)
  - Postextubation upper airway obstruction
- Respiratory pump failure
  - Thoracic wall abnormalities (flail chest, rib fractures)
  - Peripheral neurologic disorder (unilateral or bilateral phrenic nerve damage, critical care illness polyneuropathy)
  - Muscular dysfunction (neuromuscular blocking agent-associated weakness/myopathy)
  - Pulmonary hyperinflation
- Left ventricular failure
  - Left ventricular dysfunction (congestive heart failure)
  - Ischemia

Hyperinflation is one of the most common conditions and is frequently overlooked. Hyperinflation occurs in patients with acute exacerbation of severe asthma or COPD. Hyperinflation causes a shortening in the diaphragm precontraction length, which causes the diaphragm to work at a disadvantageous portion of its tension–length curve. Hyperinflation also alters the orientation of the diaphragmatic fibers medially inward and decreases the length of the zone of apposition, factors that further decrease the diaphragm's force-generating capacity.

Hyperinflation is a frequently overlooked cause of diaphragm dysfunction.

Other disorders commonly encountered in the intensive care unit that may cause abnormal respiratory muscle function, thereby hindering weaning, include undernutrition, electrolyte disturbances (hypophosphatemia, hypokalemia, hypocalcemia, hypomagnesemia), and thyroid dysfunction. Additionally, respiratory muscle atrophy has been suggested as a consequence of prolonged mechanical ventilation, when patients make no respiratory efforts over a prolonged period (several days to weeks). There are no data demonstrating that respiratory muscle atrophy occurs in humans. Data in primates, however, show a significant reduction in diaphragmatic strength after receiving continuous mechanical ventilation for 11 days.

WHEN IS THE PATIENT READY TO WEAN?

Before an attempt is made to wean a patient, certain prerequisites should be met (Table 36-2). The most important prerequisite appears to be resolution or significant improvement in the underlying cause of respiratory failure. Patients should be hemodynamically stable, with minimal or no need for vasopressor agents. The absence of sepsis or hyperthermia should be confirmed. Sedative drugs and neuromuscular blocking agents should be discontinued. Patients should be awake, alert, and able to manage secretions and protect their airway. Significant fluid, electrolyte, and metabolic disorders should be corrected before weaning attempts. Adequate gas exchange, marked by a PaO_2 to FiO_2 ratio greater than 200, FiO_2 requirements of 50% or less, and positive end-expiratory pressure 5 cmH_2O or less are desirable. Adequate respiratory muscle strength needs to be ensured (maximum inspiratory pressure or negative inspiratory force at least -25 cmH_2O).

Resolution or significant improvement in the underlying cause of respiratory failure is the most important prerequisite before weaning is attempted.

Predictors of Weaning Outcome

Determining when a patient is ready to wean from the ventilator is a complicated task. Considerable research has been devoted to finding variables that predict weaning outcome.

Pulmonary Gas Exchange

The adequacy of pulmonary gas exchange must be assessed before initiating weaning. In the past, several indices derived from arterial blood gas analysis have been used to predict weaning outcome. These indices derive from retrospective studies and, consequently, have limi-

TABLE 36-2

NECESSARY CONDITIONS TO DECIDE WHEN A PATIENT IS READY FOR WEANING

Resolution or significant improvement of the underlying cause of respiratory failure
Stable hemodynamic state
Absence of sepsis or hyperthermia
Cessation of sedative drugs
Cessation of neuromuscular blocking agents
Cessation of vasopressor agents
Patients should be awake, alert, and able to manage secretions and protect their airway
Correction of metabolic and electrolyte disorders
Adequate gas exchange
PaO_2 to FiO_2 ratio greater than 200
FiO_2 requirements less than 50%
PEEP requirements equal to or less than 5 cmH_2O
Adequate respiratory muscle strength

PaO_2, partial pressure of arterial oxygen
FiO_2, inspired fraction of oxygen
PEEP, positive end-expiratory pressure

Adequate oxygenation is essential to initiate weaning, but its predictive value is poor.

tations. An arterial blood to inspired O_2 ratio (PaO_2/FiO_2) greater than 238 had a positive predictive value of 90%, yet its negative predictive value was only 10%. In another study, an arterial/alveolar O_2 tension of 0.35 had positive and negative predictive values slightly greater than 0.5. Although adequate arterial oxygenation is essential to initiate weaning, it is clear that the predictive value of this index by itself is insufficient to predict weaning outcome.

Respiratory Muscle Strength

Muscle strength and endurance are important determinants of weaning outcome.

The strength and endurance of the respiratory system seem to be a major determinant of weaning outcome. Sahn and Lakshminarayan (1973) were among the first to describe the use of simple bedside criteria to assist decisions in discontinuing ventilatory support. In a study involving 100 patients, these investigators measured resting minute ventilation (MV), maximum voluntary ventilation (i.e., maximum sustainable ventilation over 15 s; MVV), and maximum inspiratory pressure (MIP) with a spirometer. Of these, 76 patients who had an MV less than 10 l/min, MIP of -30 cmH_2O or less, and MVV twice their resting MV who were able to complete a 2-h spontaneous breathing trial via an endotracheal tube were successfully extubated; 7 more patients with a MIP of -25 cmH_2O or less and a mean MV of 10.2 l/min were able to be extubated although they were not able to double their resting MV. By contrast, 17 patients with an MIP greater than -22 cmH_2O could not be extubated.

Application of these criteria in subsequent studies, however, did not yield comparable results. When evaluating 47 patients on mechanical ventilation, Tahvanainen found that using a MIP less than -30 cmH_2O as a weaning predictor produced a false-negative result in 11 of 11 patients and a false-positive result in 8 of 23 patients. Similarly, other authors reported poor negative and positive predictive values when evaluating other weaning parameters such as vital capacity (VC), minute ventilation (V_E), and maximum voluntary ventilation (MVV).

Factors that may account for the variability of bedside respiratory mechanics to predict outcome include different patient populations, variability in duration of mechanical ventilation, different techniques used in measuring respiratory mechanics, and inability of the measurements to appropriately assess the true cause of ventilatory dependency. For example, no matter what respiratory parameters are measured, if a patient develops an acute severe episode of heart failure or bronchospasm postextubation, respiratory failure will recur, and thus weaning will have failed. Because of the poor and variable results of bedside parameters to predict weaning outcome, investigators have turned to more complicated measurements of respiratory mechanics, such as $P_{0.1}$, gastric tonometry, and measurements of the work of breathing.

$P_{0.1}$

The airway pressure generated 100 ms after initiating an inspiratory effort against an occluded airway ($P_{0.1}$) is believed to reflect central respiratory drive and has been proposed as a useful predictor of weaning outcome. The values for normal, healthy individuals are 2 cmH_2O or less. Herrera et al. (1985) observed that 89% of patients with a $P_{0.1}$ greater than 4 cmH_2O failed weaning attempts. In patients with COPD, Sassoon and Mahutte (1993) found that patients with a $P_{0.1}$ greater than 6 cmH_2O were unable to wean from ventilatory support, but patients with a $P_{0.1}$ less than 6 cmH_2O were successfully extubated. Several studies have shown a large variation in outcome when $P_{0.1}$ is used, possibly because of its inability to predict endurance or its application to patient groups with different diseases causing respiratory failure. This technique also requires special equipment and trained personnel, which makes it less appealing.

Work of Breathing

Work of breathing can be measured by plotting the transpulmonary pressure against tidal volume. Transpulmonary pressure is calculated from the difference between pleural pressure (estimated with an endoesophageal balloon catheter) and the airway pressure. One study found that mechanical ventilation was necessary when work exceeded 1.8 kg/m²/min. Another study performed 775 measures of work and found a discriminating value of 1.34 kg/m/min to separate ventilator-dependent from ventilator-independent patients. At this level, the rate of false-negative and false-positive results was 13.8%. An additional study evaluated work of breathing in a group of 17 patients, 6 of whom required prolonged mechanical ventilation. A work index less than 1.6 kg/m²/min was observed in all patients who had a successful weaning trial; this was more accurate than conventional weaning parameters in determining weaning outcome. Furthermore, patients that went from unsuccessful to successful weaning did not show significant improvement in conventional weaning parameters but did show improvement in work of breathing measurements. There are no large prospective studies comparing this parameter against more conventional weaning parameters. The relative invasiveness and complexity of data acquisition and analysis, and the requirement for dedicated staff and equipment to perform the test make it unappealing as an effective clinical tool.

Respiratory Pattern During Spontaneous Breathing

Multiple studies have reported the role of breathing pattern in the outcome of weaning from mechanical ventilation. The development of rapid, shallow breathing, the presence of asynchronous or paradoxical thoracoabdominal movements, and marked accessory muscle recruitment during a spontaneous breathing trial herald an unsuccessful weaning trial.

Based on the premise that patients who fail weaning trials rapidly develop a high respiratory rate and a drop in tidal volume, Yang and Tobin (1991) combined measurements of frequency (f) and tidal volume (V_T) into the rapid shallow breathing index, f/V_T. They obtained data in 36 patients and noticed that an f/V_T ratio of 105 breaths/min/l best differentiated patients who weaned successfully from those who failed. They subsequently validated the rapid shallow breathing index in 64 patients, comparing it against conventional weaning indexes (Table 36-3). An f/V_T ratio less than 105 predicted a successful weaning trial (Figure 36-1). The positive and negative predictive values were 0.78 and 0.95, respectively. The predictive power of the f/V_T ratio was better than any of its components, supporting the use of this index. The f/V_T ratio is attractive because it is relatively easy to obtain and the determinant value (i.e., $\approx$100) is easy to remember. It is important to recognize that this test is more accurate in patients who have received mechanical ventilation for less than 7 days.

Patients who fail a weaning trial frequently exhibit a rapid respiratory rate and a drop in tidal volume.

An f/V_T ratio less than 105 predicts a successful weaning outcome in about 80% of patients.

In a subsequent study, Epstein (1995) attempted to define the cause of extubation failure in patients whose f/V_T predicted weaning success. He analyzed 94 consecutive patients whose f/V_T before the weaning trial predicted successful extubation. The f/V_T was measured while patients breathed unassisted for 1 min. Of the 94 patients extubated, 84 had an f/V_T less than 100 and 10 had an f/V_T of 100 or more. Extubation failure, defined as the need to reintu-

TABLE 36-3

THRESHOLD VALUES OF INDEXES USED TO PREDICT WEANING OUTCOME

INDEX	VALUE
Minute ventilation (l/min)	≤15
Respiratory frequency (breaths/min)	≤38
Tidal volume (ml)	≥325
Maximal inspiratory pressure (cmH_2O)	<−15
Dynamic compliance (ml/cmH_2O)	≥22
Static Compliance (ml/cmH_2O)	≥33
PaO_2/PAO_2 ratio	≥0.35
Frequency/tidal volume ratio (breaths/min/l)	≤105
CROP index (ml/breath/minute)	≥13

PaO_2, partial pressure of arterial oxygen; PAO_2, alveolar oxygen tension; CROP, compliance/resistance/oxygenation/mouth pressure index

SOURCE: Yang KL, Tobin MJ. A prospective study of indexes predicting the outcome of trials of weaning from mechanical ventilation. New Engl J Med 324(21):1445–1550.

FIGURE 36-1

Isopleths for the ratio of breathing frequency to tidal volume, representing different degrees of rapid shallow breathing. (From Yang KL, Tobin MJ. A prospective study of indexes predicting the outcome of trials of weaning from mechanical ventilation. N Engl J Med 1991; 324(21):1445-1450, with permission.)

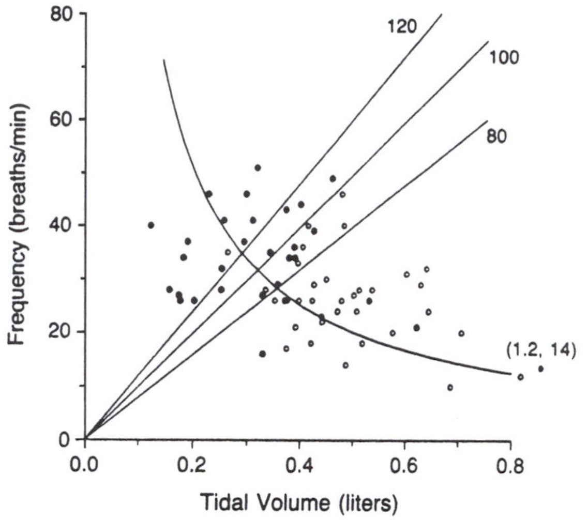

The f/V_T ratio is more accurate when an underlying respiratory process is responsible for mechanical ventilation.

The f/V_T ratio is less accurate when it does not reflect the underlying pathophysiologic cause of respiratory failure.

bate within 72 h, occurred in 14 of 84 patients in the group with f/V_T below 100 and 4 of 10 patients with f/V_T above 100 (Table 36-4). When the cause for respiratory failure was analyzed, the underlying respiratory process was responsible for extubation failure in all 4 patients with f/V_T of 100 or more. In contrast, the initial respiratory process was the cause for extubation failure in only 1 of 14 patients with an f/V_T less than 100; a new problem, such as heart failure and upper airway obstruction, were the most common causes (Table 36-5). When the author further analyzed the 57 patients in whom a respiratory process was the original cause for mechanical ventilation, the positive predictive value for their f/V_T index approached unity (Table 36-6). This study confirmed the high positive predictive value of the f/V_T index in predicting weaning outcome. It also suggested that this index may be less accurate when it does not reflect the underlying pathophysiologic cause of respiratory failure (i.e., heart failure) or when the cause is not present at the time of index measurement (i.e., upper airway obstruction due to laryngeal edema).

In a randomized, prospective trial, Ely studied 300 consecutive medical and coronary care unit ventilated patients. The intervention group ($n = 149$) underwent daily screening of respiratory function to identify those patients capable of spontaneous breathing. Patients had to satisfy five criteria to be considered for a spontaneous breathing trial (e.g., PaO_2/FiO_2 ratio <

TABLE 36-4

PREDICTIVE ACCURACY OF THE EXTUBATION f/V_T

	$f/V_T < 100$	$f/V_T \geq 100$
Extubation success	70 (TP)	6 (FN)
Extubation failure	14 (FP)	4 (TN)

	SENSITIVITY	SPECIFICITY	PPV	NPV
All patients	0.92	0.22	0.83	0.40
<6 days MV	0.93	0.08	0.82	0.20
>6 days MV	0.89	0.60	0.89	0.60

MV, mechanical ventilation; PPV, positive predictive value; NPV, negative predictive value; TP, true positives; FP, false positives; FN, false negatives; TN, true negatives

SOURCE: From Epstein SK. Etiology of extubation failure and the predictive value of the rapid shallow breathing index. Am J Respir Crit Care Med 1995;152:545–549, with permission

TABLE 36-5

CAUSES OF EXTUBATION FAILURE IN 18 PATIENTS WHO REQUIRED REINTUBATION WITHIN 72 H OF EXTUBATION

	$f/V_T \geq 100$	$f/V_T < 100$
Original respiratory process		
Alone	4	1
Plus CHF		1
CHF		
Alone		4
Plus UAO		1
New aspiration		
Alone		3
Plus encephalopathy		1
UAO		2
New pneumonia		1

CHF, congestive heart failure; UAO, upper airway obstruction; PE, pulmonary embolism; f/V_T, respiratory rate/tidal volume (rapid shallow breathing index)
SOURCE: From Epstein SK. Etiology of extubation failure and the predictive value of the rapid shallow breathing index. Am J Respir Crit Care Med 1995;152:545–549, with permission

200, PEEP < 5 cmH_2O, adequate coughing during suctioning, f/V_T ratio <105, and no need for sedative or vasopressor agents). Intervention patients meeting these criteria underwent a 2-h T-piece spontaneous breathing trial. Physicians were notified if patients successfully completed the trial (Figure 36-2). Control patients received daily screening but no other interventions. Patients assigned to the intervention group received mechanical ventilation for a median of 4.5 days versus 6 days in the control group ($p = 0.003$). The group assigned to the intervention had a significant reduction in the incidence of self-extubation, reintubation, tracheostomy, and mechanical ventilation for more than 21 days. ICU costs were significantly reduced in the intervention group.

It is important to recognize that successful weaning from ventilatory support does not ensure that a patient will be successfully extubated. These are two distinct phases in the process of liberating a patient from mechanical ventilation. This realization is particularly important because reintubation carries an increased risk of nosocomial pneumonia. Currently, there are no objective measurements to determine the outcome of extubation; therefore, clinical assessment is important in establishing which patients can be safely extubated. Important factors include the patient's level of consciousness, which should be adequate for airway protection, the presence of a gag reflex, and the ability to cough and clear the airway. Upper airway patency is one of the most difficult aspects to evaluate. Postintubation laryngeal edema can lead to respiratory failure, especially in patients with decreased respiratory reserve. Some investigators advocate the use of the "cuff-leak" test, ensuring the presence of an air leak around the endotracheal tube when the cuff is deflated and the tube is occluded. The presence of an air leak is reassuring and relatively sensitive in predicting a positive outcome from extubation, but the specificity of the test is very low. Despite this, it is clear from most studies that about 80% of patients will be extubated after a spontaneous breathing trial and the remaining 20% will require more concentrated weaning efforts; however, the majority are eventually successfully extubated.

If patients exhibit satisfactory weaning parameters, 80% will wean after a spontaneous breathing trial on a T-piece circuit.

TABLE 36-6

PREDICTIVE ACCURACY OF THE EXTUBATION f/V_T FOR EXTUBATION FAILURE RESULTING FROM THE ORIGINAL RESPIRATORY PROCESS

	SENSITIVITY	SPECIFICITY	PPV	NPV
Original pulmonary process	0.92	0.80	0.98	0.50
New or nonpulmonary process	0.92	0.67	0.96	0.50

PPV, positive predictive value; NPV, negative predictive value
SOURCE: From Epstein SK. Etiology of extubation failure and the predictive value of the rapid shallow breathing index. Am J Respir Crit Care Med 1995;152:545–549, with permission

FIGURE 36-2

Study algorithm evaluating daily screening and spontaneous breathing trial in patients on mechanical ventilation. RT, respiratory technician; PT, patient; PaO_2, arterial oxygen tension; FiO_2, inspired fraction of oxygen; PEEP, positive end-expiratory pressure; f/VT, rapid shallow breathing index; CPAP, continuous positive airway pressure; RR, respiratory rate; HR, heart rate; SBP, systolic blood pressure. (From Ely EW, Barker AM, Dunagan DP. Effect of duration of mechanical ventilation of identifying patients capable of breathing spontaneously. N Engl J Med 1996; 335:1864-1869, with permission.)

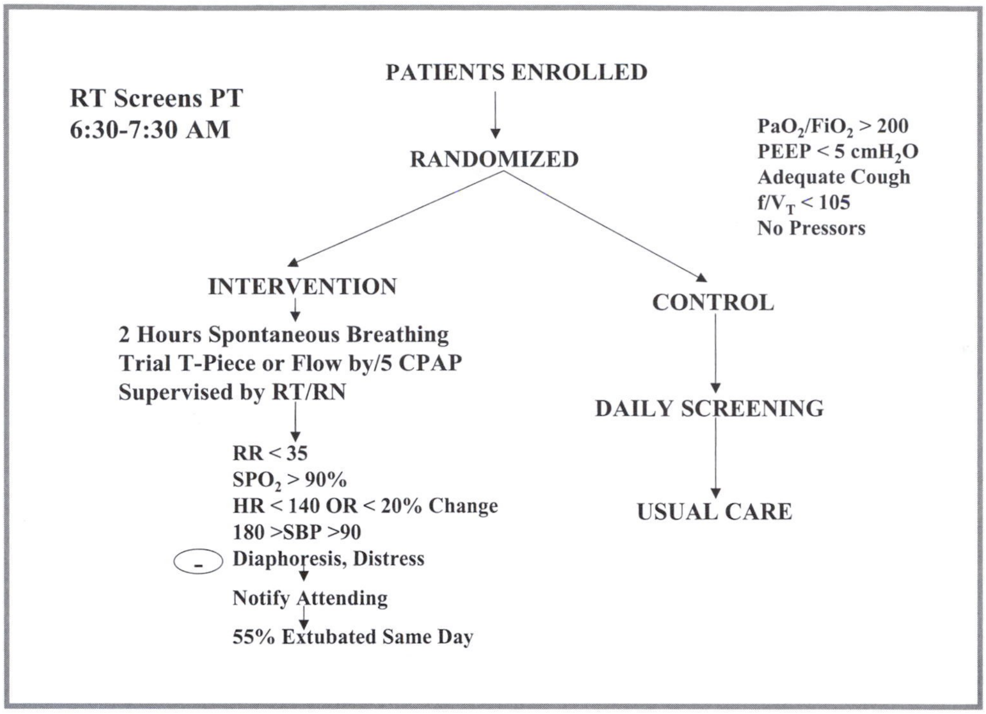

SPECIFIC WEANING METHODS

Trials of Spontaneous Breathing

Once patients show an improvement or resolution of the underlying cause of respiratory failure and fulfill the previously mentioned criteria, weaning attempts can be initiated. The abrupt discontinuation of mechanical ventilation through a T-tube system is the simplest method of weaning. A T-tube system is a continuous high flow source of oxygen delivered by corrugated tubing that is attached to the distal end of the endotracheal tube, with an additional 6-in. tail of tubing that limits the entrainment of room air oxygen. Patients who have spent relatively short periods on mechanical ventilation (less than 7 days), or in whom no problems with the resumption of unassisted breathing is expected, can be placed on a spontaneous breathing trial on a T-tube circuit. Traditionally, patients are placed on T-tube circuit for at least 2 h. If they do not develop signs of respiratory distress, such as nasal flaring, tachypnea, abdominal–rib cage paradoxical movements or tachycardia, arrhythmias, oxygen desaturation, or hypo- or hypertension during this time, they are extubated. If signs of intolerance occur, mechanical ventilation is resumed, and weaning attempts are resumed in 24 h. About 75% of the patients who undergo a T-tube weaning trial can be extubated. The 2-h duration of the spontaneous breathing trial has recently been challenged. In a study of more than 500 patients, patients underwent a traditional 120-min spontaneous breathing trial compared to a 30-minute trial. There was no significant difference within groups in the percentage of patients that were extubated, the percentage of patients that remained extubated at 48 h, and in-hospital mortality.

In difficult-to-wean patients, mechanical ventilation is gradually discontinued. Short trials of spontaneous breathing are followed by periods of rest on the ventilator in the assist-control mode. The duration of the trials is slowly increased; when patients are able to tolerate 2 h of spontaneous breathing, the weaning process is completed, and the patient can be extubated. The importance of careful observation of the patient during T-piece trials cannot be overemphasized. Resistance of the endotracheal tube imposes an additional load and increases the work of breathing during spontaneous breathing; therefore, T-piece trials are also thought to test endurance of the weaning patient.

Intermittent Mandatory Ventilation

During intermittent mandatory ventilation (IMV), or synchronized IMV (SIMV; synchronous with inspiratory effort), a specified number of volume-preset breaths are delivered to the patient each minute by the ventilator. In addition, the patient is allowed to breath spontaneously between machine-delivered breaths. This approach is still one of the most common weaning methods used in the United States. The backup respiratory rate is gradually reduced until the patient is able to tolerate a minimal backup rate (i.e., 2–4 breaths/min) for 2 h. IMV is frequently criticized because patients are generally subjected to an additional inspiratory load imposed by breathing through a demand valve. Most important, this mode has also been shown to prolong the weaning process over all other modalities (see following). It is difficult therefore to encourage the use of this mode as an appropriate weaning alternative.

The synchronized intermittent mandatory ventilation (SIMV) mode results in a prolonged weaning process when compared to all other weaning modalities.

Pressure-Support Ventilation

Pressure-support ventilation (PSV) is a pressure-targeted ventilatory mode that provides support to the patient's inspiratory effort with a preset inspiratory pressure. During PSV, the patient determines the respiratory rate. The patient's effort and the level of pressure support determine the delivered volume. Initial settings are aimed at achieving tidal volumes from 8 to 10 ml/kg and a respiratory rate between 20 and 28 breaths/min. Weaning can be accomplished by gradually reducing the level of pressure support by 3–6 cmH_2O, titrated on the basis of respiratory rate. In two prospective, randomized trials, extubation was considered when patients were able to comfortably tolerate 5–8 cmH_2O for 2 h. PSV has been shown by several authors to decrease the work of breathing imposed by the endotracheal tube and the ventilator circuit, which suggested that patients who tolerate a weaning trial at this "compensatory" pressure are ready to sustain spontaneous ventilation. There appears to be great variability in the compensatory level of pressure support between patients, and there is no reliable method to determine it. Occasionally, patients with severe obstructive disease or COPD may have problems with PSV. PSV is set to cycle at a predetermined flow, usually 25% of peak inspiratory flow; patients with COPD may require more time to reach this preset level during expiration, causing ventilator inflation during neural expiration and patient–ventilator asynchrony.

Efficacy of Different Weaning Techniques

Two recent rigorously controlled studies have prospectively compared the efficacy of three different weaning techniques: IMV, pressure support, and spontaneous breathing trials (Table 36-7). Brochard et al. (1994) found that a significantly greater number of patients could be weaned successfully after 21 days with PSV than with the other methods. This group also reported that weaning time was significantly shorter with pressure support (5.7 days) than

TABLE 36-7

COMPARISON BETWEEN BROCHARD AND ESTEBAN STUDIES EVALUATING DIFFERENT WEANING TECHNIQUES

INVESTIGATOR	WEANING TECHNIQUE	*N*	DURATION OF VENTILATION BEFORE WEANING (DAYS)	WEANING PERIOD (DAYS)
Brochard et al. (1994)	SIMV	43	11 ± 10	10 ± 8
	PSV	31	14 ± 17	6 ± 4
	T-piece	35	17 ± 31	8 ± 8
Esteban et al. (1995)	SIMV	29	6 ± 4	4 ± 3
	PSV	37	11 ± 9	4 ± 3
	T-piece	33	11 ± 7	3 ± 2

SIMV, synchronized intermittent mandatory ventilation; PSV, pressure–support ventilation

SOURCE: Modified from Esteban A, Frutos F, Tobin M, et al. A comparison of four methods of weaning patients from mechanical ventilation. Clin Pulm Med 1996;3:91–100

Daily spontaneous breathing trials lead to extubation twice as quickly as pressure-support ventilation (PSV) weaning and three times more quickly than SIMV.

with spontaneous breathing trials (8.5 days) or IMV (9.9 days). In contrast, Esteban et al. (1995) found that a once-daily trial of spontaneous breathing led to extubation twice as quickly as PSV and about three times more quickly than IMV. There was no difference between a once-daily spontaneous breathing trial and multiple daily spontaneous breathing trials (attempted at least twice daily). Some of the differences in these studies are the result of different criteria to assess tolerance to weaning and weaning completion. Esteban's group considered extubation if patients tolerated 5 cm H_2O of pressure support for 2 h compared to 8 cmH_2O in Brochard's study. During application of IMV, Esteban et al. extubated patients once they were able to tolerate a backup rate of 5 breaths/min for 2 h; in contrast, Brochard's group criteria required patients to tolerate 24 h at 4 breaths/min (a significant ventilatory challenge). Both studies similarly concluded that SIMV was less efficient in weaning patients but differed as to whether pressure support (PS) or T-piece was the superior weaning method. Overall, either PS or T-piece weaning techniques can be successful if patients are properly selected and the method is appropriately implemented.

A small percentage of all patients placed on mechanical ventilation fail to wean and require more prolonged and concentrated efforts. The medical and respiratory status of these patients should be carefully reevaluated, and efforts should be made to correct any abnormalities. Additionally, tracheostomy placement should be contemplated. The question regarding the appropriate timing for tracheostomy remains unanswered. It has been suggested that patients who are likely to require mechanical ventilation for more than 21 days should have a tracheostomy. Evidence regarding the advantages of early versus late tracheotomy and the relative advantages of tracheostomy over endotracheal tube is controversial. Overall, the most common practice is to perform a tracheostomy if a patient has been on mechanical ventilation for at least 14 days. In terms of weaning, tracheostomy has been shown to reduce the resistive work of breathing over the continued use of an endotracheal tube.

SUMMARY

Weaning from mechanical ventilation blends the art and science aspects of pulmonary and critical care medicine. Successful weaning requires knowledge of the cause of the patient's respiratory failure, a certain degree of clinical stability for the patient, and interpretation of some easily obtainable respiratory function bedside tests (Figure 36-3). These assessments,

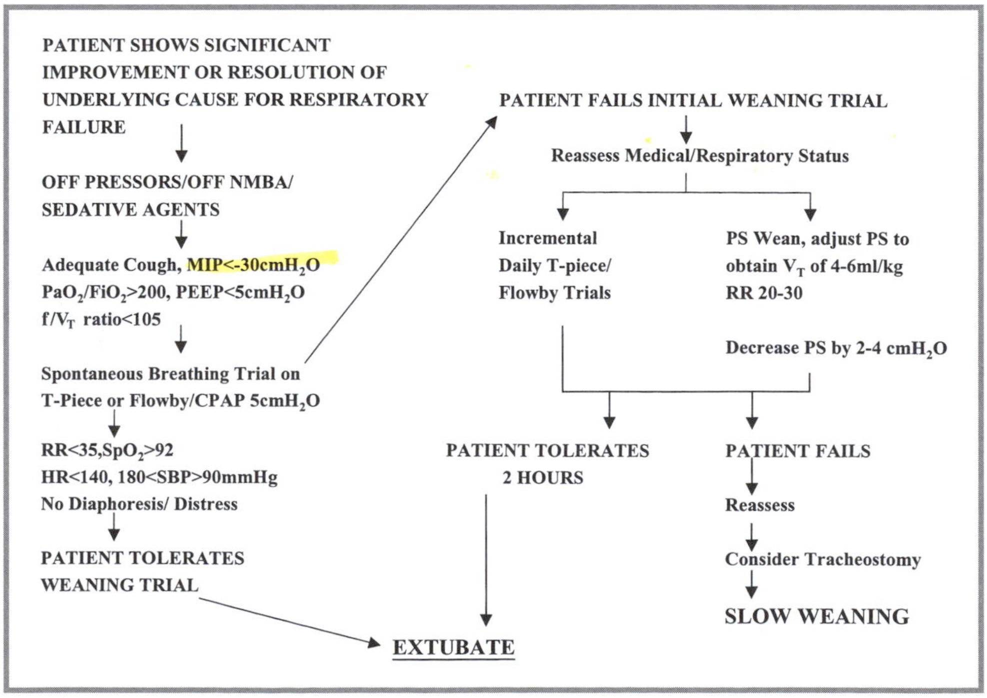

FIGURE 36-3

Weaning algorithm. NMBA, neuromuscular blocking agents; PaO_2, arterial oxygen tension; FiO_2, inspired fraction of oxygen; MIP, maximal inspiratory pressure; f/V_T, rapid shallow breathing index; CPAP, continuous positive airway pressure; PS, pressure support; RR, respiratory rate; HR, heart rate; SBP, systolic blood pressure.

in addition to careful observation of a patient's breathing pattern and tolerance of a spontaneous breathing trial on T-piece or PS, can successfully enhance weaning from mechanical ventilation.

REVIEW QUESTIONS

1. **Regarding weaning on pressure support, all the following statements are true except:**
   - A. As a weaning mode, pressure-support ventilation (PSV) has been shown to be more efficient than intermittent mandatory ventilation (IMV).
   - B. Pressure-support weans should always be started with a support level of 20 cmH_2O.
   - C. Patients with severe obstructive disease may exhibit ventilator–patient asynchrony while weaning on pressure support.
   - D. Pressure support has been shown to decrease the work of breathing secondary to the additional resistive load of the endotracheal tube.

2. **Regarding spontaneous breathing trials via T-tube system, all the following statements are correct except:**
   - A. More than 70% of the patients that are placed on a spontaneous breathing trial have a successful weaning trial.
   - B. Once-daily spontaneous breathing trials are as efficacious as intermittent spontaneous breathing trials (at least twice daily).
   - C. Spontaneous breathing trials via T-piece are associated with increased work of breathing.
   - D. The rate of reintubation is higher in patients undergoing a 30-min spontaneous breathing trial versus the conventional 120-min spontaneous breathing trial.

3. **Regarding the frequency/tidal volume (f/V_T), all the following are correct except:**
   - A. It should be measured while the patient is breathing spontaneously through a T-piece.
   - B. A determinant value less than 100 has a high positive predictive value for successful weaning.
   - C. The positive predictive value of the f/VT index is less when a respiratory process is the cause for mechanical ventilation.
   - D. The limitations of the f/VT index include its inability to predict outcome if a new condition arises after it was measured (i.e., heart failure).

4. **A frequently overlooked cause of weaning failure in mechanically ventilated patients with severe COPD is:**
   - A. Electrolyte disturbances
   - B. Critical care polyneuropathy
   - C. Malnutrition
   - D. Silent cardiac ischemia
   - E. Hyperinflation

ANSWERS

1. The answer is B. The amount of pressure support at the beginning of a weaning trial should be titrated to obtain a desired tidal volume (6–8 ml/kg) and respiratory rate (20–28 breaths/min). The pressure support required to achieve these parameters will vary depending on the respiratory system's compliance and resistance. In several studies, patients on PSV weaned twice as fast as patients on IMV. PSV decreases work of breathing due to the endotracheal tube.
2. The answer is D. A recently published study demonstrated that the rate of reintubation and mortality were not significantly different between patients who underwent a 30-min compared to a 120-min spontaneous breathing trial before extubation. The T-piece circuit is associated with an increase in work of breathing, which is why some authors believe that this weaning method also reflects the patient's endurance. In Esteban's study no difference was found between patients doing intermittent (at least twice daily) versus once-daily spontaneous breathing trials. About 70%–80% of all patients who meet basic prerequisites (resolution of underlying cause, absence of electrolyte abnormalities, absence of overt sepsis) will be successfully extubated after a spontaneous breathing trial on a T-piece circuit.
3. The answer is C. The accuracy of the f/VT index to predict weaning is very high in patients who have an underlying respiratory disturbance requiring mechanical ventilation. It diminishes when the index is not able to reflect the underlying pathophysiologic disorder (new-onset heart failure). The index should be measured while the patient is breathing spontaneously.
4. The answer is E. Although all options listed may be present in a patient with severe COPD and may be implicated in the failure to wean, a frequently overlooked (and very likely underdiagnosed) cause of weaning failure in this group of patients is hyperinflation. By altering the orientation of the diaphragm fibers and decreasing the area of apposition, hyperinflation leads to a decrement in the diaphragm's force-generating capacity.

SUGGESTED READING

Bolton CF. Muscle weakness and difficulty in weaning from the ventilator in the critical care unit. Chest 1994;106:1–2.

Brochard L, Pluskwa F, Lemaire F. Improved efficacy of spontaneous breathing with inspiratory pressure support. Am Rev Respir Dis 1989;139:411–415.

Bronchard L, Rauss A, Benito S, et al. Comparison of three methods of gradual withdrawal from ventilatory support during weaning from mechanical ventilation. Am J Respir Crit Care Med 1994; 150:739–745.

Ely EW, Baker AM, Dunagan DP. Effect of duration of mechanical ventilation of identifying patients capable of breathing spontaneously. N Eng J Med 1996;335:1864–1869.

Epstein SK. Etiology of extubation failure and the predictive value of the rapid shallow breathing index. Am J Respir Crit Care Med 1995;152:545–549.

Esteban A, Alia I, Gordo F. Weaning: What the recent studies have shown us. Clinical Pulmonary Medicine 1996;3:91–100.

Estaban A, Frutos F, Tobin M, et al. A comparison of four methods of weaning patients from mechanical ventilation. N Eng J Med 1995; 332:345–350.

Fiastro JF, Habib MP, Shon BY, et al. Comparison of standard weaning parameters and the mechanical work of breathing in mechanically ventilated patients. Chest 1988;94:232–238.

Fisher MM, Raper RF. The "cuff leak" test for extubation. Anaesthesia 1992;47:10–12.

Herrera M, Blasco J, Vanegas J. Mouth occlusion pressure ($P_{0.1}$) in acute respiratory failure. Intensive Care Med 1985;11:134–39.

Jabour ER, Rabil DM, Truwitt JD, et al. Evaluation of a new weaning index based on ventilatory endurance and the efficiency of gas exchange. Am Rev Respir Dis 1991;144:531–537.

Larminat V, Montravers P, Dureil B, et al. Alteration in swallowing reflex after extubation in intensive care unit patients. Crit Care Med 1995;23:486–489.

Lemaire F, Teboul JL, Cinsotti L, et al. Acute left ventricular dysfunction during unsuccessful weaning from mechanical ventilation. Anesthesiology 1988;69:171–179.

Lessard MR, Brochard L. Weaning from ventilatory support. Clin Chest Med 1996;17(3):475–490.

Sahn SA, Lakshminarayan S. Bedside criteria for discontinuation of mechanical ventilation. Chest 1973;63:1002–1005.

Sassoon CS, Mahutte C. Airway occlusion pressure and breathing pattern as predictors of weaning outcome. Am Rev Respir Dis 1993; 148:860–866.

Tahvaninen J, Salenpera M, Nikki P. Extubation criteria after weaning from intermittent mandatory ventilation and continuous positive airway pressure. Crit Care Med 1983;11:702–707.

Tobin MJ, Perez W, Buenther SW, et al. Pattern of breathing during successful and unsuccessful trials of weaning from mechanical ventilation. Am Rev Respir Dis 1986;134:1111–1118.

Yang KL, Tobin MJ. A prospective study of indexes predicting the outcome of trials of weaning from mechanical ventilation. N Engl J Med 1991;324(21):1445–1450.

CHAPTER 37

Scott A. Schartel

Mechanical Hemodynamic Support

CHAPTER OUTLINE

LEARNING OBJECTIVES

After studying this chapter, you should be able to:

- Discuss the indications for intraaortic balloon counterpulsation.
- Formulate a plan for the evaluation and management of ischemic limb complications related to intraaortic balloon counterpulsation.
- Discuss the use of ventricular-assist device therapy in the management of failing ventricular function.
- Compare and contrast a variety of ventricular-assist devices with regard to indications, contraindications, and complications.
- Discuss the technique of extracorporeal membrane oxygenation in the treatment of acute respiratory failure.

The mainstay of treatment for patients with inadequate hemodynamic performance is maintaining appropriate intravascular volume (preload), vascular tone (afterload), and myocardial pump function (contractility), most commonly accomplished by volume administration or diuretic therapy, pharmacologic manipulation of the vascular tone with vasodilators or vasopressors, and inotropic agents. When these measures result in an inadequate response in hemodynamic performance, mechanical circulatory support may be indicated. This chapter discusses the major mechanical circulatory support techniques currently available for use in critically ill patients, including intraaortic balloon counterpulsation (IABC) therapy, ventricular-assist devices (VADs), and extracorporeal membrane oxygenation (ECMO).

INTRAAORTIC BALLOON COUNTERPULSATION

Analysis of blood flow to the heart during the cardiac cycle reveals that the majority of the coronary artery blood flow to the left ventricle occurs during diastole, not systole, unlike flow in all other vascular beds. This phenomenon can be explained by the increased resistance to blood flow in the small intraventricular arterial branches caused by the force of ventricular contraction. Animal experiments during the 1950s and early 1960s demonstrated that delaying the systemic arterial pressure peak until diastole could augment coronary artery blood flow, which led to the development of intraaortic balloon catheters that could be used in humans. Near the end of the 1960s, clinical experiments began using intraaortic balloon

> Most of the coronary artery blood flow to the left ventricle occurs during diastole, not systole, unlike the flow in all other vascular beds.

counterpulsation (IABC) for the treatment of cardiogenic shock. Additional research and improvements in the technical aspects of IABC therapy have proved this to be a valuable therapeutic intervention in a variety of conditions.

Therapeutic Uses

Intraaortic balloon counterpulsation is usually the first choice for mechanical hemodynamic support when pharmacotherapy and the manipulation of intravascular volume are ineffective.

Intraaortic balloon counterpulsation is typically considered as the first choice for mechanical hemodynamic support in patients who have failed to respond to pharmacotherapy and the manipulation of intravascular volume. Intraaortic balloon catheterization can be instituted with a percutaneous insertion technique while the patient is in the critical care unit, cardiac catheterization laboratory, or operating room. It is less invasive and less expensive than the ventricular-assist devices discussed next and does not require a surgical incision or general anesthesia for placement.

Intraaortic balloon counterpulsation therapy requires two components that work together: the intraaortic balloon catheter, which must be placed into the patient's aorta, and an electronically controlled pumping device. The intraaortic balloon catheter has a lumen that communicates with the balloon affixed to the catheter and which is then attached to the pumping device. Depending on the size and manufacturer of the catheter, there may also be a central lumen that terminates at the distal end of the catheter. This lumen can be used to measure the blood pressure in the proximal aorta (Figure 37-1). Helium is used to inflate the in-

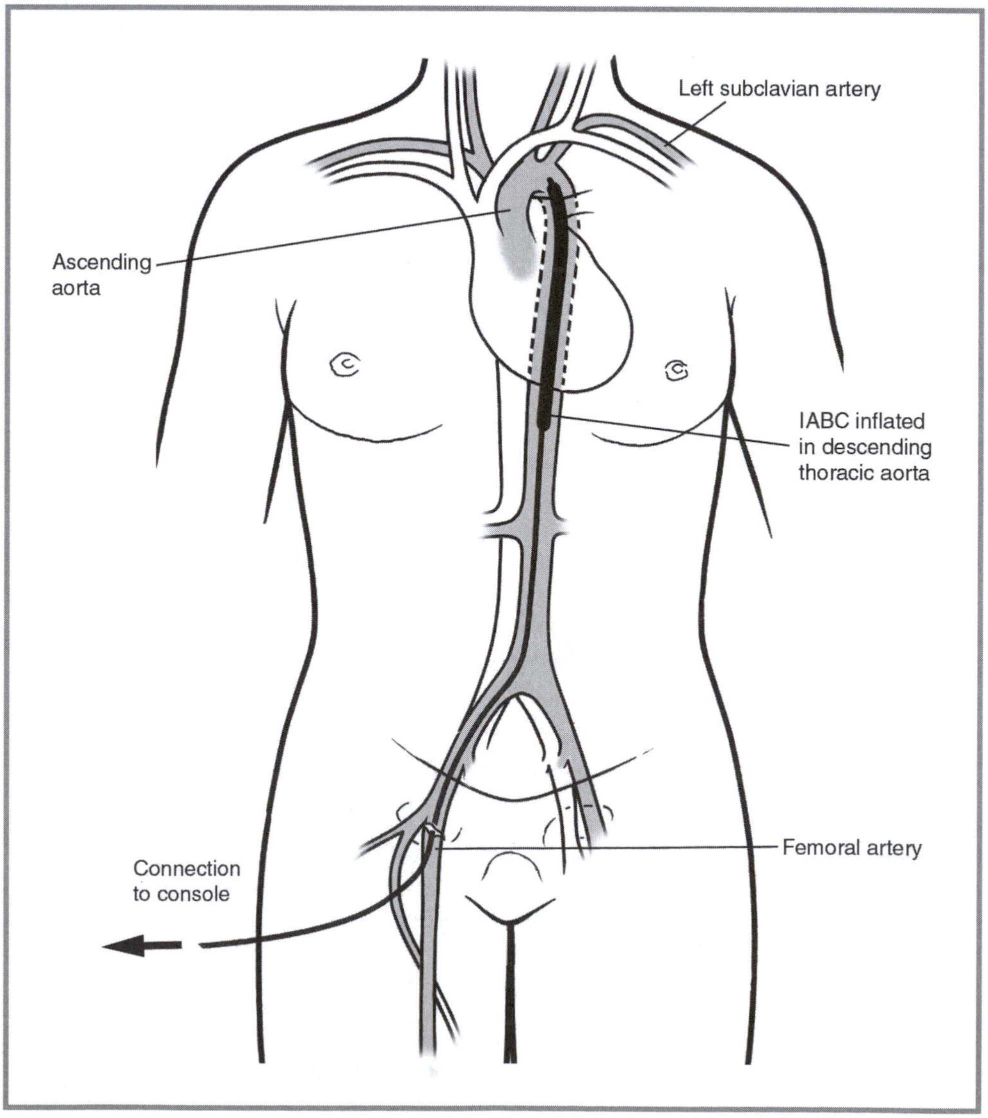

FIGURE 37-1

Intraaortic balloon catheter (IABC).

traaortic balloon because helium moves rapidly into and out of the balloon. The rapid shuttling of gas in and out of the balloon is necessary for the correct timing of balloon inflation and deflation with the cardiac cycle. Pumps within the control console provide the driving pressure necessary to inflate the balloon and vacuum to assist in balloon deflation. Balloon inflation is timed to occur with the onset of diastole and deflation to occur with the onset of systole. Information from an electrocardiographic (ECG) signal or an intraarterial pressure waveform is used to identify the specific stages of the cardiac cycle when the intraaortic balloon will be inflated or deflated by the controller. The controller allows the adjustment of the volume of balloon inflation, the frequency of balloon inflation (every beat, every second or third beat, etc.), and the trigger source (ECG, pressure waveform, fixed rate) that the controller uses to identify the inflation and deflation times.

Balloon inflation is timed to occur with the onset of diastole and deflation to occur with the onset of systole.

Early control devices required the operator to set the inflation and deflation points manually and did not function well when the patient's underlying cardiac rhythm was irregular or rapid. Currently available control consoles have sophisticated electronic circuitry that can automatically set the timing of inflation and deflation and can compensate for irregular cardiac rhythms and premature beats. This increased automation makes the operation of the console easier, but the operator must still evaluate the arterial pressure waveform to ensure that the automatically set timing is appropriate. The control console allows the operator to make adjustments in the inflation and deflation points. The balloon inflation should occur at the dicrotic notch of the aortic pressure tracing, and deflation should be seen just before the onset of the next systolic pressure upstroke. Figure 37-2 shows examples of both correct and incorrect timing.

The indications for intraaortic balloon counterpulsation (IABC) therapy can be divided into three broad classes: inadequate cardiac pump function, myocardial ischemia, and prophylactic uses. When IABC was first introduced into clinical practice, most patients who received this therapy were in cardiogenic shock. Increased experience with IABC and tech-

Indications for intraaortic balloon counterpulsation (IABC) can be divided into three broad categories: inadequate cardiac pump function, myocardial ischemia, and prophylactic uses.

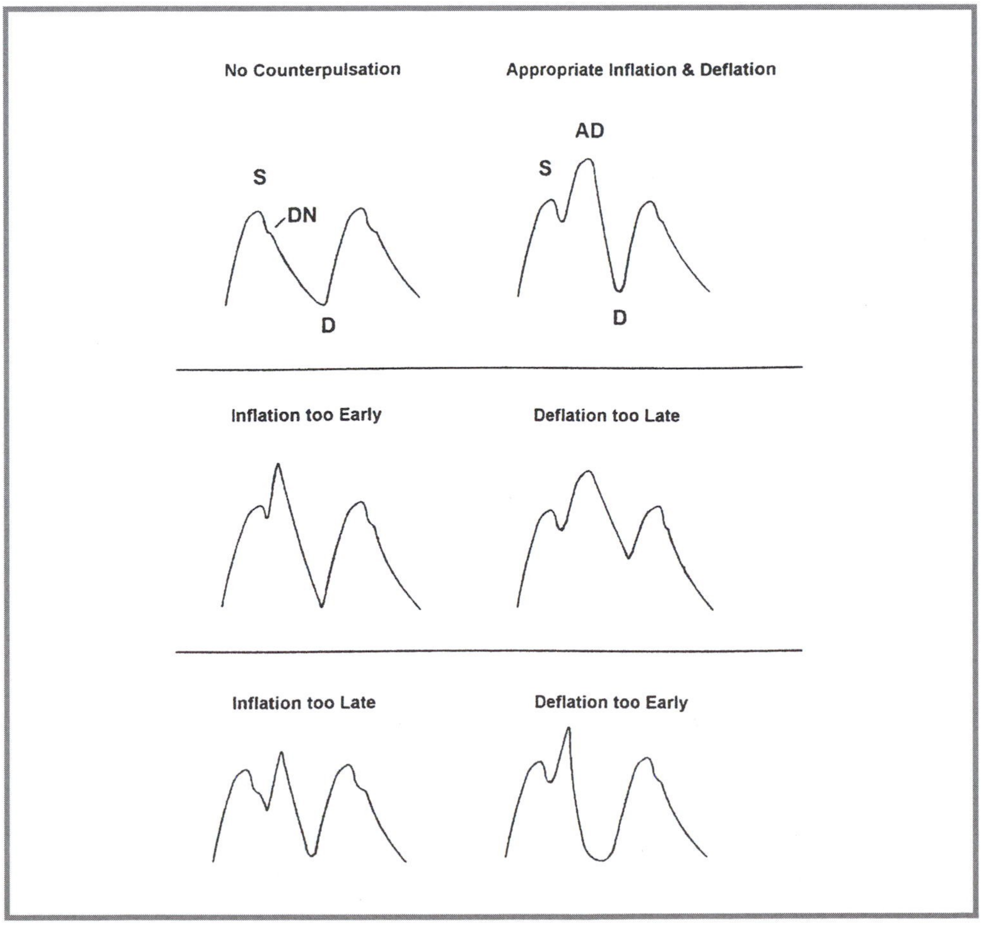

FIGURE 37-2

Arterial pressure waveforms in patient with correct IABC timing, late inflation, and early deflation. In the diagrams, counterpulsation, when present, is at a frequency of 1:2. S, systolic arterial pressure; D, diastolic arterial pressure; DN, dicrotic notch; AD, augmented diastolic pressure.

TABLE 37-1

INDICATIONS FOR INTRAAORTIC BALLOON COUNTERPULSATION

- Cardiogenic shock (failure of the heart as a pump) refractory to conventional therapy
  - Ventricular failure following myocardial infarction
  - Acute myocarditis
  - Acute mitral regurgitation with pulmonary edema and hemodynamic compromise
  - Acute ventricular septal defect
  - Cardiomyopathy (including bridge to transplant)
  - Postcardiotomy (inability to separate from cardiopulmonary bypass)
- Myocardial ischemia unrelieved with medical therapy
- Prophylactic uses
  - Support for patients with significant coronary artery disease, not amenable to revascularization, undergoing noncardiac surgery
  - Support for patients with severe valvular heart disease undergoing cardiac or noncardiac surgery
    - Left main coronary artery disease awaiting revascularization
    - Cardiomyopathy undergoing surgery (cardiac or noncardiac)
    - Support during high-risk cardiac catheterization and angioplasty

nologic advances have led to an increase in the use of IABC for the treatment of myocardial ischemia. Although the relative proportion of intraaortic balloon catheters placed for various indications varies from center to center, myocardial ischemia commonly accounts for 50% or more of indications (Table 37-1).

> The most significant contraindications to IABC are aortic insufficiency and aortic dissection or disruption.

The contraindications to IABC are mostly relative. The most significant contraindications include hemodynamically significant aortic insufficiency and aortic dissection or transection. Severe peripheral vascular disease, abdominal aortic aneurysm, prior aortoiliac-femoral surgery or bypass, sepsis, coagulopathy, or limited life expectancy related to terminal illness or malignancy are some of the relative contraindications. A decision about the use of IABC must weigh the risks of the procedure against its benefits, the risks and benefits of any alternative treatments, or no treatment.

> IABC inflation during diastole is associated with an increase in diastolic blood pressure in the proximal aorta and thus an increase in coronary artery perfusion pressure.

The inflation of the intraaortic balloon during diastole is associated with an increase in diastolic blood pressure in the proximal aorta and thus an increase in coronary artery perfusion pressure (diastolic blood pressure minus left ventricular end-diastolic pressure). The deflation of the balloon just before the onset of systole is equivalent to the removal of a volume of blood from the aorta equal to the volume of gas removed from the balloon. This decrease in central aortic volume with the onset of systole can facilitate left ventricular ejection into the aorta by reducing the left ventricular afterload. Balloon counterpulsation may also be associated with a decrease in left ventricular end-diastolic pressure. Intraaortic balloon counterpulsation is commonly associated with a small decrease in systemic systolic arterial pressure, an increase in systemic diastolic pressure, and variable changes in mean arterial pressure. In some patients the mean arterial pressure changes little while in others it increases. The net effect of IABC on systemic blood pressure is, to some extent, dependent on the reasons for institution of therapy. In hypotensive patients with cardiogenic shock, improvement in cardiac performance by IABC may result in an improvement in the systemic pressures. The elevated pulmonary artery and pulmonary capillary occlusion pressures seen in cardiogenic shock and severe myocardial ischemia may decrease if IABC improves the patient's ventricular performance or myocardial oxygen supply–demand balance. Cardiac output may increase between 500–800 ml/min. The overall beneficial effects of IABC may be limited by hypovolemia, a large aorta, an underfilled or undersized balloon, incorrect timing of balloon inflation and deflation, or frequent arrhythmias.

In theory, augmentation of diastolic blood pressure should lead to an increase in diastolic coronary artery blood flow. However, animal studies and clinical studies in humans have led to variable results. Experimental evidence that regional myocardial function improves in zones of marginal myocardial ischemic following experimental coronary occlusion has led some authors to suggest that this was indirect evidence of improvement in coronary perfusion. However, other authors using more direct measurements of coronary artery blood flow have not consistently been able to demonstrate an increase in coronary artery blood flow.

The methods used to measure or estimate coronary artery blood flow during counterpulsation therapy have included measurement of coronary artery blood flow velocity by doppler techniques (epicardial or endovascular) and the use of xeon washout techniques. In many studies the coronary blood flow distal to coronary artery lesions did not increase with IABC. One study reported that doppler blood flow velocity distal to coronary artery lesions was not changed by IABC before coronary angioplasty but did increase following successful angioplasty reduction in the coronary artery obstruction. Most studies support the theory that the relief of the signs and symptoms of myocardial ischemia by counterpulsation therapy is primarily a function of decreased myocardial oxygen demand secondary to afterload reduction induced by the counterpulsation therapy.

Myocardial ischemia refractory to maximum medical therapy is one of the major indications for the use of IABC. Institution of counterpulsation therapy frequently results in relief of the ischemia. As noted, it is likely that the reduction in myocardial oxygen demand is the most important reason for this improvement. Counterpulsation therapy alone can not provide definitive treatment for obstructive coronary artery disease but it can be an important adjunct therapy. The use of IABC may allow patients to undergo diagnostic catheterization and revascularization by either thrombolysis, coronary angioplasty, or surgical revascularization.

> The relief of signs and symptoms of myocardial ischemia by IABC is primarily a function of decreased myocardial oxygen demand secondary to afterload reduction induced by balloon deflation.

Another important indication for counterpulsation therapy is cardiogenic shock. Cardiogenic shock has many etiologies, including acute myocardial infarction, cardiomyopathy (idiopathic, ischemic, etc.), acute mitral regurgitation, acute ventricular septal defects, and other pathologic conditions leading to severe impairment of myocardial pump function. For patients with ventricular dysfunction who cannot be separated from cardiopulmonary bypass following cardiac surgery or who develop cardiogenic shock following a cardiac surgical procedure, IABC therapy may be useful.

Intraaortic balloon counterpulsation therapy is not a definitive treatment for cardiogenic shock. Counterpulsation therapy is a support modality that can provide hemodynamic support while treatment of the underlying pathophysiologic causes is instituted. For patients who have stunned myocardium following cardiac surgery, IABC can provide necessary assistance while the myocardium recovers. Many patients with cardiogenic shock complicating acute myocardial infarction show an initial benefit from IABC that diminishes over several days. In some patients it has been noted that, after an initial improvement in hemodynamic parameters, a progressive increase in mean pulmonary artery and pulmonary artery wedge pressures begins 24–48 h later; this most likely represents continuing deterioration in ventricular function in the face of continuing ischemia and infarction. Revascularization of some type (thrombolysis, angioplasty, surgery) may be necessary to preserve myocardial function in many of these patients. The use of IABC in community hospitals to stabilize a patient's condition for transfer to a hospital where revascularization procedures (angioplasty or surgery) are available has been shown to be a beneficial intervention. Aroesty and colleagues noted that without revascularization of some type, the mortality from cardiogenic shock complicating acute myocardial infarction remains as high as 85%.

> Cardiogenic shock counterpulsation therapy can provide hemodynamic support while treatment of the underlying pathophysiologic causes is instituted.

> Without revascularization of some type, the mortality from cardiogenic shock complicating acute myocardial infarction remains as high as 85%.

In the subset of patients with cardiogenic shock associated with myocardial infarction or ischemia, several patterns of response can be seen. Those patients with the best outcomes show reversal of the shock with IABC and with aggressive medical therapy may subsequently be weaned from IABC without further interventions. Another outcome group includes patients in whom the shock state is reversed during counterpulsation but who develop recurrent ischemia when attempts are made to wean from counterpulsation. The myocardium of these patients is still in jeopardy, and they require further interventions for revascularization (angioplasty, endocoronary stent placement, surgical revascularization). A third group of patients improves with counterpulsation and deteriorates when the therapy is weaned, but without signs of recurrent myocardial ischemia; these are patients with extensive myocardial damage. Use of aggressive medical therapies with inotropic agents and vasodilators may eventually allow these patients to be weaned from IABC. If medical therapy is not successful, a ventricular-assist device may be necessary to separate these patients from IABC. For these patients, heart transplantation may be necessary. The final group of patients includes those individuals who do not improve despite counterpulsation therapy. In the past, patients in this group would invariably die, but the use of ventricular-assist devices and heart transplantation has allowed some of these patients to survive.

Intraaortic balloon counterpulsation can also be employed prophylactically. Certain patients undergoing noncardiac surgical procedures may benefit from the application of IABC. Included among these patients are those with significant ischemic heart disease who are not able to undergo coronary artery revascularization before their noncardiac surgery, those with very poor ventricular function (cardiomyopathy), or those with advanced valvular heart disease. The reasons that would prevent coronary revascularization before noncardiac surgery are inoperable coronary artery disease, emergency need for the noncardiac surgery, and other factors precluding coronary artery bypass, such as severe coexisting disease. There are no controlled studies that have examined the prophylactic use of IABC in noncardiac surgery, but there are several case reports of such use. While IABC is an invasive procedure that carries with it the potential for significant complications, in selected high-risk patients it seems to be of benefit.

IABC may be beneficial as a support modality for some patients undergoing noncardiac surgery, such as those with inoperable coronary artery or valvular disease and those with cardiomyopathy.

There have also been studies on the benefit of prophylactic use of IABC in the setting of coronary angioplasty. The Second Primary Angioplasty in Myocardial Infarction (PAMI-II) Trial investigators (Stone and colleagues) reported on the results of the prophylactic use of IABC in patients with acute myocardial infarction who underwent acute coronary artery catheterization and percutaneous transluminal coronary angioplasty (PTCA). The patients who were stratified into a high-risk group based on angiographic data were randomized to receive either IABC for 36–48 h or no IABC therapy. Only patients who had no contraindication to IABC were randomized. In this study, IABC following PTCA did not decrease the rate of infarct-related coronary artery reocclusion or reinfarction, did not promote myocardial recovery, and did not change overall clinical outcome.

Intraaortic balloon counterpulsation can also be used as a short-term bridge to heart transplantation in patients with hemodynamic dysfunction not responsive to less invasive therapies. The use of IABC can allow aggressive pharmacologic therapies with subsequent separation from counterpulsation. Patients who cannot be separated from counterpulsation without deterioration in their condition may need ventricular-assist device support as a bridge to transplantation. Given that most patients will wait weeks to months for a heart transplant, the necessity for patients to remain immobile and at bedrest during counterpulsation therapy is a significant disadvantage of IABC in this group of patients.

Intraaortic Balloon Catheter Placement

Balloon counterpulsation therapy requires the placement of the balloon catheter into the descending thoracic aorta, usually accomplished by introducing the catheter via a femoral artery. Alternative sites for insertion have been described and are briefly discussed here. As with any other invasive procedure, it is important to carefully review the patient's history, physical examination, and pertinent laboratory studies. For patients about to undergo balloon catheterization, the history and physical examination should pay careful attention to signs and symptoms of peripheral vascular disease (e.g., claudication, foot ulcers, prior vascular surgical procedures, aortic aneurysm, dissection, or disruption), significant aortic regurgitation, and coagulation system problems. The pulses in the femoral, popliteal, dorsalis pedis, and posterior tibial arteries should be evaluated and the results recorded in the medical record.

In evaluating patients for IABC, the history and physical examination should pay careful attention to signs and symptoms of peripheral vascular disease, aortic insufficiency, or coagulation system abnormality.

Balloon catheters are available from a variety of manufacturers and in a variety of sizes. The catheters used for adults generally range in size from 8 to 11 Fr. in diameter and have balloon volumes of 30–40 ml. The inflated balloon should, ideally, occupy 80%–90% of the aortic diameter. The size of the catheter chosen is based on the size of the patient.

A complete discussion of the placement of an intraaortic balloon catheter is beyond the scope of this chapter, but a brief description of the technique is presented. Strict adherence to aseptic technique is essential to minimize infectious complications. The puncture site should be disinfected with an appropriate agent such as an iodophore or chlorhexadine solution. Full barrier precautions should be used with all operators wearing a surgical cap, mask, and sterile gown and gloves. Sterile drapes should be used to create a large working field. The procedure is most commonly performed under local anesthesia using a percutaneous approach to the common femoral artery. Care should be taken to ensure that the arterial puncture occurs inferior to the inguinal ligament (common femoral artery). Superior to the inguinal ligament, the artery is the external iliac artery, and bleeding from the puncture site at this level may result in retroperitoneal hemorrhage.

The common femoral artery is punctured with a needle, and a flexible guidewire is placed through the needle and advanced into the descending thoracic aorta. Fluoroscopic guidance is commonly used to identify the position of the guidewire. During intraoperative or bedside placement without fluoroscopic guidance, an external measurement of the distance from the femoral artery puncture site to the sternal notch is used as an estimate of the distance to insert the guidewire and subsequently the balloon catheter. After placement of the guidewire, the needle is removed and a series of vessel dilators are sequentially passed over the wire into the artery to enlarge the puncture site. The last free dilator is removed, and a dilator within an introducer sheath is then placed into the artery; this dilator is removed, and the balloon catheter is placed over the guidewire through the introducer sheath and advanced until the tip of the catheter is positioned just below the aortic knob on fluoroscopic examination. Confirmation of the presence of an arterial pulse in the left arm indicates that the tip of the catheter is not occluding the origin of the left subclavian artery. If the catheter was placed without fluoroscopic guidance, a chest X-ray should be obtained to identify the position of the catheter. The tip of the catheter should be seen 1–2 cm distal to the aortic knob. The femoral puncture site should be routinely checked for signs of bleeding or local infection.

When correctly positioned, the tip of the balloon catheter should be 1–2 cm below the aortic knob on radiographic examination of the chest.

Following catheter placement, the neurovascular integrity of the limb distal to the insertion site must be frequently evaluated. Periodic neurovascular checks should include palpation of peripheral pulses or assessment of the pulses by use of doppler ultrasound, determination of the temperature, color, and capillary refill in the extremity, and demonstration of intact sensory and motor function. The evaluation should include both the limb distal to the insertion site and comparison with the examination of the contralateral limb. This determination should be made every hour for the first several hours after insertion and then every 1–2 h for the duration of counterpulsation therapy. If there is any indication of ischemia, the patient should undergo further evaluation; evaluation by a vascular surgeon should be considered. Low cardiac output, hypothermia, and high-dose vasopressor therapy may also lead to decreased limb perfusion. Correcting these contributing factors may improve perfusion of the limb.

The neuromuscular integrity of the limb distal to the balloon catheter insertion site must be frequently evaluated. If there is evidence of limb ischemia, further evaluation is required and evaluation by a vascular surgeon should be considered.

It is a common practice to administer intravenous heparin to the patient by continuous infusion to prevent clot formation on the surface of the balloon or in the arterial tree distal to the balloon insertion site. The dose is adjusted to maintain an activated partial thromboplastin time (APTT) 1.5–2 fold the control value. Heparin is commonly not given to surgical patients in the early postoperative period because of the associated risk of bleeding from the surgical sites. Some physicians have advocated the use of low molecular weight dextran infusion in patients in whom heparin cannot be used, but there are no published studies demonstrating that this is beneficial.

In patients in whom femoral artery placement is not possible, usually because of peripheral vascular disease, consider alternative sites. In the operating room, following cardiac surgery, several techniques for placement of an intraaortic balloon pump via the ascending aorta into the descending thoracic aorta have been described. In one technique an end-to-side anastamosis is created between a synthetic graft and the ascending aorta. The distal end of the graft is brought through the anterior chest or abdominal wall and the balloon catheter is inserted through the graft into the aorta. This technique allows percutaneous removal of the catheter under local anesthesia. In many patients, this percutaneous removal can be accomplished in the critical care unit. The axillary artery has also been used as an alternative site for intraaortic balloon catheter placement. Axillary artery placement is generally performed with a surgical approach to the artery that allows the cannulation of the axillary artery under direct vision.

Following successful positioning of the intraaortic balloon catheter, counterpulsation therapy is instituted. The timing of the counterpulsation is adjusted as previously described. While undergoing IABC, the patient must remain at bedrest. If the catheter was placed into a femoral artery, the ipsilateral leg must remain straight to prevent kinking of the catheter or injury to the artery. The head of the bed should be kept flat or, at most, elevated to less than 30°. The patient requires good nursing care to prevent the development of pressure ulceration because of immobility.

Weaning from Counterpulsation Support

When IABC has been instituted to treat hemodynamic instability, it is common to wait until the need for pharmacologic support has substantially decreased.

Weaning from IABC can begin when the underlying disease process that led to the institution of IABC has improved. When IABC has been instituted to treat hemodynamic instability, it is common to wait until the need for pharmacologic inotropic support has substantially decreased. The specific criteria that the patient should meet before weaning is attempted varies among physicians. Some physicians advocate waiting until the patient is receiving, at most, a moderate dose of a single inotropic agent; others allow a combination of inotropic agents but require that the infusion rates be below a specific target range. Common to all approaches is the appraisal that myocardial function has improved and a demonstration that the level of pharmacologic inotropic support has been successfully reduced; this allows a margin of safety in the event of hemodynamic deterioration after the removal of the balloon catheter because pharmacologic support can be increased. In patients in whom IABC has been instituted to treat myocardial ischemia, decisions about weaning are related to the institution of medical therapy aimed at preventing or treating myocardial ischemia or interventions that improve coronary artery blood flow (angioplasty or coronary artery bypass surgery).

IABC therapy can be weaned by either decreasing the frequency of balloon inflation or by decreasing the volume of balloon inflation.

When the patient meets the criteria for weaning from IABC, two alternative strategies are available. In the first method, the frequency of balloon inflation is decreased from inflation with every heartbeat to every second, third, or fourth beat or more. Some balloon pump consoles allow counterpulsation ratios as high as 1:8. In the second method, balloon inflation continues with every heartbeat, but the volume of balloon inflation is decreased to provide less blood displacement with each inflation. Advocates of the later technique (reducing the volume within the balloon with each inflation) believe that this provides a more physiologically appropriate trial of weaning. It is the practice in the cardiothoracic surgical intensive care unit at Temple University Hospital to wean by decreasing the assist frequency from 1:1 to 1:2 to 1:3. Assist ratios of 1:3 or greater probably do not provide much hemodynamic support, and therefore trials beyond a ratio of 1:3 are not necessary. The rate at which weaning proceeds is based on the patient's overall status and the reasons for which the balloon catheter was inserted. During the period of weaning, careful assessment of the patient's clinical condition must be made to identify any deterioration in clinical status with reduction in IABC. If there is a deterioration (hemodynamic or cardiac ischemic), counterpulsation support should be increased to reverse the deterioration. With lower pumping frequencies (1:3 and above), there is an increased concern that thrombus will form on the surface of the catheter. It is our practice to limit the amount of time at a pumping frequency of 1:3 to 1–2 h; this is of special concern in patients not receiving systemic anticoagulation.

Before removal of an intraaortic balloon catheter, the patient's coagulation parameters should be in an acceptable range to assure adequate hemostasis.

Catheters that are place surgically should be removed by a surgical approach. If the balloon catheter was placed percutaneously without problems and if the puncture site appears to be below the inguinal ligament, the balloon catheter can usually be safely removed at the patient's bedside. Before removal, coagulation parameters (activated partial thromboplastin time, prothrombin time, platelet count) should be in an acceptable range to assure adequate hemostasis. For patients who have been receiving heparin therapy, the heparin should be discontinued before the assessment of the APTT. Counterpulsation is stopped, and the balloon catheter is deflated following the manufacturer's recommendations. Immediately before removal, the balloon catheter can be pulled back until it engages the introducer sheath. No attempts should be made to pull the balloon catheter into the introducer sheath because this could result in shearing off a portion of the balloon. Pressure is applied over the femoral artery distal to the puncture site to try to prevent debris or thrombus from entering the distal arterial tree; then the balloon catheter is gently withdrawn from the artery. Blood is allowed to spurt briefly from the puncture site in an attempt to flush debris out the puncture site. Pressure is then applied at the puncture site, and the distal pressure is released. The pressure should be firm enough to provide hemostasis at the puncture site but not so firm as to completely occlude the femoral artery. Continuous pressure is maintained for 30–45 min. If after 30–45 min hemostasis has been achieved, a sandbag is placed over the puncture site for an additional 6–8 h, during which time the patient must keep the leg straight.

Before placement of the sandbag and periodically during the time it is in place, the puncture site should be inspected for evidence of bleeding or hematoma formation. The distal arterial pulses in the leg should be assessed at regular intervals during and after balloon catheter removal. In the event that bleeding persists after the initial 30- to 45-min period, pressure should be held over the site for an additional 30–45 min. If a hematoma forms or if there is recurrent bleeding, consideration should be given to obtaining a noninvasive vascular assessment (duplex ultrasonography) of the involved femoral artery to identify if a pseudoaneurysm has developed. If bleeding is persistent or if pseudoaneurysm formation is noted, a vascular surgery evaluation should be obtained, as is discussed further below. Several mechanical devices can be used to provide compression of the artery after balloon catheter removal. These devices can be effective and save time for staff, but their use requires careful attention to the manufacturer's recommendations for safe use to prevent injury to the patient.

Complications of Balloon Counterpulsation

Intraaortic balloon counterpulsation is a beneficial therapy in appropriate conditions and in many patients may be a lifesaving intervention; however, it is an invasive procedure and carries with it the potential for complications from minor to life-threatening. Many studies have reported on the complications of IABC. The overall rate of complications ranges from approximately 10% to 30%, with most complications being vascular in nature, especially ischemic complications of a lower limb. Table 37-2 lists the types of complications associated with IABC.

The overall rate of complications ranges from approximately 10% to 30%, with most complications being vascular in nature, especially ischemic complications of a lower limb.

Lower limb ischemia is the predominant complication of IABC. In a retrospective review of 436 patients treated with IABC, Makhoul and colleagues reported that limb ischemia developed in 40 patients (9%) and accounted for 87% of all complications in their patients. Barnette and colleagues reported that ipsilateral limb ischemia occurred in nearly 12% of the 580 patients they reviewed. In more than 80% of these patients, the ischemia was resolved. Limb ischemia that does not resolve with treatment or which is identified or treated too late may lead to the amputation of the involved limb. The risk of limb amputation as a complication of IABC was approximately 1% in several large series. Other vascular complications such as aortic, iliac, or femoral artery dissection or rupture can also occur.

A variety of factors increase the risk of complications of IABC (Table 37-3). The most consistent risk factor has been the presence of peripheral vascular disease. Female gender, diabetes mellitus, and smoking history have also been identified in several studies. Percutaneous insertion has been found to be associated with fewer complications in many studies, although at least one group reported a lower incidence of complications with open surgical placement. The introduction of the balloon catheter without the use of an insertion sheath (sheathless insertion) may be associated with fewer complications because the diameter of

The most consistent risk factor for complications during IABC has been the presence of peripheral vascular disease.

TABLE 37-2

COMPLICATIONS OF INTRAAORTIC BALLOON COUNTERPULSATION

Vascular	Balloon rupture
Limb ischemia	Balloon catheter entrapment
Amputation	Helium embolism
Arterial dissection or rupture (femoral, iliac, aortic)	Neurologic
Embolism of atheromatous material (limb, kidney, gut, etc.)	Paraplegia
Mesenteric ischemia	Stroke
Pseudoaneurysm formation	Neuropathy
Bleeding	Thrombocytopenia
Insertion site	Infection
Retroperitoneal	Localized
Ruptured major vessel	Sepsis

TABLE 37-3

RISK FACTORS FOR COMPLICATIONS OF BALLOON PUMP THERAPY

Peripheral vascular disease	Low cardiac index
Female gender	Duration of therapy
Diabetes mellitus	Insertion via introducer sheath
Smoking history	Catheter size
Catheter size	

the balloon catheter alone is less than the diameter of the introducer sheath and therefore obstruction of the ileofemoral artery should be less. However, not all published reports have shown a benefit to sheathless insertion. The common occurrence of limb ischemia and the potentially serious problems that can develop emphasize the need for careful history and physical examination of patients undergoing balloon catheter insertion. Likewise, regular monitoring of the patients for evidence of limb ischemia during IABC is essential to allow early identification and treatment.

In patients with a clear history of severe peripheral vascular disease or physical evidence suggesting its presence in the lower extremities, an alternative site of placement should be considered. An axillary approach can be considered in both medical and surgical patients but a transthoracic approach is limited to cardiac surgical patients. Hazelrigg and colleagues published a retrospective review of 100 patients in whom transthoracic catheters were placed during cardiac surgery and reported no episodes of lower limb ischemia. They found that the incidence of mediastinal bleeding and balloon rupture was higher in these patients than in similar patients with femoral artery placement of catheters.

Once ischemia has been identified, it can usually be resolved by a therapeutic intervention. Naunheim and colleagues (in another analysis of the patients reported by Barnette and colleagues) reported that for the 69 patients with limb ischemia in their series of 580 patients, the ischemia resolved in 21 patients with catheter removal alone, in another 21 patients with surgical thrombectomy, and in 13 patients following a vascular repair. Two patients required a fasciotomy, and in 2 patients the ischemia resolved without intervention. In 10 patients (14%) the ischemia was not resolved; 6 patients died with the catheter in place without intervention, and 4 patients underwent amputations. In this study, survival was not affected by the occurrence of balloon pump-related complications.

If the patient develops ischemic vascular complications, the balloon catheter should be removed if clinical assessment suggests the patient no longer needs IABC.

If the patient develops ischemic vascular complications, the balloon catheter should be removed if clinical assessment suggests that the patient no longer needs IABC; this can be by percutaneous removal at the bedside or by surgical removal under direct vision with possible thrombectomy of the involved artery. There is no universal approach to this problem. Because many episodes of ischemia will resolve with removal of the catheter, a staged approach with percutaneous removal followed by surgical exploration if the ischemia does not resolve with catheter removal is a common approach. Because of the serious consequences that can develop from this problem, it is beneficial to consult a vascular surgeon. Some patients, especially those with evidence of significant peripheral vascular disease or severe ischemia, may benefit most from surgical removal and thrombectomy as the initial approach.

For the patient with limb ischemia who continues to require IABC, one option is to remove the catheter and place a new one into the opposite femoral artery (or an alternative site). Another alternative is to provide perfusion distal to the catheter insertion site by performing a femorofemoral arterial bypass using a conduit graft from the contralateral femoral artery to the ipsilateral femoral artery distal to the catheter insertion site.

Bleeding, another complication of IABC, can occur at the insertion site or more proximally if the catheter has injured the artery. Insertion of the balloon catheter above the inguinal ligament (external iliac artery) can cause bleeding into the retroperitoneal space because of vessel injury during insertion or when the catheter is removed. It is difficult to apply pressure over the artery at this site, and bleeding into the retroperitoneal space cannot be seen on physical examination. If there is concern that the catheter has been placed into the artery above the inguinal ligament, the catheter should be removed surgically. For a patient with an unexplained decline in hemoglobin during or after IABC therapy, evaluation for retroperitoneal hemorrhage with a CT scan should be considered.

Patients who bleed excessively after catheter removal or who develop hematomas at the insertion site are at risk for pseudoaneurysm formation, which can be diagnosed by duplex ultrasound examination. In some cases it is possible to eliminate the pseudoaneurysm by direct compression with the ultrasound probe. If direct compression is not effective, surgical repair is necessary.

Patients who bleed excessively after catheter removal or who develop hematomas at the insertion site are at risk for pseudoaneurysm formation.

Neurologic complications can also occur. Stroke has been reported and may be a more common complication with placement via the ascending aorta or aortic arch. A stroke rate of 6.2% and a transient ischemic attack rate of 1.2% were reported for ascending aortic balloon catheter placement in a retrospective review by Hazelrigg and colleagues. Stroke occurred in only 1 patient in a prospective series of 691 patients with percutaneous femoral artery placement reported by Patel and colleagues. Flushing of the central lumen of the catheter, which is located in the proximal descending aorta, can cause cerebral embolism of air, thrombus, or debris. The central lumen should not be used routinely to draw blood samples and should be flushed only if absolutely necessary. Great care should be exercised to ensure that all air bubbles have been removed from the system before the system is flushed, and only gentle pressure should be used during the flush.

Neurologic complications that can occur related to IABC include stroke, paraplegia, and peripheral neuropathy.

Paraplegia has been reported as a complication of IABC. Stavridis and colleagues found 12 published cases of paraplegia developing during or after IABC. Two main mechanisms of injury were reported: aortic dissection and spinal artery embolism. Aortic dissection or adventitial hematoma can lead to interruption of spinal cord blood supply. Local occlusion of a major anterior spinal artery by the embolism of atheromatous material from the aorta can be induced by the balloon catheter.

Another type of neurologic complication is peripheral neuropathy. Local trauma at the insertion site, either as direct nerve injury during catheter placement or as a result of nerve compression from hematoma formation, can occur. Ischemic neuropathy can develop in patients who develop impaired limb perfusion.

Infection, either local or systemic, can occur. Similar to other invasive intravascular devices, the likelihood of sepsis developing is related to the duration of catheterization. The use of sterile technique during insertion and good site care during IABC may limit this complication. Fever or sepsis in a patient with an intraaortic balloon catheter should prompt examination of the site for evidence of local infection. If there is local evidence of infection at the site or if bacteremia develops, it may be necessary to change the balloon catheter to an alternative site or, if it is no longer needed, to remove it.

Other complications of IABC include infection, rupture of the balloon catheter, helium embolism, balloon entrapment, thrombocytopenia, and embolism of atheromatous material.

Rupture of the intraaortic balloon is another possible complication, usually detected by observing the presence of blood in the helium drive line tubing. The balloon rupture is usually related to perforation of the balloon by abrasion against an atherosclerotic plaque in the aorta; this appears to be more common in smaller patients where a portion of the balloon catheter may more commonly be located in the distal thoracic or proximal abdominal aorta. The defects detected in the balloons by microscopy are usually very small pinhole perforations.

A major concern with perforation of the balloon is the risk of helium embolism. The characteristics of the balloon and drive mechanism (relatively low gas pressure during balloon inflation and large negative intraballoon pressure during deflation) favor the entrance of blood into the balloon rather than helium escape into the patient. However, a helium embolism can occur and if it travels to the cerebral circulation can result in a stroke.

Balloon rupture can be associated with balloon entrapment within the vascular tree. Numerous cases of balloon rupture and inability to remove the balloon because of entrapment have been reported. Forceful attempts at removing the trapped catheter can result in serious vascular trauma. The entrapment usually occurs because of the presence of clotted or desiccated blood within the balloon. There have been case reports of introducing thrombolytic agents into the balloon via the drive line to dissolve the clots within the balloon that are causing the entrapment.

Because of the potentially serious complications of balloon rupture an aggressive approach to management is necessary. If blood is noted in the drive line tubing, balloon inflation should be stopped immediately, and the balloon catheter should be removed. If the patient requires continued IABC, a new balloon catheter can be placed into the opposite femoral artery (or alternative site), or a guidewire exchange of the defective catheter for a new catheter can be performed. If any resistance is encountered when removing the defective catheter, the removal attempt should be stopped and a surgical removal performed. As noted, intraballoon catheter thrombolytic therapy may be a useful adjunct to surgical removal.

Thrombocytopenia is commonly seen in patients undergoing IABC. Vonderheide and colleagues published a prospective comparison of patients with acute coronary syndromes treated with heparin, some of whom had IABC. They reported that thrombocytopenia occurred in 47% of IABC patients compared with 12% of non-IABC patients. Platelet counts declined by at least 50% in 26% of the IABC group compared with only 4% of the control group. The platelet counts rose rapidly following discontinuation of the balloon pump, with normalization within 4 days. These authors also noted that for patients with prolonged counterpulsation the decline in platelet count leveled off or improved after 4 days. It is believed that increased consumption or destruction of platelets by the balloon catheter accounts for the decline; increased platelet production may explain the leveling off of the decline after 4 days.

Balloon catheters can precipitate embolism of atherosclerotic material. Patients with mobile atherosclerotic material in the aorta have been found to be at greater risk for these complications. Embolism can involve the peripheral vascular tree, the kidney, intestine, spinal cord, or other organs.

The use of IABC has also been reported to be a risk factor for the development of gastrointestinal complications including mesenteric ischemia, gastrointestinal hemorrhage, pancreatitis, and cholecystitis. Intraaortic balloon counterpulsation was not necessarily the cause of all the gastrointestinal problems reported, but rather may have served as a marker of patients who were more critically ill.

VENTRICULAR-ASSIST DEVICES

When pharmacologic therapies and intraaortic balloon counterpulsation are not successful in restoring an adequate hemodynamic condition, circulatory support with a mechanical blood pumping device can be considered.

When pharmacologic therapies and intraaortic balloon counterpulsation are not successful in restoring an adequate hemodynamic condition, circulatory support with a mechanical blood pumping device can be considered. In current practice, mechanical ventricular-assist devices (VADs) are used to treat cardiogenic shock, either as a support device until ventricular function can recover and the device can be discontinued, or as a bridge to heart transplantation. Patients who cannot be separated from cardiopulmonary bypass following a cardiac surgical procedure (postcardiotomy) because of ventricular dysfunction (left, right, or biventricular) are the largest group of patients in whom VAD therapy is used as a recovery modality. Indications and contraindications are discussed in more detail.

The choice of mechanical cardiac assist device depends on the type of ventricular support needed, the expected duration of support anticipated, and patient characteristics such as size, weight, and concomitant diseases.

A variety of options are available for ventricular assist device support. The choice of device depends on the type of ventricular support needed, the expected duration of support anticipated, and patient characteristics such as size, weight, and concomitant diseases. LVAD, RVAD, and BiVAD are used here to refer to assist devices implanted to support the left ventricle, the right ventricle, or both ventricles, respectively.

Abiomed BVS 5000

The dual-chamber, pneumatically driven Abiomed BVS 5000 can be used as an LVAD, RVAD, or BiVAD.

The Abiomed BVS 5000 Bi-Ventricular Support System (Abiomed Cardiovascular, Inc., Danvers, MA, USA) is a pneumatically powered, pulsatile, ventricular-assist device that is approved for the treatment of postcardiotomy ventricular dysfunction. It can be used as an LVAD, RVAD, or BiVAD. The device must be placed surgically and usually requires the use of cardiopulmonary bypass during the placement. Figure 37-3 illustrates the dual chamber design of the blood path within the pump, which consists of an upper collecting chamber (atrium) and a lower pumping chamber (ventricle). The device contains two tri-leaflet valves that maintain unidirectional blood flow. One valve is between the collecting chamber and

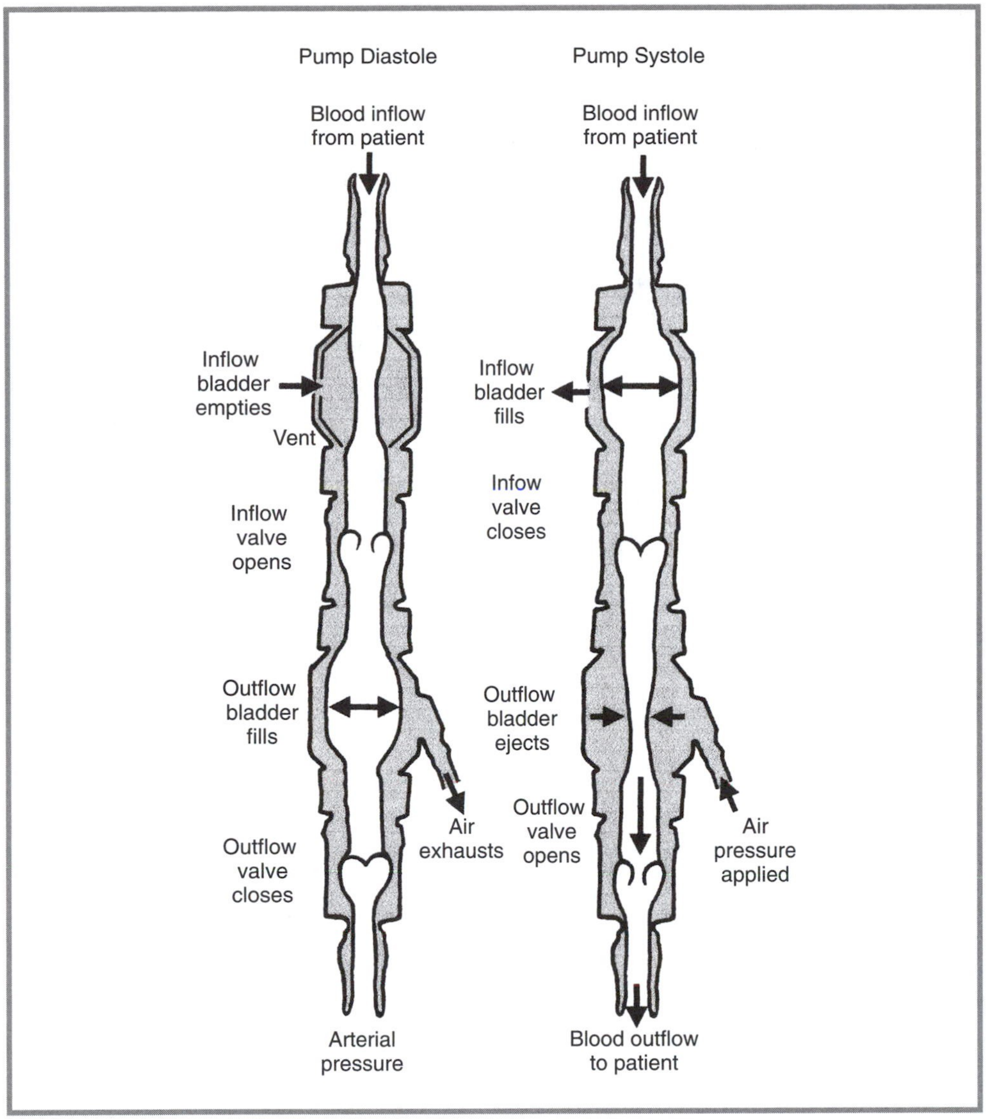

FIGURE 37-3

Cross-sectional diagram of the Abiomed® BVS 5000®. (From ABIOMED, Inc., with permission.)

the pumping chamber (the inflow valve) and the other valve is between the pumping chamber and the patient (outflow valve).

To configure the device for LVAD support, a cannula is placed into the patient's left atrium; tubing connects the cannula to the upper chamber of the device. Blood returns to the patient through tubing connected between the pumping chamber and a cannula attached to the patient's ascending aorta. This final connection involves the creation of an anastomosis between the patient's aorta and a polyester graft that is an integral part of the arterial cannula. For use as an RVAD, a cannula is placed into the patient's right atrium with the return connection being an anastomosis between the arterial cannula and the patient's pulmonary artery. The atrial and arterial cannulae are designed so that they exit the body via subcostal stab wounds, allowing for surgical closure of the chest. The cannulae have an external polyester sleeve to aid in hemostasis at the exit site and decrease the risk of infection. Biventricular support is obtained by placing both an RVAD and an LVAD. A single drive console can control two separate pumps (Figure 37-4). The drive console functions automatically and requires little operator intervention; it has a variety of alarms to alert caregivers of problems.

During VAD support, the blood flows from the patient through the atrial cannula and tubing into the upper chamber of the device. Blood collects in this chamber during the VAD systolic phase when the inflow valve is closed. During the VAD diastolic phase the inflow valve opens when the pressure in the upper chamber exceeds that in the lower chamber and

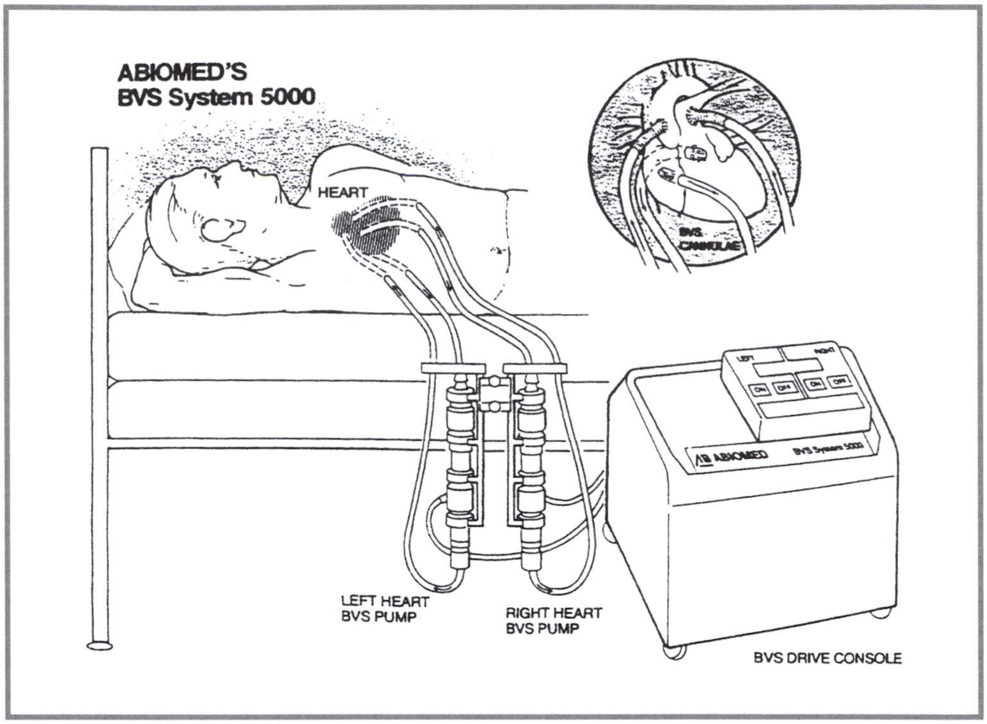

FIGURE 37-4

The Abiomed® BVS 5000® configured for biventricular support. (From ABIOMED, Inc., with permission.)

blood fills the pumping chamber. Filling of both the upper collecting chamber (atrium) and lower pumping chamber (ventricular) is passive and depends on the distance between the patient's atrium and the device. As the pumping chamber fills with blood, air is displaced into the drive console. When the drive console senses that the pumping chamber is full, the displaced air in the drive line is compressed and pushed back into the rigid shell surrounding the pumping chamber. With the external pressurization of the pumping chamber, the pressure within the pumping chamber increases, and the inflow valve closes, and the outflow valve opens, at which time blood is propelled from the device back to the patient through the arterial (aortic or pulmonary arterial) cannula. The rate of pumping is dependent on the rate at which the device fills with blood.

Use of this device can result in pulsatile flow up to 5 l/min. The control console attempts to maintain the pump stroke volume between 70 and 80 ml. Because of gravitational effects, the vertical distance between the patient and the pump controls both filling of the device (preload) and some of the resistance to pumping blood back to the patient (afterload). If the pump is too far below the patient's atrium, pump filling may be impaired because of collapse of the atrium around the cannula. Pump function may also be impaired because the height that the pump must overcome to return blood to the patient exceeds the capabilities of the drive console.

This device requires systemic anticoagulation to prevent clot formation in the pump and tubing. Anticoagulation with heparin is instituted postoperatively when bleeding related to the implantation of the pump is controlled. The manufacturer recommends that anticoagulation therapy not be delayed longer than 24 h, if possible, and suggests adjusting the heparin dose to keep the activated clotting time (ACT) between 180 and 200 s. When it is time to wean the patient from the device, the control console allows the flow rate of the pump to be limited; this allows assessment of the patient's hemodynamic status as the heart assumes more responsibility for the circulation of the blood. Removal of the device requires operative removal of the cannulae.

Jett reported the Baylor University experience with the Abiomed device in 25 patients with postcardiotomy cardiogenic shock. The complications reported were as follows: bleeding (40%), reoperation (20%), respiratory (50%), renal (30%), neurologic (30%), infection (20%), hemolysis (10%), and embolism (0%). The mean duration of support was 6.2 days.

Sixty percent of the patients were weaned from VAD support and 27% were discharged from the hospital. The patients who were discharged were New York Heart Association Functional Class I at follow-up.

Guyton and colleagues reported the results of a multicenter prospective trial of the use of the Abiomed device for postcardiotomy shock. Thirty-one patients met all criteria for inclusion in this study. The overall survival to discharge was 29%. Survival to discharge was 47% in VAD-supported patients who did not have a cardiac arrest before beginning VAD support, but only 7% for patients who had a cardiac arrest before institution of VAD support.

In the report by Guyton and colleagues, bleeding was the most common postoperative complication occurring in 76% of the patients. Other complications included respiratory failure (54%), renal failure (52%), permanent neurologic deficit (26%), hemolysis (17%), and embolism (13%). There were no reports of device-related respiratory failure, renal failure, or neurologic deficits. Three-quarters of the neurologic deficits were believed to have occurred before placement of the device. Because of the critically ill nature of these patients before institution of VAD therapy, many of these complications may have been related to postcardiotomy shock and not to the use of the device. The patients were all moribund at entry into the study; therefore, the overall outcome with the use of the device in this circumstance was favorable.

Bleeding is the most common postoperative complication reported with the Abiomed system.

HeartMate VAD

The HeartMate Vented Electric (VE) and Pneumatic (IP) left ventricular assist system (Thermo Cardiosystems, Inc., Woburn, MA, USA) are pulsatile pumps that can be used only as an LVAD (Figure 37-5). The systems are approved for VAD support as a bridge to cardiac transplantation and are contraindicated in patients with a body surface area of less than 1.5 m^2. The electric device is currently undergoing a clinical trial as a long-term treatment for end-stage cardiomyopathy in patients not suitable for heart transplantation.

There are two versions of the HeartMate device, one powered by an electrical motor within the device and the other pneumatically driven by an external drive console. The pump, characterized as a pusher plate design, consists of a titanium housing that is divided in half in-

The HeartMate ventricular-assist device can only be used as an LVAD. It has textured polyurethane and titanium surfaces to encourage the formation of a pseudoneointima that decreases the risk of thromboembolic events.

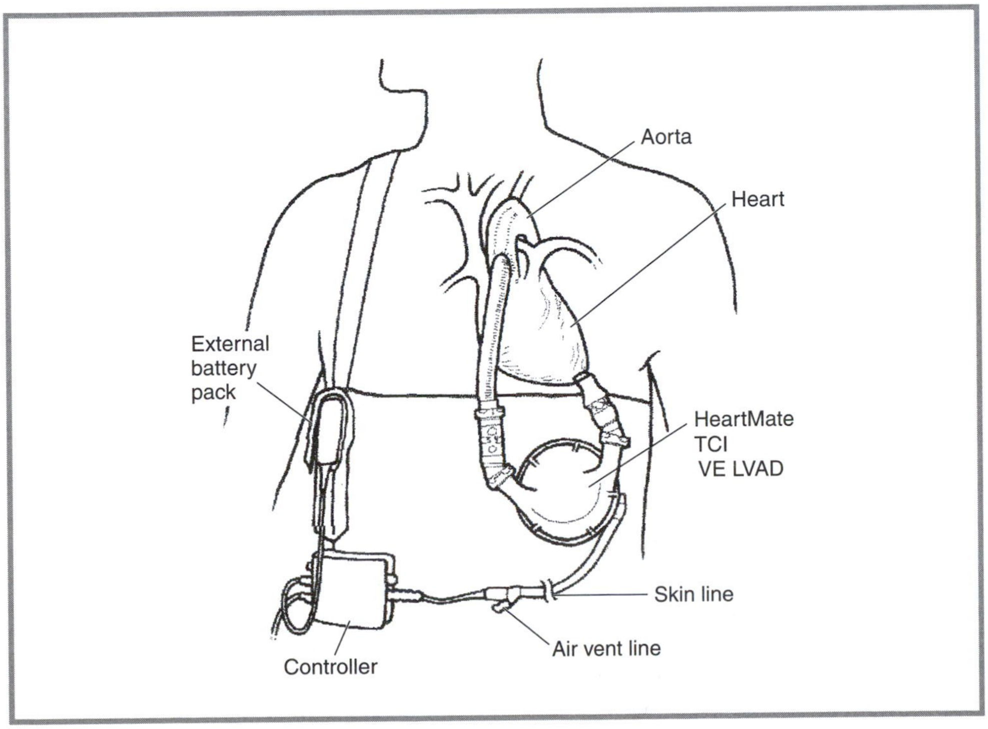

FIGURE 37-5

The TCI HeartMate (vented electric version). (Courtesy of Thermo Cardiosystems Inc.)

ternally by a textured polyurethane diaphragm attached to the pusher plate. The diaphragm divides the blood-containing portion of the pump from the drive portion (either pneumatic chamber or electric motor). Unidirectional flow is maintained by porcine xenograft inflow and outflow valves. The surface of the inlet cannula and the housing are covered with sintered titanium microspheres. The textured polyurethane and titanium surfaces encourage the deposition of a fibrin–cellular matrix from the patient's blood; this process leads to the formation of a pseudoneointima on the blood-contacting surfaces and decreases the risk of thromboembolic events.

The HeartMate device must be implanted surgically and requires cardiopulmonary bypass during the implantation. The pump is implanted in the left upper quadrant of the abdomen, either in the preperitoneal space or the intraperitoneal space. The inflow of blood from the patient to the pump is through a cannula placed into the apex of the left ventricle. Blood returns to the patient from the pump through a synthetic graft attached to the outflow valve. An anastomosis is created between the polyester outflow graft and the patient's ascending aorta to complete the circuit. In the electric device, a power cable and air vent line are brought externally through a separate skin incision. For the pneumatic device, the pneumatic drive line is brought externally in a similar fashion. The entire pump is contained within the body; only the power cable vent or pneumatic drive line passes externally. The device can generate a stroke volume of approximately 85 ml with a blood flow up to 10 l/min. The electric device is connected to an external electronic controller and power source. The power source can use household current or batteries. The pneumatic device is connected to an electronically controlled pneumatic drive console.

The device (either electric or pneumatic) can work in either a fixed rate or automatic mode. The automatic (fill-to-empty mode) is most commonly used. In this mode the pumping chamber is emptied by displacement of the pusher plate when the controller senses that the chamber is full. The two valves ensure unidirectional, antegrade blood flow. The rate of pumping in this mode is determined by the rate at which the pumping chamber fills. The device is not synchronized with the patient's intrinsic heartbeat, but the intrinsic right ventricular cardiac output is responsible for pumping blood through the pulmonary circulation into the left atrium and ventricle, from which it will enter the device. The LVAD rate is therefore indirectly related to the patient's intrinsic right heart function.

Both the electric and pneumatic HeartMate VADs can operate on batteries and thus allow the patient to ambulate.

Both the electric and pneumatic versions of the device allow patients to ambulate and both can operate on batteries. The pneumatic device, which requires that the patient remain connected to the pneumatic drive console, provides some limitation of mobility for the patient. There is also a finite period of time the pneumatic drive console can remain disconnected from an electrical outlet. The electric device can be disconnected from the power console so long as batteries are available to power the device. The batteries and controller are relatively small and can be placed in a harness the patient wears. This arrangement allows the patient to have greater freedom of movement. Both devices can also be actuated manually in the event of a controller or pneumatic console failure. In the event of a motor failure, the electric device can be connected to a pneumatic drive console and be actuated pneumatically.

Patients who receive the electric device can be discharged home when they have recovered from the implantation. The patient and support personnel (family and friends) are trained to provide routine care for the cable exit sites and to deal with VAD malfunction. Patients with the device can return to most activities of daily living, including work, school, and social activities.

The HeartMate device has been shown to have a low risk of thromboembolic events.

Poirier, in a report of the worldwide clinical results with the use of the HeartMate system, identified that the average duration of device support was 120 days (range, 24–416) in patients undergoing heart transplantation. The complication rates with both pneumatic and electric devices were similar, with bleeding, infection, and renal complications being among the most common complications. The incidence of hemolysis was low (pneumatic, 4%; electric, 0%). The device has shown a low incidence of thromboembolism in most studies. Slater and colleagues reported an incidence of 2.7% for thromboembolic events in 223 patients treated with the HeartMate as a bridge to transplant over 531.2 patient-months of LVAD support. Ninety-eight percent of the aggregate treatment months reported were without warfarin therapy. Only 23 patients received warfarin at any time during VAD support. The event rate for thromboembolism in this study was 0.011 event per patient-month of device use. Three of the patients in this study had predisposing risk factors for emboli. If those patients were excluded from the analysis, the risk of an embolic event decreased to 0.0056 events per patient-month.

Thoratec VAD

The Thoratec VAD can be used as an LVAD, RVAD, or BiVAD. The drive chamber rests externally on the patient's upper abdominal wall.

The Thoratec VAD System (Thoratec Laboratories Corporation, Pleasanton, CA, USA) is a pneumatically driven, pulsatile VAD that can be used as an LVAD, RVAD, or BiVAD. It is approved for use as a bridge to transplant or as a bridge to ventricular recovery in patients with postcardiotomy cardiogenic shock unresponsive to other therapies (Figure 37-6). The device must be placed surgically, usually with the use of cardiopulmonary bypass.

The Thoratec device consists of a seamless pumping chamber housed within a rigid polymer case. Inside the rigid case the pumping chamber is separated from the pneumatic drive chamber by a diaphragm. The membranes used for the pumping chamber are designed to minimize clot formation. Unidirectional, antegrade blood flow is maintained by two mechanical cardiac valves (modified Bjork–Shiley type) located in inflow and outflow positions. The pump has a maximum stroke volume of approximately 65 ml and can have pump flow rates from 1.3 to 7.2 l/min.

The VAD rests on the external upper abdominal wall. The cannulae that carry blood from the patient to the pump and return blood from the pump to the patient are brought externally through small incisions. Synthetic cuffs on the subcutaneous portion of the cannulae are designed to decrease the risk of infection. The blood flow from the patient is through a cannula placed in the left ventricular apex or left atrium (LVAD) or in the right atrium (RVAD). Blood returns to the patient through a cannula that terminates in a synthetic graft. An anastamosis is created between this graft and the ascending aorta (LVAD) or pulmonary artery (RVAD). As with the Abiomed device described earlier, biventricular support requires placement of two devices.

The VAD is connected to an external drive console that monitors the filling of the pumping chamber and controls the pumping actions. Blood is pumped by pressurizing the pneumatic chamber within the pump with compressed air; this displaces the diaphragm within the rigid case of the VAD and causes the blood chamber to empty. Filling of the pumping chamber with blood is assisted by the application of vacuum to the pneumatic chamber dur-

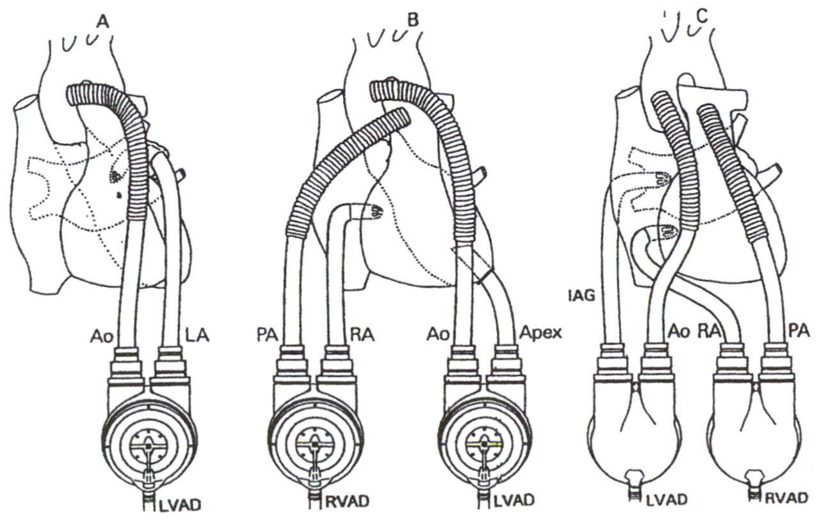

FIGURE 37-6

Configuration of the Thoratec VAD System. **(A)** The device is placed as an LVAD with outflow from the patient via a left atrial cannula. **(B)** The device is configured for BiVAD support with outflow to the LVAD via a left ventricular apex cannula. **(C)** The outflow to the LVAD is through a cannula placed into the left atrium through the intraatrial groove (this view is from behind the heart). (From Thoratec Laboratories Corporation, with permission.)

ing pump diastole. The positive and negative pressure can be adjusted by the operator on the drive console to assure optimum pump function. A single drive console can control two VADs.

While the device can function in several different control modes, most commonly it is set to function in a full-to-empty mode. In this mode the pump will empty when the sensor detects that the pumping chamber is full. This mode has a fixed stroke volume with the rate of pumping determined by the rate of filling. A fixed rate mode and an external synchronized mode are used primarily to wean patients from ventricular assist support.

The Thoratec device requires the use of systemic anticoagulation.

The Thoratec device requires the use of systemic anticoagulation because of the mechanical heart valves. Heparin is usually started in the early postoperative period when bleeding is under control. The goal of therapy is to maintain an activated partial thromboplastin time (APTT) 1.5 times control. Long-term anticoagulation is provided by administration of warfarin to maintain an international normalized ratio (INR) of 2.5–3.5. Some clinicians also use antiplatelet therapy (e.g., aspirin).

Körfer and colleagues reported on 26 patients treated with Thoratec VAD support as a bridge to heart transplantation. The most common complication noted was bleeding (35%). Neurologic complications occurred in a total of 5 patients (19%), with 3 patients (11.5%) developing irreversible neurologic disorders. Other complications were pneumonia (27%), liver failure (15%), sepsis (11.5%), cannula site infection (8%), multisystem organ failure (8%), and acute renal failure (8%). Farrar and coworkers reported a survival to transplant of 74% in patients treated with the device as an LVAD and 58% in patients treated with the device as a BiVAD. The patients with BiVAD support were more critically ill before the VAD placement.

Novacor LVAS

The electrically powered Novacor LVAS can only be used as an LVAD. The device is implanted in the anterior left upper quadrant of the abdomen.

The Novacor LVAS (Baxter Healthcare Corp., Santa Ana, CA, USA) is a pulsatile LVAD system that is approved for use as a bridge to heart transplantation. The device must be implanted surgically, usually with the use of cardiopulmonary bypass. The pump has a polyurethane pumping chamber connected to two pusher plates housed within a rigid shell. The pump has a volume of approximately 70 ml. The pumping action is provided by a pivoting solenoid (electromagnetic device) that is coupled to the pump by springs. Application of an electrical current to the solenoid causes it to pivot and flex the springs, applying pressure to the blood-containing pumping chamber and causing the ejection of blood from the pumping chamber.

The device is implanted in the anterior left upper quadrant of the abdomen (Figure 37-7). An inflow cannula is placed through the apex of the left ventricle to deliver blood to the pump. Blood returns to the patient through an anastomosis between a polyester outflow conduit and the patient's ascending aorta. Unidirectional blood flow is maintained by two bioprosthetic valves that are located at the inflow and outflow connections to the pump. Position sensors within the pump that monitor the position of various pump components are used to control the timing of the pump and monitor its function. An electrical lead from the pump passes percutaneously and is used to connect the device to the external controller and power source. A control unit regulates the operation of the pump. The electrical power for pump operation can be provided by connection to a power base connected to an electrical outlet or by a rechargeable battery pack. There is also a reserve power pack to provide a backup power supply. The device can be triggered by monitoring the fill rate (pumping will be initiated when the rate of filling decreases, indicating that the pumping chamber is full), by use of an ECG signal, or in a fixed-rate mode. The first method is most commonly used.

The most common complications reported with the Novacor LVAD were bleeding, infection, and clinically significant cerebrovascular events.

Duration of support averaged 85 days (range, 0–962 days) in a summary of the worldwide experience with the Novacor LVAS presented by Murali. Of patients in whom the device was implanted, 58% underwent heart transplantation. The most commonly reported complications were bleeding (5%–10%), infection (5%–21%), and clinically significant cerebrovascular events (20%–25%). It was noted that, after a design change in the valved conduit system, the incidence of cerebrovascular events decreased (5%–7%).

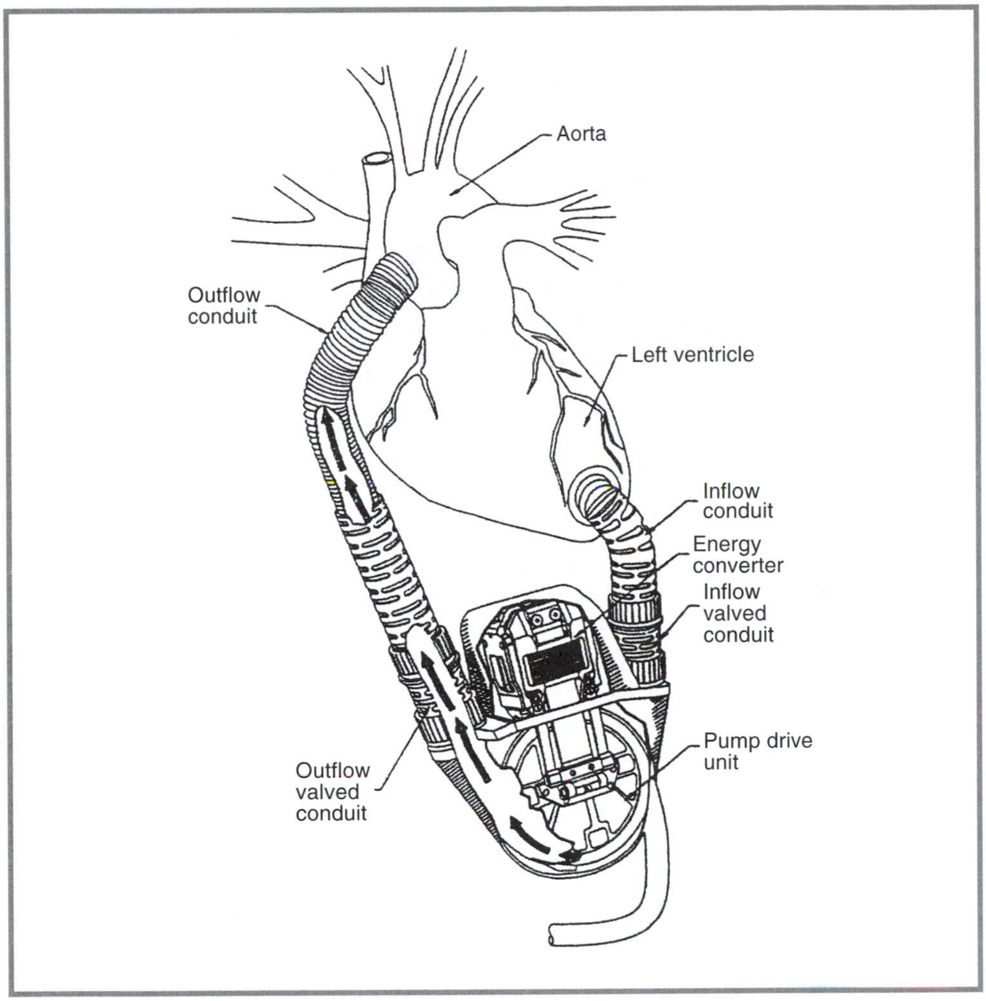

FIGURE 37-7

The Novacor LVAS.

In a series of 36 patients treated with the Novacor device by Schmid and colleagues, there was a 47% occurrence of clinically significant cerebral embolism. They reported that most patients eventually made a full neurologic recovery. Patients with the Novacor device in this report routinely received therapeutic anticoagulation using heparin or phenprocoumon. In a subset of patients who underwent transcranial doppler studies, microembolic signals were detected during 67% of the studies.

Centrifugal Pumps

The centrifugal pumps that are used during cardiopulmonary bypass have also been used to provide VAD support, especially in postcardiotomy cardiogenic shock. These pumps use a rotating pump head to cause blood flow. One pump (Bio-Medicus Bio-Pump, Medtronic, Inc., Minneapolis, MN, USA) uses a series of rotating cones powered by the rotation of a magnet in the control console to propel blood through the pump (Figure 37-8). Another design (Delfin, 3M Sarns, Ann Arbor, MI, USA) uses an impeller with fins to propel the blood. Both pumps use a sensor to determine actual pump flow because the flow at any given speed (revolutions per minute) depends on the preload and afterload of the system. The blood flow with centrifugal pumps is nonpulsatile. Neither system is approved for use as a ventricular-assist device, but there is a substantial body of literature about the use of these devices for VAD support. These pumps are commonly available in institutions that perform cardiac surgery, and before the availability of the devices discussed here, were the only type of VAD support that was available.

Centrifugal pumps, although not FDA approved for use as ventricular-assist devices, have been used to provide VAD support. These devices provide nonpulsatile blood flow.

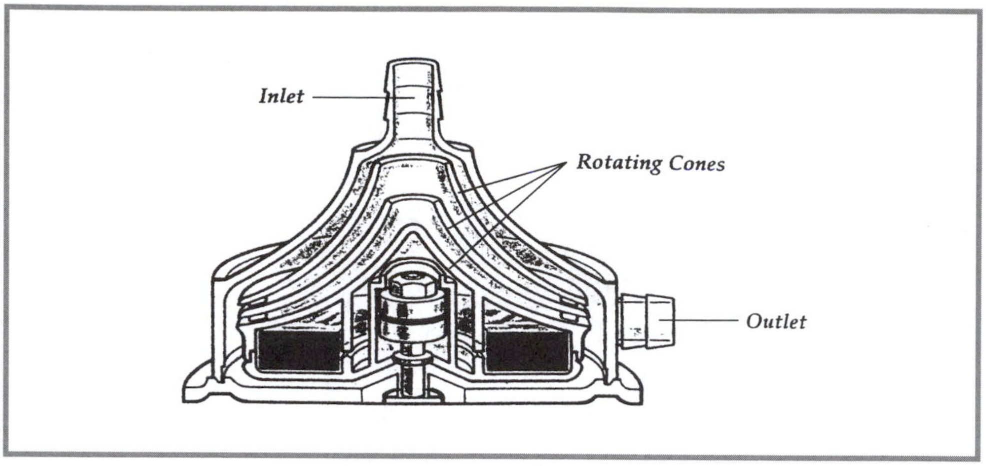

FIGURE 37-8

Cross section of the Bio-Medicus centrifugal pumphead. (From © Medtronic, with permission.)

El-Banayosy and colleagues have published their experience with the use of the Bio-Medicus pump for the treatment of cardiogenic shock. The duration of support in their patients was between 1 h and 14.4 days. They found a survival rate of 33.3% and 46.7% for patients with early and late postcardiotomy shock, respectively. For patients with cardiogenic shock resistant to other treatments following myocardial infarction, the survival rate was 27.2%. Patients with an etiology of cardiogenic shock other than these two groups had a survival of 18.1%. The major complications reported were acute renal failure and bleeding. Other complications included sepsis, multisystem organ failure, and neurologic injury. Reports of the use of the Sarns pump have demonstrated similar results and complications.

The use of anticoagulation with these pumps varies with individual centers. Some centers only use anticoagulation if the pump flows are below a certain level, and others use systemic anticoagulation when mediastinal bleeding has been controlled. Because these devices are nonpulsatile, some clinicians use concomitant IABC therapy in an attempt to achieve some pulsatile flow. Intraaortic balloon counterpulsation probably does not create true pulsatile flow. It has been reported that organ system perfusion in cardiogenic shock is better with pulsatile compared to nonpulsatile flow.

EXTRACORPOREAL MEMBRANE OXYGENATION

Extracorporeal membrane oxygenation (ECMO) therapy can provide blood oxygenation and carbon dioxide elimination when conventional management strategies have been unsuccessful.

Extracorporeal membrane oxygenation (ECMO) therapy is a technique that can provide blood oxygenation and carbon dioxide elimination for patients in whom conventional management strategies have been unsuccessful. A membrane oxygenator is used to provide oxygenation of the blood and carbon dioxide elimination. Deoxygenated blood is removed from the patient through a cannula connected to an extracorporeal circuit with a pump and membrane oxygenator, and oxygenated blood is returned to the patient through a second cannula. A centrifugal pump (as described earlier) is commonly used in this circuit. Venovenous bypass is most often employed, with placement of cannulae into the right atrium through the right internal jugular vein and into a femoral vein. Bilateral femoral vein cannulation has also been employed. In the United States, the most common pattern of flow for veno-venous ECMO involves removal of blood from the right atrium with reinfusion of the oxygenated blood through a femoral vein cannula. There is some evidence that the alternative flow pattern could result in better flow rates and oxygenation.

Ventilator management during ECMO is aimed at providing lung rest to limit further lung injury and barotrauma. Low-frequency positive pressure ventilation (either pressure-controlled or volume-controlled with low tidal volumes) with an FiO_2 less than or equal to 0.4 and peak end-expiratory pressure (PEEP) less than or equal to 10 cmH_2O is common. Routine respiratory care with bronchodilators, bronchoscopy, and, in some patients, tracheostomy is used to limit the development of atelectasis and inspisated pulmonary secretions. Fluid management is aimed at achieving the patient's dry weight by use of diuretics or ultrafiltration. Standard critical care is continued with attention to nutritional support, cardiac function, antibiotics as indicated, and other routine care. Flow-directed pulmonary artery catheterization and monitoring may provide additional information to guide fluid and hemodynamic management.

Venovenous ECMO does not provide circulatory support; therefore, in patients who also require circulatory support, a cannulation technique involving veno-arterial ECMO can be used. The arterial return can be into a femoral artery or into a carotid artery. Some centers prefer the carotid artery site to ensure that well-oxygenated blood is delivered to the proximal aorta for distribution to the major organs.

ECMO in Respiratory Failure

The role of ECMO in the management of respiratory failure refractory to conventional medical therapy remains unclear. Two randomized trials of extracorporeal treatment have failed to demonstrate any benefit. A multicenter, prospective, randomized trial (see Zapol et al.) of ECMO for the treatment of severe respiratory failure, published in 1979, reported survival rates of 9.5% in the ECMO group and 8.3% in the conventionally treated group. The difference in outcome was not statistically significant. Another prospective randomized trial that compared pressure-controlled inverse ratio ventilation to low-frequency positive pressure ventilation with extracorporeal carbon dioxide removal also demonstrated no differences in patient survival.

> The role of ECMO in the management of respiratory failure refractory to conventional medical therapy remains unclear.

The Extracorporeal Life Support Organization, which maintains a voluntary international registry of information from 119 centers, has reported the results of more than 17,000 patients treated with ECMO (see Conrad et al.) The majority of the patients (75%) were cases of neonatal respiratory distress. The overall survival for neonatal respiratory distress was 80%. The registry contains fewer cases of ECMO used in adult respiratory distress (547 patients), but the cumulative survival for adults was 47%. Survival was better for adult patients with viral pneumonia (63%), aspiration (59%), and adult respiratory distress syndrome (59%) and poorer for patients with bacterial pneumonia (35%) and pre- or posttransplant patients (25%).

> An international registry of ECMO therapy has reported an overall survival of 80% for neonatal respiratory distress and 47% for adult respiratory distress.

Complications of ECMO include bleeding, cannulation-related vascular problems, renal failure, multisystem organ failure, infection, neurologic problems, including brain death and seizures, mechanical problems with the circuit, liver dysfunction, and other problems. It is not always possible to differentiate between ECMO and the underlying disease process as a cause for many of these complications.

Results from ECMO Trials

The current status of ECMO remains unresolved. Although the only randomized study of ECMO therapy showed no benefit, it was performed more than 20 years ago and involved only 90 patients (42 receiving ECMO). The reported survival of less than 10% in both groups of patients may not reflect current survival. A more recent report (Suchyta and colleagues) of the outcome in patients with acute respiratory failure who met the entry criteria used in the randomized ECMO trial reported a survival of 45% for patients treated with conventional therapy; this demonstrates an improvement in patient outcome over the 12 years between the initial ECMO study and Suchyta's evaluation of conventional therapy in a similar group of patients. This improvement in outcome with conventional therapy must be considered when evaluating the reported outcomes from ECMO trials that make conclusions on the basis of historical controls.

The nonrandomized results from the Registry data and individual reports suggest that ECMO may be beneficial in some cases of adult respiratory failure. However, ECMO is a very resource-intensive therapy. Patients receiving ECMO require the continual presence of

ECMO is a resource-intensive therapy. Until a large, prospective, randomized trial is conducted, the role of ECMO in adults with acute respiratory failure will remain unclear.

a skilled operator capable of managing the extracorporeal circulation. The personnel and equipment costs make ECMO an expensive therapy. Until a large, prospective, randomized trial is repeated, the role of ECMO in adults with acute respiratory failure will remain unclear.

SUMMARY

Patients who develop inadequate hemodynamic function despite conventional medical therapies (diuretics or volume administration, manipulation of vascular tone, and inotropic stimulation) may benefit from the use of mechanical cardiac support. Intraaortic balloon counterpulsation is usually considered as the first-line therapy for mechanical support. IABC can also be used to treat myocardial ischemia that is refractory to conventional medical therapy. Intraaortic balloon counterpulsation, although an effective therapy in many patients, can be associated with significant adverse consequences, the most common of which are related to limb ischemia.

Patients with inadequate cardiac pump function who do not respond to IABC or who need long-term support can be considered for ventricular-assist device therapy. The choice of device depends on the expected duration of therapy, the patient's size, and whether support is needed for the left ventricle, the right ventricle, or both. Ventricular-assist device therapy is most commonly used as a bridge to heart transplantation but can also be used as a bridge to recovery in patients with cardiogenic shock where recovery of myocardial function may occur with aggressive support, such as some patients who cannot be separated from cardiopulmonary bypass or in whom cardiogenic shock has developed as a consequence of acute myocarditis or myocardial infarction. The most common complications of VAD therapy are bleeding, embolism, and infection.

Extracorporeal membrane oxygenation can be used to provide oxygenation and carbon dioxide removal in patients with respiratory failure refractory to conventional therapy. ECMO has been shown to be a beneficial therapy for the treatment of infant respiratory distress syndrome, but its role in adult respiratory distress remains unclear. Some adult patients may benefit from ECMO, but adequate data are not available to reach a clear conclusion on its role in the treatment of adults with respiratory failure.

REVIEW QUESTIONS*

1. **The indications for intraaortic balloon counterpulsation therapy include:**
   A. Cardiogenic shock following acute myocarditis
   B. Acute mitral regurgitation with pulmonary edema from papillary muscle rupture
   C. Acute ventricular septal defect developing after a myocardial infarction
   D. Acute aortic insufficiency from endocarditis

2. **A patient with an intraaortic balloon catheter placed through the right femoral artery develops evidence of limb ischemia in the right leg. Which of the following are acceptable responses to this condition?**
   A. Remove the intraaortic balloon catheter and place it through the left femoral artery
   B. Do a femoral–femoral artery bypass
   C. Obtain a vascular surgery consultation
   D. No intervention is necessary for the first 12 h

*Note: More than one answer may be correct.

3. **Advantages of the TCI HeartMate ventricular assist device include:**
   A. It can be used as LVAD, RVAD, and BiVAD.
   B. Patients do not require systemic anticoagulation.
   C. It can be used for patients with a BSA < 1.5 m^2.
   D. The textured surface of the VAD is associated with a low incidence of thromboembolism.

4. **An Abiomed BVS left ventricular-assist device was implanted in a patient who could not be separated from cardiopulmonary bypass. Which of the following are true:**
   A. This patient will not require systemic anticoagulation.
   B. The device cannot be removed until the time of heart transplantation.
   C. The patient can be discharged home after recovery from the surgery while awaiting heart transplantation.
   D. The blood chambers of the pump fill by gravity.

5. **In considering the role of extracorporeal membrane oxygenation (ECMO) therapy in treatment of acute respiratory failure, the following statements are correct:**
   - **A.** ECMO has been shown to be a beneficial therapy in the treatment of infant respiratory distress syndrome.
   - **B.** Randomized, controlled studies have shown that ECMO is a beneficial treatment for adult respiratory distress syndrome.
   - **C.** The most common type of ECMO circuit used is veno-venous ECMO.
   - **D.** Veno-venous ECMO also provides hemodynamic support in patients with ventricular failure.

ANSWERS

1. The answer is A, B, and C. Intraaortic balloon counterpulsation therapy is indicated for the treatment of myocardial ischemia or left ventricular dysfunction/failure that does not respond to medical therapy. Counterpulsation therapy can augment forward cardiac output by reducing left ventricular afterload; this is an appropriate intervention in the treatment of cardiogenic shock, acute mitral regurgitation, and acute ventricular septal defect. Counterpulsation therapy also augments diastolic blood pressure, which can improve coronary artery blood flow. Counterpulsation therapy is contraindicated in patients with significant aortic insufficiency because the counterpulsation can increase the severity of the aortic regurgitation.
2. The answer is A, B, and C. Development of limb ischemia distal to an IABC catheter is a potentially serious complication. At the earliest sign or symptom of limb ischemia, aggressive evaluation and treatment should occur. Delay in evaluation and treatment may result in permanent damage or limb loss. Early evaluation by a vascular surgeon can help in deciding the most appropriate treatment. If IABC therapy is still needed, removal of the catheter from the affected side and replacement in the opposite femoral can be considered. Femoral–femoral artery bypass surgery to provide blood flow distal to the IABC catheter insertion site is another intervention that can be used to resolve the limb ischemia.
3. The answer is B and D. The TCI HeartMate ventricular-assist device has a low incidence of thromboembolic events due to its design. The textured surface of the components that contact the blood encourage the formation of a pseudoneointima, which decreases the occurrence of thrombi. Patients with the device do not require systemic anticoagulation and are usually treated only with antiplatelet therapy (e.g., aspirin). The TCI HeartMate can only be used as a left ventricular assist device and requires a patient whose body surface area (BSA) is at least 1.5 m^2.
4. The answer is A, B, C, and D. The Abiomed BVS can be used as a bridge to recovery in patients who cannot be separated from cardiopulmonary bypass. If the ventricular function recovers, the patient can be weaned and separated from the device. The device fills passively by gravity. While the device is in place, the patient will require continuous anticoagulation and critical care.
5. The answer is A and C. ECMO is an invasive therapy that has been shown to be beneficial in the treatment of infant respiratory distress syndrome. The role of ECMO in adult patients with respiratory failure is less clear. No prospective randomized trials have shown the therapy to be beneficial in adults. Veno-venous ECMO, the most commonly described circuit configuration in adults, provides blood oxygenation and carbon dioxide removal but does not provide hemodynamic support.

SUGGESTED READING

Aroesty JM, Shawl FA. Circulatory assist devices. In: Bain DS, Grossman W (eds) Cardiac Catheterization, Angiography, and Intervention, 5th Ed. Baltimore: Williams & Wilkins, 1996:421–462.

Barnette MG, Swartz MT, Petersen GJ, et al. Vascular complications from intraaortic balloons: risk analysis. J Vasc Surg 1994;19:81–89.

Conrad SA, Rycus PT. Extracorporeal life support 1997. ASAIO J 1998:848–852.

El-Banayosy A, Posival H, Minami K, et al. Seven years experience with the centrifugal pump in patients with cardiogenic shock. Thorac Cardiovasc Surg 1999;43:347–351.

Farrar DJ, Hill JD, Pennington DG, et al. Preoperative and postoperative comparison of patients with univentricular and biventricular support with the Thoratec ventricular assist device as a bridge to cardiac transplantation. J Thorac Cardiovasc Surg 1997;113:202–209.

Guyton RA, Schonberger JPAM, Everts PAM, et al. Postcardiotomy shock: clinical evaluation of the BVS 5000 biventricular support system. Ann Thorac Surg 1993;56:346–356.

Hazelrigg SR, Auer JE, Seifert PE. Experience in 100 transthoracic balloon pumps. Ann Thorac Surg 1992;54:528–532.

Jett GK. Abiomed BVS 5000: experience and potential advantages. Ann Thorac Surg 1996;61:301–304.

Körfer R, El-Banayosy A, Posival H, et al. Mechanical circulatory support with the Thoratec assist device in patients with postcardiotomy cardiogenic shock. Ann Thorac Surg 1996;61:314–316.

Makhoul RG, Cole CW, McCann RL. Vascular complications of the intra-aortic balloon pump: an analysis of 436 patients. Am Surg 1993;59:564–568.

Murali S. Mechanical circulatory support with the Novacor LVAS: world-wide clinical results. Thorac Cardiovasc Surg 1999;47(supplement):321–325.

Naunheim KS, Swartz MT, Pennington DG, et al. Intraaortic balloon pumping in patients requiring cardiac operations: risk analysis and long-term follow-up. J Thorac Cardiovasc Surg 1992;104:1654–1661.

Patel JJ, Kopisyansky C, Boston B, et al. Prospective evaluation of complications associated with percutaneous intraaortic balloon counterpulsation. Am J Cardiol 1995;76:1205–1207.

Poirier VL. The HeartMate left ventricular assist system: worldwide clinical results. Eur J Cardio-Thorac Surg 1997:S39–S44.

Schmid C, Weynd M, Nabavi DG, et al. Cerebral and systemic embolization during left ventricular support with the Novacor N100 device. Ann Thorac Surg 1998;65:1703–1710.

Slater JP, Rose EA, Levin HR, et al. Lower thromboembolic risk without anticoagulation using advance-design left ventricular assist devices. Ann Thorac Surg 1996;62:1321–1327.

Stavridis GT, O'Riordan JB. Paraplegia as a result of intra-aortic balloon counterpulsation. J Cardiovasc Surg 1995;36:177–179.

Stone GW, Marsalese D, Brodie BR, et al. A prospective, randomized evaluation of prophylactic intraaortic balloon counterpulsation in high risk patients with acute myocardial infarction treated with primary angioplasty. J Am Coll Cardiol 1997;29:1459–1467.

Suchyta MR, Clemmer TP, Orme JF, et al. Increased survival of ARDS patients with severe hypoxemia (ECMO criteria). Chest 1991;99: 951–955.

Vonderheide RH, Thadhani R, Kuter DJ. Association of thrombocytopenia with the use of intra-aortic balloon pumps. Am J Med 1998;105:27–32.

Zapol WM, Snider MT, Hill JD, et al. Extracorporeal membrane oxygenation in severe acute respiratory failure. JAMA 1979;242(20): 2193–2196.

DAVID E. CICCOLELLA

Pharmacologic Hemodynamic Support of Shock States

CHAPTER OUTLINE

LEARNING OBJECTIVES

After studying this chapter, you should:

- Know the indications and contraindications for each medication.
- Know the clinical hemodynamic effects of each medication.
- Know the potential complications associated with each medication.
- Know the use of these agents in specific shock states.

The pharmacologic support of critically ill patients commonly includes hemodynamic support for hypotension and shock. Pharmacologic therapy is used in conjunction with other treatments such as fluids, antibiotics, and, in special situations, mechanical circulatory-assist devices. The type, dose, and number of drugs are used differently in the various causes of shock. We describe here the various categories and causes of shock as well as hemodynamic support drugs and their use in selected causes of shock.

Shock is defined as the failure of the circulatory system to maintain adequate cellular or tissue perfusion and of oxygen delivery to meet current metabolic demands, resulting in organ dysfunction, which if prolonged results in irreversible cellular damage. Although shock is more likely to exist at a mean arterial pressure of less than 60 mmHg (or a decrease in premorbid systolic blood pressure [BP] of 40 mmHg), shock is not necessarily defined by a low BP but rather as an inability to meet metabolic demands. Therefore, shock may occur at a BP of 95/70 if oxygen delivery does not meet metabolic demands.

Categories of Shock

Shock can arise from a number of different etiologies and can manifest in several different hemodynamic patterns based upon the underlying pathophysiology. One commonly used gen-

Shock may be divided into four types: hypovolemic, extracardiac obstructive, cardiogenic, and distributive.

eral shock classification describes four basic categories: hypovolemic, cardiogenic, extracardiac obstructive, and distributive shock, for which there are multiple possible underlying causes (Figure 38-1A).

Hypovolemic shock results from loss of circulatory volume due to hemorrhage or extravascular fluid losses. Cardiogenic shock results from inadequate pump function whether caused by predominant left or right myocardial infarction, acute valvular disease such as

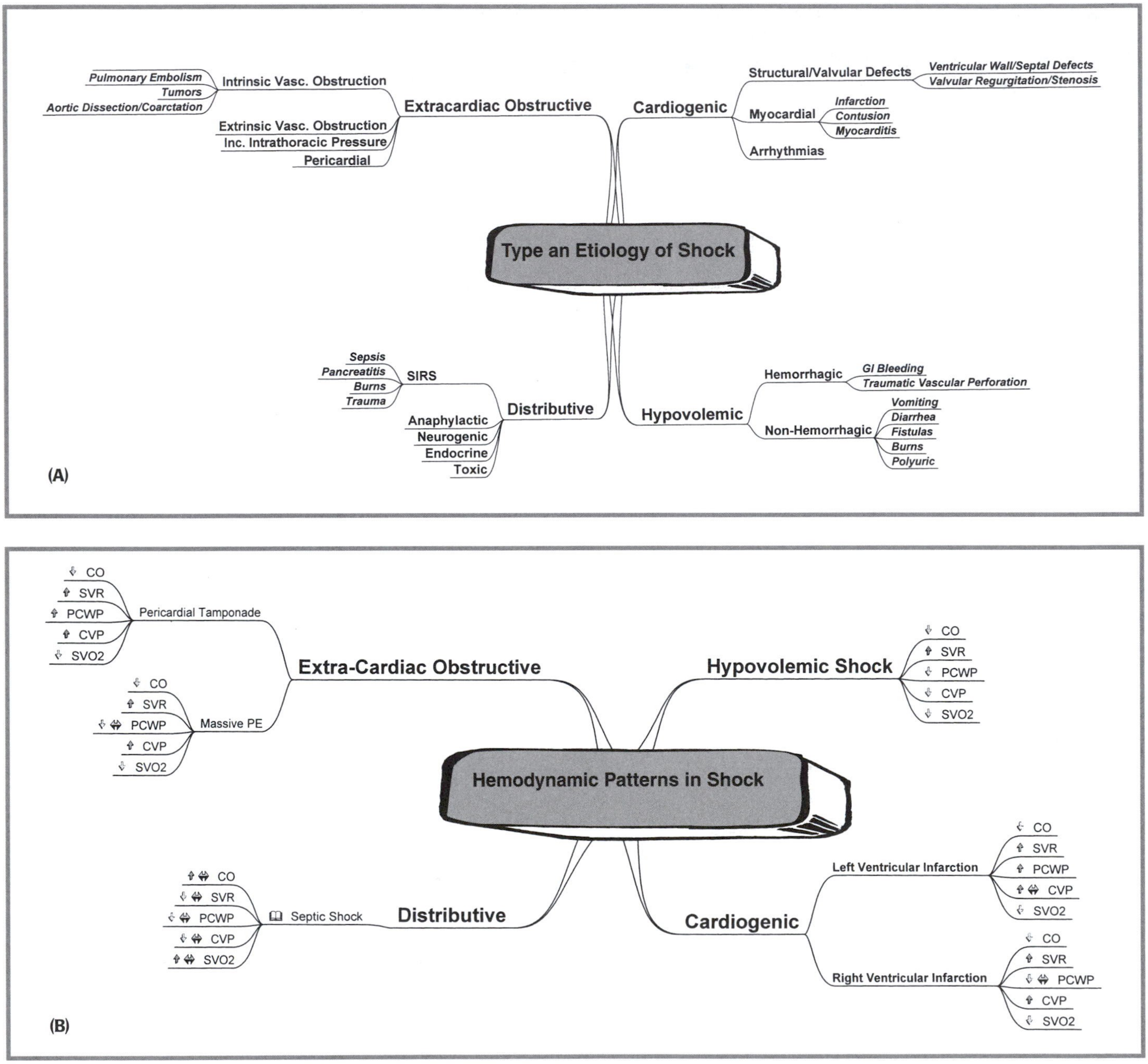

FIGURE 38-1

(A) Category and etiology of shock. The four main categories of shock and their etiologies are shown. A single etiology may occur in two or three of the shock types such as septic shock. (Information adapted from Parillo J. Approach to the patient with shock. In: Lee Goldman, Jr, Claude Bennet J (eds) *Cecil Textbook of Medicine*. Philadelphia: W.B. Saunders, 2000:495–502.) **(B)** Hemodynamic patterns in shock. The four main categories of shock and the hemodynamic patterns for some of their important causes are shown.

acute mitral regurgitation or aortic regurgitation, dysrhythmias, intracardiac obstruction, or severe cardiomyopathy. Extracardiac obstructive shock results from a mechanical impediment to blood flow caused by diseases such as pulmonary embolism, tension pneumothorax, pericardial tamponade, or aortic dissection or compression. Distributive shock results from a maldistribution of blood volume as in processes such as sepsis, anaphylaxis, spinal cord injury (e.g., spinal shock), and adrenocortical insufficiency.

In this general classification of shock, it should be noted that some of the specific causes (e.g., anaphylaxis, pancreatitis, trauma) have features of more than one of the four basic shock types. For instance, septic shock predominantly tends to be a distributive type but may include hypovolemic or cardiogenic categories. Similarly, anaphylactic shock, which is also mainly distributive, includes elements of hypovolemic shock. Moreover, a hemodynamic problem may be the result of more than one independent cause such as septic shock in the presence of a chronic ischemic cardiomyopathy. These aspects of the shock classification should be considered when evaluating any patient in the ICU for the specific cause of shock and its treatments.

Some of the specific causes of shock—anaphylaxis, pancreatitis, trauma—have features of more than one of the four shock types.

These four shock categories and their causes are associated with hemodynamic patterns that may further aid identification of the specific cause as well as the type of treatment (Figure 38-1B). Hypovolemic, cardiogenic, and extracardiac obstructive shock are associated with decreased cardiac output. In contrast, during the initial phase of septic shock, a distributive form of shock, cardiac output (CO) may be increased, and systemic vascular resistance (SVR) is decreased. Other causes of increased CO and decreased SVR include liver cirrhosis, neurogenic shock, and anaphylactic shock. The pulmonary capillary wedge pressure (PCWP) may help to further differentiate hypovolemic from cardiogenic shock.

Each of the shock types has multiple different causes.

Initial Evaluation and Diagnosis of Shock

The patient should be assessed for the etiology of shock by an initial rapid clinical evaluation based on a focused history and physical examination, followed by appropriate initial laboratory studies. Knowing the history of present illness, underlying past illnesses, medications, and other disease risk factors is especially helpful in determining the etiology. The physical examination should be directed toward evaluating traditional vital signs such as heart rate (HR) and rhythm, blood pressure, respiratory rate, and temperature, plus the adequacy of tissue or organ perfusion. Physical signs of decreased perfusion include tachycardia, hypotension, altered mental status, oliguria, tachypnea and cyanosis, and decreased skin capillary refill. Certain constellations of historical information and physical examination signs may immediately indicate or narrow down the etiology of shock; other cases may be much less obvious.

Further evaluation for the diagnosis includes laboratory studies such as serum electrolytes and anion gap, creatinine and biliary urea nitrogen (BUN), arterial blood gas (ABG); chest roentgenogram (CXR) and electrocardiogram (EKG) may be very helpful in the initial evaluation.

TREATMENT OF SHOCK

Hemodynamic Goals

In general, shock may require a combination of fluid resuscitation, specific vasopressor, inotropic, and/or vasodilator agents, or ventricular-assist devices depending upon the etiology and severity of shock. Shock results from inadequate substrate and O_2 delivery to maintain the necessary metabolic processes for proper tissue functioning. Therefore, the goals of shock treatment are to return tissue perfusion and oxygenation to an adequate level. The main determinants of tissue perfusion are cardiac output and mean arterial blood pressure (MAP). The MAP has been one method used traditionally to help assess tissue perfusion.

The treatment of shock is directed at increasing tissue perfusion and oxygen delivery through the use of fluids and vasoactive drugs, as well as mechanical ventilation and circulatory-assist devices.

Although it has its limitations, especially in certain distributive types of shock, the MAP is a simple measure to roughly determine the adequacy of tissue perfusion. MAP minus the central venous pressure (CVP) is dependent on cardiac output (CO) and systemic vascular resistance (SVR) as shown in the following equation:

$$\text{MAP} - \text{CVP} = \text{CO} \times \text{SVR} \quad (38\text{-}1)$$

which can be rearranged to

$$\text{MAP} = (\text{CO} \times \text{SVR}) + \text{CVP} \quad (38\text{-}2)$$

In this equation, we know the cardiac output is dependent on stroke volume (SV) and heart rate (HR):

$$\text{CO} = \text{SV} \times \text{HR} \quad (38\text{-}3)$$

The stroke volume, in turn, is dependent on the degree of preload, contractility, and afterload, assuming the absence of regurgitation. The preload is the cardiac chamber volume before contraction, and the afterload is the resistant load to blood ejection, of which one of the components is SVR. The main component of SVR is regulated by the systemic arterioles.

Shock may result from problems affecting one or more of the following: pump, pump rate, vascular resistance, or volume.

Circulatory support is directed at modifying CO through effects on SV and HR.

Thus, shock may result from problems with one or more of the following: the pump, the pump rate, the volume or the vascular resistance. Through clinical assessment and invasive procedures such as pulmonary artery catheterization, the volume problem should be evaluated and treated. After assessment and infusion of fluids to correct a volume problem, pharmacologic support of the circulation is directed at titrating the cardiac output through changes in cardiac stroke volume and rate and the systemic vascular resistance. Generally, the cardiac rate, which also affects preload, is not primarily modified unless it is significantly too fast or slow due to arrhythmias. Moreover, an increase in cardiac rate may be a manifestation of inadequate preload or a side effect of a vasoactive drug. However, the clinician can use different vasoactive drugs that have selective effects on these components of the circulation to improve or restore the hemodynamic status.

Initial Phase of Treatment

The initial phase of treatment involves the establishment of intravenous large-bore catheters, an arterial line for direct and continuous arterial pressure measurement, and electrocardiographic monitoring and pulse oximetry. Depending on the presumed etiology of shock (other than cardiogenic shock and pulmonary edema), a rapid intravenous fluid bolus of 0.5–1 l should be administered. More invasive procedures such as pulmonary artery catheterization and advanced studies such as echocardiography should be considered if the etiology of shock is unknown, or if the patient requires repeated intravenous fluid boluses or vasopressors.

Use of Pulmonary Artery Catheter

Placement of a pulmonary artery (PA) catheter is indicated in most cases when an initial trial of fluids is not helpful, the specific cause of shock is not known, or vasoactive drugs are required. The most useful parameters are cardiac index, pulmonary capillary wedge pressure, and systemic vascular resistance for evaluating the cause and the response to treatment. A more thorough discussion of the use of the pulmonary artery catheter is provided elsewhere in this volume.

PHARMACOLOGIC SUPPORT

Two classes of drugs are used in the treatment of shock: vasopressor/inotropic drugs and, in special situations, vasodilators.

The pharmacologic support of the circulation involves the use of a number of drugs each having a different specific effect on the cardiovascular system. Generally, two classes of drugs are used in the treatment of shock: vasopressor/inotropic drugs and the vasodilators. In shock treatment, the vasopressors/inotropic drugs are the main drugs utilized whereas the vasodilator drugs are generally used adjunctively in special circumstances. These drugs can be tailored to effect various changes in cardiac output and vascular resistance depending on their mechanism of action or receptor-binding properties (receptor type and potency) and tissue target.

Receptor Type and Actions

The vasopressor/inotropic drugs produce their effects using several different mechanisms of action that are categorized in this chapter into adrenergic receptor and nonadrenergic receptor-mediated mechanisms (Figure 38-2). The adrenergic receptor (AR) drugs mediate their effects through the alpha- and beta-receptors as well as the dopaminergic receptors present mainly on nerve terminals and effector cells in the autonomic nervous system. The nonadrenergic mechanisms are more diverse and may not be mediated by discrete receptors (e.g., the inotrope, phosphodiesterase (PDE) III inhibitors, or the vasodilator, nitroprusside).

The vasopressor/inotropic drugs used in shock treatment use either adrenergic/dopaminergic or non-adrenergic receptor.

The adrenergic receptor agonists may affect three types of receptors: α, β, and dopamine (DA).

The vasopressor/inotropic drugs utilize either adrenergic receptor-mediated mechanisms or nonadrenergic receptor-mediated mechanisms. The vasopressor/inotropic drugs using adrenergic receptor-mediated mechanisms comprise the largest group and can be further categorized into the natural catecholamines (e.g., norepinephrine), synthetic catecholamines (e.g., dobutamine), and some noncatecholamine drugs (e.g., phenylephrine). The catecholamines are removed by reuptake mechanisms and metabolized by the enzymes monoamine oxidase (MAO) and catechol-*O*-methyl transferase (COMT) but primarily by COMT. The noncatecholamine drugs using adrenergic receptor mechanisms, such as phenylephrine, are metab-

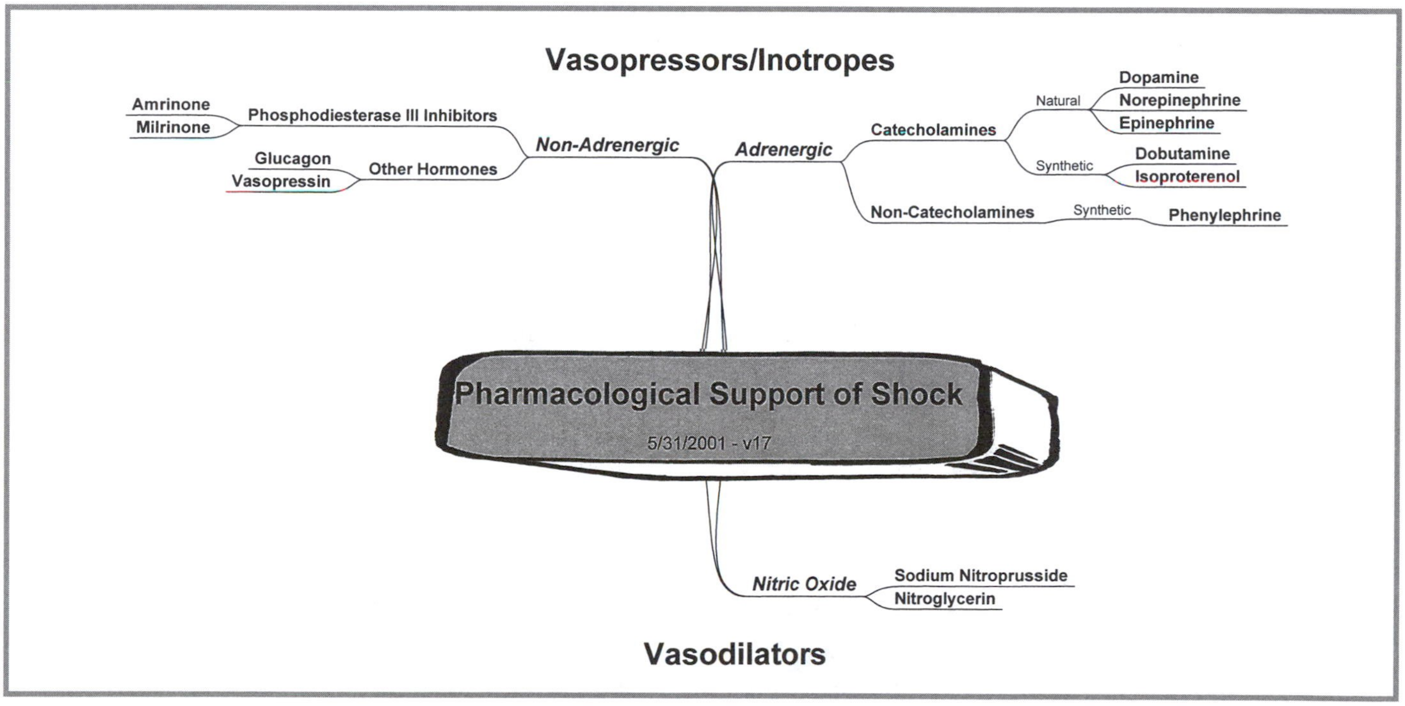

FIGURE 38-2

The drugs used in the treatment of shock are categorized as vasopressors/inotropes or vasodilators according to mechanism of action and type of drug. The vasopressor/inotrope drugs are subcategorized as adrenergic receptor or nonadrenergic receptor mechanisms. The adrenergic receptor drugs are further subcategorized as catecholamines or noncatecholamines, which may be synthetic or natural. The nonadrenergic drugs are subcategorized as phosphodiesterase inhibitors or other hormones. The vasodilators mediate their effects through the release or production of nitric oxide, an endogenous mediator of smooth muscle relaxation.

olized primarily by MAO. The type of enzymatic degradation affects the duration of drug action and interaction with other drugs such as MAO inhibitors.

An understanding of the various adrenergic receptors, including the types and effects mediated by them, is important in using the adrenergic receptor drugs effectively. In the sympathetic component of the autonomic nervous system, preganglionic nerves originate in the spinal cord and synapse with postganglionic nerves. The postganglionic nerves further extend and their nerve terminals synapse with effector cell receptors on the target tissue. The adrenergic receptors, identified as alpha- and beta-receptors, or dopaminergic receptors, identified as dopamine-1 (DA1) and dopamine-2 (DA2), are located on either or both the presynaptic terminals or the postsynaptic cell.

Generally, stimulation of the α_1-AR peripherally mediates arterial and venous vasoconstriction. In the heart, the α_1-AR also have a positive inotropic effect and a negative chronotropic effect.

Generally, the α_1-receptors are postsynaptic, whereas the α_2-receptors are mainly presynaptic but are also present on the postsynaptic membrane. The α_1-ARs in the heart have a positive effect on contractility and a negative effect on heart rate. Stimulation of both α-AR subtypes on the effector cell results in venous and arterial vasoconstriction, which varies according to their relative density. However, the presynaptic α_2-ARs inhibit release of norepinephrine depending on the stimulatory intensity and can counter the vasoconstriction. The potency of the agonists at the α_1-AR increases from dopamine to norepinephrine and then epinephrine.

The β_1-AR mediate cardiac contractility and rate. The β_2-AR mediate vasodilation.

The β_1-ARs are predominantly located in the heart, and the β_2-ARs are located in the airway and vascular smooth muscle and in glandular tissue. The β_1-ARs mediate increases in heart rate and cardiac contractility, causing increased cardiac oxygen consumption as well as decreases in atrioventricular time. The β_2-ARs mediate vasodilation.

Dopamine is an important CNS neurotransmitter that in progressively higher pharmacologic doses has effects on dopamine receptors and α- and β-adrenergic receptors.

Dopamine stimulates both DA1 and DA2 receptors depending on drug concentration. Low-dose stimulation of DA1 receptors, which vary in density according to the vascular bed, causes vascular smooth muscle relaxation and vasodilation predominantly in the mesenteric and renal vascular beds. Stimulation of the DA2 receptors on the presynaptic sympathetic nerve terminals inhibits norepinephrine release and exerts negative effects on vascular resistance.

Glucagon mediates its effect through the glucagon receptor.

Vasopressin mediates its vasoconstrictive effects by the V_1 receptor on vascular smooth muscle.

Milrinone and amrinone mediate their effects by selectively inhibiting the class III phosphodiesterases and increasing cAMP levels.

The non-adrenergic vasopressor/inotropic drugs and the vasodilators are a diverse group and may not mediate their effects through receptors. These vasopressor/inotropic drugs are not catecholamines and do not mediate their effects through adrenergic receptors; these include the hormones vasopressin and glucagon and the phosphodiesterase III inhibitors amrinone and milrinone. Glucagon mediates its effects by binding to glucagon receptors and increasing cellular cAMP levels. Vasopressin binds V_1 receptors on smooth muscle, causing contraction of vascular smooth muscle leading to vasoconstriction and other effects. Amrinone and milrinone are relatively selective inhibitors of the class III phosphodiesterase isoenzymes that regulate cyclic guanosine monophosphate (cGMP)-inhibited, cAMP hydrolysis and thereby increase intracellular cAMP levels, causing their cardiovascular effects. The vasodilators nitroprusside and nitroglycerin are considered nitrovasodilators and mediate their effects through a nitric oxide mechanism.

Specific Vasopressors, Inotropes, and Vasodilators

To use these drugs optimally in the treatment of shock, a thorough knowledge and understanding of their mechanism of action, indications, therapeutic issues, and potential adverse effects is required. Each of these drugs has a different profile of effects on cardiac contractility and rate and peripheral vascular resistance (Figure 38-3). These drug-induced changes in cardiac contractility, heart rate, and peripheral vascular resistance cause changes in hemodynamic parameters such as mean arterial pressure, cardiac output, systemic vascular resistance, and pulmonary capillary wedge pressure (Figure 38-4). These effects are discussed for each of the following drugs. The vasopressor/inotropic drugs are discussed as categorized into the adrenergic receptor-mediated drugs and nonadrenergic drugs, followed by the vasodilators.

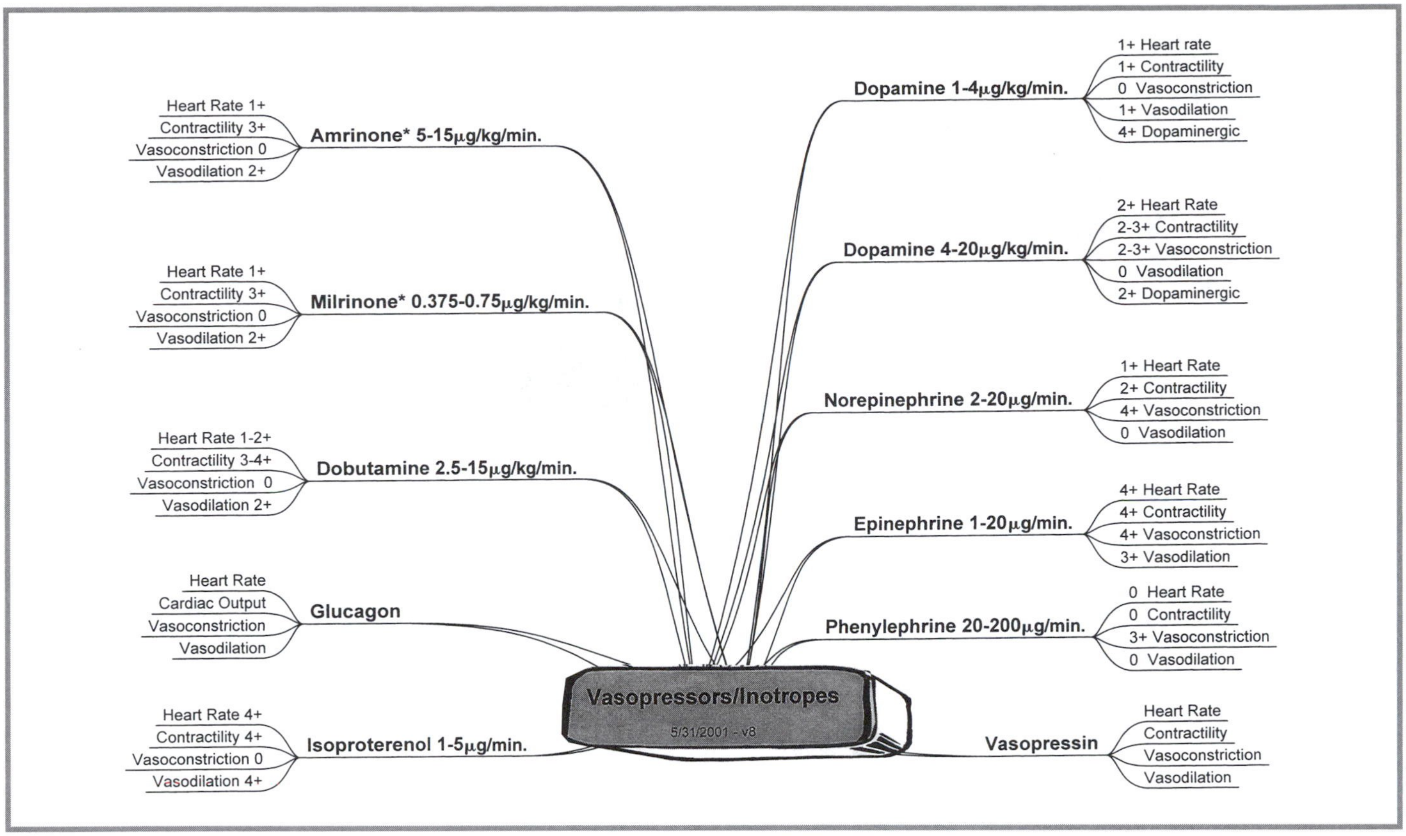

FIGURE 38-3

The effect of vasopressor/inotropic drugs on the components of the cardiovascular system are shown on a scale of 0 to 4+ for heart rate, contractility, vasoconstriction, vasodilation, and dopaminergic effects. This activity is different from the net effect of the drug produced in the patient. For example, norepinephrine has a significant effect (2+) on cardiac contractility through its β_1-adrenergic receptor, but this tends to produce no effect or only a small effect on CO because of its greater vasoconstrictor effect (4+) through its strong α_1-adrenergic activity. Note that only dopamine has dopaminergic effects and a dopaminergic category. The infusion dose is also shown for each drug. The *asterisk* for amrinone and milrinone indicates that a loading dose is needed. (Information adapted from Parillo J. Approach to the patient with shock. In: Lee Goldman, Jr. Claude Bennet J (eds) *Cecil Textbook of Medicine.* Philadelphia: W.B. Saunders, 2000: 495–502.)

Adrenergic Drugs

Dopamine

Mechanisms and Actions Dopamine is an endogenous precursor of norepinephrine and an important central and peripheral neurotransmitter. It is present in the sympathetic nerve endings as well as the adrenal medulla. Delivered in pharmacologic doses, it has important α- and β-AR and dopaminergic receptor (DA1 and DA2) effects used to modify cardiovascular hemodynamics. At pharmacologic concentrations, it has direct effects on three types of receptors: the β-ARs, both β_1 and β_2, the α-ARs, α_1 and α_2, and the dopaminergic receptors DA1 and DA2 in a dose-dependent manner. The DA1 receptors mediate vasodilation in the renal, mesenteric, coronary, and cerebral vascular beds. The DA2 receptors inhibit norepinephrine release and also induce central effects of nausea and vomiting. The DA2 receptors are stimulated at rates of 0.2–0.4 μg/kg/min. The DA1 receptors are stimulated at a concentration of 0.5–3.0 μg/kg/min. A further increase in dose causes increasing β_1-AR

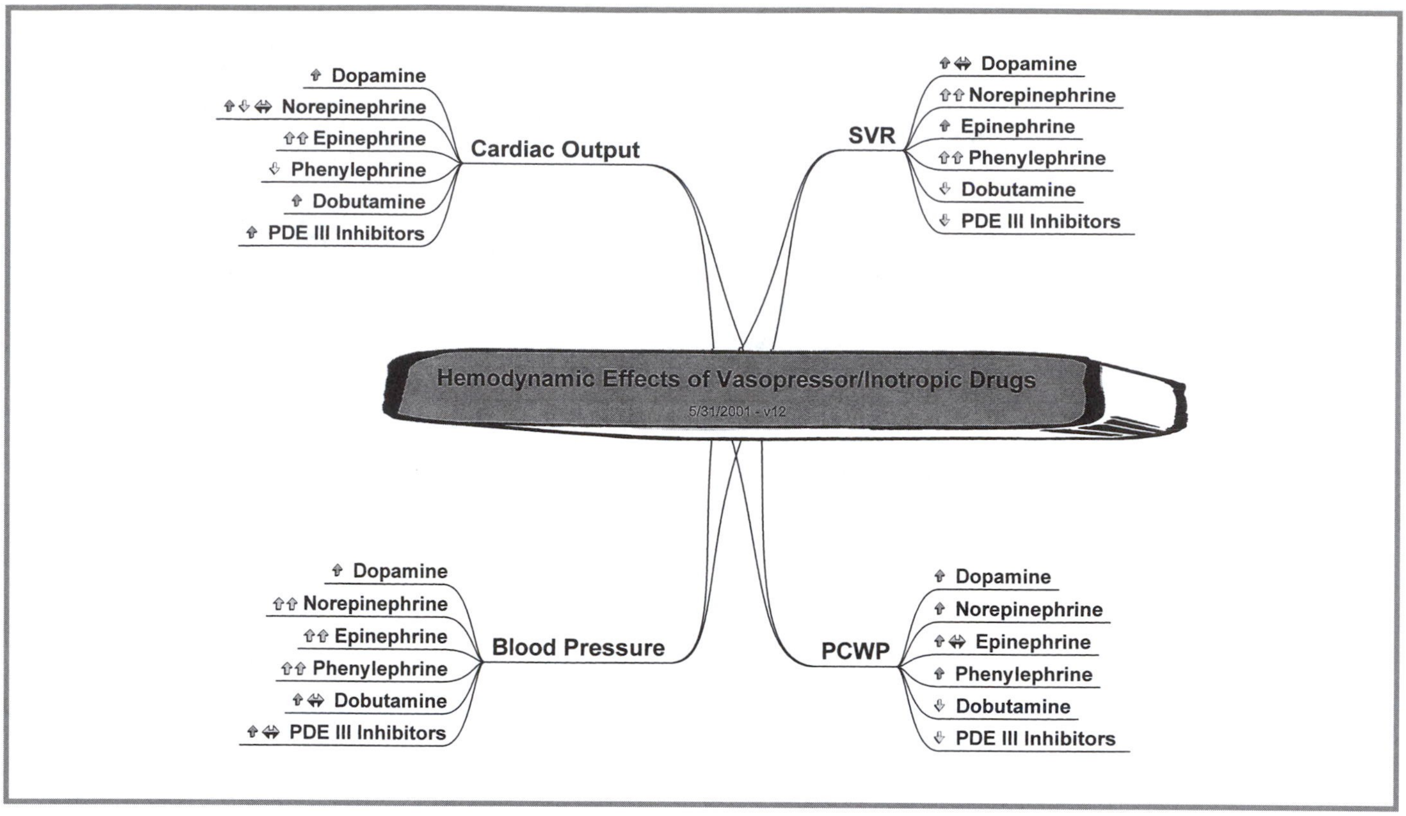

FIGURE 38-4

A general guideline of the net effect of some vasopressor/inotropic drugs on various hemodynamic parameters. The number and direction of the arrows (↑, increase; ⟷, unchanged; ↓, decreased) indicate the magnitude of the effect on each hemodynamic parameter. The net effect of each drug is partially dependent on its direct action, derived from its activity at various receptor sites (see text), as seen in Figure 38-3. For example, phenylephrine, a strong vasoconstrictor (+3) without inotropic effects (0) as seen in Figure 38-3, tends to cause a net increase in SVR and a net decrease in CO because of its strong α_1-adrenergic vasoconstrictor response. The net effect of each drug will also tend to vary depending on the clinical situation (e.g., cardiogenic shock or septic shock), the volume status, and the presence or absence of hypotension. *SVR*, systemic vascular resistance.

effects from approximately 5–10 μg/kg/min and then predominantly α-AR effects at greater than 10 μg/kg/min. The actual dose at which these effects occur varies widely in patients and therefore requires dose titration to the desired response.

Dopamine actions include positive inotropy, slight tachycardia, and an increase predominantly in systolic blood pressure (SBP) without affecting diastolic BP. Dopamine produces increases in mean arterial pressure (MAP) predominantly by increasing cardiac index (CI) and SVR at levels of approximately 5–10 μg/kg/min. The increased CI is caused mainly by increased SV and less so by increased HR. At increasingly higher doses, the α-adrenergic effects of dopamine produce further increases in SVR and pulmonary vascular resistance but less than that of norepinephrine or epinephrine. Furthermore, venous capacity is reduced through vasoconstriction, which increases pulmonary capillary wedge pressure (PCWP), especially at higher dopamine doses.

Indications for dopamine include hypotension with clinical shock, as a second-line drug for symptomatic bradycardia-associated hypotension, and for right ventricular failure with hypotension.

Indications Indications for dopamine include hypotension (SBP 70–100 mmHg) with clinical shock (e.g., cardiogenic shock with SBP 70–100 mmHg) for symptomatic bradycardia-associated hypotension as a second-line drug to atropine, and for right ventricular heart failure with hypotension. After fluid resuscitation, dopamine is the drug recommended initially for hemodynamic support in septic shock.

Therapeutic Issues and Potential Adverse Effects Dopamine can be used in patients with hypovolemia after volume replacement in cardiogenic shock states. For cardiogenic shock associated with congestive heart failure, it should be used cautiously.

Dopamine is administered as a continuous drip because it has a half-life of approximately 1 min. It is metabolized by the enzymes MAO and COMT to renally excreted products. The hemodynamic effects of dopamine may be potentiated by MAO inhibitors, requiring dose reduction to 10%, and by other medications that have similar hemodynamic effects, such as bretylium tosylate. Additionally, the concomitant administration of phenytoin and dopamine may cause hypotension. It is contraindicated in patients with pheochromocytoma as it may precipitate a hypertensive crisis. In general, the side effects of dopamine include excessive sympathomimetic-related effects, increased myocardial oxygen consumption, and increased PCWP. Extravasation of the drug may be treated with phentolamine.

Hemodynamic effects may be potentiated by MAO inhibitors, requiring dopamine dose reduction to 10%.

Norepinephrine

Actions and Mechanisms Norepinephrine is a natural precursor of epinephrine and the neurotransmitter of the postganglionic sympathetic nervous system. It is also released by the adrenal medulla. At low doses of less than 30 ng/kg/min, it typically stimulates the β_1-ARs and at higher doses has an increasing α-adrenergic receptor effect.

The effects of norepinephrine include increased MAP, increased SVR, reflex bradycardia, little change in CO, and decreased perfusion of kidney, gut, and skeletal muscle. Norepinephrine exerts its effects predominantly through both α_1- and α_2-adrenergic vascular smooth muscle receptors and cardiac β_1-ARs, making it a powerful vasoconstrictor but a less powerful inotrope to augment MAP. It has little β_2-AR vasodilator activity, resulting in unopposed α_1-AR vasoconstrictor activity and significant elevation of SVR. The vasoconstrictor effects are stronger than the contractility effects, which may increase afterload and reduce cardiac output. Moreover, the increased SVR also causes a vagally induced reflex reduction in heart rate. However, its venoconstrictor effects may also increase preload (and PCWP) through increased venous return and increase cardiac output, resulting in only a small variable negative to positive net effect on cardiac output. Therefore, the increase in MAP occurs predominantly by elevating peripheral vascular resistance. Because norepinephrine receptors are also less abundant in the coronary and cerebral vascular bed, norepinephrine tends to augment coronary blood flow, especially in shock.

Norepinephrine increases MAP mainly by increasing SVR.

Because of the opposing actions of its powerful vasoconstrictor effects and relatively weaker inotropic effects, there is little net effect on CO.

Indications Norepinephrine indications include patients with hypotensive emergencies requiring a rapid increase in MAP to maintain adequate circulatory support. Its major use is in patients with hypotensive shock and a low SVR unresponsive to volume resuscitation and other weaker inotropic/vasopressor drugs. It is used in a number of different shock conditions including septic shock, neurogenic shock, severe cardiogenic shock, right ventricular heart failure and hypotension, and massive pulmonary embolism. The most common use of norepinephrine may be in septic shock or in neurogenic shock where a low BP unresponsive to dopamine is typically found associated with a low vascular resistance. However, in severe cardiogenic shock (Figure 38-5), it is used to augment hemodynamically significant hypotension (systolic BP < 70 mmHg), but it is most useful in the rare presence of a low vascular resistance. Although its salutary effects have been noted in the treatment of cardiogenic shock, it is used as a temporizing agent for ischemic heart disease and shock until further mechanical hemodynamic support (e.g., intraaortic balloon pump) and other treatments are effective.

The major use of norepinephrine is in patients with hypotensive shock and a low vascular resistance unresponsive to other weaker inotropic/vasopressor drugs.

Norepinephrine may increase PCWP and CVP through its potent vasoconstrictor effects.

Therapeutic Issues and Potential Adverse Effects Norepinephrine is a systemic vasoconstrictor, resulting in renal and splanchnic as well as pulmonary vascular constriction, which reduces its usefulness. Because of its strong vasoconstrictor effects, especially on visceral blood flow, it should be titrated to the lowest dose that restores adequate perfu-

FIGURE 38-5

Algorithm for the initial evaluation and treatment of acute pulmonary edema, hypotension, and shock. The algorithm starts with the evaluation and determination of the potential causative problems, i.e., acute pulmonary edema, volume and/or vascular resistance, pump, or rate. Treatment, especially the use of vasoactive drugs, is then essentially based on systolic blood pressure and the presence or absence of signs/symptoms of shock. Further options to be considered are pulmonary artery catheterization, mechanical circulatory support, angiography, and other diagnostic studies and interventions (e.g., percutaneous coronary intervention [PCI]; revascularization). (Permission from American Heart Association. Guidelines 2000 for Cardiopulmonary Resuscitation and Emergency Cardiovascular Care: International Consensus on Science. Supplement to Circulation 102;8:I189.)

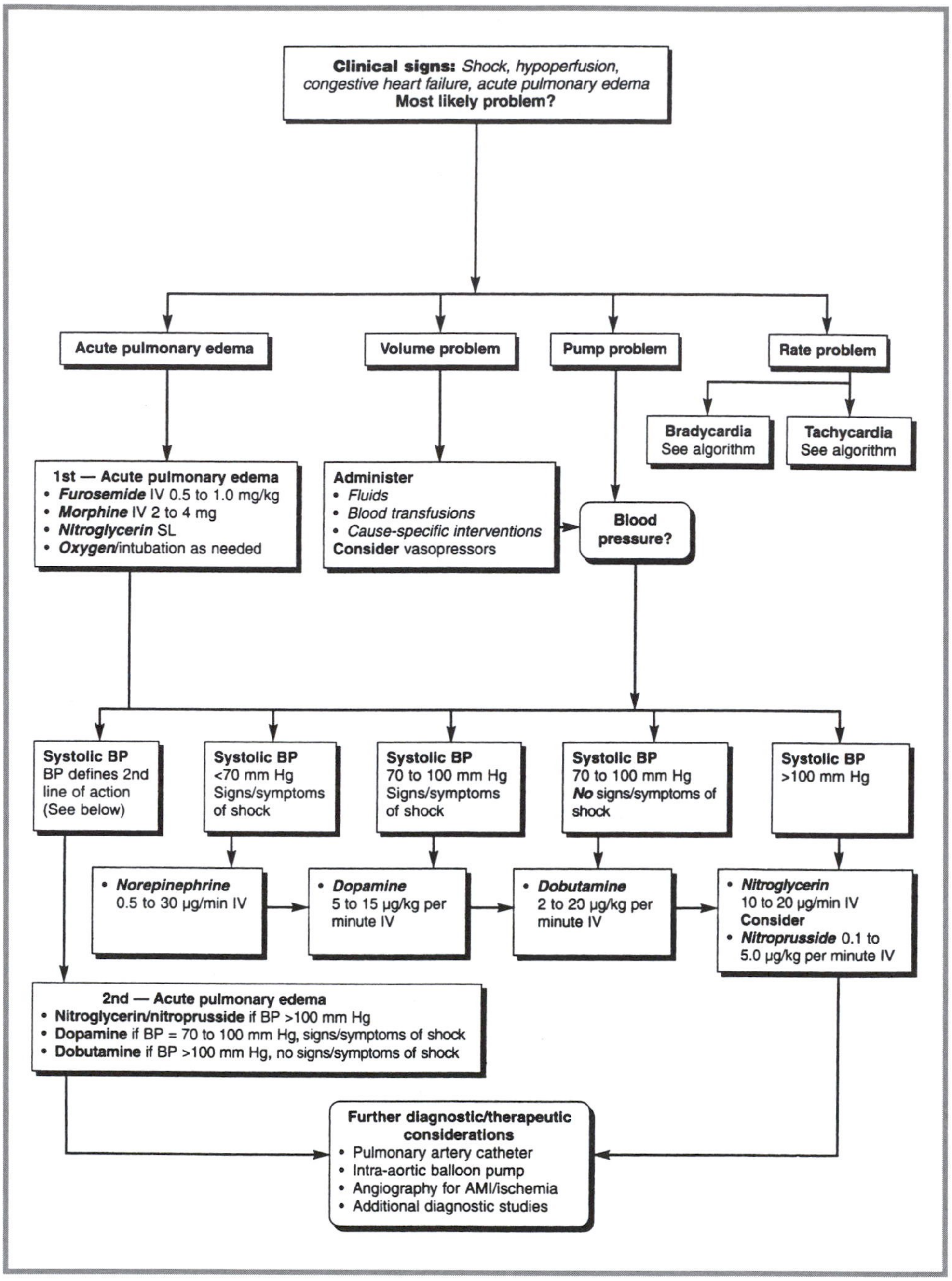

sion pressure (by clinical indices of urine output, skin perfusion, BP, and usually SVR and CO) and then replaced by a less potent vasoconstrictor as soon as possible. Norepinephrine is not recommended for use in the presence of a low intravascular volume nor in the presence of a significantly reduced cardiac function associated with an elevated SVR or PCWP. It also should be used with circumspection in the presence of pulmonary arterial hypertension.

Use norepinephrine with caution in the presence of pulmonary hypertension.

The vasopressor effect of norepinephrine is enhanced by simultaneous use of tricyclic antidepressants such as amitriptyline or by guanethidine. Unlike dopamine, MAO inhibitors do not have a marked effect on the action of norepinephrine, because MAO only metabolizes it at the sympathetic nerve terminals, and COMT metabolizes intravenously administered norepinephrine. Norepinephrine should be administered only by the central venous route because its extravasation may produce severe local tissue damage; this can be treated with liberal infiltration of the tissue with phentolamine.

The potential adverse effects include decreased skin, visceral, renal and muscle blood flow, headache, tremor, reflex bradycardia, and angina.

Dobutamine

Actions and Mechanisms Dobutamine is a catecholamine derivative, synthesized to have potent inotropic activity without peripheral vascular effect. Its salutary effects result from its administration as a racemic mixture with the levo-isomer having a strong α_1-AR effect and the dextro-isomer having strong β_1- and β_2-AR effects.

Dobutamine produces its strong inotropic effects through stimulation of both β_1- and α_1-ARs in the myocardium. It produces a net mild vasodilation through the more potent vasodilatory response, produced through peripheral vascular β_2-AR stimulation and increases in CO, and the less potent vasoconstrictor response produced by α_1-AR stimulation. Dobutamine does not stimulate dopaminergic receptors, unlike dopamine, but it does increase renal and mesenteric blood flow through augmentation of cardiac output.

Dobutamine is a synthetic catecholamine that produces strong inotropic effects and a net mild vasodilatory effect.

Indications Indications for dobutamine include patients with elevated left ventricular filling (LV) pressures and a low cardiac output state or patients with hypotension (70–100 mmHg; no signs of shock), elevated LV filling pressures, impaired LV function, and vasodilator intolerance. In conjunction with moderate volume loading, it is the main treatment for patients with hemodynamically significant right ventricular (RV) infarction.

The indications for the use of dobutamine, which produces inotropy and mild vasodilation, in patients with septic shock are less defined. The vasodilatory effects of dobutamine may cause further hypotension. In septic shock, severe cardiac dysfunction ($CI < 2.5$ l/min/m^2) may develop in a small percentage of patients, and particularly in those with elevated filling pressures, dobutamine may be helpful. However, no benefit has been shown to increasing CI to supranormal levels of O_2 delivery. Because of its vasodilatory effects, it is primarily used in conjunction with other vasopressors.

Dobutamine is best used in septic shock patients with left ventricular dysfunction ($CI < 2.5$ L/min/m^2) and elevated filling pressures.

Therapeutic Issues and Potential Adverse Effects The conventional infusion rate of dobutamine is 2–20 μg/kg/min and should be titrated according to desired response without increasing heart rate more than 10% of baseline. At doses between 5 and 15 μg/kg/min, there is a greater inotropic effect than chronotropic effect. It characteristically decreases PCWP and CVP with only a mild effect on vascular resistance. Moreover, hemodynamic monitoring is recommended for best use. Avoid use of dobutamine with systolic BP <100 mmHg and evidence of shock. It is contraindicated in poison/drug-induced shock. It is not indicated for treatment of congestive heart failure (CHF) due to diastolic dysfunction, and it is contraindicated in hypertrophic cardiomyopathy and other obstructive cardiomyopathies. In severe aortic stenosis, it may cause or worsen cardiac ischemia and not increase CO. Allergic reactions in sulfite-sensitive patients may occur from the dobutamine preparation because it contains sodium bisulfite.

Dobutamine is contraindicated in poison/drug-induced shock and in hypertrophic cardiomyopathy and other obstructive cardiomyopathies.

Dobutamine is not indicated in congestive heart failure (CHF) due to diastolic dysfunction.

Dobutamine and dopamine have been used concomitantly at moderate doses of 5.0–7.5 μg/kg/min, which maintains BP with smaller increases in PCWP or pulmonary congestion than dopamine alone. Although combination therapy does not alter mortality or survival in some patients with cardiogenic shock, its significant hemodynamic improvement and maintenance of vital organ perfusion may allow other interventions for myocardial salvage.

Adverse effects of dobutamine include cardiovascular effects and arrhythmias, BP variations, and tachycardia, which may produce myocardial ischemia. Dobutamine doses greater than 20 μg/kg/min tend to produce tachycardia, especially if the patient is hypovolemic, but doses between 2 and 20 μg/kg/min are less likely to produce tachycardia than either dopamine or isoproterenol. Myocardial ischemia may occur, especially if it produces tachycardia resulting in increased myocardial oxygen demand. Miscellaneous adverse effects include headache, tremor, nausea, and hypokalemia.

Phenylephrine

> Phenylephrine is a powerful vasoconstrictor that elevates MAP mainly through an increase in SVR.

> Phenylephrine is probably most useful as an alternative vasopressor for patients who develop tachyarrhythmias.

Actions and Mechanisms Phenylephrine is a rapid-acting, selective α_1-adrenergic agonist drug that acts as a powerful peripheral vasoconstrictor. Accordingly, phenylephrine elevates MAP mainly through an increase in SVR. Furthermore, the vasoconstriction may produce a reflex bradycardia and a small decrease in CO, which may be more marked in patients with preexisting cardiac dysfunction. Renal perfusion may also decrease.

Because phenylephrine is a vasocontrictor without direct inotropic effects and there are only a few studies on its clinical use, there have been concerns regarding the potential for reduction in CO and HR, especially in less hyperdynamic states or unrecognized cardiomyopathy (sepsis-induced cardiomyopathy). It can increase MAP in fluid-resuscitated patients in septic shock and may be especially useful in patients with tachyarrhythmias associated with β-adrenergic drugs.

There is only one small study evaluating the clinical effects of phenylephrine in septic shock patients ($n = 13$), who remained hypotensive (MAP, 57 mmHg; CI, 3.3 $l/min/m^2$) despite either low-dose dopamine or dobutamine and fluid administration. Phenylephrine was titrated to mean dosage of 3.7 μg/kg/min to maintain MAP greater than 70 mmHg, which resulted in increases in MAP, SVR, CI, SI, and urine output. Increases in oxygen consumption and delivery occurred as well. In hyperdynamic septic patients without hypotension, phenylephrine (70 μg/min) increased MAP, CI, SI and slightly decreased HR by 3 beats/min. At the same dosage in normotensive patients with cardiac disease, phenylephrine caused an increase in BP and SVR but decreased CI without change in HR.

Indications Phenylephrine is a powerful vasoconstrictor used to treat hypotension during anesthesia and occasionally for hypotension and shock in sepsis. However, phenylephrine has been studied minimally in septic shock, and thus it is difficult to determine its role in septic shock treatment. It does not have any direct inotropic properties. However, it appears it is most useful as an alternative in patients with septic shock who develop tachyarrhythmias to the other β-AR agonists. It was previously used to treat supraventricular tachycardia with hypotension.

Therapeutic Issues and Potential Adverse Effects Phenylephrine is a noncatecholamine but has a molecular structure similar to epinephrine. Unlike epinephrine, it is not metabolized by COMT but by MAO, making it short acting. Because the drug is a pure vasoconstrictor, there is a tendency for decreases in CO because of the significant afterload effect. In patients with impaired myocardial function or in valvular disease such as aortic insufficiency or mitral regurgitation, it may significantly decrease cardiac output. In septic shock, it has been used as an alternative to norepinephrine, but there is limited information on its use. The drug also decreases renal and splanchnic blood flow and may increase oxygen consumption and delivery.

Epinephrine

> Epinephrine is a naturally occurring hormone that activates both α- and β-AR.

Actions and Mechanisms Epinephrine is a naturally occurring catecholamine produced by *N*-methylation of norepinephrine in the adrenal medulla. Its production and release are regulated by sympathetic innervation of the adrenal gland. Epinephrine binds and activates β_2-, β_1-, and α-AR in a dose-dependent manner. The effects of epinephrine at low doses are more β-AR related whereas higher doses are more α-AR related. Epinephrine causes increased myocardial contraction, electrical activity, automaticity, and oxygen requirements. The increase in BP primarily results from an increase in SV and CI associated with only moderate increases in SVR and HR in sepsis.

Indications The indications for epinephrine include refractory circulatory shock; anaphylaxis with or without shock; severe allergic reactions; symptomatic bradycardia unresponsive to atropine, dopamine, and transcutaneous pacing; and cardiac arrest resulting from ventricular fibrillation (VF), pulseless ventricular tachycardia (VT), asystole, and pulseless electrical activity. After fluid infusion, it may be used, likely at higher doses, as a first- or a second-line drug after glucagon in treating β-adrenergic blocker cardiotoxicity associated with hypotension or shock and bradycardia. It is used as a third-line inotropic/vasopressor agent for septic shock after dopamine and norepinephrine. It may be particularly useful in patients with severe myocardial dysfunction.

Therapeutic Issues and Potential Adverse Effects Epinephrine may cause increased myocardial oxygen demand, ischemia, and angina induced by increased HR and BP. It may also increase lactate concentrations either by its potential effects to reduce organ perfusion or by its hypermetabolic effect. In addition to epinephrine, the treatment of anaphylaxis requires fluids, corticosteroids, and antihistamines. The potential adverse effects of epinephrine include hyperglycemia, angina, tachycardia, arrhythmias, poor cutaneous perfusion, and agitation.

Isoproterenol

Actions and Mechanisms Isoproterenol is a synthetic catecholamine produced by adding an *N*-isopropyl moiety to norepinephrine, which provides it with significant β-AR properties without affecting its α-AR properties. The drug has inotropic, chronotropic, and vasodilatory effects. The β-adrenergic properties increase myocardial contractility and rate. Indirectly, it also produces a reflex chronotropic response by decreasing SVR via its vasodilatory properties, causing significant tachycardia.

Isoproterenol is a synthetic β-adrenergic agonist with inotropic, chronotropic, and vasodilatory effects.

Isoproterenol produces a net increase in cardiac output in a euvolemic patient but a decrease in cardiac output may occur in the hypovolemic patient because of reduced venous return from vasodilation. The improvement in cardiac output is related more to increased heart rate than stroke volume. Its β_2-agonist vasodilatory properties decrease diastolic blood pressure and may also redirect blood flow from the splanchnic to the higher β_2-AR-dense skeletal muscle vascular bed.

Indications The previously broader indications for isoproterenol have been limited by the availability of safer and more effective drugs. Currently, the indications for isoproterenol include temporary control of symptomatic bradycardia (if an external pacer is not available) and for bradycardia in the denervated heart transplant patient and in torsades de pointes unresponsive to magnesium sulfate.

Indications for isoproterenol use have been narrowed by the availability of safer and more effective drugs.

Therapeutic Issues and Potential Side Effects Isoproterenol requires very careful cardiovascular monitoring, especially continuous electrocardiographic monitoring, as it may increase myocardial ischemia by increasing myocardial oxygen requirements. Accordingly, it should be avoided in adults with coronary artery disease. Symptoms of ischemia such as chest pain should lead to a quick reduction in dose. It should *not* be used for treatment of cardiac arrest, drug-induced shock, except in β-adrenergic blocker poisoning, or conditions where epinephrine is being given as it can cause ventricular fibrillation or tachycardia. It may be safely administered via a peripheral line access. MAO inhibitors or tricyclic antidepressants do not alter its effects.

Isoproterenol requires careful cardiovascular monitoring, especially electrocardiographic, as it may increase myocardial ischemia by increasing myocardial oxygen requirements.

Nonadrenergic Drugs

Amrinone and Milrinone

Actions and Mechanisms Amrinone and milrinone are part of a group of synthetic phosphodiestase III inhibitors with significant inotropic effects and less chronotropic effects but strong vasodilatory effects, thereby classifying them as ino-dilators.

Amrinone and milrinone are phosphodiesterase III inhibitors that have significant inotropic and strong vasodilatory effects.

The hemodynamic effects of increased CO associated with decreased preload and SVR are dose related and similar to dobutamine. At low doses, MAP does not decrease due to a balance between the increase in stroke volume and the reduction in SVR. High doses can cause tachycardia. These drugs decrease right atrial pressure, mean pulmonary artery pressures, and vascular resistance and dilate coronary arteries. The pulmonary vasodilator effect may help to unload the right ventricle.

Unlike catecholaminergic drugs, the hemodynamic effects of amrinone result from phosphodiesterase III inhibition causing increased cAMP concentrations and possibly other mechanisms. Accordingly, adrenergic-blocking drugs do not reverse its inotropic and vasodilator manifestations.

Indication for amrinone and milrinone is severe CHF, unresponsive to diuretics, vasodilators, and standard inotropic agents.

Indications The indication for amrinone is severe CHF unresponsive to diuretics, vasodilators, and standard inotropic agents. There have been no studies in adults evaluating the effects of amrinone in sepsis and septic shock. However, there has been one study in pediatric patients of milrinone. In septic shock, the inotropic effects of the drug may improve stroke volume, but its vasodilator effects, which decrease SVR, may worsen or prolong hypotension.

The individual variability in cardiac and vascular responses and its long half-life make it difficult to use in the unstable patient.

Therapeutic Issues and Potential Adverse Effects Maximum benefit requires a loading dose, because of the long half-life of amrinone (4–6 h), and a dose–response titration using central hemodynamic monitoring. The variability in individual cardiac and vascular responses and its long half-life make amrinone difficult to use in the unstable patient. Its vasodilator effect and long half-life may result in prolonged hypotension. Titration of an inotrope and vasodilator in cases of cardiogenic shock may be favored. It is attractive in more stable patients because of its potential to increase CO without a significant increase in HR response or myocardial O_2 demand. To start an infusion, a loading dose of amrinone at 0.75 mg/kg should be given over 10–15 min to decrease the risk of hypotension in patients with LV impairment and borderline BP, followed by a dose–response titration starting at an infusion rate of 2–5 μg/kg/min, up to 10–15 μg/kg/min. Impaired drug clearance may occur in renal or hepatic dysfunction. Because amrinone contains metabisulfate, it is contraindicated in sulfite-allergic patients.

Amrinone and milrinone may cause cardiac ischemia, hypotension, tachyarryhthmia, and thrombocytopenia.

Amrinone may cause cardiac ischemia, hypotension, tachyarrhythmias, and thrombocytopenia. The thrombocytopenia occurs within 2–3 days in 2%–4% of patients and is typically reversible (after drug discontinuation), dose dependent, and rarely associated with bleeding. Accordingly, it should be used with caution in patients with hypotension, thrombocytopenia, and restrictive cardiomyopathies. Similar to other inotropic medications, it may worsen hemodynamics in hypertrophic obstructive cardiomyopathy and is contraindicated in valvular obstructive disease. Additional potential adverse effects include gastrointestinal disturbance, liver dysfunction (enzyme elevation) with long-term use, muscle aches, fever, and ventricular irritability.

Vasopressin

Actions and Mechanisms Vasopressin, otherwise known as antidiuretic hormone (ADH), is a small peptide hormone released from the posterior pituitary that has several physiologic roles. It plays a major role in water balance and in the regulation of the cardiovascular system. It is a potent vasoconstrictor that is released in the presence of hypovolemia or hypotension and has been found to be elevated in patients with some types of shock.

Its effects are mediated through two types of receptors known as V_1 and V_2. The V_1 receptor is found in multiple tissues of the body such as bladder, liver, spleen, kidney, CNS, testes, and platelets. ADH actions are mediated mainly through renal V_2 receptors. The vasoconstrictor effects, which require higher vasopressin concentrations than its antidiuretic actions, are mediated through direct stimulation of V_1 receptors present on vascular smooth muscle. The increase in MAP has been attributable to increases in peripheral vascular resistance. Administered in supraphysiologic doses, vasopressin causes powerful vasoconstrictor effects and is more potent than angiotensin II or norepinephrine. In contrast to catecholamines such as epinephrine, the effects of vasopressin during acidosis are not altered.

Vasopressin produces powerful vasoconstrictor effects by direct stimulation of V_1 smooth muscle receptors.

Vasopressin is an alternative to epinephrine for the treatment of adult shock-refractory ventricular fibrillation.

Indications Vasopressin has been recently introduced by the American Heart Association 2000 guidelines as an alternative to epinephrine for the treatment of adult shock-refractory ventricular fibrillation. Although there are insufficient data, it is thought to be effective in patients who remain in cardiac arrest after initial treatment with epinephrine. Because vasopressin is a powerful vasoconstrictor, it also may be helpful in vasodilatory shock states, such as septic shock, that are poorly responsive to standard therapy. Although there are a few published studies on its use, it has not been considered in current guidelines for septic shock.

Vasopressin may be helpful in shock states with a vasodilatory component.

Therapeutic Issues and Potential Adverse Effects Vasopressin can produce multiple adverse effects related to smooth muscle constriction in both vascular smooth muscle and gastrointestinal, uterine, and bronchial smooth muscle. The potent vascular smooth muscle constriction may cause coronary artery constriction, resulting in cardiac ischemia and angina. Therefore, its use in alert patients with coronary artery disease is inadvisable. Other effects resulting from smooth muscle constriction include cutaneous perfusion, bronchospasm, uterine contractions, and gastrointestinal effects such as nausea and abdominal cramps. However, some clinical studies have not found any clinical evidence for cutaneous, liver, gastrointestinal, or myocardial ischemia. Moreover, vasopressin may cause platelet aggregation and increase the potential for small vessel occlusion. Its half-life is longer than that of epinephrine, approximately 10–20 min, which allows less frequent dosing.

Glucagon

Actions and Mechanisms A polypeptide hormone with multiple effects both metabolically and physiologically, glucagon has both inotropic and chronotropic effects on the heart. The cardiovascular effects of glucagon are mediated through glucagon receptors, resulting in augmentation of cAMP through adenylyl cyclase stimulation or phosphodiesterase inhibition and thereby causing cellular calcium flux. Because the effects of glucagon are not mediated by α- or β-ARs, the responses are not affected by adrenergic blockade.

Cardiovascular effects are mediated through glucagon receptors and therefore are not affected by α-adrenergic or β-adrenergic receptor blockers.

In cardiac insufficiency (CHF or cardiogenic shock), glucagon produces increased HR, CI, and O_2 delivery with minimal change in left ventricular end-diastolic pressure (LVEDP) and SVR. Glucagon infusion may increase CO by 20%. Its effects on CI and MAP, however, are less than that of dopamine, dobutamine, amrinone, or epinephrine. It has a less negative effect on myocardial O_2 consumption than norepinephrine.

Indications Glucagon is used as additional treatment of β-adrenergic blocker and calcium channel blocker toxicity. It can be used as a secondary agent to epinephrine in anaphylaxis/anaphylactic shock, especially if β-adrenergic blocking drugs are present. Glucagon has not been studied in sepsis and septic shock.

Glucagon is used for the adjuvant treatment of toxic effects of calcium channel blocker and β-adrenergic blocker toxicity.

Therapeutic Issues and Potential Adverse Effects Glucagon has been found to be superior to other drugs in the treatment of β-adrenergic blocker toxicity. Similarly, it is more effective than the phosphodiesterase inhibitors, which also enhance cAMP levels. Pharmacokinetic studies have shown that a 5-mg IV bolus of glucagon causes cardiac effects to begin in 1–5 min and to have a duration of 20–30 min. Because its half-life is approximately 20 min, the drug is started with a bolus followed by a continuous intravenous infusion.

Glucagon does have some drug interactions as well as potential adverse effects related to its physiologic role in glucose balance and in the cardiovascular, gastrointestinal, and urinary systems. It does not alter heparin effects but it does potentiate the anticoagulant effect of coumadin. The most frequent adverse effects are nausea and vomiting, which may require high-dose antiemetics, and occasionally hyperglycemia. Other adverse effects include hypokalemia, vasodilation and hypotension, and tachycardia.

Vasodilators

Actions and Mechanisms Sodium nitroprusside is a rapid-acting powerful vasodilator, mediated by both arterial and venous smooth muscle relaxation, that results in both reduced arterial resistance and an increased venous capacitance, causing a reduced preload. It produces these effects on smooth muscle through the generation of nitric oxide (NO), a physiological endogenous vasodilator. The NO activates guanylate cyclase in the vascular

Sodium nitroprusside is a rapid-acting, powerful venous and arterial vasodilator.

smooth muscle, which results in increased cellular concentrations of cGMP. Cyclic GMP reduces cellular calcium, causing smooth muscle relaxation and vasodilation.

Indications Sodium nitroprusside is primarily used in hypertensive crises, as an afterload reducing agent in both heart failure and acute pulmonary edema, and in acute mitral or aortic valve regurgitation. It is used in conjunction with other vasopressor/inotropic drugs and circulatory-assist devices such as intraaortic balloon pump (IABP) to maintain coronary blood flow in shock. The use of nitroprusside in the presence of coronary artery disease or myocardial infarction (MI), however, is controversial because it may reduce coronary blood flow and worsen ischemia. It is thought to be related to the ability of nitroglycerin to enhance flow through collateral circulation. Currently, nitroglycerin is preferred in this situation as it improves ischemia.

Therapeutic Issues and Potential Adverse Effects Sodium nitroprusside is a vasodilator with both a rapid onset of 1–2 min and a rapid offset of less than 1 min, which allows tight control of hemodynamic effects. It is recommended to start at a low dose of 0.10 μg/kg/min because it produces rapid vasodilation and hypotension, especially in the elderly and in volume-contracted patients, and then to titrate upward as high as 5–8 μg/kg/min to the desired hemodynamic effect. In congestive heart failure, a pulmonary artery catheter is required for optimal use and safety. If hypotension does occur, it usually can be reversed by stopping the infusion and administering volume as necessary. Its vasodilator actions may also cause hypoxemia by impairing the hypoxic pulmonary vasoconstrictor response, especially in those patients with pulmonary disease.

Other potential adverse effects may result from its metabolism. Sodium nitroprusside binds quickly to the sulfhydryl groups on hemoglobin, oxidizing it to methemoglobin and releasing toxic cyanide radicals of which one binds to the methemoglobin, producing cyanomethemoglobin. The other cyanide radicals are enzymatically converted by rhodanese to thiocyanate using thiosulfate and cyanocobalamin in the liver and kidney, followed by urinary excretion. However, the reaction is limited by the availability of rhodanese, thiosulfate, and cyanocobalamin.

> Cyanide and thiocyanate are toxic products of nitroprusside metabolism.

> Cyanide toxicity may manifest as metabolic acidosis, dyspnea, confusion, and headache.

Cyanide and thiocyanate are both toxic products produced during the metabolism of nitroprusside, thereby limiting its dosage of nitroprusside. The toxicity of cyanide may cause metabolic acidosis, dyspnea, confusion, and headache. The cyanide radicals are rapidly toxic by causing inactivation of the cytochrome oxidase system and impaired oxidative metabolism, resulting in anaerobic metabolism, acidosis, and eventual death if not reversed. Treatment of cyanide toxicity involves stopping the infusion and using available antidotes: sodium nitrite, sodium thiosulfate, and vitamin B_{12}. Sodium nitrite causes methemoglobin, which binds cyanide radicals, while thiosulfate is substrate for conversion of cyanide to thiocyanate.

Thiocyanate toxicity is an uncommon complication that may result in lassitude, anorexia, nausea, abdominal pain, miosis, visual blurring, mental status changes, hyperreflexia, and seizures. However, its frequency increases in the presence of impaired renal function or administration of high-dose (>3 μg/kg/min) or prolonged infusions, especially greater than 48–72 h. In these situations, monitoring of signs and symptoms and blood thiocyanate levels becomes important, as early signs of thiocyanate toxicity may occur at 5 mg/dl, but it is usually well tolerated and safe at levels less than 10 mg/dl. Thiocyanate can be removed by hemodialysis.

Nitroglycerin

> Nitroglycerin causes venodilation at low doses and both veno- and arterial vasodilation at higher doses.

Actions and Mechanisms Nitroglycerin is a powerful vasodilator that acts rapidly by increasing the formation and release of NO from vascular endothelium, causing smooth muscle relaxation. It is primarily a venodilator at low doses and both a venodilator and arteriolar vasodilator at high doses. Its venodilator effects result in mesenteric and hepatic venous pooling and a reduction in ventricular filling pressures and pulmonary congestion. Further increases in dose begin to cause arterial vasodilation with a resultant increase in cardiac output. Higher doses will result in hypotension.

The hemodynamic effects of nitroglycerin are affected not only by dose but by the volume status and cardiac function. If hypovolemia is present, nitroglycerin is likely to cause a further drop in preload and decrease CO, resulting in further hypotension. Its arterial effects are typically lost in this situation. On the other hand, in congestive heart failure, nitroglycerin reduces preload and vascular resistance, leading to a reduction in myocardial oxygen uptake and increased cardiac output.

Indications Nitroglycerin is used in patients with acute MI and congestive heart failure, large anterior wall infarction, persistent or recurrent ischemia, or hypertension for the first 24–48 h.

Therapeutic Issues and Potential Adverse Effects A major potential adverse effect of nitroglycerin is frank hypotension, including postural hypotension. The hypotension responds to volume repletion. Therefore, nitroglycerin should be used with caution in the presence of inferior wall MI and is contraindicated in patients with right ventricular infarction and ventricular filling pressure dependence. Additional adverse effects include headache, faintness, tachycardia, and paradoxical bradycardia, and impaired hypoxic pulmonary vasoconstrictor response resulting in hypoxemia. Some side effects may be related to either the alcohol or propylene glycol drug solvent.

Hypotension is a major side effect of nitroglycerin therapy.

THERAPY FOR SELECTED CLINICAL CONDITIONS

Because the mechanisms for specific causes of shock and thereby the treatment can vary significantly, this section briefly describes the pharmacologic support for some of the more common clinical disease conditions presenting to the intensive care unit. These disease conditions and their treatment are further detailed in other chapters in this book.

Hypovolemic Shock

Hypovolemic shock can result from hemorrhagic etiologies (e.g., trauma, gastrointestinal) and nonhemorrhagic etiologies (e.g., vomiting, diarrhea, GI fistulas, and third-spacing). The etiology of hypovolemic shock is usually obtainable from the history of external blood or fluid losses, physical examination, and laboratory tests such as hemoconcentration and increased BUN to creatinine ratio. Treatment of hypovolemic shock requires vascular access in the form of two large-bore peripheral lines or a central venous line for rapid infusion of blood products, colloidal solutions, or crystalloid solutions. If blood loss is occurring simultaneously, resuscitation and evaluation should be performed. Volume resuscitation should result in rapid improvement of clinical parameters of perfusion pressure such as blood pressure and pulse rate. Other parameters such as urine output improve later, and mental status may be further delayed. If significant improvement does not occur, there may be either ongoing blood or fluid volume loss or an incorrect or additional diagnoses (e.g., adrenal cortical insufficiency). The sites of blood loss need to be evaluated and repaired. To rapidly improve tissue perfusion, additional supportive measures include the temporary use of vasopressor/inotropic agents at low dosage such as dopamine, norepinephrine, or epinephrine until fluid resuscitation is adequate. However, the use of vasoactive agents in hypovolemic shock may confound the perfusion endpoints for volume resuscitation and may lead to continued hypotension due to inadequate circulatory volume.

Severe hypovolemic shock may require the temporary use of vasoactive drugs.

Extracardiac Obstructive Shock

Extracardiac obstructive shock can be caused by a wide variety of disorders and grouped into several mechanisms: extrinsic vascular obstruction (e.g., mediastinal tumors), increased intrathoracic pressure (e.g., pneumothorax), intrinsic vascular flow obstruction (e.g., pulmonary embolism, air embolism, and tumors), and pericardial disease (e.g., tamponade).

Pulmonary Embolism

Massive pulmonary embolism can cause an extracardiac obstructive pattern of shock.

In pulmonary embolism (PE), the pulmonary vascular system is obstructed, causing an impediment to blood flow and resulting in hypotension or shock, especially if massive. A massive PE causes a sudden increase in right ventricular afterload, and the right ventricle is unable to provide a commensurate increase in stroke volume to maintain BP. The hemodynamic pattern commonly produced by massive pulmonary embolus shows a decreased CO, a decreased or unchanged PCWP, but an increased CVP. The SVR and pulmonary vascular resistance (PVR) are increased, and the SVO_2 is decreased (see Figure 38-1B).

The treatment of massive pulmonary embolism involves the use of hemodynamic support, thrombolytics, or possible surgical embolectomy. The pharmacologic treatment of hypotension or shock in pulmonary embolism may include the use of fluids and vasoactive drugs. Use of a pulmonary artery catheter can help to optimize both fluid and vasoactive drug therapy.

In shock caused by pulmonary embolism, volume resuscitation may be deleterious and must be carefully titrated.

Fluid therapy should be carefully evaluated as it has the potential to further compromise right ventricular function and cardiac index. In pulmonary embolism, the right-sided filling pressures may be already high, and the addition of fluids may significantly increase these pressures causing further right ventricular distension and more hemodynamic compromise. Right ventricular distension can cause right ventricular ischemia and a decreased left ventricular compliance due to leftward interventricular septal movement. Fluid therapy should be initiated with a fluid bolus and then, if deemed hemodynamically helpful, carefully titrated with fluid while monitoring the resultant hemodynamic changes. Generally, right atrial pressures should be targeted to 15–20 mmHg while avoiding pressures greater then 20 mmHg. In acute PE, fluid loading may cause deleterious increases in the right-atrial pressure (RAP) and PCWP, causing decreased left ventricular end-diastolic pressure or volume due to interventricular septal movement and right ventricular ischemia, thereby compromising cardiac output.

If PE is unresponsive to fluid therapy, consider vasopressor/inotropic drugs such as dobutamine or norepinephrine.

If the patient does not appear to benefit from a fluid bolus, vasoactive therapy should be started. Numerous drugs have been evaluated, more so in animals than humans. Dobutamine and norepinephrine have been recommended in massive PE. Because dobutamine is an inotropic agent associated with a vasodilator effect, it may improve hemodynamics by increasing right ventricular performance or reducing pulmonary vascular resistance. Norepinephrine has been recommended by multiple authors because its positive inotropic and its vasoconstrictor effects may increase coronary artery blood flow to the right ventricle. The vasoactive drugs should be titrated to hemodynamic parameters.

Distributive Shock

Distributive shock may be caused by a number of different etiologies, which include septic shock, anaphylaxis, and neurogenic and toxic (drug overdose) shock.

Septic Shock

Septic shock generally may present in two different shock states, hypodynamic ("cold shock") and hyperdynamic ("warm shock"), depending on differences in CO and SVR. Typically, the hemodynamic parameters of hyperdynamic shock are associated with a low preload and a high CO but a low SVR. In contrast, hypodynamic shock is associated with hemodynamic parameters of a low preload and CO and a high PVR and SVR. Most septic patients present with a suboptimal preload commonly from a combination of fluid losses, caused by increased insensible losses and vascular leak, and vasodilation.

In septic shock, rapid fluid resuscitation is performed first. In severe shock a vasopressors/inotropes may be started simultaneously.

In addition to infection management, the Society of Critical Care Medicine evidence-based practice parameters for hemodynamic support of adults with sepsis recommend titration to clinical endpoints of MAP, HR, urine output (UO), skin perfusion, and mental status. They also recommend using indicators of tissue perfusion such as blood lactate concentrations and mixed venous oxygen saturation (SvO_2). However, titration to supernormal preset clinical endpoints of O_2 delivery and CI is not recommended in the patient with sepsis. Resuscitative efforts first include volume infusion to promote development of the hyperdynamic state, then vasopressors and inotropes. In those patients with persistent evidence of shock despite volume infusion, a vasopressor such as dopamine is considered the first-line drug to increase MAP, followed next by norepinephrine for a persistently low MAP. Dopamine increases CI more than norepinephrine. Norepinephrine may decrease or only mildly increase CI due to its potent vasoconstrictor effects. However, dopamine may excessively elevate HR while norepinephrine may have significantly less effect. If the patient continues to have refractory shock, epinephrine should be considered. Vasopressin has been used for the treatment of septic shock but awaits further evaluation before it is formally recommended and its place in therapy is defined.

In septic shock, rapid fluid resuscitation is performed first. In severe shock, vasopressor/inotropes may be started simultaneously.

Anaphylactic Shock

A severe, systemic allergic reaction most commonly caused by foods, bee and wasp stings, drugs, and latex, anaphylactic shock results in IgE- and IgG-4-mediated systemic release of histamine and other mediators. The clinical manifestations of anaphylaxis commonly involve two or more of the following organ systems: skin, respiratory, cardiovascular, and gastrointestinal. Cutaneous and mucosal manifestations include urticaria, conjunctivitis, and rhinitis. Gastrointestinal signs and symptoms are abdominal pain, vomiting, and diarrhea. Respiratory manifestations include upper and lower airway edema and bronchospasm. Cardiovascular manifestations include circulatory shock, commonly caused by vasodilation, and intravascular volume loss, caused by increased capillary permeability. The hemodynamic findings in anaphylaxis include a decreased or increased preload, associated with a low CO, high PVR, and a low SVR. The multiple differential diagnoses include vasovagal reactions, psychologic disorders such as panic attacks associated with paradoxical vocal dysfunction, hereditary and ACE inhibitor-induced angioedema, and scombroid poisoning.

Treatment for the multiple manifestations of anaphylactic shock includes pharmacologic therapy and important supportive measures such as early airway control, high-flow oxygen, and mechanical ventilation. Epinephrine should be administered to all patients who exhibit clinical signs of circulatory shock, airway swelling, or distinct respiratory difficulty. It is usually administered either intravenously or intramuscularly depending on its severity (profound and life-threatening) and the presence of venous access. To treat circulatory shock, administer epinephrine as the drug of choice and if multiple doses required initiate an intravenous infusion from 1 to 4 μg/min; if the patient is unresponsive to epinephrine, glucagon may be helpful especially if the patient is on beta-blockers. Normal saline, 1–4 l, should be administered rapidly if hypotension is present and the patient is slowly responsive to epinephrine.

In anaphylactic shock, epinephrine is the drug of choice; if the patient is unresponsive, glucagon may be helpful.

Neurogenic Shock

Neurogenic shock may be precipitated by general or spinal anesthesia or by cerebral or spinal cord injury resulting in sympathetic tone impairment leading to decreased MAP, preload, and CO usually without tachycardia. In fact, patients with spinal shock from traumatic spinal cord injury above T6 will tend to have bradycardia. Spinal shock, usually caused by a traumatic injury, is the complete blockade of neurotransmission in the spinal cord below the injury. The resulting fall in BP places the patient at risk for heart and brain ischemic events. The pharmacologic support of neurogenic shock depends on whether it results from a transient, reversible cause such as autonomic blockade due to anesthesia or from actual damage to the autonomic nervous system such as spinal shock, which also affects cardiac function. Patients that have decreased perfusion should be given fluids, and if inadequate perfusion continues, pharmacologic therapy should be considered. In the former, an α-adrenergic agonist is commonly used to provide BP support; in the latter, a drug with combined α-adrenergic and β-adrenergic properties, norepinephrine, is used to provide cardiac support.

Neurogenic shock may result from general or spinal anesthesia or spinal cord injury.

Cardiogenic Shock

Cardiogenic shock may result from primary myocardial dysfunction, valvular or structural abnormalities, and arrhythmias (see Figure 38-1A). Acute left ventricular failure resulting in

Cardiogenic shock has a high mortality rate, 50%–60%, and results when approximately 40% of the myocardium is infarcted.

cardiogenic shock occurs most commonly after myocardial infarction. Cardiogenic shock results when approximately 40% of the myocardium is infarcted. The incidence of shock is less than 7% but continues to have a high mortality, approximately 50%–60%.

Hemodynamically, the stroke volume decreases, causing increased left ventricular volume and dilation, leading to increased myocardial O_2 consumption and the potential for worsening ischemia (see Figure 38-1B). The reduced stroke volume decreases cardiac output, unless a compensatory tachycardia occurs, which will also increase myocardial O_2 consumption and ischemia. The decrease in CO results in increasing left ventricular pressures, causing increasing pulmonary congestion and shock. Pulmonary artery catheter pressures typically show systolic blood pressure below 100 mmHg, PCWP above 18–20 mmHg, and CI less than 2.5 $l/min/m^2$. Usually, evidence for poor perfusion is present at a systolic BP of 90 mmHg and CI of 2.2 $l/min/m^2$.

The therapy of acute pulmonary edema, hypotension, and shock is shown as an algorithm corresponding to the recent American Heart Association Guidelines 2000 (see Figure 38-5). One set of goals for hypotensive patients in cardiogenic shock is to restore MAP to at least 60 mmHg, CI to more than 2.2 $l/min/m^2$, and to maintain PCWP between 14 and 18 mmHg. The algorithmic approach to therapy is based on the most likely type of problem such as volume, pump, rate, or acute pulmonary edema and then stratified by systolic BP. In the presence of pulmonary congestion and depending on the systolic BP, diuresis is recommended while reducing preload and afterload. In a hypotensive patient with cardiogenic shock who has not developed pulmonary congestion, fluid should be cautiously administered to increase the intravascular volume. The clinician should closely monitor the patient for the development of pulmonary edema and/or coronary ischemia due to an increase in ventricular filling pressures. In the case of a cardiac pump problem, vasopressors and/or inotropic drugs are indicated according to the systolic BP. Generally, for SBP below 70 mmHg and evidence of shock, norepinephrine is indicated initially; after SBP increases to 80 mmHg or more, dopamine should be attempted, and at SBP of approximately 90 mmHg, dobutamine is added to reduce dopamine dose.

In general, vasodilators are contraindicated in cardiogenic shock. Vasodilators used in cases of congestive heart failure with normal or high systemic arterial pressures are helpful to improve stroke volume and cardiac output but are not recommended if the systemic arterial pressures or ventricular filling pressures are low because further hypotension may result. These drugs may be considered in cases where shock is caused by mitral (vasopressors contraindicated) or aortic regurgitation or aortic dissection, or in conjunction with other treatments such as intraaortic balloon pump or other vasopressor/inotropic drugs. Patients should be considered as appropriate for intraaortic balloon counterpulsation (IABP), angiography for acute myocardial infarction or ischemia, and potential procedures (percutaneous coronary intervention, revascularlization, fibrinolytics).

Right Ventricular Infarction

In the presence of inferior wall infarction, the association of hypotension with clear lungs and increased jugular venous pressures strongly indicates hemodynamically significant right ventricular infarction.

Right ventricular infarction can result in cardiogenic shock (see Figure 38-1B). This entity is more commonly associated with inferior wall infarcts than anterior wall infarcts or in isolation. On examination, the lungs are typically clear but there is jugular venous distension, sometimes associated with a Kussmaul's sign. Typically, laboratory evaluation reveals a clear chest roentgenogram, and hemodynamic parameters commonly show a decreased CO associated with elevated right-sided pressures: an increased right atrial (RA) pressure relative to PCWP and an increased right ventricular diastolic pressure but decreased PA pressure. The right ventricular infarction and resulting dysfunction produces a decrease in left ventricular preload and in turn a decreased stroke volume and cardiac output. The most common differential diagnoses includes pericardial tamponade and pulmonary embolism. Studies such as right precordial EKG, echocardiography, or ventilation–perfusion lung scanning should be considered to confirm or exclude other possible diagnoses.

Treatment of shock resulting from right ventricular infarct includes fluids and vasopressor/inotropic drugs as well as coronary reperfusion therapy (e.g., fibrinolytic therapy, percutaneous coronary intervention) and other general supportive measures (e.g., IABC, arterial vasodilators). Hemodynamic data from the pulmonary artery catheter are often used to optimize therapy. Initially, fluid therapy in the form of a single bolus should be considered carefully to optimize right ventricular preload based on clinical assessment of volume status. If there is no significant improvement, pharmacologic therapy should be considered, such as dobutamine or norepinephrine, to provide inotropy and increased coronary artery perfusion. These drugs should be titrated to clinical as well as hemodynamic indices of perfusion.

SUMMARY

Shock is defined as a failure of the circulatory system to provide adequate cellular or tissue perfusion and oxygen delivery to meet current metabolic demands, resulting in organ dysfunction and irreversible cellular damage. Shock can be classified into four categories: hypovolemic, cardiogenic, extracardiac obstructive, and distributive. Each of these four categories includes a number of different potential etiologies. The identification of the category of shock and its etiology provides for more specific treatment and potentially a better outcome. To determine the etiology of shock, a clinical (history, physical examination, and directed laboratory studies) and hemodynamic evaluation (pulmonary arterial catheterization, echocardiography) further delineate the cause and treatment.

The goal of shock treatment is to restore tissue perfusion and oxygenation. Tissue perfusion is partly related to cardiac output and systemic vascular resistance. The treatment of shock mainly utilizes vasopressor/inotropic medications, classified by adrenergic and nonadrenergic mechanisms, and, in special cases, vasodilators. Each of these drugs may also have untoward effects such as increased heart rate, splanchnic vascular bed vasoconstriction, or arrhythmias. These drugs are the tools to restore the premorbid hemodynamic state. An understanding of their mechanism of action, potency, side effects, drug interactions, and clinical effects in a particular shock state is critical to a successful outcome.

In conclusion, the pharmacotherapy of shock requires identification of the category and etiology of shock, evaluation of the hemodynamics of the shock state, and knowledge and application of the properties of each type of drug to restore tissue perfusion and oxygenation in each disease entity. Currently, new vasoactive drugs for shock are being developed with more specific hemodynamic effects and fewer potential adverse effects.

REVIEW QUESTIONS

1. **After fluid resuscitation, the drug recommended for the initial treatment of persistent hypotension in septic shock is:**
   A. Dobutamine
   B. Dopamine
   C. Norepinephrine
   D. Phenylephrine
   E. Amrinone

2. **In a euvolemic patient, administration of dobutamine (dose) generally causes:**
   A. Decreased heart rate
   B. Decreased CO
   C. Decreased or unchanged PAWP
   D. Decreased stroke volume
   E. Increased SVR

3. **A previously healthy 28-year-old man presents to the Emergency Department with spinal cord injury, occurring in the upper thoracic vertebrae (T1–T6), and develops bradycardia and hypotension. After adequate fluid administration and other ongoing treatment, the patient remains persistently hypotensive. The commonly recommended drug to use for further hemodynamic support is:**
   A. Dobutamine
   B. Nitroprusside
   C. Amrinone
   D. Norepinephrine
   E. Milrinone

4. **Which one of the following drugs causes a decrease in pulmonary capillary wedge pressure?**
   A. Dopamine
   B. Norepinephrine
   C. Epinephrine
   D. Phenylephrine
   E. Dobutamine

5. A true statement regarding norepinephrine use in cardiogenic shock caused by myocardial infarction includes:

- **A.** Norepinephrine primarily augments BP by increasing cardiac output.
- **B.** Norepinephrine is not used in hypotension due to ischemic heart disease.
- **C.** It is used for hemodynamically significant hypotension (SBP < 70 mmHg) and is more useful when SVR is low.
- **D.** Generally, it causes a marked increase in CO.
- **E.** After fluid resuscitation, norepinephrine is recommended for a patient with a systolic BP of 74 mmHg with signs and symptoms of shock.

6. Which of the following drugs may interact with the vasoactive agent dopamine?

- **A.** Phenelzine (Nardil)
- **B.** St. John's wort
- **C.** Nefazodone (Serzone)
- **D.** Nedocromil (Tilade)
- **E.** Venlafaxine (Effexor)

7. A 35-year-old woman, who is a hospital administrator, presents to the Emergency Department (accompanied by two coworkers) with a rash, facial swelling, nasal congestion, abdominal pain, and nausea approximately a half-hour after lunch. She had a small bowel of tortellini with pesto, an apple, and a caffeine-free diet cola in the hospital cafeteria. She states she has an allergy to nuts. She appears pale with facial swelling and is tachycardic with a BP of 80/48 mmHg. Her legs are elevated and given high flow oxygen. She is given epinephrine as an intravenous line is established. A normal saline fluid bolus is administered and continued at a high flow. After 5 min, her BP drops further despite treatment and flagrant shock is present. The next step is:

- **A.** Administer glucagon
- **B.** Start an epinephrine infusion
- **C.** Start a phenylephrine infusion
- **D.** Start a dopamine infusion
- **E.** Start a norepinephrine infusion

8. Match the drug to the most appropriate statement:

1.	Phenylephrine	A. First-line treatment for anaphylactic shock
2.	Amrinone	B. Treatment of beta-blocker-induced shock
3.	Norepinephrine	C. Confusion, metabolic acidosis, seizures
4.	Glucagon	D. Decrease platelets in dose-dependent fashion
5.	Isoproterenol	E. Phenytoin-induced hypotension
6.	Epinephrine	F. Treatment of hypotension after spinal cord injury
7.	Dopamine	G. Treatment of bradycardia in the denervated heart transplant
8.	Nitroprusside	H. Pure α_1-adrenergic agonist

ANSWERS

1. The answer is B. After fluid resuscitation, the drug recommended for the initial treatment of persistent hypotension in septic shock is dopamine. It increases splanchnic blood flow without vasoconstriction and at low doses increases CO. Dobutamine generally is not indicated first line in septic shock because it may cause further hypotension. It is generally indicated as an adjunctive treatment when CI is impaired (e.g., <2.5 l/min/m^2). Norepinephrine is typically used when dopamine treatment does not maintain MAP (usual maximum dose, 20 μg/kg/min) because it provides more vasoconstriction and cardiac contractility but less tachycardia. Phenylephrine has not been well studied in adult septic shock and has a tendency to decrease CI. It is best used when cardiac arrhythmias are problematic because of its lack of direct cardiovascular effects and when CI is greater than 4.0 l/min/m^2. Amrinone has not been studied in septic shock; it has significant vasodilatory properties as well as a long half-life.
2. The answer is C. Dobutamine does have beta-1 and beta-2 agonist properties, which results in inotropy but not vasoconstriction. In a euvolemic patient, dobutamine administered from 5 to 20 μg/kg/min generally results in a unchanged or increased heart rate, increased stroke volume, and cardiac output. Additionally, it causes a decrease in SVR and a decreased or unchanged PCWP and central venous pressure. Because dobutamine does not cause vasoconstriction, its use in septic shock is limited, and it is typically used in conjunction with vasoactive drugs. Furthermore, patients placed on dobutamine who are hypovolemic may experience severe hypotension.
3. The answer is D. Norepinephrine. The patient has developed neurogenic shock resulting from a spinal cord injury and spinal shock, disruption of sympathetic output, and unbalanced parasympathetic input. Spinal shock is a neurologic condition that involves injury to the autonomic system, which affects not only vascular resistance but also cardiac function, thereby requiring a combined α- and β-adrenergic agonist. Phenylephrine, a pure α-adrenergic agonist, can be used for transient, reversible forms of neurogenic shock caused by anesthesia. The other drugs, such as dobutamine, milrinone and amrinone, and nitroprusside, may cause a decreased SVR and further hypotension.
4. The answer is E. Typically, dobutamine causes a decrease in PCWP due to mild peripheral vasodilation and improved inotropic response. Dobutamine stimulates α_1- and β_1-AR in the heart and α_1- and β_2-AR in the peripheral vascular system. The β_2-AR vasodilatory response is stronger than the α_1-AR vasoconstrictor response and this results in some vasodilation. Moreover, the increased inotropic response and concomitant increase in CO also result in a decreased vascular resistance. The other drugs have significant vasocontrictor properties, resulting in arterial and/or venous vasoconstriction and causing a decrease in venous capacitance and increased blood return. For example, dopamine stimulates both α_1-AR and β_1-AR, causing an increase in vasoconstriction and increased CO. Higher doses cause further vasoconstriction resulting in more marked peripheral arterial and venoconstriction, augmenting the systemic and pulmonary vascular resistance and PCWP.
5. The answer is C. Norepinephrine is used for hemodynamically significant hypotension refractory to other sympathomimetic amines and is more useful when systemic vascular resistance is low. Although a low SVR is uncommonly found in cardiogenic shock, norepinephrine is helpful when BP is very low because it has stronger vasoconstrictor effects than dopamine and produces

less tachycardia. Furthermore, its strong inotropic properties are helpful to prevent a decrease in CO. For choice A, norepinephrine primarily augments BP by increasing peripheral vascular resistance. Although norepinephrine has potent effects on cardiac contractility, the stronger vasoconstrictor properties may actually result in decreased, unchanged, or only mildly increased cardiac output. Choice B is false because norepinephrine is used in cardiogenic shock without pulmonary edema when dobutamine and dopamine are unsatisfactory, especially in shock at SBP below 70 mmHg. D. As in choice A, typically there is only a modest change in CO, which may be negative or positive due to the balancing of its strong vasoconstrictor effects and less potent inotropic effects. E. For hypotension with a systolic BP less than 70 mmHg and signs and symptoms of shock, volume is given if preload is decreased, and norepinephrine is the recommended temporary vasoactive drug of choice. As treatment continues and blood pressure rises, norepinephrine is then substituted as soon as possible for a less intense vasoconstrictor.

6. The answer is A. Phenelzine (nardil) is a monoamine oxidase inhibitor used for treatment of depression. Dopamine is metabolized by the enzymes monoamine oxidase and catechol-*O*-methyl transferase. An inhibitor of monoamine oxidase may significantly potentiate the effects of dopamine, and it has been recommended to use 1/10th or less of the usual dose. Patients still may have exaggerated blood pressure response to dopamine days after stopping nardil. Two other MAO inhibitors used for depression are tranylcypromine (Parnate) and isocarboxazid (Marplan). Choice B is an herbal remedy marketed as a dietary supplement that has not been known to affect the pharmacology of exogenous dopamine. It appears, however, to have some antidepressant effect in controlled trials, but it may also significantly interact with other major drugs. Choices C and E are antidepressants. Serzone is a serotonin antagonist and reuptake inhibitor while Venlafaxine is both a serotonin- and norepinephrine-reuptake inhibitor. Neither of these significantly interacts with the cardiovascular effects of dopamine. However, in stable outpatients Venlafaxine has been known to cause a dose-related elevation in diastolic blood pressure. Choice D is a nonsteroidal antiinflammatory agent for treatment of mild asthma.

7. The answer is B. Administer epinephrine. The first-line treatment of anaphylactic shock is epinephrine because it has a number of beneficial effects in different organ systems derived from both its β- and α-adrenergic properties. It stimulates β-adrenergic receptors and increases intracellular cAMP levels, leading to inhibition of mast cell and basophil mediator release, bronchodilation, and inotropic and chronotropic cardiac effects. Its α-adrenergic properties cause peripheral vasoconstriction. It should be given immediately in the presence of clinical evidence for airway swelling, respiratory difficulty, or shock as delay in treatment may be fatal. It should be repeatedly administered or given as an epinephrine infusion. Moreover, rapid volume infusion, H1- and H2-receptor blockers, and corticosteroids should be given. If hypotension persists despite epinephrine, a norepinephrine or dopamine infusion should be given. Anecdotally, glucagon as a nonadrenergic agent has been useful in hypotension unresponsive to epinephrine, especially in the presence of β-adrenergic blockade. Phenylephrine is a pure α-adrenergic agonist.

8. The correct answers are:

1. Phenylephrine	Pure α_1-adrenergic agonist
2. Amrinone	Decrease platelets in dose-dependent fashion
3. Norepinephrine	Treatment of hypotension after spinal cord injury
4. Glucagon	Treatment of beta-blocker induced shock
5. Isoproterenol	Treatment of bradycardia in the denervated heart transplant
6. Epinephrine	First-line treatment for anaphylactic shock
7. Dopamine	Interacts with phenytoin causing hypotension
8. Nitroprusside	Confusion, metabolic acidosis, seizures

Phenylephrine is a noncatecholamine with adrenergic properties of α-adrenergic stimulation. Amrinone is associated with a reversible thrombocytopenia, usually developing in 2–3 days and resolving after drug cessation. Norepinephrine is used in neurogenic shock due to spinal cord injury, especially T1–T6, where sympathetic outflow is blocked resulting in bradycardia and hypotension. Glucagon is helpful in β-blocker-induced shock because of its nonadrenergic mechanism of action. It is also used in other forms of shock unresponsive to standard therapy such as anaphylactic shock. Nitroprusside is metabolized to cyanide and then converted to the less toxic product of thiocyanate. These products may accumulate during prolonged infusion, high-dose therapy, or poor renal function and cause significant side effects of anion-gap metabolic acidosis and mental status changes. Liver disease rarely is a significant contributor to accumulation of these toxic products. In critically ill patients receiving phenytoin, hypotension may occur with the administration of dopamine.

SUGGESTED READING

American Heart Association. Handbook of Emergency Cardiovascular Care. Dallas: American Heart Association, 2000.

Bone RC, Balk RA, Cerra FB, et al. Definitions for sepsis and organ failure and guidelines for the use of innovative therapies in sepsis. Chest 1992;101:1644–1655.

Cummins RO (ed) Textbook of Advanced Cardiac Life Support: 1997–99 Emergency Cardiovascular Care Programs. Dallas: American Heart Association, 1997:1-1–17-9.

Marik PE, Varon J. The hemodynamic derangements in sepsis: implications for treatment strategies. Chest 1998;114:854–860.

Parrillo JE. Approach to the patient with shock. In: Goldman L Jr, Bennett CJ (eds) Cecil Textbook of Medicine. Philadelphia: Saunders, 2000:495–502.

Parillo JE. Cardiogenic Shock. In: Goldman L, Bennett JC (eds) Cecil Textbook of Medicine. Philadelphia: Saunders, 2000:502–507.

Task Force of the American College of Critical Care Medicine, Society of Critical Care Medicine. Practice parameters for hemodynamic support of adult patients in sepsis. Crit Care Med 1999; 27(3):639–660.

The American Heart Association in Collaboration with the International Liaison Committee on Resuscitation (ILCOR). Guidelines 2000 for Cardiopulmonary Resuscitation and Emergency Cardiovascular Care: An international consensus on science. Circulation 2001; 102(8):1–380.

Wheeler AP, Bernard GR. Current concepts: treating patients with severe sepsis. N Engl J Med 1999;340:207–214.

CHAPTER 39

HENRY H. HSIA

Antiarrhythmic Drug Management

CHAPTER OUTLINE

LEARNING OBJECTIVES

After studying this chapter, you should be able to:

- Understand basic cellular electrophysiology.
- Know the classification of antiarrhythmic drugs and their electrophysiologic effects.
- Understand the potential mechanisms of clinically relevant arrhythmias.
- Identify potential pharmacologic target sites based on arrhythmia mechanisms.
- Know side-effect profiles of antiarrhythmic drugs.
- Develop a logical approach in the selection of a specific antiarrhythmic drug.

This chapter focuses on the electrophysiologic principles of antiarrhythmic drug treatment of supraventricular and ventricular arrhythmias in critically ill patients. Here we do not present a comprehensive review of individual antiarrhythmic agents but instead provide a framework for clinical approaches to antiarrhythmic drug selection based on the mechanisms of the target arrhythmia. Antiarrhythmic drugs are agents that exert their effects either directly or indirectly on cellular impulse generation or conduction. They alter cellular membrane potential by interactions with membrane receptors or ionic channels. This chapter presents an overview of antiarrhythmic drug management, including (1) a review of cellular electrophysiology, (2) a general classification of antiarrhythmic drugs, (3) a survey of arrhythmia mechanisms, and (4) clinical correlation of antiarrhythmic drug effects on the heart.

- Phase 4: resting membrane potential (−50 to −90 mV)
  K^+-dependent spontaneous depolarization
- Phase 0: action potential upstroke (V_{max})
  The slope determines the conduction velocity
  Fast Na response in atrium, ventricle and His–Purkinje fibers
  Slow Ca response in sinus node, AV node
- Phase 1: early rapid repolarization
  Inactivation of I_{Na} and K outward current
- Phase 2: plateau
  Slow Ca inward current determines the duration of AP
- Phase 3: repolarization
  Activation of outward K current determines the refractory periods

CELLULAR ELECTROPHYSIOLOGY

To optimize antiarrhythmic drug management, one must understand basic cellular electrophysiology. You may wish to review Chapter 15, which discusses the electrical properties of the cardiac cell in more detail. The resting cellular membrane potential (phase 4) of the cardiac cell is predominately determined by the potassium (K^+) electrochemical equilibrium. In the first phase of the action potential, Na^+ influx into the cell mediates the rapid upstroke (phase 0). The slope of the phase 0 upstroke (V_{max}) determines the velocity of impulse propagation. Calcium influx occurs slightly later and lasts longer, accounting for the plateau (phase 2) of the action potential, and mediates myocardial contraction. These phases are followed by K^+ efflux from the cell, leading to repolarization (phase 3) and back to the resting membrane potential (phase 4). Cells with this type of Na-dependent fast-response action potential comprise most of the heart (atrium, ventricles, His–Purkinje system, and bypass tract fiber). Other cells in the sinoatrial (SAN) and atrioventricular nodes (AVNs) have slow-

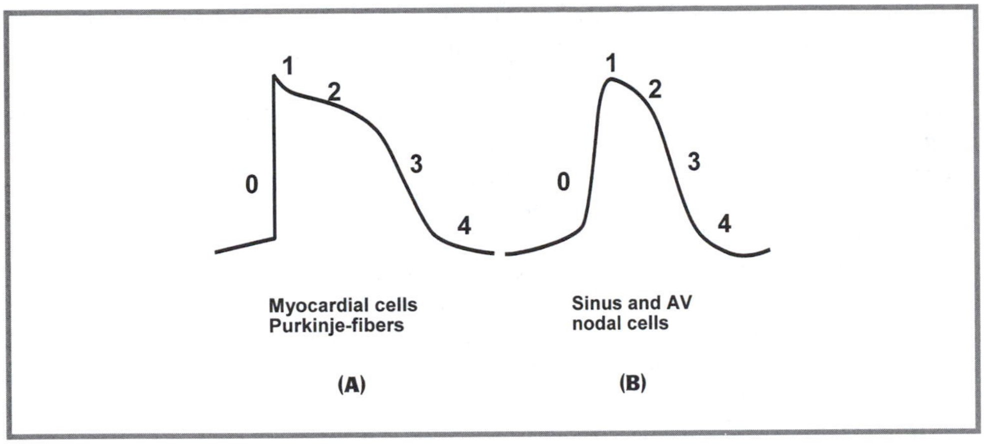

FIGURE 39-1

The cardiac action potentials. **(A)** Fast-response Na-dependent action potential in cells of atrium, ventricles, His–Purkinje system, and bypass tract myocardial fibers. **(B)** Slow-response Ca-dependent cells of the sinoatrial and atrioventricular nodes.

response action potentials, in which Ca^{2+} influx is more important than Na^+ in mediating the phase 0 upstroke of action potential (Figure 39-1).

The refractory periods determine the ability of a cell to respond to an external stimulus by depolarizing and forming an corresponding action potential for continued propagation of cardiac impulse; this is also known as excitability. Sodium ion channels are voltage dependent, and their behavior and availability are influenced by the level of membrane potentials. During phases 2 and 3 of the action potential, cells gradually resume their ability to respond as the membrane potential recovers toward the resting state. A stimulus applied early in phase 3 cannot open enough Na^+ channels to allow sufficient Na^+ influx to result in a self-sustaining action potential; the cell then is said to be in the absolute refractory period. If a stimulus arrives later, when some Na^+ channels are activated to conduct some Na^+ current but not a normal amount; this gives rise to a slower upstroke of phase 0 and is termed the relative refractory period. Stimuli occurring still later encounter essentially all available Na^+ channels and a normal action potential results (fully excitable) (Figure 39-2).

ANTIARRHYTHMIC DRUG CLASSIFICATION

Antiarrhythmic drugs modify membrane receptors or ionic channels and alter different phases of the action potential at a cellular level. This action affects rhythm formation or impulse conduction at the tissue level, which translates to clinical antiarrhythmic effects. Traditionally, antiarrhythmic drugs are classified using the Vaughan Williams classification. Singh

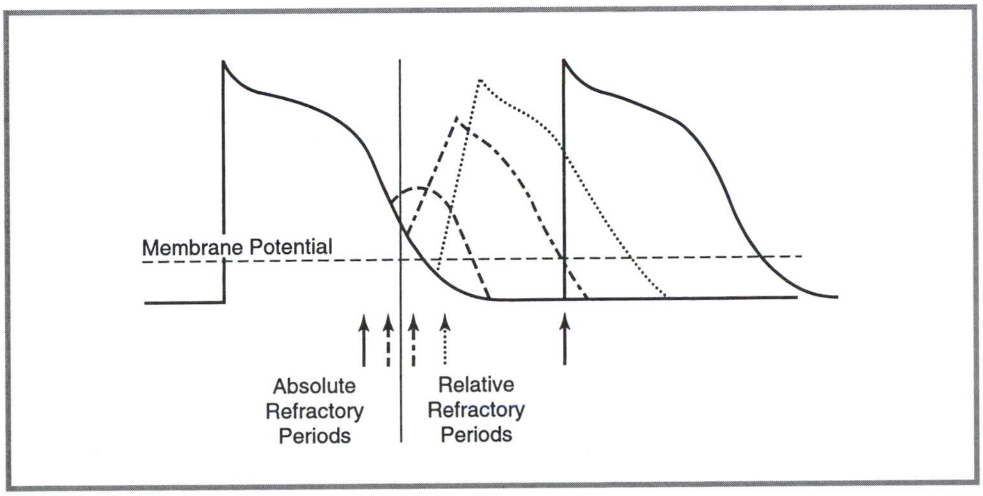

FIGURE 39-2

Effects of action potential refractory period on conduction property. A stimulus applied during the resting membrane potential phase induces a full action potential. Progressively earlier stimuli in the relative refractory period induce action potentials of smaller amplitudes and slower phase 0 upstroke and conduction velocity as fewer sodium channels are available at higher membrane potentials. No conductive action potential was generated in the absolute refractory period.

and Vaughan Williams have categorized antiarrhythmic compounds by their effect on (1) the fast sodium depolarization current, (2) the sympathetic activity of the heart, (3) the repolarization currents, and (4) the slow inward calcium current (Table 39-1).

The class I antiarrhythmic drugs antagonize the fast sodium channel, which is responsible for the initial rapid depolarization of the action potential (phase 0). They inhibit phase 0 of action potentials and slow conduction velocity that causes impulse slowing or block. Class II agents are beta-blockers, which are antiarrhythmic probably by limiting formation of the second messenger, cyclic AMP (acting mostly at phases 2 and 4). Another major category of antiarrhythmic compounds (class III) are the potassium channel antagonists. By inhibiting the potassium efflux and preventing repolarization of membrane potential back to the resting level, the duration of the action potential is increased, which translates to a prolonged cellular refractory period (phase 3). The class IV agents (calcium channel blockers) achieve their pharmacologic effects by inhibiting the slow calcium current, particularly in the atrioventricular (AV) node (Figure 39-3).

- Some drugs exert greater pharmacologic effects at a faster heart rates. The depression of Na^+ channels is greater after the channel has been used in membrane depolarizations rather than after a resting period. This property may exacerbate the proarrhythmia effects of drugs.

The class I antiarrhythmics, fast sodium channel blockers, are further divided into three subcategories based on their relative potency of sodium channel blockade. The class I-C drugs (flecainide, propafenone, encainide) have the most potent sodium channel-blocking activity among the class I agents, with significant slowing of impulse conduction and depression of phase 0 upstroke (V_{max}). This action has a propensity to bind to the activated sodium channels with slow dissociation kinetics. As heart rate increases, more activated sodium channels are available for drug binding, and greater inhibition of sodium influx results from slow dissociation. The class I-C drugs therefore exhibit considerable use-dependent (frequency-dependent) properties. The class I-B drugs (lidocaine, mexiletine) are the least potent sodium channel blockers. The I-B drugs exhibit preferential binding to "inactivated" sodium channels (at slower heart rates) with fast kinetics and thus have minimal use-dependency. Selectivity of lidocaine on ischemic myocardium has also been described and may be particularly useful in prophylactic prevention of ventricular arrhythmia in a setting of an acute ischemic syndrome or myocardial infarction. The class I-A agents, such as quinidine, procainamide, and disopyramide, demonstrate an intermediate activity and kinetics of sodium channel blockade with a modest depression of V_{max} and conduction. However, the I-A drugs also exhibit potassium blockade activity, with prolongation of action potential du-

TABLE 39-1

VAUGHAN WILLIAMS CLASSIFICATION OF ANTIARRHYTHMIC DRUGS

Class I: Fast sodium channel blockers
- IA: Moderate depression of phase 0
  - Slows conduction velocity
  - Lengthens refractory period
  - Vagolytic effects
  - Examples: quinidine, procainamide, disopyramide
- IB: Mild inhibition of phase 0 upstroke
  - Shortens APD and refractory period
  - Selective effects on diseased, ischemic tissue
  - Examples: lidocaine, tocainide, mexiletine, phenytoin, ethmozine
- IC: Most potent Na channel blockers
  - Marked depression of phase 0 upstroke; very slow conduction
  - Markedly depress His–Purkinje system conduction, widen QRS
  - Little effect on refractory period
  - Examples: flecainide, propafenone, encainide

Class II: Sympatholytic agents: beta-blockers, SAN/AVN blockers

Class III: Inhibition of repolarization
- K^+ channel blockers:
  - Prolong repolarization
  - Increase action potential duration, refractoriness
  - Examples: amiodarone, sotalol, bretylium, ibutilide

Class IV: Inhibition of slow inward Ca^{2+} channel
- Ca^{2+} channel blockers, SAN/AVN blockers

APD, action potential duration (APD); SAN, sinoatrial node; AVN, atrioventricular node

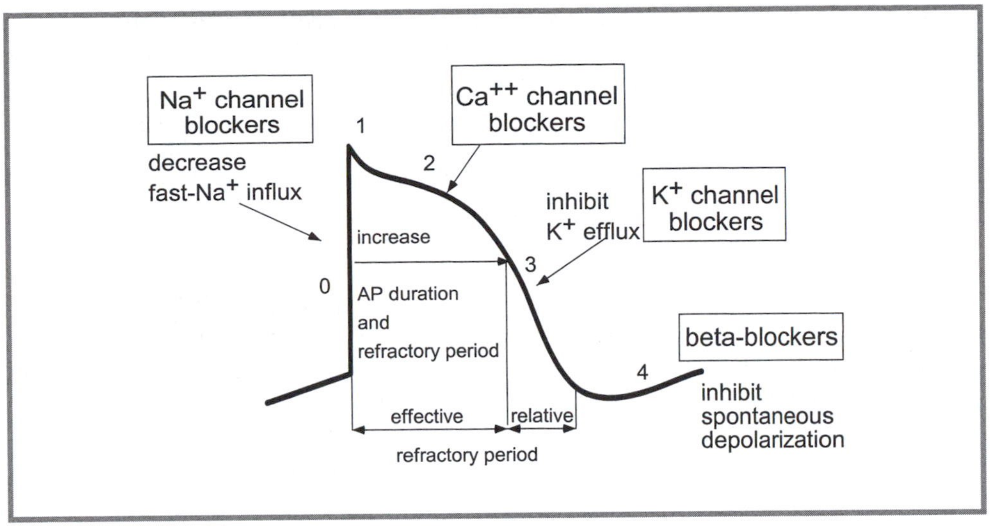

FIGURE 39-3

Antiarrhythmic drug actions on cardiac action potential. Class I drugs block the fast Na channels of the rapid phase 0 depolarization. Class IV drugs (calcium channel blockers) inhibit calcium influx of phase 2 [also block phase 0 upstroke in cells of the sinoatrial (SA) and atrioventricular (AV) nodes]. Class III drugs block potassium efflux and prevent repolarization. The action potential duration and refractory period are prolonged. Class II drugs are beta-blockers, which act mostly at phase 4.

ration and cellular refractory period. In addition, the class I-A drugs have variable anticholinergic (vagolytic) activity, which tends to facilitate conduction through the AV node and accelerates ventricular rate response during atrial fibrillation or flutter. This vagolytic effect must be considered in the determination of overall clinical actions of class I-A drugs (Figure 39-4).

The Vaughan Williams classification correlates reasonably well with specific membrane effects of the drugs. However, it provides incomplete links among the actions of antiarrhythmic agents, the mechanisms of arrhythmias, and the efficacy of therapy. From the clinical point of view, this classification has a number of shortcomings. First, it does not take into account the presence of multiple pharmacologic effects produced by a single drug. For example, quinidine has effects of both class I and class III drugs, sotalol has effects of both class II and III, and amiodarone has properties of all four classes. Second, poor concordance of response and toxicity between members of a class and among drugs within a given class can produce disparate "secondary" electrophysiologic effects; for example, the kinetics of interactions of class I drugs with sodium channels varies greatly. Although the subdivision

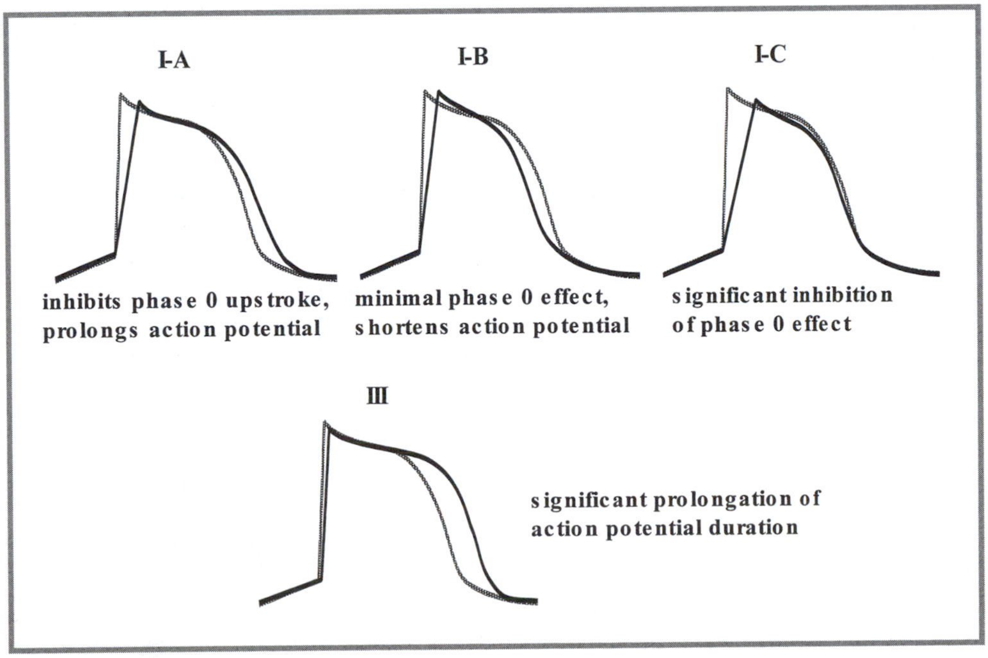

FIGURE 39-4

Differential drug effects of class I and class III antiarrhythmic agents on cardiac cellular action potentials.

of class I drugs corrects for much of these difference, the secondary vagolytic effect of class I-A drugs is not intuitively obvious. In addition, the Vaughan Williams classification does not take into consideration the effects of active metabolites, which may have a different action from their parent drugs. For example, procainamide blocks inward sodium channels and outward potassium channels, making it a class I-A drug. Its major metabolite, *N*-acetylprocainamide (NAPA), is a pure potassium channel blocker, making it a class III drug. The final pharmacologic effects of procainamide therapy depends on the relative concentration of the parent drug and the active metabolites, which is influenced by multiple factors such as renal function and genetically determined hepatic metabolism. Finally, many drugs such as digitalis or adenosine do not fall under any Vaughan Williams classification scheme.

Quinidine is the prototype of a class I-A agent. It is a typical fast sodium channel blocker with mild class III effect (prolongs refractoriness). In addition, as a group, the I-A drugs interact with muscarinic receptors, resulting in anticholinergic (vagolytic) effect. Quinidine also inhibits peripheral and myocardial α-adrenergic receptors and thus induces hypotension with intravenous administration. Its use is associated with frequent subjective side effects such as diarrhea (33%), nausea (18%), headache (13%), and dizziness (8%). The gastrointestinal (GI) effects may be less severe with the gluconate preparations. Central nervous system (CNS) toxicity, referred to as cinchonism, includes tinnitus, hearing loss, confusion, delirium, and visual disturbance, which are not uncommon, especially in elderly patients. Immune-mediated reactions, such as rash, fever, hemolytic anemia, leukopenia, hepatic toxicity, and anaphylaxis have also been reported. Overall, adverse effects preclude long-term quinidine therapy in up to 30% of patients. Significant drug interactions with digoxin, amiodarone, verapamil, and warfarin have been well documented. Prudent dosage adjustment with frequent plasma drug level monitoring is warranted. For quick reference, Table 39-2 summarizes important drug interactions.

Procainamide is a very versatile agent that may be given orally or intravenously (but rarely intramuscularly). It is the most commonly used intravenous antiarrhythmic drug in an acute setting. A good plasma level (8–10 μg/ml) can be achieved after a loading dose of 15 mg/kg administered via rapid infusion (~50 mg/min); this can be followed by a maintenance dose (1–4 mg/min or 0.11 mg/kg/min) before switching to oral drugs. Hypotension is commonly observed during IV infusion because of its vasodilator effect, and the infusion rate must be titrated to hemodynamic tolerance. Contrary to quinidine, procainamide does not increase the serum digoxin concentration. However, its clearance is significantly reduced in patients with diminished renal function. Multiple noncardiac effects that have been observed with procainamide administration include the usual GI and CNS symptoms. In addition, fever, rash, myalgia, digital vasculitis, and Raynaud's phenomenon have been reported. A potentially life-threatening pancytopenia or agranulocytosis has also been described; this may be an allergic or hypersensitivity reaction that appears days to weeks after starting procainamide. Also, 20%–30% of patients may develop clinical symptoms of a systemic lupus erythematosus (SLE) -like syndrome with positive serologic tests observed in 60%–70% of patients on chronic procainamide therapy. This phenomenon is reversible, and positive serologic tests are not necessarily a reason to discontinue drug therapy.

Disopyramide is comparable to other class I-A drugs in its antiarrhythmic actions. Its elimination is primarily via renal excretion, and the dosage must be reduced in patients with renal impairment. The most common side effects relate to the drug's potent parasympathetic, anticholinerigc property, which can cause urinary obstruction (14%), dry mouth (32%), and constipation (11%), and thus it should be avoided in elderly patients and those with glaucoma, prostatism, or myasthenia gravis. Disopyramide administration is also associated with substantial suppression of myocardial contractility (negative inotropic effect) compared to others in its class. Acute exacerbation of congestive heart failure may occur as early as 48 h following initiation of the drug, especially in those patients with a past history of heart failure (55%).

Amiodarone is an iodinated bezofuran derivative with coronary and peripheral vasodilatory properties. Its electrophysiologic and pharmacologic actions are complex. Amiodarone uniformly lengthens action potential duration and refractory periods and is usually classified as a class III antiarrhythmic potassium blocker. However, it also blocks cardiac sodium chan-

TABLE 39-2

ANTIARRHYTHMIC DRUG INTERACTIONS

DRUGS	INTERACTION WITH:	RESULTS
Quinidine	Digoxin	■ Increases digoxin level
	Type I antiarrhythmic drugs	■ Added negative inotropy and depressed conduction
	Beta-blockers	■ Enhanced hypotension, negative inotropy
	Amiodarone, sotalol	■ Torsades de pointe
	Diuretics	■ hypokalemia/torsades de pointe
	Verapamil	■ Increases quinidine level
	Nifedipine	■ Decreases quinidine level
	Warfarin	■ Enhanced anticoagulation
Procainamide	H_2 blockers	■ Increases plasma level
	Captopril	■ Enhanced immune effects
Disopyramide	Type I antiarrhythmic drugs	■ Added negative inotropy and depressed conduction
	Anticholinergic	■ Severe anticholinergic effects
Lidocaine	Beta-blockers, H_2 blockers, halothane	■ Reduces hepatic clearance, increases toxicity
Tocainide	Few interactions	
Mexiletine	Phenytoin	■ Hepatic enzyme induction; reduces plasma level
	Disopyramide	■ Negative inotropic effects
Flecainide	Agents inhibit SAN/AVN	■ SA or AV nodal conduction depression
	Negative inotropic agents	■ Severe myocardial depression
	Agents suppress HPS (IA, III)	■ Severe conduction defects
	Amiodarone	■ Increases flecainide level
Propafenone	Similar to flecainide	
	Digoxin	■ Digoxin level increases
Sotalol	Diuretic, type IA agents, amiodarone, tricyclics, phenothiazines	■ Increases risk of torsades de pointe
Amiodarone	Similar to sotalol	■ Increases risk of torsades de pointe
	Digoxin	■ Increases digoxin level
	Flecainide	■ Flecainide level increases
Verapamil	Beta-blockers, digoxin, myocardial depressants, quinidine	■ AV nodal, His–Purkinje conduction defects, sick sinus, negative inotropic effects

nels and depresses phase 0 of the action potential (Class I), as well as possessing noncompetitive α- and β-receptor antagonist (class II) and calcium channel blocking (class IV) activities. In addition, amiodarone blocks peripheral conversion of thyroxine (T_4) to triiodothyronine (T_3). It contains a significant amount of iodine (38% of its weight), and many of the effects of the drug are similar to those seen with hypothyroidism. The drug is extensively metabolized by the liver with minimal renal elimination. Amiodarone has a large volume of distribution, moderate and erratic bioavailability, and an unusually long half-life, 26–107 days (mean, ~50 days). It is lipophilic and deposits extensively into various tissues, especially those with high fat content (liver, lung, heart, skin, adipose tissue), and is not dialyzable.

Amiodarone has been used to suppress a wide spectrum of supraventricular and ventricular tachyarrhythmias. Success rates vary depending on patent population, targeted arrhythmia, underlying heart disease, and length of follow-up. In general, the efficacy of amiodarone equals or exceeds that of all other antiarrhythmic drugs. It is effective in approximately 60%–80% of supraventricular tachyarrhythmias and 40%–60% of ventricular tachyarrhythmias. Because of its long half-life and large volume of distribution, the ideal loading dose schedule remains controversial but depends on the nature of the arrhythmia and the underlying cardiac function. In general, for patients with ventricular arrhythmias, an oral loading dose of 800–1800 mg/day for a minimum of 2–3 weeks should be used. The onset of action following oral administration may require several days, and a maintenance dose of 400 mg/day is usually recommended. Due to its multiple side effects, most patients on chronic amiodarone therapy develop intolerable reactions and dosage reduction is usually required after 18–24 months. Intravenous amiodarone has recently become available for use in life-threatening arrhythmias refractory to other drugs. The onset of action after IV administration is within several hours. The initial IV loading dose, 150 mg during about 10 min, is followed by a maintenance infusion, 0.5–1.0 mg/min. Contrary to its oral route of administration, intravenous amiodarone can cause vasodilatation and has negative inotropic action (anti-adrenergic effects) and should be given with caution. For treatment of supraventricular arrhythmias, lower loading doses of 400–800 mg/day are used with an effective once-a-day maintenance dose of 100–200 mg/day. Given its long half-life, good efficacy, and easy compliance, low-dose amiodarone is considered a first-line therapy in elderly patients with atrial arrhythmias.

Adverse effects of amiodarone with long-term therapy are common, occurring in 50%–80% of patients. The frequency of side effects is dose and duration related, increasing over time, and careful follow-up is mandatory to prevent potentially serious consequences (Table 39-3). Most of the adverse effects are reversible with dose reduction or discontinuation. Fortunately, amiodarone is generally associated with a low proarrhythmia incidence, even in high-risk patients with life-threatening arrhythmias, significant structural heart disease, and ventricular dysfunction. Of all the noncardiac adverse reactions, pulmonary toxicity (up to 15%) is the most serious, usually occurring with the first 30 months of treatment and occasionally as early as 2–3 weeks. The mechanism is unclear but may be related to a hypersensitivity reaction or extensive drug/iodine deposits in the lungs. Pulmonary toxicity is associated with a 10% mortality and is uncommon in patients receiving less than 400 mg/day of amiodarone. A high degree of suspicion is essential for early diagnosis in patients who present with dyspnea, hypoxia, cough, and fever. Abnormal chest radiographic patterns of diffuse interstitial changes or alveolar infiltrates may be seen, as well as a positive gallium scan, and a reduced diffusion capacity with abnormalities on a high-resolution chest CT scan. Treatment requires drug withdrawal and supportive care; the use of steroids is controversial.

Adenosine antagonizes adenylate cyclase and decreases intracellular cyclic AMP and calcium conductance. It is a physiologic calcium antagonist and causes potent SA node and AV node depression. The clinical indications for adenosine (Adenocard®) is for acute management of narrow QRS supraventricular tachycardia (SVT) and for diagnosis of unknown wide QRS tachycardia. The advantage of its utility resides in its ultrashort half-life, less than 10 s. The adverse reactions include nausea, flushing, hypotension, bradycardia, heart block, and bronchospasm. Adenosine effects can be blocked by methylxanthines, caffeine, and theophylline.

In therapeutic concentration, digitalis has both direct and indirect cardiac effects. It directly blocks the Na/K-ATPase and causes an elevation in intracellular Na^+ concentration

TABLE 39-3

ADVERSE EFFECTS OF AMIODARONE THERAPY

Ocular:	Corneal microdeposits (95%), mostly asymptomatic
	Visual blurring (6%–14%)
	Possible optical neuritis
Dermatologic:	Photosensitivity (25%–75%)
	Blue-gray skin discoloration (5%–8%)
	Rash
Gastrointestinal:	Abnormal liver function tests (50%)
	Hepatitis (3%)
	Nausea, anorexia, constipation
Neurologic:	Peripheral neuropathy (5%), tremor (30%)
	Sleep disturbance (25%), myopathy, headache (14%)
Cardiovascular:	Symptomatic bradycardia (6%), AV block
	Heart failure (4%)
	Proarrhythmia (1%)
Thyroid:	Elevated thyroid-stimulating hormone (TSH); T3 and T4 abnormalities (25%)
	Symptomatic hypothyroidism (1%–22%), hyperthyroidism (1%–12%)
Pulmonary:	Interstitial pneumonitis (3%–15%
	Acute respiratory distress syndrome (ARDS)

that subsequently induces intracellular Ca^{2+} loading (via the Na^+/Ca^{2+} exchanger). These effects lead to enhanced myocardial contractility and reduced atrioventricular (AV) nodal conduction. The predominant indirect effects of digitalis is mediated through the parasympathetic autonomic nervous system. Digitalis enhances vagal tone on the heart and causes a reduction in sinus rate, a shortening of atrial refractory periods (increases atrial rate in atrial fibrillation or flutter), and suppression of AV nodal conduction. It slows ventricular rate response during atrial fibrillation and flutter by "indirect" vagal AV nodal block. At toxic concentrations, digitalis causes a significant intracellular Ca^{2+} overload that induces delayed afterdepolarizations (DAD) and triggered activity.

NEWER ANTIARRHYTHMIC DRUGS

Ibutilide is a new class III antiarrhythmic agent for treatment of atrial fibrillation and atrial flutter. It is effective in rapidly terminating atrial fibrillation and flutter. Under a multicenter study, the efficacy was higher for atrial flutter than fibrillation (63% versus 31%), especially in patients with a shorter duration of arrhythmia and a normal left atrial size. The major side effect is polymorphic ventricular tachycardia (torsade de pointes), which has been reported in up to 8.3% of patients receiving ibutilide. It may be considered as an alternative to electrical cardioversion under monitored condition. Other new antiarrhythmic agents include dofetilide and azimilide. Both are investigational class III agents that inhibit different K^+ channels. Dofetilide prolongs atrial and ventricular refractory periods, elevates ventricular fibrillation threshold, and exhibits reversed use-dependence with minimal negative inotropic effect. Azimilide blocks α- and β-adrenergic receptors in addition to K^+ channel blockade. Dofetilide was evaluated in the treatment of ventricular arrhythmia whereas azimilide has been studied for prevention of recurrent atrial fibrillation and supraventricular and ventricular arrhythmia.

MECHANISMS OF ARRHYTHMIAS

Because of the shortcomings of the Vaughan Williams classification, a new approach was proposed in 1991 by the Arrhythmia Task Force of the European Society of Cardiology meeting at Sicily. The Sicilian Gambit approach considers the mechanisms of arrhythmia, including the identification of vulnerable parameters that can be targeted by specific actions of antiarrhythmic agents. As described in Chapter 15, the mechanisms of arrhythmias can be divided into abnormal automaticity, triggered activity, and reentry. The abnormal automatic depolarizations result from either abnormal slopes of phase 4 action potentials or abnormal membrane threshold potentials. The treatment of abnormal automaticity should thus be focused on reducing the slopes of phase 4 depolarizations by administration of Ca^{2+} channel blockers (in the case of Ca^{2+}-dependent depolarizations) or beta-blockers (for Na^+ channel-dependent depolarizations). Arrhythmias based on triggered activity are initiated by afterdepolarizations, either early afterdepolarizations (EADs) or delayed afterdepolarizations (DADs). Polymorphic ventricular tachycardia associated with long QT intervals (either congenital or drug-induced torsade de pointes) are thought to be caused by EADs, whereas DADs are classically related to digitalis intoxication. Shortening the action potential duration (QT interval) at a fast heart rate by administration of catecholamines or pacing is the treatment of choice for torsade de pointes. For life-threatening arrhythmias associated with digitalis toxicity, the use of digitalis antibody is indicated.

The predominant clinical arrhythmias are reentrant in nature. The prerequisites of reentry include (1) an initiating event, most commonly a premature beat, (2) heterogeneous tissue properties that predispose unidirectional block with refractoriness in some part of the circuit, (3) alternative pathways for impulse propagation, and (4) critically slow conduction that allows an impulse to reenter the previously refractory part of the circuit (Figure 39-5). In general, reentry may be treated by drugs that either suppress the initiating premature beats or alter the properties of the reentrant circuit. Na^+ channel blockers (class IA, IC) may slow

- Reentry
  1. An initiating event, most commonly a premature beat
  2. Unidirectional block with refractoriness in some part of the circuit
  3. Alternative, multiple pathways
  4. Critically slow conduction in another part of the circuit

FIGURE 39-5

Critical components of a reentrant circuit: (*1*) unidirectional block, (*2*) alternative impulse pathways, and (*3*) "critically" slow conduction that reenters the previously refractory part of the circuit.

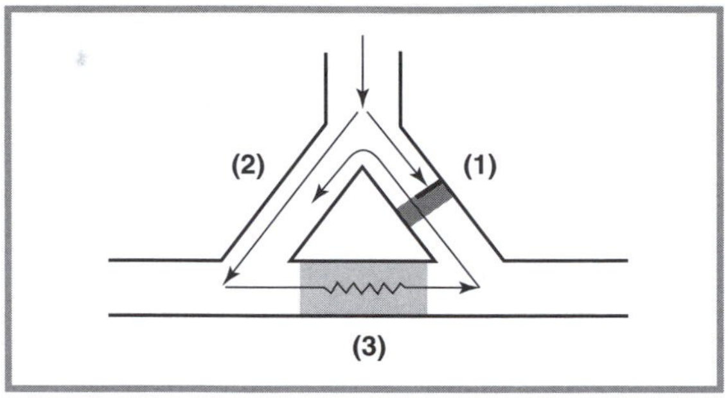

impulse conduction or cause conduction block. Along with beta-blockers or Ca^{2+} channel blockers (class II and IV), they may prevent reentry by eliminating premature beats or by creating a bidirectional block within the circuit. Some Na^{+} channel blockers (class IA) and K^{+} channel blockers (class III) can also increase refractoriness to such an extent that conduction in the circuit is insufficiently slow to allow recovery of excitability in regions where unidirectional block occurred (thus, reentry never begins) (Figure 39-6). These actions are the mechanistic basis for the selection of antiarrhythmic drugs in a clinical scenario.

GENERAL PRINCIPLES OF ANTIARRHYTHMIC THERAPY

It is essential to be familiar with the patient's underlying diagnoses and arrhythmia history. Multiple medical conditions may exist that can either induce new arrhythmias or cause exacerbation of preexisting arrhythmias. The approach to management of critically ill patients should be holistic, and various factors such as hypoxia, electrolyte imbalance, ischemia, sepsis, heart failure, renal insufficiency, or drug toxicity must be considered. The prognosis is mostly determined by the underlying cardiac or medical status.

Indications, goals, and endpoints of therapy
- Reasons to treat: alleviate symptoms, prevent sudden death
- Acute termination versus chronic preventive therapy
- Therapeutic versus palliative

An accurate diagnosis of cardiac arrhythmia is imperative. The physicians must be able to distinguish supraventricular arrhythmias versus ventricular tachyarrhythmias versus preexcited tachycardias (see Chapter 15). Indications, goals, and treatment endpoints must be clearly defined for the individual patient before initiation of antiarrhythmic therapy. The primary indication for treatment of cardiac arrhythmia is to prevent sudden death from ven-

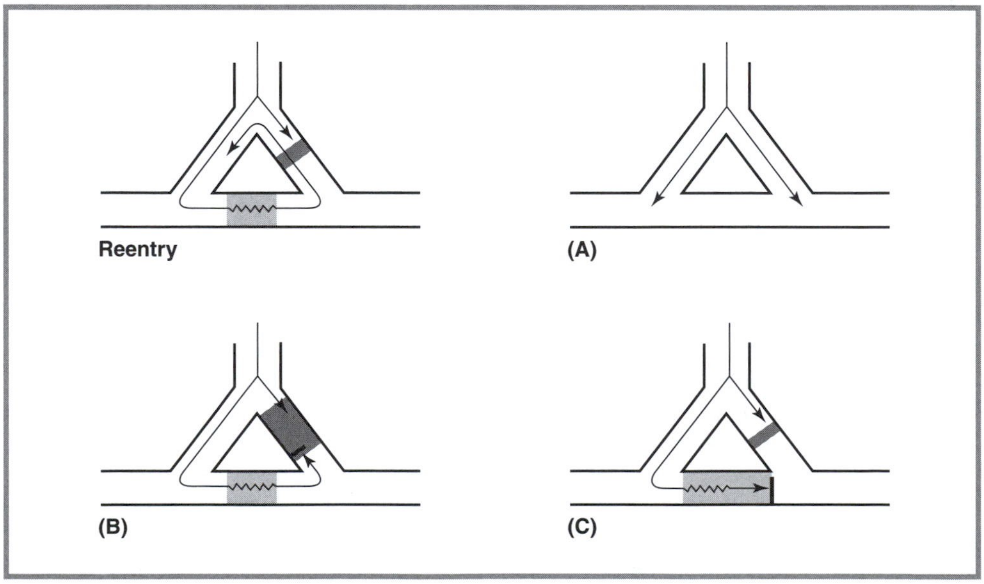

FIGURE 39-6

Antiarrhythmic drugs act on reentry by **(A)** eliminating premature triggering beats, **(B)** increasing refractoriness with insufficient recovery of excitability, and **(C)** inducing conduction block within the circuit.

tricular tachycardia (VT) or ventricular fibrillation (VF) and rarely supraventricular preexcited arrhythmias. The secondary indication is to alleviate arrhythmia symptoms. The physicians should differentiate the goals of acute treatment for arrhythmia termination from chronic treatment goals of preventing arrhythmia recurrence. Frequently, achieving a therapeutic endpoint of arrhythmia termination or prevention may not be possible or feasible. Alternative, palliative goals such as rate control during chronic atrial fibrillation or slowing of VT to improve hemodynamic tolerance may be acceptable.

In general, supraventricular tachyarrhythmias (SVT) can be categorized to AV node-dependent versus AV node-independent types based on their mechanisms (Figure 39-7). The AV node-dependent SVTs use the AV node as an integral part of the circuit, such as AV nodal reentrant tachycardia (AVNRT) or AV reciprocating tachycardia (AVRT). The AVNRT is a reentry within the AV node region involving a fast pathway and a slow pathway. The orthodromic AVRT is a reentry involving anterograde conduction down the AV node (Ca^{2+}-dependent) with AV accessory pathways/bypass tracts (Na^{+}-dependent) function as retrograde limbs of the circuit. Drugs that block impulse conduction at the AV node level (class II, IV) can terminate the arrhythmias by interrupting the anterograde limb of the reentry circuit. In AV node-independent SVTs, the mechanisms of arrhythmia reside above the AV node level and the AV node is not required for maintenance of arrhythmia. Atrial fibril-

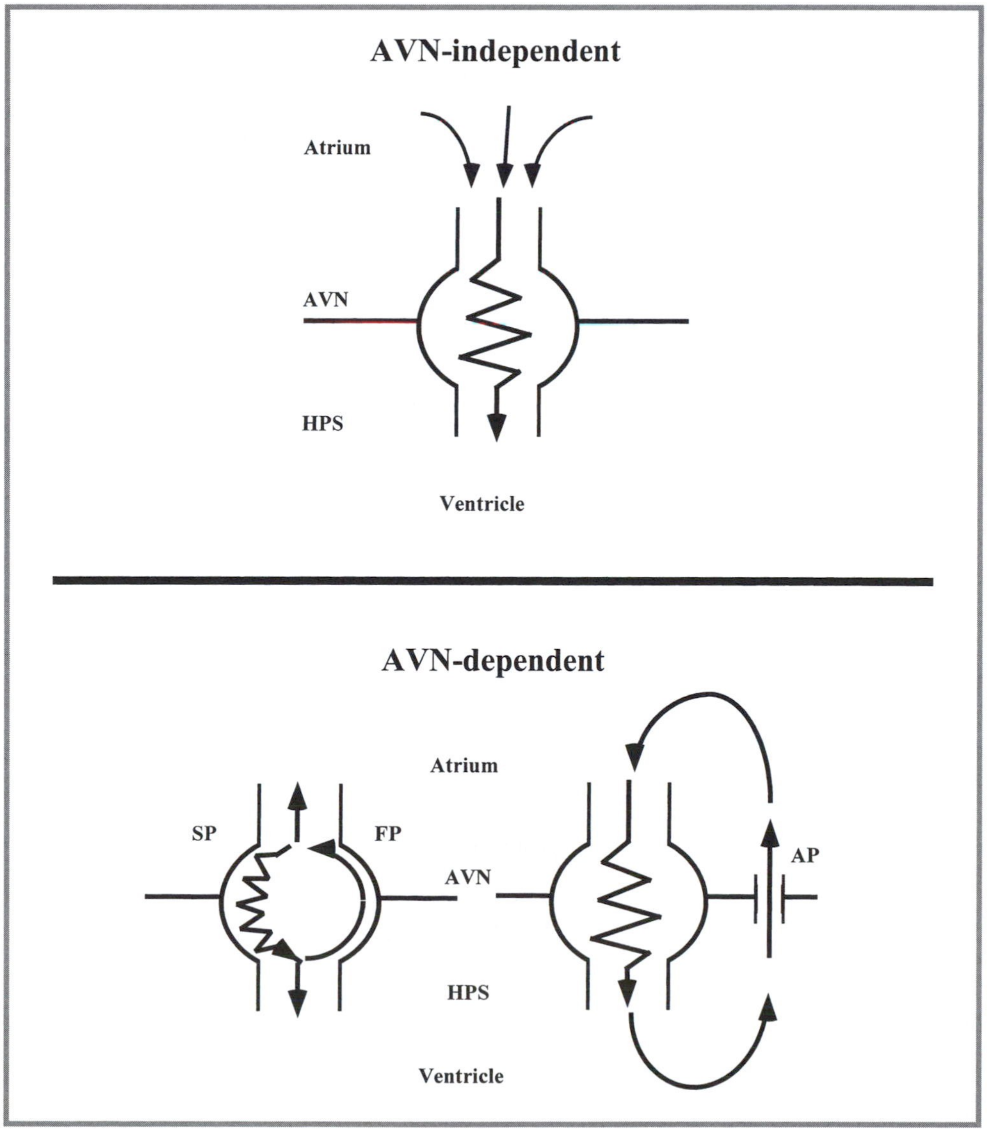

FIGURE 39-7

Classification of mechanisms of supraventricular tachycardias (SVT). The atrioventricular (AV) node is not required for maintenance of arrhythmias that originate above the AV node in *AV node-independent* SVT (*top*). The AV node-dependent SVT (*bottom*) utilizes the AV node as part of the circuit.

TABLE 39-4

ANTIARRHYTHMIC EFFICACY IN PREMATURE VENTRICULAR COMPLEX (PVC) SUPPRESSION

DRUG CLASS	EXAMPLE	RESPONSE
I-C	Encainide	70%–80%
	Flecainide	↓
III	Amiodarone	
I-C	Propafenone	
	I-A + I-B	
	↓	
	Quinidine	
I-A	Procainamide	
	Disopyramide	
	↓	
I-B	Mexiletine	
	Tocainide	
	↓	
II	Beta-blockers	
IV	Ca^{2+} channel blockers	40%

lation, atrial flutter, or atrial tachycardia are examples of AV node-independent SVTs. AV nodal blockers (class II, IV) do not affect the arrhythmia and only slow the ventricular rate response for better hemodynamics and symptomatic improvement. Direct membrane-acting drugs, such as Na^+ channel blockers or K^+ channel blockers (class I, III), act on the atrial myocardium as well as AV bypass tracts (residual myocardial fibers; Na^+-dependent). These agents are effective in both acute and chronic treatments of atrial tachyarrhythmias and SVTs involving bypass tracts. Amiodarone and Sotalol have both class III action and AV nodal blocking properties. They can be used effectively in all forms of SVTs. Unfortunately, antiarrhythmic treatment of ventricular arrhythmias is much less explicit. Although poorly defined, ventricular tachyarrhythmias (VT/VF) are thought to involve reentry (either single or multiple reentrant circuits) in ventricular myocardium. Because myocardial reentry involves Na^+-dependent tissue, class II and IV drugs are ineffective, and only direct membrane-acting agents (class I, III) should be considered in treatment of these arrhythmias.

Several factors must be considered in the selection of optimal agents: (1) antiarrhythmic efficacy (Tables 39-4 and 39-5), (2) side-effect profile, and (3) long-term drug safety and tolerance. The selection of an antiarrhythmic drug must be individualized. First and fore-

TABLE 39-5

ANTIARRHYTHMIC EFFICACY IN SUSTAINED VENTRICULAR ARRHYTHMIAS

DRUG CLASS	EXAMPLES	RESPONSE
III	Amiodarone	40%–50%
	↓	↓
III	Sotalol	
	↓	
	I-A + I-B	
	↓	
	Encainide	20%–25%
I-C	Flecainide	↓
	Propafenone	
	Quinidine	
I-A	Procainamide	
	Disopyramide	
	↓	
I-B	Mexiletine	
	Tocainide	15%
	↓	↓
II	Beta-blockers	
IV	Ca^{2+} channel blockers	5%

TABLE 39-6

SUBJECTIVE TOXICITY

DRUG CLASS	EXAMPLES	RESPONSE
I-A	Quinidine	30%–40%
I-B	Mexiletine Tocainide	↓
	↓	
I-A	Procainamide Disopyramide	
	↓	
III	Amiodarone	
	↓	
II	Beta-blockers	
	↓	
I-C	Propafenone Encainide Flecainide	10%

most, a class of drug is examined based on their actions on the targeted arrhythmia. Specific antiarrhythmic agents can then be selected after careful consideration of potential cardiovascular and noncardiovascular adverse effects (Tables 39-6 through 39-10). The side effect profiles of a drug consists of several categories that include (1) subjective toxicity, (2) end-organ toxicity, (3) negative inotropic effect, and (4) proarrhythmia. In addition, drug interactions with other agents cannot be ignored, especially in critically ill patients with multiorgan dysfunction on multiple medications (Table 39-11). Last, the long-term safety and tolerance should be considered. A once- or twice-a-day dosing regimen is far more acceptable to patients. Multiple dosing (t.i.d. or q.i.d.) results in poor compliance and potential complications because of fluctuating plasma drug levels.

Antiarrhythmic drug selection

- Antiarrhythmic efficacy
- Side-effect profile: (cardiovascular versus noncardiovascular)
  - Negative inotropic effect
  - End-organ toxicity
  - Subjective toxicity/degree of tolerance
  - Proarrhythmia
  - Drug interactions
- Long-term safety and tolerance

METHODS TO GUIDE THERAPY

Methods are needed to evaluate patient clinical response to antiarrhythmic drugs and to guide therapy. These methods are not mutually exclusive and may be complementary. For nonlethal arrhythmias, therapy guided by symptomatic assessment and plasma drug concentration is acceptable. However, empirical use of antiarrhythmic drugs with subjective evaluation for treatment of ventricular arrhythmias is potentially hazardous, especially in ICU patients with structural heart disease (see "Proarrhythmia"). Cardiology/electrophysiology consultation should be considered in these patients.

TABLE 39-7

END-ORGAN TOXICITY

DRUG CLASS	EXAMPLES	RESPONSE
III	Amiodarone	Highest
	↓	↓
I-A	Quinidine Procainamide	
	↓	
I-B	Tocainide	
	↓	
I-B	Mexiletine	
	↓	
II	Beta-blockers	
	↓	
I-C	Encainide Flecainide Propafenone	
I-B	Mexiletine	Lowest

TABLE 39-8

NEGATIVE INOTROPIC EFFECTS

DRUG CLASS	EXAMPLES	RESPONSE
I-A	Disopyramide	Worst
IV	Verapamil	
	↓	
II	Beta-blockers	
	↓	
I-C	Flecainide	
	Propafenone	
III	Sotalol	
	↓	
I-C	Encainide	
	↓	
I-A	Quinidine	
	Procainamide	
	↓	
I-B	Lidocaine	
	Mexiletine	
	Tocainide	
III	Amiodarone	
	Bretylium	Best

TABLE 39-9

PROARRHYTHMIA IN PATIENTS WITH MINIMAL HEART DISEASE AND BENIGN ARRHYTHMIAS

DRUG CLASS	EXAMPLES	RESPONSE
	Quinidine	6%–8%
I-A	Procainamide	
	Disopyramide	
	↓	
	Encainide	
I-C	Flecainide	
	Propafenone	↓
	↓	4%
I-B	Mexiletine	
	Tocainide	
	↓	
III	Amiodarone	↓
II	Beta-blockers	1%

TABLE 39-10

PROARRHYTHMIA IN PATIENTS WITH STRUCTURAL HEART DISEASE AND SUSTAINED VENTRICULAR ARRHYTHMIA

DRUG CLASS	EXAMPLES	PROARRHYTHMIA
I-C	Encainide	10%–20%
	Flecainide	
	↓	↓
I-C	Propafenone	8%–10%
	↓	
	Quinidine	
I-A	Procainamide	
	Disopyramide	
	↓	
III	Amiodarone	
I-B	Mexiletine	
	Tocainide	↓
II	Beta-blockers	2%–5%

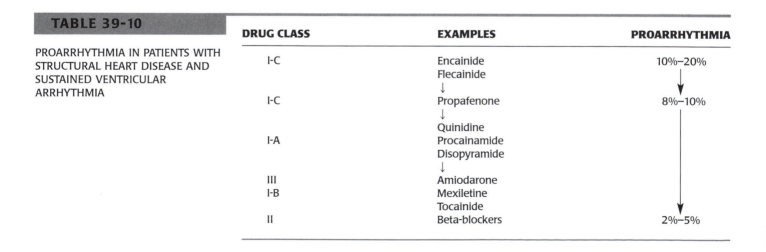

TABLE 39-11

INFLUENCE OF DISEASE STATES ON ANTIARRHYTHMIC DRUG PHARMACOKINETICS

DISEASE OR CONDITION	EFFECTS
Congestive heart failure	Reduced clearance of: Lidocaine Procainamide Flecainide Reduced volume of distribution of: Lidocaine
Liver disease	Reduced clearance of: Lidocaine Disopyramide Phenytoin Beta-blockers
Renal disease	Reduced clearance of: Disopyramide Procainamide Bretylium Flecainide Tocainide
Postmyocardial infarction	Reduced clearance of: Procainamide Altered protein binding of: Lidocaine Quinidine

The use of plasma drug concentrations to adjust drug dosage is an acceptable method with limitations; only a small number of antiarrhythmic drugs can be measured by routine clinical laboratories, and the plasma drug level does not necessarily reflect the physiologic effects on individual patients. A subtherapeutic quinidine level may represent a physiologically effective dosage in some patients. Furthermore, plasma drug level does not take into account the effects of active metabolites. For example, procainamide exhibits class I-A drug action, whereas its major metabolite from hepatic acetylation, *N*-acetylprocainamide (NAPA), is a class III agent. Using the combined procainamide + NAPA level to assess the efficacy of procainamide therapy can be misleading because the combined value reflects both class I-A and class III activities. In patients with renal insufficiency or with fast hepatic metabolism (who produce a disproportionally high NAPA level), the procainamide + NAPA level overestimates the class I-A effects. However, the combined levels are useful in estimating the risk of adverse reactions with procainamide therapy.

Electrocardiographic manifestation of drug actions: I

- PR: AV nodal conduction class II, IV
- QRS: His–Purkinje, ventricular conduction class I
- QT: action potential duration/ repolarization class III

Electrocardiographic manifestation of drug actions: II

- IA: QRS and QT interval prolongation
- IB: minimal effect on QRS and QT intervals
- IC: significant QRS prolongation, bundle branch block
- II/IV: PR interval prolongation
- III: QT interval prolongation

In addition to plasma drug levels, the overall pharmacologic effects of antiarrhythmic drugs in patients can be assessed by careful analysis of a routine 12-lead electrocardiogram. The electrocardiographic manifestations of drug actions are intuitive. The PR interval duration is determined mostly by the AV node conduction time. The QRS duration reflects the impulse conduction velocity through the ventricular myocardium, which is determined by the upstroke velocity (V_{max}) of phase 0 of action potentials. The QT interval represents the action potential duration and repolarization governed by the K^+ channels. The class I-A drugs exhibit K^+ channel inhibition in addition to Na^+ channel blockade activity. These effects produce a moderate widening of QRS duration with QT interval prolongation. The class I-C drugs are the most potent Na^+ channel blockers, with significant depression of phase 0 upstroke and conduction velocity in Na^+-dependent tissues (ventricular myocardium and His–Purkinje system); this is manifested by prolongation of QRS duration or development of bundle branch block (BBB) without alteration of ventricular repolarization. The K^+ channel blockers (Class III) cause predominately QT prolongations, whereas Class II and IV drugs affect AV nodal conduction with PR interval prolongation.

The criteria for determination of antiarrhythmic drug efficacy using either Holter monitoring or exercise testing are somewhat variable. A total elimination of nonsustained ventricular tachycardia, up to 90% reduction of couplets, and approximately 50% reduction in premature ventricular complexes (PVCs) are generally required. The roles of signal-averaged

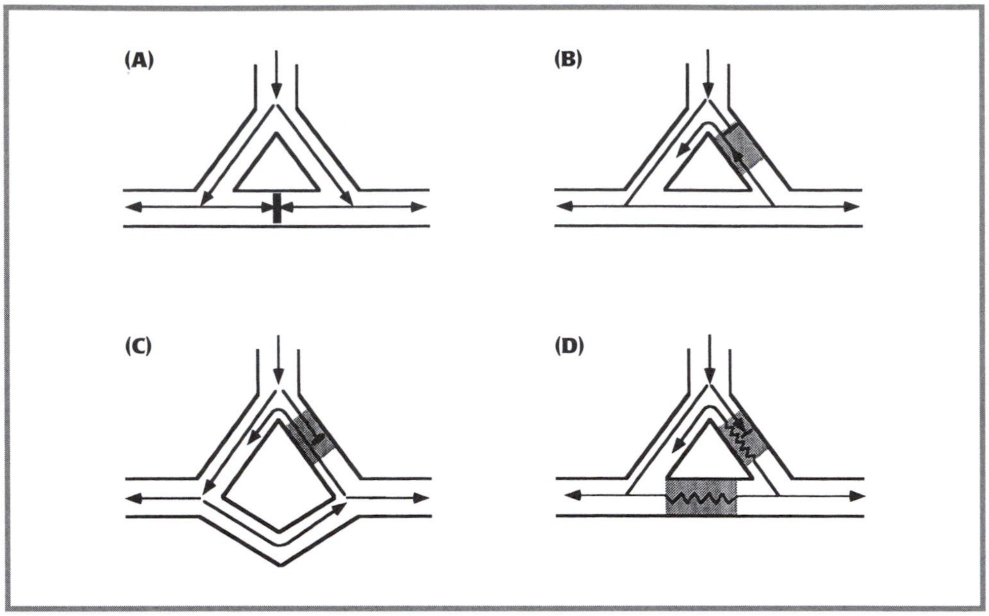

FIGURE 39-8

Mechanisms of proarrhythmia. **(A)** Baseline condition of a potential circuit; the impulse travels down both limbs of the circuit, and thus there is no reentrant arrhythmia. **(B)** Proarrhythmia caused by creation of unidirectional block (*shaded area*) at one pathway. **(C)** Proarrhythmia caused by lengthening of circuit pathway to allow sufficient recovery of excitability. **(D)** Proarrhythmia caused by further slowing of impulse conduction within the circuit.

Evaluation of clinical response to antiarrhythmic drugs
- Empiric
- Elimination of symptoms
- Plasma drug concentration
- Electrocardiographic changes
- Signal-averaged ECG
- Guided by objective criteria:
  - Ambulatory monitoring
  - Exercise testing
  - Electrophysiologic study

ECG (SAECG) and electrophysiologic study (EPS) in assessing antiarrhythmic drug responses and proarrhythmias is beyond the scope of this chapter and is less useful for daily management in an ICU setting.

PROARRHYTHMIA

The definition of proarrhythmia is a significant aggravation of arrhythmia occurring in temporal relation to the initiation of drug therapy or changes in dose. Because antiarrhythmic drugs alter the electrophysiologic characteristics of cardiac tissues, some of these changes can actually promote arrhythmia induction. The mechanisms of proarrhythmia are complex (Figure 39-8), and a number of types of proarrhythmia have been recognized (Table 39-12). The development of new arrhythmias is clearly a manifestation of proarrhythmia; this may include conversion of nonsustained ectopies to sustained tachycardia, induction of torsades de pointes with QT prolongation, or development of heart block and bradycardia. Proarrhythmia may also present as a worsening of preexisting arrhythmias. Changes in arrhythmia characteristics with more frequent recurrences, faster rate, and longer duration with less

TABLE 39-12

DEFINITION OF PROARRHYTHMIA

1. Worsening of preexisting arrhythmias
   - Increasing frequency and complexity of PVCs
   - Conversion from nonsustained to sustained arrhythmias
   - Changes in characteristics of arrhythmias: faster rate, longer duration
   - More frequent episodes, incessant arrhythmia
   - More difficult to terminate
2. Uncovering "hidden" arrhythmogenic substrate
   - Development of a new arrhythmia
   - Conversion of nonsustained to sustained arrhythmias
   - Torsade de pointes, polymorphic VT
   - Supraventricular tachycardias
3. Induction of conduction block/suppression of escape foci
   - Bradycardias
   - Sinus nodal dysfunction
   - Atrioventricular block
   - His–Purkinje block
4. Combination

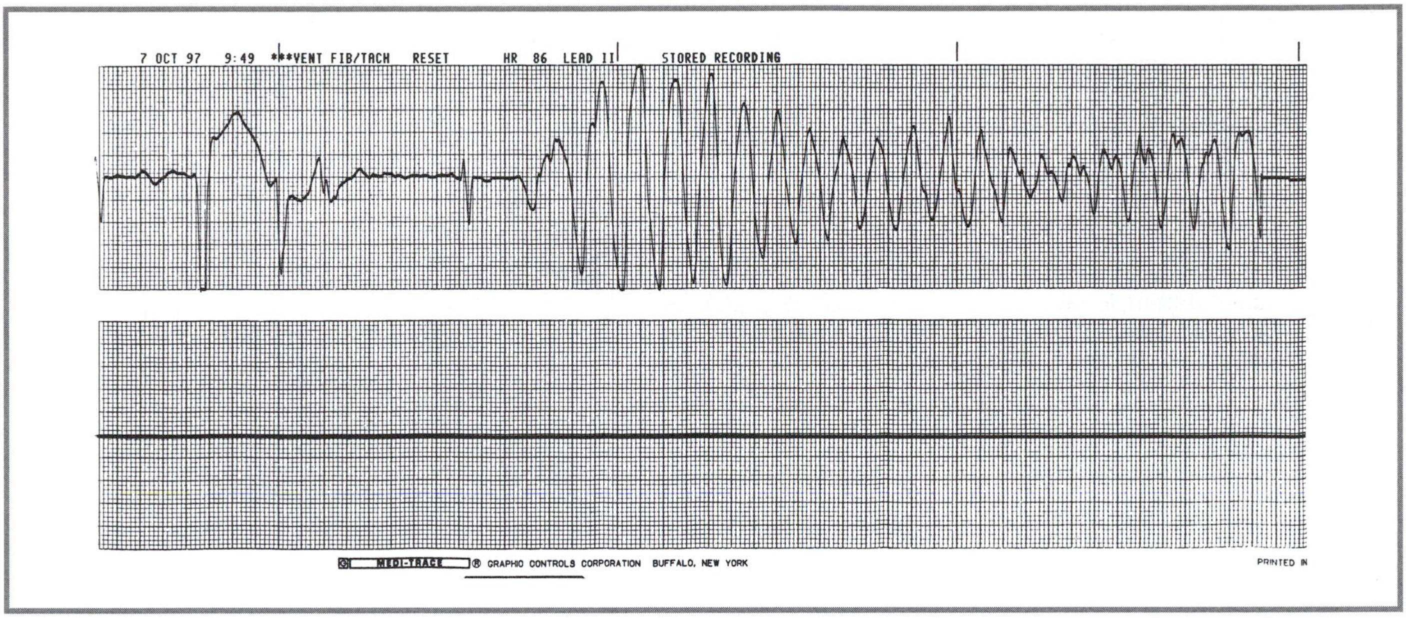

FIGURE 39-9

Torsades de pointes, the "twisting of the points," is typically used to describe polymorphic ventricular tachycardia associated with prolonged QT intervals. In this case, the QT interval was prolonged by bradycardia. A premature ventricular complex (PVC) with "R-on-T"-induced torsades de pointes.

hemodynamic stability can be problematic. Occasionally, incessant arrhythmia can develop that may be refractory to attempts of termination, by either pacing or high-energy shocks (Figure 39-9). A classic example of proarrhythmia is torsades de pointes associated with the use of class I-A or class III drugs. The development of polymorphic VT in the setting of prolonged QT interval is related to triggered activity based on early afterdepolarization (EAD) from delayed ventricular repolarizations; this is further exacerbated by hypokalemia, hypomagnesemia, and bradycardia.

Unfortunately, the time of occurrence of proarrhythmia is unpredictable. Proarrhythmia events usually occur within several days of initiation of a new drug or changing its dosage. However, it may present as an acute idiosyncratic reaction occurring within the first few doses, especially for class I-A drugs. Occurrence of proarrhythmia may be influenced by pharmacokinetics and drug metabolism, changes in substrate (new myocardial infarction or scar), ischemia, interaction with other medications, electrolyte imbalance, heart rate, and autonomic tone. The incidence of proarrhythmia has been reported to be as high as 30%–40%, depending on the methods of determination, arrhythmia presentation, individual agents, and patient-specific risk profiles (see Tables 39-9 and 39-10). Metaanalysis of trials of antiarrhythmic therapy in postinfarction patients have demonstrated an unfavorable odds ratio with increased mortality, especially with the class I agents (Figure 39-10). The risk of proarrhythmia can be estimated by careful assessment of patient clinical risk profile (Table 39-13). Proarrhythmia risk is low in patients with minimal structural heart disease who present with nonlife-threatening arrhythmias. Proarrhythmia risk is significantly elevated in patients with structural heart disease and ventricular dysfunction who present with high-grade sustained ventricular tachyarrhythmias (Figure 39-11). In hospitalized patients with multiorgan disease on many medications, the physician must be keenly aware of the risk–benefit ratio before initiating antiarrhythmic drugs. Electrocardiographic monitoring is essential in high-risk patients starting antiarrhythmic drugs. The exercise stress test may provoke proarrhythmia by sympathetic stimulation at a fast heart rate (use dependency). The role of invasive electrophysiologic study in determination of proarrhythmia risk is beyond the scope of this chapter.

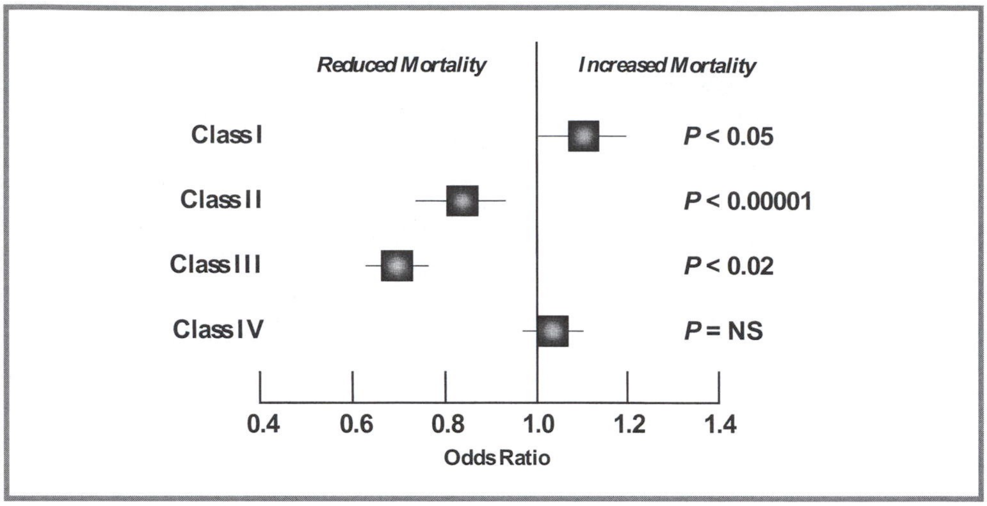

FIGURE 39-10

Metaanalysis of mortality with antiarrhythmic therapy in postinfarction patients. The overall odds ratio favors class II (beta-blockers) and class III drugs (such as amiodarone) for mortality reduction. The use of class I and class IV antiarrhythmic drugs is associated with increased mortality. (Adapted from Teo K. JAMA 1993;270(13):1589–1595, with permission.)

TABLE 39-13

PROARRHYTHMIA RISK PROFILE

1. Depressed ventricular function
2. Electrolyte imbalance
3. High dose of antiarrhythmic drug
4. In-hospital patients, multiorgan disease
5. Multiple other medications

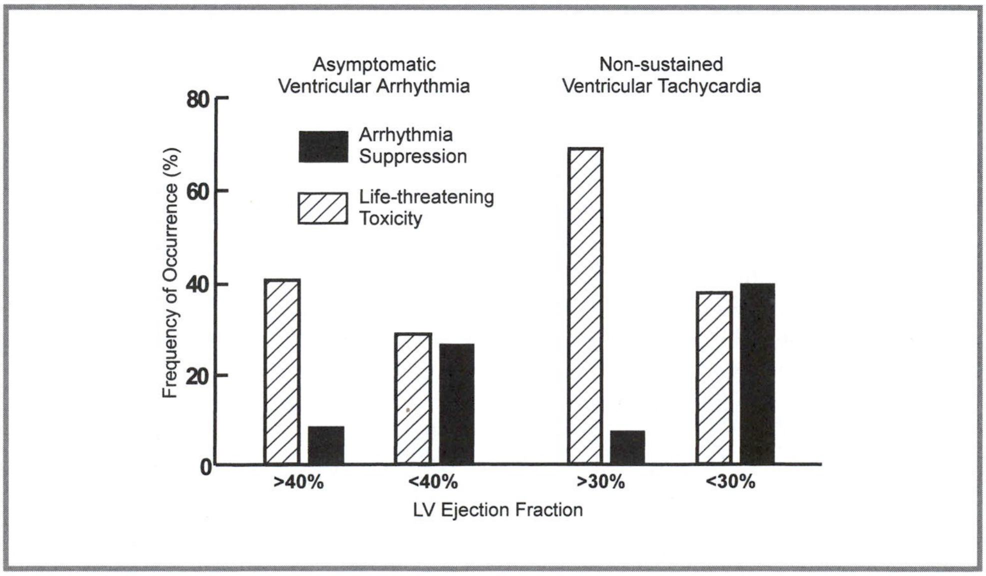

FIGURE 39-11

The relationship of proarrhythmia risk versus ventricular ejection fraction and the presenting arrhythmias. (Adapted from Pratt G. Am Heart J 1989;270(13): 1589–1595, with permission.)

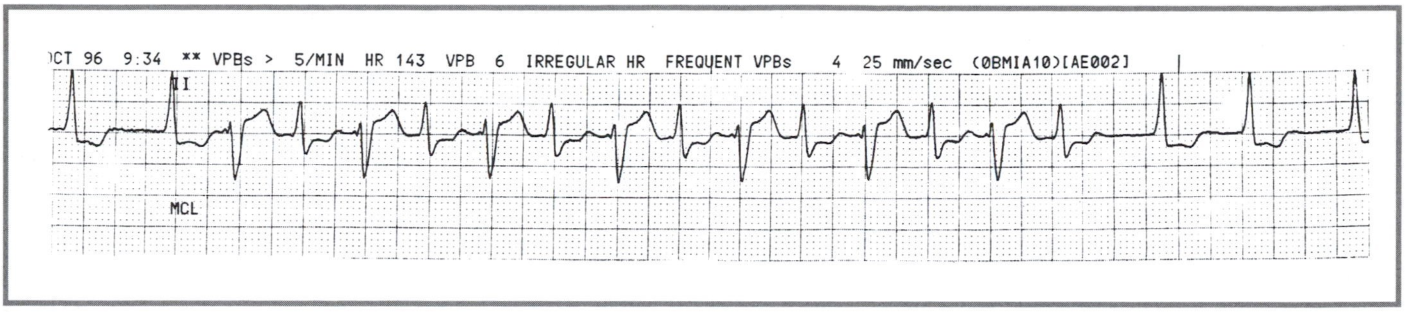

FIGURE 39-12

Bidirectional, alternating bundle branch block ventricular tachycardia (VT) is usually associated with digitalis toxicity.

It is said that any arrhythmia can develop in patients with digitalis toxicity. The key to diagnosis is a high index of suspicion. The hallmark of digitalis toxicity is ectopic arrhythmia (due to triggered activity based on DAD) with concomitant conduction blocks. The classic digitalis toxic arrhythmia is atrial tachycardia with AV block. The most common digitalis toxic arrhythmia is a ventricular arrhythmia such as bigeminy, junctional rhythm with various degree of sinus and AV nodal suppression. Occasional, bidirectional, alternating BBB VT or narrow QRS fascicular VT may occur (Figure 39-12). Serum digoxin levels are often elevated but may be within the therapeutic range in elderly patients, patients with hypokalemia, or patients with hypothyroidism. Conservative therapy by withholding digitalis with potassium/magnesium supplementation is the treatment of choice for digitalis-related arrhythmias. Phenytoin may be indicated for symptomatic digitalis toxic arrhythmias. Life-threatening arrhythmia should be treated with antidigoxin antibodies (Digibind®). Temporary pacing may be necessary in patients with symptomatic bradycardia.

- Digitalis Toxicity
  1. Triggered activity
  2. Sinus suppression with junctional rhythm
  3. Atrial tachyarrhythmias with various AV block
  4. Alternating BBB tachycardias
  5. Narrow QRS VT from Purkinje fibers

SUMMARY

An accurate arrhythmia diagnosis may imply, with variable certainty, an arrhythmia mechanism based on collation of clinical information and electrocardiographic data. Effective pharmacologic therapy requires identifying a class of drugs with the most appropriate profile to attack the most vulnerable parameter(s) of the targeted arrhythmia. Secondary assessments of both cardiovascular and noncardiovascular side effects screen for inappropriate drug interactions and minimize adverse responses. Finally, considerations of long-term safety and tolerance identify the optimal agent for the individual patient.

REVIEW QUESTIONS

1. **A 71-year-old woman with prior myocardial infarctions was admitted with congestive heart failure and paroxysmal rapid atrial fibrillation. She has had four episodes of atrial fibrillation in the last 6 months requiring hospital admissions. She has been treated with quinidine (324 mg, q8h) but continues to experience recurrent episodes with occasional heart failure exacerbation. Which would be the best antiarrhythmic drug for this patient?**
   A. Procainamide
   B. Amiodarone
   C. Beta-blocker
   D. Flecainide

2. **A 68-year-old Asian man with a nonischemic cardiomyopathy presented with recurrent dizziness and syncope. He was recently started on low-dose diuretic and procainamide (500 mg, q6h), which was initiated 1 week ago for paroxysmal atrial fibrillation. The ECG showed a widened QRS duration with corrected QT interval of 530 ms. The procainamide and NAPA levels were 7.2 and 18.8 mg/dl, respectively. What should be the first step of treatment?**
   A. Discontinuation of procainamide
   B. Implantation of a defibrillator
   C. Increasing the procainamide
   D. Holter monitor

3. **What is the best electrocardiographic parameters for assessment of physiologic effects of class I-C antiarrhythmic drugs?**
   - **A.** The PR interval
   - **B.** The height amplitude of the QRS
   - **C.** The sinus rate
   - **D.** The width of QRS
   - **E.** The QT interval

4. **Which one of the following arrhythmias is commonly associated with digitalis toxicity?**
   - **A.** Ventricular ectopies
   - **B.** Sinus bradycardia with junctional rhythm
   - **C.** Atrial tachyarrhythmias with various AV block
   - **D.** Alternating BBB tachycardias
   - **E.** All the above

5. **A 65-year-old man with coronary artery disease who underwent a coronary artery bypass grafting procedure. Two days after the surgery, the patient developed new onset of atrial fibrillation with a rapid ventricular rate. Which of the following responses is most appropriate?**
   - **A.** Start procainamide for conversion of atrial fibrillation
   - **B.** Administer digitalis
   - **C.** Administer a beta-blocker or calcium channel blocker for rate control in atrial fibrillation
   - **D.** Start amiodarone for conversion of atrial fibrillation

ANSWERS

1. The answer is B. This elderly patient has structural heart disease and ventricular dysfunction. Her atrial fibrillation is poorly tolerated and is refractory to a class I-A drug. An alternative antiarrhythmic drug is a class III agent for chronic therapy to prevent arrhythmia recurrence. In this particular patient, the best tolerated drug with the least proarrhythmia side-effect profile is amiodarone. Given her age and underlying heart diseases, low-dose amiodarone (200 mg daily) is associated with the best compliance with an acceptable risk of end-organ toxicity.
2. The answer is A. The cause of this patient's syncope and dizziness is most likely nonsustained ventricular tachyarrhythmia, especially in an elderly man with structural heart disease. His QT interval is significantly prolonged with a disproportionally elevated NAPA level (class III effect) compared to that of procainamide; this may be related to the patient's hepatic acetylation metabolism of procainamide. In addition, initiation of diuretic may predispose the patient to electrolyte imbalance and proarrhythmia aggravation. The first line of therapy is to discontinue procainamide and correct any electrolyte abnormalities.
3. The answer is D. The class I-C antiarrhythmic drugs are the most potent sodium channel blockers with significant suppression of impulse conduction velocity over the ventricular myocardium; this translates to a prolonged ventricular activation time and QRS widening. The class I-C drugs have no effect on cellular repolarization (QT interval) or AV nodal conduction (PR interval).
4. The answer is E. Digitalis toxicity can be associated with many arrhythmias. The classic digitalis toxic rhythms are atrial tachyarrhythmias with AV block and ventricular arrhythmias with alternating bundle branch block morphologies. Other forms of arrhythmias can also be observed. The key of diagnosis is a high degree of suspicion of digitalis toxicity.
5. The answer is C. For new-onset atrial fibrillation, an AV node-independent arrhythmia, direct membrane-active class I or class III agents such as procainamide or amiodarone may be used for arrhythmia conversion. However, for acute management, an AV nodal blocker should be administered first for heart rate control, especially considering the vagolytic effect of class IA drug and the slow onset of action of amiodarone. The efficacy of digitalis is low for acute rate control in the postoperative period with a high adrenergic tone.

SUGGESTED READING

Anonymous. The Sicilian gambit: a new approach to the classification of antiarrhythmic drugs based on their actions on arrhythmogenic mechanisms. Circulation 1991;84:1831–1851.

ESVEM Investigators. The ESVEM Trial: electrophysiologic study versus electrocardiographic monitoring for selection of antiarrhythmic therapy of ventricular tachyarrhythmias. Circulation 1989; 76(6):1354–1360.

Hillis LD, Lange RA, Wells PJ, Winniford MD. Manual of Clinical Problems in Cardiology. Boston: Little, Brown, 1992.

Hsia HH. Work-up and management of patients with sustained and nonsustained monomorphic ventricular tachycardias. Cardiol Clin 1993;11:21–37.

Opie L. The Heart: Physiology, Metabolism, Pharmacology, Therapy. New York: Grune & Stratton, 1987.

Podrid PJ, Kowey PR (eds) Handbook of Cardiac Arrhythmia. Baltimore: Williams & Wilkins, 1996.

Pratt CM. The inversed relationship between baseline left ventricular ejection fraction and outcome of antiarrhythmic therapy: a dangerous imbalance in the risk-benefit ratio. Am Heart J 1989;118: 433–440.

Reiser HJ, Horowitz LN (eds) Mechanism and Treatment of Cardiac Arrhythmias: Relevance of Basic Studies to Clinical Management. Munich: Urban & Schwarzenberg, 1985.

Stambler BS. Efficacy and safety of repeated intravenous doses of ibutilide for rapid conversion of atrial flutter or fibrillation. Circulation 1996;94:1613–1621.

Zipes DP, Jalife J (eds) Cardiac Electrophysiology: From Cell to Bedside. Philadelphia: Saunders, 1996.

CHAPTER 40

L.I. ARMANDO SAMUELS AND GERALD M. O'BRIEN

Dialysis

CHAPTER OUTLINE

LEARNING OBJECTIVES

After studying this chapter, you should be able to:

- Understand the physiologic principles of dialysis and renal replacement therapy.
- Be familiar with the nomenclature and modalities of dialysis and renal replacement therapy.
- Understand the complications associated with dialysis therapy.
- Recognize the general indications for dialysis therapy and the considerations in selection of a specific renal replacement modality.

Artificial renal replacement therapy for the treatment of acute renal failure was first introduced during the Korean War. Over the past two decades, technologic improvements have resulted in several treatment options that include peritoneal dialysis, hemodialysis, and continuous renal replacement therapies (CRRT). Moreover, technologic improvements in vascular catheters, semipermeable membranes, and dialytic machinery have resulted in a variety of dialysis prescription options. The clinical indications for choosing these different modalities have not been precisely defined. The choice of therapy often depends on several conditions that include availability of vascular access, types of dialysis machinery, and availability of skilled personnel. This chapter reviews the different types of renal replacement therapy and the indications and complications confronting the clinician in the ICU setting.

PHYSIOLOGIC PRINCIPLES OF DIALYTIC THERAPY

> Dialysis is the technique wherein solutes are removed from a patient's blood through the use of a semipermeable membrane.

A review of the basic mechanisms of solute and water transport across semipermeable membranes is necessary to understand the relative efficacy of the different forms of dialysis therapy. Solute transport across a semipermeable membrane occurs via two different mechanisms, diffusion and convection. With diffusion, solute movement is driven by the solute concentration gradient between the two compartments (Figure 40-1A) and is limited by the thickness and permeability of the membrane; thus, diffusive transport is more effective for molecules with a relatively lower molecular weight. In convection, solutes are dragged along with water when fluid moves from one compartment to another (Figure 40-1B). This process is called ultrafiltration and is dependent on the hydraulic permeability of the membrane

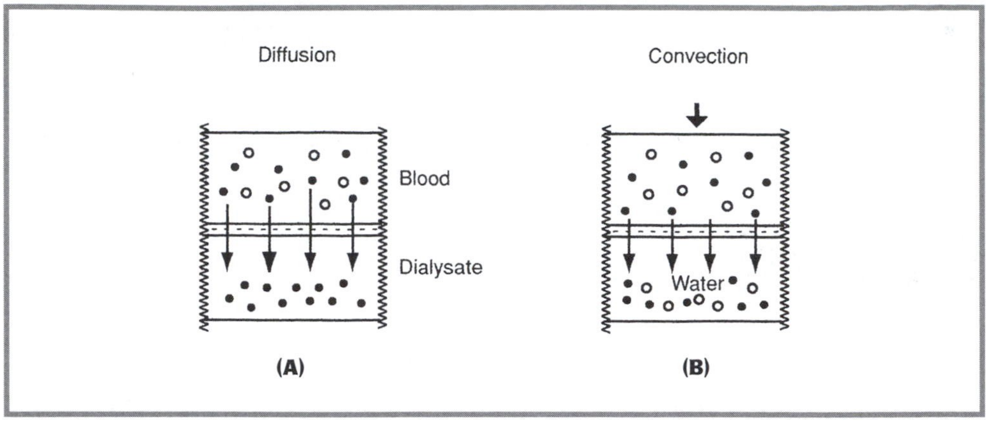

FIGURE 40-1

Basic mechanisms of solute and water transport across semipermeable membranes. **(A)** *Diffusion*. Solute movement is driven by the solute concentration gradient between the two compartments. The diffusion rate is limited by solute molecular weight and the thickness and permeability of the membrane. **(B)** *Convection*. Solutes are dragged along with water when fluid moves from one compartment to another; this is called ultrafiltration. The ultrafiltration rate is dependent on the hydraulic permeability of the membrane and the hydrostatic pressure differential between the compartments. Solute transport is dependent on the volume of ultrafiltrate and the sieving capacity of the membrane.

The diffusive transport of solute is dependent on both membrane permeability and solute molecular size. Convective transport is dependent on membrane hydrostatic permeability and transmembrane pressure gradient.

as well as the hydrostatic pressure differential between the compartments. Solute transport is dependent on the volume of ultrafiltrate and the sieving capacity of the membrane.

Dialysis Membranes

Dialysis membranes vary in composition, thickness, and their geometric design, factors that affect their ultrafiltration capacity and solute permeability. The four different types of membranes used for dialysis are (1) cellulosic, made from cotton; (2) cellulose substitute, made from cellulose acetate; (3) synthetic, made of a chemical polymer; and (4) cellulosynthetic, made from cellulose combined with a synthetic polymer (Table 40-1).

The cellulosic membranes are used most often in intermittent hemodialysis. These membranes are thin, have a relatively low hydraulic permeability and a reduced sieving capacity, and are much more dependent on diffusion for solute removal. With this type of membrane, small molecules (<20 kilodaltons, kDa) such as urea can be efficiently and rapidly removed

TABLE 40-1

COMPARISON OF DIALYTIC MEMBRANES

FILTER TYPE	CELLULOSIC	SYNTHETIC
Membrane	Cuprophan (Cellulose) Cellulose diacetate Hemophan (cellulosynthetic)	Polysulfone Polyamide Polyacrylonitrile (PAN) Polymethacrylate (PMMA)
Geometry	Hollow fiber and plate	Hollow fiber and plate
Membrane thickness	Thin	Thick
Primary mechanism	Diffusion	Convection
Hydraulic permeability	Low	High
Removal of large molecules (>10^2 kDa)	Poor (low sieving coefficient)	Good (high sieving coefficient)
Biocompatibility	Poor	Good
Primary application	Intermittent therapy	Continuous therapy
Cost	Low	High

TABLE 40-2

REPLACEMENT SOLUTION COMPOSITION

Electrolytes	Glucose
Sodium, 140–155 mmol/l	Buffers (one must be selected)
Potassium, 0–4 mmol/l	Bicarbonate
Calcium, 1.5–1.75 mm/l	Acetate
Magnesium, 0–0.75 mm/l	Lactate (converted to bicarbonate)
Chloride, 110–120 mm/l	Citrate

without excessive fluid loss. Synthetic membranes are thick and have both higher hydraulic permeability and sieving capacity than the cellulosic membranes. Synthetic membranes are more dependent on convection for solute removal and are thus more suitable for continuous therapies. The high convective component of continuous replacement therapy leads to large ultrafiltration volumes (15–20 l/day) and removal of solute over a wide range of molecular weights (10–40 kDa). A replacement solution is often needed when synthetic filters are used because plasma electrolytes (bicarbonate, sodium, calcium, and phosphate) are also removed. The composition of the replacement fluid should be individualized and appropriate for each patient, often consisting of a modified saline solution with a buffer such as acetate or bicarbonate (Table 40-2). Calcium and magnesium replacement may be needed but should not be mixed with bicarbonate solutions because they will precipitate.

RENAL REPLACEMENT MODALITIES

Intermittent Hemodialysis

Intermittent hemodialysis (IHD) is the therapy most commonly used for treatment of acute renal failure in the intensive care unit. This therapy is done in sessions lasting a few hours using a sophisticated machine and requires a specially trained nurse. Hemodialysis machines have a precise dialysate-preparing module, blood warmers, and antibubbling systems and are primarily diffusion dependent with a higher dialysate flow rate (500 ml/min) compared to blood flow (200–300 ml/min). A cellulosic membrane is most commonly used and replacement fluids are generally not needed. Blood flow runs countercurrent to the dialysate through the filter, where a rapid decrease in plasma and extracellular solute concentration occurs during a relatively short period of time (Figure 40-2). IHD is relatively inefficient in removing

Intermittent hemodialysis
- The most common dialysis prescription for acute renal failure
- Requires complex machinery
- Requires a high blood and dialysate flow rate
- Achieves a rapid decrease in plasma solute concentration

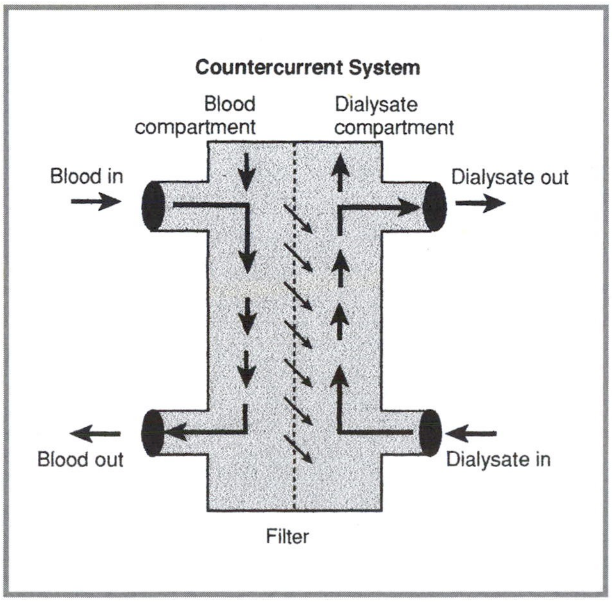

FIGURE 40-2

Blood flow runs countercurrent to the dialysate through the filter, where a rapid decrease in plasma and extracellular solute (*arrows*) concentration occurs over a relatively short period of time.

intracellular solutes because of the delay in equilibration between compartments. A sudden rebound in plasma urea concentration is generally observed a few hours after dialysis has ended. Consequently, IHD fails to achieve complete purification of body fluid.

Complications Related to IHD

Acute hypotension is the most common complication of intermittent dialysis treatments (Table 40-3). When fluid is removed from the intravascular compartment, the oncotic pressure increases, promoting refilling from the interstitium. Hypotension may develop if too much fluid is removed too fast or if mobilization of fluid from the interstitial compartment is impeded by the presence of heart failure, sepsis, or low oncotic pressure. Moreover, the rapid removal of potassium or calcium can promote cardiac dysrhythmias, which can be further exacerbated by the rapid correction of acidemia with bicarbonate-rich dialysate.

Intermittent therapies may also cause what has become known as dysequilibrium syndrome. This syndrome is thought to occur because solute is removed from the intravascular space and serum osmolality decreases faster than that of the intracellular space. Water then shifts into the brain cells, causing cerebral edema. This syndrome can manifest by causing headaches, lethargy, disorientation, and seizures.

Dialysis Membrane Biocompatability

No membrane material is completely biocompatible; however, some materials are less biocompatible than others. Cellulose membranes have the lowest biocompatibility and have been shown to induce cytokine release and compliment activation via activation of the alternative pathway when blood comes into contact with a polysaccharide membrane surface. Intense systemic complement activation leads to the release of the anaphylotoxins C3a and C5a and also results in both granulocyte and monocyte activation, with generation and release of proinflammatory reactive oxygen species, leukotrienes, and other cytokines. Thus, a potential adverse effect of hemodialysis membrane bioincompatibility, particularly in ARF patients, would include development or prolongation of systemic inflammatory response syndrome, characterized by fever, hypercatabolism, leukocytosis, and worsening of tissue injury.

Adverse reactions resulting from dialysis membrane bioincompatibility have been subclassified as either immediate (type A) or delayed (type B). Symptoms of a type A reaction occur immediately after the initiation of dialysis but may be delayed for as much as 30 min. Patients may experience a sense of impending doom, dyspnea, urticaria, itching, and abdominal pain. Cardiac arrest and even death have also been reported. Reactions occurring beyond 30 min after the initiation of dialysis therapy are more common but less severe. These delayed reactions (type B) are most commonly manifested by subjective complaints of back or chest pain. If a filter reaction is suspected, the dialysis should be stopped, and the blood in the tubing should be discarded. The patient may require anaphylaxis therapy in severe cases.

The availability of biocompatible (synthetic) membrane filters is no longer limited to continuous dialysis therapy. The high-flux membranes are also available and should be used in the critically ill patient requiring hemodialysis. However, even these membranes are not without problems. Rarely, anaphylactoid reactions are observed in patients dialyzed on polyacronylnitrile (PAN; AN69) synthetic membranes who are receiving concomitant angiotensin-converting enzyme (ACE) inhibition. The electronegative surface charges of these membranes

TABLE 40-3

COMPLICATIONS ASSOCIATED WITH INTERMITTENT HEMODIALYSIS

Severe hypotension	Hypoxemia and hypoventilation
Type A and B filter reactions	Bleeding
Dysequilibrium syndrome	Air embolism
Worsened brain edema	Cardiac arrythmias

appear to activate the kallikrein system and promote bradykinin generation. ACE inhibitors impair bradykinin degradation; thus, when they are used in combination with these membranes, circulating bradykinin levels can be increased, causing hypotension and bronchospasm. Discontinuing or substituting ACE inhibitor drugs should be considered in those patients who require dialysis using these membranes.

Continuous Renal Replacement Therapies

Continuous renal replacement therapy (CRRT) nomenclature can be at times confusing and include modalities known as CAVH (continuous arteriovenous hemofiltration), CAVHD (continuous arteriovenous hemodialysis), CAVHDF (continuous arteriovenous hemofiltration), CVVH (continuous veno-venous hemofiltration), CVVHD (continuous veno-venous hemodialysis), CVVHDF (continuous veno-venous hemodiafiltration), and SCUF (slow continuous ultrafiltration). All these modalities employ the use of synthetic, highly permeable membranes and differ with regard to how the circulatory system is accessed as well as their principal method of solute removal (Table 40-4).

Continuous renal replacement therapies

- Employs synthetic, highly permeable membranes
- Employs low blood flow rate
- Achieves slow decrease in plasma solute concentration
- Better tolerated in patients who are hemodynamically unstable
- Heparin dosing should be adjusted to maintain minimal elevations in the partial thromboplastin time (PTT)

CAVH and CAVHD

Both these modalities depend on the patient's mean arterial pressure as the driving force for blood flow across the membrane (Figure 40-3). Vascular access requires two large-bore (8 Fr.) catheters, one arterial and the other venous, which are placed in the femoral vessels. The technique is relatively simple and driven by the arteriovenous pressure differential, which obviates the need for a blood pump and complicated machinery. In CAVH the blood flow rate ranges between 50 and 100 ml/min depending on the mean arterial pressure (Figure 40-3B). Solute removal is achieved by convective clearance, resulting in an ultrafiltrate between 5 and 10 ml/min.

In addition to ultrafiltration, CAVHD also employs diffusive solute clearance with the addition of dialysis. The blood and dialysate flow through the filter in countercurrent directions so that the existing gradient across the membrane can be maintained at all times (Figure 40-3C). The dialysate flow rate is set between 15 and 30 ml/min on an IV pump. The slow blood flow allows total equilibration of solute between the blood and the dialysate. The effluent dialysate is collected and measured hourly. The amount of ultrafiltrate is then calculated by subtracting the hourly dialysate volume (960 ml) from the total effluent volume. By changing the vertical distance between the filter and the collection bag, the volume of ultrafiltrate can be increased or decreased passively by using a siphon effect. Euvolemia can be maintained only if the ultrafiltrate is replaced volume for volume with replacement fluid on an hourly basis. More commonly, the patient is kept in a negative fluid balance by administering the hourly volume of ultrafiltrate minus 50–100 ml.

TABLE 40-4

CONTINUOUS REPLACEMENT THERAPIES

	IHD	PD	SCUF	CAVH	CVVH	CAVHD	CVVHD
Vascular access	AV	None	AV/VV	AV	VV	AV	VV
Pump	Yes	None	Sometimes	None	Yes	None	Yes
Blood flow (ml/min)	300	–	50	100	150	100	150
Dialysate flow (ml/min)	500	33[a]	None	None	None	16	16
Urea clearance (ml/min)	225	8.5[a]	1.7	10	17	27	30

IHD, intermittent hemodialysis; PD, peritoneal dialysis; SCUF, slow continuous filtration; CAVH, continuous arteriovenous hemofiltration; CVVH, continuous veno-venous filtration; CAVHD, continuous arteriovenous hemofiltration; CVVHD, continuous veno-venous hemodialysis

[a] Value is dependent on exchange rate. Numbers shown are based on an exchange rate of 2 l every hour

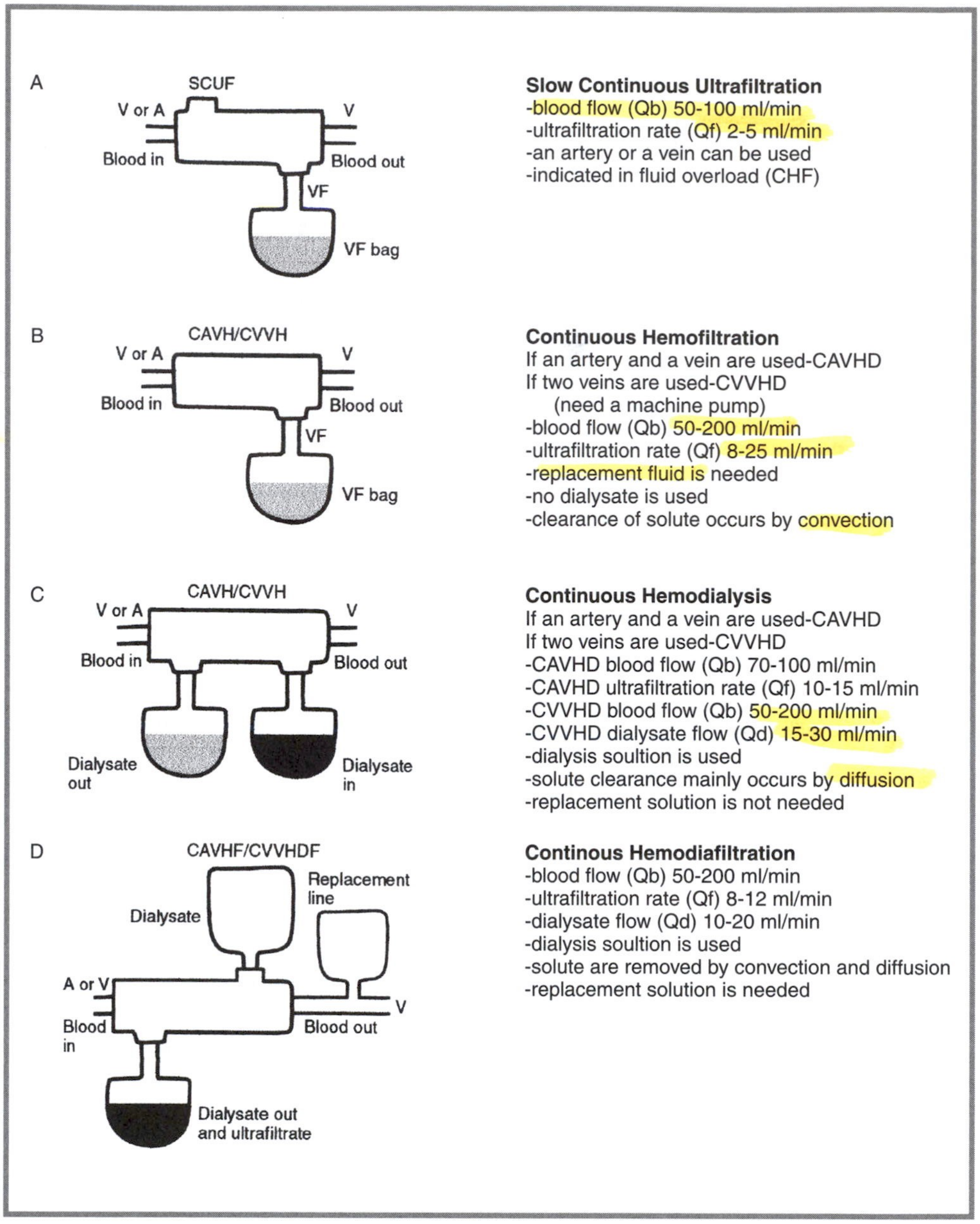
A
SCUF
V or A
V
Blood in
Blood out
VF
VF bag
Slow Continuous Ultrafiltration
-blood flow (Qb) 50-100 ml/min
-ultrafiltration rate (Qf) 2-5 ml/min
-an artery or a vein can be used
-indicated in fluid overload (CHF)
B
CAVH/CVVH
V or A
V
Blood in
Blood out
VF
VF bag
Continuous Hemofiltration
If an artery and a vein are used-CAVHD
If two veins are used-CVVHD
(need a machine pump)
-blood flow (Qb) 50-200 ml/min
-ultrafiltration rate (Qf) 8-25 ml/min
-replacement fluid is needed
-no dialysate is used
-clearance of solute occurs by convection
C
CAVH/CVVH
V or A
V
Blood in
Blood out
Dialysate out
Dialysate in
Continuous Hemodialysis
If an artery and a vein are used-CAVHD
If two veins are used-CVVHD
-CAVHD blood flow (Qb) 70-100 ml/min
-CAVHD ultrafiltration rate (Qf) 10-15 ml/min
-CVVHD blood flow (Qb) 50-200 ml/min
-CVVHD dialysate flow (Qd) 15-30 ml/min
-dialysis soultion is used
-solute clearance mainly occurs by diffusion
-replacement solution is not needed
D
CAVHF/CVVHDF
Replacement line
Dialysate
A or V
V
Blood in
Blood out
Dialysate out and ultrafiltrate
Continous Hemodiafiltration
-blood flow (Qb) 50-200 ml/min
-ultrafiltration rate (Qf) 8-12 ml/min
-dialysate flow (Qd) 10-20 ml/min
-dialysis soultion is used
-solute are removed by convection and diffusion
-replacement solution is needed

FIGURE 40-3

The nomenclature and circuitry of continuous renal replacement therapies. In CAVH (continuous arteriovenous hemofiltration), CAVHD (continuous arteriovenous hemodialysis), and CAVHDF (continuous arteriovenous hemofiltration), the trans-membrane gradient is dependent on the difference between the venous (V) and arterial (A) pressure. In CVVH (continuous veno-venous hemofiltration), CVVHD (continuous veno-venous hemodialysis), and CVVHDF (continuous veno-venous hemodiafiltration), a perfusion pump on the venous (*blood in*) is required to maintain the transmembrane pressure gradient.

CVVH and CVVHD

These modalities are different from the previously mentioned ones in that only a single large central vein is cannulated with a double lumen dialysis catheter. One port opening mid-catheter (A) supplies blood to the filter and the other port (V) at the tip of the catheter is used to return blood to the patient (Figure 40-3B,C). This procedure requires special dialysis equipment with a pump that permits continuous blood flow (100–150 ml/min). These pumps provide continuous flow for patients with poor arterial access but add to the cost and complexity of an otherwise simple technique. CVVHD is similar to CAVHD except for the extracorporal use of blood pumps.

SCUF

Slow continuous ultrafiltration (SCUF) is similar to CVVH or CAVH, but the primary goal is removal of fluid and not solute (Figure 40-3A). The usual blood flow ranges between 50 and 100 ml/min, adjusted to achieve an ultrafiltrate volume of 2–5 ml/min, and replacement fluid is generally not needed. This modality is useful for patients with heart failure.

Specific Problems of Continuous Renal Replacement Therapies

Vascular Access

A vascular access is achieved at the bedside by percutaneously placing a noncuffed double lumen catheter into a central vein. These catheters can be inserted in either the femoral, internal jugular, or subclavian veins at the bedside. The size of the catheters most commonly used for dialysis are 11.5 Fr. × 8 in. (20 cm) or 11.5 Fr. × 6 in. (15 cm) (duo-flow, double lumen catheter). These catheters provide a blood flow that varies between 250 and 350 ml/min. The subclavian vein should be avoided because venous stenosis may develop that can compromise use of the ipsilateral arm if the patient requires permanent vascular access. Before starting dialysis, proper position of catheters should be confirmed by chest X-ray. It is recommended that all noncuffed catheters be changed at least every 3 weeks. Catheters used for femoral venous access should be at least 19 cm in length and should not be kept in place for more than 5 days because of the high risk of infection.

Circuit Clotting and Anticoagulation

Patency of the extracorporeal circuit and the integrity of the dialysis membrane are important in maintaining the efficacy of renal replacement therapy. Filter integrity is less problematic in IHD compared to CRRT because IHD is done over a shorter period of time with higher blood flows. The exposure of blood and plasma to the filter membrane results in the activation of the coagulation factors, clotting, and ultimately filter failure. Heparin is used commonly to achieve regional anticoagulation and prolong filter life. A loading dose of 5–10 U/kg and a maintenance dose rate of 3–12 U/kg/h are usually infused prefilter (arterial access side) (see Figure 40-3). Regulating anticoagulation to maintain the permeability of the filter can be one of the most difficult problems in CRRT. Anticoagulation has been reported to cause bleeding in 5%–26% of patients on CRRT. The heparin dosage should be reduced to maintain minimal elevations in the partial thromboplastin time (PTT). Other efforts to prolong filter life include infusing the replacement fluid prefilter to in effect predilute the blood. Factors that may impact the longevity of the filter include a reduced blood flow in the extracorporal circuit and hypercoagulable disorders such as disseminated intravascular coagulation (DIC), heparin-induced thrombocytopenia (HIT), and antithrombin III deficiency.

The viability of the filter needs to be monitored; it typically lasts from 1 to 4 days. When clots are visible in the tubing or filter, the filter must be replaced as the efficiency of the filter has been compromised. The ratio of urea in the dialysate to that of the blood (FUN/BUN) is a useful predictor of imminent filter failure. Under normal conditions, the concentration of the urea in the dialysate should be equal to the concentration of urea in plasma and this ratio should be equal to 1. As the efficacy of the filter decreases, the FUN/BUN ratio approaches 0. When the FUN/BUN ratio is less than 0.6, the filter should be changed.

Hypothermia and Filter Reactions

A mild reduction in core temperature often occurs among patients receiving CRRT; this appears to be more prevalent with replacement of large volumes of ultrafiltrate. Simple rewarming of replacement fluid may prevent or reduce the degree of hypothermia.

PERITONEAL DIALYSIS

Despite the advances in hemodialysis, peritoneal dialysis (PD) represents a viable renal replacement alternative. In this type of dialysis, the peritoneum is used as the semipermeable membrane. Here, 1–3 l of dextrose- and salt-containing solution is introduced into the peri-

Peritoneal dialysis
- Employs the peritoneal cavity as a dialysis membrane
- Dialysate is instilled into the peritoneal cavity and then drained
- Requires placement of peritoneal catheter
- Efficiency is dependent on cycle length

toneal cavity and is allowed to dwell for 1–6 h. Diffusive clearance occurs because of the concentration gradient that exists between the peritoneal capillary network and the dialysate. The ultrafiltration rate (convective clearance) is dependent on the concentration of the glucose (1.5%, 2.5%, or 4.25%) in the dialysate; the higher the glucose concentration, the better the ultrafiltration. Shortening the dwell times to 1 h and thus increasing the cycle frequency can increase the ultrafiltrate volume. However, because of a lower efficiency, PD may not adequately remove sufficient waste products for patients who are hypercatabolic.

Peritoneal dialysis has been largely abandoned in the ICU as a treatment of acute renal failure in favor of extracorporeal dialytic modalities. PD requires surgical placement of a peritoneal catheter and may be contraindicated for patients suffering from burns or abdominal sepsis or for those with a history of abdominal surgery. Moreover, this modality is limited in the ICU because of its impact on respiration. The increment of the abdominal pressure caused by the PD fluid may limit diaphragmatic excursion and compromise ventilation among patients with respiratory insufficiency. Despite these disadvantages, PD may be more appropriate in certain circumstances. It may be useful for patients with severe congestive heart failure or severe hypotension because dialysis is not dependent on extracorporeal blood flow. It also does not require anticoagulation, and thus it can be used safely for patients who have a high risk of bleeding or when heparin is contraindicated.

GENERAL INDICATIONS FOR INITIATING DIALYSIS IN THE ICU

General indications for initiating dialysis therapy:
- Therapy is indicated for patients who manifest clinical evidence of uremia or biochemical evidence of solute or fluid imbalance.

General indications for dialysis therapy are listed in Table 40-5. There is no consensus on the optimal timing for the initiation of dialysis therapy in the critically ill patient with acute renal failure; renal replacement therapy is usually considered for patients who manifest clinical evidence of uremia (pericarditis, encephalopathy, hemorrhage) or biochemical evidence of solute or fluid imbalance. Dialysis is usualy not initiated in end-stage renal disease (ESRD) until the creatinine clearance is less than 10 ml/min. Extrapolation of this criterion to critically ill patients in the ICU is fraught with danger because acute renal failure is a non-steady-state process with daily fluctuations in body water, catabolic rate, and urea production. Biochemical disturbances such as hyperkalemia, marked acidosis, uremia, and fluid overload are the most common renal-related indications for renal replacement therapy.

Renal Indications

Hyperkalemia

The most common cause of hyperkalemia in the ICU is a decrease in renal excretion. The kidney has a large capacity to excrete potassium, and patients usually become hyperkalemic only when the GFR is less than 10 ml/min. Nonrenal causes of hyperkalemia are the result of shifts in potassium from the intracellular to the extracellular space that may occur among patients who are hyperosmolar, or have rhabdomyolysis syndromes, tumor lysis syndrome,

TABLE 40-5

INDICATIONS FOR DIALYSIS IN THE INTENSIVE CARE UNIT

Renal	Nonrenal
Hyperkalemia ($K^+ > 6.5$)	Toxic ingestion
Acidemia	Volume overload secondary to:
Uremia (pericarditis, encephalopathy, GI bleeding)	Hyperalimentation
Volume overload secondary to renal failure	Heart failure with pulmonary edema
	Liver failure
	Hypertransfusion

inorganic acidosis, and acute fluoride intoxication. Hyperkalemia resulting from increased potassium intake is unusual if renal function is normal. However, patients who receive rapid IV or oral potassium administration can develop hyperkalemia. Falsely elevated potassium levels can be seen in thrombocytosis (platelet counts >500,000/ml), leukocytosis (leukocyte counts >100,000/ml), or when blood is collected while using a tourniquet and contracting the muscle to increase blood return.

Acidosis

Patients with severe acidosis resulting from acute renal failure may benefit from dialysis. The use of exogenous bicarbonate therapy to control acidemia is controversial and has been found to be detrimental in certain situations. Rapid correction of acidosis can be accomplished with intermittent hemodialysis by using a bicarbonate-rich dialysate (35–38 mEq/l), which allows back diffusion across the membrane into the blood. However, the clinician should be aware that metabolic alkalosis may occur at the end of IHD, which can promote hypokalemia and symptomatic hypocalcemia.

Uremia

A blood urea nitrogen (BUN) greater than 100 mg/dl usually indicates a severely decreased glomerular filtration rate (GFR <10 ml/min). However, many nonrenal conditions can elevate BUN to this level. In general, urea is a poor index of GFR because it is filtered and then reabsorbed by the renal tubule. Among patients with a reduction in circulating blood volume or low renal perfusion, the BUN can become markedly elevated compared with creatinine. Other conditions such as gastrointestinal hemorrhage, corticosteroid use, and excessive protein ingestion [total parenteral nutrition (TPN), or enteric nutrition] may cause high levels of circulating urea that are often the result of catabolic mechanisms.

Hypervolemia

There is evidence that volume overload may be an independent risk factor for mortality in patients in the ICU. It is not uncommon for critically ill patients to have in excess of 10 l of extravascular fluid. The rate of volume removal should be monitored closely without compromising hemodynamic stability. Once the optimal volume status has been achieved, RRT can be prescribed according to the anticipated fluid administration requirements (intravenous fluids, TPN, antibiotics) and guided by the objective measurements of intravascular volume and mean arterial blood pressure.

Nonrenal Indications

Toxins or Drug Removal

Hemodialysis can be used to treat life-threatening intoxications. The removal of a toxin or drug by hemodialysis depends on biochemical properties that include protein binding, water and lipid solubility, state of ionization, and molecular size. Moreover, hemodialysis can correct the metabolic acidosis that results from certain toxins (methanol, aspirin, and ethylene glycol). Hemoperfusion is a form of dialysis in which a resin-containing cartridge is used to bind the offending toxin (Table 40-6).

Hyperalimentation

Protein-caloric malnutrition has been implicated as one of the factors that contribute to the high mortality among critically ill patients with acute renal failure. Nutritional depletion has been associated with increased nosocomial infections, reduced or delayed wound healing,

TABLE 40-6

DIALYSIS FOR TOXIC INGESTIONS: INDICATIONS FOR HEMODIALYSIS AND/OR HEMOPERFUSION

DRUG	LEVEL
Amphetamine	–
Barbiturates	5 mg/dl
Glutethimide	4 mg/dl
Methaqualone	4 mg/dl
Aspirin	80 mg/dl
Theophylline[a]	30–40 mg/dl
Methanol	50 mg/dl
Ethylene glycol	50 mg/dl
Lithium	2.5 mEq/l

[a] Hemoperfusion is preferred

tissue repair, and muscle weakness, all of which may complicate weaning from the ventilator. Frequently, aggressive nutritional support can be provided only if dialysis is used to compensate for the large amounts of fluid associated with parenteral nutrition administration.

Congestive Heart Failure (CHF)

Among patients with severe heart failure, the low cardiac output and resulting renal hypoperfusion may lead to an increase in the levels of circulating renin, angiotensin, aldosterone, catecholamines, and antidiuretic hormone (ADH). These pathophysiologic events serve to further increase sodium and fluid retention, and the patient may become refractory to inotropic agents and diuretics. Isolated ultrafiltration (intermittent or SCUF) can be used effectively to reduce fluid retention in these patients. Some of these patients may exhibit an improvement in their heart failure and a return of renal function. For others, this technique can buy time until a more definitive therapy such as heart transplantation is available.

Liver Failure

Patients with liver failure may have azotemia resulting from a variety of pathophysiologic abnormalities such as prerenal azotemia, acute tubular necrosis, acute interstitial nephritis, glomerular diseases (IgA nephropathy, cryoglobulinemia, and glomerulonephritis), as well as hepatorenal syndrome. Hepatorenal syndrome is a condition characterized by reduction of renal function solely due to liver failure. Hepatorenal syndrome is usually a diagnosis of exclusion as these patients have no evidence of intrinsic renal disease and do not respond to volume expansion. The urinary sodium is very low, as well as the fraction excretion of sodium. CVVHD is often the therapy of choice for patients awaiting liver transplantation because these patients are often hemodynamically unstable. The utilization of heparin to maintain patency of the extracorporeal circuit should be done cautiously as many of these patients have bleeding disorders. In some patients with severe coagulopathy, CVVHD can be performed without heparin.

Systemic Inflammatory Response

The inflammatory mediators such as interleukin 1 and 6 and tumor necrosis factor (TNF) that are released during systemic inflammatory response (SIRS) are believed to induce multiple organ failure and perpetuate the systemic inflammatory state. The synthetic highly permeable filters allow passage of these cytokines and may adsorb others. Some investigators have proposed that CRRT may be beneficial if used preemptively for patients with sepsis, acute respiratory distress syndrome, and pancreatitis. CRRT for these conditions remains investigational and is not currently recommended in the absence of other indications.

TABLE 40-7

INTERMITTENT HEMODIALYSIS

ADVANTAGES	DISADVANTAGES
Rapid correction of hyperkalemia	Hypotension is common
High ultrafiltration capacity	Dysequilibrium syndrome
Efficient drug/toxin removal	Complex machine
Allows time for dialysis independence	Technical personnel required
Can be used without anticoagulation	Poor solute control

CHOICE OF RENAL REPLACEMENT THERAPY IN THE CRITICALY ILL PATIENT

The choice of dialytic therapy is often dependent on the (1) clinical indication for dialysis, (2) the presence of other organ system dysfunction, (3) availability of vascular access, (4) the technical support and training of personnel, and (5) anticipated duration of dialysis therapy (Figure 40-4). The advantages and disadvantages of each of these modalities are presented in Tables 40-7 through 40-9. There is only limited information comparing the efficacy of CRRT versus IHD in the treatment of acute renal failure (ARF) in the critically ill pa-

Choice of RTT in the critically ill patient:

- Recurrent hypotension has been strongly associated with a delay in functional renal recovery.

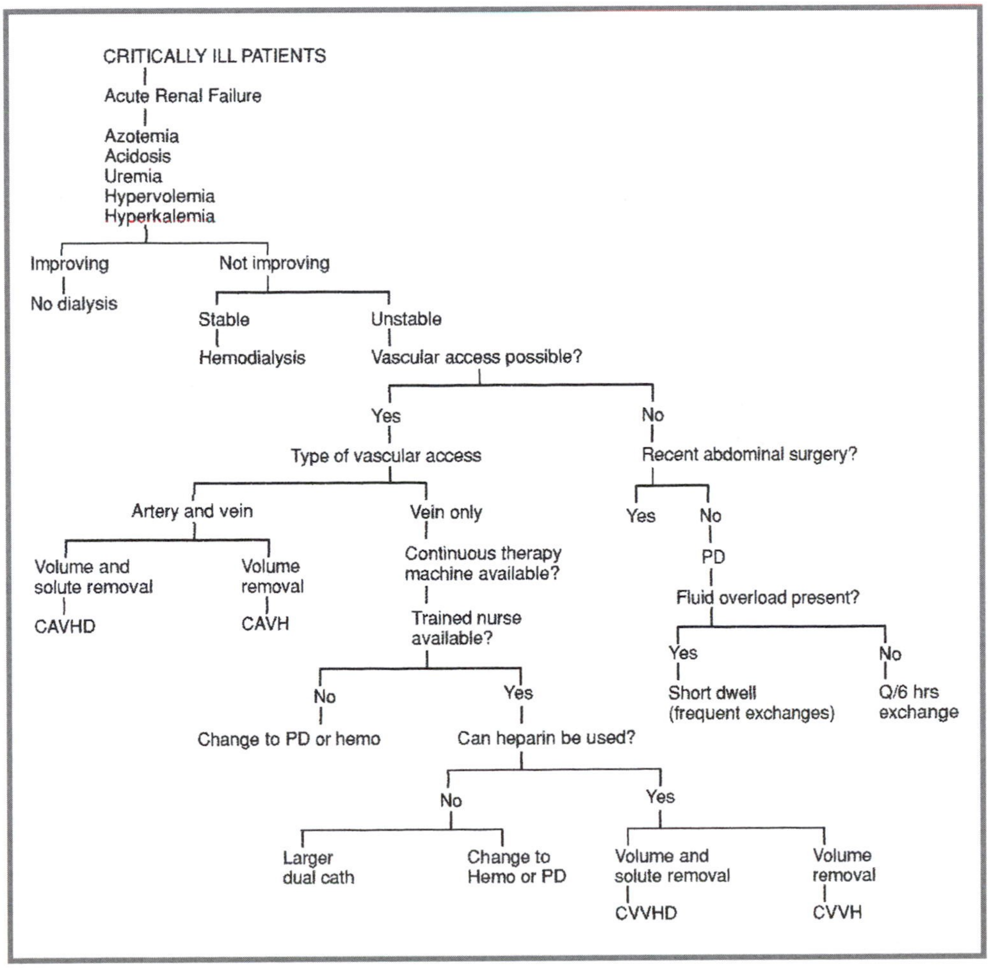

FIGURE 40-4

Algorithmic approach to renal replacement therapeutic (RTT) management of the critically ill patient with acute renal failure. *PD*, peritoneal dialysis.

TABLE 40-8

CONTINUOUS HEMODIALYSIS

ADVANTAGES	DISADVANTAGES
Technically simple	Frequent filter clotting
Hemodynamically well tolerated	Anticoagulation often necessary
High membrane sieving and adsorptive capacity	Large amounts of dialysate and replacement fluid needed
No solute concentration rebound	Requires 1:1 nursing staffing
Stability of total body solute and fluid balance	

tient. If the indications for dialysis were hyperkalemia or toxic ingestion, then IHD would be the most effective prescription. On the other hand, the majority of patients in the ICU have some degree of hemodynamic instability that makes intermittent hemodialysis risky. Recurrent hypotension has been strongly associated with delay in functional renal recovery by further aggravating hypoperfusion-mediated renal ischemic injury. Continuous renal replacement therapy is generally better tolerated in hemodynamically unstable patients because the removal of solutes and water is slower and achieved over a prolonged period of time, allowing increased time for mobilization of fluid from the extravascular compartment. Moreover, the rapid compartmental shifts of electrolyte and solute concentration can be avoided. One disadvantage to CRRT is that continuous anticoagulation is required, whereas intermittent hemodialysis can be done without the use of heparin in many cases.

SUMMARY

Renal replacement therapy (RRT) for the critically ill patient has evolved differently than therapy for patients with end-stage renal disease. Despite significant advances in therapy, the associated mortality from acute renal failure among patients with multiple organ dysfunction remains high, and the clinical impact of CRRT on patient outcome remains unclear. Precise indications for RTT prescription for the critically ill patient and the timing for initiation of RTT have yet to be clearly defined. Consideration as to which form of RTT is best should be given to the available resources, the clinical situation, and the needs of the individual patient.

TABLE 40-9

PERITONEAL DIALYSIS

ADVANTAGES	DISADVANTAGES
No machines needed	Low efficiency
No need for anticoagulation	Risk of peritoneal access
Hemodynamically well tolerated	Respiratory compromise
No need for vascular access	Protein losses
Easy monitoring	

REVIEW QUESTIONS

1. **Solutes are removed during dialysis by which of the following mechanisms?**
   A. Diffusion
   B. Convection
   C. A and B

2. **A patient develops chest and back pain, dyspnea, and hypotension 5 min after starting dialysis therapy. What is the most likely diagnosis?**
   A. Acute allergic reaction to heparin sulfate
   B. Dissecting aortic aneurysm
   C. First-use dialysis syndrome
   D. Acute myocardial infarction

3. **Synthetic membranes interact less with plasma components than cellulose membranes.**
   A. True
   B. False

4. **Which of the following continuous renal replacement therapies does not require a pump?**
   A. CVVHD
   B. CVVH
   C. CAVHD
   D. CVVHDF

5. **Which of the following is the most common complication of dialytic therapy?**
   A. Air embolism
   B. Hypotension
   C. Headache
   D. Heparin-induced thrombocytopenia

6. **A 40-year-old diabetic is admitted to the ICU with acute on chronic renal failure and sepsis. The decision to initiate dialysis therapy is made. Which of the following vascular access sites is the least appropriate for the placement of the dialysis catheter?**
   A. Femoral vein
   B. Subclavian vein
   C. Right internal jugular vein
   D. Left internal jugular vein

7. **A 32-year-old male patient is admitted to the ICU with a BP of 110/60 mmHg, HR of 100/min, and RR of 30. His serum creatinine is 8.0 mg/dl, hematocrit is 30%, and platelets are 40,000. The patient was receiving heparin for DVT prophylaxis and is suspected of having heparin-induced thrombocytopenia. The most appropriate dialysis modality for this patient would be:**
   A. CVVHD
   B. CAVHD
   C. Intermittent hemodialysis

8. **A 25-year-old patient with HIV nephropathy is admitted to the intensive care unit with a serum potassium level of 8 mEq/dl. The best dialytic modality for this patient is:**
   A. CVVHD
   B. Intermittent hemodialysis
   C. Peritoneal dialysis
   D. CAVHD

9. **A 41-year-old man with a dilated cardiomyopathy and left ventricular ejection fraction of 7% is admitted to the ICU with oliguric renal failure that is refractory to diuretics and a serum creatinine of 7 mg/dl. Which dialytic modality would be the least appropriate?**
   A. CVVHD
   B. Intermittent hemodialysis
   C. Peritoneal dialysis
   D. CAVHD

10. **A 52-year-old male patient with end-stage liver disease awaiting liver transplantation is admitted to the ICU with hepatic encephalopathy, hypotension, and oliguric renal failure. On admission, temperature is 38°C, BP is 80/50, RR is 30/min, and HR is 110/min. On physical exam he is lethargic but arousable. His abdomen is distended with a fluid wave and there is 3+ edema. His serum BUN and creatinine are 106 and 3.0 mg/dl, respectively. His prothrombin time is 29 (INR of 3.0). Which form of dialytic therapy would be the most appropriate?**
    A. CVVHD
    B. Peritoneal dialysis
    C. Intermittent dialysis
    D. CAVHD

ANSWERS

1. The answer is C. Solutes are removed through a semipermeanble membrane by two mechanisms, diffusion and convection. In diffusion, the movement of solute from one compartment to another is driven by an electrochemical gradient. Smaller molecules have more kinetic energy and are preferentially removed according to the size of the concentration gradient. Larger molecules are removed inefficiently or not at all. Solute movement continues until equilibrium is reached between the compartments. With convection, solutes are dragged from one compartment to the other along with fluid. The membrane only stops molecules larger than the membrane pore size and larger molecules are removed more efficiently. Dialysis uses a combination of both convection and diffusion.
2. The answer is C. First-use dialysis reaction is the result of the activation of leukocytes and plasma proteins with a fresh dialysis filter membrane.
3. The answer is A. Cellulose membranes (cellulose and cellulose acetate) are much less biocompatible and are more likely to result in complement and leukocyte activation. Although synthetic membranes are more biocompatible, they are more costly.
4. The answer is B. Hypotension is the most common complication of dialysis therapy. Hypotension may develop if too much fluid is removed too fast or if mobilization of fluid from the interstitial compartment is impeded by the presence of heart failure, sepsis, or low oncotic pressure.
5. The answer is C. In CVVH (continuous veno-venous hemofiltration), CVVHD (continuous veno-venous hemodialysis), and CVVHDF (continuous veno-venous hemodiafiltration), a roller pump on the venous (blood-in) line creates hydrostatic pressure, which drives the solvent through the membrane and is required to maintain the transmembrane pressure gradient.
6. The answer is B. The subclavian vein is not a preferred catheterization site because catheter kinking and compromised blood flow may occur in this location. Subclavian catheters also have a greater risk of causing stenosis and thrombosis, which may affect the effluent branches of the superior vena cava, innominate vein, and brachiocephalic truncus. Catheterization of the internal jugular vein is far less likely to cause thromboses and stenoses, but the site is more prone to infection, particularly in patients with a tracheostomy. Femoral access is preferred because spontaneous reductions of blood flow through the catheter occur less frequently in the femoral vein compared to the jugular and subclavian sites. Improved blood flow improves filter life and hemodialysis efficacy.
7. The answer is C. Because of the low blood flow during continuous renal replacement therapy, anticoagulation is generally necessary to minimize clot formation in the dialysis filter, maintain filter patency, extend filter life, and improve filtration. Heparinization is usually necessary in all but the most coagulopathic states and is associated with the development of heparin-induced thrombocytopenia (HIT). Higher blood flows are present during intermittent hemodyalysis, and thus filter clotting is less of a problem.
8. The answer is B. Hyperkalemia frequently accompanies acute renal failure, crush injury, or any massive tissue destruction. Rapid removal of potassium is required, which is not possible with slow continuous hemodialysis or peritoneal dialysis.
9. The answer is C. Intermittent hemodialysis rapidly removes intravascular fluid by ultrafiltration, which is followed by delayed refilling from extravascular spaces. This intravascular hypovolemia is poorly tolerated in patients with systolic dysfunction, and the increased vasoconstriction leads to activation of the renin-angiotensin system, further aggravating renal dysfunction and heart failure. Slow continuous hemofiltration avoids the roller coaster periods and beneficially affects cardiac function even in end-stage, diuretic-resistant cardiomyopathy. As preload declines and ventricular filling pressures improve, the patient achieves a more favorable point on the Starling curve. Improvement in cardiac function often results in improved renal function and diuretic sensitivity. Slow ultrafiltration techniques are most suitable as initial treatment of congestive heart failure resistant to conventional medical therapy or in emergent situations of sudden cardiac decompensation. Peritoneal dialysis is better suited as long-term maintenance therapy for those patients who are not candidates for heart transplantation.
10. The answer is A. Continuous renal replacement therapy is preferred in patients suffering from acute hepatic failure with elevated intracranial pressure (ICP), which is the major cause of death in these patients with stage IV hepatic encephalopathy. CRRT can be used as a bridge for liver transplantation in acute on chronic hepatic failure or hepatorenal syndrome. Because the mean arterial pressure (MAP) and serum osmolality remain relatively stable during CRRT, cardiovascular stability is achieved in patients with cirrhosis renal failure.

SUGGESTED READING

Briglia A. Acute renal failure in the intensive care unit. Therapy overview, patient risk stratification, complications of renal replacement, and special circumstances. Clin Chest Med 1999;20(2): 347–366.

Daugirdas JT, Ing TS. Handbook of Dialysis. Philadelphia: Lippincott-Raven, 1983.

Henrich WL. Hemofiltration in multiple organ failure. In Principles & Practice of Dialysis, 2nd Ed. Baltimore: Williams & Wilkins, 1988.

Meyer MM. Renal replacement therapies. Crit Care Clin 2000;16(1): 29–58.

CHAPTER 41

CATHY LITTY AND JAY HERMAN

Use of Blood Products

CHAPTER OUTLINE

LEARNING OBJECTIVES

After studying this chapter, you should be able to:

- Describe the composition of the different products extracted from whole blood.
- Recognize the risk of viral transmission associated with blood product transfusion.
- Assess the impact of anemia, particularly in critical care patients and patients with cardiovascular disease.
- Recognize the clinical threshold for blood transfusion in different patient populations.
- Use specific blood products, such as fresh-frozen plasma, cryoprecipitate, and platelets, for particular clinical indications.
- Identify the clinical indications for plasmapheresis in specific diseases such as thrombotic thrombocytopenic purpura.

Physicians who work in the intensive care unit (ICU) almost certainly will transfuse blood components to many patients. All transfusing physicians should have an understanding of the blood donation process and the products that are made from the donation. Risk of transfusion-transmitted viruses is often uppermost in the minds of patients and their families. This chapter reviews the most important aspects of blood product transfusion in critically ill patients.

BLOOD DONOR SCREENING

Before an individual donates blood, a detailed health history is taken. The objectives of questioning are twofold. Some questions are asked to screen for conditions that would make donation unsafe for the donor. Other questions search for behaviors that would put an individual at risk for infectious diseases or might jeopardize the future transfusion recipient. Although every donation undergoes a battery of tests, this prescreening protects the blood supply from donors who may be in the window period, defined as the period before a positive test can be detected but during which the donor can become infectious for a transfusion-transmitted viral disease. The safety of the blood supply has experienced drastic improvements in the

Before an individual donates blood, a detailed health history is taken.

Risk of human immunodeficiency virus (HIV) in the blood supply is currently estimated to be 1 in 676,000 units transfused. The risk of hepatitis C transmission is better than 1 in 103,000 units of transfused blood.

past decade, as tests used to screen for infection have improved in quality and number and health history questions have been expanded to screen for behaviors that would put donors at risk to be in the window period for infectious diseases. The risk of human immunodeficiency virus (HIV) in the blood supply currently is estimated to be 1 in 676,000 units transfused and the risk of hepatitis C transmission to be more than 1 in 103,000 units transfused. The composite transfusion transmitted viral risk is approximately 1 in 34,000.

WHOLE BLOOD AND ITS COMPONENTS

A whole blood donation of 500 ml yields a number of components. It is usually separated into packed red blood cells (PRBC), a plasma concentrate (PC), and the plasma portion that is frozen into fresh-frozen plasma (FFP).

Apheresis platelets are sometimes referred to as single donor platelets, and whole blood-derived platelets are referred to as random donor platelets.

A whole blood donation of 500 ± 50 ml may yield a number of components. The blood is usually separated into packed red blood cells (PRBCs), a platelet concentrate (PC), and the plasma portion that is rapidly frozen into fresh-frozen plasma (FFP). The red cells and platelets from one donation are designated as one unit. The plasma may be further processed into cryoprecipitate. Platelets can be collected via apheresis, a process whereby only platelets are collected, and the other components are returned to the donor after centrifugation. The apheresis product is equivalent in dose to approximately five whole blood-derived platelet products. Apheresis platelets are sometimes referred to as single donor platelets, and whole blood-derived platelets may often be referred to as random donor platelets. The PRBCs commonly available today are suspended in about 20 ml of the original plasma, an anticoagulant, and an additive solution to ensure that the product has a 42-day shelf life at refrigerator temperatures (1°–6°C). The final volume is between 300 and 350 ml with a hematocrit of about 60%. The platelet concentrate is stored at room temperature (20°–24°C) and expires in 5 days, and the FFP is frozen (at −18°C or below) and can be used up to 12 months. See Table 41-1 for the components that can be derived from a whole blood donation.

Virally mediated infectious diseases are not the only complications of transfusing blood and components.

Virally mediated infectious diseases are not the only complications of transfusing blood and blood components. Various reactions, both hemolytic and nonhemolytic in type, as well as bacterial contamination may occur. These topics are not discussed here but may be found in any textbook of transfusion medicine. When transfusion is necessary, it is often lifesaving. It is important, however, to know when to transfuse each blood component, because if a transfusion is unwarranted even a small risk is too large to take.

RED BLOOD CELLS

The indication for transfusing packed red blood cells is to increase oxygen-carrying capacity.

The indication for transfusing PRBCs is to increase oxygen-carrying capacity. If volume is the only deficit, this can be addressed with crystalloid or colloid solutions and red cell transfusions are not required. The oxygen-carrying capacity in the healthy state is four times higher than the oxygen requirement; thus, a sizable reserve exists, and it is never necessary to transfuse a patient to a normal level.

Adverse Effects of Anemia

Anemia itself causes decreased blood viscosity.

In acute anemia, the body attempts to maintain oxygen delivery to the tissues, particularly in the myocardium, where there is little reserve, by increasing cardiac output. Adrenergic stimulation causes vasoconstriction on the venous side of the cardiovascular system, thereby increasing the volume of blood returning to the right side of the heart (i.e., preload). This increase in returning blood volume causes more distension of the cardiac muscle and results in enhanced contractility. Hypoxia and acidemia cause vasodilation on the arterial side, decreasing systemic vascular resistance. Anemia itself may cause decreased blood viscosity. The decrease in systemic vascular resistance and viscosity leads to afterload reduction. Aug-

TABLE 41-1

COMPONENTS DERIVED FROM A WHOLE BLOOD DONATION

Packed red blood cells (PRBC)	Fresh-frozen plasma (FFP)
Platelet concentrate (PC)	Cryoprecipitate (CRYO)

mented contractility and decreased afterload increase the stroke volume to maintain or increase cardiac output. Tachycardia is a sign that these other mechanisms are either at their maximum or are not possible because of the patient's underlying condition. The Bohr effect plays a role when systemic acidosis accompanies acute blood loss. The acidosis causes hemoglobin to decrease its affinity for oxygen, thus releasing more oxygen at the tissue level.

A phosphorylated sugar acid called 2,3-diphosphoglycerate (2,3-DPG) is produced in all cells but is present in large quantities only in the red blood cell. This compound binds to the β-subunits of deoxyhemoglobin and stabilizes them. In the face of chronic anemia, red blood cells increase their synthesis of 2,3-DPG, further stabilizing the deoxygenated form of hemoglobin and thus allowing more oxygen to be released from the red blood cells at the tissue level. This mechanism does not affect the ability of red blood cells to take up oxygen in the lungs. (A more complete discussion of the oxyhemoglobin dissociation curve and the effects of 2,3-DPG can be found in most textbooks of transfusion medicine or hematology.) The increase in 2,3-DPG is seen when the patient's hemoglobin falls below 9 g/dl and becomes more marked when the hemoglobin level is below 6.5 g/dl. In the patient with chronic anemia, this compensatory mechanism exists in addition to adjustments in cardiac output.

Only in the red blood cell is 2,3-diphosphoglycerate (2,3-DPG) present in large quantities.

Left ventricular dysfunction may interfere with a patient's ability to employ cardiac compensation in anemia. The medications that the patient is taking may also interfere with the heart's ability to respond. Beta-blockers are just one example. In patients with hypovolemic anemia, a decrease in red cell mass is accompanied by a fall in total blood volume, which may cause plasma volume to be equivalently reduced. Peripheral blood measurements of hematocrit and hemoglobin may then be artificially high. In the hypovolemic patient, early transfusion may be necessary to avoid the risk of underestimating the need for red blood cells, especially in the patient with compromised cardiac status, when fluid resuscitation is not effective. In chronic anemia, an expanded plasma volume may have the opposite effect on the measured hematocrit and hemoglobin. It is important to consider this fact before transfusion, especially in patients whose cardiac status may put them at risk for fluid overload. When determining when to transfuse, considerations include the patient's cardiac status, the duration of the anemia, and whether there is an increased oxygen requirement, as in pain or fever. Impaired pulmonary function and peripheral vascular disease may further impair compensation by the body by limiting hemoglobin ability to bind oxygen or vasculature ability to alter preload or afterload.

Left ventricular dysfunction, medications, impaired pulmonary function, and peripheral vascular disease may impair the ability of the body to compensate for anemia.

Clinical Thresholds for Blood Transfusions

During the 1980s, a growing awareness of the link between viral transmission and transfusion of blood components led to the adoption of a more thoughtful approach to transfusion. In 1988, the National Institutes of Health convened a consensus conference, whose participants recommended a more conservative approach to transfusion, stating that the commonly used transfusion trigger of 10 g/dl was too high. In addition, they concluded that there was no evidence that mild to moderate anemia contributed to perioperative morbidity. In 1992, the American College of Physicians recommended letting the hemoglobin in normovolemic patients decline to a level of 7 g/dl before transfusing. In 1994, guidelines for blood utilization established by the American Association of Blood Banks recommended transfusion in a normovolemic patient only when they became symptomatic, regardless of the hemoglobin, and preoperatively for a hemoglobin of less than or equal to 8 g/dl. In 1996, the American Society of Anesthesiologists Task Force also published transfusion guidelines, which stated that perioperative or peripartum RBC transfusion is rarely indicated when the hemoglobin concentration is greater than 10 g/dl and is almost always indicated when the hemoglobin is less than 6 g/dl. They also stated that the decision to transfuse in patients with hemoglobins of 6–10 g/dl should be based primarily on the patient's individual risks for complications.

Growing awareness of the link between viral transmission and transfusion of blood products has led to a more thoughtful approach to transfusion.

Transfusion in a normovolemic patient should only occur when the patient is symptomatic, regardless of the hemoglobin, and preoperatively for hemoglobin levels $\leq$ 8 g/dl.

Jehovah's Witnesses are a religious group whose members rarely accept transfusions, including autologous transfusions. Because they accept all other modern medical treatments, comparisons of their outcomes are a good measure of the efficacy of transfusion. Unfortunately, available studies are retrospective reviews, which limits the ability to draw conclusions. In 1993 a review of 16 prior studies of surgical patients found a mortality rate of less

Low preoperative hemoglobin or substantial operative blood loss increases morbidity and mortality significantly more in patients with underlying cardiovascular disease.

than 2% in patients who refused blood. Another such review, which included medical and surgical case reports published in 1994, concluded that survival without transfusion is possible with hemoglobin levels as low as 5 g/dl. The authors acknowledged that the data had significant limitations, and that there were three deaths with higher hemoglobin levels in patients who had cardiac surgery, implying that these patients had preexisting cardiac disease. In 1996, the largest analysis of the impact of severe anemia in Jehovah's Witnesses undergoing surgery (1958 patients) was reported. It showed that low preoperative hemoglobin or substantial operative blood loss increased morbidity and mortality significantly more in patients with cardiovascular disease. The difference became apparent at hemoglobin concentrations of 10 g/dl and increased as the hemoglobin level decreased.

Over the past 15 years, it has become clear that a lower level of hemoglobin can be tolerated than was previously considered safe before concern about the risks of transfusion heightened. A greater consideration of the patient's status before transfusion is necessary. There is, however, a group of patients that may not tolerate severe anemia. Patients vary in their ability to compensate for anemia, and in these patients it is unclear how low the hemoglobin can safely be allowed to fall. The appropriate course at this time is to examine the risks versus the benefits and to transfuse patients based upon the clinical needs at the time. The impact of this information is especially important in the ICU where many patients have underlying diseases, as well as deviations in volume status, that interfere with their ability to compensate for both acute and chronic anemia.

The appropriate course is to consider the risks versus the benefits of transfusion and to transfuse on the basis of clinical needs at the time.

Transfusion in Critically Ill Patients

Critically ill patients are not specifically addressed in the consensus papers from the organizations that have published guidelines. Recently, the Canadian Critical Care Trials Group made assessments on transfusion strategy for patients in the ICU. Two of these studies were prospective comparisons in which patients were randomized to one of two groups. In the first, which was actually a pilot study from the same group who performed the second, 69 patients were included, all normovolemic. The groups had different transfusion triggers; one was transfused at hemoglobin levels below 7 g/dl and maintained at 7–9 g/dl, and the other was transfused at hemoglobin levels below 10 g/dl and maintained at 10–12 g/dl. There were no differences between the two groups in mortality or development of organ dysfunction. In the more restrictive group, only 15% (5 of 33) had ischemic heart disease or congestive heart failure, making it hard to ascertain whether cardiac disease warrants an altered strategy.

The second larger study included 838 patients, also all normovolemic. Less than 25% in either group had baseline cardiovascular disease. The same groups of liberal versus restrictive transfusion strategies were used as was done in the pilot study. The 30-day mortality was similar in the two groups; however, the mortality rate during hospitalization was lower in the restrictive group. Complications of myocardial infarction and pulmonary edema were actually higher in the liberal group. Although these studies strongly support the idea that transfusing at 10 g/dl is unnecessary, questions about patients with volume disturbances or severe cardiac disease were not answered.

Critically ill patients with cardiovascular disease or those who have undergone high-risk cardiovascular procedures do not tolerate anemia and have increased mortality rates if not transfused.

In 1997, the same Canadian Critical Care Trials Group performed a cohort study rather than a prospective randomized trial as in the two publications already described. This study demonstrated that severely ill patients with cardiovascular disease or patients who had undergone high-risk cardiovascular procedures did not tolerate anemia and had an increased mortality rate if not transfused. Moderate levels of anemia were tolerated in critically ill patients who did not have cardiovascular disease. Based on this finding, one might speculate that volume overload in the more liberally transfused patients in the 1999 study contributed to the higher incidence of myocardial infarction and pulmonary edema.

Transfusion in Sickle Cell Anemia

In sickle cell disease, a number of variables affect the decision to transfuse.

In sickle cell disease, an even greater number of variables affect the decision to transfuse. In this condition a genetic polymorphism of hemoglobin (Hgb S) causes RBCs to assume a sickle shape under low oxygen tensions, which leads to the occlusion of small blood vessels. Multiple tissues and organs may be affected, and bone pain, stroke, acute chest syndrome, hepatic failure, or priapism can result. Although simple transfusion does not usually ameliorate vasoocclusive episodes, transfusion of red blood cells is sometimes desirable to increase the oxygen-carrying capacity and decrease erythropoietic drive. Decreasing the stimulus on the patient's bone marrow to make red cells will lower the amount of abnormal cells released into the circulation.

Decreasing the stimulus on the patient's bone marrow to make red cells will lower the amount of abnormal cells released into the circulation.

All patients with sickle cell disease have some degree of anemia. Because the patient adjusts to this degree of chronic anemia, transfusion is not indicated even at a level far below that which would trigger transfusion in a patient who was acutely bleeding. In certain instances, such as bleeding, infection, splenic sequestration, or hemolysis, an acute anemia is superimposed upon the chronic anemia. A simple transfusion may be required if the patient is experiencing excessive fatigue, difficulty in breathing, tachycardia, postural hypotension, or other symptoms of anemia.

Simple transfusion may be required if the patient experiences excessive fatigue, difficulty in breathing, tachycardia, postural hypotension, or other signs of anemia.

The abnormal red cells in sickle cell disease also exhibit hyperviscosity, which worsens at higher hematocrits. Adverse effects of hyperviscosity may be seen even at hematocrits in the 50%–60% range in these patients. Transfusing red cells at this point will increase the total hematocrit while the Hgb S remains constant. The viscosity may increase; thus oxygen delivery does not improve even though oxygen-carrying capacity has been increased.

Erythrocytopheresis, or red cell exchange, is a superior method to treat the ICU patient with sickle cell complications such as acute chest syndrome. It affords removal of hemoglobin S, in addition to the transfusion of normal red blood cells. The normal red cells are more deformable and may actually bypass partial occlusions already in the microvasculature. This procedure may result in dramatic improvement in acute chest syndrome and acute or impending cerebrovascular episodes. Moreover, red cell exchange in lieu of chronic transfusion regimens has the advantage of avoiding the effects of iron overload that are commonly seen in sickle cell patients. Patients are unlikely to experience iron-induced organ toxicity until a level greater than 500 mg/kg of body weight accumulates. To perform this procedure with commonly used apheresis machinery, larger-bore catheters are needed than with simple transfusion; these must be dual lumen and stiff enough to withstand the high flow rates used in this procedure.

Erythrocytopheresis, or red cell exchange, is a superior method to treat the ICU patient with sickle cell complications such as acute chest syndrome.

A common problem in patients with sickle cell disease is that they have been frequently transfused in the past and have developed red cell alloantibodies, specifically, antibodies to the antigens present on the red cell surface. There are a number of antigen systems in addition to ABO that are immunogenic. The Cooperative Study of Sickle Cell Disease from 1990 of 1814 patients found that the overall rate of red cell alloimmunization was 18.6%, and that the rate increased with increasing numbers of transfusions. Children whose first transfusion occurred at an age of less than 10 years had a lower rate than expected based on the number of transfusions. Of those patients with antibodies to red cell antigens, 55% had more than one. There is a genetic difference in the frequency of certain red cell antigens in different groups. In the United States, patients with sickle cell anemia are African-Americans, and most donors are of European ancestry. This phenotypic difference in red cell antigens is a significant factor that contributes to alloimmunization. The problem of multiple antibodies is especially serious because they are often made to antigens common in the donor population. Often the provision of compatible blood in a crisis is delayed.

Patients with sickle cell disease have been frequently transfused in the past and have developed red cell alloantibodies.

The phenotype differences in red cell antigens secondary to race are a significant factor contributing to alloimmunization.

Prevention of alloimmunization is possible if patients are not transfused with genetically mismatched blood. Because of racial differences, providing blood from patients of the same ethnic origin would improve the situation. In addition, blood can be phenotyped, tested for the presence or absence of certain antigens, and then matched to the recipient for as many antigens as are possible. In centers where these programs exist, coordination between the physicians transfusing the blood and the blood bank personnel is essential.

Leukoreduction and Irradiation of Red Blood Cells

Leukoreduction of blood became practical in the late 1980s when filters became available that could remove 99.9% of the white blood cells (WBCs) from donated units of blood. The residual count of WBCs could be reduced in a unit of PRBCs from a factor of 10^8 to less than 5×10^6. Leukoreduction has a number of benefits, including a reduced risk of cytomegalovirus (CMV) transmission because white cells are a site of CMV latency. Although

Leukoreduction has a number of benefits, including a reduced risk of cytomegalovirus (CMV) transmission because white blood cells are a site of CMV latency.

many studies show clear reductions in CMV transmission due to leukoreduction by all methods including filtration, its use in place of CMV screening of donors does still have some controversy. The American Association of Blood Banks states that current data support the conclusion that leukocyte reduction to a level of WBCs below 5×10^6 reduces transfusion-transmitted CMV in a manner equivalent to CMV testing. The U.S. Food and Drug Administration, (FDA), however, contends that there is not yet enough evidence with leukocyte reduction to label the product CMV safe. It is important to note that the FDA does not regulate CMV test kits to the same level as other tests for transfusion-transmitted viruses because this is an elective donor screening test as opposed to a required donor screening test. The false-negative rate is accepted to be 1%–4%.

Leukoreduction also works to prevent primary alloimmunization to HLA antigens when the patient has not yet made antibodies secondary to a previous transfusion or pregnancy.

Leukoreduction also works to prevent primary alloimmunization to HLA antigens in a patient who has not yet made antibodies to a previous transfusion or pregnancy. These antibodies are triggered by HLA class II antigens on B lymphocytes, monocytes, and dendritic cells. Once HLA alloimmunization has occurred, the patient may destroy the class I antigens present on platelets, resulting in a refractory state to platelet transfusions. If the afferent limb of the immune response is interrupted by not exposing the patient to class II antigens, the patient will not make antibody by exposure to class I antigens that are present on platelets. Patients who require platelet transfusion but have many antibodies may require extensive matching; when these patients have rare types, much difficulty may arise in finding compatible products.

Leukoreduction also alleviates febrile nonhemolytic transfusion reactions.

Leukoreduction also alleviates febrile nonhemolytic transfusion reactions. Although these reactions are relatively benign, they are not without discomfort to the patient or cost. With the presence of a fever, a transfusion reaction workup is initiated in the blood bank to rule out hemolysis. Often, if the reaction starts before the entire blood component is transfused, the remainder of the product is wasted. Some components are in short supply and may be difficult to replace.

A choice now exists as to which type of leukoreduced product to transfuse, based on filtration at the bedside, in the blood bank, or at the blood center before storage. When filtration is performed at the blood center, the product is called prestorage leukoreduced RBCs. The filter can be manufactured into the blood collection bag set. There are a number of advantages to this product. The reductions in WBCs that manufacturers claim are often generated under controlled conditions may be impossible to duplicate on the patient floors of a general hospital. Conditions that seem to adversely affect the efficiency of leukocyte removal are slow filtration rate and room temperature. One study showed significantly higher residual WBC contamination in units filtered over 2 h, similar to the rate at which a unit is actually transfused, as opposed to those filtered by gravity over 10 min. Another study compared filtration of RBCs at 4°C and 37°C. Significantly fewer WBCs remained in the units filtered at the colder temperature, which of course would not be practical in a unit of RBCs hanging at the patient's bedside. With storage, WBCs are known to fragment. It has been shown that WBC fragments are inefficiently removed by filtering. Thus, the earlier in the life of the product that filtration takes place, the better.

Immunocompromised patients who are not able to destroy foreign T lymphocytes are at increased risk for transfusion-associated graft-versus-host disease.

Immunocompromised patients may not be able to destroy foreign T lymphocytes, which are infused along with transfusion of cellular components (red cells and platelets). These patients are then at risk for transfusion-associated graft-versus-host disease (TA-GVHD), where the foreign T cells engraft and lead to the initiation of a cellular immune response against the host; this is clinically similar to graft-versus-host disease in bone marrow transplant recipients in whom high fevers, rash, and gastrointestinal and liver involvement are seen. The important difference, however, is that the bone marrow, which is spared in transplant patients because it is the graft, is part of the host in a transfusion recipient. Therefore, in this situation, pancytopenia is prominent, and the mortality rate is in excess of 90%.

There is one situation in which an immunocompetent patient is at risk for TA-GVHD, namely, when the donor of the component is homozygous for an HLA haplotype that is shared with a recipient who is heterozygous for the same haplotype. A haplotype is composed of the genes for the HLA-related antigens A, B, C and D which are inherited in a group as if they were a single gene. The recipient thus does not recognize the transfused cells as foreign because both haplotypes in the donor match one of the recipient's haplo-

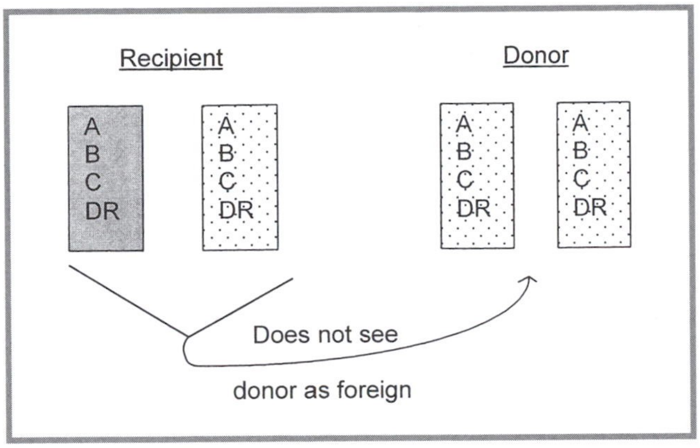

FIGURE 41-1

A, B, C, and *DR* are antigens designated as shown. For simplicity, two different haplotypes are represented here by *shading* and *dots*.

types. Because the foreign cells are not eliminated, they may engraft and lead to the same sequelae as in an immunocompromised patient (Figure 41-1). The HLA system exhibits extreme polymorphism, a rare occurrence, but one that is most likely to occur in recipient–donor pairs who are blood relatives.

Irradiating cellular blood products is the only method recognized to prevent TA-GVHD, and irradiation is only performed in the blood bank for this indication. The threshold number of T lymphocytes needed to initiate this disease is not known, and leukoreduction by filtration is not appropriate for its prevention. Irradiation is accomplished with a cesium-137 or cobalt source and will render the lymphocytes incapable of replication. Some blood banks have their own irradiators, and this procedure can be performed just before the component is issued. Blood banks that do not have their own irradiator must order the irradiated blood products from the blood supplier and will need some advance notice. Once red cells are irradiated, their shelf life is shortened to 28 days or the original date of expiration, whichever comes first, because there is accelerated storage damage to the cells.

Irradiating cellular blood products is the only method recognized to prevent transfusion-associated graft-versus-host disease.

The patient groups that are candidates for the specialized components described are listed in Table 41-2. Table 41-3 lists thresholds of lymphocyte numbers currently recognized for the various complications just discussed.

TABLE 41-2

CANDIDATES FOR SPECIALIZED BLOOD COMPONENTS

Candidates for irradiated cellular components to prevent TA-GVHD

- ❒ Fetuses receiving intrauterine transfusions
- ❒ Low birth weight premature neonates (<1200 g)
- ❒ Neonates who have received intrauterine transfusions
- ❒ Patients with immunodeficiency syndromes
- ❒ Bone marrow transplant patients
- ❒ Certain patients with hematologic malignancies
- ❒ Recipients of cellular components from directed donors who are blood relatives
- ❒ Selected others

Candidates for CMV safe cellular components (seronegative or leukoreduced)

- ❒ Newborns less than 1200 g born to mothers who are CMV seronegative or unknown
- ❒ Intrauterine transfusions in pregnant women who are CMV seronegative or unknown
- ❒ Seronegative recipients of bone marrow/organ transplants from donors who are also seronegative
- ❒ Seronegative candidates for bone marrow transplant
- ❒ AIDS patients who are CMV seronegative

Candidates for leukoreduced cellular components to avoid HLA alloimmunization

- ❒ HLA antibody-negative patients with conditions that include thrombocytopenia which will lead to dependence on platelet transfusion
- ❒ HLA antibody-negative patients with malignancies where chemotherapy will lead to dependence on platelet transfusion
- ❒ Candidate for future bone marrow transplant
- ❒ Candidate for future renal (or other organ) transplant

TA-GVHD, transfusion-associated graft-versus-host disease; CMV, cytomegalovirus; AIDS, acquired immunodeficiency disease; HLA, human leukocyte antigen

TABLE 41-3

THRESHOLDS FOR LEUKOCYTE REDUCTION LEVELS

Prevention of febrile nonhemolytic transfusion reactions	Less than 5×10^8
Prevention of CMV infection	Less than 5×10^6
Prevention of HLA alloimmunization	Less than 5×10^6
Prevention of TA-GVHD	?? (Lower than can be accomplished by leukoreduction)

CMV, cytomegalovirus; HLA, human leukocyte antigen; TA-GVHD, transfusion-associated graft-versus-host disease

PLATELET CONCENTRATES

Platelet Shelf Life

Platelet concentrates have a shelf life of only 5 days.

Platelet concentrates (PC), whether apheresis platelets or whole blood-derived platelets, have a shelf life of only 5 days. Because this product must be stored at 22°C, it is more prone to bacterial growth than refrigerated red cells. The FDA has approved storage for this time period because low-level bacterial inocula show significant growth after 5 days. Thus, if bacteria enter the unit at the time of collection, they can grow to a clinically significant concentration in the PC by the time of transfusion. The results may vary from a subclinical transient bacteremia to a fever mistaken for a transfusion reaction, catheter sepsis, or to a fatal septic reaction.

Apheresis Platelets (Single Donor)

Platelet transfusions may be given as single donor or random donor platelets.

Platelet transfusion is often the cause of confusion because of the two product choices, the variable biologic response, and the question of how much to transfuse. It is common to refer to apheresis platelets as single-donor platelets (SDP) and whole blood-derived platelets as random-donor platelets (RDP). Much confusion exists as to the distinction of single donor versus random donor. Randomly assigned SDPs are just as random as RDPs, and a single RDP that is sufficient for infants and small children is still a single-donor exposure. Because of their short shelf life, many blood banks do not keep large amounts of unassigned platelets in their inventory. When there is a specific need for apheresis platelets, waiting for them to be delivered from the blood supplier for an urgent transfusion is not in the best interests of the patient. Differences in the two types are summarized in Table 41-4. Because there is variation in donor platelet counts, the products are not standardized by the number of platelets. The American Association of Blood Banks (AABB) publishes standards that require whole blood-derived platelets to have at least 5.5×10^{10} platelets and apheresis platelets to have at least 3.0×10^{11} platelets in at least 75% of components prepared; see Table 41-5 for comparisons.

Apheresis platelets, however, are called for in many instances in which the patient needs a specialized product. Some patients have become refractory to platelet transfusions due to antibodies they have made to HLA class I antigens that exist on platelets (see preceding discussion). Even though leukoreducing blood products assists in the prevention of HLA alloimmunization, many patients have received nonleukoreduced products previously or have

TABLE 41-4

COMPARISON OF APHERESIS PLATELETS AND WHOLE BLOOD-DERIVED PLATELETS

	APHERESIS	WHOLE BLOOD-DERIVED
Advantages	Single-donor exposure Platelet-matching possible Prestorage leukoreduction available	Maximal availability Dose osculation possible Blood collection by product
Disadvantages	Limited Availability Variable platelet content Inconvenient for donor	Multiple-donor exposures Cannot match for refractory patients When leukoreduced, cytokines already present

TABLE 41-5

PLATELET PRODUCT CONTENTS[a]

	APHERESIS	WHOLE BLOOD DERIVED
Platelet content (average)	4×10^{11}	$8–9 \times 10^{10}$
Leukocytes	$<1 \times 10^5$ (with modern equipment)	Approximately 7×10^7
Volume	200–300 ml	Approximately 50 ml

[a] American Association of Blood Banks (AABB) standards

become alloimmunized to HLA antigens because of prior pregnancies. Once a patient has formed these antibodies, further leukoreduction can do nothing to alleviate the problem.

Apheresis platelets may be typed for HLA antigens and then matched to the patient. Because of the extreme polymorphism of this system it is often impossible to find a match for the four antigens that exist on the platelet surface, and cross-reactive antigens are sometimes adequate. Also, it is possible to avoid HLA antigens on donor platelets that correspond to the antibodies the patient has and to get a good response to the transfusion even though the type of the donor is not perfectly matched to that of the recipient. It is also possible to cross-match a sample from the unit of platelets with the patient's serum. A compatible cross match implies that the antibodies in the patient do not correspond to antigens present on that donor's platelets.

Leukoreduction of Platelets

Leukoreduction of platelets also aids in the prevention of febrile, nonhemolytic transfusion reactions.

Leukoreduction of platelets also aids in the prevention of febrile, nonhemolytic transfusion reactions, much the same as in red blood cell transfusions. There is a difference, however, in the cause of febrile reactions between the two products. Due to the storage temperature of platelets (20°–24°C), monocytes, which have a long storage life, remain active and secrete cytokines into the plasma portion of the platelet concentrate. Cytokines are soluble glycoproteins that act over short distances, react with cell-surface receptors, and activate intracellular pathways. They are produced in many cells in addition to the monocytes, including lymphocytes, fibroblasts, and endothelial cells. Cytokines have many important roles in the body, such as hematopoiesis and maintenance of immunocompetence; those belonging to the proinflammatory subset, however, may lead to the uncomfortable symptoms in many febrile platelet reactions. Table 41-6 shows the cytokines that are seen in platelet concentrates and some of their actions. With platelet transfusion, hemolysis is not likely when fever is seen, but the reaction may be confused with sepsis. Patients receiving platelets are often patients with malignancy on chemotherapy or with bone marrow failure. In these neutropenic patients, it is wise to avoid fever.

Cytokines and Plasma Concentrates

A number of studies have shown high concentrations of cytokines in the plasma of platelet concentrates.

A number of studies have demonstrated the presence of cytokines in high concentrations in the plasma in which platelet concentrates are suspended and lower cytokine concentrations with the early removal of white cells. Leukoreduction of an older platelet concentrate will remove the white cells but not the cytokines once they are present. Apheresis platelets may be leukoreduced as they are collected by modern techniques. Prestorage leukodepletion of red cells is accomplished by filtration. The filter may be in line with the tubing of the bag set into which the donation is collected or sterilely attached at the time of component manufacturing. It is much harder to accomplish this with whole blood-derived platelets because bag sets with two in-line filters are not as widely used. In the future, as more innovations are made to the bags we draw blood into, we will not need to solely rely on apheresis platelets to have the advantage of prestorage leukoreduced platelets. Now, however, most leukoreduction of whole blood-derived platelets is accomplished with a filter at the bedside or at the time of pooling in the blood bank.

TABLE 41-6

CYTOKINES PRODUCED BY MONOCYTES IN PLATELET CONCENTRATES

NAME	EXAMPLES OF FUNCTIONS
Interleukin-1β (IL-1β)	Pyrogen: causes hypotension
Interleukin-6 (IL-6)	Pyrogen: essential for immunoglobulin production
Interleukin-8 (IL-8)	Neutrophil chemotactic and activating factor
Tumor necrosis factor-σ (TNF-σ)	Pyrogen: causes hypotension

Indications and Dosing of Platelet Transfusions

Certain conditions result in increased consumption of platelets: fever, hypersplenism, DIC, certain drugs, and bleeding.

One unit of whole blood-derived platelets per 10 kg of body weight is considered an adequate dose for children. It has become standard to transfuse pools of six in adults; however, it may be more appropriate to tailor that dose for individual patients because of the large variation in size of adult patients. It is recommended that adults weighing more than 120 pounds should receive a dose of approximately 6×10^{11} platelets. Certain conditions result in increased consumption of platelets. Fever, hypersplenism, disseminated intravascular coagulation (DIC), certain drugs, and bleeding may all have this effect and require larger doses of platelets. A study of thrombocytopenic children showed that a count of about 40,000/μl was needed to achieve hemostasis when the patient was bleeding.

Patients are usually transfused prophylactically when the platelet count is 20,000/μl or less.

In determining when to transfuse the nonbleeding patient, the same dilemma of transfusion trigger exists as observed with red cell transfusion. The platelet count commonly used as the threshold for prophylactic transfusion is 20,000/μl. Unfortunately, this number originates from experience gained in the 1960s before the knowledge that aspirin inhibits platelet function. Many stable thrombocytopenic patients tolerate lower counts. More restrictive guidelines based on a study of patients with acute leukemia published in 1991 uses an approach tailored to patient factors. The authors suggest transfusing all patients at or below platelet counts of 5,000/μl, transfusing at platelet counts of 10,000/μl when the patient is febrile or has minor hemorrhagic manifestations, between 10,000 and 20,000/μl platelet counts when there are coagulation disorders or heparin therapy, and at or above 20,000/μl platelet counts with major bleeding complications. An approach such as this may be especially advisable in aplastic anemia patients who need to be maintained without excessive risk of alloimmunization to facilitate a potentially lifesaving bone marrow transplant. A multicenter controlled trial of leukemic patients recently published compared transfusion thresholds of 10,000/μl and 20,000/μl, except in cases of fever and minor bleeding, and concluded that the lower threshold was adequate. This study did not let patient platelet counts decline as low as 5,000/μl. In the ICU, keep in mind that many patients do have clinical factors that make bleeding a risk and may have an alternate diagnosis that should be considered as a cause of thrombocytopenia.

To determine the effectiveness of platelet transfusion, posttransfusion platelet counts should be obtained 10 min to 1 h after transfusion.

To correct for patient size and the amount of platelets transfused, the corrected platelet count (CCI) is calculated.

A CCI of 7,000–10,000/μl is considered an adequate response.

Once the decision to transfuse is made, it is important to assess whether the transfusion is effective. Measuring the posttransfusion platelet increment at 10 min to 1 h after transfusion is a common method of deterring the effects of platelet transfusion. It is important to determine first if the patient has splenomegaly, fever/sepsis, or DIC, factors that increase platelet consumption. To correct for patient size and amount of platelets transfused, the corrected count increment (CCI) is calculated (Figure 41-2). A CCI of at least 7,000–10,000/μl is considered an adequate response. When factors that would cause increased consumption are ruled out, a poor response is the result of antibody-mediated destruction, as seen in refractory patients.

Platelets are irradiated to prevent TA-GVHD for the same indications discussed in the red cell section (see Table 41-2 for selected patient groups). Because the shelf life of the platelet component is only 5 days, irradiation does not shorten the shelf life as it does in PRBCs.

FRESH-FROZEN PLASMA

Fresh-frozen plasma (FFP) is by definition the plasma portion, which is separated from the whole blood donation and frozen within 8 h. The requirement to freeze within this time pe-

$$CCI = \frac{(\text{Platelet count}_{post} - \text{platelet count}_{pre}) \times \text{body surface area (in m}^2)}{\text{Number of platelets transfused (in multiples of }10^{11})}$$

FIGURE 41-2

Formula to calculate the corrected count increment (CCI) with platelet transfusion. A CCI of at least 7,000–10,000/μl is considered an adequate response.

riod exists because clotting factors V and VIII are heat labile and degrade quickly at higher temperatures. No standard volume is possible for units of FFP. The volume depends on the amount of plasma present in the original unit of whole blood as well as whether a unit of random donor platelets was also produced, because the platelets must be suspended in a small amount of plasma. There is also biologic variation among factor levels in donors so that the actual factor activity of specific FFP factors cannot be standardized from one unit to the next. Due to this variation, as well as variation in patient size, it may be necessary to transfuse patients with 2–4 units of FFP for adequate clotting factor replacement.

Fresh-frozen plasma (FFP) is the plasma portion that is separated from a whole blood donation and frozen within 8 h.

Because there is significant biologic variation in factor levels between donors, the actual factor activity of a specific agent cannot be standardized from one unit to the next.

Indications for FFP Administration

FFP is used to treat coagulation factor deficiencies when there is not an available factor concentrate, or when there are multiple coagulation factor deficiencies. Multiple factor deficiencies are most likely to be seen in the ICU setting in patients with liver disease. Dilutional coagulopathy secondary to massive transfusion with replacement of more than one plasma volume with red blood cells and crystalloid solutions is also likely in the ICU setting. Patients transfused with large volumes of packed cells and crystalloid during fluid resuscitation secondary to massive blood loss have a relative deficiency of functional platelets and very little plasma. It is likely that thrombocytopenia and coagulation deficiencies will result.

FFP is used to treat coagulation factor deficiencies when there is not an available factor concentrate or when multiple coagulation factor deficiencies exist.

FFP is not needed to treat prolongations in the prothrombin time (PT) or activated partial thromboplastin time (APTT) until they are increased more than 1.5 times the normal. Mild prolongations are likely to occur before factor levels are too low for hemostasis; this is also true for patients about to undergo minor procedures, such as thoracentesis, paracentesis, or liver biopsy, who have mild prolongations. When a patient has received excess amounts of warfarin-containing compounds, the resulting deficiency of vitamin K-dependent factors can be treated with vitamin K alone. This treatment may require 10 h to be fully effective, so if a patient is actively bleeding or requires emergency surgery, it will be necessary to give FFP transfusion.

FFP is not needed to treat prolongations in the PT or APTT until they have increased more than 1.5 times normal.

Thrombotic Thrombocytopenic Purpura

Another situation that might arise in the ICU patient is thrombotic thrombocytopenic purpura (TTP). TTP presents with clinical features of thrombocytopenia, (often severe), microangiopathic hemolytic anemia, neurologic symptoms, fever, and occasionally renal dysfunction. Schistocytes are seen on the blood smear as a result of widespread platelet thrombi in the circulation causing a microangiopathic process, and unusually large multimers of von Willebrand's factor develop that may lead to thrombus formation. As a result of hemolysis, marked elevations in lactate dehydrogenase (LDH) are usually seen. Two recent studies showed that a deficiency of von Willebrand's factor-cleaving protease was most likely the cause of the large multimers and the ensuing disease process. In the acute form of the disease, both studies showed an inhibitor (IgG antibody) to be present in the majority of patients. In one study, patients with a familial form of TTP were included and were found to lack the von Willebrand's factor-cleaving protease but not to have the inhibitor. Thus, two forms of the disease exist, a familial form in which there is a genetic basis to the deficiency and an acute form where some external factor elicits an autoantibody mediator inhibitor that causes the deficiency.

TTP had a mortality rate greater than 90% until the early 1980s when plasmapheresis with FFP as the replacement fluid became the first line of treatment. Plasmapheresis should

In TTP, plasmapheresis should commence on an emergency basis and continue daily with at least 1 plasma volume of FFP until platelet count normalizes, and signs of hemolysis remit.

commence on an emergency basis and continue daily with at least one plasma volume of FFP until platelet count normalizes and signs of hemolysis remit. A number of studies in the late 1970s and early 1980s showed improved survival when plasmapheresis with FFP was used. The results of some early case reports were complicated with mixtures of other treatment modalities such as steroids, splenectomy, and antiplatelet agents. There were some, however, that separated out other treatments and showed a clear benefit with early and aggressive treatment of this type. The same catheter concerns exist as for red cell exchange in sickle cell anemia. Patients who fail to respond to treatment with FFP or relapse soon after such treatment sometimes do better with cryosupernatant instead of FFP. The cryosupernatant fraction of plasma is what remains after cryoprecipitate is produced (see discussion that follows on cryoprecipitate). Because cryoprecipitate contains von Willebrand's factor, the remaining plasma is thus deficient and will have fewer ultralong multimers as well. The von Willebrand's factor-cleaving protease remains.

New Plasma Products

SD-plasma is a new pooled product made from donor plasma treated by the solvent detergent method to inactivate viruses.

Although FFP presently is the standard of care for factor replacement, the availability of new alternatives may change this in the future. In May 1998, the FDA licensed SD-plasma, which is a pooled product made from donor plasma treated by the solvent detergent method of viral inactivation for 4 h. Because this product is pooled, the dosing of the factors is more standard from unit to unit and a constant volume of 200 ml makes up each unit. The solvent detergent method is the same inactivation process that has been used for factor concentrate products since 1985. It kills all lipid-enveloped viruses including human immunodeficiency virus (HIV) as well as hepatitis B and C viruses. Hepatitis A and parvovirus B19 are not lipid enveloped, but there are high levels of antibodies to these agents in the product, which are thought to be protective; these also are not agents that cause significant transfusion-transmitted disease. There has been some criticism of this product because of the pooling process. If a new infectious disease agent emerges and is not lipid enveloped, it is likely to be transmitted to more patients via a blood product that is pooled. This concern is only theoretical at this point, however. The history of the mutatibility of HIV and HCV makes new subtypes of these viruses a greater concern. The solvent detergent process would be effective in preventing disease due to this occurrence.

Delayed-release plasma is FFP stored and not released until the donor returns 3–4 months after donation to be retested to ensure the original product is not contaminated by transmissible infectious agents.

Some blood centers have begun to manufacture another product called delayed-release plasma. Instead of viral inactivation, this FFP is stored and not released until the donor comes back 3–4 months later and is retested to ensure that the original product was not from a donor in the window period. This practice avoids the pooling process but only protects from viruses for which we can currently test. A new lipid-enveloped virus or a mutation in a lipid-enveloped virus may thus be missed but killed by the solvent detergent process. The biggest problem with the delayed-release method is that most donors do not return within the donation interval, and if the component is needed, it may have to be released as FFP. Most likely, it will not be possible to meet the nation's plasma supply needs with this product.

Cryoprecipitate

Cryoprecipitate (CRYO) contains factor VIII, von Willebrand's factor, fibrinogen, factor VIII, and fibronectin.

Cryoprecipitate (CRYO) is a concentrate of high molecular weight proteins that precipitate in the cold. It is produced from FFP by thawing to 1°–6°C and concentrating the cold-insoluble portion; it contains factor VIII, von Willebrand's factor, fibrinogen, factor XIII, and fibronectin. The most common use of CRYO in the ICU is for patients with disseminated intravascular coagulation who are consuming large amounts of their own fibrinogen and require replacement.

Hemophilia A is no longer treated with CRYO because there are many factor VIII concentrates available, including recombinant. Severe von Willebrand syndrome may be treated with CRYO as it contains von Willebrand's factor. Mild cases are usually treated with a synthetic analogue of vasopressin, called desmopressin acetate (DDAVP), a pharmacologic agent that enhances release of von Willebrand's factor from endothelial cells. This product is contraindicated in type IIb. When individuals with von Willebrand syndrome require major surgery, or the factor deficiency leads to major bleeding episodes, the dosing of CRYO is quite variable from patient to patient, and a physician with experience should be involved in the case.

SUMMARY

Although safety of the blood supply has increased dramatically in the past 10–15 years, there are well-recognized complications to transfusion. Issues such as cost and availability of products that are donated and often in short supply are also important to consider. In the ICU, however, use of blood components is often lifesaving and of urgent necessity. It is important for the clinician who practices in this arena to be aware of the varied product choices and their appropriate use.

REVIEW QUESTIONS

1. **Erythrocytophoresis or red cell exchange has been advocated in the treatment of patients with sickle cell disease complications, such as acute chest syndrome. All the following statements regarding red cell exchange are correct, except:**
   - **A.** It is generally performed using an apheresis machine.
   - **B.** It requires the insertion of a large-bore, double lumen catheter to perform the exchange.
   - **C.** It allows for removal of hemoglobin S, while transfusing normal red blood cells.
   - **D.** It carries an increased risk of iron overload.

2. **Leukoreduction of packed red blood cells is a process that removes 99.9% of the white blood cells from donated units of blood. All the following statements regarding leukoreduction are correct, except:**
   - **A.** It prevents primary alloimmunization to HLA antigens in patients who have not yet made antibodies to a previous transfusion.
   - **B.** It markedly decreases the risk of CMV transmission.
   - **C.** Leukoreduction is the preferred method to prevent transfusion-associated graft-versus-host disease.
   - **D.** It decreases the incidence of febrile nonhemolytic transfusions.

3. **All the following statements regarding platelet transfusion are correct, except:**
   - **A.** A platelet count greater than 40,000/μl is needed to achieve hemostasis in bleeding patients.
   - **B.** A corrected count increment of 2,000–4,000/μl is considered appropriate in most patients.
   - **C.** Platelets must be irradiated to prevent transfusion-associated graft-versus-host disease.
   - **D.** According to recent studies, in afebrile, nonbleeding patients, a threshold of 10,000 platelets/μl is considered adequate.

4. **A 62-year-old patient with a known history of hypertension, hepatitis C, and paroxysmal atrial fibrillation presents to the emergency department (ED) complaining of hematemesis. He takes warfarin and sotalol for atrial fibrillation and hydrochlorothiazide for hypertension. His atrial fibrillation has been under control since he was started on sotalol 4 weeks ago. At that time, he also underwent a coronary angiogram that did not evidence coronary artery disease. The patient states that he noticed the onset of black, tarry stools 2 days before his admission to the ED. Shortly before being brought to the ED, he became nauseated and vomited about one cup of bright red blood. Upon admission to the ED, he is in no distress, his blood pressure is 124/68, his heart rate is 98, his respiratory rate is 14, and his temperature is 37°C. An electrocardiogram shows normal sinus rhythm. His physical exam is unremarkable, except for mild pedal edema. Laboratory results show hemoglobin of 8.5 and platelet count of 54,000/μl. The international normalized ratio (INR) for prothrombin time (PT) is 6.5 (therapeutic range, 2–3) and the activated partial thromboplastin time (PTT) is 48 (1.6 times normal). Based on this, your initial approach should include the following:**
   - **A.** Vitamin K 10 mg IM; transfuse 6 units of platelets; transfuse 2 units of packed red blood cells to keep hemoglobin around 10 mg/dl
   - **B.** Vitamin K 10 mg IM; transfuse 2 units of packed red blood cells to keep hemoglobin around 10 mg/dl
   - **C.** Fresh-frozen plasma 4–6 units; transfuse 6 units of platelets
   - **D.** Fresh-frozen plasma 4–6 units; vitamin K

ANSWERS

1. The answer is D. Erythrocytophoresis or red cell exchange has been successfully used in the treatment of complications of sickle cell disease such as the acute chest syndrome and cerebrovascular accidents. It is accomplished using a conventional apheresis machine. It requires the insertion of a large-bore, double lumen intravascular catheter to withstand the high flow rates used during the procedure. The procedure decreases the percentage of hemoglobin S and transfuses fresh, normal red blood cells. Normal cells are more deformable and may even bypass partial occlusions in the microvasculature. Red cell exchange, as opposed to chronic transfusions, is not associated with an increased risk of iron deposition.
2. The answer is C. Leukoreduction is a process that, by means of a filter, removes 99.9% of the blood cells from a donated unit of blood. This process has been shown to reduce the transmission of CMV (white cells are the preferred site for CMV latency), decrease the incidence of febrile nonhemolytic transfusion reactions, and prevent HLA alloimmunization in patients without previous exposure to blood products. Transfusion-associated graft-versus-host disease (TA-GVHD) is a syndrome seen in immunosuppressed patients who are not able to destroy foreign T lymphocytes infused along with other blood products. These foreign T lymphocytes will attack the immunosuppressed patient's bone marrow and cause pancytopenia and possibly death. Leukoreduction is not sufficient to eliminate the small amounts of T lymphocytes that cause TA-GVHD; in these cases, blood products must be irradiated to prevent this syndrome.
3. The answer is B. According to recent studies, a transfusion threshold of 10,000 platelets/μg/l is considered adequate in nonbleeding patients. One study suggested that 5,000 platelets/μl might be an adequate threshold level in stable thrombocytopenic patients without fever or signs of bleeding; this contrasts with the old 20,000 platelet/μl standard. As with white blood cells, platelets have to be irradiated to prevent transfusion-associated graft-versus-host disease. A corrected count increment (see Figure 41-2) of at least 7,000–10,000 is considered adequate after platelet transfusion. A corrected count increment of 2,000 suggests platelet consumption or destruction, which may be seen in patients with fever or alloantibodies to platelets.
4. The answer is D. The patient in Question 4 has an upper gastrointestinal bleed. The INR is elevated; the PTT shows a moderate elevation; and the platelet count is decreased. In this patient, these laboratory results are consistent with initial disseminated coagulopathy and the effects of warfarin. The reduction in platelets could also be attributed to the patient's history of hepatitis C, especially if there is any evidence of cirrhosis. Vital signs are stable. Warfarin should be withheld. The patient should be treated with fresh-frozen plasma to reverse the INR. Although vitamin K can be given, it takes about 6–10 h for its effect to take place. There is no indication to transfuse platelets as the platelet count is above 40,000/μl. Without a history of cardiac disease, the patient is likely to tolerate moderate levels of anemia. Also, the patient's hemodynamic status does not warrant volume infusion.

SUGGESTED READING

Chambers LA, Herman JH. Considerations in the selection of a platelet component: apheresis versus whole blood derived. Transfus Med Rev 1999;13(4):311–322.

Goodnough LT, Brecher ME, Kanter MH, AuBuchon JP. Review article. Transfusion medicine. Part 1: Blood transfusion. N Engl J Med 1999;340:438–447.

Goodnough LT, Brecher ME, Kanter MH, AuBuchon JP. Review Article. Transfusion medicine. Part 2: Blood conservation. N Engl J Med 1999;340:525–533.

Litty C. A review: Transfusion reactions. Immunohematology 1996;12: 72–79.

Mintz PD (ed) Transfusion Therapy: Clinical Principles and Practice. Bethesda: American Association of Blood Banks, 1999.

Mollison PL, Engelfriet CP, Contreras M (eds) Blood Transfusion in Clinical Medicine, 9th Ed. London: Blackwell, 1993.

Rossi EC, Simon TL, Moss GS, Gould SA (eds) Principles of Transfusion Medicine, 2nd Ed. Philadelphia: Williams & Wilkins, 1996.

Smith DM, Lipton KS. Leukocyte reduction for the prevention of transfusion-transmitted cytomegalovirus (TT-CMV). AABB Bulletin 97-2. Bethesda: American Association of Blood Banks, 1997.

Vengelen-Tyler V (Ed). Technical Manual, 12th Ed. Bethesda: American Association of Blood Banks, 1996.

CHAPTER 42

FREDERIC H. KAUFFMAN

Advanced Cardiopulmonary Resuscitation

CHAPTER OUTLINE

LEARNING OBJECTIVES

After studying this chapter, you should be able to:

- Describe the evolution of various CPR techniques, including open and closed chest resuscitation.
- Describe the epidemiology of sudden cardiac death.
- List the various etiologies of sudden cardiac arrest.
- Describe the research-validated mechanisms by which blood flows in a forward direction during CPR.
- Correlate coronary and cerebral perfusion pressures with survival and clinical outcome.
- Describe several techniques by which CPR can be performed, along with pros and cons for each technique.
- List the techniques for assessment and support of the airway, breathing, and circulation.
- Recite the algorithms for the treatment of asystole, pulseless electrical activity, ventricular fibrillation, ventricular tachycardia, and the bradycardic rhythms.
- Alter properly the resuscitation techniques for victims of cardiac arrest associated with hypothermia, near-drowning, trauma, electrical shock/lightning, and pregnancy.

A BRIEF HISTORY OF BASIC CARDIOPULMONARY RESUSCITATION

Death, an inevitable reality for all of us, has not always been viewed as a potentially reversible event. Before the Renaissance, the views espoused by Galen in the second century A.D. were deemed the final, inviolable authority on all matters related to health, disease, and death. Galen taught that life began with the first beat of the heart and ended with the last beat (brought about by the cessation of flow of the vital spirit held within breath), never again to be started; death was permanent and irreversible.

The great awakening of intellectual curiosity during the Renaissance included matters related to medicine. However, religion still had a stronghold on all matters of death, and attempts at resuscitation were viewed as against the laws and will of God. By the eighteenth century, the scientific method was established, and the potential reversibility of death began to be explored. The stage was set for the first documented cases of resuscitation, along with the scientific inquiry to support its development.

During the early eighteenth and mideighteenth century, when accounts of artificial resuscitation techniques began to surface, common causes of sudden death included trauma, smoke inhalation from fires, drowning, and infectious diseases. Sudden cardiac death was not the norm for the day. One of the initial accounts of mouth-to-mouth resuscitation occurred during this time in a man overcome by smoke inhalation from a coal fire; he had no spontaneous respirations or pulse but was revived successfully and returned to his job a few days later. Later in that same century rescue societies were developed in many cities, and a concerted effort begun to develop a successful method of resuscitation from sudden death. Recommendations at that time included patient warming, placing the head below the feet, and stimulating the abdomen and feet to remove swallowed and aspirated fluids, rectal and oral stimulation via fumigation techniques, mouth-to-mouth or bellows-supported respirations, and bloodletting. By the midnineteenth century the obstructing role of the flaccid tongue during resuscitation became known, along with the need to intervene as soon as possible after arrest. Multiple methods of respiratory support were proposed at the time, but by the beginning of the twentieth century the American Red Cross endorsed the technique developed by Edward Schafer: intermittent pressure was placed on the back of the prone victim. By the early 1930s a new method, developed by Holger Nielsen, was endorsed by the Red Cross: with the victim in the prone position, back pressure was alternated with bilateral arm lifts.

In the 1940s, James Elam demonstrated the effectiveness in mouth-to-nose ventilation in supporting patient oxygenation. His experience with polio victims who had suffered respiratory paralysis convinced him that there was a better method of respiratory support than the Nielsen method. By the late 1950s, research by Elam and Peter Safar using postoperative patients and curarized volunteers conclusively demonstrated the superiority and adequacy of mouth-to-mouth resuscitation in providing ventilatory and oxygenation support in the setting of respiratory insufficiency. The technique of "expired air breathing" was endorsed in the *Journal of the American Medical Association* in 1958, and efforts to disseminate this information began.

The first accounts of chest compression and its success in the setting of cardiac arrest occurred in the late nineteenth and early twentieth centuries. The technique, however, did not catch on in the medical community until it was "rediscovered" in the late 1950s by William Kouwenhoven and his team at Johns Hopkins University. It was observed that the application of defibrillator paddles to the chest of a dog in ventricular fibrillation transiently in-

CASE STUDY: PART 1

A 58-year-old male businessman with a past history of hypertension and diabetes mellitus suddenly collapsed at his office while speaking to a group of business executives. Shortly before the meeting he complained of an uncomfortable sensation in his chest but thought that it was "just heartburn." After collapsing, he was attended to immediately by a colleague who was trained in basic life support. The victim was ashen in color, was not breathing, and did not respond to shaking or verbal stimuli. The colleague asked another executive to call 911, then opened the airway with a head tilt and noted no evidence of breathing. He gave two slow breaths to the victim via mouth-to-mouth respiration, and then felt for a carotid pulse. Finding no pulse, he initiated chest compressions alternating with mouth-to-mouth respirations until the ambulance squad arrived and assumed care of the patient.

creased arterial blood pressure, and with continued application of the paddles, that the length of time available to achieve successful defibrillation could be lengthened significantly. Through trial and error they determined that compression with the heel of the hand could achieve similar results, and that optimal arterial pressures were obtained with compressions over the lower third of the sternum to a depth of 1.5–2 in. at a rate of 60–80 per minute. In an article in the *Journal of the American Medical Association* in 1960 Kouwenhoven and colleagues reported the use of chest compressions in 20 patients who suffered cardiac arrest, most resulting from complications of anesthesia; 14 of the 20 survived. Up until that time, open cardiac massage was the standard of care. Shortly thereafter, the techniques of mouth-to-mouth respiration and external chest compression were joined, and as such, modern basic cardiopulmonary resuscitation (CPR) techniques were born.

EPIDEMIOLOGY OF SUDDEN DEATH

Understanding sudden death and the potential for intervention begins not with treatment algorithms but rather with collection and analysis of data regarding factors associated with sudden death. Such epidemiologic data allow health care providers to understand better just what is being treated and promotes the efficient study of potentially effective clinical interventions. Table 42-1 lists some traditional epidemiologic data that are collected and studied.

Epidemiologic study begins with establishing strict definitions of terms. A consensus definition established by the Utstein II international workshop in 1991 defines sudden death as "cessation of cardiac mechanical activity, confirmed by the absence of a detectable pulse, unresponsiveness, and apnea or agonal, gasping respiration." Ischemic heart disease is the most common cardiac condition predisposing to sudden death. Other less common causes in adults include primary dysrhythmias not associated with ischemic disease, pulmonary disease, cerebrovascular disease, and toxins.

Sudden death is defined as "cessation of cardiac mechanical activity, confirmed by the absence of a detectable pulse, unresponsiveness, and apnea or agonal, gasping respiration."

Ischemic heart disease is the most common cause of sudden death.

Ischemic heart disease increased substantially in the United States in the early twentieth century. By the 1940s, cardiovascular disease was the leading cause of death in adults, but perhaps as a result of diet and lifestyle changes, smoking cessation, and treatment of hypertension, there has been a significant decline in the incidence of cardiac arrest in the United States. Currently, however, nearly 1 million deaths annually are attributable to cardiovascular disease, and one-third of these occur in sudden fashion outside the hospital setting. Approximately 50% of these deaths occur in patients older than 65 years of age and nearly half occur in women. Successful resuscitation from sudden death occurring outside the hospital setting is, unfortunately, unusual. Nationally, it is estimated that survival from out-of-hospital cardiac arrest reaches only 3%–5%, and in some large cities it is even less. Through intensive educational programs and community training, however, some midsize cities now boast survival rates as high as 18%.

Exactly why sudden cardiac arrest should occur at a given moment in a given individual is rarely known. Typically, such individuals have identifiable risk factors for the development of cardiac disease that have been present for a significant period of time. Superimposed upon these relatively static factors may be transient factors that can suddenly trigger the events leading to sudden death. For example, in a patient with underlying hypertension

TABLE 42-1

EPIDEMIOLOGIC DATA ASSOCIATED WITH SUDDEN DEATH

Demography	Comorbid illnesses
Age	Hypercholesterolemia
Sex	Diabetes mellitus
Race	Physiologic associations
Behavior	Atherosclerosis
Smoking	Dysrhythmias
Stress	Favorable interventions
	Early defibrillation

TABLE 42-2

POTENTIAL TRANSIENT TRIGGERS THAT MAY LEAD TO SUDDEN DEATH

Transient ischemia and reperfusion	Electrolyte abnormalities
Hypoxia	Autonomic and neurohumoral alterations
Hypotension	Toxins
Acidosis	

and coronary artery disease, transient ischemia and reperfusion may be the triggering factor leading to dysrhythmia and death. Table 42-2 lists other potential transient triggering factors leading to sudden cardiac death.

Obviously, not all risk factors for the development of cardiac disease can be modified. All forms of underlying cardiac disease have been associated with sudden death syndrome. The most significant risk factors in this category include known coronary artery disease and a history of sudden death in the family. In addition, the presence of known dysthrhythmias represents risk for sudden death. Increasing age increases the rate of cardiac arrest exponentially, and sudden death risk is greater in males than in females for any given age. Race also plays a role in sudden death. African-Americans have a higher rate of sudden death than whites, most likely because of higher rates of hypertension, diabetes mellitus, and renal disease. Fortunately, some risk factors for the development of sudden death are potentially modifiable. Obviously, prevention of sudden death is much preferable to treatment. Table 42-3 lists potentially modifiable risk factors for sudden death.

Survival rates for out-of-hospital sudden death range from 0% to 18%.

Survival rates from sudden death vary considerably, from nearly 0% to 18% overall. Many factors influence and enhance survival rate within a community. Population modification of the foregoing risk factors, in and of itself, can have a positive influence. In addition, community education regarding CPR certification and rapid notification of the Emergency Medical Services (EMS) system, coupled with prompt institution of CPR and defibrillation, can enhance survival. Other factors, not all of which can be modified, that influence survival from sudden death include witnessed versus unwitnessed cardiac arrest, race, age, sex, initial rhythm, and amplitude of ventricular fibrillation. Lack of uniform reporting of data regarding out-of-hospital cardiac arrest has led to difficulties in evaluating data and resuscitation techniques between communities. The Utstein template for uniform reporting of data from out-of-hospital sudden death, recommended in *Circulation* in 1991 by Cummins et al., has become an accepted mode of data collection and reporting, thereby facilitating overall and subgroup analysis of epidemiologic and therapeutic modalities.

Positive predictors of successful resuscitation are listed in Table 42-4. Witnessed cardiac arrest consistently has been determined to be a predictor of increased survival, as has the initiation of bystander CPR before EMS arrival at the scene. Unfortunately, only 20%–30% of sudden death victims in most communities have CPR performed by bystanders at the scene. In addition, the chance of survival falls precipitously as time passes, once again emphasizing the need for prompt basic and advanced life support efforts to be initiated as soon as possible. Finally, victims who present with ventricular tachycardia or ventricular fibrillation are two to three times more likely to survive than patients presenting in pulseless electrical activity or asystole.

TABLE 42-3

MODIFIABLE RISK FACTORS FOR SUDDEN DEATH

Smoking	Lack of exercise
Hypertension	Drug use, especially cocaine
Hyperlipidemia	Diabetes mellitus
Obesity	Renal disease

TABLE 42-4

POSITIVE PREDICTORS OF SURVIVAL FROM SUDDEN DEATH

Witnessed cardiac arrest	Initial rhythm ventricular tachycardia or ventricular fibrillation
Initiation of bystander CPR	Young age
Short treatment intervals	

ETIOLOGY OF SUDDEN DEATH

As noted, approximately 300,000 cases of sudden death occur each year in the United States, and nearly 80% of these deaths are attributable to underlying coronary artery disease. Autopsy studies indicate that 40%–70% of victims have evidence of healed myocardial infarction, and acute myocardial infarction is found in approximately 30% of victims. Other less frequently found cardiac and vascular etiologies of sudden death include coronary artery vasculitis, congenital cardiac abnormalities, left ventricular hypertrophy, congestive heart failure, myocarditis, infiltrative disorders of the myocardium, valvular heart disease, conduction system disease, pericardial tamponade, aneurysm rupture, aortic dissection.

Various respiratory diseases (e.g., asthma, bronchial obstruction, pulmonary infarction, pulmonary infections) may be associated with sudden death, with hypoxia and catecholamine excess playing important causative roles. Acute neurologic events may also result in sudden death. The abnormal depolarization and repolarization electrocardiogram (EKG) findings in patients with subarachnoid hemorrhage or large cerebral infarctions are well described and may result from altered autonomic nervous system regulation. Sympathetic overactivity, giving rise to cardiac dysrhythmias, may be the cause of sudden death associated with seizure activity. Electrolyte disturbances associated with various endocrine disorders are also potential culprits for sudden death, giving rise to lethal dysrhythmias. Examples include prolonged QT syndrome seen with hypothyroidism, hypokalemia in Cushing's Syndrome, and hyperkalemia in adrenal insufficiency. Toxins as causative factors in sudden death have received increasing publicity in recent years. Typically, the involved toxins cause lethal ventricular dysrhythmias. Examples include cocaine, inhalant drugs such as toluene, anabolic steroids, and chloroform. Finally, overwhelming infection may give rise to sudden death within 24 h of presentation; examples include bacterial meningitis, endocarditis, myocarditis, and Chagas disease.

MECHANISMS OF BLOOD FLOW DURING STANDARD CPR

It makes intuitive sense that if CPR is to have a successful outcome, with return of cardiac and neurologic function, forward blood flow to the heart and brain during CPR would be beneficial. Indeed, optimizing coronary and cerebral perfusion pressures is central to successful resuscitation and is described further in the next section. To optimize these factors, we must first understand the forces behind the forward flow of blood during CPR.

Debate continues as to the nature of the pump during external chest compressions. Three basic theories have evolved: the cardiac compression pump, the intrathoracic pressure pump, and a combination of the first two theories. The standard theory proposed for many years was the cardiac compression pump theory. It states that intrathoracic pressures do not rise during external chest compression. Rather, external compression compresses the heart directly between the sternum and vertebral column, thereby squeezing blood out of the heart and forward into the peripheral circulation, including the coronary and cerebral vasculature. In this theory, the cardiac valves remain competent, thereby preventing retrograde flow of blood during compression and decompression. During decompression the heart refills with blood, and the cycle repeats itself as compression is again instituted. It is presumed that air moves freely in and out of the lungs, thereby preventing a rise in intrathoracic pressure during chest compression and allowing air to return to the lungs during cardiac decompression.

Beginning in the 1960s, suspicion arose as to the proposed cardiac compression pump theory of forward blood flow. It was noted in dogs that external chest compressions did not result in a pressure gradient between arterial and venous systems. Such a gradient would be required for blood to flow by a direct compression mechanism. In the 1970s and early 1980s, cyclic fluctuations in intrathoracic and vascular pressures during chest compressions were demonstrated. It was suggested that forward blood flow during CPR was caused by alterations in intrathoracic pressure being transmitted to the vascular system. During chest compression, intrathoracic pressure rises and alveolar collapse occurs. In addition, retrograde venous flow is prevented by collapse of venous structures at the thoracic inlet. The cardiac valves are not competent and not necessary to explain forward flow. During chest decompression there is a fall in intrathoracic pressure, with venous return of blood to the thoracic structures. The heart, rather than being directly compressed and decompressed as with the cardiac compression pump theory, actually acts as a passive conduit responding to changes in intrathoracic pressure.

Changes in intrathoracic pressures account for most, and possibly all, forward blood flow during cardiopulmonary resuscitation (CPR).

Since then, many elegant techniques have been developed to measure intrathoracic pressure during CPR, evaluate cardiac and aortic dimensions, and evaluate competency of the cardiac valves. Currently, most investigators believe that the bulk of evidence supports the intrathoracic pressure pump theory, though direct cardiac compression may play some role, albeit minor, in the generation of forward blood flow during CPR.

CORONARY AND CEREBRAL PERFUSION PRESSURES

CPR provides only 10%–30% of normal myocardial blood flow, and only 30%–40% of normal cerebral blood flow.

Chest compression during CPR is intended to provide vital organ perfusion to sustain viability until native cardiovascular activity is restored. Research has indicated, however, that regional organ perfusion achieved during CPR is substantially less than what occurs with normal sinus rhythm. Standard closed chest CPR techniques provide, at best, only 30%–40% of normal cerebral blood flow and only 10%–30% of normal myocardial blood flow. In addition, there is almost no perfusion of peripheral structures. It is critical to evaluate the questions of minimal heart and cerebral perfusion required not only for return of spontaneous circulation but also for provision of acceptable neurologic recovery. Maximization of cerebral and myocardial perfusion, thereby enhancing survival, is a major challenge to resuscitation researchers.

Estimation of myocardial perfusion during CPR is best achieved via measurements of coronary artery perfusion pressure. Work by Crile and Dolley in the early 1900s led to the concept that a minimum coronary perfusion pressure in experimental models of cardiac arrest was necessary for successful resuscitation to occur. This concept was reaffirmed by studies done in the 1960s and 1970s, with an understanding that a minimum aortic diastolic pressure of approximately 40 mm Hg was necessary for return of spontaneous circulation. As a result, the role of alpha-adrenergic agents in resuscitation was better defined, giving rise to an increase in peripheral vasoconstriction and a subsequent rise in aortic diastolic pressure. Selective alpha-blockade resulted in the inability to raise aortic diastolic pressures with epinephrine. With selective beta-blockade, the ability to raise aortic diastolic pressure with epinephrine was retained. Further work refined the concept of coronary perfusion by demonstrating that forward blood flow more precisely was related to the difference between aortic diastolic pressure and right atrial pressure, this difference representing an arteriovenous gradient responsible for organ perfusion. Raessler, Kern, and colleagues have elucidated not only what happens during the relaxation, or diastolic, phase of CPR, but also during the compression, or systolic phase. Investigation into the entire cardiac cycle has revealed that diastolic pressure gradients account for the majority of forward blood flow and myocardial perfusion during CPR, and that retrograde coronary flow often occurs during the compression phase. In addition, the correlation between coronary perfusion pressure and myocardial blood flow has been well established, with laboratory-documented increases in myocardial perfusion as coronary perfusion pressure increases. Finally, as would be expected, coronary artery stenoses compromise myocardial perfusion during CPR in experimental animals, and research indicates that stenoses deemed insignificant under normal physiologic conditions play a compromising role in the setting of CPR.

Fortunately, the rises in myocardial perfusion associated with rises in coronary perfusion pressures also translate into increased success in defibrillation, short-term survival, and long-term survival. Thus, maximization of coronary perfusion, a goal of resuscitation, can be studied objectively and lead to improvements in CPR techniques and pharmacologic interventions.

Unfortunately, most victims of cardiac arrest do not survive. Interestingly enough, most victims of cardiac arrest undergoing external CPR have coronary perfusion pressures less than 10 mmHg. Those victims who do survive typically have much higher coronary perfusion pressures, generally greater than 15 mmHg. This correlation between coronary perfusion pressure and survival persists both in the laboratory and in human clinical situations. As such, coronary perfusion pressure seems to be a predictor of survival during CPR, and pressures greater than 15 mmHg seem to be an important goal of research and clinical efforts.

Minimum coronary perfusion pressure required for survival is ~15 mmHg.

Predictably, much research has occurred in an attempt to develop optimal dosing regimens and newer drugs that further enhance coronary perfusion pressure. Epinephrine has been the standard alpha-agonist used in cardiac arrest. Optimal dosing has been the study of much research, with high hopes for so-called high-dose epinephrine to produce higher coronary perfusion pressures and survival. Multiple human trials of high-dose epinephrine in adults have failed to demonstrate a survival advantage, however, perhaps because of an offset of the balance between myocardial oxygen demand and consumption compared to increases in coronary perfusion pressure. Other alpha-agonists studied in cardiac arrest have included norepinephrine, phenylephrine, and methoxamine; no consensus yet exists as to coronary perfusion pressures and survival data associated with these drugs.

Avoidance of ischemic neurologic injury during CPR and after successful return of spontaneous circulation is necessary to avoid significant morbidity and mortality. Cerebral blood flow is closely correlated to the difference between carotid artery pressure and intracranial cerebrospinal fluid pressure. Initially during CPR carotid artery pressure equals intrathoracic aortic pressure. With time, however, there is a fall in carotid pressure, known as carotid collapse, which correlates with a parallel fall in cerebral blood flow. Alpha-agonists reverse this decline in carotid pressure.

Experimental evidence in dogs suggests that standard techniques of CPR generate cerebral blood flow of 30 ml/min/100 g and that this degree of flow is adequate to maintain cerebral oxygen consumption and ATP levels at prearrest levels for approximately 1 h. Animals resuscitated under such conditions appear to be neurologically intact. For these conditions to be met, cerebral perfusion pressures of approximately 30 mmHg are required, which in turn require mean aortic pressures of 55–60 mmHg.

Data are less available in humans due to obvious technical limitations of directly measuring cerebral perfusion pressure and cerebral blood flow during CPR. Typical aortic pressures generated during CPR, however, probably yield adequate mean pressure levels to generate cerebral perfusion pressures up to 20 mmHg. Such levels probably support cerebral blood flow for up to 15 min under standard conditions, consistent with the fact that early CPR, coupled with early return of spontaneous circulation, frequently results in good neurologic recovery from cardiac arrest.

High-dose epinephrine fails to increase survival in adult cardiac arrest. Standard CPR techniques can support cerebral blood flow for ~15 min.

CLOSED CPR TECHNIQUES

Much research has attempted to improve results of current standard techniques of CPR in terms of generation of coronary perfusion pressure, rates of return of spontaneous circulation, and overall survival to neurologically acceptable states of function. We briefly discuss some of the alternative methods studied.

CASE STUDY: PART 2

Upon arrival of the ambulance crew, the executive performing CPR told what happened. He stated that a full cardiorespiratory arrest took place, and that since institution of CPR no vital signs have returned. The emergency medical technician (EMT) reassessed the airway in the head tilt–chin lift position and confirmed lack of spontaneous air movement. Using a bag-valve-mask device after placing an oral airway, he administered oxygen and confirmed air movement into the lungs. After confirming pulselessness in the victim, the EMT continued with one-person CPR. His assistant placed an 18-gauge needle in the left antecubital fossa without difficulty and began IV administration of normal saline solution as CPR continued.

Increased forced of compression does, indeed, produce an increase in coronary perfusion pressure. Overly aggressive chest compressions, however, are not without hazard. Increasing coronary perfusion pressure comes at the expense of CPR-induced injury and mortality. Thus, chest compression forces that result in depressions greater than the recommended 1.5–2 in. are not warranted.

High-impulse CPR, a technique whereby the rate of chest compression is increased, yields increased mean aortic diastolic pressures and, consequently, increased coronary perfusion pressures. Though true survival data are not available, the increase in coronary perfusion pressure warranted the recommended increase in compression rate from 60/minute to 80–100/min.

Interposed abdominal compression CPR is a three-person technique with the proposed hemodynamic advantages of raising coronary perfusion pressure, along with myocardial perfusion pressure and blood flow. Most animal studies support the concept, but human clinical experience has been less straightforward. Measurements of coronary perfusion pressure have yielded inconsistent results. Preliminary clinical outcome studies have suggested a possible role for in-hospital cardiac arrest. However, the technique has potential for patient injury, especially in the abdomen, along with pulmonary aspiration if the airway is not properly protected. Interposed abdominal compression CPR is a promising technique, but as yet insufficient data exist as to its safety and efficacy.

No "alternative methods" of closed chest CPR have demonstrated significantly improved survival data compared to standard CPR techniques.

Active compression-decompression CPR is often referred to as the "plunger" technique. The device used allows active suction to be applied to the chest during the relaxation phase of CPR. Laboratory models of cardiac arrest suggest an improvement in coronary perfusion pressure using this technique. To date adequate hemodynamic data in humans are not available, and use of the device still is considered experimental.

Another promising adjunct for CPR is the use of the perithoracic pneumatic vest, which alters intrathoracic pressure in rhythmic fashion in conjunction with asynchronous ventilation. Early clinical studies have demonstrated significant increases in coronary perfusion pressures.

AIRWAY, VENTILATION, AND OXYGENATION

It is not just for purposes of convenience and ease of recall that the initial response to any emergency begins with the ABCs. Failure to manage properly the airway and breathing of a cardiac arrest victim, while doing everything correctly to maintain circulatory support, results in a dead patient. Resuscitation begins with the airway, as does periodic reassessment of the patient during times of clinical change. The importance of the ABCs, in that order, can not be overemphasized.

Only airway management in the setting of full respiratory arrest is addressed here. Chapter 1 also discusses in great depth many of the techniques presented here. When an arrest victim is encountered, first rule out the readily reversible cause of respiratory arrest due to airway obstruction. Witnesses to the arrest may provide invaluable information. For example, the victim who collapses while eating dinner after placing their hands to the anterior neck almost certainly has arrested due to foreign body obstruction. In acute airway obstruction, regardless of cause, the highest priority is to open the airway. In the absence of foreign body obstruction, most likely the flaccid tongue is occluding the posterior pharynx. Loss of tone of the supporting submandibular muscles makes at least partial airway obstruction in this setting almost universal. The head tilt, coupled with the chin lift or jaw thrust, is a simple but potentially lifesaving technique. In the setting of trauma the cervical spine must be maintained in a neutral position to avoid cervical injury; thus, the head is not tilted but the chin lift or jaw thrust can be used safely.

The flaccid tongue is the most common cause of airway obstruction in the victim of sudden death.

The head tilt, coupled with the chin lift or jaw thrust, is the initial airway procedure of choice in the noninjured adult victim of sudden death.

The airway is inspected to exclude obstruction for foreign body, and if present, a foreign body should be removed with protected fingers or suction. If spontaneous respirations begin, maintenance of a patent airway is essential. In the absence of return of respirations, and in the absence of an obvious foreign body, airway adjuncts, such as the oraopharyngeal or nasopharyngeal airway, may assist in establishing airway patency. Ventilation is attempted via one of several techniques: mouth-to-mouth, mouth-to-mask, or bag-valve-mask with 100% oxygen. If air does not enter the chest easily, and if the chest does not rise, airway obstruction once again must be suspected. The head and neck are repositioned, and ventilation is again attempted. If ventilation still is not achieved, reversal of airway obstruction is attempted utilizing the Heimlich maneuver or back blows. If ventilation is achieved, pulselessness is confirmed, and chest compressions instituted. Definitive airway support and protection, however, still have not been accomplished. Optimal oxygenation and ventilation are best achieved via endotracheal intubation. The American Heart Association lists the following as indications for endotracheal intubation: cardiac arrest with ongoing chest compressions, inability of a conscious patient to ventilate adequately, inability of the patient to protect the airway (coma, areflexia, or cardiac arrest), or inability of the rescuer to ventilate the unconscious patient with conventional methods. As a matter of course, cricoid pressure should be applied in adults before intubation to help prevent aspiration of gastric contents and should be maintained until the endotracheal tube cuff is inflated and proper tube position established.

In the setting of sudden death, if a patent airway and ventilation cannot be achieved, foreign body obstruction must be assumed to be the etiology for respiratory failure.

Definitive airway support for the victim of sudden death requires endotracheal intubation.

VASCULAR ACCESS AND CIRCULATORY SUPPORT

Once the airway has been established, ventilation accomplished, and oxygenation begun, pulselessness is confirmed, and chest compressions begun. Continuous monitoring of all functions is necessary, with ongoing cardiac monitoring to assess initial rhythm and any changes in rhythm. It is essential that cardiac rhythm be assessed at the earliest possible moment because immediate defibrillation is of highest priority if ventricular fibrillation or pulseless ventricular tachycardia are present.

Intravenous access must be established for optimal fluid therapy and drug administration as necessary, but all is not lost if intravenous access is delayed or difficult to establish. Atropine, lidocaine, and epinephrine can be administered via the endotracheal tube in the absence of intravascular access. A 35-mm through-the-needle intracatheter is threaded down the endotracheal tube, and 2 to 2.5 times the usual drug dose is injected, followed by a 10-ml flush of normal saline down the catheter and several forceful ventilations via the endotracheal tube.

Atropine, epinephrine, and lidocaine can be administered via the endotracheal tube.

It is not surprising that drug delivery to the central circulation from a peripheral venous site of administration is greatly delayed compared to normal physiologic conditions. Direct central vein cannulation is preferable for drug delivery. There are disadvantages of this approach, however; central line access takes longer than peripheral vein access and may inter-

Central lines provide more rapid drug delivery to the central circulation compared to peripheral lines.

CASE STUDY: PART 3

Next, the assistant placed "quick-look paddles" on the victim's chest and determined that the patient's cardiac rhythm was asystole. She proceeded with endotracheal intubation, confirmed the rhythm and that 100% oxygen was being administered, and then administered 1 mg epinephrine intravenously while her colleague continued CPR.

TABLE 42-5

POSSIBLE CAUSES OF ASYSTOLE

Hypoxia	Acidosis
Hyperkalemia	Toxins
Hypokalemia	Profound hypothermia

fere with airway management and chest compression. Central techniques also are not without hazard due to the potential for pneumothorax, puncture of associated arterial or neurologic structures, and lack of ready access for bleeding control. The American Heart Association balances these issues and recommends that "cannulation of a peripheral venous access site is the procedure of choice even during CPR because of the speed, ease, and safety with which it can usually be performed." I agree that peripheral access is the procedure of choice in the field and for many resuscitations in the hospital during the initial phases. However, I view cardiorespiratory arrest as the ultimate complication, which should be managed as aggressively as possible; maximizing drug delivery and effect is essential, in my opinion, and often outweighs the potential disadvantages of central venous cannulation.

The following are prudent guidelines to follow, in my opinion: (1) begin with easy peripheral cannulation so that drugs can be administered as rapidly as possible; (2) utilize femoral vein access with a long catheter to achieve delivery of drug above the diaphragm if well-trained individuals are not available to proceed with direct central vein access; (3) if well-trained personnel with significant expertise are available, proceed quickly with central vein access; and (4) choose internal jugular vein or supraclavicular subclavian vein access as the central line of choice to minimize potential complication and interference with airway management and chest compression.

ASYSTOLE TREATMENT

When CPR has been initiated, intubation with oxygen administration accomplished along with intravenous access, and the rhythm determined to be asystole, prompt therapy is essential. Possible causes of asystole are listed in Table 42-5.

Asystole should be considered an end-stage arrhythmia and must be treated rapidly. Transcutaneous pacing should be instituted immediately in conjunction with drug therapy if it is to be used at all; clearly, waiting until drug therapy has failed to begin transcutaneous pacing is too late. Little evidence supports a significant positive effect for transcutaneous pacing in asystole, even after early initiation, however.

Drugs used for the treatment of asystole include epinephrine and atropine.

Drug therapy for asystole consists of epinephrine 1 mg IV every 3–5 min, followed by atropine 1 mg IV every 3–5 min to a total dose of 0.03–0.04 mg/kg. Sodium bicarbonate 1 mEq/kg should be considered in known cases of severe preexisting metabolic acidosis or hyperkalemia and in cases of cyclic antidepressant drug overdose associated with cardiac arrest. Much has been reported recently about the dose of epinephrine and the basic science in support of high-dose epinephrine (generally defined as 0.1–0.2 mg/kg). Suffice it to say that three large randomized clinical trials comparing standard-dose to high dose-epinephrine failed to demonstrate a significant resuscitation benefit coupled with a survival benefit with

CASE STUDY: PART 4

Epinephrine therapy resulted in a bradyasystolic rhythm, with ventricular escape beats every 15 s. Atropine 1 mg was administered intravenously with restoration of sinus rhythm at a rate of 60 beats/min. Despite restoration of the rhythm, no pulse was felt, and CPR was continued. Intravenous fluids were run wide open, bilateral breath sounds were confirmed with bag-valve-mask respiratory support, and neck veins were determined to be flat. The IV epinephrine dose was repeated.

TABLE 42-6

CAUSES OF PULSELESS ELECTRICAL ACTIVITY

Hypovolemia	Toxins (cyclic antidepressants, digoxin, beta-blockers, calcium channel blockers)
Hypoxia	Hyperkalemia
Cardiac tamponade	Severe acidosis
Tension pneumothorax	Massive myocardial infarction
Hypothermia	
Massive pulmonary embolism	

high-dose epinephrine. Its potential role in pediatrics, and in young adults with primary respiratory arrest, has yet to be evaluated by rigorous clinical trial.

PULSELESS ELECTRICAL ACTIVITY TREATMENT

Pulseless electrical activity is defined as the presence of electrical cardiac activity on the monitor in the absence of palpable pulse or blood pressure via traditional means of measurement. The study of ultrasound during pulseless electrical activity has demonstrated that some cases actually have evidence of mechanical myocardial contraction but that there is not enough forward force to produce a palpable pulse or blood pressure. As with asystole, causative and potentially correctable reasons should be considered for the development of pulseless electrical activity (Table 42-6). Pulseless electrical activity is commonly encountered in the victim of penetrating trauma, and in my experience this rhythm often can be converted to a more stable rhythm because of potentially correctable causes in trauma patients. The so-called medical patient with pulseless electrical activity is a much more difficult case to stabilize.

Drugs used for the treatment of pulseless electrical activity include epinephrine and atropine.

Always look for correctable causes of asystole and pulseless electrical activity.

Though epinephrine and atropine are the first-line drugs for the management of pulseless electrical activity, determination and treatment of underlying cause(s) provide the cornerstone of therapy without which the patient will not survive.

VENTRICULAR FIBRILLATION TREATMENT

The presence of ventricular fibrillation represents the greatest likelihood for patient survival, assuming that prompt intervention takes place. Time is of the essence in this situation, and immediate defibrillation should take top priority. Defibrillation should be attempted initially at 200 joules, and, if there is no change in rhythm, defibrillation should be repeated immediately at 200–300 joules. If ventricular fibrillation persists, defibrillation at 360 joules should be attempted. If the patient remains in ventricular fibrillation after three attempts at defibrillation, CPR should be continued, airway management optimized, and epinephrine administered at the above-noted doses. Defibrillation should then be reattempted at 360 joules, and if unsuccessful, second-line drugs administered alternating with defibrillation. These sec-

The most important aspect to the treatment of ventricular fibrillation is rapid (and successive, if necessary) defibrillation.

CASE STUDY: PART 5

Two minutes after the second dose of epinephrine was administered, the cardiac monitor revealed ventricular fibrillation. The patient was immediately defibrillated at 200 joules without success; a second attempt at defibrillation at 300 joules resulted in restoration of sinus rhythm at 50 beats/min with frequent PVCs; this time, there was a palpable pulse with a blood pressure of 70/40 mmHg.

TABLE 42-7

CONTINUOUS INFUSION DOSES FOR VENTRICULAR FIBRILLATION

Lidocaine: 2–4 mg/min
Bretylium: 1–2 mg/min
Procainamide: 1–4 mg/min

ond-line drugs include lidocaine 1–1.5 mg/kg IV, repeated in 3–5 min, to a maximum dose of 3 mg; bretylium 5 mg/kg IV, followed by 10 mg/kg after 5 min; procainamide 30 mg/min to a maximum of 17 mg/kg for refractory ventricular fibrillation; and magnesium sulfate 1–2 g IV for torsades de pointes, severe suspected hypomagnesemia, or refractory ventricular fibrillation.

If spontaneous circulation returns at any point during the above management, airway, breathing, and vital signs should be reassessed and managed as indicated. Ventricular ectopy should be suppressed, unless otherwise contraindicated, by maintenance drips of the medication(s) that appeared to be successful in terminating the rhythm in association with defibrillation (see Table 42-7).

BRADYCARDIA TREATMENT

Management of bradycardia is dictated by the clinical condition of the patient, not the absolute pulse rate.

The case study indicates that treatment of bradycardias in the prior setting of cardiac arrest is determine by clinical evaluation, or looking at the patient. In the presence of any of the serious signs or symptoms noted in Table 42-8 and related directly to the bradycardia itself, heart rate must be increased; this is accomplished via the sequential use of atropine 0.5–1 mg IV every 3 min to clinical response or a total dose of 0.03–0.04 mg/kg, transcutaneous pacing, dopamine 5–20 μg/kg/min, and epinephrine 2–10 μg/min. Cardiac transplant patients, who have denervated hearts, will not respond to atropine and should be treated initially with transcutaneous pacing or catecholamine infusion. Finally, lidocaine should not be given in bradycardic patients with ventricular escape mechanisms because this may terminate the very electrical activity that is keeping the patient alive.

In the absence of symptomatic bradycardia, and in the presence of type II second-degree AV block or third-degree AV block, preparation for transvenous pacemaker insertion should be started due to the potential for worsening degrees of heart block. In the absence of such situations, the patient can be monitored and observed without acute intervention.

VENTRICULAR TACHYCARDIA TREATMENT

As with bradycardic rhythms, the presence of ventricular tachycardia on the monitor requires the clinician to look at the patient. Not all patients with prolonged ventricular tachycardia develop unstable vital signs. In the unstable patient, or the patient without vital signs who develops ventricular tachycardia, treatment should proceed identical to the treatment for the victim of ventricular fibrillation. In the stable patient, therapy is initiated with lidocaine 1–1.5 mg/kg IV, followed by lidocaine 0.5–0.75 mg/kg IV every 5–10 min to a maximum dose of 3 mg/kg. If unsuccessful, the next treatment is procainamide 30 mg/min to a maximum dose of 17 mg/kg. If still unsuccessful, bretylium 5–10 mg/kg is administered. If the

Unstable ventricular tachycardia is treated in identical fashion as ventricular fibrillation.

CASE STUDY: PART 6

The patient's pulse decreased to 40 beats/min, and blood pressure of 70/40 is barely audible. Atropine 1 mg IV was administered, and the pulse increased to 75 beats/min. Repeat blood pressure is now 110/60 mmHg. The PVCs continue.

TABLE 42-8

SERIOUS SIGNS AND SYMPTOMS RELATED TO BRADYCARDIA

Chest pain	Hypotension
Dyspnea	Pulmonary edema
Altered level of consciousness	Myocardial infarction

patient remains in ventricular tachycardia, synchronized cardioversion should be considered. As with ventricular fibrillation, continuos maintenance doses of these drugs should be administered, based on which appeared to terminate ventricular tachycardia (see Table 42-7).

SPECIAL RESUSCITATION SITUATIONS

Hypothermia

Chapter 25 provides an extensive review of the management of hypothermic patients, including caveats of resuscitation in the setting of cardiorespiratory arrest. A few points are worth emphasizing here.

1. Prevention of further heat loss is essential, especially in the wet victim who loses significant heat due to the enhanced conductivity of water compared to air.
2. Excessive jostling of the patient may precipitate ventricular fibrillation.
3. Careful intubation is a safe procedure and should be done by the most experience person available.
4. Active core rewarming techniques are indicated in the profoundly hypothermic, unstable patient.
5. Drugs and defibrillation techniques rarely work in the profoundly hypothermic patient; emphasis should be placed on rewarming, with reservation of standard procedures until rewarming is achieved.
6. CPR should be withheld in the hypothermic patient with an organized rhythm whose clinical status corresponds to the degree of hypothermia; aggressive rewarming should be the treatment of first priority; chest compressions may convert the bradycardic patient to a patient with ventricular fibrillation.
7. Patients should not be pronounced dead until adequate rewarming has taken place.

Near-Drowning

Victims of near-drowning should be assumed to have associated neck injuries, and airway management should proceed with this caution in mind. It is imperative to restore ventilation and oxygenation as rapidly as possible. Care must always be taken to protect the rescuer(s) during removal of the patient from the water. Once the patient is in shallow water or on land, rescue breathing should be initiated. The Heimlich maneuver should not be used unless upper airway obstruction from a foreign body is suspected. Generally only a minimum of water is aspirated, and laryngospasm prevents aspiration all together in approximately 10% of vic-

CASE STUDY: PART 7

The patient's pulse and blood pressure remained stable over the next 2 min. As an IV drip of lidocaine was being prepared for administration after a bolus of lidocaine, the cardiac rhythm suddenly reverted to ventricular tachycardia. There was no palpable pulse. Immediate defibrillation at 200 Joules restoreed sinus rhythm, a pulse of 80/min, and blood pressure of 138/70 mmHg. The lidocaine bolus of 1.5 mg/kg was given, followed by a lidocaine drip at 3 mg/min. The victim's pulse and blood pressure remain stable over the next several minutes. There was no return of ventricular ectopy, and the patient was transported to the nearest hospital emergency department for further care.

tims. The Heimlich maneuver as such is of little benefit and in fact may promote the aspiration of gastric contents.

Victims of near-drowning should be resuscitated using the basic principles of advanced life support. Many such victims also have associated hypothermia due to submersion, which frequently plays a protective function in maintaining organ system viability despite prolonged periods of cardiorespiratory arrest. The principles of hypothermic resuscitation should be followed as outlined in Chapter 25.

Failed Field Advanced Cardiac Life Support Resuscitation

In this age of cost cutting in medical care, it seems reasonable to assess clinical strategies for patients with extremely poor prognoses. One such group is those victims of cardiorespiratory arrest who have failed lengthy out-of-hospital resuscitation based upon Advanced Cardiac Life Support (ACLS) guidelines. Depending on the level of sophistication of the local prehospital system, this scenario may or may not be common in a given emergency department.

Data support the concept that failed prehospital Advanced Cardiac Life Support (ACLS) resuscitation represents a medically futile state.

Two extensive studies in the past decade have addressed this issue with similar results: the first by Kellerman and colleagues and the second by Gray and colleagues, published in the *Annals of Emergency Medicine* and the *New England Journal of Medicine*, respectively. Both reports described medically futile outcomes in resuscitative efforts performed on victims of cardiac arrest who failed to regain spontaneous circulation after full out-of-hospital resuscitation efforts. Placing the issue of medical student and resident education aside, these studies support the notion that continued resuscitative efforts in these futile situations simply increase health care cost and patient agony without any hope of patient benefit. There are important caveats, however. Victims of hypothermic-induced cardiac arrest must continue to be resuscitated until core rewarming has been achieved; failure to recognize correctable causes of arrest in the field may be amenable to hospital resuscitation; and the pregnant victim of cardiac arrest actually represents two patients, not just one, and aggressive maternal resuscitation, even in the setting of maternal medical futility, is necessary if an attempt at fetal survival is the goal. As such, it is my opinion that strict policies governing cessation of resuscitative efforts for victims of failed out-of-hospital resuscitation are not in order; rather, sound individualized clinical judgment, coupled with an understanding of medical futility, makes the most sense both for the patient and for society.

The Controversy over Closed CPR Versus Open Cardiac Massage

Open cardiac massage clearly provides for marked increases in coronary perfusion pressure, significantly above those produced by closed techniques, although survival advantage declines with increasing time from induction of arrest. Case reports exist whereby cardiac arrest victims unable to be resuscitated by closed techniques have survived open chest cardiac massage. Such success appears limited to the first 15–20 min post arrest, after which open chest cardiac massage appears to have little to no value. Finally, before the introduction in 1960 of closed chest CPR, open chest cardiac massage was the standard of care for resuscitation. Successful resuscitation rates were much higher than current values for closed CPR, although most patients studied before 1960 were victims of cardiac arrest associated with surgery.

Why was closed CPR so readily accepted and open cardiac massage discarded? For one thing, the appeal of the closed technique was its universality. Lay persons and health professionals alike could be taught the technique of standard CPR. The open technique was messy, bloody, and poorly applicable to the prehospital setting. Bodies were not judged to be "violated" by the closed technique. Opening the chest and restarting the heart was only the first step; now, the proper surgeon needed to be immediately available to finish the resuscitation and operative closure. Finally, worries about bloodborne pathogens now abound, and closed CPR , from that perspective, is less risky.

When the hemodynamics of closed versus open techniques are compared, the hemodynamics of open chest cardiac massage clearly are superior. Among others, the following have been demonstrated in various models to be significantly superior via the open technique: aortic systolic and diastolic pressures, coronary perfusion pressure, myocardial blood flow, and cerebral blood flow. The fundamental question is whether such hemodynamic improvements translate into significant survival improvements.

Open cardiac massage produces significantly better hemodynamic data compared to closed CPR.

Many laboratory models of cardiac arrest have been designed to help address this issue. The overwhelming evidence supports the concept that, in animals in which cardiac arrest has been initiated, not only does open chest cardiac massage improve hemodynamics, but it also improves immediate resuscitation rates, short-term survival, long-term survival, and neurologic recovery. There appears to be a limited "window of opportunity" after which open cardiac massage still improves hemodynamics but not ultimate survival; this window appears to be within the first 15–20 min of cardiac arrest.

If open cardiac massage is to be used successfully, it must be initiated early in the resuscitation process (probably within the first 15–20 min of cardiac arrest).

Designing clinical trials of open versus closed techniques within this time frame represents a major challenge. Animal trials clearly support the importance of such research, however. To date, adequate trials based upon what we have learned from animal models of cardiac arrest are quite limited, and there is no definitive answer to the question of the utility in humans. To make the issue even more complicated, new technology, such as cardiopulmonary bypass and ventricular-assist devices, is based upon the concepts already known concerning the hemodynamics of open chest cardiac massage.

In summary, then, should we continue what may be suboptimal closed techniques in the setting of cardiac arrest? The answer lies within clinical research that, unfortunately, cannot answer the question very soon. The newer technologic developments are of great interest, but like the emergency thoracotomy required for direct cardiac massage, they can be criticized for lack of universal availability and propensity for increased risk of transmission of bloodborne pathogens to the health care provider. What is indisputable is the laboratory evidence supporting the need for study of open chest techniques. The challenge is in the development and study of limited, readily learned, invasive techniques that can be used in the hospital setting outside the operating room and perhaps in the prehospital setting as well. One such device, utilizing a minimal chest incision and a simple piece of equipment for direct cardiac compression within the chest, is about to undergo human trials. It is clear that open techniques make logical sense but need further evaluation. It is also clear that if they are to be used, they must be used relatively early after cardiac arrest and not as a last-ditch effort. As with many aspects in medicine, we may come full circle in our management of cardiac arrest.

SUMMARY

The approach to cardiorespiratory arrest initially often involves a single rescuer who initiates the health care delivery system, resulting in a team approach to the resuscitation efforts. Standard protocols exist regarding management of very specific clinical scenarios as pertain to respiratory and cardiac status. Ongoing research of currently accepted dogma is essential to continued resuscitative improvements, with special emphasis given to rediscovered, yet more invasive, techniques of cardiac resuscitation. One thing appears clear, however; technology will never replace sound clinical judgment and the necessity to stabilize the ABCs.

REVIEW QUESTIONS

1. **The definition of sudden death includes which of the following?**
   - A. Absence of a detectable pulse
   - B. Unresponsiveness
   - C. Agonal or apneic respirations
   - D. All the above

2. **The most common clinical condition predisposing to sudden death is:**
   - A. Nonischemic-related cardiac dysrhythmias
   - B. Underlying cerebrovascular disease
   - C. Ischemic heart disease
   - D. Hypertension

3. **Positive predictors of successful resuscitation from cardiac arrest can be attributed to which of the following factors?**
   - A. Establishment of coronary perfusion pressure of at least 15 mmHg
   - B. Adequate perfusion pressures to both central and peripheral structures
   - C. Maintenance of normal levels of cerebral perfusion during CPR
   - D. None of the above

4. **The use of high-dose epinephrine in the setting of cardiac arrest:**
   - A. Has been proven to be of clinical benefit for children but not adults.
   - B. Is defined as 1 mg/kg body weight.
   - C. Is indicated as first-line therapy for both asystole and refractory ventricular fibrillation.
   - D. Has not been proven to be of significant clinical benefit in adults.

5. **Which of the following statements is/are true regarding cardiac arrest in the setting of profound hypothermia?**
   - A. Excessive jostling of the patient may precipitate ventricular fibrillation.
   - B. Intubation may precipitate ventricular fibrillation and should not be performed.
   - C. Defibrillation rarely is successful.
   - D. Chest compression should be performed in the presence of marked bradycardia but no palpable pulse.

ANSWERS

1. The answer is D. In 1991, a consensus definition of sudden death was established by the Utstein II international workshop. Such strict definition was necessary for meaningful epidemiologic studies to be performed.
2. The answer is C. Ischemic heart disease is the most common condition that predisposes to sudden death. Other less common conditions include answers A and B. Since the 1940s there has been a decline in the incidence of cardiac arrest in the United States, attributable to diet changes, smoking cessation, and the treatment of hypertension.
3. The answer is A. Successful resuscitation from cardiac arrest requires return of spontaneous circulation and avoidance of ischemic neurologic injury. Both experimental and clinical data support the need to generate coronary perfusion pressures of at least 15 mmHg for spontaneous circulation to be restored. Direct measurement of cerebral perfusion in humans has obvious technical limitations, but extrapolation of available data suggests that generation of cerebral perfusion pressures of 20 mmHg is possible during the first 15 min of standard CPR. Peripheral structures receive almost no perfusion during CPR.
4. The answer is D. High-dose epinephrine is defined as 0.1–0.2 mg/kg. Laboratory studies have suggested a possible clinical benefit, but such survival benefits have not been substantiated in large human trials of cardiac arrest. Large trials evaluating its potential use in children have not been done.
5. The answer is A and C. The mainstay of successful resuscitation in the setting of profound hypothermia is core rewarming. Ventricular fibrillation in this setting is exceedingly difficult to treat and may be precipitated by unnecessary jostling of the patient; defibrillation rarely works before adequate rewarming. Careful intubation is a safe procedure, and, as in all instances of cardiac resuscitation, airway management is essential to survival. Even bradycardic rhythms may be able to provide adequate levels of coronary and cerebral perfusion in this setting, even if palpable pulses cannot be felt due to peripheral vasoconstriction. The use of chest compressions may convert an organized rhythm into ventricular fibrillation.

SUGGESTED READING

Brown CG, Martin DR, Pepe PE, et al. A comparison of standard dose and high dose epinephrine in cardiac arrest outside the hospital. N Engl J Med 1992;327:1051–1055.

Callaham M, Madsen CD, Barton CW, et al. A randomized clinical trial of high dose epinephrine and norepinephrine versus standars dose epinephrine in pre-hospital cardiac arrest. JAMA 1992;268:2667–2671.

Cummins RO (ed) Textbook of Advanced Cardiac Life Support. Dallas: American Heart Association, 1994.

Cummins RO, Chamberlain D, Abramson N, et al. Recommended guidelines for uniform reporting of data from out-of-hospital cardiac arrest: the Utstein style. Circulation 1991;84:960–965.

Gray WA, Capone RJ, Most AS. Unsuccessful emergency medical resuscitation: are continued efforts in the emergency department justified? N Engl J Med 1991;325:1393–1398.

Gueugniaud PY, Mols P, Goldstein P, et al. A comparison of repeated high doses and repeated standard doses of epinephrine for cardiac arrest outside the hospital. European Epinephrine Study Group. N Engl J Med 1998;339:1595–1601.

Kellermann AL, Staves DR, Hackman BB. In-hospital resuscitation following unsuccessful prehospital advanced cardiac life support: "heroic efforts" or an exercise in futility? Ann Emerg Med 1988; 17:589–594.

Paradis NA, Halperin HR, Nowak RM (eds) Cardiac Arrest: The Science and Practice of Resuscitation Medicine. Baltimore: Williams & Wilkins, 1996.

Stiell IG, Hebert PC, Weitzman BN, et al. High dose epinephrine in adult cardiac arrest. N Engl J Med 1992;327:1045–1050.

CHAPTER 43

WISSAM CHATILA

Antimicrobials

CHAPTER OUTLINE

LEARNING OBJECTIVES

After studying this chapter, you should be able to:

- Recognize the different classes of antimicrobials and their mechanisms of action.
- Identify the spectrum of coverage for specific antimicrobials.
- Describe possible adverse effects and drug interactions caused by antimicrobials.
- Select appropriate antimicrobials for various pathogens.

Patients in the intensive care unit (ICU) are often infected with multiresistant organisms.

Judicious use of empiric antimicrobial therapy is needed to minimize emergence of resistant organisms.

The intensive care unit (ICU) is a special environment that often harbors a considerable number of highly resistant organisms. Critically ill patients are frequently exposed to broad-spectrum antibiotics and invasive procedures that make them more susceptible either to be colonized by exogenous organisms or to have overgrowth of resistant endogenous strains. As newer antimicrobials are introduced, many organisms have demonstrated the capability to develop resistance to these newer agents; thus, it is common to find intensivists facing the challenge of treating highly selected organisms while trying to minimize emergence of other antibiotic-resistant organisms.

Empiric antibiotic therapy is frequently used in the intensive care unit, but it is a double-edged sword. Early institution of adequate antimicrobial coverage in critically ill patients with documented infections improves their outcome. On the other hand, overuse of antibiotics in noninfectious situations or incorrect choice of the empiric coverage may be associated with development of resistant organisms, resulting in more refractory infections later. In general, clinicians start with broad-spectrum antibiotics for empiric coverage. Nevertheless, broad-spectrum antibiotics are not all equivalent, and they still must be tailored according to several factors. Once an infection is suspected, and after obtaining appropriate diagnostic testing, three factors should guide the choice of antibiotic: suspected source of infection, severity of the illness, and local (hospital or ICU) microbiologic flora. The ideal empiric coverage should be an antibiotic, or combination of agents, efficient with good tissue penetration, bactericidal, and tolerable without significant toxicity. The sicker the patient, the broader the coverage should be, to minimize the risk of treatment failures.

Furthermore, knowing the source of infection, whether lower respiratory tract, intraabdominal, or central nervous system, streamlines the coverage.

When comparable antibiotics are available, the choice is often driven by cost. A review of selected characteristics of antibiotics commonly used in the intensive care unit follows, grouped according to their class. Because almost all antibiotics used in ICUs are given via the parenteral route, antimicrobials described in this chapter mostly are those given intravenously.

ANTIBACTERIAL ANTIBIOTICS

There has been a significant increase in the number of antibiotics during the last decade. Almost all classes of antimicrobials have expanded, giving clinicians a wide variety of broad-spectrum agents from which to choose: antipseudomonal and extended-spectrum penicillins were added to the natural penicillins and the aminopenicillins, more third-generation and newer fourth-generation cephalosporins were introduced, ciprofloxacin is competing against a myriad of fluoroquinolones, and erythromycin is no longer the only macrolide available. In addition, agents of newer classes of antibiotics are joining the older ones in the fight against emerging resistant organisms.

Mechanisms of Action and Resistance

The underlying mechanisms for bacterial killing and growth inhibition differ among the various classes of antibiotics. Depending on their site and mode of action, antimicrobials are divided into bactericidal and bacteriostatic agents. Some antimicrobials are bactericidal for some strains while being bacteriostatic for others. Moreover, agents are divided according to their mode of action: some have a concentration-dependent killing effect, while others have a time-dependent killing effect. In the first group, there is a clear relationship between serum drug concentrations and the killing effect, and thus delivering an adequate dose to reach expected levels at the site of infection is crucial for good response. On the other hand, the latter group of antimicrobials relies on time of exposure of the bacteria to that antibiotic; the longer the exposure to the antibiotic, the greater the killing effect. Thus, for time-dependent killing drugs, their effectiveness is not related to their concentration above the minimal inhibitory concentration (MIC), but rather to the time span above MIC; accordingly, adjusting the dosing interval is as important as giving the adequate dose. In addition, some antimicrobials exhibit two important properties: postantibiotic effect (PAE) and synergy. The PAE is a period of suppression of bacterial growth after exposure to the antimicrobial concentrations above the MIC. Synergy occurs when the combination of two drugs results in greater killing than that of their cumulative effect when given separately.

> Some antibiotics may be bactericidal for some strains while being bacteriostatic for others.

> Knowing the pharmacologic properties and mechanisms of action of antimicrobials permits their optimal use and dosing. When giving combination antibiotic therapy, choose agents that have synergistic effects and minimal drug interaction.

Although newer antimicrobials continue to be added to our armamentarium, various bacteria have developed or acquired resistance to commonly used agents. The mechanism to develop or to transmit resistance varies among organisms: antimicrobial inactivation, modification of the antimicrobial target, alteration in permeability to the antimicrobial agent, and modification of biosynthetic pathways targeted by the antibiotic.

β-Lactams

β-Lactam antibiotics, by binding to a variety of penicillin-binding proteins (PBPs) found on inner cell membranes of certain bacteria, activate endogenous bacterial autolysins and cause cell lysis. The activity of an antimicrobial corresponds to the type of PBP and to the degree of affinity to a particular PBP. Formation of β-lactamase enzymes, which hydrolyze β-lactam antibiotics, is the most common mechanism of bacterial resistance among nosocomial gram-negative organisms. Gram-positive and gram-negative β-lactamases are different; gram-positive β-lactamases are either inducible or constitutive and are often plasmid mediated. In contrast, gram-negative β-lactamases are more diverse: they are either encoded on bacterial chromosomes, plasmid mediated, or carried on transposons. Other bacteria escape autolysis by changing the permeability of their outer membranes to antimicrobials or altering their PBPs.

> β-Lactam antibiotics activate bacterial autolysins by binding to specific penicillin-binding proteins (PBPs) on the cell membranes of bacteria. A variety of bacterial β-lactamases target and inactivate these β-lactam antibiotics, accounting for their resistance.

Cephalosporins have the same mechanism of action as penicillins and are similarly susceptible to β-lactamases. Some cephalosporins (e.g., ceftazidine) can induce production of β-lactamases in *Pseudomonas aeroginosa*, *Enterobacter* species, and *Citrobacter* species that will affect all other β-lactam antibiotics. Pharmaceutical companies were able to generate a newer generation of penicillins and cephalosporins by modifying their side chains, thus increasing their affinity to PBPs and permeability through the outer cell membrane. It is the side chain that affects the coverage spectrum of these agents and confers some of their properties, including their pharmacokinetics and side effects. Newer β-lactams include the carbapenems (imipenem, meropenem) and the β-lactam/β-lactamase inhibitor combination (ampicillin-sulbactam, ticarcillin-clavulanate, piperacillin-tazobactam). Although the carbapenems contain the β-lactam rings, they have special stereochemical characteristics that make them resistant to hydrolysis by most β-lactamases; consequently, carbapenems have the widest spectrum of all other β-lactam antibiotics. Similarly, combining β-lactamase inhibitors with other β-lactams has extended their spectrum of activity; but β-lactamase inhibitors are not all equipotent. Tazobactam has the greatest β-lactamase inhibiting potency. Aztreonam is a monobactam that binds exclusively to PBPs of gram-negative organisms; hence, it is completely ineffective against all gram-positive bacteria. Aztreonam is not hydrolyzed by many β-lactamases, but bacteria have developed resistance against it by blocking its uptake into the inner cell membrane or altering their PBPs.

Aminoglycosides

Aminoglycosides exert their bactericidal activity by interfering with bacterial protein synthesis during aerobic metabolism. These agents are potent antibacterials because of both their concentration-dependent killing effect and their time-dependent PAE on gram-positive as well as gram-negative organisms. Not all agents in this group are equivalent in potency, because they differ in their susceptibility to aminoglycoside-inactivating enzymes and their permeability to cell walls.

Fluoroquinolones

Fluoroquinolones affect the genetic controls of most gram-negative, gram-positive, and some intracellular bacteria. They inhibit DNA gyrase of susceptible organisms, leading to a bactericidal effect. They may have a synergistic effect with some β-lactam antibiotics. The observed resistance to quinolones has been explained by mutations in the DNA gyrase gene that lead to alteration in the target of the quinolones.

Glycopeptides (Vancomycin)

Of the two glycopeptides that have been used clinically, vancomycin and teicoplanin, only vancomycin is available in the United States. Vancomycin exerts its activity by inhibiting cell wall synthesis of gram-positive organisms. Unfortunately, the incidence of vancomycin resistance is on the rise, posing a major threat for many hospitals because of the lack of comparable agents. Two newer agents, linezolid and quinupristin-dalfopristin, from different classes of antibiotics, have been recently introduced and appear to be promising alternatives against these emerging gram-positive bacteria; nevertheless, the antibiotic arsenal against these organisms is alarmingly void compared to available gram-negative coverage. Among the gram-positive bacteria that are resistant to vancomycin, *Enterococcus* species are by far the most common, and although they are not as intrinsically virulent as other gram-positive cocci, they are strikingly resistant to many antibiotics. *Enterococcus* species carry vancomycin-resistant genes on self-transferable plasmids and transposons that encode for altered vancomycin targets, thus inhibiting vancomycin binding to the cell wall.

Macrolides (Erythromycin, Azithromycin) and Clindamycin

Macrolides share the same mechanism of action as clindamycin but have a different spectrum of coverage. They inhibit bacterial growth by interfering with protein synthesis and are bacteriostatic. Unlike erythromycin, the newer macrolides, clarithromycin and azithromycin, can penetrate the cell membrane of gram-negative bacilli and thus have a broader spectrum of coverage compared to erythromycin. Resistance to macrolides and clindamycin is carried on a plasmid, resulting in alteration of their ribosomal binding site.

Sulfonamides

Sulfonamides exert a bacteriostatic effect by interfering with the substrate metabolism of bacteria. They inhibit enzymes involved in the formation of folic acid and act synergistically with trimethoprin to block purine synthesis. The combination of these two agents, trimethoprin-sulfamethoxazole (Bactrim), has a net bactericidal effect when bacteria are sensitive to both, and the two agents are synergistic to other antimicrobials. Various mechanisms account for trimethoprin-sulfamethoxazole resistance: altering or overproducing dihydrofolate reductase enzyme, which is plasmid mediated and is the most important mechanism, leaving the tetrahydrofolate pathway to synthesize thymidine, and decreasing cell permeability. Resistance to trimethoprin-sulfamethoxazole is increasing; in some reports, 40% of ICU gram-negative flora is resistant these two agents.

Tetracyclines

The primary mode of action of tetracyclines is inhibition of protein synthesis, and the observed resistance mainly results from a decrease in cell wall permeability to the drug. The use of tetracycline has become limited in the ICU because of the growing number of resistant organisms.

Nitroimidazoles (Metronidazole)

Metronidazole is the only nitroimidazole available in the United States. It is bactericidal and acts by inhibiting DNA synthesis. Resistance to metronidazole results from its reduced intracellular uptake; fortunately, it is rare.

Antituberculous Antibiotics

Among all antituberculous drugs, the most active antimicrobials are isoniazid and rifampin because of their bactericidal effect. Because of the slow rate of growth of mycobacteria, these agents need to be administered over a prolonged period of time and in combination therapy when a tuberculous infection is suspected.

Streptogramins (Quinupristin-Dalfopristin) and Oxazolidinones (Linezolid)

Quinupristin-dalfopristin and linezolid constitute the antibiotics recently approved for the treatment of vancomycin-resistant infections. All three agents are bacteriostatic individually, by inhibiting protein synthesis, but quinupristin and dalfopristin have a synergistic effect and are combined into one bactericidal end product.

Spectrum of Coverage

Penicillins

In many ICUs, penicillin G, ampicillin, and even the penicillinase-resistant penicillins (nafcillin, cloxacillin) have fallen out of favor as first-line empiric therapy because of the high incidence of resistance to these agents. Certain exceptions may exist; ampicillin is recommended for the treatment of acute meningitis, together with a cephalosporin $\pm$ vancomycin, in patients with defective cell immunity, due to high risk of *Listeria monocytogenes* infection. Nafcillin may be considered as initial therapy for suspected staphylococcal infections only if the local ICU flora has a very low incidence for methicillin-resistant coagulase-negative or coagulase-positive staphylococci. Once the organism and its sensitivity have been identified, these penicillins are the drug of choice for infections caused by susceptible streptococci, staphylococci, clostridia, *Neisseria*, and other anaerobes.

In contrast, the new generation of penicillins, especially the β-lactam/β-lactamase inhibitor combination, is often used for empiric coverage. Antipseudomonal penicillins (carbenicillin, ticarcillin) retained their gram-positive spectrum and have an excellent gram-negative activity, including that against *Pseudomonas aeruginosa*. Extended-spectrum penicillins (piperacillin, azlocillin, mezlocillin) gained activity against more enteric gram-negative aerobic and anaerobic bacteria, including against *Bacteroides fragilis*, in addition to the activity of antipseudomonal penicillins. Both antipseudomonal and extended-spectrum penicillins are not very β-lactamase stable and have been combined with β-lactamase inhibitors (ticarcillin-clavulanic acid, piperacillin-tazobactam). Among the β-lactam/β-lactamase inhibitor class, piperacillin-tazobactam stands out because of a greater antibacterial effect of piperacillin and the greater β-lactamase-inhibiting potency of tazobactam. Nonetheless, *Klebsiella*, *Acinetobacter*, and *Pseudomonas* are being reported in some ICUs that are more resistant against all penicillins; therefore, these newer agents are given in combination with aminoglycosides or fluoroquinolones when highly resistant organisms are suspected.

Cephalosporins

Older-generation β-lactam antibiotics (penicillins and cephalosporins) are active against gram-positive organisms. Newer β-lactam generations, β-lactam/β-lactamase inhibitors, and carbapenems have a wider range of coverage and are often used for empiric therapy, especially when resistant organisms are suspected.

First-generation cephalosporins (cefazolin, cephalexin) have good activity against streptococcal species and methicillin-sensitive *Staphylococcus aureus* (MSSA). Second-generation cephalosporins (cefuroxime, cefoxitin, cefotetan) gained some gram-negative coverage while maintaining adequate gram-positive coverage. Cefuroxime is very active against MSSA and streptococcal species and is β-lactamase stable. The third generation is characterized by two types of agents: antipseudomonal cephalosporins (ceftazidime, cefoperazone), and broad-spectrum cephalosporins (cefotaxime, ceftriaxone). The antipseudomonal activity of ceftazidine is greater than the activity of cefoperazone. Although the activity of ceftazidime is strong against gram-negative organisms, it induces resistance to many β-lactams, especially in the *Enterobacter* species, so it is not recommended to be used as a monotherapy when such gram-negative infections are suspected. Both cefotaxime and ceftriaxone have excellent activity against streptococcal species and gram-negative coverage, but their activity against MSSA is moderate. Because of their broad coverage, cefotaxime and ceftriaxone are widely used as first-line empiric therapy for nosocomial infections and in particular for bacterial meningitis due to their excellent cerebrospinal fluid (CSF) levels. In contrast, first- and second-generation cephalosporins are seldom used as the drugs of choice to treat nosocomial infections. Recently, a new fourth generation of cephalosporin (cefipime) has been introduced with characteristics of both antipseudomonal and broad-spectrum third-generation cephalosporins. Cefipime appears to be very effective and β-lactamase stable against *Klebsiella*, *Enterobacter*, and other aerobic gram-negative rods and has activity similar to ceftazidine against *Pseudomonas aeruginosa*. Cefipime also has an excellent activity against streptococcal species and moderate activity against MSSA. Unlike third-generation cephalosporins, CSF penetration of cefipime is less; hence, it should not substitute for cefotaxime or ceftriaxone to treat acute bacterial meningitis.

Carbapenems

Carbapenems (imipenem, meropenem) have the most broad-spectrum coverage available. Except for methicillin-resistant *Staphylococcus aureus* (MRSA) and *Enterococcus faecium* (gram-positive cocci), and *Stenotrophomonas maltophilia* and *Pseudomonas cepacia* (gram-negative rods), carbapenems inhibit almost all anaerobic bacteria and gram-positive and gram-negative aerobes. Despite their wide coverage, impenem and meropenem are not used usually as first-choice empiric therapy; rather, they are reserved for suspected resistant or polymicrobial infections. Meropenem is no more active than imipenem but may be preferred in some ICUs because of its lower incidence of seizures compared to imipenem.

Monobactams (Aztreonam)

The only available monobactam is aztreonam. Aztreonam has no activity against gram-positive species and anaerobes. It has good activity against gram-negative aerobic pathogens including *Pseudomonas aeruginosa*; its spectrum resembles that of aminoglycosides. Aztreonam is not used as a monotherapy unless susceptibility is documented. It is often given for double coverage of serious gram-negative infections, or it is used as a substitute for aminoglycosides, particularly in patients at high risk for toxicity from these latter agents.

Aminoglycosides

Aminoglycosides (gentamicin, tobramycin, amikacin, neomycin, netilmicin, streptomycin) are well known for their excellent activity against gram-negative aerobic bacteria. They have a synergistic inhibitory effect against MSSA and MRSA when combined with an effective β-lactam antibiotic. Limitation to the use of aminoglycosides is related to their toxicity rather than to their activity. Nonetheless, in view of the high prevalence of resistant gram-negative bacteria in some ICUs, aminoglycosides continue to be indispensable because of their strong activity against some of these organisms. For suspected pseudomonal infections, tobramycin is preferred by some because it is more potent than gentamicin, and for suspected multiresistant infections, amikacin is the aminoglycoside of choice because it is less susceptible to inactivating enzymes. Streptomycin is limited to the treatment of tuberculosis and other uncommon infections, and neomycin is limited for topical application and for the treatment of hepatic encephalopathy.

Aminoglycosides are used exclusively in gram-negative infection to enhance the activity of β-lactam antibiotics against refractory infections, including some resistant gram-positive organisms.

Fluoroquinolones

This group of antimicrobials has recently expanded dramatically. Early quinolones (nalidixic acid, oxolinic acid) were limited to treatment of urinary tract infection because of their limited tissue penetration. Currently, intensivists have numerous potent intravenous broad-spectrum quinolones to chose from (ciprofloxacin, levofloxacin, trovafloxacin, gatifloxacin). Except for *Pseudomonas cepacia* and *Stenotrophomonas maltophilia*, these antimicrobials are remarkable for their excellent activity against gram-negative bacteria and intracellular organisms (*Chlamydia*, *Legionella*, *Mycoplasma*, and some mycobacterial species). Compared to the newer quinolones, ciprofloxacin remains the most potent against *P. aeruginosa*, even against some *Pseudomonas* that are resistant to aminoglycosides. The newer quinolones, levofloxacin and trovafloxacin, gained more activity against gram-positive bacteria including enterococcus species, some penicillin-resistant streptococcal species, and MSSA. Trovafloxacin is unique among the quinolones because of its wider coverage; it is a potent inhibitor of gram-negative anaerobes and has some activity against resistant gram-positive organisms including MRSA and Vancomycin resistant enterococcus (VRE). Quinolones were used to treat urinary tract infections and are still excellent drugs because of their elevated urine concentrations, but trovafloxacin is an exception; trovafloxacin is not eliminated by the kidneys, and thus it should not be first choice for treatment of such infections. Trouafloxacin now is restricted only to serious infections requiring hospitalization because of suspected hepatotoxicity. Quinolones are good substitutes for aminoglycosides, and based on their broad-spectrum coverage, newer quinolones could be used as empiric monotherapy for certain ICU infections or in combination with other antimicrobials if highly resistant organisms are suspected.

Fluoroquinolones are remarkable for their broad coverage, including atypical intracellular organisms, and are preferred over aminoglycosides for gram-negative infections because of their safety profile.

Glycopeptides (Vancomycin)

Vancomycin and teicoplanin are active only against gram-positive organisms. Vancomycin has a higher intrinsic activity against coagulase-negative staphylococci. Vancomycin, introduced around 40 years ago, has been the only drug available for effective treatment of resistant gram-positive organisms including MRSA and certain enterococcus species. Unfortunately, the use of broad-spectrum antimicrobials and vancomycin has led to a drastic increase in resistance to vancomycin. Results from the National Nosocomial Infections

Vancomycin-resistant strains of *Enterococcus* are on the rise in many ICUs and are potential reservoirs for resistance gene transmission to *Staphylococcus* strains.

Surveillance (NNIS) revealed that enterococcal vancomycin resistance increased from 0.4% to 13.6% in nosocomial infections over 3–5 years. In the past few years, several centers have reported strains of staphylococci with intermediate levels (MIC, 4–8 μg/ml) of resistance to vancomycin and teicoplanin; these were named glycopeptide-intermediate *Staphylococcus aureus* (GISA). Nonetheless, whenever MRSA infections are suspected in an ICU endemic with MRSA, vancomycin must be included in the empiric therapy. Last, vancomycin also has an important role in the treatment of resistant or severe *Clostridium difficile* colitis.

Sulfonamides

Sulfonamides are less effective compared to the available broad-spectrum antibiotics, and except under certain circumstances, they are not first-line therapy in the ICU. Sulfamethoxazole (SMX) is combined with trimethoprin (TMP) because of its in vitro synergistic activity. Sulfonamides inhibit a variety of aerobic gram-positive and negative bacteria, *Nocardia*, *Actinomyces*, protozoa (*Toxoplasma*, *Pneumocystis carinii*), and *Chlamydia*. TMP-SMX (Bactrim, Septra) use in ICUs is often limited to patients known to have susceptible organisms, or to immunocompromised patients suspected to have protozoal infections. On the other hand, SMX/TMP may be given as an adjunctive therapy for certain resistant nosocomial infections, such as against *Stenotrophomonas maltophilia* and *Staphylococcus* infections, because of its synergistic activity.

Macrolides (Erythromycin, Azithromycin)

The two newer macrolides, azithromycin and clarithromycin, have surpassed the spectrum of erythromycin; however, only azithromycin is available in intravenous formulation. All three agents cover gram-positive and gram-negative bacteria along with atypical organisms (*Legionella*, *Mycoplasma*, *Chlamydia*). They are usually drugs of choice for penicillin-allergic patients. The newer macrolides have the advantage over erythromycin of lower side effects, more favorable pharmacokinetics, and enhanced potency against atypical organisms as well as *Mycobacterium avium intracellulare* (MAI), *Helicobacter pylori*, *Moraxella catarrhalis*, and *Neisseria gonorrhoeae*. Even with the added properties of azithromycin, it is not preferred as first-line therapy in ICUs because of its unpredictable coverage against both gram-positive and gram-negative resistant bacteria. During a *Legionella* nosocomial outbreak, azithromycin, or a fluoroquinolone, should be included in the antimicrobial regimen.

Clindamycin and Metronidazole

Clindamycin and metronidazole are well known for their potent activity against gram-positive (*Peptostreptococcus*) and gram-negative (*Bacteroides fragilis* group) anaerobic organisms. Clindamycin also inhibits MSSA and other streptococcal species as well as toxoplasmosis and actinomycosis, accounting for its use for treatment of serious anaerobic infections above the diaphragm. *Clostridium difficile* and a small percentage of *Bacteroides* species, which are found most frequently below the diaphragm, are resistant to clindamycin but not to metronidazole; accordingly, metronidazole is the preferable agent for the treatment of anaerobic abdominal and genital infections. In the ICU, both agents are competing with the extended-spectrum penicillins (piperacillin, ticarcillin) for suspected anaerobic infections, but metronidazole maintains the lead for the treatment of *Clostridium difficile* infections.

> In general, for suspected anaerobic infections below the diaphragm, metronidazole is the preferable agent.

Tetracyclines

Doxycycline and minocycline are available for intravenous injection. Tetracyclines inhibit numerous gram-positive and gram-negative organisms, but in view of increased resistance, their use in ICUs is limited to atypical infections (*Borrelia*, *Brucella*, *Chlamydia*, *Coxiella*, *Rickettsia*).

Quinupristin-Dalfopristin and Linezolid

Quinupristin-dalfopristin (Synercid) and linezolid may be effective in the treatment of vancomycin-resistant *Enterococcus faecium* infections, when no alternative treatment is available, and treatment of *Staphylococcus aureus* and *Streptococcus* species causing skin infections and nosocomial pneumonias. The clinical efficacy of quinupristin-dalfopristin for vancomycin-resistant infection has ranged from 52% to 70%. These agents have no gram-negative coverage.

Chloramphenicol

The new emergence of resistant gram-positive organisms (such as MRSA and methicillin-resistant coagulase-negative staphylococci, vancomycin resistant enterococcus (VRE), and penicillin-resistant pneumococci) is becoming a serious threat in clinical practice because of limited alternative therapy. Chloramphenicol, an old antibiotic that was abandoned because of its toxicity, and tetracyclines are returning to the ICU as another approach to treat some of these multiresistant organisms.

Pharmacology and Adverse Effects

Although it is simple to find antibiotic dosage in many books, care should be taken to individualize the therapy in the ICU because of critical illness-altered physiology and drug interactions. Most references give the dosing according to severity of infection, and as discussed earlier, one should rather guide the therapy by the susceptibility of the suspected organisms. Successful treatment is determined not only by availability of potent antibacterials but also by tolerability to these drugs. Maximizing therapeutic effects of a certain regimen while minimizing its toxicity can be executed by tailoring drug dosing according to principles of pharmacokinetics (bioavailability, volume of distribution, and clearance) and pharmacodynamics (relationship between drug movement and pharmacologic response).

Treat infections according to organism susceptibility rather than severity of the patient's illness. Be aware of factors that may alter the pharmacokinetics of your antibiotic of choice, such as renal insufficiency, severe malnutrition, and drug interactions.

The rational approach to dosing that relies on pharmacology can be summarized as follows: (1) the volume of distribution determines the loading dose; (2) the elimination rate, that is, clearance (excretion and metabolism), at a steady state determines the maintenance dose; (3) three to five half-lives are needed to attain steady-state plasma levels; and (4) adverse drug events are preventable by optimizing their levels and considering drug interaction. Almost all critically ill patients are inflicted with one or more system dysfunction that may affect protein binding, volume of distribution, and clearance. Drug interactions can increase or decrease drug effects, thus possibly increasing the risk for toxicity or therapeutic failure. Careful consideration of these factors should eliminate most adverse reactions but not those caused by hypersensitivity reactions, alteration in the normal bacterial flora, or idiosyncratic events, which are reactions not often related to dose or concentration. In the ICU setting, except for specific infections, the parenteral route is always used to deliver antibiotics to maximize their bioavailability.

Penicillins

Penicillins are nonuniform regarding their protein binding, and the volume of distribution is inversely related to the degree of protein binding. Their half-life is relatively short (0.3–1.5 h), requiring frequent doses per day, and most are renally excreted (50%–90%), requiring dose adjustment in renal failure but not in hepatic failure. Nafcillin is an exception in this class because it is cleared by the liver. Shortening the dosing interval as well as increasing the dose should be considered when the volume of distribution is significantly increased.

Nafcillin is the only penicillin cleared by hepatic metabolism.

Side Effects Penicillins are relatively safe agents, and their dose-related toxicity is of less concern than their hypersensitivity reactions; allergic reactions to penicillins have been reported to occur in 0.7%–10.0% of patients, but severe life-threatening reactions are rare (1 per 100,000 cases treated). The real inconvenience of allergic reactions, after they have been documented and treated, derives from cross-reactivity with all other penicillins, cephalosporins, and carbapenems (imipenem), which precludes the use of these antibacterials. Allergic reactions may be manifested as a simple rash, urticaria, serum sickness, exfoliative dermatitis, and anaphylaxis. Even interstitial nephritis, usually seen after prolonged and large doses of methicillin, may be immunologically mediated as a form of delayed hypersensitivity. If penicillins are the only effective therapy available, skin testing and desensitization should be performed before administration of these agents. Dose-related side effects observed with some penicillins include salt and volume overload (ticarcillin), neurotoxicity (penicillin G), and bleeding secondary to impaired platelet aggregation (ticarcillin). Reversible neutropenia (methicillin), thrombocytopenia, and hypokalemia and *Clostridium difficile* colitis are other nondose-related adverse reactions that may be seen with these antibiotics.

Hypersensitivity reactions are the most common side effects of cephalosporins and penicillins. There is a certain degree of cross-reactivity between these two classes and carbapenems; in the event of serious allergic reaction to one of the three classes, antibiotics from the other two classes should be avoided.

Drug Interactions Probenecid competes with the renal tubular secretion of penicillins and has been used to potentiate therapy. Mezlocillin and azlocillin reduce the clearance of cefotaxime and azlocillin may increase levels of ciprofloxacin. Nafcillin inhibits efficacy of warfarin and reduces cyclosporine levels.

Cephalosporins

Like penicillins, there is a significant variation within the cephalosporins in their degree of protein binding and volume of distribution. Although most are renally excreted, hepatic metabolism and biliary elimination are important clearance mechanisms for some agents in this group (cefoperazone, cefoxitin, ceftriaxone). Doses of most cephalosporins should be adjusted in the presence of hepatic or renal insufficiency.

Side Effects Cephalosporins are also similar to penicillins in regard to their adverse reactions. Hypersensitivity reactions are the most common side effects. Associated coagulation abnormalities, gastrointestinal symptoms, phlebitis, fever (<1%), anaphylactic reactions (<0.02%), and overgrowth of resistant organisms and toxigenic *Clostridium difficile* also occur. Studies have reported 1%–20% allergy cross-reactivity between penicillins and cephalosporins. Patients who had a severe allergic reaction to penicillins should not be given cephalosporins because they are at risk to develop a similar reaction, and penicillin skin testing does not predict cephalosporin anaphylactic reactions.

Drug Interactions Probenecid decreases the renal clearance of many cephalosporins (cefazolin, cefotaxime, cefuroxime). A group of cephalosporins containing the 1-*N*-methyl-5-tetrathiozolethiol (NMTT) side chain (cefamandole, cefotetan, cefoperazone) have an additive anticoagulant effect to warfarin causing excessive bleeding.

Carbapenems

Imipenem is metabolized in the renal tubules and is combined with cilastatin, an inhibitor of dehydropeptidase I, causing a reduction in its renal toxicity and a reduction in its metabolic clearance by the renal tubules. Meropenem is not degraded by the renal peptidase and does not require cilastatin. Both carbapenems have a half-life of 1 h and are renally excreted. Imipenem is 20% protein bound and penetrates into the neurons, which may explain its epileptogenic potential.

Side Effects As with other β-lactams, hypersensitivity reactions are the most common adverse reactions, and cross-reactivity with penicillins have been reported. Among the β-lactams, carbapenems are unique in their potential to induce seizures (0.2%); seizures are likely related to carbapenem overdosing in patients with risk factors including old age, preexisting central nervous system disease, and renal failure. Meropenem is known to have a less epileptogenic potential than imipenem.

Drug Interactions Concurrent therapy of imipenem with ganciclovir or theophylline may increase risk for seizures.

Aztreonam The pharmacokinetic properties of aztreonam are similar to other β-lactams. Its serum half-life is 1.7 h, and it is excreted mostly in the urine; its elimination decreases in renal failure.

Side Effects Interestingly, aztreonam produces fewer hypersensitivity reactions and has no allergy cross-reactivity with penicillins or other β-lactams. Nausea, vomiting, rash, and isolated rise in transaminases have been reported, but most reactions occur at the site of injection.

Aminoglycosides

Aminoglycosides are hydrophilic and polycationic compounds. Protein binding of aminoglycosides is low; they diffuse mainly into extracellular fluids and have a large volume of distribution (25%–30% of ideal body weight), increasing with protein depletion. Aminoglycosides are not metabolized and are cleared almost exclusively by glomerular filtration. Therefore, dosing should be adjusted according to the milieu they are being administered into and to renal function because of their narrow therapeutic window. Because of their toxicity profile, monitoring of aminoglycoside levels is important. The concentration-dependent killing and PAE of aminoglycoside, together with the fact that their uptake across the brush border of proximal renal tubular cells is saturable, have shifted aminoglycoside dosing frequency from intermittent dosing to once daily. Although there are enough data to suggest that once-daily administration of aminoglycosides is as effective as intermittent administration, and possibly less nephrotoxic and ototoxic, there is limited information on such a practice in patients with renal insufficiency, women who are pregnant, and subgroups of critically ill patients, such as those with neutropenia, burns, sepsis, and endocarditis. Until future studies clarify the role of once-daily dosing, intermittent administration of these drugs is recommended for these latter conditions.

Side Effects Aminoglycosides are known for their dose-related nephrotoxicity, ototoxicity, and neuromuscular paralysis. Fortunately, these adverse reactions vary widely and are reversible. Nephrotoxicity ranges from being asymptomatic with enzymuria to acute renal failure, which has been associated with the elevated trough serum aminoglycoside levels and potentiated by hypotension, exposure to other nephrotoxic drugs, female sex, and liver disease. Ototoxicity of aminoglycosides includes vestibular damage, causing vertigo, and cochlear damage, causing hearing loss. Neuromuscular paralysis is likely to appear with concurrent administration of neuromuscular blocking agents or with coexisting neuromuscular pathology. Other infrequent dose-independent adverse reactions include allergic reactions and *C. difficile* colitis.

> Aminoglycosides have a narrow therapeutic window and are well known for their nephrotoxicity and ototoxicity. Once-daily dosing may be the preferable dosing interval to maximize killing and decrease adverse effects.

Drug Interactions Aminoglycosides have an additive renal toxicity when given with other nephrotoxic drugs (cephalothin, amphotericin B, cisplatin, vancomycin, cyclosporine), an additive ototoxicity with ethacrynic acid and possibly with furosemide, and a cumulative effect with nondepolarizing muscle relaxant (vecuronium, atracurium). Nonsteroidal anti-inflammatory drugs (NSAIDs) reduce the renal clearance of aminoglycosides, hence raising their trough levels.

Fluoroquinolones

Except for trovafloxacin, quinolones are eliminated mostly by urinary excretion and to a smaller extent by biliary secretion. They have a relatively long half-life (>4 h), and their plasma protein binding ranges from 20% to 40%. Although the dose of trovafloxacin should be adjusted for patients with liver disease, adequate doses for patients with hepatic insufficiency are not well documented, even for older quinolones. Care is needed when prescribing trovafloxacin to a patient with liver disease because it has been associated with liver enzyme abnormalities, hepatitis, liver necrosis, and pancreatitis.

Side Effects Side effects include gastrointestinal symptoms (nausea, anorexia, vomiting, diarrhea), photosensitivity (skin reactions), and neurologic symptoms (dizziness, headaches, agitation, seizures). Quinolones are pregnancy category C (may interfere with skeletal formation), and their safety has not been established in the pediatric age group.

Drug Interactions Quinolones inhibit hepatic metabolism of many drugs (theophylline, cyclosporine, midazolam, NSAIDs, warfarin) by inhibiting cytochrome P-4501A2, thus interfering with their clearance and increasing their effect. Although minerals, antacids, sucralfate, and morphine sulfate reduce the absorption of quinolones, they do not interfere with the bioavailability of intravenously administered quinolones. Cimetidine, but not ranitidine, decreases the metabolism and increases the level of ciprofloxacin.

Vancomycin

Vancomycin is not absorbed after oral ingestion but is given orally to treat *Clostridium difficile.* It is also given intraperitoneally in dialysis fluid to treat gram-positive peritonitis in patients on chronic peritoneal dialysis. Vancomycin pharmacology and reactions in this section are those of systemic intravenous therapy. Peak serum levels are achieved 2 h after administration, and its volume of distribution is approximately 40%. Vancomycin is principally eliminated by glomerular filtration and has a variable half-life (3–13 h), and about 55% is bound to serum proteins. Obtaining vancomycin plasma levels is somewhat controversial because there is no evidence that this practice reduces vancomycin toxicity or improves outcome. Dosage nomograms for vancomycin are available and may obviate the need for frequent vancomycin levels. Vancomycin is not removed by conventional hemodialysis, and weekly infusions in end-stage renal disease usually assure adequate peaks and troughs; nonetheless, slow removal of vancomycin may occur during continuous veno-venous hemodialysis (CVVHD). When there is doubt about serum vancomycin concentrations, such as for patients with unstable renal disease, significant hepatic insufficiency, or on CVVHD, levels should be obtained to maintain adequate therapeutic levels.

Side Effects Red-man or red-neck syndrome is an anaphylactoid reaction to vancomycin related to the rapidity of its infusion and is not considered to be a hypersensitivity reaction. Flushing of the upper body, pruritus, angioedema, and in rare cases progression to shock result from histamine release and are prevented by slow administration of vancomycin or by antihistamines. Allergic reactions also occur and should be differentiated from the red-neck syndrome because management of the two conditions is dissimilar. Nephrotoxicity, ototoxicity, thrombophlebitis, and blood dyscrasias have also been reported. It is unclear whether vancomycin is nephrotoxic when used alone; it is likely that it produces additive renal injury when combined with other nephrotoxins. Of more concern is the ototoxicity caused by vancomycin because of its possible irreversibility. Tinnitus and dizziness have preceded hearing loss despite discontinuation of vancomycin. Risk factors to develop ototoxicity include renal failure, old age, and elevated peak vancomycin levels.

Drug Interactions Possible increases in ototoxicity and nephrotoxicity can occur when vancomycin is coadministered with aminoglycosides.

Sulfonamides and Trimethoprim

Trimethoprim has a good tissue penetration and a large volume of distribution that exceeds that of sulfamethoxazole. TMP, SMX, and their metabolites (from hepatic metabolism) are excreted by the kidneys. They are combined in a dose ratio of 1:5 (TMP:SMX), and because the volume of distribution of SMX is much lower than that of TMP, their plasma ratio becomes 1:20 at peak levels, the optimal ratio for synergistic activity. Silver sulfadiazine and mafenide are topical sulfonamides used in the ICU for the prevention of burn-related infections. Silver sulfadiazine is minimally absorbed, but mafenide is more soluble and is readily absorbed, a contributor to its antibacterial activity and side effects.

Side Effects Skin rashes due to hypersensitivity reactions are common. Through its action on the folic acid pathway, TMP interferes with vitamin replacement in patients with megaloblastic anemia and may induce severe but reversible bone marrow suppression; hence, its relative contraindication in patients who are predisposed to have megaloblastic anemia (pregnant, patients on phenytoin, primidone, or barbiturates).

Drug Interactions TMP can increase the effect of digoxin, phenytoin, procainamide, sulfonylureas, warfarin, and zidovudine by either decreasing their renal elimination or decreasing their metabolisms. An increase in myelosuppression of methotrexate, neurotoxicity of amantadine, and nephrotoxicity of cyclosporine have been observed when coadministered with TMP. In addition TMP-SMX may reduce cyclosporine serum levels.

Macrolides (Erythromycin and Azithromycin)

Clarithromycin is not available for parenteral administration. Azithromycin has replaced erythromycin in many ICUs because of its favorable pharmacokinetics, minimal adverse effects, insignificant drug interactions, and lower infusion volume. Macrolides are lipid soluble and distribute extensively into tissues; erythromycin volume of distribution is 0.6 l/kg, and that of azithromycin is 23 l/kg. The half-life of erythromycin is 1.4 h, and that of azithromycin is 68 h, allowing its use as a daily drug. Erythromycin is minimally excreted in the urine and has poor CSF penetration. Hepatic failure interferes with erythromycin metabolism more than renal disease; thus, dose adjustment is to be considered in the former condition. On the other hand, azithromycin is excreted unchanged in the feces.

> Erythromycin decreases the metabolism of many drugs, thus increasing their effects and possibly their toxicities; azithromycin, which has trivial side effects and drug interactions, has outflanked erythromycin.

Side Effects Gastrointestinal reactions and thrombophlebitis are common side effects during erythromycin therapy; however, incidence is lower with the newer macrolides. Hypersensitivity reactions, cholestatic hepatitis, and reversible deafness are rare but more serious adverse reactions of erythromycin. Hepatitis is related to the estolate salt preparation of erythromycin and not to intravenous therapy with erythromycin lactobionate or gluceptate; therefore, a history of hepatitis after oral erythromycin is not a contraindication for the use of intravenous erythromycin or azithromycin. Expectedly, some patients who developed hypersensitivity reactions to azithromycin, including anaphylaxis, and who were treated had relapse of their allergic symptoms after discontinuation of therapy despite no further exposure to azithromycin, which is likely caused by its slow release from tissues.

Drug Interactions Erythromycin induces liver microsomal enzymes and decreases the oxidative metabolism of many drugs. These effects are observed to a lesser degree with clarithromycin and not at all with azithromycin. Erythromycin increases the effects, hence causing possible toxicity, of the following drugs: carbamazepine, valproic acid, phenytoin, theophylline, warfarin, cyclosporine, digoxin, cisapride, lovastatin, methylprednisolone, midazolam, zidovudine, bromocriptine, and ergotamine. Careful observation is required when erythromycin is given with these drugs, especially when it is coadministered with cimetidine, which increases the level of erythromycin.

ANTIFUNGAL DRUGS

Fungal infections are commonly seen in some ICUs because of their selected patient populations and overuse of broad-spectrum antibiotics. Compared with antibacterials and antivirals, antifungals did not witness the same rate of proliferation. Amphotericin B remains the most potent antifungal used to treat most serious deep mycotic infections and fungemias.

> Amphotericin B remains the most potent antifungal agent and is reserved for life-threatening and resistant fungal infections because of its grave toxicities.

Newer azole antifungal agents are either reserved for less severe infections or used in combination with amphotericin B.

Mechanisms of Action and Resistance

Amphotericin B alters the cell membrane permeability of susceptible fungi, resulting in cell lysis and increased uptake of 5-flucytosine (another synthetic antifungal) that inhibits fungal growth. Similarly, azole antifungal agents (ketoconazole, fluconazole, itraconazole) exert their action by inhibiting cell wall synthesis and causing cell lysis. Resistance against amphotericin B is uncommon and is usually not considered the prime reason for failure except in certain subgroups of patients, such as bone marrow transplant patients, in whom it occurs with selected organisms, such as *Candida glabrata*. In contrast, acquired resistance to ketoconazole and fluconazole has been reported with chronic therapy, mainly against certain fungal species such as *Candida albicans*.

Spectrum of Coverage

Amphotericin B

Amphotericin B has a broad antifungal activity covering *Cryptococcus neoformans*, *Blastomyces dermatitis*, *Histoplasma capsulatum*, *Coccidioides immitis*, *Sporotrichium schenkii*, the various *Candida* species (*albicans*, *tropicalis*, *glabrata*), *Aspergillus* species (*niger*, *flavus*, *fumigatus*), and the zygomycoses (*Mucor*, *Absidia*, *Rhizopus*). Chromomycosis are resistant to amphotericin B but may be suppressed by the combination of amphotericin and 5-flucytosine. This additive effect has been also observed when amphotericin B is combined with 5-flucytosine against other fungal infections; this led to recommending this combined therapy for cryptococcal meningitis and possibly for severe candidal and aspergillus infections. However, the same has not been reported when amphotericin B was added to the azoles. For that reason, some clinicians are reluctant to use amphotericin B with itraconazole or fluconazole. Alternatively, the newer lipid formulations of amphotericin B (see pharmacology of amphotericin B) may substitute the combination of amphotericin B-flucytosine for refractory fungal infections. The lipid formulations of amphotericin B are indicated for the treatment of patients who are unresponsive or intolerant to therapy with the traditional amphotericin B (amphotericin B deoxycholate) because the lipid formulations have been shown to reduce the incidence of nephrotoxicity and possibly to improve the therapeutic efficacy of amphotericin B.

Fluconazole

Fluconazole is also a broad-spectrum antifungal having activity against most *Candida* species, *Cryptococcus neoformans*, *Histoplasma capsulatum*, *Coccidioides immitis*, *Blastomyces dermatitis*, *Sporotrichium schenkii*, and others. In contrast to amphotericin B, some *Candida* species (*krusei*), *Aspergillus* species, and the mucormycosis may be resistant to fluconazole. Fluconazole has been proven as an effective alternative therapy to amphotericin B in the treatment of less severe cryptococcal meningitis as well as some uncomplicated systemic and urinary tract fungal infections. It has also been used as maintenance therapy after fungal meningitis in immunocompromised patients.

Ketoconazole

Ketoconazole has an antifungal coverage similar to that of fluconazole but is less frequently used in the ICU because of its unfavorable pharmacokinetics and its availability in oral formulation only. Ketoconazole is mostly reserved for treatment of blastomycosis, histoplasmosis, coccidiomycosis, and paracoccidiomycosis in noncritically ill patients.

Itraconazole

Itraconazole is more potent than ketoconazole and has a better activity against some *Aspergillus* species and sporotrichosis. Itraconazole is the preferred treatment for nonmeningeal aspergillosis, disseminated blastomycosis, disseminated histoplasmosis, pulmonary paracoccidioides, and sporotrichosis.

Pharmacology and Adverse Effects

Amphotericin B

Amphotericin B has been delivered intrathecally, intraperitoneally, as bladder irrigation, as an aerosol, and intravenously. The discussion in this section is limited to intravenous administration. There are two preparations of amphotericin B; the older formulation is a colloidal preparation at a dosage of 0.5 mg/kg/day. The second formulation is a lipophilic preparation made by incorporating the parent compound into lipid complexes (liposomal amphotericin B, amphotericin B colloidal dispersion known as ABCD, and amphotericin B lipid complex known as ABLC) at 3–5 mg/kg/day, resulting in increased delivery of amphotericin B to fungal cells and decreased free toxic amphotericin. In addition, lipid formulations bypass the kidneys and allow higher hepatocytes and erythrocytes penetration, thus allowing for a larger dose of amphotericin B to be administered while minimizing their toxic effects. The metabolism of both traditional and lipid complex amphotericin B is not influenced by renal or hepatic function.

Side Effects Because of possible severe febrile reactions, malaise, generalized aches, and vomiting, a test dose of 1 mg of amphotericin and premedications with acetaminophen, antiemetic, and antihistamine are given. Some patients require meperidine and hydrocortisone for severe infusion-related toxicity. Other reported adverse reactions to amphotericin B include hypertension, hypotension, hypothermia, anemia, neurotoxicity, cardiotoxicity, and renal failure with severe hypokalemia and hypomagnesemia. Nephrotoxicity is potentiated by sodium depletion, and sodium loading has been found to attenuate renal injury caused by amphotericin. Lipid formulations cause less nephrotoxicity and local infusion reactions, but unfortunately their costs are prohibitive for indiscriminate use.

Drug Interactions An additive renal toxicity effect may occur with other nephrotoxic drugs, such as cyclosporine and aminoglycosides. Ticarcillin can potentiate the hypokalemia caused by amphotericin B. The combination of amphotericin B and the antineoplastic agent cytosine arabinoside has been associated with parkinsonism.

Fluconazole

Fluconazole (100–400 mg/day) is available in both oral and intravenous formulation. It is unique among the azoles by its excellent bioavailability after oral administration and by its high penetration across the blood–brain barrier. Fluconazole is minimally bound to plasma protein, hence its low potential for drug interactions, and is excreted almost exclusively unchanged by glomerular filtration.

Side Effects Fluconazole is well tolerated with minimal adverse effects. A reversible transaminitis has been reported, and gastrointestinal upset is the most common adverse event.

Drug Interaction Among the azoles, fluconazole has the weakest inhibitory effect on human microsomal P-450 enzymes; nevertheless, increased levels of cyclosporine and phenytoin and an exaggerated effect of coumadin have been observed. Moreover, the half-life of fluconazole is significantly reduced with coadministration of rifampin.

Ketoconazole

Ketoconazole is only available in oral preparation, and although food does not interfere with its absorption, gastric acidity should be normal for adequate absorption of the drug; any cause of achlorhydria will cause malabsorption of ketoconazole. Ketoconazole is 99% protein bound with negligible penetration into the cerebrospinal fluid. It is metabolized by the liver, then eliminated by biliary excretion.

Side Effects Most adverse effects of ketoconazole are gastrointestinal and endocrinologic in nature, and they include anorexia, nausea, vomiting, impotence, gynecomastia, menstrual irregularities, decreased synthesis of cortisol, and alopecia. In addition, up to 10% of patients receiving ketoconazole have a transaminitis and rarely develop fulminant hepatitis ($<0.01\%$).

Drug Interactions Antacids, including H2-blockers, sucralfate, and proton pump inhibitors, inhibit absorption of ketoconazole. On the other hand, ketoconazole alters the metabolism of a myriad of drugs including antibiotics, antivirals, antiepileptics, cardiac medications, and immunosuppressants. Careful consideration for drug interaction when ketoconazole is administered during polypharmacology is crucial to avoid iatrogenic catastrophes.

Itraconazole

Itraconazole shares many properties with ketoconazole in its pharmacology, adverse reactions, and drug interactions because both agents inhibit metabolism through the cytochrome P-450 isoenzyme 3A4; itraconazole is less potent compared to ketoconazole, thus has a more favorable pharmacologic and toxic profile. The absorption of the oral formulation of itraconazole may be variable and erratic; therefore, there may be a need to follow drug levels. Moreover, although itraconazole plasma levels may be much lower than those of ketoconazole, itraconazole has a much longer half-life (15–42 h), a much higher tissue penetration, and a bioactive hepatic metabolite, resulting in a superior therapeutic profile.

ANTIVIRAL DRUGS

The ongoing fight against human immunodeficiency virus (HIV) disease has spawned a large number of effective retroviral and antiviral agents. In addition, and with the recent understanding of viral immunology, newer agents that augment the host response, such as interferons and exogenous antibodies, have been also introduced to control various viral infections. Both immunomodulators and HIV retroviral agents are usually introduced in an outpatient setting rather than for critically ill patients. This section briefly reviews antiviral agents more relevant to the ICU patient and excludes retroviral HIV therapy.

Mechanisms of Action and Resistance

Antivirals are limited in their activity and are virustatic rather than virucidal. They exhibit their antiviral activity by inhibiting viral attachment to the cell, viral macromolecular synthesis, progeny virion assembly, or by uncoating the viral genome. The majority of the available antiviral agents used in the ICU are nucleoside analogues (acyclovir, ganciclovir, ribavarin), targeting either DNA or RNA polymerases and blocking their genomic synthesis. Other agents, such as amantadine and rimantadine, inhibit viral replication by uncoating the organism and releasing its genome in lysosomes. DNA polymerases of different viruses differ in their susceptibility to the inhibition by antivirals; however, resistance results from either reduced phosphorylation of the antiviral agent and mutations in DNA polymerases (acyclovir, ganciclovir) or reduced intracellular uptake of the agent (ganciclovir). Clinically, 8% of herpes simplex virus (HSV) are resistant to acyclovir, and 8% of cytomegalovirus (CMV) are resistant to ganciclovir in immunosuppressed patients, with the frequency of resistance increasing after prolonged exposure to both agents. In contrast to other antivirals, emergence of resistance in susceptible respiratory syncytial virus (RSV) strains against ribavarin has not been documented.

Spectrum of Coverage

Acyclovir and Valacyclovir

Acyclovir and valacyclovir, which is completely converted to acyclovir after oral administration, are indicated for herpesvirus infections. They are more potent against HSV-1 and

HSV-2 than against varicella zoster virus (VZV), and are least active against CMV. Acyclovir is the drug of choice for the treatment of HSV encephalitis, varicella (chickenpox), and recurrent herpes zoster (shingles) infections. It is effective in reducing the incidence of HSV and VZV infections in seropositive transplantation patients and possibly in treating viscerally disseminated HSV infections. Acyclovir inhibits Epstein–Barr virus (EBV) but does not affect persistent or latent infections, and its usefulness to treat severe EBV complications (hepatitis, lymphoproliferative disease) is unclear.

Ganciclovir

Ganciclovir is used for the treatment and prophylaxis of CMV infections, mostly in immunocompromised patients. It is less potent against HSV and VZV, and 10- to 100-fold more potent against CMV than acyclovir, but is limited to serious infections because of its toxicity. Except for central nervous system CMV infections, in general, there is a consistent clinical improvement in AIDS patients and solid organ transplant patients with CMV pneumonia and gastrointestinal infections. In bone marrow transplant recipients, improved mortality from CMV pneumonia is observed only if ganciclovir is given with immunoglobulin.

Amantadine and Rimantadine

Amantadine and rimantadine, a methylated analogue of amantadine with similar efficacy, are limited to prevention and treatment of influenza A infections. They are recommended in hospitals and in ICUs mostly as prophylaxis during nosocomial influenza A outbreaks, but they have not been shown to alter the outcome of influenza A infections in critically ill patients with underlying lung disease (obstructive airway disease, interstitial lung disease) or in patients with life-threatening primary influenza A pneumonia.

Ribavarin

Ribavarin has in vitro activity against influenza A, B, parainfluenza, respiratory syncytial virus (RSV), Lassa virus, and bunyaviruses. Ribavarin is effective in uncomplicated RSV respiratory infections; however, in critically ill immunocompromised patients with RSV pneumonia, aerosolized ribavarin requires the addition of immunoglobulin to improve outcome. Moreover, ribavarin is recommended for the treatment of complicated Lassa fever, hemorrhagic fevers with renal syndrome, and hantavirus pulmonary syndrome. Its role against severe parainfluenza, measles, vaccinia, and adenovirus infections is uncertain.

Zanamivir and Oseltamivir

Zanamivir and oseltamivir have been recently introduced to the United States market for the treatment of influenza A and B. Both agents are effective for treatment and prophylaxis of acute influenza, but their role in the ICU is not yet defined. Clinical studies should determine their effect on outcome of patients with significant pulmonary disease complicated by influenza infections or patients with severe primary influenza pneumonia.

Pharmacology and Adverse Effects

Acyclovir and Valacyclovir

The bioavailability of acyclovir is only 15%–30% after oral administration but is three to five times greater after oral intake of valacyclovir. Acyclovir is available in intravenous formulation, distributes widely in body fluids, and is less than 20% bound to protein. Acyclovir is mostly cleared by the kidneys and is hemodialyzable.

Toxicity from acyclovir is often related to high levels of the drug in the presence of renal insufficiency.

Side Effects Intravenous acyclovir has been associated with reversible neurotoxicity (confusion, delirium, seizures, extrapyramidal signs, autonomic instability) and renal insufficiency from either crystalline obstructive nephropathy or interstitial nephritis. Patients who develop neurotoxicity tend to have renal failure and high acyclovir serum levels.

Drug Interactions Neurotoxicity and nephrotoxicity may be potentiated by administration of other neurotoxic (seizures during concurrent therapy with ciprofloxacin) and nephrotoxic (cyclosporine) agents while on acyclovir.

Ganciclovir

Ganciclovir has adequate tissue and CSF penetration and negligible protein binding after intravenous administration. Ganciclovir intravitreal implants are effective to treat CMV retinitis and cause no systemic toxicity. Ganciclovir is exclusively excreted via the kidneys, and 60% cleared after hemodialysis.

Side Effects Ganciclovir has a low therapeutic to toxic ratio. It is known for its reversible myelosuppression (neutropenia, thrombocytopenia), which occurs more commonly in AIDS patients as compared to transplant recipients. Neurotoxicity (headaches, confusion, psychosis, seizures, and coma), nephrotoxicity, fever, hepatic abnormalities, and gastrointestinal symptoms are also common. Ganciclovir is teratogenic, embryotoxic, and carcinogenic in animals and possibly humans.

Drug Interactions Ganciclovir raises the concentration of other retroviral drugs and possibly cyclosporine. Nephrotoxic agents may alter ganciclovir clearance and increase its toxicity.

Ribavarin

Ribavarin is available in oral, intravenous, and aerosolized preparations. Plasma ribavarin concentrations are much higher after intravenous delivery compared to oral and aerosol administration, but respiratory secretion levels after aerosol therapy far exceed ribavarin infusion. Distribution and elimination of ribavarin is complex; ribavarin concentrates in erythrocytes and is cleared through renal and hepatic metabolism

Side Effects Systemic ribavarin has neurologic (headaches, lethargy), gastrointestinal, and hematologic adverse effects. Anemia, which may require dose adjustment, is reversible and may be due to either extravascular hemolysis or bone marrow suppression. Aerosolized ribavarin has not been associated with adverse hematologic effects.

Drug Interactions Adverse drug interactions have not been described with ribavarin therapy.

SUMMARY

Antimicrobials are indispensable in the ICU but are not a panacea for all infections. Preventive measures against nosocomial infections and judicious use of antimicrobials are pivotal to minimize complications that often overwhelm vulnerable critically ill patients. When faced with refractory febrile illnesses and suspected malignant infectious diseases, and before inundating patients with antimicrobials, common sense and clinical judgement require ample knowledge of antimicrobial pharmacology to avoid causing iatrogenic injuries and breeding resistant organisms. Failing antiinfectious therapy is not always indicative of ineffective antimicrobials and should prompt investigation to ensure optimal drug dosing, absence of superinfections, and exclusion of drainable abscesses before changing the antibiotics.

REVIEW QUESTIONS

1. **A 60-year-old man with a history of rheumatoid arthritis maintained on prednisone presents with high-grade temperature, productive cough, and diffuse bilateral patchy infiltrates on chest radiograph. You decide to start antibiotics for the treatment of a community-acquired pneumonia. An appropriate antibiotic therapy for this patient is:**
   - **A.** Clindamycin or metronidazole
   - **B.** Levofloxacin or azithromycin
   - **C.** Imipenem or cefepime
   - **D.** Trimethoprin/sulfamethoxazole or aztreonam

2. **Dose adjustment of the majority of penicillins and carbapenems should be made:**
   - **A.** In patients with renal failure
   - **B.** In patients with hepatic failure
   - **C.** In patients receiving warfarin or cyclosporine
   - **D.** In malnourished patients
   - **E.** In patients allergic to penicillins

3. **For a patient diagnosed with staphylococcal bacteremia:**
   - **A.** Vancomycin is the treatment of choice regardless of drug susceptibility.
   - **B.** Vancomycin with or without gentamicin should be used only if the patient is known to have a penicillin allergy or MRSA.
   - **C.** Oxacillin with gentamicin is the treatment of choice, even if the organism is an MRSA.
   - **D.** Vancomycin is as effective as oxacillin for MSSA.

4. **A patient with an abdominal sepsis who is being treated with metronidazole, gentamicin, and ampicillin starts to develop progressive renal failure. The most appropriate step in managing his antibiotic therapy is to:**
   - **A.** Adjust the doses of gentamicin, ampicillin, and metronidazole
   - **B.** Discontinue gentamicin and continue ampicillin and metronidazole
   - **C.** Continue metronidazole and substitute cefotaxime for gentamicin and ampicillin
   - **D.** Continue metronidazole and substitute aztreonam for gentamicin and vancomycin for ampicillin

5. **Acyclovir and valacyclovir are indicated for the treatment of:**
   - **A.** Life-threatening CMV infections
   - **B.** EBV hepatitis
   - **C.** Suspected HSV encephalitis
   - **D.** Influenza A pneumonia

6. **The different lipid formulations of amphotericin B:**
   - **A.** All have similar tissue penetration
   - **B.** Have been shown to be more effective than amphotericin B deoxycholate in the treatment of all fungal infections
   - **C.** Allow the administration of more amphotericin B with less nephrotoxicity
   - **D.** Need dose adjustment in the presence of renal insufficiency
   - **E.** Should be used with other azole antifungal for synergy in life-threatening yeast infections

7. **A patient with chronic obstructive pulmonary disease was admitted to the intensive care unit for treatment of theophylline toxicity and right lower lobe pneumonia. The most appropriate antibiotic for this patient is:**
   - **A.** Cefuroxime
   - **B.** Ciprofloxacin
   - **C.** Erythromycin
   - **D.** Vancomycin
   - **E.** Imipenem

8. **The concentration-dependent killing effect of antibiotics:**
   - **A.** Is only seen in antibiotics that have synergy with other agents
   - **B.** Does not occur in commonly used antibiotics
   - **C.** Relies on time of exposure of bacteria to the antibiotic
   - **D.** Indicates that the higher the serum antibiotic concentration, the more the killing effect

ANSWERS

1. The answer is B. The patient is on prednisone and is at risk to have *Legionella* pneumonia, which could not be excluded based on his presentation and findings. Among the listed antibiotics, levofloxacin or azithromycin are appropriate to cover atypical infections. Although some of the remaining antibiotics are potent and allow for broad-spectrum coverage, they do not cover for *Legionella* infection, which is suspected in this patient.
2. The answer is A. Except for nafcillin, penicillins and carbapenems are excreted by the kidney, and their dose should be adjusted in the presence of renal insufficiency.
3. The answer is B. Nafcillin (or oxacillin) is the treatment of choice for staphylococcal infections unless the organism is resistant, e.g., MRSA, or the patient is allergic to penicillins. Vancomycin is less effective than nafcillin to treat MSSA.
4. The answer is C. The patient's renal failure may be caused by acute tubular necrosis from either his sepsis or aminoglycoside or by interstitial nephritis from ampicillin. Because the progression of his renal failure may be in part iatrogenic, and in the presence of many other alternative nonnephrotoxic antibiotics, the most appropriate approach to this patient is to discontinue ampicillin and gentamicin while maintaining the same antibacterial coverage with another agent such as a third-generation cephalosporin or a fluoroquinolone.
5. The answer is C. Ganciclovir is indicated for serious CMV infections. There is no documented benefit from treating EBV hepatitis with acyclovir, which is also ineffective against influenza infections.
6. The answer is C. Lipid formulations of amphotericin B are dissimilar regarding their tissue penetration and so far have not been shown to improve outcome compared to the traditional amphotericin B for all patients. However, clearly they have the advantage of delivering more drug to the site of infection with less toxicity. Synergy has not been documented between amphotericin and the azoles.

7. The answer is A. Ciprofloxacin and erythromycin increase levels of theophylline and hence may exacerbate the patient's theophylline toxicity. Imipenem is epileptogenic and also may induce seizures in this predisposed patient because of underlying theophylline toxicity. Vancomycin is not an appropriate antibiotic for community-acquired pneumonia unless MRSA is documented.

8. The answer is D. Antibiotics that have a concentration-dependent killing effect, such as aminoglycosides, are commonly used in the ICU and rely on concentration above MIC to exert their effect.

SUGGESTED READING

Aoki FY. Principles of Antimicrobial Therapy and the Clinical Pharmacology of Antimicrobial Drugs. Principles of Critical Care, 2nd Ed. New York: McGraw-Hill, 1998.

Hayden FG. Antiviral drugs (other than antiretrovirals). In: Mandell XX (ed) Principles and Practice in Infectious Diseases, 5th Ed. New York: Churchill Livingstone, 2000.

Patel R. Antifungal agents. Part I. Amphotericin B preparations and flucytosine. Mayo Clin Proc 1998;73:1205–1225.

Terrell CL. Antifungal agents. Part II. The azoles. May Clin Proc 1999; 74:78–100.

CHAPTER 44

RODGER E. BARNETTE AND GERARD J. CRINER

Use of Analgesics and Sedatives in Critical Care

CHAPTER OUTLINE

LEARNING OBJECTIVES

After studying this chapter, you should be able to:

- Understand the pharmacokinetics and pharmacodynamics of various sedative/hypnotics and analgesics.
- Be aware of the action of sedative/hypnotics and analgesics on central γ-aminobutyric acid (GABA) and opioid receptor systems.
- Understand the need for routine and effective sedation and analgesia in the critically ill patient.
- Make recommendations regarding the use and dose of sedative/hypnotics and analgesics in the critically ill.
- Recognize that agitation has multiple etiologies and should be investigated as fully as possible prior to treatment.
- Recognize that an agitated patient should not be allowed to cause self-injury or injury to health care personnel.

Most patients admitted to an intensive care unit (ICU) struggle with anxiety, fear, apprehension, and loss of control. In addition, critically ill patients often undergo a variety of diagnostic and therapeutic interventions, most of which are associated with physical discomfort or pain. In some patients, there will be an indication for the use of neuromuscular blocking agents; patients receiving these agents will be completely unable to communicate, so the need for adequate and consistent sedation, anxiolysis, and analgesia will be even more important. Fortunately, a variety of agents and techniques are available to alleviate both pain and anxiety. To safely utilize these methods of pain control and anxiolysis, however, the clinician must possess current knowledge regarding the advantages, disadvantages, and potential side effects of each of these agents.

A number of pharmaceutical agents, originally used exclusively in the operating room by anesthetists, are now used in the ICU. This transfer of new agents is appropriate given that indications for these pharmaceuticals in the ICU are often identical to their indications in the operating room. Prolonged periods of unpleasant and often painful diagnostic or therapeutic modalities should be appropriately treated with analgesics, sedatives, anesthetics, and often paralytics, regardless of the location of the patient.

However, several significant differences set apart the use of potent pharmaceutical agents in the ICU from their use in the operating room. First, in the ICU, these agents are administered to critically ill patients with significant, often multiple, organ system dysfunction. These patients are receiving multiple medications including nutritional support, are often mechanically ventilated, and may have profound alterations in drug metabolism and recep-

TABLE 44-1

DIFFERENCES BETWEEN PATIENT POPULATION IN THE OPERATING ROOM AND ICU THAT AFFECT ANALGESIC AND SEDATIVE DRUG CHOICES

OPERATING ROOM (CLINICAL STUDIES)	ICU (CLINICAL USE)
Younger patients	Older patients
Essentially healthy (usually one surgical issue)	Critically ill (multiple issues; ± multiple organ system dysfunction)
Few or no medications	Multiple medications
Usually well nourished	May be malnourished (± nutritional support)
Short-term mechanical ventilation	Long-term mechanical ventilation
Normal pharmacokinetics	Alterations in elimination half-life
Normal pharmacodynamics	Alterations in drug metabolism
	Changes in receptor function and volume of distribution and clearance.

tor regulation and function. These patients are not the usual population of relatively healthy, young surgical patients chosen for clinical studies involving new anesthetic or paralytic agents (Table 44-1). Elimination half-life, volume of distribution, and drug clearance may be markedly altered in the critically ill population. Second, in the ICU these agents are often administered over days to weeks, whereas in the operating room they are utilized for much shorter periods of time. Finally, many of these agents are administered by continuous infusion in the ICU, while in the operating room administration is often by intermittent injection.

> Alterations in the administration and pharmacokinetics of drugs used in intensive care unit (ICU) patients may lead to a propensity for prolonged action and, in some instances, an increased incidence and severity of side effects.

Because of these differences, initial information regarding new sedative or paralytic agents is often irrelevant to the care of critically ill patients. Additionally, alterations in the administration and pharmacokinetics of drugs used in ICU patients may lead to a propensity for prolonged action and, in some instances, an increased incidence and severity of side effects. These issues must be borne in mind whenever consideration is given to using a relatively new agent, devised for short-term use in the operative patient, in critically ill ICU patients.

ANALGESICS

Pain control in the ICU is of paramount importance. Control of pain with parenteral narcotics, nonsteroidal antiinflammatory agents, and a variety of regional techniques are all satisfactory methods to alleviate patient pain. However, not all pain experienced by critically ill patients is related to diagnostic or therapeutic procedures. It may be related to the disease process, and thus it is important to attempt to understand the etiology of pain before treatment. Adequate evaluation of pain and consideration regarding its significance are crucial.

> Pain is a fiercely subjective experience, and thus any rating system is inexact.

Rating systems, such as the commonly used visual analogue scale or the McGill pain questionnaire, are available for assessment of the intensity of pain but are infrequently used in the clinical setting. Pain is a fiercely subjective experience, and thus any rating system will be inexact. Pain usually consists of two components. There is a constant nociceptive component secondary to the injury or surgery, and there is acute incident pain related to the patient's coughing, deep breathing, or getting out of bed. Complaints regarding pain and discomfort should be given serious attention, and effective control measures should be instituted as rapidly as possible. Patients who are not able to communicate because of endotracheal intubation, sedation, or administration of neuromuscular blocking agents may manifest pain by agitation or changes in heart rate, blood pressure, or respiratory pattern.

> Patients who are not able to communicate because of endotracheal intubation, sedation, or administration of neuromuscular blocking agents may manifest pain by agitation or changes in heart rate, blood pressure, or respiratory pattern.

> Concern regarding addiction and abuse have historically led to inappropriate undermedication and withholding of opioids.

A past history of narcotic abuse or concerns about causing addiction should not be given undue weight by the physician. Concern regarding addiction and abuse have historically led to inappropriate undermedication and withholding of opioids. Conversely, in more than 30% of patients who have been intubated for prolonged periods and received narcotics and benzodiazepines in excess of recommended daily doses, an acute withdrawal state has been described. When administering these types of agents for prolonged time periods, careful titration and avoidance of rapid drug weaning is necessary.

Opioids

There are five classes of opioid receptors: mu (μ), kappa (κ), delta (δ), sigma (σ), and epsilon (ϵ). Of these receptor classes, the μ, κ, and δ receptors are firmly established and have identifiable subtypes. Most of the opioids used in clinical medicine today cause effects at peripheral, spinal, or central sites and mediate their effect largely through the μ receptor. Nalbuphine hydrochloride and butorphanol tartrate are agonists/antagonists and are clinically relevant exceptions. Naloxone, a competitive antagonist, is nonselective for receptor type and is used in a variety of settings to reverse narcotic effects.

In critically ill patients, the clearance of narcotics is often decreased. Because the volume of distribution often changes, the elimination half-life is variably affected (Table 44-2). Therefore administration of these agents must be titrated to clinical effect with careful attention to cardiovascular and respiratory function. There appears to be no difference in the magnitude of side effects associated with μ-receptor-selective opioids when parenterally administered at equianalgesic steady-state concentrations. Issues related to ventilatory depression, sedation, hypoxemia, pruritus, hypotension, increased common bile duct pressure, and nausea are common to all μ-selective agents.

There appears to be no difference in the magnitude of side effects associated with μ-receptor selective opioids when parenterally administered at equianalgesic steady-state concentrations. Issues related to ventilatory depression, sedation, hypoxemia, pruritus, hypotension, increased common bile duct pressure, and nausea are common to all μ-selective agents.

According to several recent surveys, morphine is the narcotic most frequently administered in the critical care setting. Morphine acts through stimulation of peripheral and central receptor systems; however, central effects predominate following parenteral administration. Although morphine may cause histamine release at higher doses, it has the advantage of being well known, inexpensive, and easy to administer. Morphine-6-glucuronide is a potent metabolite that is eliminated by the kidney. It is thought to be responsible for the increased sensitivity to morphine observed in patients with renal failure; for this reason, morphine should be administered cautiously to these patients.

Morphine may be administered intermittently, by continuous intravenous infusion, or via a patient-controlled analgesia device. In a well-staffed and intensively monitored location such as the ICU, there should be no need to administer narcotics on a regular basis via the intramuscular route. Morphine may also be administered via neuraxial technique, as discussed next. There is good evidence that morphine has peripheral actions. It has been shown to have local analgesic actions in animal and clinical studies, although this method of administration has found little clinical application in the critically ill patients.

In a well-staffed and intensively monitored location such as the ICU, there should be no need to administer narcotics on a regular basis via the intramuscular route.

Fentanyl is a narcotic with 50 to 100 times the potency of morphine. It has a rapid onset of action and no active metabolites. It is a μ-selective agonist with little effect on other opiate receptors and produces profound dose-dependent analgesia. At high doses, it can produce loss of consciousness and muscle rigidity. It has a rapid redistribution half-life, measured in minutes, and for that reason is usually administered by continuous infusion in critically ill patients. With high doses, or prolonged administration, there will be saturation of lipophilic redistribution sites, accumulation of drug, and extended clinical effects. Once the lipophilic redistribution sites are saturated, the duration of action of fentanyl is determined by an elim-

TABLE 44-2

OPIOID USE IN CRITICALLY ILL ADULT PATIENTS

OPIOID	ROUTES OF ADMINISTRATION	ELIMINATION HALF-LIFE (h)	INTERMITTENT OR BOLUS DOSE (IV)	CONTINUOUS INFUSION RATE (IV)
Morphine	IV, IM, SC, continuous infusion, PCA	2–4	2–5 mg	1–5 mg/h
Fentanyl	IV, continuous infusion, skin patch	3–6	25–100 μg	50–150 μg/h
Meperidine	IV, IM, SC, PCA	3–4	12.5–50 mg	N/A
Nalbuphine	IV, IM	5	5–10 mg	N/A
Butorphanol	IV, IM	2.5–3.5	1.5–3 mg	N/A

IV, intravenous; IM, intramuscular; SC, subcutaneous; PCA, patient-controlled analgesia; N/A, not available

The executive summary of practice parameters published by the Society of Critical Care Medicine for the administration of intravenous analgesia and sedation in critically ill adults recommends 1–2 μg/kg/h for fentanyl. Although these may be appropriate initiation doses, titration to effect will be necessary in most patients.

ination half-life of approximately 3–6 h. The elderly (>60 years of age) may have a prolonged terminal half-life that is roughly two to three times that of younger individuals. Prolonged elimination or decreased metabolism of fentanyl may be observed in patients with significant hepatic dysfunction. Fentanyl does not cause histamine release, does not cross-react in patients with morphine allergy, and its pharmacokinetics are not altered by renal failure. It has been recommended as the analgesic agent of choice in critically ill, hemodynamically unstable patients. Similar to morphine it may also be administered via a neuraxial technique. The executive summary of practice parameters published by the Society of Critical Care Medicine for the administration of intravenous analgesia and sedation in critically ill adults recommends 1–2 μg/kg/h for fentanyl. These doses may be appropriate for initiation, but titration to effect will be necessary in most patients.

Meperidine has a rapid onset of action when administered intravenously. It binds to both the μ and κ receptors. Through its effect on the κ receptor, it acts as a potent suppressor of shivering and thereby prevents shivering-induced increased metabolic demand. Normeperidine, a metabolite, may accumulate in patients with renal failure and is a convulsant. Meperidine at doses greater than 5 mg/kg has been associated with myocardial depression, and for that reason this agent has never been used as part of an anesthetic technique involving high-dose narcotic administration. For all these reasons, meperidine is used infrequently in the critically ill patient.

Mixed agonist-antagonist opioids such as nalbuphine and butorphanol have an effect at the μ receptor but are less potent than agents such as morphine or fentanyl. In the presence of a potent opioid, these agents may act as μ-receptor antagonists while exerting an agonist effect on other classes of narcotic receptors. For example, nalbuphine has the characteristics of a μ antagonist when given following morphine administration, but has an agonist effect at the κ receptor. Like meperidine, it has a significant suppressive effect on shivering, presumably mediated via the κ receptor.

Lower efficacy opioids, such as nalbuphine and butorphanol, partially depress respiratory drive as opposed to higher efficacy narcotics, which in large doses may completely suppress it. For this reason lower efficacy agents may be combined with more potent opioids, in postoperative settings, to moderate opioid side effects while not completely negating the antinociceptive effect.

Additional potent μ agonists are available, such as alfentanil, sufentanil, and remifentanil. These agents are used primarily in anesthetic care, are expensive, and have little documented advantage over fentanyl. The one exception is remifentanil, which, because of an ester functional group, is susceptible to hydrolysis by blood and tissue esterases; this results in a very rapid breakdown of the drug. These agents have not yet found routine application in the ICU.

Patient-Controlled Analgesia

Patient-controlled analgesia (PCA) allows for consistent therapeutic narcotic blood levels by enabling the patient to time analgesic drug administration and the unit dose, while safeguarding a lockout time between doses and total cumulative dose allowable; parameters set by the physician.

Initial doses for a morphine PCA in an adult patient would be a bolus dose, 1–5 mg; unit dose, 0.5–2.0 mg; lockout time, 10 min between doses; and cumulative 4 h dose, 20 mg.

Patient-controlled analgesia (PCA) is an important analgesic delivery technique. All narcotics have threshold plasma concentrations at which they are effective. PCA allows for consistent therapeutic narcotic blood levels by enabling the patient to time analgesic drug administration. Dose, lockout time between doses, and total cumulative dose are set by the physician. This technique may involve both continuous infusion and concomitant patient control of the interval between unit doses. It is used to provide pain relief following surgery, in patients with cancer, and in the critically ill. However, in many critically ill patients, this technique is not appropriate because of agitation, primary or secondary changes in cognitive function, or severity of illness. Initial doses for a morphine PCA in an adult patient would be a bolus dose of 1–5 mg; unit dose of 0.5–2.0 mg; lockout time of 10 min between doses; and a cumulative 4 h dose of 20 mg.

Nonsteroidal Antiinflammatory Drugs

The nonsteroidal agent ketorolac tromethamine is available in parenteral form. Like other nonsteroidal antiinflammatory drugs (NSAIDs), its primary mode of action is inhibition of prostaglandin-mediated amplification of pain pathways. Ketorolac at 10–30 mg intramuscularly has been reported to have the analgesic equivalence of 10 mg of morphine. Ketorolac is also commonly injected intravenously; the dosage is 15–30 mg every 4–6 h. It is recommended that the duration of therapy not exceed 5 days.

Ketorolac at 10–30 mg intramuscularly has been reported to have the analgesic equivalence of 10 mg morphine.

Ketorolac has the usual NSAIDs-related adverse effects; it can cause or exacerbate peptic ulcers and gastrointestinal bleeding and is contraindicated in patients with these problems. Antiplatelet effects are a concern and, as with many NSAIDs, are usually reversible within 24–48 h. There may be effects on renal function because NSAIDs block prostaglandin-mediated autoregulation of renal blood flow. Thus, this agent should be avoided in patients with advanced renal impairment or those at increased risk for acute renal injury; hypovolemia should be corrected before its administration. Because this agent does not have the side effects commonly seen with the narcotics, it may be a useful adjunct to therapy in combination with opioids. It should not be administered to patients with allergies to aspirin or other NSAIDs.

Regional Techniques

Neuraxial

Neuraxial blockade refers to spinal or epidural anesthesia or analgesia. Neuraxial administration of a local anesthetic, a narcotic, an alpha-2 agonist such as clonidine, or a combination of these agents can dramatically reduce or eliminate pain in the thorax, abdomen, or lower extremities.

The narcotics most commonly administered via the neuraxial method are morphine and fentanyl.

Epidural Local Anesthetic Intermittent or continuous administration of a local anesthetic via an epidural catheter blocks sympathetic, motor, and sensory neurons and thus provides complete anesthesia or profound analgesia without the risk of narcotic-mediated respiratory depression. This technique is commonly used in the operating room and labor suite. Distribution of the local anesthetic and subsequent pain relief are dependent on correct placement of the catheter and the concentration and volume of local anesthetic injected. Long-acting agents such as bupivicaine or ropivicaine are commonly used. A bolus injection is usual, followed by a continuous infusion. Contraindications to this technique include local skin lesions, sepsis, coagulation defects, or a history of recent drug administration that could adversely alter coagulation. Complications of epidurals stem from incorrect catheter placement and subsequent drug administration. Intrathecal injection of local anesthetic can cause total spinal blockade and profound hypotension; intravenous administration can lead to seizures and cardiac arrest. Infection or hematoma formation in the epidural space are extremely rare complications with appropriate technique and selection of patients.

Complications of epidurals stem from incorrect catheter placement and subsequent drug administration. Intrathecal injection of local anesthetic can cause total spinal blockade and profound hypotension; intravenous administration can lead to seizures and cardiac arrest.

Spinal and Epidural Narcotics Analgesia after neuraxial administration of narcotics occurs through action on opioid receptors located in the dorsal horn of the spinal cord. Both intrathecal and epidural opiates act on the presynaptic and postsynaptic neurons in the substantia gelatinosa. Relatively small doses of intrathecal and epidural narcotics produce profound analgesia with no autonomic, sensory, or motor blockade. The potency, onset of action, duration of effect, and likelihood of side effects are related to lipid solubility and narcotic concentration within the cerebrospinal fluid (CSF). The narcotics most commonly administered via the neuraxial method are morphine and fentanyl.

Intrathecal administration of narcotics produces a drug concentration within the CSF that is agent specific and dose dependent. Fentanyl, because of its high lipid solubility, is absorbed rapidly into the spinal cord. Morphine penetrates the cord more slowly, and considerable amounts of the drug remain in the CSF with the potential for direct action. When morphine is used, the onset of drug effect is slower than with fentanyl, but pain reduction may last for 18–24 h following a single injection.

Epidural administration of narcotics involves larger doses of drug. Following diffusion of a small percentage of the administered dose across the dura, the action of the narcotic is mediated in the same way as via the intrathecal route. However, vascular absorption by the extensive venous plexus in the epidural space leads to blood levels that can be similar to those of an equivalent intramuscular dose. It is possible that the profound pain relief experienced with the use of epidural narcotics reflects a synergistic action of spinal and central receptor systems. The beneficial effects of this technique postoperatively have been reported to include better pain control, less sedation, earlier mobilization, and a decreased time to recovery.

Side effects are related to the presence of opioids in the CSF or blood, are dose dependent, and can be seen with any narcotic. Morphine, because of its water solubility and greater concentration in the CSF, has a higher incidence of side effects than fentanyl. Although numerous side effects have been described, the four classic effects are nausea and vomiting, pruritus, urinary retention, and respiratory depression. Respiratory depression, the most serious and feared side effect, may occur within minutes of injection or be delayed for several hours. Clinically relevant early respiratory depression has not been reported with morphine. The incidence of respiratory depression requiring some type of intervention is reported to be approximately 1%.

Delayed respiratory depression is typically related to the neuraxial administration of morphine and results from transport via the CSF to central opioid receptors in the ventral medulla. This area of the central nervous system is critically important in the regulation of normal respiration. Delayed respiratory depression usually occurs 6–12 h following neuraxial administration of morphine and may be manifested by progressive bradypnea, hypercapnia, and a depressed level of consciousness. Protocols for detection and treatment of respiratory depression should be developed and consistently followed at all institutions utilizing neuraxial narcotics.

All side effects seen with the intrathecal and epidural administration of narcotics are mediated via opioid receptors. Therefore, treatment involves parenteral administration of an opioid antagonist or an opioid agonist/antagonist. Side effects are easily treated in this manner. Pain relief has been variably reported to be maintained or antagonized in a dose-dependent fashion. For that reason, naloxone should be titrated to effect, unless profound respiratory depression is present, as the goal is reversal of side effects with preservation of pain control. For nonlife-threatening side effects, 10–50 μg of naloxone would be an appropriate initial adult dose. Repetitive administration of naloxone, a naloxone infusion, or oral administration of naltrexone, a long-acting opioid antagonist, may be necessary as side effects can recur. Reversal of nausea and pruritus, with maintenance of analgesia, is also possible if an agonist/antagonist such as nalbuphine (initial adult dose, 5 mg) is administered.

Addition of a narcotic to a local anesthetic and administration via an epidural can result in profound pain relief and obviate the need for any parenteral narcotics. Epidural administration of an opioid with or without a local anesthetic has been found to be efficacious following thoracotomy in patients with marginal pulmonary function and following abdominal surgery in patients with sleep apnea.

Epidural administration of local anesthetics or opioids allows, in most instances, repetitive dosing or a continuous infusion, as an epidural catheter is usually placed in the lumbar or thoracic epidural space. Administration of narcotics directly into the CSF via a spinal technique is equally effective, but an indwelling catheter is not usually used in the intensive care unit.

Nerve Blocks

Peripheral nerve blocks may be useful in controlling postoperative pain depending on the site of surgery. In thoracic surgery, blockade of the intercostal nerves with a local anesthetic, either at the time of surgery or percutaneously in the ICU, will reduce pain and the likelihood of respiratory depression by decreasing the need for parenteral narcotics. Bupivicaine 0.5% in doses of 2–3 ml per intercostal nerve can be placed at the level of incision and two levels above and below the incision. Discomfort from thoracostomy tubes can be alleviated by intercostal nerve blockade at the level of insertion.

Interpleural anesthesia allows multiple intercostal nerves to be blocked without multiple needle injections. This technique involves placement of an interpleural catheter, which may be introduced percutaneously or at the time of surgery. The patient's position is an important factor in the action of the local anesthetic and clinical result. With the patient in the supine position, a continuous infusion of a local anesthetic "bathes" the posterior pleural space and results in continuous blockade of multiple intercostal nerves. Use of this technique may be limited by loss of local anesthetic if a thoracostomy tube is in place. A related technique involves placement of a catheter in an extrapleural position. Following an intrathoracic procedure a catheter is introduced superficial to the parietal pleura and parallel to the vertebral bodies. Infusion of local anesthetic into the catheter results in blockade of multiple intercostal nerves. One advantage to this technique is avoidance of drug loss via the thoracostomy tube. Pneumothorax and the systemic toxicity of local anesthetics are potential complications associated with these nerve blocks.

The term cryoanalgesia refers to a method of pain relief achieved through the application of extreme cold to a peripheral nerve. This technique produces a prolonged period of analgesia, from several weeks to up to 6 months, but does not anatomically disrupt the nerve and thus allows for eventual return of nerve function. Clinically, it has found greatest application in blockade of the intercostal nerve(s) internally, usually just before thoracotomy closure.

The term cryoanalgesia refers to a method of pain relief achieved through the application of extreme cold to a peripheral nerve.

SEDATIVE/HYPNOTICS

Critically ill patients frequently require anxiolytics or sedatives to modify distress and mental discomfort and to facilitate compliance with life-sustaining treatment (Table 44-3).

The adequacy of sedation is most often assessed clinically. Sedation scales may be untested for reliability or validity (The Ramsay scale), may be validated only in pediatric populations (The Comfort scale), or may be relatively new and not widely known (The Motor Activity Assessment Scale). The bispectral index, a new noninvasive technology for monitoring anesthetic effect, offers the hope of an objective method of assessing and monitoring sedation. It correlates well with the level of responsiveness and may one day find applicability within the ICU.

Critically ill patients frequently require anxiolytics or sedatives to modify distress, for mental discomfort, and to facilitate compliance with life-sustaining treatment.

Benzodiazepines

The ideal sedative/hypnotic would be inexpensive, have anxiolytic and analgesic properties, a rapid onset of action, a short half-life with no accumulation of active metabolites, and insignificant cardiovascular and respiratory effects. Although the perfect agent does not yet exist, the group of drugs known as benzodiazepines (BZDs) is closest to the ideal. Because these drugs are used daily in the ICU, it is helpful to have some understanding of their mechanism of action.

The discovery in 1977 of specific membrane-binding sites for the benzodiazepines was the initial step into the insight we now have regarding how these drugs function. Benzodiazepines exert their pharmacologic actions by enhancing γ-aminobutyric acid (GABA)-

Benzodiazepines exert their pharmacologic actions by enhancing γ-aminobutyric acid (GABA) mediated inhibition of neuronal transmission.

TABLE 44-3

SEDATIVE/HYPNOTIC USE IN CRITICALLY ILL ADULT PATIENTS

AGENT	ROUTES OF ADMINISTRATION	ELIMINATION HALF-LIFE (h)	INTERMITTENT DOSE	INFUSION RATE (μg/kg/MIN)	ACTIVE METABOLITE	ONSET
Diazepam	IV	20–70	2–10 mg q2–4 h	N/A	Desmethyldiazepam	Slow
Midazolam	IV, continuous infusion	1–4	1–4 mg q1–3 h	0.25–2.0	1-Hydroxymidazolam; 4-hydroxymidazolam	Fast
Lorazepam	IV, continuous infusion	10–20	1–4 mg q1–6 h	0.2–0.5	No	Slow
Propofol	Continuous infusion	1–7 (rapid awakening secondary to redistribution)	N/A	10–100	No	Fast

FIGURE 44-1

The action of various agonists on the γ-aminobutyric acid (GABA) receptor complex results in an increased affinity of the receptor for GABA and increases the average time the channel remains open.

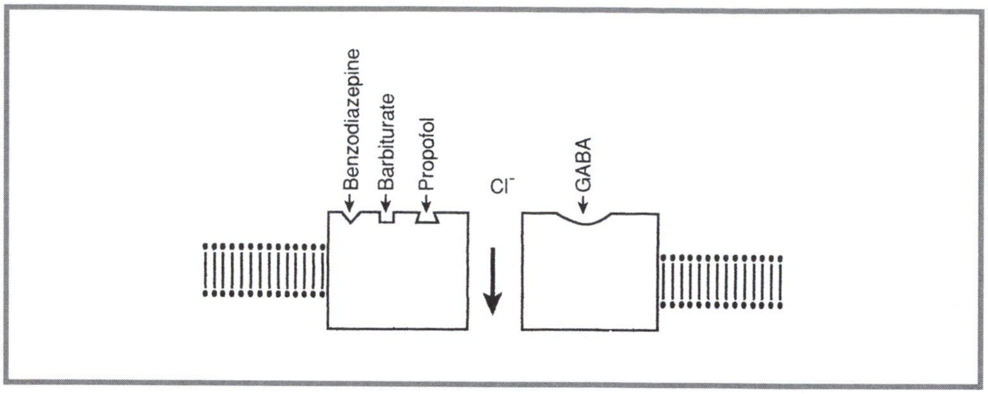

mediated inhibition of neuronal transmission. The GABA receptor–chloride ionophore complex is composed of multisubunit proteins that when activated form a selective channel, allowing chloride to enter the cell (Figure 44-1). This free flow of chloride hyperpolarizes the neuron and inhibits neural transmission. A number of drugs modulate GABA receptor-regulated chloride channels. BZDs, barbiturates, and propofol react with discrete, modulatory receptor sites within the GABA receptor–chloride channel complex. The end result of BZD action on the GABA receptor is to increase the affinity of the receptor for GABA and to produce a modest increase in the average time the channel stays open. Benzodiazepines thus facilitate the inhibitory effect of GABA on neuronal transmission at limbic, thalamic, hypothalamic, and spinal levels, resulting in sedation, amnesia, anxiolysis, and muscle spasm reduction; they have no analgesic effects.

> Benzodiazepines (BZDs) thus facilitate the inhibitory effect of GABA on neuronal transmission at limbic, thalamic, hypothalamic, and spinal levels, resulting in sedation, amnesia, anxiolysis, and muscle spasm reduction; they have no analgesic effects.

It should be pointed out that the GABA receptor–chloride channel complex is unusual in that it has the ability to respond not only to agonists (BZD, barbiturates, propofol) and competitive antagonists (flumazenil) but also to inverse agonists (picrotoxin, bicuculline). The action of an inverse agonist is to decrease the inhibitory effect of GABA. In animal experimentation, these inverse agonists have prominent convulsant effects. The competitive antagonist flumazenil will reverse the action of agonists and inverse agonists by binding tightly to the BZD receptor yet will produce no clinical effect itself. Thus, evidence strongly suggests that there is an agonist–antagonist–inverse agonist continuum in terms of the action of various substances on this receptor complex. This information regarding benzodiazepine receptor kinetics gives insight into the withdrawal symptoms described with this class of agents. All clinically available BZDs interact with the GABA receptor complex in a qualitatively similar fashion.

> Clinically, in the critical care setting, BZDs are used for anxiolysis, sedation, treatment of alcohol withdrawal, and often as initial therapy for control of agitation.

Clinically, in the critical care setting, BZDs are used for anxiolysis, sedation, treatment of alcohol withdrawal, and often as initial therapy for control of agitation. Any of the BZDs can be associated with a paradoxical or disinhibitory reaction, causing the patient to become uncooperative or agitated. The three BZDs used most frequently in the critical care setting are diazepam, lorazepam, and midazolam. All may be administered intravenously and any of them can cause dose-dependent respiratory depression and decreased blood pressure secondary to a central sympatholytic effect. The time course and intensity of their clinical effects will vary, depending in part on the sensitivity of the patient, the amount of drug, and whether administered as a bolus or via continuous infusion. The other clinical differences noted between the different agents in this class are due to variations in the rates at which the agents penetrate the CNS and their metabolic profiles.

> Diazepam, with a half-life of 30 h for the parent compound, up to 200 h for active metabolites, and decreased clearance in the critically ill, is used less frequently than in the past.

Diazepam, with a half-life of 30 h for the parent compound, up to 200 h for active metabolites, and decreased clearance in the critically ill, is used less frequently than in the past. After a single dose of diazepam, its pharmacologically active metabolite, desmethyldiazepam, is usually not present in sufficient concentration to have prolonged clinical effect. During prolonged administration, production of desmethyldiazepam can be extensive and, because of its longer half-life, can exceed the concentration of the parent compound. It is technically difficult to administer diazepam via continuous infusion as a dedicated line and syringe pump are required. However, because it is inexpensive, has a rapid onset of action, and, when used intermittently, has a relatively short clinical effect, it still has a valuable role in treatment of the critically ill.

Midazolam, a water-soluble agent with a half-life of 1.5–3 h, was the first BZD to be administered via continuous intravenous infusion. Like diazepam it is highly lipophilic and for that reason has a rapid onset of clinical effect. Midazolam has found wide application as a short-acting sedative for endoscopic procedures, angiography, and cardioversion. In patients with inadequate intravascular volume or compromised cardiac function, rapid administration may lead to hemodynamic instability and respiratory depression. Midazolam is eliminated almost exclusively by hepatic hydroxylation and then conjugated with glucuronic acid; its major metabolite is α-hydroxy-midazolam.

Midazolam has found wide application as a short-acting sedative for endoscopic procedures, angiography, and cardioversion.

In spite of a short half-life, prolonged sedation in critically ill patients has been reported with midazolam. An increase in the volume of distribution and a prolongation in elimination half-life have been demonstrated in critically ill patients and contribute to this effect. Midazolam has a hepatic extraction ratio of 30%–70%, and a decrease in hepatic blood flow could reduce its clearance. Additionally, conjugated metabolites have been found to have substantial pharmacologic effect and may accumulate with prolonged administration and in patients with renal failure.

Lorazepam may also be administered via continuous infusion now that solubility issues have been resolved. Lorazepam has a half-life of 10–20 h but has no active metabolites. Because lorazepam is less lipid soluble than midazolam or diazepam, maximum effects may not be seen for 15–30 min. Although this may be a disadvantage in patients who need rapid sedation, cardiovascular changes are usually less. Although lorazepam has a longer half-life than midazolam, its duration of effect is shorter following cessation of continuous infusion, and it is generally believed to be more cost-effective for long-term sedation. The greater duration of effect with midazolam in critically ill patients is attributed to altered drug kinetics and accumulation of active metabolites. A continuous infusion of any BZD administered for an extended period of time should be tapered rather than abruptly discontinued. The executive summary of the Society of Critical Care Medicine practice parameters for the administration of intravenous analgesia and sedation in critically ill adults recommends 0.044 mg/kg every 2–4 h for lorazepam as an appropriate initiation dose; however, titration to clinical effect is necessary in every patient.

Because lorazepam is less lipid soluble than midazolam or diazepam, maximum effects may not be seen for 15–30 min.

The executive summary of the Society of Critical Care Medicine practice parameters for the administration of intravenous analgesia and sedation in critically ill adults recommends 0.044 mg/kg every 2–4 h for lorazepam as an appropriate initiation dose; however, titration to clinical effect is necessary in every patient.

Hepatic biotransformation accounts for the majority of BZD clearance. The two principal pathways involved are oxidation (diazepam, midazolam), and glucuronide conjugation (lorazepam). The oxidative pathway is most susceptible to impairment in the elderly or cirrhotic patient, which has led to the recommendation that lorazepam be considered the BZD of choice in these patients.

The oxidative pathway is most susceptible to impairment in the elderly or cirrhotic patient, which has led to the recommendation that lorazepam be considered the BZD of choice in these patients.

Zolpidem (Ambien), a compound structurally dissimilar to the BZDs, exerts its effect via action on the BZD recognition site of the GABA receptor complex. It is indicated in the short-term treatment of insomnia and causes less sleep disturbance compared to the BZDs. It is available in tablet form only.

Flumazenil, an imidazobenzodiazepine derivative, binds in a competitive and reversible manner to the BZD receptor on the GABA receptor–chloride ionophore complex. Administration of 1 mg or less usually reverses the effects of the BZDs and may be useful following iatrogenic oversedation. A dose of up to 3 mg is appropriate to emergently reverse a drug overdose involving the BZDs. The clinical effects of this agent are evident within minutes of administration. Resedation may occur within several hours or less depending on which BZD and what amount is being antagonized. Convulsions are the most common serious adverse effect reported and usually occur in patients who are chronically dependent on BZDs, use them to control seizures, or have ingested large doses of other drugs.

Propofol

Propofol, an alkyl phenol derivative, is a short-acting intravenous anesthetic agent. It has a rapid onset of action but a brief duration of effect due to a short redistribution half-life; this rapid redistribution occurs because propofol is extremely lipophilic. Propofol is formulated in an oil–water emulsion consisting of propofol, soybean oil, glycerol, and egg phosphatide; the agent is contraindicated in patients with hypersensitivity to any of its components. Although it may be administered as a bolus for short procedures, such as endotracheal intubation or cardioversion, it is usually administered as a continuous infusion for sedation in intubated, mechanically ventilated patients. The central venous route of administration is recommended as it may cause pain on injection into a peripheral vein. Because of its effect on cardiac output and a reduction in systemic vascular resistance, hypotension may be seen with propofol use. For that reason, it should be used with caution in patients with hypotension, hypovolemia, or other forms of cardiovascular instability. As it is a respiratory depressant and will blunt protective airway reflexes, it should be used with extreme caution in patients who are not intubated and mechanically ventilated.

Propofol has been used with success for prolonged periods of time. It is safe, has a short duration of action, and may allow more effective patient ventilator synchrony than is possible with other sedative/hypnotics. Because propofol mediates its effect via the GABA receptor complex, it does have some amnestic and anticonvulsant effects. However, single-drug therapy with propofol has been associated with patient recall during therapeutic paralysis in a surgical ICU, and thus it seems best to administer other sedatives or narcotics with it. When combined with opioids, the deep sedation possible with propofol infusion may obviate the need for neuromuscular blockade.

When combined with opioids, the deep sedation possible with propofol infusion may obviate the need for neuromuscular blockade.

There is a risk of inducing seizure activity following the abrupt cessation of a propofol infusion after prolonged use, presumably a result of the development of tolerance or down-regulation of the central GABA receptor. For this reason, it seems prudent to wean this agent if it has been used for an extended period of time.

Propofol provides approximately 1.1 kcal/ml, which should be taken into account when it is administered in association with enteral or parenteral nutrition. Long-term administration may result in elevations in serum triglycerides, amylase, and lipase; a chemical pancreatitis may occur. When using propofol over an extended period, a serum triglyceride level should be obtained two or three times per week. Strict aseptic technique must be followed because propofol has been reported to support the rapid growth of microorganisms.

Ketamine

Ketamine, a rapid-acting, dissociative anesthetic agent with analgesic properties, also has central sympathomimetic effects that may be efficacious in agitated patients with bronchospasm or hemodynamic instability. However, it is unlikely to add significantly to the effects of standard asthma treatment. Ketamine also has potential for direct negative inotropic effects, which preclude its use in patients with severely impaired left ventricular function. It should be administered with a BZD to prevent psychomimetic reactions. The combination of ketamine and midazolam may avoid the inhibition of intestinal motility that is commonly observed with sedation regimens which include opioids.

Inhalational Agents

Inhalational anesthetic agents administered via ventilator-mounted vaporizers may be used for sedation in the ICU. Rapid reversal of sedation is due to excretion of the drug via the respiratory tract and is one of the attractive features of inhalational agents in this setting. The use of these drugs holds promise, but more work is needed regarding long-term administration in critically ill patients. Halogenated inhalational agents may also be used in the critical care setting to treat status asthmaticus, status epilepticus, and for emergent control of intracranial and systemic hypertension.

Control of Agitation

Agitation is common among the critically ill and its etiology is multifactorial; ideally, it requires a definitive diagnosis before initiation of therapy. It is important to realize that sedating a patient experiencing pain without first providing adequate analgesia will induce agitation.

Agitation is common among the critically ill, and its etiology is multifactorial (Table 44-4). Ideally, agitation should have a definitive diagnosis before initiation of therapy. It is important to realize that sedating a patient experiencing pain without first providing adequate anal-

TABLE 44-4

CAUSES OF AGITATION IN THE CRITICALLY ILL

Sepsis	Subdural hematoma
Seizures	Hypertensive encephalopathy
Meningitis/encephalitis	Anxiety disorders
Delirium tremens	Cerebrovascular accident
Drug reactions	Thyroid disease
Hepatic encephalopathy	Uremic encephalopathy
Hypoglycemia	Hypoxia/hypercapnia
Hyponatremia	Steroid psychosis
Intracranial bleed	ICU psychosis

ICU, intensive care unit

gesia will induce agitation. If a cause for agitation is found, therapy will, at least in part, involve treatment of the underlying cause. If no cause for agitation is found, there is still a need to treat the patient to prevent self-injury or injury to health care professionals. If nonspecific agitation cannot be adequately controlled with BZDs alone, other drugs are used, either alone or in combination with the BZDs.

Haloperidol

Intravenous haloperidol has become a mainstay in the management of agitation in the intensive care unit, despite a lack of approval by the FDA for this route of administration. This agent is potent, has a rapid onset of action, and has few negative effects on respiration or hemodynamics. Thus, it can be used in spontaneously breathing patients who are not intubated or on mechanical ventilation.

Haloperidol is a neuroleptic with an onset of action of 5–20 min and a terminal half-life of 20–50 h. The appropriate dose of haloperidol is in dispute, although a wide range of recommendations exist. A reasonable starting dose is 2–5 mg, with a doubling of the dose every 10–20 min until sedation is achieved. The suggested maximum single dose of haloperidol is 40 mg. The drug is metabolized in the liver and has no active metabolites.

A reasonable starting dose is 2–5 mg, initially with a doubling of the dose every 10–20 min until sedation is achieved. The suggested maximum single dose of haloperidol is 40 mg.

Although extrapyramidal side effects are observed less frequently when haloperidol is administered intravenously, they still can occur. Akathisia should be considered in patients who continue to move in a repetitive manner despite adequate treatment. Lorazepam or dopaminergic agents such as bromocriptine may be helpful in this setting. Neuroleptic malignant syndrome (NMS) is a potentially fatal reaction to neuroleptic agents. Haloperidol or the phenothiazines, alone or in combination, may trigger NMS. The signs and symptoms include muscle rigidity, hyperthermia, tachycardia, hypertension, rhabdomyolysis, mental status changes, and acidosis. NMS may be confused with malignant hyperthermia, pheochromocytoma, thyroid storm, or sepsis. Therapy of NMS includes discontinuation of the offending agents, administration of intravenous dantrolene or a neuromuscular blocking agent, and bromocriptine. The administration of haloperidol may also rarely be associated with torsades de pointes and laryngospasm.

Haloperidol may be used alone, or in combination with lorazepam. A reasonable initial dose in an adult patient is haloperidol 5 mg and lorazepam 0.5 mg, in association with a one-time administration of opioid. The dose of haloperidol and lorazepam is then repeated or increased every 20–30 min until the patient is sedated. Once sedation is achieved with this type of combination therapy, subsequent doses and scheduling of each medication and intervals of administration depend on the recurrence of agitation.

Haloperidol may be used alone, or in combination with lorazepam. A reasonable initial dose in an adult patient is haloperidol 5 mg and lorazepam 0.5 mg, in association with a one-time administration of opioid.

Intermittent doses of analgesics or a continuous narcotic infusion may be combined with the sedative/hypnotics to control agitation. It is important to note that the combination of sedative/hypnotics and analgesics is synergistic rather than simply additive. For that reason, the combination of an analgesic with one or more sedative-hypnotic agents may allow for a greater likelihood of successful sedation, uncomplicated by significant cardiovascular side affects. Careful titration to effect should mitigate the potential for oversedation.

It is important to note that the combination of sedative/hypnotics and analgesics is synergistic rather than simply additive.

If control of agitation is still needed after intermittent administration of a BZD alone or in combination with analgesics and/or haloperidol, other choices are available; these include, but are not limited to, continuous infusions of lorazepam, midazolam, propofol, or ketamine.

Mechanical ventilation, with or without the use of neuromuscular blocking agents, may be necessary on occasion in an individual patient.

SUMMARY

Most patients admitted to an intensive care unit will receive some combination of sedative/hypnotics and analgesics. There is no reason to allow critically ill patients to experience fear, anxiety, or pain. Often, multiple agents and techniques are employed. An understanding of how critical illness affects the pharmacokinetics and pharmacodynamics of these agents is vital. Although multiple tools are available to assess the degree of this emotional and physical discomfort, they lack routine clinical applicability in the care of the critically ill.

Morphine is the agent of choice for analgesia in the critically ill patient. If hemodynamic instability or allergy to morphine exists, fentanyl is an excellent alternative analgesic. Lorazepam is the sedative/hypnotic agent recommended for anxiolysis or sedation. It may be administered by intermittent injection or continuous infusion. Midazolam or propofol are reasonable alternative choices.

Agitation has multiple etiologies and should be investigated fully. Appropriate diagnosis will lead to appropriate care; however, treatment of agitation is crucial in prevention of injury to the patient and health care personnel. Haloperidol with or without concomitant administration of a benzodiazepine is an appropriate first choice.

REVIEW QUESTIONS*

1. **The following opioids have significant action at the μ and κ receptors:**
   - **A.** Morphine
   - **B.** Meperidine
   - **C.** Fentanyl
   - **D.** Nalbuphine

2. **The following are potential causes of agitation in the critically ill patient:**
   - **A.** Sepsis
   - **B.** Alcohol withdrawal
   - **C.** Hypoglycemia
   - **D.** Hypertensive encephalopathy

3. **Which of the following are potential side effects of the epidural or spinal administration of narcotics?**
   - **A.** Nausea and vomiting
   - **B.** Pruritus
   - **C.** Urinary retention
   - **D.** Respiratory depression

4. **Which of the following sedative/hypnotics have active metabolites?**
   - **A.** Diazepam
   - **B.** Propofol
   - **C.** Midazolam
   - **D.** Lorazepam

5. **The intravenous administration of haloperidol may be associated with:**
   - **A.** Neuroleptic malignant syndrome
   - **B.** Torsades de pointes
   - **C.** Laryngospasm
   - **D.** Hypokalemia

*Note: More than one answer may be correct.

ANSWERS

1. The answer is B and D. There are five classes of opioid receptors; mu (μ), kappa (κ), delta (δ), sigma (σ), and epsilon (ϵ). Morphine and fentanyl mediate their effect largely through the μ receptor. Nalbuphine hydrochloride is considered an agonist/antagonist because, although it has an weak intrinsic agonist effect at the μ receptor, it acts as an antagonist in the presence of a potent μ receptor agonist such as morphine. Meperidine and nalbuphine both act on the κ receptor in addition to their action on the μ receptor. κ receptor agonists suppress shivering and thereby avoid increasing metabolic demand.
2. The answer is A, B, C, D. All these conditions may lead to agitation. If a cause for agitation is found, therapy will, at least in part, involve treatment of the underlying cause. While that treatment is ongoing it is important to note that there may still be a need to treat the patient with sedatives and analgesics, or haloperidol, to prevent self-injury or injury to health care personnel.

3. The answer is A, B, C, D. Although there are a number of side effects described with the epidural or spinal administration of opioids, the four symptoms named (nausea and vomiting, pruritus, urinary retention, and respiratory depression) are considered the classic side effects. All these side effects are mediated by opioid action and can be effectively treated with naloxone. Titration with naloxone is recommended in an attempt to maintain pain relief while reversing nonemergent side effects. Profound respiratory depression is rare and should be treated immediately.
4. The answer is A and C. Diazepam and midazolam have potent, active metabolites, which, to some extent, has limited their use in the critically ill patient. Although lorazepam has a longer elimination half-life than midazolam, its duration of effect has been reported to be shorter following discontinuation of a continuous infusion. The prolonged effect of midazolam is believed due to altered drug kinetics and an accumulation of active metabolites in critically ill patients. Propofol has no active metabolites and is rapidly redistributed to lipophilic sites following discontinuation of administration.
5. The answer is A, B, C. Neuroleptic malignant syndrome, torsades de pointes, and laryngospasm are considered rare but potential complications of the intravenous administration of haloperidol.

SUGGESTED READING

Cammarano WB, Pittet JF, Weitz S, et al. Acute withdrawal syndrome related to the administration of analgesic and sedative medications in adult intensive care unit patients. Crit Care Med 1998;26:676–684.

Chaney MA. Side effects of intrathecal and epidural opioids. Can J Anaesth 1995;42:891–903.

Devlin JW, Boleski G, Mlynarek M, et al. Motor activity assessment scale: a valid and reliable sedation scale for use with mechanically ventilated patients in an adult surgical intensive care unit. Crit Care Med 1999; 27:1271–1275.

Marinella MA. Propofol for sedation in the intensive care unit: essentials for the clinician. Respir Med 1997;91:505–510.

Morgan D, Cook CD, Smith MA, Picker MJ. An examination of the interactions between the antinociceptive effects of morphine and various opioids: the role of intrinsic efficacy and stimulus intensity. Anesth Analg 1999;88:407–413.

Pasternak GW. Pharmacological mechanisms of opioid analgesics. Clin Neuropharmacol 1993;16:1–18.

Shapiro B, Warren J, Egol A, et al. Practice parameters for intravenous analgesia and sedation for adult patients in the intensive care unit: an executive summary. Crit Care Med 1995;23:1596–1600.

Wagner BKJ, O'Hara DA. Pharmacokinetics and pharmacodynamics of sedatives and analgesics in the treatment of agitated critically ill patients. Clin Pharmacokinet 1997;33:426–453.

Wagner BKJ, Zavotsky KE, Sweeney JB, Palmeri BA, Hammond JS. Patient recall of therapeutic paralysis in a surgical critical care unit. Pharmacotherapy 1998;18:358–363.

Wang JJ, Tai S, Lee ST, Liu YC. A comparison among nalbuphine, meperidine and placebo for treating postanesthetic shivering. Anesth Analg 1999;88:686–689.

Watling SM, Dasta JF, Seidl EC. Sedatives, analgesics, and paralytics in the ICU. Ann Pharmacother 1997;31:148–153.

Zorumski CF, Isenberg KE: Insights into the structure and function of GABA-benzodiazepine receptors: ion channels and psychiatry. Am J Psychiatry 1991;148:162–173.

CHAPTER 45

WALTER A. WYNKOOP AND GILBERT E. D'ALONZO

Prophylactic Regimens in the Intensive Care Unit

CHAPTER OUTLINE

LEARNING OBJECTIVES

After studying this chapter, you should be able to:

- Identify risk factors associated with the development of deep vein thrombosis and its consequence, pulmonary embolism.
- Understand the indications for medical, mechanical, and inferior vena cava filter prophylaxis and describe the available methods for each.
- Identify the major physiologic mechanism associated with stress-induced gastritis and ulceration and identify the risk factors associated with this condition.
- Know the methods used for prophylaxis of stress-induced gastritis and ulceration and the potential complications of the medical therapies used for this condition.
- Identify the nosocomial infections common in the intensive care unit and the causative organisms responsible.
- Discuss the various risk factors associated with the development of infection in critically ill patients.
- Employ a variety of effective prophylactic regimens to prevent pneumonia, line sepsis, and urinary tract infection in critically ill patients.

DEEP VENOUS THROMBOSIS PROPHYLAXIS

The prevention of deep vein thrombosis of the lower extremities, by definition, will reduce the frequency of pulmonary embolism. Pulmonary embolism is not a disease; it is merely a complication of deep vein thrombosis. Therefore, if venous thrombosis can be prevented, pulmonary embolism will be prevented.

A number of clinical conditions, diseases, and laboratory findings have been associated with an apparent predisposition to the development of deep vein thrombosis. For most intensive care unit patients, one or more of these conditions exist. Many of these so-called risk factors have been found to be associated with one or more of the thrombogenic alterations responsible for the development of a hypercoagulable state, namely, venostasis, vascular intimal injury, or both. Risk factors are cumulative in their effect, with generally more than one factor present (Table 45-1). Thromboembolic risk after surgical and nonsurgical trauma is related to the severity, site, and extent of the trauma, the length of the surgery, the age of the patient, a previous thromboembolic episode, and the length of immobilization. Five in-

TABLE 45-1

RISK FACTORS FOR DEEP VENOUS THROMBOSIS

Clinical conditions	Systemic lupus erythematosus
Immobilization	Polycythemia
Obesity	Homocystinemia
Trauma: surgical and nonsurgical	Paroxysmal nocturnal hemaglobinuria
Previous thrombosis	Nephrotic syndrome
Contraceptives: oral estrogens	Paraplegia
Pregnancy and postpartum state	Stroke
Warfarin and heparin	Laboratory findings
Central venous catheter	Antithrombin-III deficiency
Diseases	Protein C deficiency
Heart failure and myocardial infarction	Protein S deficiency
Cancer	Lupus anticoagulant
Serious infection with septicemia	Anticardiolipin antibodies
Bechet's disease	Factor V Leiden mutation

dependent risk factors for thrombosis have been identified: older age, need for blood transfusions or surgery, fracture of the pelvis or leg, and spinal cord injury. The posttraumatic setting is a paradigm for the hypercoagulable state. Increased coagulability as a result of tissue thromboplastin release into the blood, vessel endothelial damage, stasis of blood flow resulting from immobilization, and reduced fibrinolysis have all been identified. A practical guide for determining the risk of venous thromboembolism in surgery or trauma patients is found in Table 45-2.

Indications

Most patients who die of pulmonary embolism die rapidly; therefore, no treatment modality can have an impact comparable to appropriate deep vein thrombosis prophylaxis. The use of appropriate prophylaxis in high-risk patient groups will reduce the incidence of deep vein thrombosis significantly. The ideal preventative method should be effective, safe, free of clinically relevant side effects, easily administered and monitored, and cost-effective for the specific patient. Either pharmacologic or mechanical methods may be used, and sometimes a combination of methods must be employed for a specific patient. There is no single method that is appropriate or efficacious for every clinical situation.

> Pulmonary embolism is potentially fatal; therefore, the best therapy is prevention.

A strategy for the prevention of deep vein thrombosis according to risk category is shown in Table 45-2. The general approach to prophylaxis is to use the simplest and usually a single modality in patients with low or medium risk and double modalities or special interventions in patients at high risk.

Methods

A variety of preventative measures have proven effective in reducing lower extremity deep vein thrombosis in critically ill patients. The methods can be divided into medical, mechanical, and inferior vena cava filters.

Medical Prophylaxis

Low-Dose Unfractionated Heparin The method of prophylaxis most frequently used in both medical and surgical patients is low-dose subcutaneous unfractionated heparin (LDUH). Heparin, in conjunction with antithrombin III, inhibits thrombin, kallikrein, and factors Xa, IXa, XIa, and XIIa. Simply put, heparin accelerates the activity of antithrombin III, which then inhibits the conversion of prothrombin to thrombin, and in the absence of active thrombosis, this action occurs at low doses of heparin, below the doses that interfere with other aspects of the coagulation process. At low doses, heparin inhibits thrombus formation with a minimal risk for bleeding as compared to full anticoagulation. Low-dose unfractionated heparin is indicated for those medical patients who are at moderate to high risk

> Low-dose unfractionated heparin (LDUH) can be used as monotherapy for the prophylaxis of thromboembolism in all but the highest risk patients.

TABLE 45-2

INCIDENCE OF THROMBOEMBOLIC EVENTS AFTER SURGERY OR TRAUMA OR WITH CERTAIN MEDICAL CONDITIONS, AND RECOMMENDED DEEP VENOUS THROMBOSIS PROPHYLAXIS

RISK GROUP AND THROMBOEMBOLIC INCIDENCE	RECOMMENDATION
Low risk	
Under 40 years old	Early ambulation *and* graduated compression stockings
Minor surgery (>60-min duration)	
Bedridden, uncomplicated	
Medical patients, pregnancy	
Event/incidence, %	
Distal DVT: 2–6	
Proximal DVT: 0.4–1	
PE: 0.2–1	
Fatal PE: 0.002	
Moderate risk[a]	
Over 40 years old	
Abdominal, pelvic, thoracic surgery	Early ambulation *and* LDUH or LMWH or IPC[b]
Myocardial infarction, cardiomyopathy, previous thromboembolism	
Event/incidence, %	
Distal DVT: 8–40	
Proximal DVT: 1–8	
PE: 1–8	
Fatal PE: 0.1–0.4	
High risk[a]	
Elderly	IPC and LDUH *or* LMWH and early ambulation
Extended surgery duration	
Hip and major knee surgery	
Fractured hip	
Extensive trauma, including soft tissue injury and multiple fractures[c]	
Stroke	
Event/incidence, %	For elective hip and major knee surgery, use low-dose warfarin or adjusted-dose heparin or LMWH and IPC with early ambulation
Distal DVT: 40–80	
Proximal DVT: 10–20	
PE: 5–10	
Fatal PE: 1–5	

DVT, deep venous thrombosis; PE, pulmonary embolism; LDUH, low-dose unfractionated heparin; LMWH, low molecular weight heparin; IPC, intermittent pneumatic compression

[a] Risk is increased further by the following factors: obesity, prolonged bedrest, estrogens, and venous varicosities

[b] Intermittent pneumatic compression is the prophylactic method of choice for neurosurgery, ophthalmologic surgery, certain urologic procedures, or when the bleeding risk is considered to be high

[c] Consider early placement of a vena cava filter

for deep vein thrombosis formation. Often, LDUH is used in combination with sequential compression devices applied to the lower extremities in patients who are critically ill and who may be at highest risk for thrombus formation. LDUH has been shown to be effective at preventing thrombus formation in patients who undergo general surgery, including thoracoabdominal and gynecologic procedures. However, this form of prophylaxis has not proved to be equally effective in all patient groups. For example, limitations have been recognized in patients who undergo major orthopedic procedures, particularly repair of femoral fractures and reconstructive operations of the hips and knees, and heparin is inadequate after prostate surgery and cystectomy. LDUH is contraindicated in patients who are having ophthalmologic or brain surgery.

There appears to be no clear consensus on the correct dose of heparin. Most clinical situations involving patients at low or moderate risk for venous thrombosis require no more than 5,000 units of LDUH every 12 h by subcutaneous administration. The administration of 10,000–15,000 units per day in divided doses, either every 12 h or every 8 h, has been employed in most clinical trials. LDUH at 5,000 units every 8 h in general surgical patients appears more efficacious in preventing deep vein thrombosis without increasing the occurrence of wound hematoma. The benefits of LDUH are its proven efficacy, ease of administration, and relatively low cost. Its risks are low, with estimates of serious bleeding less than 1% and of heparin-induced thrombocytopenia less than 3%. Laboratory tests of coagulation status are not monitored; however, periodic platelet counts must be performed in patients who receive this form of prophylaxis over an extended period of time.

Prophylaxic LDUH is safe, with less than 1% risk of serious bleeding.

Low Molecular Weight Heparin Low molecular weight heparin (LMWH) is derived from unfractionated heparin and exerts its antithrombotic effects primarily through inhibition of factor Xa. The advantages of LMWH stem from its pharmacokinetics. LMWH has an active half-life that is twice as long as that of unfractionated heparin with a four times greater bioavailability, allowing for once-daily dosing. LMWH may have a reduced tendency to induce bleeding and perhaps a lower incidence of heparin-induced thrombocytopenia. LMWH is more expensive than LDUH. Effectiveness has been shown in patients undergoing general surgery or hip and knee surgery, and for those patients who have suffered a thrombotic stroke.

Low molecular weight heparin (LMWH) is recommended for patients at high risk for thromboembolism.

There are several different LMWH. The prophylactic dose of enoxaparin sodium depends on the clinical situation. For patients who are having abdominal surgery, 40 mg is administered subcutaneously each day with the initial dose given 2 h before surgery. For patients who are undergoing hip or knee replacement surgery, the prophylactic dose of enoxaparin sodium is 30 mg every 12 h, administered by subcutaneous injection. The initial dose should be given 12–24 h after surgery, provided that hemostasis has been established. An alternative prophylactic measure using enoxaparin sodium for hip replacement surgery is a dose of 40 mg once daily subcutaneously, given initially 12 h before surgery, with either 30 mg every 12 h or 40 mg once daily being administered following surgery. The risks of LMWH are similar to unfractionated heparin. It is not recommended in patients with active bleeding or in documented cases of heparin-induced thrombocytopenia. Additionally, when LMWH is used concomitantly with epidural or spinal anesthesia, one must be aware of the risk of epidural or spinal hematoma. Caution regarding its use in these patients is therefore recommended.

Dalteparin sodium is another LMWH. For patients undergoing abdominal surgery, the recommended dose of dalteparin sodium is 2500 IU administered subcutaneously once daily starting 1–2 h before surgery with repeat dosing on a daily basis thereafter. Similarly, for patients undergoing hip replacement surgery, dalteparin is administered 2 h before surgery, and the second dose of 2500 IU is administered subcutaneously the evening of the day of surgery, at least 6 h after the first dose. Thereafter, 5000 IU is administered subcutaneously once daily.

Ardeparin sodium, another LMWH, can be used for the prevention of deep vein thrombosis in patients undergoing knee replacement surgery. The recommended subcutaneous dose of ardeparin sodium is 50 units per kilogram of body weight every 12 h with treatment beginning the evening of the day of surgery or the following morning.

Danaparoid sodium is another antithrombotic agent that can be used for prophylaxis against the formation of deep vein thrombosis in patients who are undergoing elective hip replacement surgery. This medication is not a low molecular weight heparin but is actually a glycosaminoglycan. This particular antithrombotic acts in a way similar to that of LMWH. Danaparoid prevents fibrin formation by inhibiting the formation of thrombin by antifactor Xa and IIa activity. Danaparoid sodium is administered by subcutaneous injection beginning 1–4 h preoperatively at 750 units and then continued twice daily until the risk of thrombosis formation has diminished. Danaparoid sodium seems to have less effect on platelets, with a lower incidence of heparin-induced thrombocytopenia. It has been shown to have a low cross-reactivity with antiplatelet antibodies in individuals who have developed heparin-induced thrombocytopenia in the past. Therefore, danaparoid sodium is used in individuals who require thrombosis prophylaxis and who cannot tolerate unfractionated heparin or low molecular weight heparin because of prior development of thrombocytopenia.

Danaproid is useful in patients with a history of heparin-induced thrombocytopenia.

Low-Dose Warfarin Low-dose warfarin is another prophylactic option for patients undergoing elective total hip or knee replacement surgery, patients undergoing surgery for fractured hips, and certain general surgery patients, particularly those that are at highest risk for the development of deep vein thrombosis. However, the use of warfarin is more cumbersome than heparin because it requires some dosage titration and monitoring of laboratory tests of coagulation status. Furthermore, certain drug interactions are relevant. Warfarin works by inhibiting the production of vitamin K-dependent coagulation factors, namely VII, IX, and X, and prothrombin, as well as the naturally occurring anticoagulants protein C and protein S. When long-term prophylaxis is indicated in chronic high-risk patients, warfarin therapy may be appropriate.

The initial dose of warfarin is 10 mg orally followed by a daily dose of 2 mg. Then, the dosage is adjusted to achieve a prothrombin time with an international normalized ratio (INR) of 2–3. Warfarin has been used at 1 mg/day to reduce the risk of catheter-associated deep vein thrombosis formation. This dose normally does not alter the INR above that of control.

The use of warfarin is associated with a higher risk of bleeding. There are numerous endogenous and exogenous factors, including a large variety of medications that are associated with either increasing or decreasing the anticoagulant effect of warfarin. A keen awareness of these factors is required when warfarin therapy is used.

Mechanical Prophylaxis

Intermittent Pneumatic Compression Devices Intermitted pneumatic compression devices (IPCD) are applied to the legs and provide rhythmic external compression with 35–40 mmHg pressure for about 10 s every 1–2 min. In addition to mechanically accelerating blood flow, these devices may enhance blood fibrinolytic activity. The proposed mechanism is a reduction in plasminogen activator inhibitor-1, with a resultant increase in local tissue plasminogen activator activity. Either alone or in combination with LMWH, IPCD are effective prophylaxis for deep vein thrombosis in patients undergoing general surgery, major knee and hip surgery, open urologic procedures, and gynecologic surgery. These devices have been shown to be useful prophylactic measures in patients with moderate to high thrombotic risk and as adjunctive therapy in the highest risk population. Obviously, IPCD do not increase the risk for bleeding, but they should not be used in patients with compromised arterial circulation. These devices are generally well accepted by the patient, are comfortable, and can be removed easily for physical therapy or ambulation.

Intermittent pneumatic compression devices (IPCD) are effective prophylaxis for deep vein thrombosis in patients undergoing surgery.

Graded Compression Stockings Graded compression elastic stockings can improve venous return from the lower extremities, and when properly fitted and worn preoperatively, they provide a safe, simple, and inexpensive method for preventing deep vein thrombosis, especially in low-risk patients. These stockings apply graduated compression, that is, compression that is greatest in the lower part of the calf and steadily diminishes up the leg. When used in combination with low-dose unfractionated heparin, intermittent pneumatic compression and graded compression elastic stockings enhance each other's effectiveness at reducing the incidence of lower extremity deep vein thrombosis during a variety of surgical interventions.

Inferior Vena Cava Filters

Inferior vena cava filters have been shown to substantially reduce the risk of fatal pulmonary embolism in certain clinical scenarios, namely, documented iliofemoral vein thrombosis and a contraindication to anticoagulation, documented pulmonary embolism during full anticoagulation, a large free-floating thrombus, and a high-risk condition for fatal pulmonary embolism. Such high-risk conditions include patients with severe cardiopulmonary disease. Furthermore, IVC filters can be placed in individuals who do not have ilial vein thrombosis but are at high risk for the development of thrombosis and require long-term prophylaxis. Such patients include those who have paraplegia or who have a very high-risk for both thromboembolism and hemorrhage.

STRESS GASTRITIS AND ULCER PROPHYLAXIS

In 1938, Cushing described an association between head injury and gastrointestinal hemorrhage. A similar association between severe burns and duodenal ulceration was described by Curling in 1942. These discoveries were followed by an understanding of the protective process or mucosal barrier associated with the gastric or duodenal epithelium, which maintains its integrity despite constant assault from what the individual eats and hydrochloric acid and pepsin. In the past, it was not uncommon for major gastrointestinal hemorrhage to occur in seriously ill people. However, over the past 10–20 years, the incidence of upper gastrointestinal hemorrhage in seriously ill patients has dramatically declined, because of the widespread use of histamine blockers, antacids, and enteral feeding, all of which are likely responsible for this improvement. Early gastric alkalinization trials with histamine blockers and antacids clearly demonstrated efficacy in reducing stress-related mucosal damage, both gastritis and ulceration. More recent research has concentrated on finding medications that are even more efficacious, less costly, and with fewer adverse reactions.

The incidence of stress gastritis and ulceration in the intensive care unit varies from as low as 6% to as high as 100% when endoscopy is used to identify its presence. Rates of overt bleeding and hemodynamically significant bleeding requiring blood product transfusions are 10%–20% and 2%–5%, respectively. Mortality in patients who have hemodynamically significant bleeding approaches 50%, but fortunately this occurrence is now rare. Most gastric erosions in critically ill patients are clinically silent. Gastric perforation can occur, and the incidence of nosocomial septicemia related to stress-related mucosal damage remains unknown.

Overt stress-induced gastrointestinal bleeding occurs in 10%–20% of intensive care unit (ICU) patients.

Pathophysiology

The gastric mucosa is composed of epithelial cells with tight junctions capable of secreting bicarbonate as well as mucus (Figure 45-1). Theories behind the pathogenesis of stress-related mucosal damage relate to disruption of these tight junctions, destruction of the underlying epithelial cells, and impairment of blood flow necessary for mucosal and bicarbonate production, as well as epithelial regeneration. Endogenous prostaglandins play a role by stimulating blood flow, enhancing the regeneration of epithelial cells, inducing mucus and bicarbonate production, and by suppressing gastric acid production. Although gastric acid is crucial to the development of stress gastritis and ulceration, shock with decreased mucosal blood flow actually decreases acid production, but this reduction in blood flow leads to a decreased synthesis of mucus, bicarbonate, and a variety of prostaglandins, and to epithelial cell regeneration. Therefore, this reduction in mucosal blood flow is thought to be essential to the development of stress-related gastric mucosal damage. However, in certain clinical conditions such as burns, central nervous system trauma, and severe infection, gastric acid secretion may be markedly increased.

Indications

Not all patients in the intensive care unit require stress ulcer prophylaxis. Historically, a variety of clinical conditions have been considered high risk for stress ulcer-related bleeding

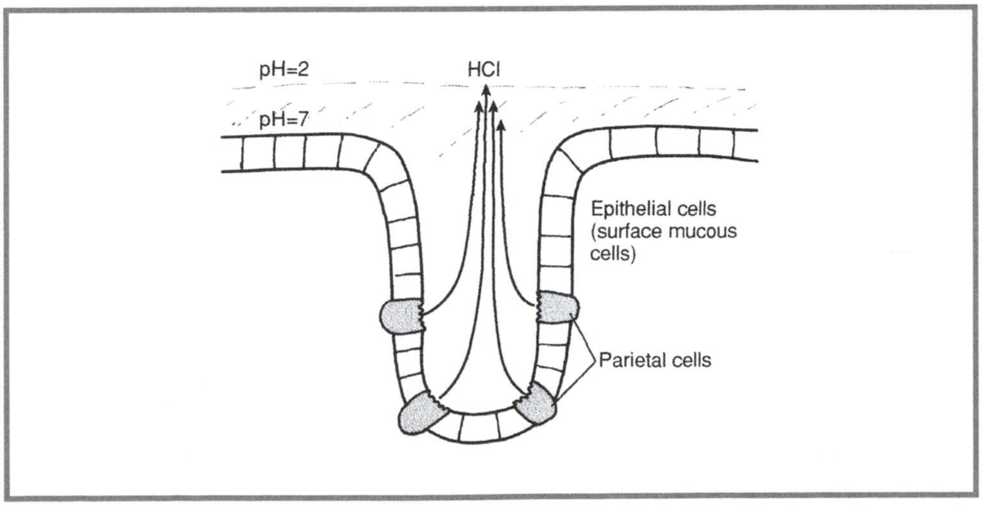

FIGURE 45-1

Production of HCl by parietal cells in the gastric mucosa and transport to the gastric lumen. A protective layer of mucus preserves a pH of 7 near the cell surface, whereas the intraluminal pH is 2. (Adapted from DelValle J, Lucey MR, Yamada T. Gastric secretion. In: Textbook of Gastroenterology, 2nd Ed. Philadelphia: Lippincott, 1995:219.)

prophylaxis. These conditions include head injury, thermal injury involving at least 30% of the body surface area, emergent or major surgery, severe multisystem trauma, shock and multiorgan failure, coagulopathy, mechanical ventilation for longer than 48 h, ongoing therapy with a variety of ulcerogenic drugs, and a history of ulcer-related bleeding. More recently, a very large trial conducted to study the indications for the use of stress gastritis prophylaxis identified two important independent risk factors, namely, respiratory failure requiring mechanical ventilation for more than 24 h and coagulopathy. For patients who are eating normally or receiving near-target rates of enteral tube feedings, gastric acid suppression has no benefit, especially for nonventilated patients.

Patients with coagulopathy and requiring mechanical ventilation benefit highly from stress-induced gastritis prophylaxis.

Endoscopically, stress ulcerations are superficial erosions in the gastric mucosa, distinctly different from the lesions of peptic ulcer disease, which are deeper craters that can erode through the entire width of the gastric wall. Sometimes not just erosions but actual ulcerations are associated with this condition. These gastric ulcers are generally found on the lesser curvature of the fundus of the stomach; they are often associated with clinically relevant hemorrhage. Rarely, hemorrhage from an exposed artery in the ulcer crater may occur.

Gastric acid suppression has been associated with a slight increased risk of nosocomial pneumonia. This risk likely results from the increased gastric growth of bacteria and subsequent aspiration, particularly in individuals that have gastric feeding tubes in place. This risk can be eliminated if stress ulceration prophylaxis is not given when not needed. Furthermore, by elevating the head of the patient to 30°, the risk of gastric content reflux and potential aspiration is minimized. Others advocate the use of enteral feedings as a way of not only reducing stress ulceration but also minimizing this further risk of nosocomial pneumonia.

Methods

Stress ulceration is generally asymptomatic. Therefore, prophylactic efficacy for medications has been evaluated by the incidence of clinically recognized bleeding. Therapies that have been recognized as effective for reducing the incidence of overt bleeding from stress ulceration include antacids, histamine-2-blockers, sucralfate, proton pump inhibitors, prostaglandin inhibitors, and enteral feeding.

The principal mechanism for the development of stress-related mucosal damage is impaired mucosal blood flow. Therefore, the most important preventative strategy includes measures that preserve an adequate mesenteric blood flow. The best strategy is to maintain appropriate systemic blood pressure, hemoglobin, and cardiac output so that oxygen transport to the bowel is optimal.

Decreased gastric mucosal blood flow is the primary casual factor of stress-induced gastritis.

Antacids

Knowing the role of hydrochloric acid in the development of stress-related mucosal damage led to the hypothesis that antacids could be given to neutralize gastric acid and thus reduce the incidence and severity of stress gastritis and ulceration. When the gastric pH was kept above 4 by antacid therapy, this form of prophylaxis was deemed successful. However, large volumes of antacid therapy are frequently required, and an intensive degree of work by nurses is required to accomplish this feat. Furthermore, diarrhea is a bothersome adverse event. Considering these negatives, there is no advantage to using antacids over other therapies that neutralize gastric acid, such as histamine-2-blockers and sucralfate. Furthermore, antacids that include aluminum, magnesium, or calcium reduce the absorption of a variety of different medications, including digoxin, iron, prednisone, phenytoin, thyroxine, and multivitamins. For these reasons, antacids are rarely used for stress gastritis and ulceration prophylaxis in the intensive care unit.

Antacids are rarely used for stress-induced gastritis prophylaxis.

Sucralfate

Sucralfate is a product of sucrose octasulfate and aluminum hydroxide. Its therapeutic action appears to be related to its ability to bind to exposed epithelial cells and ulcer craters, forming a protective barrier. It may also work by stimulating prostaglandin synthesis, enhancing the absorption of pepsin and stimulating epidermal growth factor. The medication is administered either orally or via a nasogastric tube at a dose of 1 g every 6 h. This medication is safe, inexpensive, and easy to administer, requiring less volume than antacid therapy. Sucralfate has been shown to be as effective as antacid therapy and histamine-2 blocker therapy, and more recent data have suggested that there is a decreased incidence of nosocomial pneumonia when compared to these other medications. A disadvantage of sucralfate is that it potentially can interfere with the absorption of a large variety of medications, including cimetidine, ciprofloxacin, coumadin, warfarin, phenytoin, ranitidine, theophylline, and ketoconazole. Therefore, these medications must be given at least 2 h before the enteral administration of sucralfate. Obviously, this disadvantage does not apply when these medications are administered parenterally. Because sucralfate requires acid for dissolution and tissue binding, it is ineffective if administered concurrently with antihistamines or histamine-2-blockers.

Sucralfate prevents stress-induced gastritis and is not associated with the development of nosocomial pneumonia.

Enteral Nutrition

Enteral feedings have been shown to reduce the risk of stress ulcer bleeding and at the same time to provide daily nutritional requirements. It is thought that nutritional feeding neutralizes gastric acid, but it also maintains the integrity of the mucosa of the gastrointestinal tract. If enteral feedings are being used, other protective measures are not necessary for the majority of patients, with the exception of very high risk patients, to prevent the development of stress ulceration.

Histamine-2 Receptor Antagonists

Perhaps the most popular method of preventing stress-related mucosal injury is to inhibit gastric acid production with histamine-2 receptor blockers. All histamine antagonists are equally effective in reducing the incidence of stress ulcer bleeding. In the critically ill patient, these medications are often given intravenously, although oral therapy is just as effective. Several different histamine-2 receptor blockers are available, including cimetidine, ranitidine, and famotidine. Famotidine administered twice daily has been shown to be as effective as the continuous infusion of cimetidine and ranitidine and superior to bolus therapy of either drug. Therefore, famotidine 20 mg intravenously every 12 h is considered the histamine-2 receptor antagonist of choice.

Histamine receptor blocker therapies are highly effective and safe for the prevention of stress-induced gastritis.

Histamine-2 blockers do have side effects and potential drug interactions. Certain agents can induce thrombocytopenia, and cimetidine decreases the hepatic metabolism of a large number of medications. Famotidine seems to have the lowest adverse-effect profile.

Proton Pump Inhibitors

Orally administered proton pump inhibitors, omeprazole and lansoprazole, theoretically should reduce the risk of bleeding from stress-related mucosal damage. However, there are no data to suggest that these therapies are helpful in critically ill patients. They are both used in the treatment of peptic ulcer disease, gastroesophageal reflux disease, and erosive esophagitis.

Prostaglandins

Misoprostol, a prostaglandin, has both antisecretory and mucosal protective properties. Therefore, it reduces gastric acid secretion and protects the gastroduodenal mucosa from ulceration. Furthermore, this medication likely increases mucosal bicarbonate and actual mucosal mucus production and may stimulate the production of new mucosal epithelial cells. Misoprostol's efficacy at preventing stress ulcer bleeding is unclear. It has been used to protect against gastric ulcer formation in patients taking nonsteroidal antiinflammatory drugs.

NOSOCOMIAL INFECTION PROPHYLAXIS

Recently, the results of a very large European trial that evaluated the prevalence of infection in the intensive care unit reported that approximately 20% of the patients had intensive care unit-acquired infection. The majority had infection of the lower respiratory tract, followed by urinary tract infections and bacteremia. Seven risk factors for the development of infection in the intensive care unit were identified:

1. Length of stay greater than 48 h
2. Mechanical ventilation
3. Surgery or trauma
4. Central venous line catheterization
5. Pulmonary artery catheterization
6. Urinary catheterization
7. Stress ulcer prophylaxis

When infection was present, the likelihood of death also increased, but the study identified that nearly 30% of the patients could have had their infection prevented through programs that stress surveillance.

Nosocomial Pneumonia

Nosocomial, or hospital-acquired, pneumonia in the intensive care unit is common, accounting for approximately half of all nosocomial infections in critically ill patients. Also, it is the most fatal of the nosocomial infections, with a mortality of approximately 50% despite aggressive therapy and a large variety of newer antibiotics. Nosocomial pneumonia generally occurs by aspiration of oropharyngeal contents into the airways, but it can also occur by bacterial spread from another focus. Risk factors for the development of nosocomial pneumonia that have been identified include aspiration of bacteria from the oropharynx, colonization of the oropharynx with virulent nosocomial pathogens, the supine position, the presence of a nasogastric tube, and possibly reflux of bacteria from gastric colonization. In healthy adults, there is a certain bacterial colonization picture involving the oropharynx. This picture changes in patients who have been hospitalized only a few days, where the predominant bacteria change from anaerobic bacteria, such as *Bacteroides melaninogenicus*, to a variety of aerobic gram-negative rods and *Staphylococcus*. The gram-negative rods include *Pseudomonas, Proteus, Haemophilus, Escherichia coli*, and *Acinetobacter*. *Legionella* and *Pneumococcus* also may be found.

The major pathogens in nosocomial pneumonia are *Staphylococcus aureus* and a variety of enteric gram-negative rods.

In seriously ill patients, in an attempt to reduce the incidence of stress-induced mucosal injury, a variety of medications are employed to reduce the acid pH of the stomach. When gastric acidity is suppressed, the bacteria that normally inhabit the oropharynx and are found in the saliva can survive in the stomach. This gastric colonization provides another reservoir for bacteria that eventually find its way up the esophagus and into the airways of the lungs. With the presence of a nasogastric tube, even while the patient has an endotracheal tube in place, there is a facilitated pathway from the stomach to the lungs.

Currently, major issues in nosocomial pneumonia focus on the problems associated with documenting true infection and isolating the responsible pathogens. However, this section focuses on preventive interventions only. Patients who are at high risk for stress ulceration should receive preventative therapies. The use of sucralfate, which does not decrease gastric pH, carries the lowest risk of nosocomial pneumonia; however, if histamine-2 receptor antagonist therapy is required, then this should be reserved for those patients who need it the most, namely, patients with coagulopathy or those who have been intubated for more than 48 h. Nasogastric tubes should be left in place only so long as necessary, and when in place, the patient should be maintained in the semirecumbent position to minimize esophageal reflux and subsequent aspiration. Patients who are able and encouraged to perform incentive spirometry frequently have a lower risk for the development of nosocomial pneumonia. Therefore, minimizing sedation so that pulmonary toilet maneuvers, including an effective cough,

Maintaining the semirecumbent position, following pulmonary toilet measures, and minimizing sedation all reduce the risk of nosocomial pneumonia.

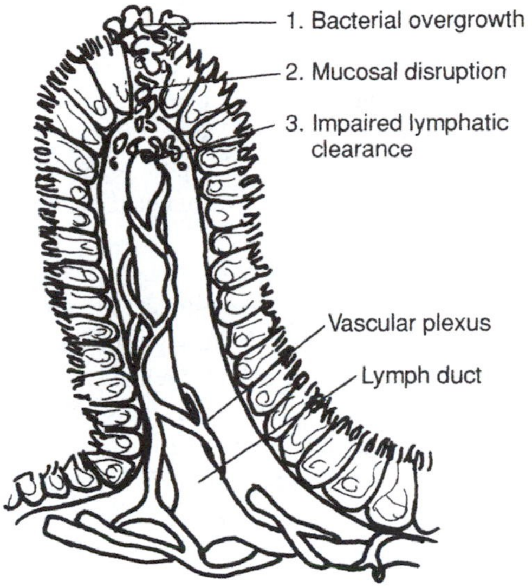

FIGURE 45-2

Intestinal mucosal disruption followed by bacterial translocation. Impaired lymphatic clearance subsequently allows bacterial vascular penetration.

can be accomplished is an important prophylactic measure. The topical application of an antimicrobial paste to the oral mucosa has been shown to prevent colonization of the oropharynx with potential pathogenic organisms. One preparation is methylcellulose paste containing 2% polymyxin, 2% tobramycin, and 2% amphotericin B, which can be applied to the inside of the mouth with a gloved finger every 6 h.

As mentioned, a bacteremic etiology of nosocomial pneumonia must be recognized. The bacteremia may come from a variety of sources, including intravenous line or arterial line sepsis and from translocation of bacteria through the bowel (Figure 45-2). In critically ill patients, a variety of protective mechanisms that limit the movement of bacteria from the bowel into the bloodstream become defective. Therefore, translocation of bacteria can occur. With bowel microbial overgrowth and disruption of the surface mucosa, bowel microbes can leak into the bloodstream, and in the absence of effective lymphatic protective mechanisms, bacteremia can occur. With bacteremia, nosocomial pneumonia can occur. Therefore, selective digestive decontamination has been used to reduce the incidence of nosocomial infection, including pneumonia. This method includes not only the use of the oral cavity paste as just described, but the administration of a solution containing polymyxin E, tobramycin, and amphotericin B into the bowel itself. Within 1 week, decontamination occurs, and this prophylactic method can be continued while the patient is in the intensive care unit. Despite favorable results in published studies, this intervention has not been well accepted by physicians.

Finally, if mechanical ventilation can be performed in a noninvasive manner, that is, without an endotracheal tube, then the incidence of nosocomial pneumonia is less. A variety of methods are used for noninvasive mechanical ventilation in critically ill patients.

Vascular Catheter Sepsis

Central venous catheterization and pulmonary artery catheterization are independent risk factors for nosocomial infection in the intensive care unit. Vascular catheters are responsible for up to 15% of all hospital-acquired infections. Nosocomial septicemia can double the length of stay in the intensive care unit and can substantially increase the chance of death. Catheter bacterial colonization is probably very common, but when the denseness of the infection is large enough on the catheter, and the patient demonstrates the findings of infection, then a catheter-related infection can be diagnosed. When the same condition exists, and the bacteria are found in the blood, then catheter-related septicemia is diagnosed. Often, the diagnosis of catheter-related infection is one of exclusion because the catheter site often does not demonstrate any signs of local infection. Catheter-related infection usually is suspected when the patient manifests an unexplained fever and an indwelling vascular catheter has been in place for more than 48 h. The presence of erythema at the catheter site often heightens the suspicion, and rarely pus can be found. Risk factors for catheter-related infection include its site, with femoral catheters having the highest rate of infection and subclavian catheters the lowest, and the duration of catheterization. Negative risk factors include a rigid aseptic insertion technique and careful sterile dressing changing techniques. Catheters impregnated with antibiotics, particularly when placed using a tunneled technique, have the lowest incidence of infection.

Catheter-related infections, by definition, require the recovery of more than 15 colony-forming units (cfu) from the catheter tip while simultaneously recovering the same organism from the blood. The roll plate technique for culturing catheter tips is an acceptable method for evaluating catheter-related infections. A catheter-related infection is defined as greater than 15 cfu from the catheter tip and no organisms in the blood, whereas a catheter-related septicemia is defined as more than 15 cfu from the catheter tip and the same organism in the blood. Septicemia from another site can be suspected if there are fewer than 15 cfu from the catheter tip and the same organism in the blood. The most common organisms cultured are coagulase-negative *Staphylococcus, Staphylococcus aureus*, gram-negative rods, and, less commonly, *Candida* species.

Most catheter-related infections are caused by gram-negative rods and *Staphylococcus* species.

Most people believe that the catheter-related infection originates from the skin. More recently, the bowel has been implicated. With translocation of bacteria from the bowel into the bloodstream in the presence of a foreign body, such as a catheter, colonization of the catheter tip can occur with subsequent infection developing. It is likely that both the skin and the bowel play a role in the etiology of catheter-related infection.

Strict aseptic catheter insertion technique minimizes the risk of line sepsis.

Several practices may be employed to reduce the incidence of catheter-related infection. When a vascular catheter is inserted, standard aseptic technique is employed. Vigorous scrubbing of the skin at the insertion site is the best way to remove surface microorganisms. A povidone-iodine solution is used as a scrub for approximately 1 min before the insertion of the catheter. A polymicrobial ointment is often applied to the catheter site after insertion, but this practice has not been shown to reduce the incidence of catheter-related infection. Once the catheter is inserted, either a standard dressing using sterile gauze or an occlusive dressing made of transparent polyurethane or colloid gels is used to cover the catheter. The occlusive dressings have the advantage of allowing catheter site inspection without removing the dressing, but they do promote microbial colonization on the underlying skin. Occlusive dressings that are more permeable to water vapor are less likely to promote skin colonization; however, gauze dressings are much less expensive. Finally, the routine replacement of indwelling vascular catheters cannot be recommended. Whether the catheter is replaced over a guidewire, or a new site is selected, the incidence of catheter-related infection does not change; however, when the catheter site is changed, there is a risk for catheter-associated complications.

There are certain indications for replacing vascular catheters. Obviously, when the catheter site is erythematous and pus is identified, then the catheter should be removed, and a new insertion site should be selected. When a catheter has been inserted emergently without strict aseptic technique, then either a guidewire exchange or a withdrawal and new site selection for catheterization should be considered. When catheter-related infection is suspected, the use of a guidewire exchange technique is acceptable. Finally, when a cultured catheter reveals more than 15 cfu, and the catheter was replaced over a guidewire, then a new catheter insertion site should be selected, and the old catheter site should be discontinued.

Finally, infection can be introduced to the body from catheter flushing, so minimizing catheter flushing is likely to reduce nosocomial infection.

Urinary Tract Infection

Urinary catheters are responsible for nearly all nosocomial urinary tract infections.

Urinary tract infection accounts for 15%–30% of all nosocomial infection, and it accounts for approximately 15% of nosocomial infection in the intensive care unit. Of these, 80% are associated with indwelling urinary catheters. Bacteriuria is the accepted precursor of urinary tract infection and potentially urosepsis. Risk factors for bacteriuria include diabetes mellitus, colonization of the catheter and drainage bag, and duration of urinary catheterization. There is a 5% per day increase in bacteriuria with urinary catheterization with rates as high as 50% by 5 days. Bacterial migration along the catheter is the presumed mechanism for the link between catheters and urinary tract infections. Also, the protective lining of the bladder, which in part involves *Lactobacillus* organisms, seems to be disrupted in patients who have chronic urinary bladder catheterization and who are chronically ill.

The common pathogens responsible for nosocomial urinary tract infections include *Escherichia coli*, *Enterococcus* species, *Pseudomonas aeruginosa*, *Klebsiella pneumoniae*, and others. *Candida* species are also part of this picture. With long-term catheterization, both *Staphylococcus epidermidis* and *Staphylococcus aureus* can be the cause of the urinary tract infection. The diagnosis is made by urine culture with colony count, with a traditional threshold of 10^5 colony-forming units per milliliter.

Prophylaxis for intensive care urinary tract infections should include the following: the strict adherence to aseptic technique when the urinary catheter is inserted; when necessary, the use of antimicrobial-impregnated catheters; and appropriate daily catheter care which includes the prevention of contamination of the collecting system.

SUMMARY

Currently available prophylactic regimens can reduce the risk of deep vein thrombosis and pulmonary embolism by 50%–70%. Medications can be employed with only minimal risk, namely, bleeding. Deep vein thrombosis prophylaxis should be tailored to the individual's estimated risk assessment.

Stress-induced gastric mucosal injury such that bleeding becomes clinically relevant is rarely encountered because the use of prophylactic measures has dramatically increased; however, many patients who receive stress ulceration prophylaxis likely do not need these medications. Prophylaxis should be directed to those patients who are at highest risk for the development of stress-related mucosal bleeding. Many prophylactic regimens are effective, but famotidine 20 mg intravenously every 12 h or sucralfate 1 g every 6 h appears to be the safest and the most cost-effective medication.

More than 20% of patients admitted to the intensive care unit develop some form of nosocomial infection. Pneumonia, vascular catheter-related infection, and urinary tract infection are the three major nosocomial infections against which we must guard. With meticulous care and certain prophylactic techniques, the rate of each of these infections can be reduced by at least 30%.

REVIEW QUESTIONS

1. **In patients at the highest risk for thromboembolic disease, who are not given deep venous thrombosis (DVT) prophylaxis, the rate of fatal pulmonary embolism is as high as:**
   - **A.** 1:20
   - **B.** 1:200
   - **C.** 1:2,000
   - **D.** 1:20,000

2. **Which of the following interventions has been shown to decrease the rate of nosocomial pneumonia?**
   - **A.** Elevating the head of the bed
   - **B.** Minimizing nasogastric tubes
   - **C.** Noninvasive mechanical ventilation instead of endotracheal intubation and mechanical ventilation
   - **D.** Minimizing sedation
   - **E.** All the above

3. **Which of the following is not a reason to change or remove a central venous catheter?**
   - **A.** Erythema at the insertion site
   - **B.** Fever/leukocytosis without an obvious source
   - **C.** A catheter in place for 8 days
   - **D.** A catheter that was placed emergently without aseptic technique

4. **Urinary tract infections account for 15% of all ICU nosocomial infections. Of these, 80% are catheter related. Proven methods of prophylaxis include:**
   - **A.** Strict aseptic insertion
   - **B.** Antimicrobial-impregnated catheters
   - **C.** Prevention of contamination of the collecting system
   - **D.** Prevention of reflux of urine from the collecting system into the bladder
   - **E.** All the above

5. **True or False: Prophylactic doses of low molecular weight heparin (LMWH) or unfractionated heparin can increase the risk of clinically significant bleeding.**

6. **Which of the following is not a risk factor for clinically significant stress gastritis?**
   - **A.** Mechanical ventilation
   - **B.** Coagulopathy
   - **C.** Acute head injury
   - **D.** Myocardial infarction

7. **All the following are acceptable forms of deep venous thrombosis prophylaxis in patients at moderate risk except:**
   - **A.** Low molecular weight heparin
   - **B.** Intermittent pneumatic compression devices
   - **C.** Low-dose unfractionated heparin
   - **D.** Graded compression stockings

ANSWERS

1. The answer is A. Patients at the highest risk for thromboembolism include those with stroke, spinal cord injury, the elderly, victims of multiple trauma, and lower extremity fractures and surgery. In this group, the risk of fatal pulmonary embolism is between 1% and 5% if no prophylaxis is given. Additionally, the overall risk of pulmonary embolism is 5%–10%, and the risk of proximal DVT is 10%–20%. Given this potential for morbidity and mortality, it is imperative to prophylax accordingly with coumadin, low molecular weight heparin, or a combination of low-dose unfractionated heparin plus intermittent pneumatic compression stockings.
2. The answer is E. Nosocomial pneumonia is the most common ICU-acquired infection; it also carries the highest morbidity (about 50%). Proven prophylactic methods include elevating the head of the bed 30°–45° to reduce reflux and aspiration, minimizing the use of nasogastric tubes, which can be a conduit for aspiration and a source of sinusitis, minimizing sedation to allow for pulmonary toilet, and, whenever possible, using noninvasive positive pressure ventilation instead of endotracheal intubation and mechanical ventilation. Using these methods can reduce the risk of nosocomial pneumonia by as much as 30%.
3. The answer is C. Line-related sepsis accounts for approximately 15% of all ICU acquired infections, doubles the ICU length of stay, and adds to overall mortality. In light of this, many physicians favor changing central venous catheters on a regular basis such as every 3–7 days. This method of prevention has never been shown to be superior to changing lines only when clinically indicated. This practice also exposes the patient to the potential for procedure-related complications. Proven indications for changing a central venous catheter to a new site include erythema or pus at the insertion site, or when the catheter tip ultimately grows more than 15 colony-forming units of bacteria. Lines should be changed over a wire when fever and leukocytosis are present without an obvious source, or when a line was placed emergently without adequate aseptic technique.
4. The answer is E. Urinary tract infections account for 15% of all ICU-acquired infections. Of these, more than 80% are related to urinary catheters. Prophylaxis therefore centers around the proper care and insertion of these catheters. Methods to decrease infection rates include aseptic insertion technique, consideration of antimicrobial-impregnated catheters, prevention of contamination of the collecting system, and, when feasible, removal of the catheter. Employing these methods can reduce the risk of infection by as much as 30% over historical controls.
5. The answer is False. Prophylactic doses of low molecular weight heparin or low-dose unfractionated heparin are exceptionally safe. Clinically significant bleeding resulting in hemodynamic instability or the need for blood transfusion is extremely rare, occurring in less than 1% of all treated patients. When considering the patient population in which these agents are being used (potential mortality as great as 5%), this becomes a clearly favorable intervention in patients at moderate to high risk for thromboembolism.
6. The answer is D. Stress gastritis is relatively common in the ICU. Clinically significant gastritis resulting in hemodynamic instability or the need for blood transfusion is less common, with an incidence of 10%–20%. Studies of which patients are at risk for clinically significant stress gastritis found only four significant causes: head trauma, burns over 30% of the body, coagulopathy, and the need for mechanical ventilation for more than 24–48 h. Myocardial infarction can lead to gastritis but has not been shown to result in clinically significant stress gastritis.
7. The answer is D. Patients at moderate risk for thromboembolic disease include patients more than 40 years of age, undergoing moderate nonorthopedic surgery, with a history of prior deep venous thrombosis, or with a cardiomyopathy or myocardial infarction. These patients clearly benefit from deep venous thrombosis prophylaxis with low molecular weight heparin or low-dose unfractionated heparin. In this group, intermittent pneumatic compression devices are also acceptable, particularly in neurosurgical patients for whom heparin may be contraindicated. Graded compression stockings are only modestly effective at deep venous thrombosis prophylaxis and therefore are reserved for those patients with only a low risk for thromboembolic disease.

SUGGESTED READING

Deep Venous Thrombosis:

Becker DM, Philbrick JT, Selby B. Inferior vena cava filters. Indications, safety, effectiveness. Arch Intern Med 1992;152:1985–1994.

Clagett GP, Anderson FA, Heit JA, et al. Prevention of venous thromboembolism. Chest 1998;114:5315–5605.

Thromboembolic Risk Factors (THRIFT) Consensus Group. Risk of and prophylaxis for venous thromboembolism in hospitalized patients. Br Med J 1992;305:567–574.

Stress-Induced Gastritis and Ulceration:

Ben-Menachem T, Fogel R, Patel RV, et al. Prophylaxis for stress-related gastric hemorrhage in the medical intensive care unit. Ann Intern Med 1994;121:568–575.

Binder HJ. Selective summaries: stress erosive gastritis: what is optimal thrapy and who should undergo it? Gastroenterology 1995; 109:626–632.

Cook DJ, Fuller MB, Guyatt GH. Risk factors for gastrointestinal bleeding in critically ill patients. N Engl J Med 1994;330:377–381.

Cook DJ, Reeve BK, Guyatt GH. Stress ulcer prophylaxis in critically ill patients. JAMA 1996;275:308–314.

Cook DJ, Laine LA, Guyatt GH, et al. Nosocomial pneumonia and the role of gastric pH. Chest 1991;100:7–13.

Heyland DK, Cook DJ, Jaeschke R, et al. Selective decontamination of the digestive tract. An overview. Chest 1994;105:1221–1229.

Maier RV, Mitchell D, Gentiello L. Optimal therapy for stress gastritis. Ann Surg 1994;220:353–363.

Martin LF, Booth FV, Reines HD, et al. Stress ulcers and organ failure in intubated patients in surgical intensive care units. Ann Surg 1992;215:332–337.

O'Keefe GE, Gentilb LM, Maier RV. Incidence of infectious complications associated with the use of H2-receptor antagonists in critically ill trauma patients. Ann Surg 1998;227:120–125.

Nosocomial Infections:

General

Emori TG, Gaynes RP. An overview of nosocomial infections, including the role of the microbiology laboratory. Clin Microbiol Rev 1993;6:428–442.

Garner JS, Jarvis WR, Emori TG, et al. CDC definitions for nosocomial infections, 1988. Am J Infect Control 1988;16:128–140.

Haley RW, Culvar DH, White JW, et al. The efficacy of infection surveillance and control programs in preventing nosocomial infections in US hospitals. Am J Epidemiol 1985;121:182–205.

Vincent JL, Bihari DJ, Suter PM, et al. The prevalence of nosocomial infection in intensive care units in Europe: results of the European Prevalence of Infection in Intensive Care (EPIC) study. JAMA 1995;274:639–644.

Pneumonia

Driks MR, Craven DE, Celli BR, et al. Nosocomial pneumonia in intubated patients given sucralfate as compared with antacids or histamine type-2 blockers. N Engl J Med 1987;317:1376–1382.

Estes RJ, Meduri GU. The pathogenesis of ventilator-associated pneumonia: I. Mechanisms of bacterial transcolonization and airway inoculation. Intensive Care Med 1995;21:365–383.

Fiddian-Green RG, Baker S. Nosocomial pneumonia in the critically ill: product of aspiration or translocation? Crit Care Med 1991; 19:763–769.

Griffin JG, Meduri GU. New approaches in the diagnosis of nosocomial pneumonia. Surg Clin North Am 1994;78:1091–1122.

Lode HM, Schaberg T, Raffenberg M, et al. Nosocomial pneumonia in the critical care unit. Crit Care Clin 1998;14:119–133.

Meduri GU, Johanson WG (eds) International Consensus Conference: clinical investigation of ventilator-associated pneumonia. Chest 1992;102(suppl 1):551S–588S.

Meduri GU, Mauldin GL, Wunderink RG, et al. Causes of fever and pulmonary densities in patients with clinical manifestations of ventilator-associated pneumonia. Chest 1994;106:221–235.

Catheter Sepsis

Bjornson HS. Pathogenesis, prevention, and management of catheter-associated infections. New Horiz 1993;1:271–278.

Cunha BA. Intravenous line infections. Crit Care Clin 1998;14:339–346.

Eyer S, Brummit C, Crossley K, et al. Catheter related sepsis: prospective, randomized study of three methods of long term catheter maintenance. Crit Care Med 1990;18:1073–1079.

Intravenous Nurses Society. Intravenous Nursing Standards of Practice. Belmont, MA: Intravenous Nurses Society, 1990.

Maki DG, Stolz SM, Wheeler S, et al. Prevention of central venous catheter related bloodstream infection by use of an antiseptic impregnated catheter. A randomized, controlled trial. Ann Intern Med 1997;127:257–266.

Norwood S, Ruby A, Civetta J, Cortes V. Catheter-related infections and associated septicemia. Chest 1991;99:968–975.

Perucca R. Intravenous monitoring and catheter care. In: Terry J, Baranowski L, Lonsway RA, Hedrick C (eds) Intravenous Therapy. Philadelphia: Saunders, 1995:392–399.

Timsit JF, Brunell F, Cheval C, et al. Use of tunneled femoral catheters to prevent catheter-related infection. Ann Intern Med 1999; 130:729–735.

Urosepsis

Amin M. Antibacterial prophylaxis in urology: a review. Am J Med 1992;92(suppl 4A):114–117.

Cunnin CM. Detection, Prevention and Management of Urinary Tract Infections, 4th Ed. Philadelphia: Lea & Febiger, 1987.

Daifuku R, Stamm WE. Bacterial adherence to bladder uroepithelial cells in catheter-associated urinary tract infection. N Engl J Med 1986;314:1208–1213.

Paradisi F, Giampaolo C, Mangani V. Urosepsis in the critical care unit. Crit Care Clin 1998;14:165–180.

Sobel JD. Pathogenesis of urinary tract infections: host defenses. Infect Dis Clin North Am 1987;1:751–772.

Tambyah P, Halverson KT, Maki DG. A prospective study of pathogenesis of catheter-associated urinary tract infections. Mayo Clin Proc 1999;74:131–136.

Warren JW. Catheter-associated urinary tract infections. Infect Dis Clin North Am 1987;1:823–854.

Wong ES. New aspects of urinary tract infections. Clin Crit Care Med 1987;12:25–38.

CHAPTER 46

RODGER E. BARNETTE AND GERARD J. CRINER

Use of Neuromuscular Blocking Agents in the Intensive Care Unit

CHAPTER OUTLINE

LEARNING OBJECTIVES

After studying this chapter, you should be able to:

- Understand the pharmacokinetics and pharmacodynamics of various neuromuscular blocking (NMB) agents.
- Know the complications associated with the prolonged use of NMB agents in the critically ill patient.
- Recognize the potential for interaction among commonly used drugs and NMB agents.
- Make recommendations regarding the use and dose of NMB agents in the critically ill.
- Understand the need for routine monitoring of neuromuscular function in the critically ill patient receiving NMB agents.
- Understand the need for routine and effective sedation and analgesia in the critically ill patient receiving NMB agents.

In the mid-1980s, the two intermediate-duration neuromuscular blocking (NMB) agents atracurium and vecuronium were introduced into practice; within a few years, these accounted for the majority of NMB agent use in critically ill patients. In association with the introduction of these new agents, there was an expansion of the indications for muscle paralysis in this country, which was at least partially related to new ventilatory modes and technologic advances that necessitated cooperative, sedate, or immobile patients. These new indications for an immobile patient, coupled with an expanded knowledge of available NMB agents, led to a dramatic increase in the use of muscle paralysis in the intensive care unit (ICU). In association with that increased use came a growing awareness of the potential for severe complications and side effects.

It cannot be stressed too heavily that neuromuscular blocking (NMB) agents do not have sedative, amnesic, or analgesic effects.

It cannot be stressed too heavily that NMB agents do not have sedative, amnesic, or analgesic effects. Therefore, it is mandatory to administer, concurrently with NMB agents, medications that have those effects. Adequate dosing with a combination of benzodiazepine and narcotic is optimal. Propofol infusions in the dosages commonly used in the ICU may lack amnesic action and provide no analgesia. In this chapter we review the pharmacology, indications for use, monitoring, and complications of NMB agents used in the management of critically ill patients techniques.

PHYSIOLOGY OF NEUROMUSCULAR BLOCKADE

Transmission of the nerve cell action potential across the synaptic cleft and initiation of a muscle cell action potential is accomplished in the following manner. Acetylcholine is synthesized from acetate and choline and stored in vesicles in the motor nerve ending in close proximity to the nerve cell membrane and opposite the area of the muscle cell with the highest density of nicotinic acetylcholine receptors. A nerve cell action potential initiates an influx of calcium, which allows exocytotic release of acetylcholine into the synaptic cleft. Acetylcholine then diffuses across the synapse and interacts with acetylcholine receptors (Figure 46-1).

The nicotinic acetylcholine receptor is present at three locations: postsynaptic junctional, extrajunctional, and a presynaptic receptor on the nerve ending. The postsynaptic junctional receptors are present in high density at a specialized area of muscle membrane located at the juncture of the primary and secondary synaptic clefts, close to the nerve ending. These receptors are composed of five protein subunits that span the muscle cell membrane. Arranged in a tubelike structure, the receptor complex allows passage of ions through the muscle cell membrane and down their respective concentration gradients when properly stimulated. The two alpha-subunits carry recognition sites for agonists and antagonists. Both alpha-subunits must bind acetylcholine simultaneously to induce a conformational change in receptor structure. With the opening of this five-subunit receptor, sodium and calcium move into the muscle cell, potassium moves out of the cell, and a miniature end-plate potential is generated. If an adequate number of receptors are stimulated, miniature end-plate potentials summarize to exceed the threshold potential and generate an action potential. The action potential activates the adjacent voltage-dependent sodium channels and spreads throughout the muscle fiber, triggering the contraction process. Stimulation of presynaptic receptors causes mobilization of additional acetylcholine for future neuromuscular transmission. Extrajunctional receptors are a concern to the clinician only if they proliferate because of dysfunction of nerve or muscle. Acetylcholine, after diffusing off the receptor, is rapidly hydrolyzed by the enzyme acetylcholinesterase, which is present within the synaptic cleft.

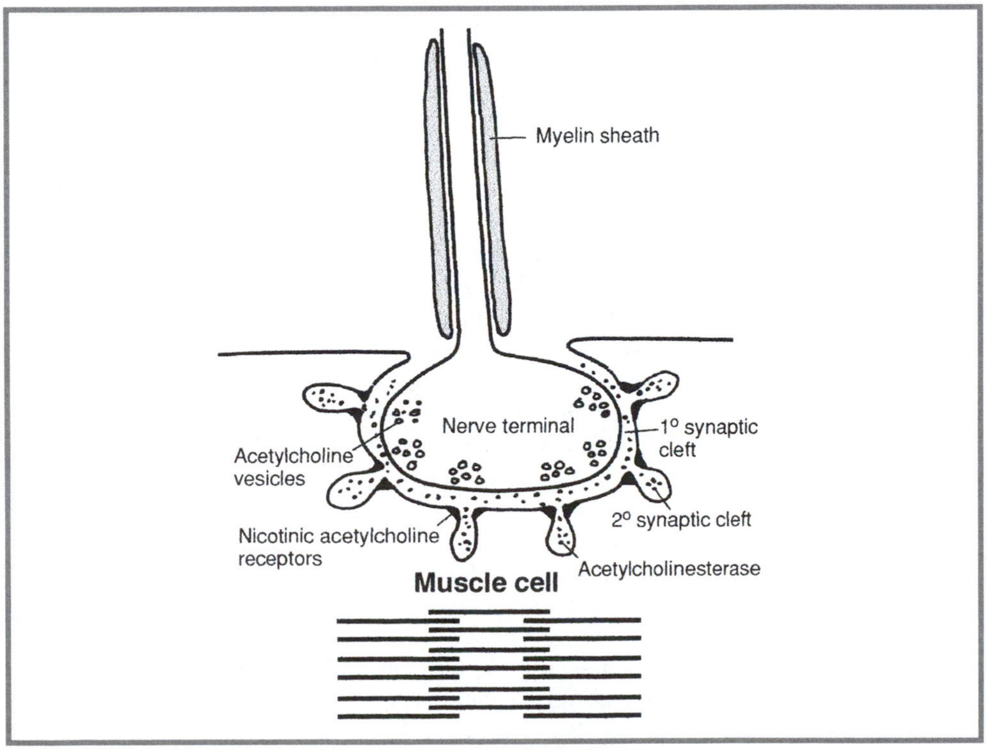

FIGURE 46-1

Schematic diagram of neuromuscular junction.

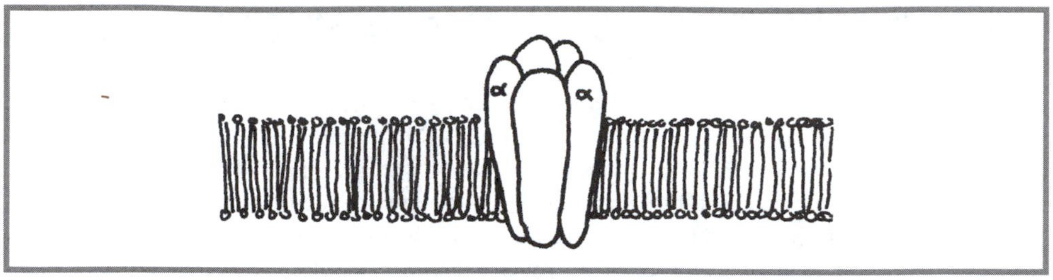

FIGURE 46-2

The nicotinic acetylcholine receptor is composed of five subunits. Both alpha subunits must bind acetylcholine simultaneously to open the ion channel.

Depolarization of the muscle membrane must occur for muscle contraction to take place. Nondepolarizing NMB agents prevent depolarization of the muscle membrane and thus cause muscle paralysis, primarily by competitive inhibition at one or both of the alpha-subunits of the postsynaptic nicotinic acetylcholine receptor (Figure 46-2).

Depolarizing NMB agents also bind to both alpha subunits to exert an effect, but they act as agonists. Because these drugs have a longer duration of action than acetylcholine, the muscle, following an initial contraction (fasciculation), remains persistently depolarized and flaccid.

It should be noted that there exists a wide margin of safety in the number of postsynaptic nicotinic acetylcholine receptors. Only a small fraction of receptors needs to be stimulated to produce depolarization and muscle contraction. For that reason, 70%–75% of postsynaptic receptors must be occupied by nondepolarizing NMB agents before clinical blockade is detectable. Clinically relevant neuromuscular paralysis thus occurs over a narrow range of receptor occupancy (i.e., 70%–100%).

TYPES AND CLASSES OF NMB AGENTS

Depolarizing NMB Agents

Succinylcholine is the only depolarizing NMB agent utilized clinically within the United States.

Succinylcholine is the only depolarizing NMB agent utilized clinically within the United States. It has a very short time to onset, a short duration of action, and is inexpensive. When administered to adults in an intravenous dose of 1–1.5 mg/kg, onset occurs in 60–90 s; spontaneous ventilation is resumed in 8–9 min. It is used most often in situations that require rapid control of the airway. Once the airway has been successfully controlled, if there is an ongoing need for neuromuscular blockade, a nondepolarizing agent is administered (Table 46-1).

In patients who have suffered denervation injuries, massive increases in the number of extrajunctional nicotinic acetylcholine receptors can result in life-threatening hyperkalemia if succinylcholine is administered.

The side effects of succinylcholine include a transient, but potentially hazardous, increase in serum potassium levels. This increase in serum potassium is mediated by the simultaneous opening of large numbers of nicotinic acetylcholine receptors and is on the order of approximately 0.5 mEq/dl. In patients with normal nicotinic acetylcholine receptor density, this becomes a concern only if high levels of potassium exist at the time of drug administration, as might be the case in a patient with renal failure. However, in patients who have suffered denervation injuries, massive increases in the number of extrajunctional nicotinic acetylcholine receptors can result in life-threatening hyperkalemia if succinylcholine is administered. Both upper and lower motor neuron lesions are contraindications to the use of succinylcholine, depending on time from injury. Succinylcholine should not be administered to patients beyond 48 h from time of injury and remains contraindicated for 6–12 months. Direct muscle injury, extensive burns, and a recent history of chronic administration of nondepolarizing NMB agents are also contraindications. Cardiac arrest, secondary to hyperkalemia following succinylcholine administration, has been reported in ICU patients with no risk factors other than immobilization due to confinement.

Succinylcholine is one of the classic triggers for malignant hyperthermia and should not be administered to patients with a history, or family history, of this disorder.

Succinylcholine is one of the classic triggers for malignant hyperthermia and should not be administered to patients with a history, or family history, of this disorder. Other possible side effects include increased intraocular, intracranial, and intragastric pressure. Diffuse muscle pain may occur following succinylcholine administration.

TABLE 46-1

NMB AGENTS USED IN ICU CLINICAL PRACTICE

CLASS	AGENT	BOLUS OR INTERMITTENT INJECTION IN ADULTS (MG/KG)	ONSET (MIN)	DURATION OF ACTION	INFUSION RATE (mg/kg/h)	RECOVERY TIME (MIN)
Depolarizing	Succinylcholine	1–1.5	1–1.5	Ultrashort	N/A	7–9
Nondepolarizing (aminosteroid)	Pancuronium	0.1 every 90–min	3–5	Long	N/A	60–100
Nondepolarizing (aminosteroid)	Vecuronium	0.1 every 35–40 min	2–3	Intermediate	0.05–0.1	20–40
Nondepolarizing (aminosteroid)	Pipecuronium	0.09–0.1 every 90–100 min	3–5	Long	N/A	60–120
Nondepolarizing (aminosteroid)	Rocuronium	0.6–1.0 every 25–30 min	1–1.5	Intermediate	N/A	30–60
Nondepolarizing (benzylisoquinolinium)	Atracurium	0.4–0.5 every 25–30 min	2–3	Intermediate	0.4–1.0	30–45
Nondepolarizing (benzylisoquinolinium)	Cisatracurium	0.15–0.2 every 25–30 min	2–3	Intermediate	0.03–0.6	40–45
Nondepolarizing (benzylisoquinolinium)	Mivacurium	0.15–0.25 every 15–20 min	1.5–3	Short	N/A	15–20
Nondepolarizing (benzylisoquinolinium)	Doxacurium	0.025 every 90–100 min	4–6	Long	N/A	100–160

Nondepolarizing NMB Agents

The nondepolarizing compounds used commonly within both the operating theatre and the critical care unit are organized by structure into two major groups: the aminosteroid compounds and the benzylisoquinolinium compounds. Agents in both groups are quaternary ammonium compounds that contain a positively charged nitrogen atom capable of binding to the alpha-subunit(s) of the nicotinic acetylcholine receptor (Figure 46-3).

Aminosteroid Compounds

The aminosteroid compounds contain a steroid skeleton within their structure. Pancuronium, vecuronium, pipecuronium, and rocuronium are members of this group.

Pancuronium is a synthetic NMB agent that has classically been administered by intermittent injection because of its relatively long duration of action (approximately 100 min following an intubation dose of 0.1 mg/kg). The vagolytic action of pancuronium causes an increase in heart rate, and for that reason it may be unsuitable in patients with coronary artery disease. Excretion is accomplished primarily by renal routes, although hepatic elimination plays a role; it is contraindicated in patients with significant organ dysfunction. Pancuronium has an active metabolite, 3-hydroxypancuronium, with 30%–50% of the potency of the parent compound.

The vagolytic action of pancuronium causes an increase in heart rate, and for that reason, it may be unsuitable in patients with coronary artery disease.

A great deal has been learned about the use of vecuronium in critical care since its introduction in 1984. It is a NMB agent with an intermediate duration of action, often administered by continuous infusion. After a single dose of 0.1 mg/kg, it has a duration of effect of 30–40 min. Vecuronuim has a safe cardiovascular profile and does not affect heart rate or blood pressure. Like pancuronium, it has an active metabolite, 3-desacetylvecuronium, with 80% of the potency of the parent compound. This agent, its metabolism, and its complications are described later in greater detail.

Vecuronium has a safe cardiovascular profile and does not affect heart rate or blood pressure.

Pipecuronium and rocuronium are newer members of this group and have not as yet found routine use among intensivists. Pipecuronium is a long-acting agent similar to pancuronium in structure, potency, and duration of effect but without the vagolytic actions of pancuronium. It also is primarily eliminated via the renal route. There appears to be little difference,

FIGURE 46-3

Acetylcholine, succinylcholine, atracurium, and vecuronium.

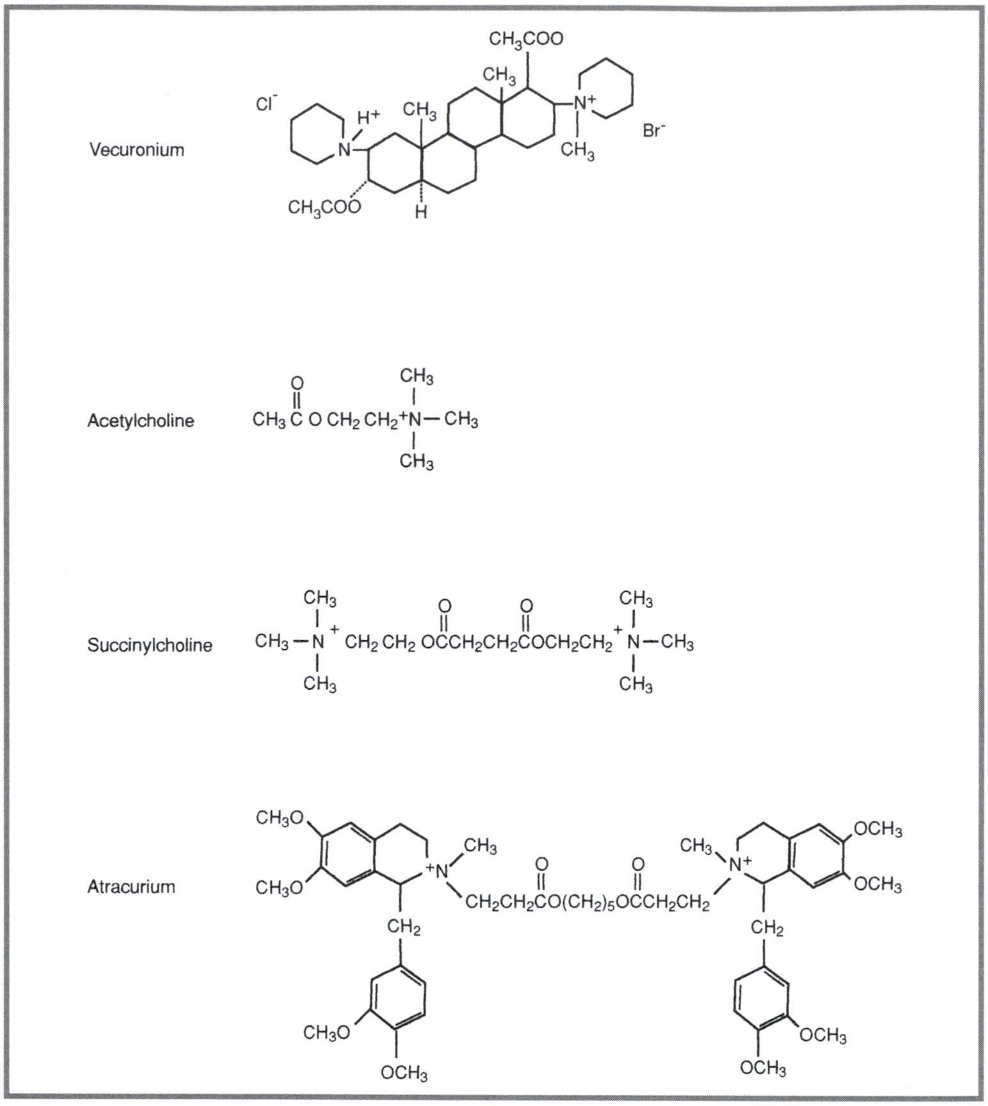

other than cost, in long-term administration of pancuronium versus pipecuronium in the critical care setting.

Rocuronium is intermediate in duration of action (30–60 min). Although similar to vecuronium in pharmacokinetics, it has a more rapid onset of action and a lack of active metabolites. Its time to onset makes it the most attractive alternative to succinylcholine when a nondepolarizing NMB agent is indicated for rapid tracheal intubation. When administered continuously over several days in critically ill patients, plasma clearance decreases, volume of distribution increases, and terminal half-life is prolonged.

Benzylisoquinolinium Compounds

This group includes D-tubocurarine, metocurine, atracurium, doxacurium, mivacurium, and cisatracurium. These agents are esters, and metabolism via ester hydrolysis occurs, to some extent, with each member of the group; some (atracurium, cisatracurium) also undergo a nonorgan-based degradation known as Hofmann elimination. Histamine release, and its effect on cardiac and respiratory function, has been a relatively consistent concern over the years with this group of agents.

Both D-tubocurarine and metocurine have been available for decades and found extensive use within the operating room before the introduction of pancuronium. Bolus administration of these agents can cause significant release of histamine and secondary cardiovascular changes. Both have elimination half-lives greater than 100 min and are primarily cleared by the kidney.

Atracurium is a NMB agent with an intermediate duration of action. Histamine release occurs with bolus administration and can be associated with skin flushing, hypotension, or bronchospasm. This agent is usually administered by continuous infusion in a critical care setting. Atracurium is best known for its rapid spontaneous metabolism, which is largely independent of organ function. It has no active metabolites. Atracurium is metabolized by Hofmann elimination (nonenzymatic degradation at normal body temperature and pH) and ester hydrolysis to yield laudanosine and a monoacrylate metabolite. Concern has been expressed regarding its metabolite, laudanosine, which has been reported to cause seizure activity in animal models. The initial lack of enthusiasm for use of this agent in the ICU may have been the result of fear regarding a possible association between atracurium administration and seizure activity in humans. However, there appears to be no clinical relevance to this concern.

Atracurium is best known for its rapid spontaneous metabolism, which is largely independent of organ function.

Cisatracurium besylate is a purified form of one of the isomers of atracurium. Cisatracurium has a neuromuscular blocking profile similar to that of atracurium with the following exceptions. It is approximately three times more potent than atracurium, has a slower onset of action, and is devoid of the dose-related histamine-releasing effects that plague atracurium. Its rapidity of metabolism, independent of organ function, mirrors that of atracurium. Mean recovery time, comparable to that of atracurium, is approximately 45 min following cessation of infusion. Potential dose-related side effects, such as the accumulation of laudanosine, would be even less likely than with atracurium, because a lesser amount of agent is administered. Cisatracurium has become preferred over atracurium in the critically ill patient because of its lack of histamine release, increased potency, and decreased cost. The safety of cisatracurium and its lack of active metabolites make it a reasonable choice for use in critically ill patients.

Cisatracurium besylate is a purified form of one of the isomers of atracurium.

Doxacurium is a long-acting NMB agent, devoid of histamine-releasing side effects. It is similar to pancuronium in its elimination half-life and dependence on renal clearance but does not cause tachycardia or have other hemodynamic effects. Doxacurium has a slow onset of action and a long duration of effect. It is used infrequently in a critical care setting, and there is limited information regarding administration by infusion.

Mivacurium is a short-acting agent that is rapidly hydrolyzed by plasma cholinesterase. This agent has limited utility in the intensive care unit due to its relatively slow onset, short duration of action, and expense.

INDICATIONS FOR ADMINISTRATION OF NMB AGENTS

Indications for administration of NMB agents can be categorized as short term, to facilitate procedures, or long term, as therapeutic interventions.

Indications for administration of NMB agents can be categorized as short term, to facilitate procedures, or long term, as therapeutic interventions.

In patients with respiratory failure and in patients who need urgent or rapid control of the airway, these drugs are often used to facilitate endotracheal intubation. Additionally, some diagnostic studies, such as magnetic resonance imaging or computed axial tomography, may require absolute immobility for successful completion (Table 46-2). To ensure patient safety

TABLE 46-2

INDICATIONS FOR USE OF NEUROMUSCULAR BLOCKING (NMB) AGENTS

SHORT TERM	LONG TERM
Endotracheal intubation	Facilitation of medical ventilation (synchrony, inverse ratio ventilation, permissive hypercapnia)
Diagnostic studies	Tetanus
Therapeutic procedures	Infant respiratory distress syndrome (RDS)
Patient transport	ARDS, adult respiratory distress syndrome (ARDS)
	Agitation (with concurrent sedative and analgesic treatment)
	Ventilatory support in association with increased intracranial pressure

and successful completion of a diagnostic or therapeutic procedure, such as bronchoscopy, endoscopy, or transesophageal echocardiography, short-term use of NMB agents may be indicated. Additionally, in some settings, patient transport may be an appropriate indication. In these settings, the duration of use is measured in minutes or perhaps hours, and airway control and some form of assisted ventilation is mandatory.

Facilitation of mechanical ventilation is the most common indication for long-term administration of NMB agents.

Facilitation of mechanical ventilation is the most common indication for long-term administration of NMB agents. These agents may allow improvement in the interface between patients and new ventilatory modes, such as inverse ratio ventilation or permissive hypercapnia. Additional indications include the treatment of tetanus, infant respiratory distress syndrome, acute respiratory distress syndrome (ARDS), and adult patients requiring high inspired oxygen concentrations in association with the prone position.

In critically ill patients with neurologic dysfunction and increased intracranial pressure, NMB agents allow suctioning of airway secretions without provoking coughing or dysnchrony with the ventilator. Either of these responses to routine pulmonary toilet could increase intracranial pressure to potentially dangerous levels.

Indications for use of NMB agents in critically ill patients have historically included agitation. Clearly, it is not always possible to adequately sedate a patient without compromising cardiovascular stability. In such a situation, the use of a NMB agent coupled with amnesic doses of benzodiazapines and analgesics would be appropriate. It is important to point out, however, that there are many different combinations of sedative/hypnotics and analgesics available. Personnel in the ICU should be familiar with as many of these combinations as possible to avoid unnecessary neuromuscular paralysis (see Chapter 44). Unfortunately, many critical care practitioners receive inadequate training in the use of sedative/hypnotics, analgesics, and NMB agents, and thus utilize muscle paralysis before exhausting other means of treating their patients.

Once the decision has been made to administer a NMB agent, consideration needs to be given to the most appropriate choice. In patients with significant organ system dysfunction, consideration should be given to metabolism and elimination pathways. Many clinicians make decisions based on their perception of the likelihood of complications; these issues are discussed in greater detail later. It is important to note that as the likelihood and severity of complications has become more widely known, a consensus has been reached that NMB agents should be used only as a last option following failure of sedation/analgesia regimens. Moreover, NMB agents should be used for the minimum time possible.

COMPLICATIONS FROM PROLONGED USE OF NMB AGENTS

Overall, in critically ill adults, there is approximately a 10% incidence of prolonged neuromuscular weakness, of varying duration, following the use of these agents.

Reports of prolonged muscle weakness or paralysis associated with administration of new NMB agents appeared with increasing frequency beginning in the late 1980s. A variety of etiologic mechanisms were proposed. One broad approach to categorizing these reports divided causative factors into pharmacokinetic based, usually persisting for days to weeks, and neuromuscular function based, persisting for weeks to months. Overall, in critically ill adults, there is approximately a 10% incidence of prolonged neuromuscular weakness, of varying duration, following the use of these agents.

Pharmacokinetic Causes

In some instances, a prolonged effect of NMB agents is caused by therapeutic overdose.

In some instances, a prolonged effect of NMB agents is due to therapeutic overdose. A minority of critical care practitioners monitor the degree of neuromuscular blockade, and when monitoring occurs, the findings may be misinterpreted. If monitoring is not performed, or performed improperly, critically ill patients are at increased risk for relative or absolute drug overdose even if state-of-the-art administration guidelines are followed. Patients with prolonged paralysis have often received significantly more muscle relaxant than patients whose recovery was not prolonged. Overdosing of muscle relaxants may be avoided, and an adequate degree of paralysis maintained, by titrating administration of NMB agents with appropriate monitoring of neuromuscular function.

Hepatic and/or renal dysfunction has been implicated as a cause of prolonged drug effect following the discontinuation of NMB agents. The prolonged duration of action of vecuronium in critically ill patients with renal failure has been well documented; this has been ascribed to the inability, in patients with renal failure, to excrete the pharmacologically active metabolite, 3-desacetylvecuronium. The association of renal failure and the prolonged action of vecuronium has been further linked with the presence of metabolic acidosis and elevated magnesium concentrations.

Hepatic and/or renal dysfunction has been implicated as a cause of prolonged drug effect following the discontinuation of NMB agents.

Recently, the pharmacokinetics and pharmacodynamics of 3-desacetylvecuronium have been clarified. It appears that 3-desacetylvecuronium has 80% of the potency of vecuronium and that the liver, not the kidney, is the primary organ of elimination for this metabolite. The reason that patients with chronic renal failure have a markedly decreased clearance of 3-desacetylvecuronium, and thus prolonged drug effect, is related to an associated decrement in hepatic function. The uremia of renal failure has been implicated as a cause of this decreased hepatic clearance. Renal failure thus secondarily prolongs neuromuscular blockade by markedly decreasing hepatic clearance of 3-desacetylvecuronium. Vecuronium and 3-desacetylvecuronium are not removed by hemodialysis.

Interestingly, the action of 3-desacetylvecuronium is clinically relevant even in patients with normal hepatic and renal function and has been found to contribute to the cumulative effect associated with repetitive vecuronium dosing. This cumulative effect further illustrates the need for routine and competent monitoring of neuromuscular function. Although the issue of active metabolites is commonly associated with vecuronium, it has been observed with other aminosteroid NMB agents.

Severe electrolyte disorders (e.g., hypermagnesemia, hypocalcemia, hypophosphatemia, hypokalemia) may produce weakness alone or in combination with NMB agents. Additionally, a number of drugs may potentiate neuromuscular blockade: clindamycin, metronidazole, tetracycline, furosemide, anticholinesterase drugs, and many antiarrhythmic agents. In addition, corticosteroids are known to interact with nondepolarizing agents.

Severe electrolyte disorders (e.g., hypermagnesemia, hypocalcemia, hypophosphatemia, hypokalemia) may produce weakness alone or in combination with NMB agents. Additionally, a number of drugs may potentiate neuromuscular blockade: clindamycin, metronidazole, tetracycline, furosemide, anticholinesterase drugs, and many antiarrhythmic agents. In addition, corticosteroids are known to interact with nondepolarizing agents.

Neuromuscular Causes

Not all instances of prolonged effect of NMB agents are explained by overdose or alterations in pharmacokinetics (Table 46-3). Another major pattern of prolonged paralysis is that of acute myopathy, which becomes apparent only as transmission resumes across the neuromuscular junction. There also appears to be a broad category of persistent paralysis that is secondary to physiologic disruption of neuromuscular transmission.

Another major pattern of prolonged paralysis is that of acute myopathy, which becomes apparent only as transmission resumes across the neuromuscular junction.

The acute myopathy described following prolonged use of NMB agents in critical care has been documented in multiple case reports and patient series. This myopathy is usually described in critically ill patients with nonneuromuscular disorders who have been treated for longer than 24–48 h with a NMB agent. Increasing duration of therapy and total cumulative dose may increase the likelihood of this complication, as will simultaneous administration of corticosteroids. The association of NMB agents and corticosteroids is believed responsible for the 30%–40% incidence of myopathy in intubated paralyzed asthmatics.

This acute myopathy is associated with a variable increase in creatin phosphokinase (CPK), myoglobinuria (which may lead to acute renal failure), and weakness, which in its most extreme form is manifested as flaccid paralysis and areflexia.

This acute myopathy is associated with a variable increase in creatine phosphokinase (CPK), myoglobinuria (which may lead to acute renal failure), and weakness, which in its

TABLE 46-3

CATEGORIES OF PROLONGED PARALYSIS FOLLOWING USE OF NMB AGENTS

1. Overdose and/or the presence of active metabolites
2. Acute myopathy
3. An uncharacterized neuromuscular transmission deficit(s) or a deficit in muscle proteins that support muscle action potential generation
4. One or more of the above in combination
5. Any of the above in association with other neuromuscular complications of critical illness including interactions with drugs that affect neuromuscular function

most extreme form is manifested as flaccid paralysis and areflexia. Cognition and sensation are normal in these patients. Proximal musculature may be more severely affected than distal, and recovery is slow. Prolonged physical therapy and an extended stay at a rehabilitation center are often necessary.

The characteristic pathology involves atrophy of type I and type II fibers with preservation of muscle cell structure, no inflammation, and loss of thick myosin filaments. In animal studies involving steroid administration and surgical denervation of musculature, a severe myopathy with similar pathologic lesions of the thick myosin filaments has been described. The common factor appears to be some type of denervation (anatomic or pharmacologic) in association with the parenteral administration of large doses of steroids.

This myopathy was initially reported with the aminosteroid NMB agents, which accounted for the majority of therapeutic paralysis in the late 1980s and early 1990s. However, as nonsteroidal NMB agent use increased, it became clear that they also cause complications. Atracurium, cisatracurium, and doxacurium have each been associated with the development of myopathy. Apparently the initial lack of association with prolonged paralysis resulted from a lesser experience with this group of drugs rather than specific properties of the benzylisoquinolinium NMB agents.

In addition to an acute myopathy, there is the distinct possibility of an as yet uncharacterized neuromuscular transmission deficit(s).

In addition to an acute myopathy, there is the distinct possibility of an as yet uncharacterized neuromuscular transmission deficit(s). In some patients, neuromuscular junction dysfunction has been documented with nerve conduction studies. Unfortunately, this information is not meaningful unless plasma levels of the parent compound and its metabolites are measured and found to be clinically irrelevant. Otherwise, it is difficult to separate overdose or accumulation of active metabolites from a pathophysiologic alteration in neuromuscular transmission.

Although not all reports regarding persistent neuromuscular blockade resolve the issue of residual drug effect, it is probable that in some patients there is a persistent dysregulation of the nicotinic acetylcholine receptor following prolonged exposure to NMB agents. Many ICU patients demonstrate increasing requirements for NMB agents to maintain a constant level of blockade. A relationship between this observation and an increase in nicotinic acetylcholine receptors has been postulated. Also, infusions of D-tubocurarine have been demonstrated to accentuate burn-induced upregulation of postsynaptic nicotinic acetylcholine receptors. Given what we know regarding the effects of agonist and antagonist therapy on the much-studied cardiac beta receptors, it seems quite likely that similar changes will be found involving the nicotinic acetylcholine receptor or some other muscle protein involved in generating the muscle action potential. It is possible that changes in the nicotinic acetylcholine receptor density, function, or ability to propagate excitation to muscle membranes are common to many if not all patients with prolonged muscle weakness following NMB agent administration.

Other reports of neuromuscular dysfunction following the use of NMB drugs implicate disuse atrophy, critical illness polyneuropathy, or toxic neuromyopathy. Part of the difficulty in evaluating these reports is that it is likely more than one pathologic process is active. The polyneuropathy of critical illness is not uncommonly seen in patients with sepsis, systemic inflammatory response syndrome (SIRS), and multiple organ failure. It is also common for patients with these disease entities to receive NMB drugs. It should not surprise us if there are reports of patients with both critical illness polyneuropathy and severe complications secondary to the use of NMB agents. Additionally, a recent study involving an animal model of sepsis implicated cross-reactive antibodies (initially produced against bacteria) in the downregulation of nicotinic acetylcholine receptors, leading to impaired neuromuscular function. Thus, in some situations sepsis may play a role in the development of neuromuscular dysfunction.

In summary, it seems that most reports of prolonged paralysis can be categorized in one of five groups: (1) overdose and or the presence of active metabolites; (2) acute myopathy; (3) an uncharacterized neuromuscular transmission deficit or a deficit in muscle proteins that support muscle action potential generation; (4) one or more of these in combination; or (5) any of these in association with other neuromuscular complications of critical illness, including interactions with drugs that affect neuromuscular function.

CLINICAL USE OF NMB AGENTS

An appropriate indication must exist for the use of a NMB agent. Long-term utilization of NMB agents to control agitation, assure immobility, or allow synchronization with the ventilator should not be undertaken unless an attempt to control the patient with combinations of sedative/hypnotics and analgesics has been attempted. It has been the experience of the authors that NMB agents are often utilized for control of agitation following an inadequate trial of analgesics and sedative/hypnotics. The combination of various sedative/hypnotics with analgesics has the useful property of synergism and allows a much lower dose of each individual agent than would be possible if their effects were simply additive. This approach is analogous to using multiple chemotherapeutic agents for cancer treatment; it allows maximization of individual drug effect while minimizing unwanted side effects. Involvement of an anesthesiologist may be helpful in tailoring an appropriate combination of sedative/hypnotics and analgesics; in the operating room, this technique of using small amounts of various agents to maximize their effect, while minimizing the side effects of each agent, is known as balanced anesthesia. Some patients will require administration of NMB drugs for control of agitation, but with appropriate use of sedative/hypnotics and analgesics, this number can be minimized.

An appropriate indication must exist for the use of a NMB agent.

NMB agents are often utilized for control of agitation following an inadequate trial of analgesics and sedative/hypnotics.

The choice of NMB agent and the method of its administration should be considered. It is premature to state that one particular NMB agent, or even one particular class of agent, is clearly superior to another. However, in patients with severe organ dysfunction some benzylisoquinolinium agents appear to have an advantage over the aminosteroid compounds based solely on pharmacokinetics. There does not appear to be strong evidence favoring one class of agent over another in regard to complications. NMB agents may be administered by intermittent injection or continuous intravenous infusion. Some clinicians believe that intermittent bolus administration may place a patient at lesser risk because it allows monitoring and titration of drug in addition to periods of normal neuromuscular function. However, there is no clear evidence that one method of administration is superior to another.

It is premature to state that one particular NMB agent or even one particular class of agent is clearly superior to another.

If use of a NMB agent is instituted, it should be utilized for the shortest possible time. Discontinuation of NMB agent administration should occur at least every 24 h as this may decrease the incidence of complications; it will certainly help prevent overdose or accumulation of active metabolites and allow early recognition of prolonged blockade. It also permits a daily physical and neurologic examination and allows the intensivist to repetitively evaluate the need for continuation of this agent. In addition, this allows for daily screening of respiratory function, which may allow for earlier discontinuation of mechanical ventilation.

Discontinuation of NMB agent administration should occur at least every 24 h as this may decrease the incidence of complications. It will certainly help prevent overdose or accumulation of active metabolites and allow early recognition of prolonged blockade.

Care of the Patient Receiving NMB Agents

In addition to the complications noted above, there are potential problems common to all patients who receive NMB drugs long-term. There is an increased incidence of pulmonary embolus in patients receiving NMB agents, which may result from the severity of illness of these patients or their marked degree of immobility. Prophylactic measures should be routinely employed in an attempt to prevent this complication. Issues regarding eye care and protection, prevention of soft tissue injury and pressure necrosis, and adequate sedation should be adequately and consistently addressed in all patients receiving NMB agents. These patients cannot move or communicate with health care personnel in any way. Hypoxemia will result from loss of airway, disconnection from the ventilator, or ventilator malfunction. Therefore, all monitoring devices and alarm systems must be operational, and any alarm must be investigated immediately. An adequate and up-to-date nursing care policy and protocol is an extremely important tool that will help ensure consistency of care. In-service training of ICU nursing personnel at regular intervals is also crucial to the care of patients receiving NMB agents.

Patients receiving NMB agents have an increased incidence of pulmonary embolus.

Issues regarding eye care and protection, prevention of soft tissue injury and pressure necrosis, and adequate sedation should be adequately and consistently addressed in all patients receiving NMB agents.

Monitoring of the Patient Receiving NMB Agents

When the effective dose of a particular drug varies among patients, some type of assessment of therapy must take place. This assessment may simply entail observing for an appropriate clinical response; if that is not forthcoming, and if there are no significant side effects, then additional medication is administered. If there are potential adverse effects, the clinician may choose to measure drug levels or to monitor for adverse effects through some form of clinical observation. Because only a few medical centers are capable of accurate measurement of plasma levels of NMB agents and their active metabolites, we must use some clinical measurement of drug effect in an attempt to achieve neuromuscular blockade while minimizing adverse sequelae.

Neuromuscular function is usually evaluated in the intensive care unit by a nerve stimulator.

Neuromuscular function is usually evaluated in the intensive care unit by a nerve stimulator. The ratio of a single twitch to that of a control twitch reflects the extent of receptor occupancy, in that muscle, by a nondepolarizing NMB agent (i.e., 80% reduction in twitch height is equivalent to 80% blockade). When using train-of-four (TOF) stimulation, four electric stimuli are administered to a peripheral nerve in rapid sequence. Usually the response of the adductor pollicis brevis muscle (adduction of thumb) to percutaneous supramaximal stimulation of the ulnar nerve is chosen for TOF monitoring. However, other sites and other types of monitoring may be useful in the critical care arena. Successive twitches disappear as progressively greater degrees of neuromuscular blockade are achieved. Good correlation exists between the degree of neuromuscular blockade and the number of responses to TOF stimulation. Over the range of 75%–100% blockade, the fourth, third, second, and first twitch become inappreciable, in that order; spontaneous recovery occurs predictably in reverse order (Figure 46-4).

Emphasis must be placed on appropriate training in the use of a twitch monitor. Although TOF stimulation is a relatively simple procedure, there are potential problems associated with its performance. Two common problems are imprecise placement of the electrodes and failure to recognize the variation in response to TOF stimulation that is due to increased tissue thickness between electrodes and nerve (often seen in edematous patients). Placement of the electrodes at the level of the wrist and over the ulnar arterial pulse (the ulnar nerve is adjacent to the artery) is helpful. Wrapping an edematous extremity for several minutes before TOF stimulation can be useful in solving the second problem. Ongoing training and quality assurance activities should be instituted to maintain an acceptable level of expertise in the use of NMB agents and TOF monitoring.

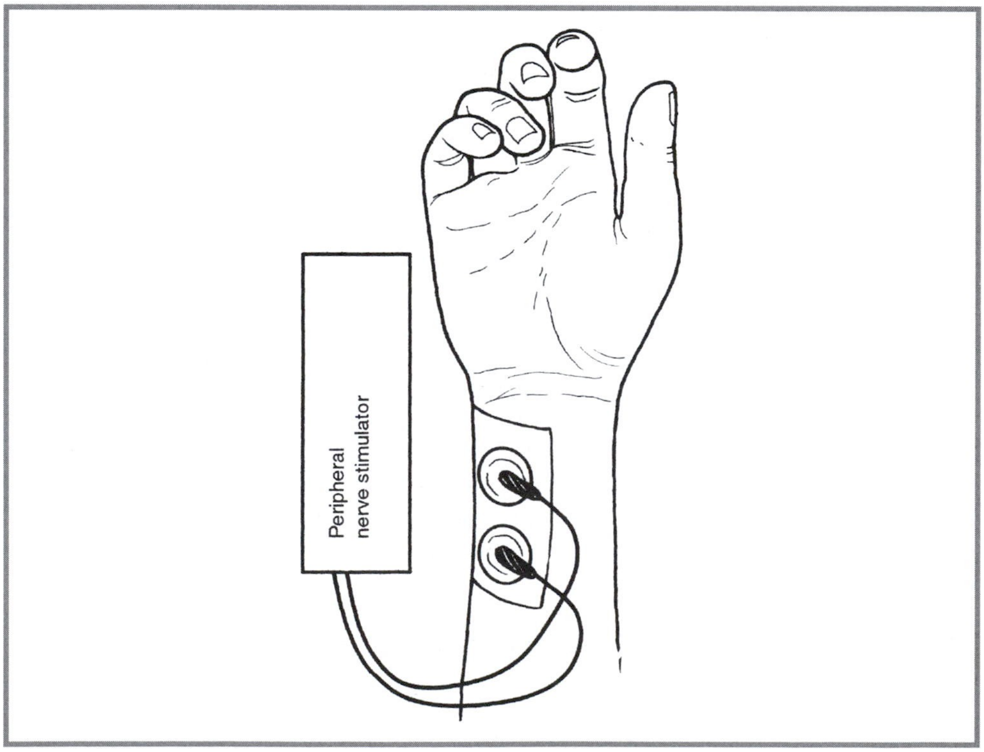

FIGURE 46-4

Proper placement of train-of-four (TOF) twitch monitor electrodes over ulnar nerve.

The diaphragm is the most resistant of all muscles to the action of neuromuscular blocking agents, requiring 1.4–2.0 times as much agent as the adductor pollicis brevis muscle for identical degrees of paralysis. Because the diaphragm will continue to show activity in the face of complete blockade, as measured by ulnar nerve TOF stimulation, more sensitive techniques may be employed. In the operating room, where access to the ulnar nerve is at times limited, it has long been known that TOF stimulation may be applied to the facial nerve and the response monitored at the orbicularis oculi muscle. When TOF stimulation of the facial nerve is compared to stimulation of the ulnar nerve, onset of neuromuscular blockade and time to recovery are similar at the diaphragm and the orbicularis oculi muscle but not at the adductor pollicis brevis muscle. Therefore, the response of the orbicularis oculi to facial nerve stimulation depicts the degree of neuromuscular block of the diaphragm better than the response of the adductor pollicis to ulnar nerve stimulation and is perhaps more clinically relevant in the critically ill.

Ablation of more than three twitches to TOF stimulation at the ulnar nerve is usually unnecessary in the critically ill patient. However, if it is deemed essential to stop all diaphragmatic motion, it will be necessary to increase the degree of neuromuscular blockade to the point where there is no response to TOF stimulation, regardless of monitoring site. Thus, when diaphragmatic paralysis is required, a dilemma in monitoring occurs. In such situations use of the posttetanic count rather than TOF stimulation may enable the critical care practitioner to estimate the amount of time necessary for recovery from neuromuscular blockade and thus more appropriately titrate drug administration. Posttetanic count requires administration of a tetanic stimulus (50 Hz for 5 s) followed a few seconds later by a TOF pattern. It allows accurate prediction of the duration of no response to TOF stimulation because mobilization of acetylcholine from reserve stores will outlast the period of tetanic stimulation (posttetanic facilitation). In the absence of organ dysfunction a positive response to a posttetanic TOF stimulation in a patient receiving vecuronium usually indicates that routine TOF monitoring will be possible within 20 min. Monitoring the degree of neuromuscular blockade with a twitch monitor is reasonable, cost effective and likely to lessen the possibility of prolonged muscle weakness or persistent paralysis.

Ablation of greater than three twitches to TOF stimulation at the ulnar nerve is usually unnecessary in the critically ill patient.

Monitoring the degree of neuromuscular blockade with a twitch monitor is reasonable, cost-effective, and likely to lessen the possibility of prolonged muscle weakness or persistent paralysis.

SUMMARY

A small percentage of critically ill patients will be administered a neuromuscular blocking (NMB) agent for an extended period of time. These agents have a significant profile of adverse effects and should be used with great caution, for the shortest possible period of time, and only if various combinations of sedatives and analgesics have failed to achieve a cooperative patient. Adequate monitoring and cessation of NMB agent administration every 24 h are recommended. It is vital that all personnel involved in the care of patients receiving NMB agents understand their actions, potential complications, and the methods that can be utilized to avoid or decrease the likelihood of a prolonged effect.

NMB agents have a significant profile of adverse effects and should be used with great caution, for the shortest possible period of time, and only if various combinations of sedatives and analgesics have failed to achieve a cooperative patient.

REVIEW QUESTIONS*

1. **Neuromuscular blocking agents:**
   - **A.** Act in part by direct interference with the actin and myosin filaments
   - **B.** Have both analgesic and amnestic effects
   - **C.** In sufficient doses will completely paralyze smooth muscle
   - **D.** Exert an effect via recognition sites on the alpha subunits of the nicotinic acetylcholine receptor

2. **Vecuronium bromide:**
   - **A.** Is a nondepolarizing neuromuscular blocking agent
   - **B.** Has been associated with the development of myopathy following long-term use in the critically ill patient
   - **C.** Is classified as intermediate in duration of action
   - **D.** Is eliminated via the hepatic and renal routes

*Note: More than one answer may be correct.

3. **Cisatracurium:**
   - **A.** Is an isomer of atracurium
   - **B.** Is classified as an aminosteroid
   - **C.** Is more potent than atracurium
   - **D.** Is primarily eliminated via the hepatic route

4. **Which of the following potentiate the action of neuromuscular blocking agents?**
   - **A.** Hypermagnesemia
   - **B.** Hypokalemia
   - **C.** Hypocalcemia
   - **D.** Hyperphosphatemia

5. **Reasonable maneuvers to minimize the potential for prolonged paralysis following the long-term use of neuromuscular blocking agents in the critically ill patient include:**
   - **A.** Stopping administration of the neuromuscular blocking agent at least once every 24 h
   - **B.** Using only neuromuscular blocking agents from the amino steroid group
   - **C.** Monitoring drug effect with a train-of-four twitch monitor
   - **D.** Administering neuromuscular blocking agents via continuous infusion

ANSWERS

1. The answer is D. The postsynaptic nicotinic acetylcholine receptors are present in high density at a specialized area of the skeletal muscle membrane located at the juncture of the primary and secondary synaptic clefts. The two alpha subunits carry the recognition sites for agonist and antagonist drug action. Neuromuscular blocking agents have no analgesic or amnestic effects.
2. The answer is A, B, C, and D. Vecuronium bromide is a nondepolarizing neuromuscular blocking agent with an intermediate duration of action. It has been associated with the development of myopathy following long-term use in critically ill patients. The likelihood of developing such a myopathy is increased with the concurrent administration of corticosteroids. Metabolism and elimination are dependent on hepatic and renal routes.
3. The answer is A and C. Cisatracurium besylate is a purified form of one of the isomers of atracurium and is a benzylisoquinolinium compound. It is approximately three times more potent than atracurium, and its metabolism is independent of organ function.
4. The answer is A, B, and C. Severe electrolyte disorders, such as, hypermagnesemia, hypocalcemia, hypophosphatemia, and hypokalemia may produce weakness alone or in combination with neuromuscular blocking agents.
5. The answer is A and C. Prolonged paralysis has been described with neuromuscular blocking agents from the amino steroid and benzylisoquinolinium groups. Several clinical studies have indicated that monitoring of drug effect with a train-of-four nerve stimulator, cessation of drug administration every 24 h, and intermittent injection, rather than continuous infusion, may reduce the likelihood of prolonged paralysis.

SUGGESTED READING

Barohn RJ, Jackson CE, Rogers SJ, et al. Prolonged paralysis due to nondepolarizing neuromuscular blocking agents and corticosteroids. Muscle Nerve 1994;17:647–654.

Caldwell JE, Szenohradszky J, Segredo V, et al. The pharmacodynamics and pharmacokinetics of the metabolite 3-desacetylvecuronium (ORG 7268) and its parent compound, vecuronium, in human volunteers. JPET 1994:270;1216–1222.

Gooch JL. AAEM case report # 29: prolonged paralysis after neuromuscular blockade. Muscle Nerve 1995;18:937–942.

Hoyt JW. Persistent paralysis in critically ill patients after the use of neuromuscular blocking agents. New Horiz 1994;2:48–55.

Lee C. Intensive care unit neuromuscular syndrome? Anesthesiology 1995;83:237–240.

Lopez DM, Singer LP, Weingarten-Arams JS, et al. Use of neuromuscular blocking agents and sedation in pediatric patients and associated prolonged neuromuscular weakness. Pharm Ther 1999;24: 290–296.

Martyn JAJ, White DA, Gronert GA, et al. Up-and-down regulation of skeletal muscle acetylcholine receptors. Anesthesiology 1992;76: 822–843.

Rich MM, Teener JW, Raps EC, et al. Muscle is electrically inexcitable in acute quadriplegic myopathy. Neurology 1996;46:731–736.

Standaert FG. Doughnuts and holes: molecules and muscle relaxants. Semin Anaesth 1994;13:286–296.

Tsukagoshi H, Morita T, Takahashi K, et al. Cecal ligation and puncture peritonitis model shows decreased nicotinic acetylcholine receptor numbers in rat muscle. Anesthesiology 1999;91:448–460.

Wagner BKJ, Zavotsky KE, Sweeney JB, et al. Patient recall of therapeutic paralysis in a surgical critical care unit. Pharmacotherapy 1998;18:358–363.

Watling SM, Dasta JF. Prolonged paralysis in intensive care unit patients after the use of neuromuscular blocking agents: a review of the literature. Crit Care Med 1994;22:884–893.

CHAPTER 47

Kathleen J. Brennan

Hypertensive Crisis

CHAPTER OUTLINE

LEARNING OBJECTIVES

After studying this chapter, you should be able to:

- Understand the difference between malignant hypertension, hypertensive emergency, and hypertensive urgency.
- Understand the pathophysiology of a hypertensive crisis.
- Evaluate and diagnose a hypertensive crisis using history, physical examination findings, and laboratory studies.
- Know the various classes of drugs to treat hypertensive crisis, their mechanisms of action, and their use in treating hypertensive emergencies.
- Recognize the secondary causes of hypertensive emergencies and the drugs used in their treatment.

Hypertension is a common disease, affecting about 60 million people in the United States alone. Hypertensive crisis, defined as a severe elevation in systemic blood pressure, has an annual incidence of 1% in the general population but accounts for 27% of emergency room admissions. Hypertensive crisis can be divided into hypertensive emergency and hypertensive urgency. Hypertensive emergency is defined as a severe elevation in blood pressure accompanied by signs of end-organ damage (brain, heart, or kidneys). Hypertensive emergencies require rapid control of blood pressure, usually with intravenous medications and intensive care monitoring. Hypertensive urgencies are elevations in blood pressure, without acute end-organ damage, that can usually be treated with oral medications. The main distinction between hypertensive emergency and urgency is the presence of end-organ damage, not the magnitude of elevation in blood pressure. The term malignant hypertension is used to describe a hypertensive emergency with associated encephalopathy.

A hypertensive emergency is elevated blood pressure with signs of end-organ damage. It requires immediate therapy

Hypertensive urgency is elevated blood pressure without signs of end-organ damage. It can be treated with oral antihypertensive medications.

The most common presentation of a hypertensive emergency is a patient with a history of hypertension, already prescribed antihypertensive medication, who is poorly controlled or noncompliant on current therapy. However, there are several other causes of hypertensive emergencies (Table 47-1). If untreated, hypertensive crisis is ultimately fatal. The development of effective antihypertensive pharmacologic therapy has resulted in successful treatment even in patients with severe end-organ damage.

The difference between hypertensive emergency and urgency is the presence of end-organ damage and not the amount by which blood pressure is elevated.

TABLE 47-1

CAUSES OF HYPERTENSIVE EMERGENCIES

- Essential or accelerated hypertension
- Acute aortic dissection
- Preeclampsia and eclampsia
- Acute myocardial infarction or ischemia
- Pheochromocytoma (excess catecholamines)
- Acute renal failure
  - Renal parenchymal disease (glomerulonephritis)
  - Renovascular
- Drugs
  - Cocaine
  - Amphetamines
  - Clonidine withdrawal
  - Monoamine oxidase inhibitor interactions

PATHOPHYSIOLOGY

A hypertensive emergency is the result of several factors that involve changes in systemic vascular resistance, overproduction of renin and other vasoconstrictors, and disruption of blood flow autoregulation in renal and cerebral vascular beds (Figure 47-1). The overproduction of renin leads to an increase in blood pressure via angiotensin II. Studies have found malignant hypertensive patients to have high plasma renin activity. Overproduction of renin also leads to intravascular volume depletion. Loss of autoregulation in vascular beds, coupled with continued release of vasoconstricting substances and volume loss, results in progressive increases in systemic vascular resistance and eventual organ ischemia and necrosis (end-organ damage). Other effects that play a role in this process include thrombocytopenia and intravascular hemolysis.

> The development of hypertensive crisis is a combination of increased humeral vasoconstrictors, loss of vascular autoregulation, and volume depletion.

Important risk factors in the development of hypertensive emergencies include use of birth control pills, smoking, and untreated or poorly controlled hypertension.

DIAGNOSIS AND TREATMENT

> Evaluation of patients with hypertensive emergency should include a complete medical history including previous renal problems, coronary artery disease, hypertension, and peripheral vascular disease.

The diagnosis of hypertensive emergency is made by finding extreme elevations of blood pressure accompanied by physical and laboratory evidence of end-organ damage. Frequent complaints on presentation include headache, visual symptoms, weight loss, and shortness of breath. In the evaluation of hypertensive emergency, a careful history should be taken with

FIGURE 47-1

Pathophysiology of the development of hypertension.

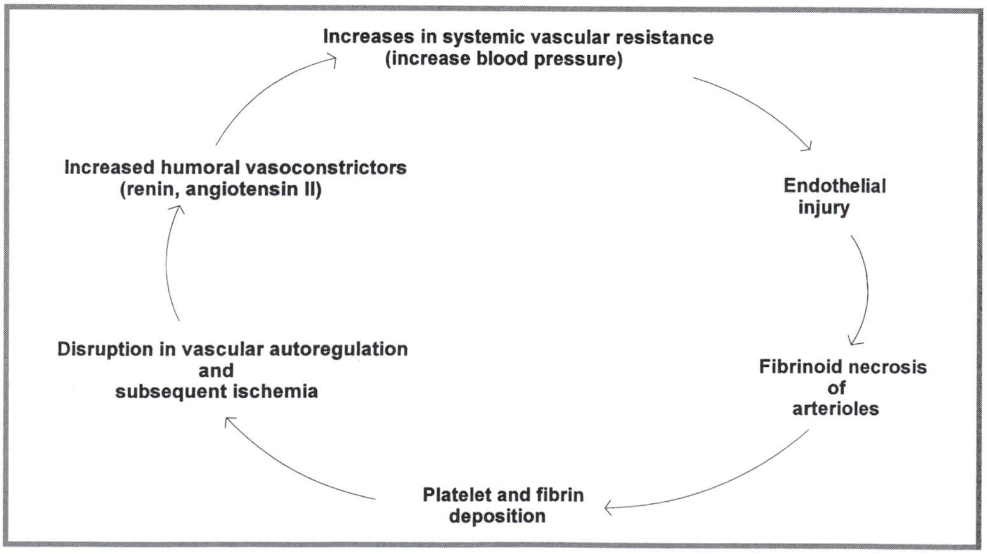

emphasis on prior medical conditions such as hypertension, renal problems, coronary artery disease, peripheral vascular disease, and prior episodes of hypertensive crisis. A detailed history of current medications (prescribed and over-the-counter, including herbal products and nutritional supplements) should be obtained as well as information concerning the use of illicit drugs such as amphetamines, cocaine, and PCP (pentachlorophenol). The patient should be asked about usual blood pressure values.

A complete drug history should include prescribed and over-the-counter medications and illicit drug use.

On physical examination, blood pressure should be measured in both arms using the appropriate size blood pressure cuff while the patient is sitting and standing. While the pupils are fully dilated, a complete funduscopic exam should be done, looking for papilledema, retinal exudates, hemorrhages, or retinopathy. The physical exam should include a careful evaluation of the lungs and heart for signs of pulmonary edema and heart failure. A complete neurologic evaluation assessing level of consciousness, reflexes, and muscle strength is also required. Laboratory testing should include a complete blood count and differential, electrolytes, blood urea nitrogen, creatinine, and urinalysis. A peripheral smear with schistocytes and target cells indicates a microangiopathic hemolytic anemia. Certain changes in serum electrolyes, blood urea nitrogen, and creatinine can suggest the presence of hypovolemia and renal dysfunction. An electrocardiogram and chest X-ray should be done in all patients. Table 47-2 lists important history, physical examination, and laboratory findings in the workup of a patient who is in hypertensive crisis.

Blood pressure should be taken in both upper extremities. A funduscopic examination should be done to rule out papilledema.

If a neurologic process is suspected, a CT or MRI of the head should be included in the initial evaluation.

Computerized tomography (CT scan) or magnetic resonance image (MRI) of the head should be included in the initial hypertensive evaluation if a neurologic process is suspected after taking a history and performing a physical examination. Further evaluation of left heart function can be assessed by performing an echocardiogram if left ventricular dysfunction is suspected or if the patient has signs consistent with myocardial ischemia. Renal ultrasound by doppler technique is recommended if renal artery stenosis is suspected. In cases of suspected aortic dissection or aneurysmal dilatation, a CT scan with contrast or a MRI of the chest and abdomen should be done to identify the location and extent of the process.

Hypertensive patients with suspected left ventricular dysfunction or ischemia can be assessed with an echocardiogram.

In cases of suspected aortic dissection or aneurysmal dilation, initial studies should include a contrast CT or MRI of the chest and abdomen to determine location.

The ultimate treatment goal during a hypertensive emergency is to control systemic blood pressure to prevent further end-organ damage. Initially, intravenous antihypertensive medications should be used to reduce diastolic blood pressure by 15%–20% over a period of 30–60 min. However, in aortic dissection or aneurysm, a 20% reduction in diastolic blood pressure should be achieved in 5–10 min. Once diastolic blood pressure has been reduced by 20% using intravenous medications, oral antihypertensive medication can be instituted and intravenous therapy can be tapered off. In hypertensive urgency, where the goal is to re-

During a hypertensive emergency, diastolic blood pressure should be reduced by 15% over a period of 30 min, except in the case of aortic dissection or aneurysmal dilatation where this reduction should be achieved in at least 15 min.

TABLE 47-2

INITIAL EVALUATION OF HYPERTENSIVE EMERGENCY

History	
Medical:	Hypertension, coronary artery disease, renal disease, peripheral vascular disease, cerebral vascular disease
Medications:	Prescribed (assess compliance)
	Over-the-counter medications (antihistamines and herbal products)
	Illicit drugs: amphetamines, cocaine
Physical examination	
Blood pressure: in both upper extremities while patient sitting and standing	
HEENT: assess for papilledema (increased intracranial pressure), retinal hemorrhages, and exudates	
Lungs: bilateral crackles as sign of pulmonary edema	
Cardiac: extra heart sounds such as an S_3 that signify heart failure	
Abdomen: bruits that can signify partial occlusion of a renal artery	
Extremities: peripheral edema due to left ventricular failure	
Neurologic: weakness; assess mental status to exclude hypertensive encephalopathy	
Laboratory studies	
Electrolytes: blood urea nitrogen, creatinine to rule out renal insufficiency	
Complete blood count urinalysis	
Electrocardiogram to assess cardiac ischemia	
Chest X-ray for evaluation of pulmonary edema	
CT scan or MRI of the head to rule out cerebral ischemia or bleeding	
CT scan or MRI of the chest to rule out aortic dissection	
Echocardiogram to assess left ventricular function	

Hypertensive urgency can be treated with oral antihypertensive therapy, and control should be achieved over several hours.

Patients with hypertensive emergency require frequent blood pressure monitoring either with an automatic blood pressure cuff or an indwelling arterial line. Other support, such as mechanical ventilation, Swan–Ganz catheter, or hemodialysis, may also be required.

duce blood pressure over 24 h, oral medication can be used for initial blood pressure reduction.

Patients presenting in hypertensive crisis usually require accurate and frequent blood pressure monitoring, which can be done with a noninvasive automatic blood pressure cuff or by measuring blood pressure directly using an indwelling peripheral arterial line (i.e., radial arterial line). Patients presenting with alterations in mental status or pulmonary edema may require intubation and assisted mechanical ventilation. Placement of a Swan–Ganz catheter may be needed to assess volume status and aid in fluid management. Patients who present with hypertension due to renal parenchymal disease or who present in renal failure may require hemodialysis.

PHARMACOLOGIC AGENTS FOR HYPERTENSIVE CRISIS

Selection of a pharmacologic agent in hypertensive crisis depends on the rapidity with which blood pressure control needs to be achieved and a number of associated medical conditions. Intravenous medications are usually preferred when rapid blood pressure control is necessary. This section reviews the various classes and examples of antihypertensive drugs used to treat hypertensive emergency (Table 47-3).

Direct Vasodilators

Sodium Nitroprusside

Nitroprusside is a direct arterial and venous vasodilator with an immediate onset of action and short half-life. It is the agent of choice in the treatment of hypertensive emergency.

Nitroprusside is metabolized in the liver to cyanide and thiocyanate. These toxic metabolites rapidly accumulate in patients on high doses or those with renal or hepatic disease.

Nitroprusside can inhibit hypoxia-induced pulmonary vasoconstriction and lead to arterial hypoxemia.

Intravenous sodium nitroprusside has become the agent of choice in the treatment of hypertensive crisis. It has an immediate onset of action and a short plasma half-life. Sodium nitroprusside is an arterial and venous vasodilator. Cardiac output and myocardial blood flow remain unchanged. Cerebral blood flow may decrease. Renal blood flow remains unchanged, and plasma renin activity can increase. Nitroprusside is initially metabolized in the liver to cyanide and then to thiocyanate. These toxic metabolites can accumulate with use of high doses or if medication is continued for long periods and are especially pronounced in patients with hepatic or renal disease. Nitroprusside is usually started at a dose of 0.5 μg/kg/min and titrated in increments of 0.5–10 μg/kg/min until blood pressure is effectively controlled.

Nitroprusside has the advantage of a rapid onset of action and can be easily titrated. However, this process requires monitoring in an intensive care setting, and the medication is degraded on exposure to light so it must be wrapped in a special fashion. Adverse effects include nausea, vomiting, retching, and light-headedness. Nitroprusside can alter pulmonary blood flow, which can result in higher perfusion to poorly oxygenated alveolar areas of the lung, thereby increasing intrapulmonary shunting and arterial hypoxcemia. Patients should be converted to oral blood pressure medications when their blood pressure has been controlled.

Nitroglycerin

Nitroglycerin dilates coronary arterioles, large and small arteries, and venules. It reduces preload and causes coronary vasodilation. It is the drug of choice in myocardial infarction. Tolerance may develop with prolonged use.

Nitroglycerin is absorbed by plastic tubing. Its side effects include headache, tachycardia, flushing, nausea, and vomiting.

Nitroglycerin has long been used as a therapy for the treatment of hypertensive crisis in patients with cardiac ischemia. Nitroglycerin dilates coronary arterioles, arteries, and venules. It is a very potent venodilator that lowers blood pressure by reducing preload and cardiac output. Nitroglycerin reduces cerebral and renal blood flow and therefore should be avoided in patients with increased intracranial pressure or aortic or subaortic stenosis. Nitroglycerin is absorbed by plastic tubing and containers. Its adverse effects include headache, tachycardia, flushing, nausea, and vomiting. Tolerance to nitroglycerin may develop with prolonged use.

Nitroglycerin has a rapid onset of action with a peak effect achieved in 2–5 min. The effects of nitroglycerin persist 5–10 min after the drug is abruptly discontinued. The initial intravenous dose of nitroglycerin is 5–10 μg/min. Nitroglycerin is considered the drug of choice in hypertension secondary to acute myocardial infarction.

TABLE 47-3

CLASSES OF ANTIHYPERTENSIVE MEDICATIONS USED IN HYPERTENSIVE EMERGENCY

DRUGS	USUAL DOSE	RECOMMENDED USES
Direct vasodilators		
Nitroprusside	IV 0.25–10 μg/kg/min and titrate up in increments of 0.5–1.0 μg/kg/min	Hypertensive crisis, intracranial hemorrhage, cerebral infarction, myocardial infarction
Nitroglycerine	IV 5–100 μg/min	Acute myocardial infarction, left ventricular failure
Hydralazine	10 mg IV then 5–20 mg every 20–30 min (maximum 50 mg)	Eclampsia
Beta-blockers		
Esmolol	250–500 μg/kg loading dose over 1 min then infuse 50–100 mg/kg/min	Aortic dissection
Labetolol (alpha and beta blocker)	IV bolus 20 mg then 20–80 mg every 10 min IV infusion 0.5–2 mg/min	Hypertensive encephalopathy, intracranial hemorrhage, cerebral infarction, myocardial infarction, aortic dissection, acute renal failure, eclampsia
Calcium antagonists		
Nicardipine	IV 5–15 mg/h	Myocardial infarction, acute renal failure, eclampsia
Verapamil		Aortic dissection when beta-blockers contraindicated
Diltiazem	5–20 μg bolus (repeat every 5–30 min) IV 5–10 μg/h (increase by 5 μg every 30 min)	
Angiotension-converting enzyme inhibitors		
Enalapril	0.625 to 1.25 mg IV initial dose, then 1–25.0 mg IV every 6 h	Acute left ventricular failure
Central agents		
Clonidine	0.2 mg initially PO (a patch form is available)	Hypertensive urgency
Miscellaneous		
Fenoldopam	0.1 μg/kg/min and increase by 0.05 μg/kg/min	Renal failure

Hydralazine

Hydralazine is a direct arteriolar vasodilator and is indicated in eclampsia. Hydralazine is associated with development of a lupus-like reaction, arthritis, drug fever, and rash.

Hydralazine is a direct arteriolar vasodilator with a short onset of action and a relatively long plasma half-life. The peak effect of hydralazine is observed in 5–15 min with a duration of action of 2–6 h. Hydralazine is metabolized in the liver, but about 8% is excreted unchanged in the urine. In patients with renal insufficiency, hydralazine doses may be reduced due to a longer elimination time. Hydralazine can induce reflex tachycardia and sudden drops in blood pressure. It is not recommended in patients with ischemic heart disease and aortic dissection. Hydralazine has also been associated with the development of systemic lupus erythematosus-like reaction, rheumatoid arthritis, drug fever, rash, gastrointestinal complaints, and peripheral neuropathies. In most cases, removal of the drug is curative. Hydralazine causes sodium and water retention and is indicated for use in pregnancy-induced hypertension (preeclampsia and eclampsia).

Diazoxide

Diazoxide is an arterial vasodilator. It is contraindicated in patients with coronary artery disease, myocardial ischemia, or aortic dissection because it can induce a reflex tachycardia.

Diazoxide, a potent arterial vasodilator, is rarely used in the treatment of hypertensive emergency. The effects of diazoxide are seen within minutes following an intravenous bolus of 50–100 mg. Boluses can be repeated every 15 min to a total dose of 600 mg or until blood pressure is lowered to the desired level. The effects of diazoxide can last for up to 12 h, and large boluses can produce rapid and extreme falls in blood pressure. Diazoxide is associated with a reflex tachycardia that can induce angina or myocardial ischemia, and it is contraindicated in patients with coronary artery disease, angina, myocardial infarction, aortic dissection, and intercerebral hemorrhage.

Beta-Blockers

Labetalol

Labetalol is both an alpha- and a beta-blocker and has both an intravenous and oral form. It produces vasodilation without a change in cardiac output.

Labetalol is a competitive selective alpha-1 and a noncardioselective competitive beta-blocker (beta-1 and beta-2). Labetalol acts on both alpha- and beta-receptors to produce vasodilation without stimulation of cardiac output. Labetalol also has an additional direct vasodilatory effect. Labetalol has both intravenous (infusion and bolus) and oral forms. Intravenous labetolol has an onset of action that begins in 5 min with a peak effect seen in 5–30 min and a duration of action of 4 h. Labetalol is usually administered as a 20-mg bolus, which can be followed either by a repeated bolus every 10–15 min or, more commonly, by an intravenous infusion at 0.5–2 mg/min. It is then titrated to achieve blood pressure control. Labetalol is metabolized in the liver, so doses should be reduced in patients with liver failure. Less than 5% of labetolol is excreted in the urine.

Labetalol is useful in the treatment of hypertensive emergency caused by aortic dissection or myocardial ischemia.

Labetalol produces a decrease in systemic arterial pressure and total peripheral vascular resistance. Cardiac output remains stable, and cerebral, renal, and coronary blood flow are maintained. There is a decrease in pulmonary artery pressure and pulmonary capillary wedge pressure. Labetalol is especially useful in cases of malignant hypertension accompanied by myocardial ischemia or aortic dissection. However, because of its effects on beta-receptors, it can decrease forced expiratory volume in one second (FEV_1) in patients with chronic obstructive pulmonary disease or asthma and should not be used in cases where beta-blockers are contraindicated.

Esmolol

Esmolol is a short-acting beta-1-adrenergic selective blocking agent useful in treating hypertension associated with myocardial infarction.

Esmolol is a short-acting beta-1-adrenergic selective blocking agent. It has a rapid onset of action and a short half-life. Esmolol had been used to treat supraventricular arrhythmias. It has been shown to be effective in treating hypertension associated with myocardial infarction and postoperative hypertension.

Angiotensin-Converting Enzyme Inhibitors

Angiotensin-converting enzyme inhibitors (ACE inhibitors) decrease total peripheral vascular resistance while causing little change in heart rate, cardiac output, or pulmonary artery wedge pressure. ACE inhibitors decrease blood pressure by decreasing systemic concentrations of angiotensin II, inhibiting local vascular effects of angiotensin II, and increasing concentrations of bradykinin, a vasodilator. Unfortunately, the response to ACE inhibitors is variable because effectiveness depends on the patient's plasma volume and renin activity. ACE inhibitors should be used with caution in cases of bilateral renal artery stenosis.

Enalaprilat is the most common ACE inhibitor used in treatment of hypertensive emergency. Enalaprilat has an onset of action of 10–60 min and a duration of action of 2–6 h. It is given as an IV bolus of 1–25 mg every 6 h after an initial dose of 0.625–1.25 mg.

Captopril, another ACE inhibitor, is useful in reducing blood pressure but only comes in an oral form.

Dopamine Agonists

Fenoldopam

Fenoldopam is a short-acting dopamine (DA_1) agonist that produces renal vasodilation. Fenoldopam acts on dopamine receptors in the proximal and distal tubules, resulting in inhibition of sodium reabsorption and increased diuresis and sodium wasting. It has a rapid onset of action and is metabolized in the liver with no active metabolites. Fenoldopam has been found to be comparable in effectiveness to sodium nitroprusside in the treatment of hypertensive crisis. Unlike nitroprusside, fenoldopam improves creatinine clearance and sodium excretion in patients with renal insufficiency and hypertension. Because of these renal effects, fenoldopam is a useful drug in the treatment of hypertensive patients with renal insufficiency.

Fenoldopam, a dopamine agonist, acts on dopamine receptors to produce renal vasodilation. It also improves creatinine clearance and sodium excretion. Fenoldopam is useful in the treatment of hypertension with coexisting renal insufficiency.

After an initial intravenous dose of 0.1 μg/kg/min, peak effects of fenoldopam are seen in 15 min. The duration of action is 30–60 min. To date there has been no associated rebound hypertension once the drug is discontinued.

Calcium Channel Blockers

Calcium channel blockers reduce cardiac contractility and produce vasodilation in both the coronary and systemic blood vessels. Calcium channel blockers act by inhibiting calcium uptake, and they interfere with excitation contraction coupling in smooth muscle. The original calcium channel blockers—verapamil, nifedipine, and diltiazem—are not usually considered effective therapy in the treatment of hypertensive emergency.

The original calcium channel blockers—verapamil, nifedipine, and cardizem—are not usually considered as first-line therapy in hypertensive emergency.

Verapamil, while effectively reducing blood pressure, can also slow the heart rate, prolong the PR interval, and precipitate heart block in doses necessary to effectively control blood pressure. Verapamil is contraindicated in the treatment of hypertensive emergency in patients with preexisting cardiac conduction problems. Although nifedipine is an effective treatment for chronic essential hypertension, it is associated with rapid falls in blood pressure that can lead to renal, cerebral, and cardiac infarctions. Because of the possibility of severe hypotension, nifedipine is not recommended in the treatment of malignant hypertension.

Nicardipine, an intravenous calcium channel blocker, is easily titratable and not associated with rapid blood pressure swings. Nicardipine reduces both cardiac and cerebral ischemia; its action is similar to nitroprusside in lowering blood pressure. It has also been shown to produce cerebral vasodilation and can therefore increase intracranial pressure. Side effects of nicardipine are nausea, vomiting, headache, and hypotension. The initial intravenous dose is 5 mg/h, and it can be increased by 1–2.5 mg/h every 15 min to a maximum dose of 15 mg/h. Nicardipine has an onset and duration of action of 15 min and 5 h, respectively. Nicardipine is contraindicated in patients with cerebral edema or with an intracranial mass.

Nicardipine, a calcium channel antagonist, may decrease cerebral vasospasm in cases of subarachnoid hemorrhage. It is contraindicated in patients with cerebral edema or intracranial space-occupying lesions.

Alpha-Adrenergic Blockers

Clonidine

Clonidine is an effective agent in treating hypertensive urgency but is not used for hypertensive emergency. It is contraindicated in hypertensive encephalopathy because of its sedating effects.

Clonidine is a centrally acting alpha-2-adrenergic agonist. It is now available in a transdermal patch and is useful in the treatment of hypertensive urgency and other situations in which urgent blood pressure control is not required. A side effect of clonidine is sedation, so its use is contraindicated during hypertensive encephalopathy.

SPECIAL CONSIDERATIONS

Cerebrovascular Emergencies and Hypertensive Encephalopathy

Hypertensive encephalopathy can occur with a sudden increase of systemic blood pressure. It is characterized by alterations in mental status and grade III or IV retinopathy on funduscopic exam.

Hypertensive encephalopathy is a severe complication of systemic hypertension, and carries a poor prognosis. Encephalopathy occurs in patients who have a sudden increase in systemic blood pressure. It is characterized by severe headache, nausea, vomiting, and alterations in mental status ranging from lethargy to coma. Focal neurologic findings may be seen, such as cranial nerve palsies, aphasia, and blindness. Funduscopic exam reveals advanced retinopathy (Keith–Wagener–Barker grades III and IV), retinal hemorrhages, exudates, cotton wool spots, and papilledema.

Treatment of hypertensive encephalopathy is aimed at reducing mean blood pressure by 20%.

Treatment of hypertensive encephalopathy is aimed at a prompt reduction of blood pressure. Mean arterial blood pressure should be lowered by 20%. Current recommended agents to lower blood pressure include the direct vasodilators nitroprusside and nitroglycerin. Patients require intensive care monitoring. Once the blood pressure has sufficiently been reduced, clinical improvement should be seen. Blood pressure can be further reduced over the next 48 h, and patients switched to oral medications.

Hypertension Associated with Thrombotic Strokes or Subarachnoid Hemorrhage

Chronic hypertension results in arterial intimal and medial thickening, sclerotic plaques, and luminal narrowing. These changes result in increased cerebrovascular resistance and produce a functional abnormality in cerebral vessel autoregulation. This change can be reversed by antihypertensive therapy. In normal individuals, the brain maintains cerebral blood flow (CBF) over a wide range of blood pressure. Cerebrovascular autoregulation is maintained by delicate and regular changes in vasoconstriction and vasodilation. The usual autoregulatory range is between 50 and 150 mmHg. When systemic arterial blood pressure drops below 50 mmHg, CBF decreases. Alternately, when blood pressure rises above 150 mmHg, CBF and cerebral blood volume increase. Chronically elevated blood pressure shifts the autoregulatory curve to the right. Acute severe increases in blood pressure can result in cerebral edema due to increased microvascular pressure, vessel damage, and necrosis with subsequent vascular leakage.

When systemic blood pressure is greater than 150 mmHg, cerebral blood flow (CBF) increases. Chronic elevations in systemic blood pressure result in alterations in the brain's ability to autoregulate CBF, producing a shift to the right in the curve.

Optimal therapy for patients presenting with hypertensive emergency caused by cerebrovascular accidents is unclear. Immediately preceding a stroke, systemic pressure rises, along with CBF. One theory is that increased systemic blood pressure allows improved perfusion to the ischemic area. No studies have shown that hypertension has increased mortality during the acute phase of stroke, and normalization of blood pressure in acute strokes may actually worsen the damage. The risks of severe elevations in systemic blood pressure need to be balanced against the risk of worsening cerebral ischemia caused by excessive reductions in blood pressure. Current recommendations suggest treatment of patients with diastolic pressures above 120 mmHg, with the goal being a 20% reduction in mean blood pressure (or a diastolic blood pressure between 100 and 110 mmHg).

Optimal therapy for patients presenting with thrombotic strokes or intracerebral hemorrhage is not known.

Current recommendations suggest treatment if diastolic pressure is greater than 120 mmHg, with a goal of a 20% reduction in mean blood pressure.

Patients with large intracerebral hemorrhages have been shown to benefit from judicious lowering of their systolic blood pressure to less than 200 mmHg or the diastolic pressure to less than 120 mmHg. Short-acting agents that do not have CNS effects are preferred to maintain better control over blood pressure changes. Nitroprusside, while having a rapid onset of action and a short half-life, is known to increase intracerebral pressure. A suitable alternate choice is labetolol. Nicardipine has also been used in treatment of subarachnoid bleeding to reduce cerebral vasospasm.

Acute Aortic Dissection

Acute aortic dissection and aneurysmal dilatation can present as a hypertensive emergency. Rapid blood pressure control is required to reduce aortic stress. Reduction in the force of left ventricular contraction will reduce the rate of rise in blood pressure. In cases of aortic dissection and distension, the drugs of choice include an alpha- and beta-blocker such as labetalol, or a combination of beta-blocker and vasodilator such as esmolol and nitroprusside. Drugs such as nicardipine and fenoldopam can be substituted if there is concern over nitroprusside's toxicity.

Treatment of aortic dissection requires a prompt reduction in blood pressure to reduce aortic wall stress. Treatment of choice includes labetalol or a combination of a beta-blocker and a vasodilator.

Along with blood pressure reduction, a cardiothoracic or vascular surgery consultation should be requested. Aortic dissections are categorized as either type A (dissections involving the ascending aorta) or type B (dissections of the descending aorta). All type A dissections require surgical intervention. Uncomplicated distal dissections are treated medically with antihypertensive agents. Distal dissections with signs of leakage of blood from the aorta, or compromised blood flow to a limb or organ, are usually treated with surgery. Both surgical and medical treatment of distal dissections have similar survival rates at 75%.

All type A dissections (dissections of the ascending aorta) require surgical intervention. Type B dissections (distal or descending aorta), if uncomplicated, are managed medically. Blood flow compromise to a limb or organ or leakage of blood into the abdomen requires surgical intervention.

Preeclampsia

Pregnancy-induced hypertension can range from mild to severe and does not resolve until delivery. Patients with preeclampsia are volume depleted and vasoconstricted. Other signs associated with preeclampsia include proteinuria, peripheral edema, and alterations in coagulation pathways and in liver function. Eventually, preeclampsia can lead to seizures (eclampsia).

Treatment of eclampsia includes magnesium for seizure prevention and hydralazine for blood pressure control.

Therapy is aimed at volume reexpansion, control of seizures, and treatment of hypertension. In patients with severe elevations in blood pressure (diastolic blood pressure >100 mmHg), hydralazine is the parenteral drug of choice in patients with preeclampsia because it has a long history of safe use in pregnancy. For treatment of mild hypertension (diastolic blood pressure <95), the National High Blood Pressure Education Program (NHBPEP) recommends methyldopa (a centrally acting alpha-agonist). In cases of hypertensive emergency where diastolic blood pressure exceeds 110 mmHg or systolic pressure is greater than 180 mmHg, intravenous antihypertensives such as nitroprusside, labetalol, or nicardipine can be used, and the patient can be changed to hydralazine once blood pressure is controlled. Sodium nitroprusside can only be used for a few hours because of fetal cyanide toxicity, and it is usually reserved for cases where fetal delivery will occur soon. A target for the diastolic blood pressure is approximately 90 mmHg. Magnesium is also used in patients with preeclampsia as prophylaxis against seizures.

Cardiac Causes of Hypertensive Emergency

Left ventricular failure and pulmonary edema are the result of severe elevations in systemic vascular pressure. Treatment is aimed at rapid reduction in preload and afterload to improve cardiac output. Nitroprusside and nitroglycerin are both effective agents, with supplemental oxygen and morphine sulfate, if needed. ACE inhibitors can be used once blood pressure is stable. Beta-blockers may worsen cardiac function and therefore are generally not indicated. Along with reducing blood pressure, management should include diuretics to facilitate fluid removal.

Severe elevations in systemic blood pressure can result in left ventricular failure and pulmonary edema. Treatment is aimed at rapidly reducing preload and afterload. Nitroprusside or nitroglycerine are effective agents to reduce blood pressure. Other therapies include diuretics, oxygen, and morphine sulfate.

In cases of hypertension complicated by myocardial infarction or cardiac ischemia, nitroglycerin is the drug of choice. Nitroglycerin dilates coronary vessels and reduces myocardial oxygen consumption. Other agents that can be used are beta-blockers such as esmolol or labetalol.

SUMMARY

Hypertensive crisis is an emergency that requires aggressive management to control blood pressure and is associated with significant morbidity and mortality. Hypertensive emergencies, defined as severe elevation in blood pressure associated with end-organ damage, require rapid blood pressure control, usually within minutes. Blood pressure reduction can be achieved over hours in cases of hypertensive urgency. Intensive care monitoring of blood pressure is usually required to prevent rapid and profound falls in blood pressure, especially with use of several of the rapid-acting intravenous agents.

REVIEW QUESTIONS

1. **Hypertensive emergency is distinguished from hypertensive urgency by:**
   A. Greater elevations in blood pressure
   B. Evidence of end-organ damage
   C. A history of cocaine use
   D. Diastolic blood pressure greater than 120 mmHg

2. **A 68-year-old man with a history of hypertension and diabetes presents with sudden right-sided weakness and dysphagia that had developed over the last 24 h. His current medications include an oral hypoglycemic and diltiazem. On physical exam, blood pressure is 220/140 in both upper extremities with a heart rate of 95 beats/min and a respiratory rate of 16 breaths/min. Laboratory tests are all normal. EKG is normal. Further management of this patient would include all the following except:**
   A. CT of the head
   B. Pulse oximetry and airway assessment
   C. IV antihypertensive agent to reduce blood pressure to within normal range
   D. Blood pressure monitoring

3. **Nitroprusside does all the following except:**
   A. Has a rapid onset of action and short half-life
   B. Acts only on arterial smooth muscle to reduce blood pressure
   C. Is light sensitive
   D. Has toxic metabolites that can limit use

4. **The antihypertensive drug of choice in preeclampsia when diastolic blood pressure is >100 mmHg is:**
   A. Clonidine
   B. Enalapril
   C. Hydralazine
   D. Nitroglycerine

5. **Which of the following is true:**
   A. Hypertensive encephalopathy is characterized by changes in mental status and findings of advanced retinopathy.
   B. In cases of cerebral ischemia, blood pressure reduction is advised if the diastolic blood pressure exceeds 90 mmHg.
   C. Most patients who present with hypertensive emergency have no prior diagnosis of blood pressure problems.
   D. Labetalol is a beta-2-selective adrenergic blocking agent.

ANSWERS

1. The answer is B. Both hypertensive urgency and emergency are characterized by extreme elevations in blood pressure. However, patients with a hypertensive emergency also have evidence of end-organ damage, unlike patients with hypertensive urgency. The organs most commonly affected are the heart, brain, and kidneys. Patients with hypertensive emergency require blood pressure be reduced over the course of 30 min to 1 h. Although cocaine use is associated with episodes of hypertensive emergency and urgency, it does not distinguish one from the other.
2. The answer is C. For a patient presenting with hypertensive emergency due to a cerebral event, the initial workup should include a CT of the head to assess for bleeding or cerebral edema, frequent blood pressure monitoring, and pulse oximetry and airway assessment. Antihypertensive agents should be used to reduce the patient's blood pressure as diastolic pressure is well above 120 mmHg. However, blood pressure should NEVER be reduced to normal levels because this may affect blood flow to the affected area and worsen symptoms.
3. The answer is B. Nitroprusside is a rapid-acting drug that produces both arterial and venule vasodilation. It has a half-life of minutes, making it easily titratable. The medication is light sensitive and is broken down into cyanide and thiocyanate. These toxic metabolites can accumulate to toxic levels, especially in patients with renal failure or in those who require high doses for an extended period of time.
4. The answer is C. Hydralazine is the parenteral drug of choice in patients with preeclampsia and diastolic blood pressure >100 mmHg. It is a direct vasodilator and has a long history of safety and efficacy in treatment of preeclampsia. Other possible agents include labetalol. Methyldopa, a centrally acting alpha-agonist, is useful in

treatment of mild hypertension (diastolic blood pressure <95 mmHg). Agents to be avoided include calcium agonists, because of possible synergistic effects with magnesium, and ACE inhibitors or angiotensin II blockers. Both ACE inhibitors and angiotensin II receptor blockers have been associated with fetal abnormalities.

5. The answer is A. The only true statement is that hypertensive encephalopathy is characterized by changes in mental status and findings of advanced retinopathy along with elevated blood pressure. In treating hypertension associated with cerebral ischemia, blood pressure reduction is advised once the diastolic blood pressure exceeds 120 mmHg. The majority of patients presenting with hypertensive emergency have a prior history of hypertension and are usually noncompliant or poorly controlled on their current medications. Labetalol is a noncardioselective beta (beta-1 and beta-2) blocker and a selective alpha-1-blocker. Labetalol produces vasodilation without stimulation of cardiac output.

SUGGESTED READING

Calhoun DA, Oparil S. Treatment of hypertensive crisis. N Engl J Med 1990;323:1177–1183.

Joint National Committee on Detection, Evaluation, and Treatment of High Blood Pressure. The Sixth Report of the Joint National Committee on Prevention, Detection, Evaluation, and Treatment of High Blood Pressure. Clinical Guidelines and Evidence Reports November 1997. Arch Intern Med 157(21):2413–46.

Kitiyakra C, Guzman NJ. Malignant hypertension and hypertensive emergencies. J Am Soc Nephrol 1998;9(1):133–420.

Varon J, Marik, PE. The diagnosis and management of hypertensive crisis. Chest 2000;118:214–227.

PART IV

Appendices

Commonly Used Parenteral Medications and Dosage Recommendations for Adult Therapeutics

GENERIC NAME

Caution: The dosage of a particular medication may require modification based on a patient's age, renal status, liver function, or concomitant drug therapy. The reader is encouraged to consult reliable sources for indications, adverse effects, precautions, drug interactions, and other pharmacologic issues.

Acetazolamide	IV 250 mg q 6–12 h Titrate to effect on metabolic akalosis
Adenoside	IV bolus 6 mg followed in 2–10 min with 12 mg If not converted, may use additional 12 mg (total dose, 30 mg)
Alpha acid aminocaproic	IV 5 g initially, then 1 g/h Titrate to coagulation effect for excessive fibrinolysis
Aminophylline	IV 5–6 mg/kg loading dose, then 0.3–0.9 mg/kg/h Titrate to bronchodilatory effect and therapeutic blood level of 10–20 μg/ml or 1 mg/l
Amiodarone	IV 5–10 mg/kg loading dose, then 5 μg/kg/min for refractory ventricular arrhythmias
Amrinone	IV bolus 0.75 mg/kg, then 5–10 μg/kg/min
Anistreplase	IV bolus 30 μg
Aprotinin	IV bolus 10^6 units, then 1 g/h
Atenolol	IV bolus 5 mg followed by second 5 mg dose in 10 min, then po drug administration
Atracurium	IV bolus 0.3–0.5 mg/kg, then 7–10 μg/kg/min Titrate to peripheral nerve stimulation
Atropine	IV bolus 0.5–1 mg for bradycardia, repeat q 3–5 min (max 3 mg), 2–2.5 mg via endotracheal tube
Bretylium	IV loading dose 5–10 mg/kg over 10 min for VT, then infuse 0.5–2 mg/min IV bolus 5 mg/kg for VF, repeat q 5 min at 10 mg/kg to max 35 mg/kg
Bumetanide	IV bolus 0.5–4 mg, then IV 0.5–1 mg q 6 h
Calcium chloride	IV slow push 2–4 mg/kg, then same dose q 10 min as required

Chlorpromazine	IV 1–5 mg q 6 h
Cimetidine	IV 300 mg q 6 h; IV infusion 40–50 mg/h In renal failure 300 mg q 8–12 h
Cisatracurium	IV bolus 0.1–0.2 mg/kg, then infuse 3 μg/kg/min
Clonidine	IV bolus 150 μg, then infuse 2–3 μg/min/m^2
Cyclosporine	IV initially 2 mg/kg/day Constant infusion to desired blood level
Desmopressin	IV 1–2 μg q 12 h as an antidiuretic IV 0.3 μg/kg over 30 min q 8 h, as needed for platelet dysfunction
Dantrolene	IV bolus 1 mg/kg, repeat q 10 min until symptoms clear or max dose 10 mg/kg, then infuse 0.75–1 mg/kg q 4–6 h for several days post-crisis; po 1–2 mg/kg q 6–8 h
Dexamethasone	IV initially 10 mg, then 4 mg q 6 h for cerebral edema
Diazepam	IV 5–10 mg; repeat q 5–15 min as needed (max 20 mg) but protect airway and maintain blood pressure
Diazoxide	IV bolus 50–300 mg
Digoxin	IV loading 10–15 μg/kg (about 1 mg) in divided doses of 50% initially and remainder in two divided doses q 2–6 h apart, then 0.125–0.25 mg/day; Monitor level
Diltiazem	IV bolus 0.25 mg/kg (max 25 mg), repeat 0.35 mg/kg if necessary Then infuse 5–20 mg/h and titrate to ventricular rate
Diphenhydramine	IV bolus 25–50 mg, repeat q 30–60 min to response, then q 6 h
Dobutamine	IV infusion 2–20 μg/kg/min titrated to hemodynamic effect
Dopamine	IV infusion 5–30 μg/kg/min titrated to hemodynamic effect
Doxapram	IV bolus 0.5–2 mg/kg over 5–10 min, repeat bolus q 1–2 h as needed IV infusion 1–3 mg/min, titrate to effect on breathing
Edrophonium	IV 10 mg challenge
Enalaprilat	IV 1.25 mg over 15 min q 6 h; IV 0.625 mg when used with a diuretic Titrate IV by 1.25 mg at 12–24 h intervals to max 5 mg q 6 h
Enoxaparin	SQ 30 mg q 12 h
Epinephrine	IV 0.05–2.0 μg/kg/min, titrate to BP effect SQ 0.3 cc 1:1000 solution or 0.01 mg/kg not to exceed 0.3 mg
Esmolol	IV bolus 500 μg/kg over 1 min IV infusion 50 μg/kg/min Titrate 25–300 μg/kg/min to HR and BP effect
Ethacrynic acid	IV bolus 0.5–1 mg/kg or 50 mg; repeat or increase to no higher then 100 mg in 2–4 h, then q 4–6 h as needed
Etomidate	IV bolus 0.2–0.3 mg/kg; repeat 0.15–0.2 mg/kg at 5-min intervals to 0.5 mg/kg max
Famotidine	IV 20 mg q 12 h; 20 mg q 24 h in renal failure
Fentanyl	IV bolus 3 μg/kg; IV infusion 0.02–0.05 μg/kg/min titrated to desired CNS effect
Flumazenil	IV for sedation reversal 0.2 mg over 15 s and repeat in 1 min to max dose of 1 mg or wakefulness IV for overdose 0.2 mg over 30 s, then 0.3 mg, then 0.5 mg q 1 min to max dose of 5 mg or wakefulness; may need to readminister q 20 min; watch for benzo withdrawal
Furosemide	IV bolus 10–400 mg; dose >200 mg are infused slowly IV infusion 0.25–0.4 mg/kg/h titrated to increase urine output
Glucagon	IV bolus 1–5 mg over 15 min; then infusion 1–10 mg/h Titrate to glucose effect or hemodynamics
Haloperidol	IV bolus 0.5–20 mg, may double dose q 30 min to a max dose 160 mg daily in q 6 h divided doses

Heparin	SQ 5,000 units q 12 h for DVT prophylaxis
	IV bolus 5,000–10,000 units or 50–100 units/kg, then 80 units/kg/h but adjust to anticoagulate effect desired
Hydralazine	IV bolus 10–50 mg q 3–6 h adjusted to hemodynamic effect
Hydrocortisone	IV 100 mg q 6–8 h
Hydromorphone	IV 0.5 mg q 10–15 min to max 0.02 mg/kg, then 1–2 mg q 1–6 h prn; or infuse 5–20 μg/kg/h
Insulin, regular	IV load 1–10 units (0.1 unit/kg), then 0.5–12 units/h (0.1 unit/kg/h) titrated to blood sugar
Isoproterenol	IV infusion 2–20 μg/min titrated to HR and BP effects
Ketorolac	IV load 30–60 mg, then 15–30 mg q 6 h, not to exceed 120 mg/day (do not use more than 5 days)
Labetalol	IV bolus 10–20 mg, then 20–40 mg q 10 min to BP effect to max 300 mg
	IV infusion 2–3 mg/min, titrate to BP effect
Levothyroxine	IV 12.5–50 μg/day to max 200 μg/day
Lidocaine	IV loading dose 1–1.5 mg/kg, then 0.5–1.5 mg/kg q 3–5 min until arrhythmias stabilized or max 3 mg/kg, then infused at 1–4 mg/min
Lorazepam	IV 0.5–4 mg, then repeat after 10 min 1–2 mg as needed for agitation
Magnesium SO_4	IV 1–2 g over 1 h for moderate and 3–4 g over 2 h for severe hypomagnesiemia
	IV infusion 0.5–1 g/h when indicated; 1 g $MgSO_4$ = 8 mEq Mg^{2+}
Mannitol	IV 0.25–1 g/kg, 20% solution over 30–60 min, then 0.25–0.5 g/kg over 15 min q 4 h; adjust repeat doses to control ICP
	IV infusion 20% solution at 10–20 ml/h
Meperidine	IV 25–100 mg q 3–4 h as needed
Methyldopa	IV 250–1000 mg q 6 h
Methylprednisolone	IV bolus 2 mg/kg then 40 mg q 6 h × 24–48 h for status asthmaticus
	IV bolus 30 mg/kg, then infuse 5.4 mg/kg/h for 23 h for spinal cord injury
Metoclopramide	IV 10 mg q 6–8 h
Metoprolol	IV post MI 5 mg, repeat q 2–5 min to max 15 mg as hemodynamically tolerated
	IV 5–10 mg q 4–6 h as maintenance
Midazolam	IV bolus 0.5–4 mg q 10 min to 20 mg max for rapid sedation
	IV infusion 0.5–15 mg/h, titrate by 1 mg q 30 min to desired effect
Mivacurium	IV bolus 0.15 mg/kg, IV infusion 5–10 μg/kg/min
	Titrate to peripheral nerve stimulation
Morphine	IV bolus 0.03–0.2 mg/kg q 1–2 h
	IV infusion 0.05–0.3 mg/kg/h
Naloxone	IV bolus 0.4–2 mg q 2–3 min up to 10 mg max
	IV infusion 0.1–0.8 mg/h
Neostigmine	IV 2.5–5 mg with IV atropine 0.5–1 mg to reverse neuromuscular blockade and avoid undesired muscarinic effects (bradycardia)
	IV or IM 0.5 mg (1 ml 1:2000 solution) in myasthenia gravis diagnosis
Nicardipine	IV 5 mg/h, increase q 15 min to max 15 mg/h
Nitroglycerin	IV infusion 5–10 μg/min with rapid titration, 10 μg/min q 10 min, to chest pain and blood pressure control (usual range, 5–400 μg/min)

Nitroprusside	IV infusion 0.5–10 μg/kg/min Titrate to desired hemodynamics by increasing dose 0.5–1 μg/kg/min q 5–15 min
Norepinephrine	IV infusion 0.1 μg/kg/min and increase by 0.1 μg/kg/min every 5–10 min up to 3 μg/kg/min to hemodynamic response (usual dose, 5–20 μg/min)
Octreotide acetate	IV or SQ 50 μg q 12–24 h IV infusion 25 μg/h
Pancuronium	IV bolus 0.07–0.1 mg/kg (4–10 mg) over 15–30 s IV maintenance 0.03–0.04 mg/kg (2–4 mg) q 2–3 h IV infusion 0.02–0.04 mg/kg/h to max 0.6 mg/kg/h Titrate to peripheral stimulation
Pentobarbitol	IV loading dose 5–10 mg/kg over 1–2 h, then 1–2 mg/kg/h to a therapeutic level of 20–40 μg/ml
Phenobarbital	IV 10–20 mg/kg at a rate of 50 mg/min, then 3–6 mg/kg/day to a therapeutic level of 10–40 μg/ml
Phentolamine	IV bolus 5–10 mg q 5–15 min, then IV infusion 1–5 mg/min to desired hemodynamic effect
Phenylephrine	IV bolus 0.1–0.5 mg IV infusion 10–100 μg/min to max 15 μg/kg/min Titrate to desired BP effect
Phenytoin	IV loading 18–20 mg/kg at 50 mg/min for seizure, then IV 300–400 mg daily in divided doses q 8–12 h IV 100 mg q 3–5 min to max 1000 mg for arrhythmia, then 100–250 mg IV q 12 h
Physostigmine	IV 0.5–1 mg over 5 min
Procainamide	IV loading 50–100 mg q 5 min up to 1–1.5 g or 12–17 mg/kg over 1 h IV infusion 1–5 mg/min
Progesterone	IM 100 mg q d as a respiratory stimulant
Propanolol	IV bolus up to 0.15 mg/kg over 20 min, or 1 mg q 2–5 min to max 10 mg to HR effect IV infusion 3 mg/h
Propofol	IV bolus 1.5–3 mg/kg IV infusion 0.30–130 μg/kg/min; 3–8 mg/h
Protamine	IV 1 mg will neutralize 90–115 USP units of heparin; max 50 mg; generally 0.75 mg for each 100 heparin units
Pyridostigmine	IV 10–20 mg for paralysis reversal, pretreat with IV atropine 0.5–1 mg to prevent bradycardia
Ranitidine	IV 50 mg q 6–8 h IV infusion 6.25–12.5 mg/h
Streptokinase	MI: IV bolus 1.5 million IU over 60 min DVT/PE IV loading dose 250,000 IU over 30 min; then IV infusion 100,000 IU/h for 24–72 h (PE, 24 h; DVT, 48–72 h)
Succinylcholine	IV bolus 1–1.5 mg/kg and 0.5 mg/kg q 10–30 min
Terbutaline	SQ 0.25 mg q 2–4 h
Thiopental	IV load 0.5–1 mg/kg (sedation); 3–6 mg/kg (anesthesia) IV infusion 1–5 mg/min or 4–8 mg/kg/h
tPA (tissue plasminogen activator)	MI: pts > 67 kg IV bolus 15 mg, then 50 mg over 30 min, then 35 mg over 60 min MI: pts <67 kg IV bolus 15 mg, then 0.75 mg/kg over 30 min, then 0.5 mg/kg over 60 min DVT/PE$_i$ IV 100 mg over 2 h
Trimethaphan	IV infusion 0.5–5 mg/min, titrate to hemodynamic effect

Urokinase	IV load 4400 U/kg over 10 min IV infusion 4400 U/kg/h for 12–24 h (PE, 12 h; DVT, 24–72 h)
Vasopressin (aqueous)	Diabetes insipidus: IV load 10 units IV infusion 0.2–0.3 U/min, max 60 U/h GI bleed: IV bolus 10–20 U over 10–30 min IV infusion 0.05–0.3 U/min, max 0.9 U/min
Vecuronium	IV bolus 0.075–0.1 mg/kg over 15–30 s IV infusion 1 μg/kg/min and titrate to peripheral nerve stimulation
Verapamil	IV load 1 mg/min, max 20 mg IV infusion 1–5 μg/kg/min titrate to HR and BP effect
Vitamin K	IM or SQ 2.5 mg–10 mg daily as needed

COMMON ICU PARENTERAL MEDICATIONS

BRAND NAME	GENERIC NAME
Abbokinase	urokinase
Adenocard	adenosine
Adivan	lorazepam
Adrenalin	epinephrine
Aldomet	methyldopa
Alteplase	tpa
Amicar	alpha aminocaproic acid
Amidate	etomidate
Anectine	succinylcholine
Antilirium	physostigmine
Aprasolina	hydralazine
Aquamephyton	vitamin K
Arfonad	trimethaphan
Benedryc	diphenhydramine
Brevibloc	esmolol
Bumex	bumetanide
Cardene	nicardipine
Cardizem	diltiazem
Carodarone	amrinone
Catapres	clonidine
Dantrium	dantrolene
DDAVP	desmopressin
Decadron	dexamethasone
Demerol	meperidine
Diamox	acetazolamide
Dilantin	phenytoin
Dilaudid	hydromorphone
Diprivan	propofol
Dobutrex	dobutamine
Dopram	doxapram
Edocrin	ethacrynic acid
Eminase	antistreplase
Haldol	haloperidol
Inderol	propranolol
Inocor	amrinone
Intropin	dopamine
Isoptin	verapamil
Isuprel	isoproterenol
Levophed	norepinephrine
Lopressor	metoprolol
Mestinon	pyridostigmine
Mivacron	mivacurium
Mucomyst	acetylcysteine
Narcan	naloxone
Nembutal	pentobarbital
Nimbex	cisatracurium

BRAND NAME	GENERIC NAME
Neo-synephrine	phenylephrine
Norcuron	vecuronium
Normodyne	labetalol
Pavulon	pancuronium
Pentothal	thiopental
Pepsid	famotidine
Pitressin	vasopressin
Proglycem	diazoxide
Pronestyl	procainamide
Regitine	phantolamine
Reglan	metoclopramide
Romazicon	flumazenil
Sandimmune	cyclosporine
Strepitase	streptokinase
Sublimaze	fentanyl
Tagamet	cimetidine
Tenormin	atenolol
Tensilon	edrophonium
Thorazinc	chlorpromazine
Toradol	ketorolac
Tracrium	atracurium
Trasylol	aprotinin
Valium	diazepam
Vasotec	enalaprilat
Ventolin	albuterol
Versed	midazolam
Xylocaine	lidocaine
Zantac	ranitidine

REFERENCES

Gora-Harper ML. The Injectable Drug Reference. Society of Critical Care Medicine. Princeton: Bio-scientific Resources, Inc., 1998.

Susla GM, Masur H, Cunnion RE, et al. (eds) Handbook of Critical Care Drug Therapy. New York: Churchill Livingstone, 1994.

Commonly Used Calculations

RESPIRATORY

Alveolar Gas Equation

$$PAO_2 = (P_B - PH_2O)\ FiO_2 - PaCO_2 \left(FiO_2 + \frac{1 - FiO_2}{R} \right)$$

Alveolar-Arterial Oxygen Difference (A-a Gradient)

$P\ (A\text{-}a)\ O_2 = PAO_2 - PaO_2$

Normal values = 2.5 + 0.2 (age)

Alveolar Volume

$V_A = V_T - V_D$

Alveolar Ventilation

$V_A = V_E - V_D$

Relationship of Partial Pressure of CO_2 to $\dot{V}_A$ and $\dot{V}CO_2$

$$PaCO_2 = \frac{K(\dot{V}CO_2)}{\dot{V}_A} \qquad K = 0.863$$

$$\dot{V}_A = \dot{V}_E - V_D$$

$$PaCO_2 = \frac{0.863\ (\dot{V}CO_2)}{\dot{V}_E - \dot{V}_D}$$

VENTILATOR MONITORING

Total Compliance (C)

$$C = \frac{\Delta V}{\Delta Pao} \text{ or } \frac{I}{E}$$

Normal Values = >60 ml/cmH_2O

Static Compliance (C_{STATIC})

$$C_{STATIC} = \frac{V_T - V_{LOST}}{P_{PLATEAU} - PEEP_{TOTAL}} \quad \text{or} \quad \frac{V_{T\ CORRECTED}}{P_{PLATEAU} - PEEP_{TOTAL}}$$

Normal Values = >60 ml/cmH_2O

V_{LOST} = Volume Lost in Ventilator Tubing = (PIP − $PEEP_{TOTAL}$) C_{TUBING}

Corrected V_T = V_T Exhaled − V_{LOST}

Dynamic Compliance ($C_{DYNAMIC}$)

$$C_{DYNAMIC} = \frac{V_T - V_{LOST}}{PIP - PEEP_{TOTAL}} \quad \text{or} \quad \frac{V_{T\ CORRECTED}}{PIP - PEEP_{TOTAL}}$$

Airway Resistance (Raw)

$$Raw = \frac{P_{PEAK} - P_{PLATEAU}}{\dot{V}}$$

Inspiratory Flow Rate (V_I)

$$\dot{V}_I = \frac{V_T}{T_I}$$

Inspiratory Time (V_T)

$$T_I = \frac{V_T}{\dot{V}_I}$$

Total Cycle Time (TCT)

$$TCT = \frac{60\ s/min}{f}$$

Expiratory Time (T_E)

T_E = TCT − T_I

Physiologic Deadspace

$V_{D\ ALVEOLUS} = V_{D\ PHYSIOLOGIC} + V_{D\ ANATOMIC}$

Bohr Equation of Deadspace

$$V_D/V_T = \frac{PaCO_2 - P_ECO_2}{PaCO_2}$$

Normal Values = 0.2 − 0.3

Calculations Used to Adjust Ventilator Settings

Adjusting V_T

(Mechanical Ventilation) $$\text{Desired } V_T = \frac{(PaCO_{2\ ACTUAL})\ (V_{T\ ACTUAL})}{PaCO_{2\ DESIRED}}$$

Adjusting f

(Mechanical Ventilation) $$\text{Desired } f = \frac{(PaCO_{2\ ACTUAL})\ (f_{ACTUAL})}{PaCO_{2\ DESIRED}}$$

Adjusting FiO_2

(Mechanical Ventilation) $\text{Desired } F_iO_2 = \dfrac{(FiO_{2\ \text{ACTUAL}})\,(PaO_{2\ \text{DESIRED}})}{PaO_{2\ \text{ACTUAL}}}$

OTHER PULMONARY CALCULATIONS

Response to Bronchodilator (FEV_1)

$$\%\,\Delta\, FEV_1 = \frac{(\text{Post } FEV_1) - (\text{Pre } FEV_1)}{\text{Pre } FEV_1} \times 100$$

Smoking Pack-Years

Pack-Years = (Packs/Day)(Years Smoked)

METABOLIC EQUATIONS

Energy Expenditure

Harris Benedict Equation of Resting Energy Expenditure (Kcal/Day)

Males $REE = 66 + (13.7 \times (Wtg\ (Kg)) + (5 \times Htg)\ (cm)) - (6.8 \times Age(Yrs))$

Female $REE = 655 + (9.6 \times Wtg\ (Kg)) + (1.8 \times Htg\ (cm)) - (4.7 \times Age/Yrs))$

Weir Equation Modified Energy Expenditure (Kcal/Day)

$REE = (3.94 \times \dot{V}O_2\ (ml/min)) + (1.11 \times \dot{V}CO_2\ (ml/min))$

Nitrogen Balance

Nitrogen Balance = Nitrogen Intake − Nitrogen Excreted

$$= \frac{\text{Protein Calories (kcal/day)}}{25} - \text{Urine Nitrogen (g/day)} - 5\text{(g/day)}$$

Body Surface Area (BSA)

$BSA = [Htg\ (cm)]^{0.718} \times [Wtg\ (kg)]^{0.427} \times 74.49$

CARDIOVASCULAR CALCULATIONS

Cardiac Output

$CO = HR \times SV$

Cardiac Index

$$C_I = \frac{CO}{BSA}$$

Fick Equation for Cardiac Index

$$C_I = \frac{O_2 \text{ Consumption}}{\text{Arterial-Venous } O_2 \text{ Content}}$$

$$C_I = \frac{\dot{V}O_2 \times 10}{\text{Hgb (gm/dl)} \times 1.36 \times (SpO_2 - S\overline{V}O_2)}$$ Normal = 2.5 − 4.2 l/min/m^2

Pulse Pressure = Systolic (SP) − Diastolic (DP) Pressures

Systemic Mean Arterial Pressure (MAP) = $\frac{SP + 2\,(DP)}{3}$ Normal = 70–105 mmHg

Stroke Volume (SV) SV = CO/HR = ml/beat Normal = 30–65 ml/beat

Systemic Vascular Resistance

$$SVR = \frac{MAP - CVP}{CO} \times 80$$ Normal Value = 770–1500 dynes s cm^{-5}

Systemic Vascular Resistance Index

$$SVRI = \frac{MAP - CVP}{CI} \times 80$$

Mean Pulmonary Arterial Pressure

$$\overline{PAP} = \frac{\text{PA Systolic} + 2\,(\text{PA Diastolic})}{3}$$ Normal 5–10 mmHg

Pulmonary Vascular Resistance

$$PVR = \frac{\overline{PAP} - PAWP}{CO} \times 80$$ Normal Value = 150–250 dyne s cm^{-5}

Pulmonary Vascular Resistance Index

$$PVRI = \frac{\overline{PAP} - PAWP}{CI} \times 80$$

Oxygen Delivery

$DO_2 = CaO_2 \times CO$ Normal = 800–1200 ml/min

Arterial Oxygen Content

$CaO_2 = SaO_2\,(Hb)\,(1.36) + PaO_2\,(0.003)$ Normal = 20 ml O_2/dl blood

Mixed Venous Oxygen Content

$C\overline{V}O_2 = S\dot{V}O_2\,(Hb)\,(1.36) + P\overline{V}O_2\,(0.003)$ Normal = 15 ml O_2/dl blood

Arterial-Venous Oxygen Content Difference

$A - \overline{V}\ O_2$ Difference $= CaO_2 - C\overline{v}O_2$

End Pulmonary Capillary Oxygen Content

$CcO_2 = Hb\ (1.36)\ (1.0) + P_AO_2\ (0.003)$

Shunt Equation

$$\frac{Q_S}{Q_T} = \frac{CcO_2 - CaO_2}{CcO_2 - CVO_2}$$ Normal Values: <5%

Oxygen Extraction Ratio

$$ER = \frac{CaO_2 - C\bar{v}O_2}{CaO_2}$$ Normal Values = 25%

Oxygen Consumption

$\dot{V}O_2 = CO\ (CaO_2 - C\bar{v}O_2)$ Normal Value = 225–275 ml/min

NEUROLOGIC CALCULATIONS

Cerebral Perfusion Pressure

$CPP = MAP - ICP$

Cerebral Blood Flow

$$CBF = \frac{MAP - ICP}{CVR}$$

RENAL CALCULATIONS

OLIGURIA

	PRERENAL	ARF	POSTRENAL
U_{NA} (mmol/L)	<20	>40	Variable
U_{OSMOL} (mmol/kg H_2O)	>500	<350	Variable
FENA	<1	>1	Variable
Urinalysis	Normal	Muddy brown casts	Crystals WBC, RBC
U/P_{CR}	>40	>20	Variable

Estimated Glomerular Filtration Rate (GFR)

$$\textbf{Males} = \frac{(140 - \text{Age}) \times \text{Lean Body Wtg (kg)}}{P_{CREAT} \times 72}$$

Females = 0.85 (Male Estimate)

$$\textbf{Measured GFR} = \frac{\text{Creatinine Urine (g/dl)} \times \dfrac{\text{Urine Volume (ml/day)}}{\text{1440 (min/day)}}}{\text{Creatinine Plasma (mg/dl)}}$$

$$\textbf{FENA} = \frac{U_{NA}(\text{mmol/l})}{S_{NA}\ (\text{mmol/l})} \times \frac{S_{CR}\ (\mu\text{mol/l})}{U_{CR}\ (\mu\text{mol/l})} \times 100$$

SODIUM ABNORMALITIES

Hyponatremia

Calculated Na Deficit (mmol) = $0.6 \times$ wtg (kg) $\times (140 - \text{Na}) + 140$
(Volume Deficit in liters)

Correction for Serum Triglycerides and Protein

$\%\ \text{Serum } H_2O = 99 - 1.03\ (\text{lipids g/l}) = 0.073 \times \text{Protein (g/l)}$

$$\text{Corrected Na} = \text{Measured Na} \times \frac{0.93}{\%\ \text{Serum } H_2O}$$

Corrections for Serum Glucose

Corrected Na = Glucose (mmol/l) + Serum Na (mmol/l)

Hypernatremia

$$\text{Calculated Water Deficit} = 0.6 \times \text{Wtg (kg)} \times \frac{(\text{Na} - 1)}{(140)}$$

ACID–BASE DISORDERS

Anion Gap = $[Na^+] - [CL^-] - [HCO_3^-]$ Normal: 9–13 mEq/l

Calculated Serum Osmolality $= 2\,[Na^+] + \dfrac{[\text{Glucose}]}{18} + \dfrac{[\text{BUN}]}{2.8}$

Normal: $275\text{–}290\ \dfrac{\text{mOsm}}{\text{kg}}$

Osmolar Gap = Serum Osmolality Measured − Serum Osmolality Calculated

Normal = 0–5 mOsm/kg

DISORDER	PRIMARY	COMPENSATION	MAGNITUDE OF COMPENSATION
Metabolic acidosis	$HCO_3^- \downarrow$	$PaCO_2 \downarrow$	$\Delta\ PaCO_2 = 1.0 - 1.4 \times \Delta\ [HCO_3^-]$
Metabolic alkalosis	$HCO_3^- \uparrow$	$PaCO_2 \uparrow$	$\Delta\ PaCO_2 = 0.5\text{–}1.0 \times \Delta\ [+\ HCO_3^-]$
Respiratory acidosis	$PaCO_2 \downarrow$	$HCO_3^- \downarrow$	
		Acute	$\Delta\ HCO_3^- = 0.1\ (\Delta\ PaCO_2)$
		Chronic	$\Delta\ HCO_3^- = 0.35\ (\Delta\ PaCO_2)$
Respiratory alkalosis	$PaCO_2 \downarrow$	$HCO_3^- \downarrow$	
		Acute	$\Delta\ HCO_3^- = 0.2\ (\Delta\ 0.5\ (\Delta\ PaCO_2))$
		Chronic	$\Delta\ HCO_3^- = 0.5\ (\Delta\ PaCO_2)$

Creatinine Clearance $= \dfrac{\text{Urine Creatinine}}{\text{Serum Creatinine}} \times \begin{matrix}\text{Urine Volume}\\ \text{(ml/min)}\end{matrix} \times \dfrac{1.73}{\text{BSA}^{(m2)}}$

GLASGOW COMA SCALE (GCS)

GCS = Eyes (1–4) + Motor (1–6) + Verbal (1–8)

PARAMETER	SCORE
Eyes opening	
Spontaneous	4
To speech	3
To pain	2
None	1
Motor Response	
To commands	6
Localizes	5
Withdraws	4
Abnormal flexion	3
Abnormal extension	2
None	1
Verbal response	
Oriental	5
Confused, converses	4
Inappropriate words	3
Incomprehensible sounds	2
None	1
Normal value: 15	

APACHE II SEVERITY OF DISEASE CLASSIFICATION

A. Acute Physiologic Scores

PHYSIOLOGIC VARIABLE	HIGH ABNORMAL RANGE				LOW ABNORMAL RANGE				
	+4	+3	+2	+1	0	+1	+2	+3	+4
Temperature – (rectal(°C))	≥41°	39°–40.9°		38.5°–38.9°	36°–38.4°	34°–35.9°	32°–33.9°	32°–33.9°	≤29.9
Mean arterial pressure – (mmHg)	≥180	130–159	110–129		70–109		50–69		≤49
Heart rate (ventricular response)	≥50	140–179	110–139		70–109		55–69	40–54	≤39
Respiratory rate (nonventilated or ventilated)	≥500	35–49		25–34	12–24	10–11	6–9		≤5
Oxygenation: A-aDO_2 or PaO_2 (mmHg)	≥500	350–499	200–349		<200				
a. $FiO_2 > 0.5$ record A-aDO_2									
b. $FiO_2 < 0.5$ record only PaO_2					$PO_2 > 70$	PO, 61–70		PO_2 55–60	$PO_2 < 55$
Arterial pH	≥7.7	7.6–7.69		7.5–7.59	7.33–7.49		7.25–7.32	7.15–7.24	<7.15
Serum sodium (mMol/l)	≥180	160–179	155–159	150–154	130–149		120–129	111–119	≤110
Serum potassium (mMol/l)	≥7	6–6.9		5.5–5.9	3.5–5.4	3–3.4	2.5–2.9		≤2.5
Serum creatnine (mg/100 ml, double point score for acute renal failure)	≥3.5	2–3.4	1.5–1.9		0.6–1.4		<0.6		
Hematocrit (%)	≥60		50–59.9	46–49.9	30–45.9		20–29.9		<20
White blood count (total/mm³ in 1,000s)	≥40		20–39.9	15–19.9	3–14.9		1–2.9		<1
Glasgow coma score (GCS): Score = 15 minus actual GCS									
Total acute physiology score (APS): Sum of the 12 individual variable points									
Serum HCO_3 (venous-mMol/L)[Not preferred, use if no ABGs]	≥52	41–51.9		32–40.0	22–31.9		18–21.9	15–17.9	<15

B. Age Points

Assign points to age as follows:

AGE (YRS)	POINTS
≤44	0
45–64	2
55–64	3
65–74	5
≥75	6

C. Chronic Health Points

If the patient has a history of severe organ system insufficiency or is immunocompromised assign points as follows:

a. For nonoperative or emergency postoperative patients – 5 points or;
b. For elective postoperative patients – 2 points

Definitions

Organ insufficiency of immunocompromised state must have been evident before this hospital admission and conform to the following criteria:

LIVER: Biopsy-proven cirrhosis and documented portal hypertension; episodes of past upper GI bleeding attributed to portal hypertension; or prior episodes of hepatic failure/encephalopathy/coma.
CARDIOVASCULAR: New York Heart Association Class IV
RESPIRATORY: Chronic restrictive, obstructive, or vascular disease resulting in severe exercise restriction, i.e., unable to climb stairs or perform household duties; or documented chronic hypoxia, hypercapnia, secondary polycythemia, severe pulmonary hypertension (>40 mmHg) or respirator dependency.
RENAL: Receiving chronic dialysis patient
IMMUNOCOMPROMISED: The patient has received therapy that suppresses resistance to infection, e.g., immunosuppression, chemotherapy, radiation, long-term or recent high-dose steroids, or has a disease that is sufficiently advanced to suppress resistance to infection, e.g., leukemia, lymphoma, AIDS.

APACHE II SCORE
Sum of A + B + C
A APS Points
B Age Points
C Chronic Health Points
Total APACHE II

DEFINITION OF ABBREVIATIONS USED IN CALCULATIONS

P_AO_2	Alveolar oxygen tension
PB	Barometric pressure
P H_2O	Water vapor
$PaCO_2$	Arterial carbon dioxide tension
PaO_2	Arterial oxygen tension
FiO_2	Fractional concentration of inspired oxygen
R	1.25
$\dot{V}_A$	Alveolar volume
V_T	Tidal volume
$\dot{V}_D$	Deadspace volume
$\dot{V}_E$	Minute ventilation
C	Compliance
PaO	Airway pressure
E	Elastance
C_{STATIC}	Static compliance
PIP	Peak inspiratory pressure
PEEP	Positive end-expiratory pressure
$PEEP_{TOTAL}$	Applied and intrinsic PEEP
Raw	Airway resistance
$P_{PLATEAU}$	Plateau airway pressure
$\dot{V}$	Flow
$\dot{V}_I$	Inspiratory flow rate
T_I	Inspiratory time
TCT	Total cycle time
TE	Expiratory time
P_ECO_2	Expired carbon dioxide tension
FEV_1	Forced expiratory volume in one second
REE	Resting energy expenditure
HR	Heart rate
SV	Stroke volume
CI	Cardiac index
CO	Cardiac output
BSA	Body surface area
MAP	Mean arterial pressure
SP	Systolic pressure
DP	Diastolic pressure
CVP	Central venous pressure
PAWP	Pulmonary artery wedge pressure
SVR	Systemic vascular resistance
SVRI	Systemic vascular resistance index
PAP	Pulmonary arterial pressure
PVRI	Pulmonary vascular resistance index
$\dot{D}O_2$	Oxygen delivery
CaO_2	Arterial oxygen content
$C\bar{V}O_2$	Venous oxygen content
CcO_2	End pulmonary capillary oxygen content
ER	Extraction ratio
$\dot{V}O_2$	Oxygen consumption
CPP	Cerebral perfusion pressure
ICP	Intracranial pressure
CBF	Cerebral blood flow
CVR	Cerebral vascular resistance
UVA	Urine sodium
SNA	Serum sodium
SCR	Serum creatinine
CR	Urine creatinine
U_{OSMOL}	Urine osmolality
FENA	Fractional excretion of sodium
U/P_{CR}	Urine/plasm creatinine
GFR	Glomerular filtration rate

REFERENCES

Formulas Appendix. In: Kirby RR, Taylor RW, Civelta JM (eds) Handbook of Critical Care, 2nd Ed. Philadelphia: Lippincott-Raven, 1997.

Calculations Commonly Used in Critical Care. In: Rippe JM, Irwin RS, Fink MP, Cerro FB (eds) Intensive Care Medicine, 3rd Ed. Boston: Little Brown, 1996.

Index

E

F

G

Q

R